SRB's Clinical Methods in
SURGERY

VIDEO LIST FOR QR CODES

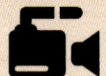 *Access the Videos by Scanning the QR Code Inside*

S.No.	Video Title	Chapter No.	Page No.
1.	General Examination	1	11
2.	Examination of Ulcer	3	64
3.	Examination of Swelling	4	94
4.	Examination in Peripheral Vascular Disease	6	158
5.	Examination of Varicose Veins	7	184
6.	Examination of Lymphatic System	8	205
7.	Examination of Oral Lesions-Ulcer	11	239
8.	Examination of Salivary Glands	14	282
9.	Examination of Neck Swelling	15	299
10.	Examination of Thyroid	16	321
11.	Examination of Breast	17	342
12.	Examination of Hernia	18	370
13.	Examination of Scrotal Swelling	19	390
14.	Examination of Abdominal Mass	23	448

SRB's Clinical Methods in SURGERY

As per the Competency-based Medical Education Curriculum (NMC)

Fourth Edition

Sriram Bhat M
MS (General Surgery) FRCS (Glasgow)
Professor and Head
Department of Surgery
Kasturba Medical College
Mangalore, Karnataka, India
Honorary Surgeon
Government Wenlock District Hospital
Mangalore, Dakshina Kannada, Karnataka, India
meera_sriram2003@yahoo.com

Forewords
CR Ballal
Narayanaswamy Srinivasan
Harish Rao
Sribatsa Kumar Mohapatra

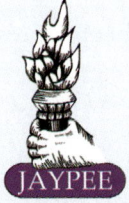

JAYPEE BROTHERS MEDICAL PUBLISHERS
The Health Sciences Publisher
New Delhi | London

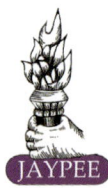

Jaypee Brothers Medical Publishers (P) Ltd

Headquarters
Jaypee Brothers Medical Publishers (P) Ltd
EMCA House, 23/23-B
Ansari Road, Daryaganj
New Delhi 110 002, India
Landline: +91-11-23272143, +91-11-23272703
+91-11-23282021, +91-11-23245672
Email: jaypee@jaypeebrothers.com

Corporate Office
Jaypee Brothers Medical Publishers (P) Ltd
4838/24, Ansari Road, Daryaganj
New Delhi 110 002, India
Phone: +91-11-43574357
Fax: +91-11-43574314
Email: jaypee@jaypeebrothers.com

Overseas Office
J.P. Medical Ltd
83 Victoria Street, London
SW1H 0HW (UK)
Phone: +44 20 3170 8910
Fax: +44 (0)20 3008 6180
Email: info@jpmedpub.com

Website: www.jaypeebrothers.com
Website: www.jaypeedigital.com

© 2023, Jaypee Brothers Medical Publishers

The views and opinions expressed in this book are solely those of the original contributor(s)/author(s) and do not necessarily represent those of editor(s) and publisher of the book.

All rights reserved. No part of this publication may be reproduced, stored or transmitted in any form or by any means, electronic, mechanical, photocopying, recording or otherwise, without the prior permission in writing of the publishers.

All brand names and product names used in this book are trade names, service marks, trademarks or registered trademarks of their respective owners. The publisher is not associated with any product or vendor mentioned in this book.

Medical knowledge and practice change constantly. This book is designed to provide accurate, authoritative information about the subject matter in question. However, readers are advised to check the most current information available on procedures included and check information from the manufacturer of each product to be administered, to verify the recommended dose, formula, method and duration of administration, adverse effects and contraindications. It is the responsibility of the practitioner to take all appropriate safety precautions. Neither the publisher nor the author(s)/editor(s) assume any liability for any injury and/or damage to persons or property arising from or related to use of material in this book.

This book is sold on the understanding that the publisher is not engaged in providing professional medical services. If such advice or services are required, the services of a competent medical professional should be sought.

Every effort has been made where necessary to contact holders of copyright to obtain permission to reproduce copyright material. If any have been inadvertently overlooked, the publisher will be pleased to make the necessary arrangements at the first opportunity.

Inquiries for bulk sales may be solicited at: jaypee@jaypeebrothers.com

SRB's Clinical Methods in Surgery

First Edition: 2010
Second Edition: 2015
Third Edition: 2019
Fourth Edition: **2023**

ISBN: 978-93-5465-868-6

Printed at Nutech Print Services India

Dedicated to...

College where I had my undergraduation, postgraduation and surgical professional career till date, i.e.,

**Kasturba Medical College and
Government Wenlock District Hospital, Mangalore, Karnataka, India**

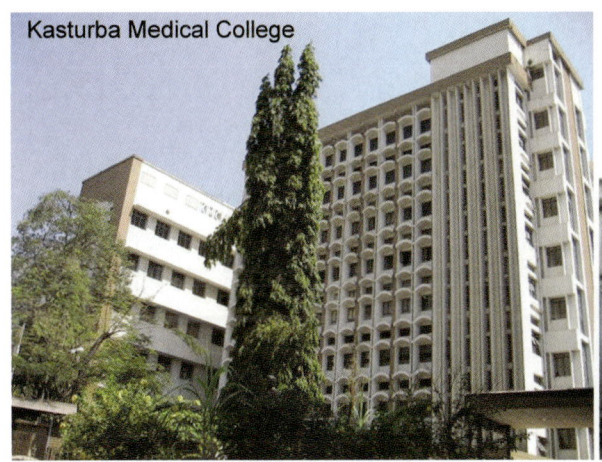
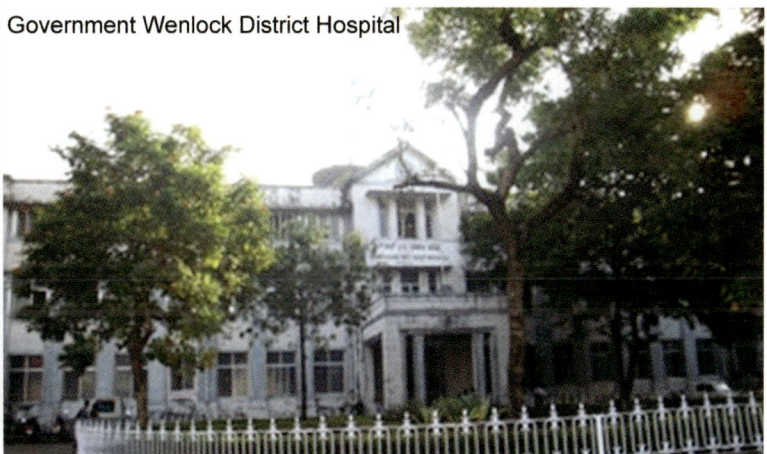

*and
My beloved wife Dr Meera Sriram and my daughter Miss Ananya*

Contributors

Bhargav Vyas MS (General Surgery)
Assistant Professor
Department of Surgery
Kasturba Medical College
Mangalore, Karnataka, India

Meera Karanth P (Meera Sriram) MD
Gynecologist
Light House Poly Clinic
Mangalore, Karnataka, India
She has contributed Chapter 24—Approaches and Examination in Rectal and Vaginal Problems

Narayanaswamy Srinivasan MS FRCS (Glasgow)
Medical Superintendent
Fathima Institute of Medical Sciences
Kadapa, Andhra Pradesh, India
Former Dean and Director
Bangalore Medical College and Research Institute
Bengaluru, Karnataka, India
His innovative invention—'Srinivasan costal sign' is published in this book

Sribatsa Kumar Mohapatra MS FRCS DNB
Veer Surendra Sai Medical College
Burla, Odisha, India
He has contributed his new approaches in breast and abdomen examination—an innovative triple ABC technique (Sribatsa Mohapatra Clinical Technique) for clinical breast examination (CBE) for breast disorders and a cricketing approach to the abdomen and stethoscope sign in acute appendicitis.

Foreword

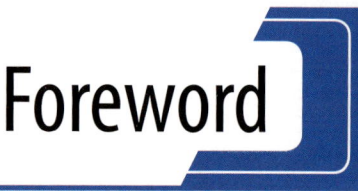

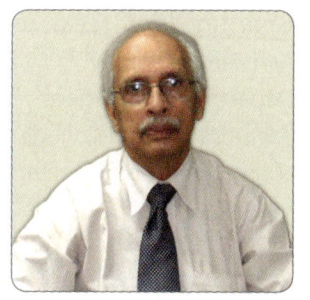

Dr Sriram Bhat M, Professor of Surgery, Kasturba Medical College (KMC), Mangalore, Karnataka, India, is a very popular teacher and I have known him for more than three decades. He has always been interested in teaching and his emphasis was on the fundamentals of good clinical examination. At a time when imaging and other methods of investigations are becoming popular than methodical and a well-executed clinical examination, a well-written book on clinical surgery is most welcome. Dr Bhat has tried to emphasize as very systemic examination so that one could arrive at a working diagnosis at the end of a good history and physical examination. The value of this book has been enhanced by a very large number of highly illustrative pictorial descriptions. Unfortunately, the number and the variety of patients in many teaching hospitals across the country are unfavorable as far as undergraduates and postgraduates are concerned. I am sure, this book will find a place in the armamentarium of all the students.

Dr Bhat is already the author of a popular textbook of surgery. I have no hesitation to believe that on clinical surgery will be equally popular.

CR Ballal MS
Professor Emeritus
Department of Surgery
Mangalore, Karnataka, India

Foreword

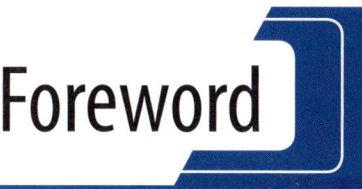

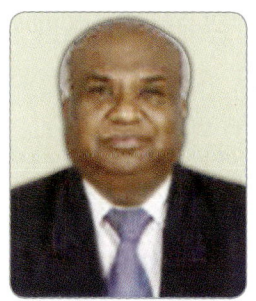

When Professor *Sriram Bhat M,* from Kasturba Medical College (KMC), Mangalore, Karnataka, India, has requested me to write a foreword for the current edition of his clinical book *SRB's Clinical Methods in Surgery,* I readily accepted it because I know him since few years if not personally because of his popular well-known book *SRB's Manual of Surgery* and *SRB's Clinical Methods in Surgery,* first edition and regular communications through phone and e-mail.

This book carries its own merit by lucid presentation, detailed methods of clinical examinations with excellent clinical photographs and illustrations. Even though present era is of imaging, this book stresses the need for proper clinical examination to clinch the proper diagnosis, treatment plans and during follow-up. This book has covered all topics including clinical examination in orthopedics. As by his request, I have given permission to publish the sign which I have invented, i.e., *'Srinivasan costal sign'* and I also felt it is my honor to get the sign published in *SRB's Clinical Methods in Surgery,* current edition.

This book will become probably an essential one to all undergraduates and postgraduates to get a clear idea of clinical methods. Accompanying online videos contain clinical examinations of all important topics with background voice explanation of the author.

This is also very useful to practicing clinicians and surgeons worldwide to understand the surgical conditions and to achieve proper clinical diagnosis.

I appreciate dedication and determination of Professor Sriram Bhat M in bringing out the current edition of *SRB's Clinical Methods in Surgery* and wish him a grand success and also recommend this clinical book to all undergraduates, postgraduates and clinicians to make use of it in clinical practice or learning or in examinations.

Narayanaswamy Srinivasan MS FRCS (Glasgow)
Medical Superintendent
Fathima Institute of Medical Sciences
Kadapa, Andhra Pradesh, India
Former Dean and Director
Bangalore Medical College and Research Institute
Bengaluru, Karnataka, India

Foreword

"Observe, record, tabulate, and communicate. Use your five senses. Learn to see, learn to hear, learn to feel, learn to smell, and know that by practice alone you can become an expert".

—*Sir William Osler*

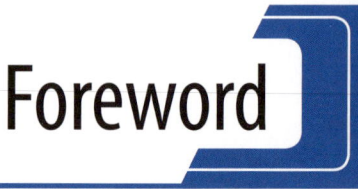

Great advice from a doyen of the past. Today, in the age of ultrasound, CT, MRI and PET scans, clinical examination seems redundant. Yet with all the available sophistry, we seem to be making more mistakes than in the past. We have made diagnosis a costly exercise. In our mad rush towards super-specialization, the art of history taking and eliciting clinical signs is rapidly fading. Yet many times, it is not the scans that help us come to the conclusion nor battery of tests but simple old-fashioned clinical examination.

Dr Sriram Bhat M has been working tirelessly to preserve and perpetuate this art for the past several years. The result is this new and improved version of his clinical textbook. I am sure enthusiasts of this subject will delight in reading and learning from this book. It is a great privilege to be writing the foreword for this book that is virtually a Bible amongst surgical students both in India and abroad. The text is lucidly written, explanations are brought to current levels of knowledge and the illustrations and photographs are of superb quality. This book is a must read for the undergraduates and postgraduates of surgery so that they can be better clinicians.

"From inability to leave well alone; from too much zeal for the new and contempt for what is old; from putting knowledge before wisdom and science before art, and cleverness before common sense; from treating patients as cases; and from making the cure of the disease more grievous than the endurance of the same, Good Lord, deliver us".

—*Sir Robert Hutchinson*

There in lies the gist of what this book is trying to do. For the sake of clinical surgery I wish this book all the best and many many reprints in the coming years.

Harish Rao MS
Professor and Ex-Head
Department of Surgery
Kasturba Medical College
Mangalore, Karnataka, India

Foreword

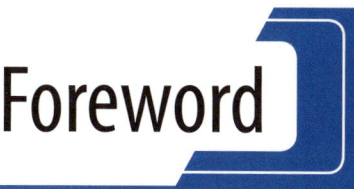

"Diagnosis is not the end but the beginning of practice" – said **Martin Fischer**. This is an ideal advice by a legend.

When **Professor Sriram Bhat M** requested me to write foreword to his upcoming current edition of the *SRB's Clinical Methods in Surgery*, I certainly accepted. I know him very well through his different books in surgical fields which are authentic, informative and very useful. His book, *SRB's Clinical Methods in Surgery* is exceptionally methodical and it gives in detail methodology to approach a patient clinically with history taking, clinical examination and final clinical diagnosis with differential diagnoses. I had great opportunity to express my views in few topics. This book has covered all clinical examination methods with analytical approach, topic-wise with brief ideas about different clinical conditions. It also includes X-rays, instruments and surgical pathology which are useful for students during their practical examination.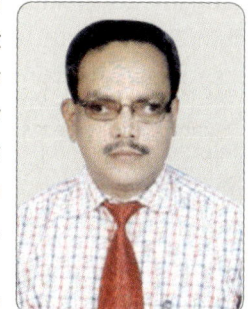

I would say it is an outstanding and remarkable contribution by Professor Sriram Bhat and I have no hesitation in recommending this book to all undergraduate and postgraduate students, and medical teachers engaged in knowledge transfer. It is said no stones should be left unturned for a proper diagnosis, and this book gives the clues in a simple way of how to turn those difficult stones. This book will be very useful to practicing surgeons as a clinical guide.

I affectionately and wholeheartedly wish Professor Bhat a great success in this endeavor.

Sribatsa Kumar Mohapatra
MBBS MS Dip NB FRCS (Edin)
Professor of Surgery
Veer Surendra Sai Institute of
Medical Sciences and Research
Burla, Odisha, India

Preface to the Fourth Edition

It is now four years *third edition of SRB's Clinical Methods in Surgery* has released with good acceptance from students and faculties altogether. But I sincerely thought further editions are sure a need due to change in trend of examination pattern and incoming new CBME syllabus. I did a lot of changes in the upcoming fourth edition. Unnecessary lengthy discussions are removed. Most of the subjects topics in each chapter are put in table format briefly, so that students can quickly go through the clinical conditions whenever needed in the ward or outpatient room. Relevant CBME numbers are highlighted in each chapter. Many photos are deleted to avoid repetitions; many are replaced with new one. Text and illustrations are made in such a way that those students while reading will have continuous flow of thoughts with lucid language. Important clinical topics are added with newer high definition clinical video demonstrations of examining the patients which will be very useful to students to understand the clinical methods of examination of the patient. Differential diagnoses are discussed in each topic in an orderly passion. X-rays, instruments, pathology specimens are discussed. Orthopedic topics in relation to clinical examination are briefly covered.

Clinical knowledge is essential knowledge in treating surgical patients in spite of availability of high technology investigations. Final decision of treatment and probability of outcome is decided purely by analysis, clinical applications and correlations. Old quote is—*"Never let the skin stand between you and the diagnosis"* which means clinical examination is so important in finalising the clinical diagnosis and taking decision.

I hope this newer edition of the clinical book will be very useful to practicing surgeons, all students including undergraduate and postgraduates and all surgical faculties of different teaching institutions.

Healthy constructive criticisms by beloved readers are very well accepted to improve the quality of the book.

Sriram Bhat Muguli

Preface to the First Edition

It was my long time dream to bring out a good surgical clinical book for undergraduates, postgraduates and practicing surgeons. Even though I have written surgical manual for students of MBBS, Dental and Nursing category, I had an aspiration to write an adequate sufficient clinical book which can cover all category of students who need to learn clinical surgery properly. I have covered every aspect of clinical surgery with good illustrations in all chapters. This contains methods of basic clinical surgery for medical students. Clinical approaches, clinical analysis and clinical diagnosis with differential diagnosis are discussed in each chapter. However, therapeutic aspects, controversies and recent advances are not a part of this book. Students who want to learn in detail in these aspects are requested to refer to my textbook *SRB's Manual of Surgery,* 3rd edition or any other surgical books of their choice. I have taken enough care to discuss different clinical methods and signs. I have also referred standard clinical books and surgery books prior to writing this book. Many methods and signs which are old are well accepted but still many methods are controversial. But whatever given in this are commonly followed one; individual opinions and controversies are not highlighted here.

I hope this book will be useful for all those who are keen to learn clinical surgery.

I sincerely appreciate everyone who has helped me. I thank M/s Jaypee Brothers Medical Publishers (P) Ltd, New Delhi, for their support to bring out this book.

Any constructive criticisms are most welcome.

Sriram Bhat M

Acknowledgments

I am happy to bring out the *fourth edition* of *SRB's Clinical Methods in Surgery* after four years of the previous edition. This is due to constant help and support of many.

I thank our Chancellor, Dr Ramdas M Pai; Mrs Vasanthi Pai, Trustee, MAHE Trust, Manipal; Dr Ranjan Pai, CEO, MEMG; Pro-Chancellor Dr HS Ballal; Vice-Chancellor of Manipal Academy of Higher Education (MAHE), Lt. Gen. Dr MD Venkatesh, Pro-Vice-Chancellor, Dr Venkatraya Prabhu, and Dr Dilip G Naik.

My immense thanks to my beloved Dean-Professor, Unnikrishnan; Associated Deans Professor, Shrikala Baliga; Professor Suresh Kumar Shetty, Professor Pramod Kumar.

I thank my beloved teacher, a great clinician and senior surgeon, Professor Dr CR Ballal, Mangalore for accepting my request to give foreword to this clinical book. I owe a lot to him.

I thank Professor Narayanaswamy Srinivasan, Former Dean and Director, Bangalore Medical College and Research Institute, Bengaluru, Karnataka, Presently Medical Superintendent, Fathima Institute of Medical Sciences, Kadapa, Andhra Pradesh for writing foreword to this book and contributing to the book with 'Srinivasan costal sign'.

I always remember my senior teachers, Professor Suresh Kamath and Professor K Prakash Rao, Dr Jayaprakash Rao for their constant help. I thank Professor GG Laxman Prabhu, Urologist, Kasturba Medical College, Mangalore, Karnataka.

I thank Professor Dr Sribatsa Kumar Mohapatra, Veer Surendra Sai Institute of Medical Sciences and Research, Burla, Odisha, contributed his new approaches in breast and abdomen examination—An innovative triple ABC technique (Sribatsa Mohapatra Clinical Technique) for clinical breast examination (CBE) for breast disorders and A cricketing approach to the abdomen.

I thank Professor Ramlingam, Kamineni Institute of Medical Sciences, Narketpally for contributing with many photographs. I thank many other senior consultants and professors in different medical colleges across the country for contributing towards this in the form of opinions, photos and corrections.

I thank many professors and teachers, who guided, corrected, helped me and contributed in different forms like clinical photos towards this edition of the book.

Earlier and current Professors, Department of Surgery, Kasturba Medical College, Mangalore namely Dr BM Nayak, Dr Thangam Varghese, Dr Jayaram Shenoy, Dr Anand Kini, Dr Harish Rao, Dr Ramachandra Pai, Dr SP Rai, Dr Yogish Kumar, Dr Shivananda Prabhu H, Dr Rajesh Ballal, Dr Manohar Pai and Dr Ashfaque Mohammad are always supportive for my work and are worth to be remembered always.

I am grateful to all my teachers and colleagues in surgery department who directly or indirectly helped me to bring out book.

I need thank specifically—Dr Bhargav Vyas AN, my Assistant Professor, Department of Surgery, Kasturba Medical College, Mangalore, Dr Balodi Divya Maheshbhai, Senior Resident and Dr Gopal, Postgraduate, who have helped me with real affection in all editing, collecting photos, taking videos. I really owe them a lot.

I appreciate District Medical Officer and Resident Medical Officer of Government Wenlock District Hospital, Mangalore for their kind help.

I will never forget my close associates Dr Ganapathy, Director, Mangala Hospital, Kadri, Mangalore; Dr Ashok Pandith, Consultant Urologist, Yenepoya Speciality Hospital, Kodialbail, Mangalore for their affectionate help and encouragement in all my endeavors. They always stood with me in my difficulties.

I thank Dr Poornachandra Tejashri, Dr Shibumon MM, Dr Rahul Bhat, Dr Kalpana Sridhar, Dr Keshava Prasad, Dr Sunilkumar Shetty, Dr Sunil Matt, Dr Jawahar BK, Dr Achaleshwar Dayal, Dr Ashok Hegde, Dr Devidas Shetty, Dr Venkatesh Sanjeeva, Dr Sunil, Dr Harish Nayak, Dr Subraya Kamath and Dr Nandakishore, for their help in various aspects.

I thank my friends Dr Manjunath Shenoy, Urologist; Dr Jagadish for his contributions to photos and X-rays and opinion on dental and faciomaxillary topics; Dr Harsharaj, Orthopedician, Mangalore, and Dr Ishwarakeerthi, Spine specialist, Mangalore for their help. I thank Dr Balasaraswathy, Consultant Dermatologist, Mangalore for providing rare photos.

My wife Dr Meera Karanth helped me day and night in editing this new book and without her help this could not have been possible. My beloved daughter Ananya helped me in drawing and diagrams artistically. I enjoy her love and affection towards me.

I thank all my students especially postgraduates of surgery department who were helping regularly in bringing out this second edition.

Words are not sufficient to remember all my patients who are the main material for the book. I pray for their good health always.

I am very grateful to the whole team of M/s Jaypee Brothers Medical Publishers (P) Ltd, New Delhi, India, who helped and guided me, Shri Jitendar P Vij (Group Chairman), Mr Ankit Vij (Managing Director), Mr MS Mani (Group President), Dr Madhu Choudhary (Director–Educational Publishing), Ms Pooja Bhandari (Production Head), Ms Sunita Katla (Executive Assistant to Group Chairman and Publishing Manager), Ms Samina Khan (Executive Assistant to Director–Educational Publishing), Dr Aditya Tayal (Development Editor), Mr Rajesh Sharma (Production Coordinator), Ms Seema Dogra (Cover Visualizer), Ms Geeta Shirvastava (Proofreader), Mr Deep Kumar Dogra (Typesetter), Mr Gopal Singh (Graphic Designer) and their team members, for all their support to work in this project and make it a success. Without their cooperation, I could not have completed this project.

Contents

Section 1: Examination in General Surgery

1. Introduction to Clinical Approach and Examination 1
- Clinical methods   1
- Symptoms and signs   3
- History taking   3
- Chief complaints   4
- History of present illness   5
- Past history   5
- Personal history   5
- Family history and genetic history   6
- Other relevant history   7
- Assessment of specific symptoms and signs   7
- Physical examination   11
- Examination of skin and mucous membrane   17
- Examination of nails   20
- Skin changes and eruptions   23
- Texture of the skin   26
- Pigmented lesions in the skin   27
- Hair   27
- Edema   28
- Visible veins   31
- Examination of pulse   33
- Blood pressure   34
- Respiration   36
- Eyes   36
- Nose   38
- Ears   38
- Fever/rise in temperature   38
- Tongue   39
- Crepitus   40
- Local examination   40
- Systemic examination   41
- Final diagnosis   41
- Levels of evidences   42
- ECOG performance status   42
- Karnofsky performance status   42

2. Investigations 43
- Types of investigation   43
- Cellular study   44
- Biopsy   44
- Endoscopic examination   47
- X-ray and imaging   47
- Examination by exploration   53
- Preanesthetic assessment   53
- Examination of feces   55
- Examination of urine   55

3. Examination and Clinical Approach of an Ulcer 57
- Definition   57
- Parts of an ulcer   57
- Life history of an ulcer   59
- History   62
- General examination   64
- Local examination of an ulcer   64
- Other ulcers   85

4. Examination and Clinical Approach of a Swelling/Lump 88
- History   88
- General examination   94
- Local examination   94
- Relevant systemic examination   115
- Proper clinical diagnosis   115
- Relevant investigations   116
- Differential diagnosis   116

5. Examination and Clinical Approach of Sinus and Fistula 143
- Sinus   143
- Fistula   143
- Clinical features of sinus/fistula   144
- History   145
- General examination   146
- Local examination   146
- Investigations   148

6. Examination and Clinical Approach in Arterial Diseases 153
- History   153
- Chief complaints   154
- General examination   158
- Local examination   158
- Systemic examination   171
- Investigations for arterial diseases   173
- Limb ischemia   175
- Diseases of the arteries   175
- Acute arterial occlusion   176

7. Examination and Clinical Approach in Venous Diseases 181
- History   182
- General examination   184
- Local examination   184
- Investigations for varicose veins   196
- Surgical anatomy of lower limb veins   197

8. **Examination and Clinical Approach to Lymphatic System** 201
   - Chief complaints 203
   - General examination 205
   - Local examination 205
   - Investigations 214
   - Diseases of lymphatic systems 216

9. **Examination and Clinical Approach to Peripheral Nervous System** 220
   - History 220
   - Examination 221
   - Local examination 221
   - Relevant investigations 229
   - Peripheral nerve injuries 229
   - Brachial plexus injury 229

10. **Examination and Clinical Approach in Diseases of Muscles, Tendons and Fasciae** 234
    - History 234
    - General examination 234
    - Local examination 234

11. **Clinical Approach and Examination of Oral Cavity** 238
    - History 238
    - General examination 239
    - Local examination 239
    - Examination of cervical lymph nodes 258
    - Systemic examination 258
    - Investigations 258
    - Other malignant conditions of oral cavity 262
    - Benign conditions in oral cavity 262
    - Premalignant conditions of oral cavity 263
    - Differential diagnosis of tongue ulcers 263
    - Stomatitis 264

12. **Clinical Approach and Examination of Jaw** 266
    - History 267
    - General examination 267
    - Local examination 267
    - Investigations for jaw disease 270

13. **Clinical Approach and Examinations of Pharynx, Larynx, Nasal Cavities and Paranasal Sinuses** 275
    - Examination of pharynx 275
    - Examination of larynx 276
    - Examination of nasal cavities and paranasal air sinuses 278

14. **Clinical Approaches and Examination of Salivary Glands** 280
    - History 280
    - General examination 282
    - Local examination 282
    - Investigations for salivary diseases 293
    - Salivary neoplasms 294

15. **Clinical Approaches and Examination of Neck** 298
    - History 298
    - General examination 299
    - Local examination 299
    - Systemic examination 311
    - Investigations 312
    - Classification of neck swellings 312
    - Cold abscess 313
    - Secondaries in neck lymph nodes 313
    - Thoracic outlet syndrome 314

16. **Clinical Approach and Examination of Thyroid** 317
    - General examination 321
    - Local examination 325
    - Systemic examination 332

17. **Clinical Approaches and Examination of Breast** 340
    - History 340
    - General examination 342
    - Local examination of breasts 343
    - Investigations in carcinoma breast/breast lump 360
    - Differential diagnosis 361
    - Benign and inflammatory conditions of breast 363

18. **Clinical Approaches and Examination of Hernia** 366
    - History 368
    - General examination 370
    - Local examination 370
    - Investigations 377
    - Hernia 378
    - Boundaries and anatomy of the inguinal canal 378
    - Types of indirect inguinal hernia 379
    - Direct hernia 379
    - Differences between indirect inguinal and direct inguinal hernias 381
    - Incisional hernia 382
    - Femoral hernia 383

19. **Clinical Approaches and Examination of Inguinoscrotal and Scrotal Swelling** 387
    - History 387
    - General Examination 390
    - Local Examination 390
    - Investigations 397

20. **Approaches and Examination of Male External Genitalia** 403
    - History 403
    - General examination 404

- Local examination 405
- Disorders of penis 407

Section 2: Examination in Abdominal and Related Conditions

21. Approaches and Examinations in Chronic Abdominal Conditions 411
- History 411
- General examination 414
- Local examination 414
- Systemic examinations 424
- Investigations 425
- Different chronic abdominal conditions 428

22. Approaches and Examination of Acute Abdomen 432
- History 432
- General examination 434
- Local examination of abdomen 435
- Systemic examination 439
- Investigations 439
- Acute appendicitis 440
- Intestinal obstruction 443
- Other acute abdomen conditions 445

23. Approaches and Clinical Examination of Mass Abdomen 446
- History 446
- General examination 448
- Local abdominal examination 448
- Differential diagnosis 460
- Diseases of the umbilicus and abdominal wall 469

24. Approaches and Examination in Rectal and Vaginal Problems 472
- History 472
- Examination of the anorectum 475
- Vaginal examination 482
- Anorectal diseases 484

25. Approaches and Examination in Dysphagia 488
- History 488
- General examination 489
- Dysphagia 489
- Diseases of esophagus 491

Section 3: Examination in Specialized Areas

26. Approaches and Clinical Examination in Urinary Diseases.. 493
- Definitions of various terms 493
- Hematuria 493
- Retention of urine 494
- Increased urinary frequency 495
- History 495
- General examination 497
- Local examination 497
- Systemic examination 499
- Examination of urine 500
- Investigations 500
- Diseases of the kidney 503
- Conditions of urinary bladder, prostate, urethra 506

27. Approaches and Examination in Hand Diseases 511
- History 511
- Examination 511
- Investigations 514
- Hand infections 515
- Hand injuries 516
- Syndactyly 516

28. Approaches and Examination in Foot Diseases 517
- History 517
- Examination 517
- Investigations 518
- Diseases of the foot 518

29. Approaches and Examination of Face and Head 520
- Cleft disorders 520
- Examination of cranial nerves 522

30. Approaches and Examination in Intracranial Diseases 524
- History 524
- General examination 524
- Nervous system examination 524
- Examination of cranial nerves 524
- Investigations 526
- Intracranial diseases 526

31. Approaches and Examination of Chest Diseases 529
- History 529
- General examination 529
- Local examination 529
- Investigations 530
- Different chest diseases 530

Section 4: Examination in Trauma

32. Approaches and Examination in Head Injuries..................... 533
- History 533
- Examination 533
- Local examination 534
- Investigations 534

33. **Approaches and Examination in Chest Injuries** 537
    - History   537
    - Examination   537
    - Investigations   537
    - Chest injuries   538

34. **Approaches and Examination in Abdominal Injuries** 540
    - General examination   540
    - Investigations   541

Section 5: Clinical Methods in Orthopedics

35. **Approaches and Examination of Bone and Joint Injuries** 545
    - History   545
    - Examination   546
    - Investigations   547
    - Fracture   548
    - Dislocation   549

36. **Approaches and Examinations in Injuries of Various Joints** 550
    - Examination in injuries around shoulder joint and arm   550
    - Examination in injuries of elbow joint and forearm   553
    - Examination in injuries of wrist and hand   556
    - Examination in injuries to pelvis   558
    - Examination in injuries of hip and thigh   560
    - Examination in injuries of knee joint and leg bones   563
    - Examination in injuries of ankle joint and foot   568

37. **Approaches and Examination in Bone Diseases** 571
    - History   571
    - Examination   571
    - Investigations   573

38. **Approaches and Examination of Pathological Joint** 578
    - History   578
    - Examination   579
    - Investigation   580

39. **Approaches and Examinations in Pathologies of Individual Joints** 582
    - Examination of pathological shoulder joint   582
    - Examination of pathological elbow joint   585
    - Examination of pathological wrist and joints of hand   588
    - Examination of pathological hip joint   588
    - Examination in pathological knee joint   594
    - Examination of pathological ankle joint and foot   597

40. **Approaches and Examinations in Spine Injuries and Diseases** 599
    - Spinal injuries   599
    - Local examination   599
    - Fracture spine   601
    - Spinal cord injuries   601
    - Spinal diseases   602
    - Investigations   607

Section 6: Miscellaneous

41. **Instruments** 611
    - Forceps   611
    - Clamps   613
    - Retractors   614
    - Scissors   616
    - Suction instruments   617
    - Drains   617
    - Catheters   618
    - Urethral dilators   619
    - Nasogastric tube/Ryle's tube   619
    - Surgical needles   620
    - Tracheostomy and endotracheal tubes and related instruments   622
    - Other instruments   623

42. **X-rays** 626
    - Plain X-ray abdomen   626
    - Chest X-rays   629
    - X-ray bones   630
    - Other plain X-rays   630

43. **Surgical Pathology** 635

    Index *641*

Competency Table

Number	The student should be able to	Core (Y/N)	Chapter number	Page Number
SU1.3	Describe basic concepts of perioperative care	Y	2	43
SU6.1	Define and describe the etiology and pathogenesis of surgical infections	Y	3, 4, 5, 27, 28	57, 88, 143, 511, 517
SU6.2	Enumerate prophylactic and therapeutic antibiotics plan appropriate management	Y	3	57
SU9.1	Choose appropriate biochemical, microbiological, pathological, imaging investigations and interpret the investigative data in a surgical patient	Y	2, 42, 43	43, 624, 633
SU9.2	Biological basis for early detection of cancer and multidisciplinary approach in management of cancer	Y	2, 42	43, 624
SU9.3	Communicate the results of surgical investigations and counsel the patient appropriately	Y	2	43
SU14.2	Describe surgical approaches, incisions and the use of appropriate instruments in surgery in general	Y	41	609
SU14.3	Describe the materials and methods used for surgical wound closure and anastomosis (sutures, knots and needles)	Y	41	609
SU17.4	Describe pathophysiology, mechanism of head injuries	Y	32	533
SU17.5	Describe clinical features for neurological assessment and GCS in head injuries	Y	32	533
SU17.6	Chose appropriate investigations and discuss the principles of management of head injuries	Y	32	533
SU17.7	Describe the clinical features of soft tissue injuries. Chose appropriate investigations and discuss the principles of management	Y	10	234
SU17.8	Describe the pathophysiology of chest injuries	Y	33, 34	537, 540
SU17.9	Describe the clinical features and principles of management of chest injuries	Y	33, 34	537, 540
SU17.10	Demonstrate airway maintenance. Recognize and manage tension pneumothorax, hemothorax and flail chest in simulated environment	Y	33, 34	537, 540
SU18.1	Describe the pathogenesis, clinical features and management of various cutaneous and subcutaneous infections	Y	4	88
SU18.2	Classify skin tumors Differentiate different skin tumors and discuss their management	Y	4	88
SU18.3	Describe and demonstrate the clinical examination of surgical patient including swelling and order relevant investigation for diagnosis. Describe and discuss appropriate treatment plan	Y	4	88
SU19.1	Describe the etiology and classification of cleft lip and palate	Y	12, 29	266, 520
SU19.2	Describe the principles of reconstruction of cleft lip and palate	Y	12, 29	266, 520
SU20.1	Describe etiopathogenesis of oral cancer symptoms and signs of oropharyngeal cancer	Y	11	238
SU20.2	Enumerate the appropriate investigations and discuss the principles of treatment	Y	11	238
SU21.1	Describe surgical anatomy of the salivary glands, pathology, and clinical presentation of disorders of salivary glands	Y	14	280
SU21.2	Enumerate the appropriate investigations and describe the principles of treatment of disorders of salivary glands	Y	14	280
SU22.1	Describe the applied anatomy and physiology of thyroid	Y	16	317
SU22.2	Describe the etiopathogenesis of thyroidal swellings	Y	16	317

Competency Table

Number	The student should be able to	Core (Y/N)	Chapter number	Page Number
SU22.3	Demonstrate and document the correct clinical examination of thyroid swellings and discus the differential diagnosis and their management	Y	16	317
SU22.4	Describe the clinical features, classification and principles of management of thyroid cancer	Y	16	317
SU22.5	Describe the applied anatomy of parathyroid	Y	16	317
SU22.6	Describe and discuss the clinical features of hypo - and hyperparathyroidism and the principles of their management	Y	16	317
SU24.1	Describe the clinical features, principles of investigation, prognosis and management of pancreatitis	Y	21, 22	411, 432
SU24.2	Describe the clinical features, principles of investigation, prognosis and management of pancreatic endocrine tumors	Y	21	411
SU24.3	Describe the principles of investigation and management of pancreatic disorders including pancreatitis and endocrine tumors	Y	21, 22	411, 432
SU25.1	Describe applied anatomy and appropriate investigations for breast disease	Y	17	340
SU25.2	Describe the etiopathogenesis, clinical features and principles of management of benign breast disease including infections of the breast	Y	17	340
SU25.3	Describe the etiopathogenesis, clinical features, investigations and principles of treatment of benign and malignant tumors of breast	Y	17	340
SU25.4	Counsel the patient and obtain informed consent for treatment of malignant conditions of the breast	Y	17	340
SU25.5	Demonstrate the correct technique to palpate the breast for breast swelling in a mannequin or equivalent	Y	17	340
SU26.3	Describe the clinical features of mediastinal diseases and the principles of management	Y	31	529
SU26.4	Describe the etiology, pathogenesis, clinical features of tumors of lung and the principles of management	Y	31	529
SU27.1	Describe the etiopathogenesis, clinical features, investigations and principles of treatment of occlusive arterial disease	Y	6	153
SU27.2	Demonstrate the correct examination of the vascular system and enumerate and describe the investigation of vascular disease	Y	6	153
SU27.3	Describe clinical features, investigations and principles of management of vasospastic disorders	Y	6	153
SU27.4	Describe the types of gangrene and principles of amputation	Y	6	153
SU27.5	Describe the applied anatomy of venous system of lower limb	Y	7	181
SU27.6	Describe pathophysiology, clinical features, investigations and principles of management of DVT and varicose veins	Y	7	181
SU27.7	Describe pathophysiology, clinical features, investigations and principles of management of lymph edema, lymphangitis and lymphomas	Y	8	201
SU27.8	Demonstrate the correct examination of the lymphatic system	Y	8	201
SU28.5	Describe the applied anatomy and physiology of esophagus	Y	25	488
SU28.6	Describe the clinical features, investigations and principles of management of benign and malignant disorders of esophagus	Y	25	488
SU28.7	Describe the applied anatomy and physiology of stomach	Y	21	411
SU28.8	Describe and discuss the etiology, the clinical features, investigations and principles of management of congenital hypertrophic pyloric stenosis, peptic ulcer disease, carcinoma stomach	Y	21	411
SU28.9	Demonstrate the correct technique of examination of a patient with disorders of the stomach	Y	21, 22	411, 432
SU28.10	Describe the applied anatomy of liver. Describe the clinical features, investigations and principles of management of liver abscess, hydatid disease, injuries and tumors of the liver	Y	21, 22	411, 432

Number	The student should be able to	Core (Y/N)	Chapter number	Page Number
SU28.12	Describe the applied anatomy of biliary system. Describe the clinical features, investigations and principles of management of diseases of biliary system	Y	21	411
SU28.13	Describe the applied anatomy of small and large intestine	Y	21	411
SU28.15	Describe the clinical features, investigations and principles of management of diseases of Appendix including appendicitis and its complications	Y	22	432
SU28.16	Describe applied anatomy including congenital anomalies of the rectum and anal canal	Y	24	472
SU28.17	Describe the clinical features, investigations and principles of management of common anorectal diseases	Y	24	472
SU28.18	Describe and demonstrate clinical examination of abdomen. Order relevant investigations. Describe and discuss appropriate treatment plan	Y	22, 23	432, 446
SU29.1	Describe the causes, investigations and principles of management of hematuria	Y	26	493
SU29.2	Describe the clinical features, investigations and principles of management of congenital anomalies of genitourinary system	Y	26	493
SU29.3	Describe the clinical features, investigations and principles of management of urinary tract infections	Y	26	493
SU29.4	Describe the clinical features, investigations and principles of management of hydronephrosis	Y	26	493
SU29.5	Describe the clinical features, investigations and principles of management of renal calculi	Y	26	493
SU29.6	Describe the clinical features, investigations and principles of management of renal tumors	Y	26	493
SU29.7	Describe the principles of management of acute and chronic retention of urine	Y	26	493
SU29.8	Describe the clinical features, investigations and principles of management of bladder cancer	Y	26	493
SU29.9	Describe the clinical features, investigations and principles of management of disorders of prostate	Y	26	493
SU29.10	Demonstrate a digital rectal examination of the prostate in a mannequin or equivalent	Y	26	493
SU29.11	Describe clinical features, investigations and management of urethral strictures	Y	26	493
SU30.1	Describe the clinical features, investigations and principles of management of phimosis, paraphimosis and carcinoma penis	Y	20	403
SU30.2	Describe the applied anatomy clinical features, investigations and principles of management of undescended testis	Y	19	387
SU30.3	Describe the applied anatomy clinical features, investigations and principles of management of epidydimo-orchitis	Y	19	387
SU30.4	Describe the applied anatomy clinical features, investigations and principles of management of varicocele	Y	19	387
SU30.5	Describe the applied anatomy, clinical features, investigations and principles of management of hydrocele	Y	19	387
SU30.6	Describe classification, clinical features, investigations and principles of management of tumors of testis	Y	19	387
Integrations				
AN10.6	Explain the anatomical basis of clinical features of Erb's palsy and Klumpke's paralysis	N	8, 9	201, 220
AN10.7	Explain anatomical basis of enlarged axillary lymph nodes	N	8	201
AN12.8	Describe anatomical basis of clawhand	Y	9	220
AN12.10	Explain infection of fascial spaces of palm	N	10, 27	234, 511
AN12.11	Identify, describe and demonstrate important muscle groups of dorsal forearm with attachments, nerve supply and actions	Y	9, 10	220, 234
AN12.12	Identify and describe origin, course, relations, branches (or tributaries), termination of important nerves and vessels of back of forearm	Y	9	220

Competency Table

Number	The student should be able to	Core (Y/N)	Chapter number	Page Number
AN12.13	Describe the anatomical basis of wrist drop	Y	9	220
AN12.14	Identify and describe compartments deep to extensor retinaculum	Y	10	234
AN15.3	Describe and demonstrate boundaries, floor, roof and contents of femoral triangle	Y	18	366
AN15.4	Explain anatomical basis of psoas abscess and femoral hernia	N	18	366
AN18.3	Explain the anatomical basis of foot drop	Y	9	220
AN19.3	Explain the concept of "peripheral heart"	Y	7	181
AN20.4	Explain anatomical basis of enlarged inguinal lymph nodes	N	8	201
AN20.5	Explain anatomical basis of varicose veins and deep vein thrombosis	Y	7	181
AN20.9	Identify and demonstrate palpation of vessels (femoral, popliteal, dorsalis pedis, post tibial), mid inguinal point, surface projection of: femoral nerve, saphenous opening, sciatic, tibial, common peroneal and deep peroneal nerve, great and small saphenous veins	Y	6, 7	153, 181
AN23.7	Mention the extent, relations and applied anatomy of lymphatic duct	Y	8	201
AN28.10	Explain the anatomical basis of Frey's syndrome	N	14	280
AN29.2	Explain anatomical basis of Erb's and Klumpke's palsy	Y	9	220
AN30.1	Describe the cranial fossae and identify related structures	Y	12, 13, 30	266, 275, 524
AN30.2	Describe and identify major foramina with structures passing through them	Y	12, 13, 30	266, 275, 524
AN33.2	Describe and demonstrate attachments, direction of fibers, nerve supply and actions of muscles of mastication	Y	12, 13	266, 275
AN33.4	Explain the clinical significance of pterygoid venous plexus	Y	12, 13	266, 275
AN33.5	Describe the features of dislocation of temporomandibular joint	N	12, 13	266, 275
AN34.1	Describe and demonstrate the morphology, relations and nerve supply of submandibular salivary gland and submandibular ganglion	Y	14	280
AN34.2	Describe the basis of formation of submandibular stones	N	14	280
AN35.5	Describe and demonstrate extent, drainage and applied anatomy of cervical lymph nodes	Y	8, 15	201, 298
AN35.9	Describe the clinical features of compression of subclavian artery and lower trunk of brachial plexus by cervical rib	N	15	298
AN43.5	Demonstrate; 1) Testing of muscles of facial expression, extraocular muscles, muscles of mastication, 2) Palpation of carotid arteries, facial artery, superficial temporal artery, 3) Location of internal and external jugular veins, 4) Location of hyoid bone, thyroid cartilage and cricoid cartilage with their vertebral levels	Y	15	298
AN44.1	Describe and demonstrate the planes (transpyloric, transtubercular, subcostal, lateral vertical, linea alba, linea semilunaris), regions and quadrants of abdomen	Y	23	446
AN44.4	Describe and demonstrate extent, boundaries, contents of inguinal canal including Hesselbach's triangle	Y	18	366
AN44.5	Explain the anatomical basis of inguinal hernia	Y	18	366
AN44.6	Describe and demonstrate attachments of muscles of anterior abdominal wall	Y	23	446
AN46.4	Explain the anatomical basis of varicocele	N	19	387
AN46.5	Explain the anatomical basis of phimosis and circumcision	N	20	403
AN47.1	Describe and identify boundaries and recesses of lesser and greater sac	Y	21	411
AN47.2	Name and identify various peritoneal folds and pouches with its explanation	Y	21	411
AN47.3	Explain anatomical basis of ascites and peritonitis	N	22	432
AN47.4	Explain anatomical basis of subphrenic abscess	N	22	432
AN47.5	Describe and demonstrate major viscera of abdomen under following headings (anatomical position, external and internal features, important peritoneal and other relations, blood supply, nerve supply, lymphatic drainage and applied aspects)	Y	21, 23	411, 446

Number	The student should be able to	Core (Y/N)	Chapter number	Page Number
AN47.7	Mention the clinical importance of Calot's triangle	N	21	411
AN48.8	Mention the structures palpable during vaginal and rectal examination	N	24	472
AN52.6	Describe the development and congenital anomalies of foregut, midgut and hindgut	Y	21	411
AN52.7	Describe the development of urinary system	Y	26	493
AN55.1	Demonstrate the surface marking of regions and planes of abdomen, superficial inguinal ring, deep inguinal ring, McBurney's point, renal angle and Murphy's point	Y	23	446
AN55.2	Demonstrate the surface projections of stomach, liver, fundus of gallbladder, spleen, duodenum, pancreas, ileocecal junction, Kidneys and root of mesentery	Y	21, 23	411, 446
PA19.1	Enumerate the causes and describe the differentiating features of lymphadenopathy	Y	8, 15	201, 298
PA19.2	Describe the pathogenesis and pathology of tuberculous lymphadenitis	Y	8, 15	201, 298
PA19.4	Describe and discuss the pathogenesis pathology and the differentiating features of Hodgkin's and non-Hodgkin's lymphoma	Y	8	201
PA19.5	Identify and describe the features of Hodgkin's lymphoma in a gross and microscopic specimen	Y	8	201
PA19.6	Enumerate and differentiate the causes of splenomegaly	Y	21, 23	411, 446
PA24.4	Describe and etiology and pathogenesis and pathologic features of carcinoma of the stomach	Y	21, 23	411, 446
PA24.5	Describe and etiology and pathogenesis and pathologic features of tuberculosis of the intestine	N	21	411
PA24.6	Describe and etiology and pathogenesis and pathologic and distinguishing features of inflammatory bowel disease	Y	21	411
PA24.7	Describe the etiology and pathogenesis and pathologic and distinguishing features of carcinoma of the colon	Y	21, 23	411, 446
PA25.2	Describe the pathophysiology and pathologic changes seen in hepatic failure and their clinical manifestations, complications and consequences	Y	21	411
PA25.4	Describe the pathophysiology, pathology and progression of alcoholic liver disease including cirrhosis	Y	21, 23	411, 446
PA25.5	Describe the etiology, pathogenesis and complications of portal hypertension	Y	21	411
PA29.2	Describe the pathogenesis, pathology, presenting and distinguishing features, diagnostic tests, progression and spread of carcinoma of the penis	Y	20	403
PA29.3	Describe the pathogenesis, pathology, hormonal dependency, presenting and distinguishing features, urologic findings and diagnostic tests of benign prostatic hyperplasia	Y	26	493
PA29.4	Describe the pathogenesis, pathology, hormonal dependency, presenting and distinguishing features, diagnostic tests, progression and spread of carcinoma of the prostate	Y	26	493
PA29.5	Describe the etiology, pathogenesis, pathology and progression of prostatitis	N	26	493
PA32.6	Describe the etiology, pathogenesis, manifestations, laboratory, morphologic features, complications and metastases of pancreatic cancer	N	23	446
MI7.1	Describe the etio-pathogenesis and discuss the laboratory diagnosis of infections of genitourinary system	Y	26	493
AS3.1	Describe the principles of preoperative evaluation	Y	2	43
AS3.2	Elicit, present and document an appropriate history including medication history in a patient undergoing surgery as it pertains to a preoperative anesthetic evaluation	Y	2	43
AS3.3	Demonstrate and document an appropriate clinical examination in a patient undergoing General Surgery	Y	1	1
AS3.4	Choose and interpret appropriate testing for patients undergoing surgery	Y	1, 2	1, 43
AS3.5	Determine the readiness for General Surgery in a patient based on the preoperative evaluation	Y	2	43
IM5.8	Describe and discuss the pathophysiology, clinical evolution and complications of cholelithiasis and cholecystitis	Y	22, 23	432, 446

Competency Table

Number	The student should be able to	Core (Y/N)	Chapter number	Page Number
IM12.9	Order and interpret diagnostic testing based on the clinical diagnosis including CBC, thyroid function tests and ECG and radio iodine uptake and scan	Y	2	43
IM13.7	Elicit document and present a history that will help establish the etiology of cancer and includes the appropriate risk factors, duration and evolution	Y	1	1
IM15.5	Perform, demonstrate and document a physical examination based on the history that includes general examination, volume assessment and appropriate abdominal examination	Y	22	432
PE21.14	Recognize common surgical conditions of the abdomen and genitourinary system and enumerate the indications for referral including acute and subacute intestinal obstruction, appendicitis pancreatitis perforation intussusception, phimosis, undescended testis, chordee, hypospadiasis, torsion testis, hernia hydrocele, vulval synechiae	Y	20	403
OR4.1	Describe and discuss the clinical features, investigation and principles of management of tuberculosis affecting major joints (Hip, Knee) including cold abscess and caries spine	Y	40	598

Section 1: Examination in General Surgery

CHAPTER 1

Introduction to Clinical Approach and Examination

Competency: AS3.3; AS3.4; IM13.7.

Clinical examination is an art. It is an important basic essential part in surgical learning. Surgery is categorized as *clinical surgery; surgical principles and operative surgery*. So surgery is not just cutting. It involves proper clinical analysis; and application of principles while treating patients surgically.

Clinical observation has been a part of medicine since Egyptian, Babylonian, Chinese and Indian physicians began examining the body thousands of years ago. Clinical reasoning and bedside diagnosis first played a role in ancient Greece when Hippocrates began measuring body temperature, evaluating the patient's pulse and palpating the abdomen.

A clinician should be good in theoretical knowledge as well as a master in practical knowledge, as both go hand in hand. Without theoretical knowledge of a disease it is like sailing in an unchartered sea; having book knowledge without patients to treat is like not seeing the sea at all— *William Osler*.

Five essential qualities to be a good surgeon are:
He should acquire
1. *Lady's finger* (should be gentle in handling patients and tissues)
2. *Lion's heart* (being brave to take decisions)
3. *Eagle's eye* (carefully watching changes occurring in the patient during treatment)
4. *Horse's leg* (immense stamina to withstand long hours of surgery)
5. *Camel's belly* (ability to carry on without food for hours)

Clinician is the one who listens patiently; who sees carefully; who feels evidentially; who hears silently.

A clinician should show '*empathy*' towards patient (ability to understand what the patient is undergoing through); have self-confidence/positive attitude thereby can impart confidence in the patient; and should be honest while treating the patient.

Note:
- The 'patient' word is derived from Latin—Pati means 'to suffer'.
- All patients in a surgical ward need not undergo or need surgery. Conditions like cellulitis, amebic colitis or acute pancreatitis commonly do not require surgery but treated by surgeons.

- A surgeon should be a good clinician and physician all together to impart proper treatment to his patients. Even though there are many subspecialties in surgery now, basic clinical surgery remains the same. It is the pillar of surgical basics.
- Clinical examination has mystical power. *History and examination skills still remain at the very core of clinical practice.*
- "Clinical examination skills will gradually atrophy and become redundant if not rejuvenated and stressed upon. Technology should become an extension of what we are doing rather than a replacement". Investigations are just one more piece of evidence that has to be interpreted by a doctor—Asghar Rastegar MD.

Case taking or case analysis includes:
Clinical methods in detail
Clinical diagnosis by analyzing the proper adequate clinical findings
3/4th of the diagnosis can be arrived by proper history taking and systematic examinations (only) along with relevant investigations. Investigations are basic and along with relevant imaging (to know the anatomical nature, extent or spread) and biopsy (histological/pathological/histochemistry) for tissue diagnosis
Proper history and clinical examination is the basis which helps to decide for further needed evaluation methods

CLINICAL METHODS

(Word 'clinical methods'—was used in *September 1897*, by *Sir Robert Hutchison* from London who was founder and author of the famous Hutchison's clinical methods book) **(Figs. 1-1 to 1-3)**.

Clinical methods are schematically divided as

History taking: It is very important part. Careful detail history taking many times gives clue about the exact disease. 70–80% of diagnosis can be made by proper history taking.

Physical examination: It includes general examination; inspection of the part (diseased or suspected) which is

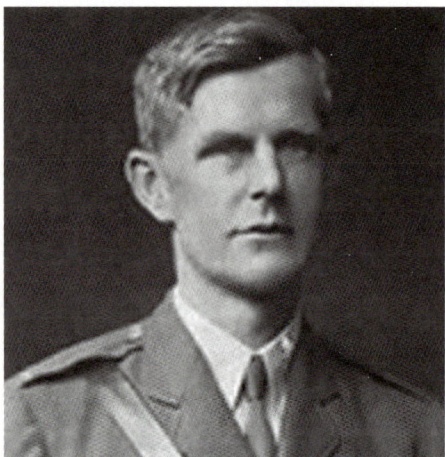

Fig. 1-1 Sir Henry Wade—Surgeon, Scientist, Soldier. He said *"The wards are the greatest of all laboratories"*.

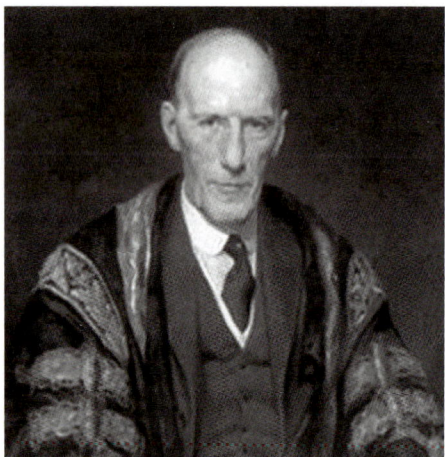

Fig. 1-2 Sir Robert Hutchison (London) who coined and used the word 'clinical methods'.

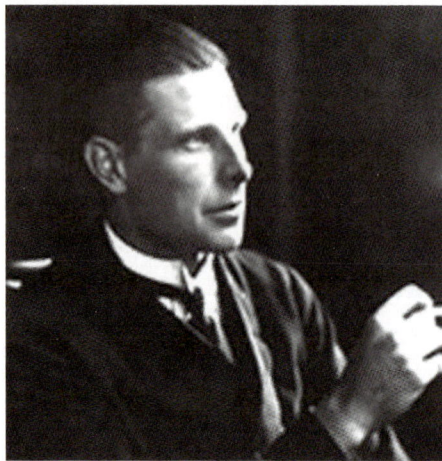

Fig. 1-3 *Sir Henry Hamilton Bailey*; he was a British surgeon and excellent clinician; he wrote Clinical book "Demonstration of Physical Signs in Clinical Surgery" in 1927 and textbook "A Short Practice of Surgery" in 1932. Finest illustrations which he provided in his books were with the help of his photographer wife Vera Gillender. He lost his left index finger due to infection while doing surgery; it is observed in the photos in his book of clinical examination. He died of obstructed carcinoma colon.

proper observation prior to palpation for specific findings; palpation is done only once inspection is completed in detail; percussion done in specific areas like abdomen and chest; auscultation for altered or specific sounds in particular region.

Investigations: Investigations are done to arrive into final diagnosis by various methods like X-ray, CT scan, ultrasound, blood tests and so on. Types of investigations are decided based on the clinical suspicion of the disease.

Final diagnosis: It is to plan the therapy, predict the outcome.

Treatment: Treatment plan or protocol which often differs for individual patient. Postoperative/post-therapy management. Progress of the patient.

Follow-up: Management after discharge and further treatment which is often needed after treatment.

CLINICAL PEARLS

- You see but you do not observe—will be a downtrend in clinical practice.
- Never trust general impression but concentrate on details.
- There is nothing like firsthand evidence.
- The world is full of obvious things which nobody by any chance observes.
- Do not try to twist the facts to suit the theories rather, theories should suit the facts.
- Uncommon manifestations of common diseases are more common than common manifestations of uncommon diseases.
- If we make rare diagnosis, it will rarely be correct.
- You see only what you look for and you recognize only what you know.
- The least indicated procedures lead to most complications.
- There is something more important than all medicine—the *human touch*.
- "Always listen to the patient, they might be telling you the diagnosis." *Attr. William Osler*.
- The first part of any examination is to observe. Learn to observe. Look before you lay on hands. You may get valuable information from the facies, skin coloration, gait, handshake and personal hygiene.
- 25%—one will learn from teachers—guidance; 25%— by your own effort; 50%—by repetitive methods and gaining experience.
- Learn what is essential; Learn what is important; Learn what is helpful; Learn to ask why? And why not? Learn also—when to do? And when not do?
- You are answerable for every word you speak and every act you do.
- *History and clinical examination has no alternative. It is still— the powerful and loving art*.

Remember you are the master but also do not forget that *you are not the only master*; there are others enough alike you with equal potentials.

One should be inspirational, hard working, competitive, should think outside the box, always learning, with calm, cool, courage, compassion, confidant, with proper communication.

When you are an eagle, fly like an eagle even though you are surrounded by Turkeys—Iann MacLennan.

Surgery should not be glamour but it should be a dedicated profession.

Surgeon should be artist, innovator, teacher, superb operator with skill, planning, thinking, understanding merits and demerits, and execution of the skill.

'To be a good doctor one must first be a good human'

SYMPTOMS AND SIGNS

- Two important parts in clinical methods are *symptoms and signs*.
- *Symptom* is the one patient complains of. It is the subjective sensation of the patient.
- *Sign* is the one which clinician elicits. It is an indication of existence of an objective evidence of a disease.
- Even though both *symptoms and signs are complimentary to each other*, sign by and large often becomes more relevant.

Sign

- *Sign* is an indication of existence of an objective evidence of a disease, i.e. such evidence is perceptible to the examining physician, as opposed to the subjective sensation (symptoms) of the patient.
- Usually many signs are observed, confirmed by clinical methods like mobility, fixity, fluctuation, transillumination and clinical conclusion is arrived at.
- Sometimes by one sign diagnosis is clinched, and so called as *diagnostic sign*. Blumberg sign (release sign—while releasing the pressed fingers over the abdomen rebound tenderness is elicited) is diagnostic of peritonitis.
- **Pathognomonic sign** (patho = disease, gnoma = signature, pathognomonic = signature of the disease): Specially distinctive or characteristic sign of a disease or pathological condition on which a diagnosis can be made. Hernial sac which is resonant on percussion and reduces with gurgling is pathognomonic of enterocele.
- **Accessory sign** (Assident sign): Any nonpathognomonic sign of disease, which adds on to the surety of the diagnosis when present.
- **Antecedent sign**: Any precursory indication of an attack of disease. These signs are to be identified at the earliest.

HISTORY TAKING

Clinician should spend adequate time for detailed history taking from the patient. Clinician should show no hurry during conversation; hear sympathetically; behave patiently with the patient; keeping a pleasant face with a smile; should show good bedside (examination table) manners to gain confidence from patients; clinician should avoid harsh words while conversing with patients and relatives. Patient should be made comfortable while taking history. Successful history taking should make patient to completely open out towards the matter needed.

If the patient is a child or patient is dumb, then history is given by the mother or close relative who takes care of the individual. Name and relation of the person who is giving history should be noted down.

History taking should be done in an order and every history should be documented properly. In critical patients it is better to have video documentation of the history taking and explaining the relatives towards the risk involved and therapeutic aspects.

History taking is the first step as—*gathering information; it is a sensitive, respectful, nonjudgmental, confidential thorough interview between patient and the clinician*.

General History

Name

Correct name of the patient should be asked and noted down. It is better to remember each patient by name while doing rounds, at least up to the discharge from the hospital. This helps to build a zone of comfort with the doctor for the patient. It may be helpful to keep a pocket note book to write down in short about the details of the patient. Asking patients name gives the identity; creates cordial relationship; achieve patient's cooperation.

Age

- Noting the age of the patient is important.
- Certain diseases are specific to certain age group. Cleft lip and palate; phimosis, meningocele, cystic hygroma, exists since birth. Congenital anomalies occur in young age group.
- Branchial cyst even though of congenital origin occurs in later age group in 2nd or 3rd decade.
- Certain tumors like Wilm's tumor (kidney) and neuroblastoma occur in early childhood.
- Sarcomas develop in adolescents. Usually carcinomas occur after middle age. But malignancies can occur at any age group.
- Benign prostatic hyperplasia occurs in old age often causing retention of urine.
- Polio, acute osteomyelitis and arthritis and tuberculosis occur in children.

Congenital dislocation of hip (CDH)	< 5 years
Legg-Calve-Perthe's disease	5–10 years
Slipped femoral epiphysis	10–15 years
Secondary osteoarthritis	Up to 25–30 years
Primary osteoarthritis	45 years and later

Sex

Certain diseases occur only in one particular sex other than gender specific diseases. Hemophilia occurs only in males but females can be carriers. Thyroid diseases are more common in females. Carcinoma lung, stomach, kidney are more common in males but can occur in females. Gallstones, hysteria, mobile kidney, carcinoma breast are common in females.

Religion

Carcinoma penis is not seen in Muslims and Jews due to their religious practice of early circumcision in childhood. Duodenal ulcer perforation is common in Muslims during fasting month of Ramzan. Carcinoma breast is common in Parsees.

Residence

Complete postal address and method of communication must be taken down. Many diseases have got geographical distribution. Hydatid disease is common in Australia, Iran, Greece, etc; schistosomiasis is common in Egypt; trypanosomiasis is common in Africa; amebiasis is common in tropical countries; leprosy in West Bengal; gallstones in Bihar and north east India; peptic ulcer in South India; endemic goiter in mountain region [Republic of Guatemala country at the ranges of Andes Mountain and Republic of Panama used to have high prevalence (38%) of endemic goiter due to iodine deficiency until iodized salt usage has standardized]; madura foot in Madurai; kangri cancer in Kashmir **(Figs. 1-4A to C)**; filariasis in Surat, Orissa; guinea worm infestation in Tamil Nadu, north Gujarat, Rajasthan.

Occupation

- Some diseases are common in people with certain occupations. Varicose veins are common in people who stand for long hours like bus conductors, garden workers, watchmen, traffic policemen, barbers, surgeons, and nurses, etc.
- Sportsmen are more prone to injuries to ankle, knee and elbow.
- Certain malignancies can occur as occupational disease. High-risk of leukemia is present in people exposed to ionizing radiation and working in nuclear reactors. Aromatic amines, benzenes, asbestos, nickel, arsenic, coal tar, petroleum are carcinogens (can cause cancers). Carcinoma urinary bladder is more common in workers in aniline dye factories.
- Exposure to ultraviolet radiation can cause skin cancers.
- Vibrating tools can cause Raynaud's phenomenon and osteoporosis of wrist bones.
- Certain *adventitious bursae* can develop due to friction—like housemaid's knee (prepatellar bursitis); clergyman's knee (infrapatellar bursitis); student's elbow (olecranon bursitis).
- Inguinal hernia can occur in heavy weight lifters, hookworm infestation is common in farmers; plumbers may develop lead poisoning; carbon monoxide poisoning can occur in automobile workers; pneumoconiosis in silica workers; jaundice in trinitrotoluene workers.

Social Status

Tuberculosis is common in low socioeconomic group; peptic ulcer disease is common in high socioeconomic group. *Social status* is classified as:
- Class I—professionals;
- Class II—executive and higher management;
- Class III—lower management and clerical;
- Class IV—skilled laborers;
- Class V—unskilled laborers.

■ CHIEF COMPLAINTS

Main complaints of the patient are mentioned in the chronological order of occurrence. Complaints of same duration should be narrated in the order of severity. For example:
- Lump in the breast—6 months.
- Ulcer in the swelling of breast—2 months.
- Pain in the breast—1 month.
- Fever—1 month.

Proper leading questions should be avoided but sometimes are necessary to elicit clear relevant history. But this should be used only after proper initial detailed history. History should be elicited in language which the patient is comfortable. One should not elicit diagnosis from the patient. Negative reply of the patient is also very relevant and so it should not be ignored.

Main complaint gives the idea as which system in the body is grossly affected. For example—constipation and diarrhea in gastrointestinal disease; pain in right iliac fossa in

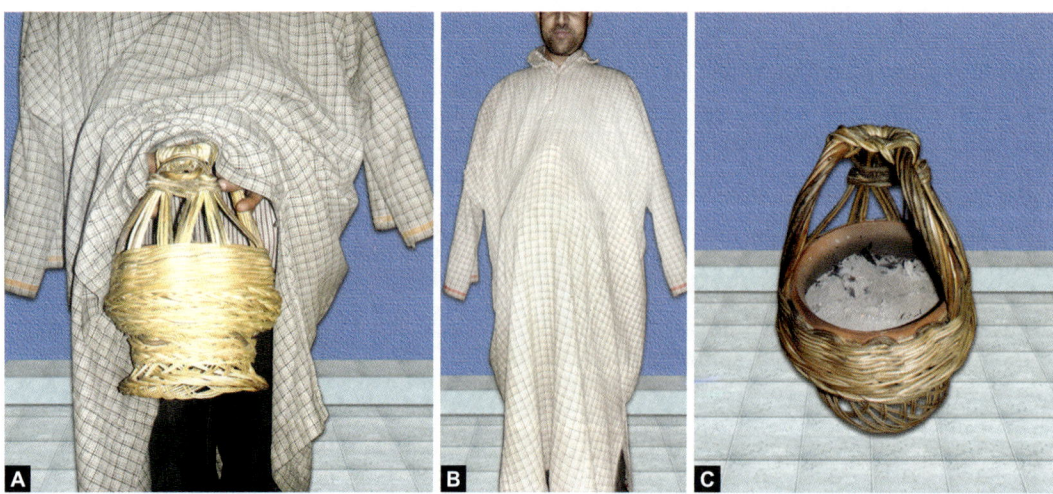

Figs. 1-4A to C Kangri is a special device used in Kashmir to warm the body to tolerate extreme cold; pot with hot charcoal is placed in a bamboo basket which is kept close to the abdomen under the clothes so as to keep the body warm. Kangri cancer is common in Kashmir; it is squamous cell carcinoma in lower abdomen.

appendicitis; hematuria (blood passage in urine) in urinary stones or tumors.

■ HISTORY OF PRESENT ILLNESS

It is detailed history in relation to onset of the present disease until date. It should be in order of occurrence. Each symptom should be questioned/enquired in detail before going to next part of the history.

Mode of Onset of Symptom

It may be gradual, or sudden or initially slow but later progress rapidly. History suggestive of whether it is related to any trauma or any earlier disease should be asked.

Progress of the Disease

Whether the symptoms are decreasing or increasing; in severity gradual or rapid; or waxing and waning should be asked (increase-decrease-increase). For example—pain due to ureteric stone is colic and often intermittent; pain of acute appendicitis is progressive and persisting. Pain of intussusception (telescoping one segment of the bowel to adjacent segment) appears and disappears. Pain of salivary calculus is waxing and waning.

Related Symptoms Suggestive of Complications of the Disease

Though patient may not be able to reveal these should be specifically asked for by leading questions. For example—history suggestive of melena or steatorrhea in jaundice; history of hematemesis in acid peptic disease; difficulty in swallowing in thyroid disease.

Associated Symptoms

Patient may or may not reveal any changes in weight; if not revealed direct enquiry into the weight gain or loss to be made as it is very important aspect to be noted in gastrointestinal, visceral and advanced malignancies.

Often history like back pain, headache, visual problems, disability may require to be elicited carefully which in fact patient may presume them as not relevant.

Note: Detailed enquiry of specific symptoms like pain, fever, loss of weight, vomiting, jaundice and constipation should be made (discussed under *"specific symptoms"* later in this chapter).

■ PAST HISTORY

Old (earlier) diseases should be detailed in order. Often patient may not know the name of the disease which he had earlier. History suggestive of specific disease should be elicited like tuberculosis, syphilis, leprosy, bronchial asthma, diabetes mellitus, and tropical diseases. When such disease has occurred; detailed history of treatment taken; response to treatment should be asked for. Often patient might have got hospitalized for the treatment which should be asked in detail like place where he is hospitalized; duration; type of treatment (type of drugs, injections, etc.). Earlier treatment summary/prescriptions if present should be taken and studied for reference.

History of earlier surgery/trauma; its detail like duration of hospital stay, recovery period, any postoperative complications, drain placed or not, response of surgery, whether patient is relieved of symptoms completely or partially should be asked for any operative notes available for reference.

History of taking chemotherapy earlier (for malignancies or tuberculosis or leprosy), their side effects if any should be asked for. Detailed chemotherapy regime in malignancy and going through earlier documentation are also important.

Previous history of radiotherapy, its detail, number of days, type, dose, complications, and response to radiotherapy should be asked for.

Long-term drug intake should be asked if any in all patients. Examples—steroids (for asthma, joint diseases, ulcerative colitis, etc; dose, type—tablet or inhalation); hormone intake like thyroxine, oral contraceptives; antithyroid drugs like carbimazole or propylthiouracil; psychiatric drugs; analgesics like diclofenac or ibuprofen; oral antidiabetics or insulin; antihypertensives; anticoagulants like warfarin. Side effects, duration of intake and relevant documents should be collected and analyzed.

History of allergy to any drugs like penicillins, septran, analgesics and other antibiotics should be asked. Type of allergy—rashes, anaphylaxis, edema, utricaria or acute problems should be asked for. Allergy to food or other allergens should be noted. Allergy to egg and certain diets are not uncommon.

■ PERSONAL HISTORY

History of personal habits like smoking beedi or cigarettes with duration/frequency/number of beedi or cigarettes per day; history of drinking alcohol with duration, quantity, whether addicted, whether associated with alcohol-induced problems should be noted.

Diet

Vegetarian or nonvegetarian; spicy or bland; more carbohydrate (rice) or protein or fatty diet—should be asked for. Type of diet is also relevant in many diseases like atherosclerosis, diabetes. History of tapioca intake should be taken especially in people from Kerala which is commonly associated with chronic pancreatitis.

Drinking Habits

Alcohol Intake

A problem drinker is one whose physical, social and mental well-being is harmed by drinking. *One unit* of alcohol equals to 8 grams of alcohol in 290 mL of 4% beer. *Teetotaler* is one who has not taken alcohol in last one year.

Occasional drinker is one not taken alcohol in last one month. *Light drinker* is one who drinks alcohol <25 units per week in males; <15 units in females. **Moderate drinker** is the one who drinks alcohol 25–35 units/week in males; 15–25 units in females. **Heavy drinker** is the one who drinks alcohol 36–50 units/week in males; 26–35 units in females. **Very heavy drinker** is the one who drinks alcohol >50 units/week in males; >35 units/week in females.

Alcohol abuse leads into medical, psychiatric and social problems. Consumption of more than 21 units of alcohol per week for women; more than 28 units per week for a man is harmful. Alcohol addiction is a syndrome with withdrawal symptoms (tremor, sweating, anxiousness); symptoms are relieved by drinking; drinking in the morning; increase in quantity of the alcohol intake gradually with tolerance for more quantity; stereotyped pattern of drinking; craving for alcohol; impossible to achieve abstinence; avoiding other activities.

Alcohol causes medical problems like peptic ulcer with bleeding, cirrhosis of liver with its consequences, gynecomastia, testicular atrophy, neuropathy, pancreatitis, diabetes, osteoporosis, nutritional deficiencies, accidents; *psychiatric problems* like anxiousness, delirium, panic attacks, blackouts, confusion, dementia; *social problems* like accidents, crime, debt, violence, loss of job, family problems.

Other Drinking Habits

Drinking tea, coffee, soft drinks (cococola, pepsi, sprite, etc.); quantity, frequency should be asked for. Drinking in more quantity of any of these beverages is harmful to health especially gastrointestinal tract. Drinking more hot tea may cause carcinoma esophagus.

Smoking

Light smoker—one packet of cigarette/day for 2–10 years. *Moderate smoker*—1–10 packets of cigarettes/day. Chronic *heavy smoker* is 10–20 packets of cigarettes/day for 2–10 years. Use of beedies for smoking is equally bad and dangerous to health **(Fig. 1-5)**.

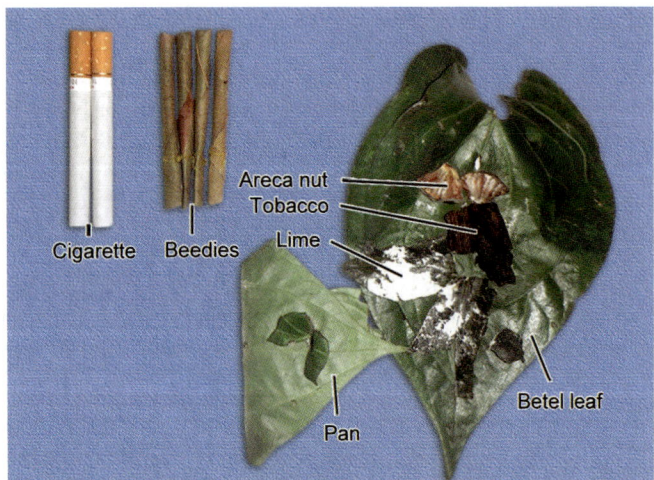

Fig. 1-5 Smoking cigarette, beedies, chewing pan can cause carcinoma lung, oral cavity, etc.

Other Habits

Eating betel nut and leaves—pan, supari, slaked lime and tobacco; snuff inhalation; hookah, chilam smoking; history of contact with sexual workers (can cause sexually transmitted diseases like HIV, syphilis, gonorrhea) should be asked for. Use of protective sex in such situation is important. History of taking narcotics is also important. Tablets, powders, injections are used for narcotic drug intake. Multiple injection pricks may be evident in these patients. Smoking, alcohol and narcotic intake, pan chewing are **addictions**.

Appetite and Weight

Weight gain or loss; increased appetite or loss of appetite are important. Increased appetite is seen in bulemia or some hormone disorders. Appetite is decreased in anorexia nervosa and in tuberculosis, sepsis, malignancies. Feeling fullness and satisfied after intake of small quantity of food is called as *early satiety*. It is suggestive of gastric carcinoma or other gastrointestinal malignancies or infections.

Bowel and Micturition Habits

Frequency in bowel habits, passing blood or mucus, tenesmus and constipation should be asked for. Frequency in urination (number/day and number/night), hematuria, burning and pain during urination should be enquired.

Sleep Habits

Whether patient gets proper sleep, duration of sleep hours or sleeplessness (insomnia) or lethargic; feeling sleepy during day and working time should be asked for. Often patient interprets sleepy nature for tiredness. It should be clearly clarified as tiredness may be due to anemia, renal failure, specific diseases like malignancy, tuberculosis, jaundice. Patient may be taking sleeping tablets for insomnia. Name and dose of the drug should be noted down. Alcohol withdrawal also often causes sleeplessness, irritability, etc.

In Females

A detailed menstrual history should be noted. Time of attaining menarche/menopause/regularity of the cycle/presence of pain/dysmenorrhea/white discharge/date of last menstrual period are noted in detail. Pregnancy history with number of pregnancies/abortions/normal delivery or cesarean section (LSCS)/last child birth should be noted. Any complications during pregnancy and need of any blood transfusions should be asked for.

FAMILY HISTORY AND GENETIC HISTORY

Many diseases run in family. Examples are—piles; breast cancer; diabetes mellitus; tuberculosis; bleeding disorders; hypertension, etc. If any of the family member is suffering from any disease; its detail, type, therapy for the same, whether he has undergone any surgery for the same should be mentioned in detail. Number of siblings and their health details should also be taken.

Tuberculosis as infectious disease, carcinoma breast as familial, hemorrhoids, hypertension and diabetes mellitus as hereditary can occur in family members.

Marital status, number of children their ages and work/education; number brothers/sisters to patient (whether they are suffering from any diseases); parents and their details in relation to health should be asked for. Details about patient's maternal or paternal relatives (uncles) and whether they are suffering from any illnesses should be asked for.

OTHER RELEVANT HISTORY

In younger age group history of immunization for different diseases like poliomyelitis, tetanus, diphtheria, hepatitis is taken. History suggestive of allergy/reactions during earlier drug intake; history of long-term drug therapy like insulin, steroids, antidiabetics, antihypertensives, diuretics, hormones, etc. should be noted. History suggestive of bleeding disorders (hemophilia in males, other coagulopathies, acquired bleeding disorders due to chronic liver disease) should be asked for.

ASSESSMENT OF SPECIFIC SYMPTOMS AND SIGNS

Pain

Pain is the commonest symptom which patient complains to a clinician. Latin word *'poena'* means penalty/punishment. Pain is the one patient feels (symptom and is subjective); tenderness (sign) is the one surgeon/clinician elicits during examination.

Pain is the **nature's warning** to say that something is not well within the body; though we look upon it as a curse but actually it is a boon.

Tenderness sometimes (occasionally) can be a symptom as the patient feels the pain while he himself palpates the painful area; but it is usually recorded as 'pain present while palpating or feeling by the patient himself'.

'Rebound tenderness' is the term used when the patient experiences more pain on release of pressure from the diseased area (usually used in abdomen).

Types of Pain

Superficial pain: It is usually sharp localized pain, due to irritation of peripheral nerve endings in superficial tissue by chemical/mechanical/thermal/electrical injury. It is due to irritation of nerve roots or trunks or endings by pressure or infiltration or inflammation. It is usually well localized, sharp and short duration (acute onset) unlike deep pain. It can cause increased systolic blood pressure and heart rate and pupillary dilatation. When superficial pain is very severe; there will be generalized vasoconstriction of skin, skeletal muscles, brain and gastrointestinal tract due to autonomic reaction.

Segmental pain: It occurs due to irritation of particular nerve trunk/root; located in particular dermatome of the body supplied by the sensory nerve trunk or root.

Deep pain: It is due to irritation of deeper structures like muscles/tendons/bones/joints/viscera. It is vague and diffuse when compared to superficial pain. It is often referred to common segmental areas of representation. Often spasm of skeletal muscle of same spinal cord segment can occur.

Deep pain has either autonomic (organ pain) or somatic (deeper tissue pain) pathways to reach brain. It is dull aching or colicky or crushing or discomfort. Its localization is vague as representation in spinal column is common for skin and deeper structures. Deep pain is often associated with nausea, tiredness, sweating, pallor, decrease in blood pressure and heart rate (bradycardia). Skeletal muscles supplied by the same spinal cord segment may develop involuntary spasm due to deep pain.

Psychogenic pain: It may be functional/emotional/hysterical.

Other types of pain: Due to thalamic/spinothalamic diseases/*causalgia* [intense burning pain along the distribution of the partially injured (and healed) nerve] pain develops along the distribution.

Central pain: Central pain is the one which originates from the brain. It can be functional due to emotional or anxiety status or hysteria. It can be thalamic or spinothalamic lesions or originating from gray matter or hyperexcitability status of the brain even after etiology of pain is no more existing. Due to irritation of the central nervous system, there develops irritability, weakness, sleeplessness, loss of appetite, tachycardia.

Expression of the *pain* is related to the pain threshold. When, in certain area severe pain is present; pain in less severe area is masked. If pain threshold is less, pain intensity will be severe; if pain threshold is more, then pain may be less severe. Often to small extent body develops adaptation to pain. In acute pain, where patient is in shock (like in trauma/road traffic accidents) pain will not be felt for certain (shorter) period immediately after the event. It is due to sudden activation of sympathetic system as defence.

Features of Pain

Exact site, type and character, origin, time of onset, mode of onset, progression and end, duration, severity, movements of pain, aggravating or relieving factors and associated symptoms should be asked for.

Common features of pain	*Specific features of pain*
• Site • Type and character—vague, burning, gnawing, crushing, dull, pricking, continuous, intermittent, colicky, waxing and waning, scalding, rest pain, claudication pain, throbbing, pins and needles, shooting, distension, twisting, constricting, stabbing, etc.	• *Movements of pain*—radiation pain; referred pain; shifting pain; migration of pain • *Precipitating/aggravating factors* • *Relieving factors* • *Pain in relation to exercise,* exertion, meals, urination, etc.

Contd...

Contd...

Common features of pain	Specific features of pain
• *Origin*—dramatic, acute, chronic • *Time of onset* • *Duration* • *Mode of onset*—sudden and persisting or sudden with a decline or insidious and gradual • *Progress*—steadily increasing or slowly gradually declining or gradually progressing or rapidly progressing or fluctuating • *End*—sudden declining and cessation or gradually decreasing or crescendo and later sudden cessation • *Severity*—mild, moderate, severe	• Associated symptoms • *Hunger pain* occurs in duodenal ulcer on empty stomach usually wakes the patient at early morning compulsing him to take some food to relieve his pain • *Migraine* [(Greek) a type of primary severe headache on one side of the head often familial precipitated by certain stimuli and physical activities associated with nausea, vomiting, visual disturbances, an aura (usually visual just before an attack) and sensitivity to light, sound and smell] occurs usually at early morning often at regular intervals like weekly or during menstruation

Specific Points in History in Relation to Pain

Original Site of Pain

Original site of the pain gives fair idea of the anatomical location of the origin of pain. It is very important in identifying probable site of pathology/cause. Pain in the epigastrium means pain is probably originating from stomach/duodenum/pancreas/left lobe of liver; pain in right hypochondrium means pain could be originating from gallbladder/liver; pain in groin means it could be due to hernia/lymph nodes/cord structures. One should also confirm whether pain is *superficial* (abdominal wall or surface in the skin or subcutaneous) or *deep* (intra-abdominal/intrathoracic/deep in the muscle or bone). *Patient should point the site of the pain with one finger (index finger)*. Often pain may be in one site or multiple sites; if it is in multiple sites one should confirm where exactly pain started first and severity in each sites. In acute appendicitis original site of pain is in umbilicus; but later it shifts to right iliac fossa.

Time and Mode of Onset of Pain

It may be *sudden onset, rapidly progressive* in acute appendicitis; it is of *insidious onset* and of long duration with episodic nature in chronic peptic ulcer; pain after trauma means very important and may be an emergency like internal organ injuries (liver, spleen, and kidney) or due to fracture bone.

Time of occurrence of pain is often important in diagnosing the condition. In duodenal ulcer, *hunger pain* occurring in early morning or later evening is typical. *Migraine* occurs in early morning; frontal sinusitis induced headache occurs few hours *after getting up. Cyclical mastalgia* occurs premenstrually and gets relieved in oestrogenic phase. *Mittelschmerz* occurs between 12–14 days of menstruation is actually ovulatory pain in females. *Dysmenorrhea* presents as spasmodic pain in both iliac fossa often with low back pain; it occurs few days prior to menstruation and is relieved by menstruation.

Mode of onset may be *dramatic* wherein pain begins in few seconds reaches peak in minutes with severe intensity. It is seen in perforated duodenal ulcer, ruptured abdominal aortic aneurysm, torsion of ovarian cyst or of testis or mobile spleen. It may be *acute onset* if pain reaches its peak in hours usually due to acute inflammation like cellulitis, abscess, paronychia etc. In *chronic onset* pain begins insidiously reaches to its peak only few weeks to months from the onset—like pain of osteoarthritis (joint pain), pain due to spondylosis.

Type/Nature of Pain

It may be superficial/deep; localized or diffuse; dull ache or sharp severe/pricking/bursting/vague aching (continuous mild pain), throbbing, scalding (burning sensation particularly felt during urination in cystitis, pyelonephritis, urethritis), pins and needles pricking sensation (in peripheral nerve injury or irritation), shooting pain (seen in intervertebral disc prolapse and sciatica—pain shoots along the course of nerve), stabbing pain (sudden, severe, sharp, episodic—seen in perforated duodenal ulcer), distension pain (a feeling of restricted or distended like in paralytic ileus or intestinal obstruction), colicky pain (due to muscular contraction in a hollow tube in an attempt to obviate the obstruction by forcing the content out, which is gripping, and episodic associated with vomiting and sweating seen in intestinal colic, ureteric colic of stone, biliary colic of stone), twisting pain (of bowel volvulus/twisted ovarian cyst/torsion testis), constricting pain (around the chest by angina), etc.

Often patient perceives pain in different way; in such situation detailed history is needed to find right type of pain.

Colicky pain is sudden in onset, *gripping nature* (gripping nature is *most important* in colicky pain) which begins suddenly, and disappears suddenly. It has got two features; it comes and goes in a sinusoidal pattern; it is migrating constrictive and gripping in nature; it is due to spasmodic contraction of the hollow tube as forcible attempt to push the contents across the constriction or obstruction. Patient develops tachycardia, vomiting and sweating. It is either intestinal or ureteric or biliary or salivary (salivary calculus) or Fallopian tube or uterine in origin.

Distension pain is encircling and restricting the wall like of bowel/bladder, capsulated neoplasm or fascial compartment (leg/forearm/thigh/arm). It may cause tightness/bursting sensation.

Constricting pain occurs in chest, abdomen, limbs or head; it is like a iron band tightening in the part. Example is constricting pain of angina pectoris.

Stabbing pain is sudden, severe, sharp and for a short period.

Severity of the Pain

Pain may be *mild/moderate/severe (agonizing, terrible)*. Severe pain wakes the patient suddenly from his sleep; stops him working further; makes him to roll around the bed; makes him restless and anxious; prevents him from getting proper sleep.

Severe pain is common in acute appendicitis, acute pancreatitis, ureteric colic, perforation of bowel, acute peritonitis, intestinal obstruction, acute abscess.

Type and severity of the pain depends on the etiology for the pain and extent of the disease. It may be due to inflammation, abscess formation, nerve irritation, distension of organ, stretching of fascia or capsule, obstruction or infiltration by neoplasm.

Progression of Pain

It may be persistent and progressive; or initially mild, gradually increases, later gradually subsides; fluctuation in intensity—whether increases and decreases in intensity at regular intervals or quickly reaches maximum and remains like that.

Pain progresses to maximum and may remain like that or it reaches maximum and suddenly or slowly disappear completely or severity may progress with waxing and waning (fluctuating pain) variably or pain progresses to peak, disappears fully and may reappear with original severity. In duodenal ulcer perforation initially severe pain appears for certain period later pain reduces but eventually becomes more severe. Initially leak of acid chemical into the peritoneal cavity causes pain which gets diluted by peritoneal fluid leads into reduction in pain but once bacterial peritonitis develops there is reappearance of severe pain.

Duration of Pain

Duration of pain should be mentioned in minutes/hours/days/weeks/months/years. It can be acute/subacute/chronic. Exacerbations of pain with period of remissions are common which should be mentioned. It is often seen in peptic ulcer, osteoarthritis. Colicky pain lasts usually for a minute in each episode; anginal pain lasts for 3–5 minutes; but an acute pain of pancreatitis persists.

Periodicity of Pain

Pain appears, persists for few weeks and then disappears for few weeks and again reappears. Such periodicity is often observed in chronic peptic ulcer; trigeminal neuralgia. Peptic ulcer pain may be seasonal. Migraine headache occurs once in few weeks or during menstruation in females.

Precipitating/Aggravating Factors

Abdominal pain may get worsened by taking food like in gastric ulcer. Pain due to appendicitis, ureteric stone aggravates in change of position, walking, jolting. Pain of urinary bladder stone aggravates in standing position. In reflux esophagitis pain increases while bending. Pain in pancreatitis increases on lying down. Pain in intervertebral disc prolapse aggravates by lifting the weight. Pain in sigmoid diverticulitis may increase by exercise or movement. Pain in gastritis aggravates by taking nonsteroidal anti-inflammatory drugs (NSAIDs). Peritonitis pain increases by coughing, deep breathing and moving abdomen. Ischemic claudication pain aggravates by walking. Cardiac angina aggravates by exertion.

Relieving Factors of Pain

Pain reduces by certain methods and so patient uses those methods to relieve the pain. Hunger pain of early morning in duodenal ulcer is relieved by taking food. Pain of pancreatitis is relieved in sitting and bending forward position. Propped up position relieves pain of reflux esophagitis. In acute peritonitis, pain reduces temporarily by lying still.

Associated Symptoms

Acute pain may be associated with pallor, sweating and vomiting. Migraine pain with vomiting and visual disturbances; intestinal/ureteric colic with sweating, vomiting and cold periphery; acute pyelonephritis and urinary infections with chills/rigors and fever; ureteric colic with hematuria; biliary colic with jaundice and pale stool are other examples of such association. Ruptured ectopic pregnancy, aortic aneurysm have severe pain with severe pallor.

Pain May Move from One Place to Other

Radiation of pain: It is extension of pain from original site to another site with persisting of pain at original site. This radiating pain is of same character of original site. Penetration of duodenal ulcer posteriorly causes pain both in epigastrium and back—is an example. Pain of pancreatitis radiates back. In ureteric colic pain radiates from loin to groin; frequently to testis in male. In myocardial infarction, pain develops in the left side chest which eventually radiates towards left side neck and left upper limb.

Referred pain: Pain is not felt at the site of the disease but felt at distant site. It is due to common area of representation in brain for visceral and somatic components and inability of brain to differentiate between two sites. Diaphragmatic irritation causes referred pain at the tip of shoulder as the segmental supply of diaphragm (phrenic nerve C4, C5) and shoulder (cutaneous supply—C4, C5 through supraclavicular nerves) is same. Hip joint pathology may cause referred pain in knee joint—through articular branches of femoral, obturator and sciatic nerves. Other examples—referred pain in ear from carcinoma tongue through lingual and auriculotemporal nerve; referred pain in the epigastrium from the heart; referred pain in the abdomen from pleura; referred pain over the testis from the ureter. Foregut pain refers to upper abdomen in the midline; midgut in the middle of the umbilical region; hindgut to lower abdomen in the midline. It is through the corresponding somatic area of the skin in relation to corresponding visceral nerve distribution.

Shifting of pain: Origin of pain is at one site; later pain shifts to another site and pain at original site disappears. Pain when begins in viscera, it is felt at the same somatic segmental area in the body; but once parietal layer is involved by inflammation/pathology pain is felt at the anatomical site.

Example is pain of acute appendicitis where original visceral pain is at the umbilicus (T9 and T10 segments supply both umbilicus and appendix) which shifts later to right iliac fossa when once the parietal peritoneum of that area is inflamed.

Migration of pain: It is a feature of spreading inflammation from one site to adjacent/distant site. In perforated duodenal ulcer duodenal content later spills over the right paracolic gutter and so pain from epigastrium shifts downwards with spread of peritonitis; in perforated/burst appendicitis initial right iliac fossa pain migrates towards left iliac fossa indicating spreading of peritonitis (peritonitis initially localized becomes generalized).

Grading of pain:
It is done using pain scale. It is compared to a 10 cm line numbered 0 to 10. This is called as visual analog scale (VAS).
- *Minimum* is 0 means no pain;
- 2 is *mild*;
- 4 is *discomforting*;
- 6 is *distressing*;
- 8 is *intense*;
- 10 is the *worst excruciating pain*.

Hiccup (Singultus)

It is spasmodic contraction of diaphragm. It is *commonly idiopathic* which subsides on its own.

Types

- **Postoperative hiccup is common.** It is due to increased abdominal pressure, pushing the under surface of the diaphragm upwards. It may be due to paralytic ileus, gastric dilatation, and intestinal obstruction.
- **Peritonitis involving diaphragmatic surface can cause hiccup.**
- **Renal failure (usually advanced one) causes hiccup.** Typical facial look, brown dry tongue with typical pallor; edema face and feet may be obvious. Blood urea, serum creatinine and electrolytes should be done.

Vomiting

Vomiting is a common symptom heard in clinical practice.

Causes of vomiting:

General:
- Acute infection
- Renal failure
- Acidosis
- Diabetic ketosis, hypercalcemia
- Pregnancy
- Food poisoning
- Hyperparathyroidism
- Labyrinthitis

Gastrointestinal:
- Acute gastritis
- Pyloric stenosis
- Carcinoma stomach
- Intestinal obstruction
- Mesenteric ischemia
- Acute gastric dilatation
- Acute abdomen like peritonitis, pancreatitis, cholecystitis
- Paralytic ileus
- Intestinal, ureteric, biliary colic

Central nervous system:
- Intracranial space occupying diseases like tumor, abscess
- Intracranial hemorrhage
- Stroke
- Meningitis, encephalitis
- Migraine

Psychogenic—anorexia nervosa

Drug induced:
- Alcohol
- Anesthetic drugs
- Chloroquine
- Nonsteroidal anti-inflammatory drugs (NSAIDs)
- Poisonous drugs
- Morphine, digitalis

Reflex:
- Glaucoma
- Travelling sickness
- Colicky abdomen like ureteric stone

Vomiting may be:
- One/multiple episodes
- Continuous/intermittent
- Mild/severe
- Projectile/regurgitant (effortless)
- Of short duration—acute cause/long duration—chronic cause
- Slight quantity/moderate quantity/profuse quantity

Vomitus may be:
- Watery—gastric juice—acidic
- Ingested food
- Blood—recent fresh blood; old, dark, clotted blood; coffee ground—altered blood and blood clot (red wine and iron preparations can create coffee ground vomitus)
- Bile—greenish yellow (green tinge of bile can be better made by diluting it with water)
- Dark green colored—upper small bowel obstruction
- Feculent, brown with smell—lower small bowel obstruction (vomited tea mimics feculent)
- Fecal (frank)—in gastrocolic fistula
- Acute onset/insidious onset

Vomiting is graded as follows:
0 – None;
1 – One episode of vomiting in 24 hours;
2 – 2–5 episodes/24 hours;
3 – >6 episodes/24 hours;
4 – Needs parenteral fluid/nutrition.

It may be due to—pregnancy, traveling sickness, labyrinthitis, gastritis, peptic ulcer, migraine, meningitis, intracranial tumor, ureteric colic, pyloric stenosis, carcinoma stomach (pylorus), intestinal obstruction, intracranial space occupying diseases, acute peritonitis, cholecystitis, pancreatitis, metabolic causes like diabetic ketosis, and drug induced.

- Color, quantity, smell of the vomitus should be asked. Coffee ground colored vomitus is seen in upper GI bleed. When bled blood comes in contact with gastric juice, hemoglobin forms acid hematin coloring content blackish or dark brown. Vomitus may contain frank blood/clots.
- Presence of undigested material should be asked for.
- Esophageal obstruction by achalasia cardia or stricture causes regurgitation.
- Nonbilious vomiting means obstruction proximal to sphincter of Oddi.
- Bilious vomiting occurs in small bowel obstruction; which may be either yellow or green colored.
- Fecal content in the vomitus suggests ileal/large bowel obstruction. Feculent vomiting is also seen in gastrocolic fistula. Content is brown in color with fecal odor.
- *Hematemesis* is vomiting bright red or dark blood. *Melemesis* is vomiting of altered blood (coffee ground); bled blood in the stomach stays for long time here

for gastric acid to convert hemoglobin into hematin. Hematemesis should be distinguished from hemoptysis.

Nausea

It is sense (feel) of vomiting. It may or may not end up with vomiting. It can be none (0); nausea present but able to eat (1); oral intake is reduced (2); No oral intake, on IV fluids (3).

Itching (Pruritus)

It is due to local or general causes. Multiple scratch marks are often obvious.

It may be due to:
- *Skin diseases*: Utricaria, eczema, scabies (Psoriasis will not cause itching).
- *Local causes*: Clothing, washing soap, washing powder, fungal, parasites like fleas, scabies; vaginal and rectal discharge.
- *Systemic causes:* Obstructive jaundice due to bile acid irritation, Hodgkin's disease, leukemia, uremia, allergy/hypersensitivity, drug reactions, diabetes mellitus, etc.
- *Allergic reactions:* Drugs can cause itching.

Fatigue

It is subjective sensation of weakness (asthenia/lethargy). It is graded as none (0); fatigue over baseline (1); moderate fatigue (2); severe (3); bedridden (4).

Anorexia

It is loss of appetite: it is seen in anorexia nervosa, gastrointestinal (GI) cancers, tuberculosis, debilitating illness like sepsis. Anorexia is graded as none (0); loss of appetite (1); significant reduction in oral intake (2); unable to take orally requiring IV fluids (3).

Satiety is sense of fullness after completion of meals. It is normal. *Early satiety* **is a feature of GI malignancy; patient feels full and satisfied with small quantity of food.**

Flatulence and Regurgitation

- *Flatulence* is frequent belching more than normal.
- *Regurgitation* is effortless return of food into the mouth. It is associated with powerful involuntary contractions of abdominal muscles. It is seen esophageal/OG junction obstructions like carcinoma and achalasia cardia.
- *Heartburn* is burning sensation behind the sternum due to acid reflux into the esophagus.

Defecation

Frequency, physical characters of the stool, pain during defecation should be asked for. Stool may be brown/black/pale/white/silvery in *color*. It may be hard/soft/watery in *consistency*. It may be bulky/pellets/string or tape like. It may contain *blood;* blood may be mixed with stool or on the surface of the stool or may appear after passing stool. Stool may be mixed with mucus or pus. *Pain* may be before or after defecation or throughout the defecation.

Constipation

It is defined as having bowel movement fewer than three times per week; with hard, dry, small sized stool; difficult to evacuate. It is *graded* as none (0); needs diet modification (1); needs laxatives (2); needs manual evacuation or enema (3); due to obstruction (4).
- **Constipation can *be relative* wherein patient can pass flatus but not feces; *or absolute* wherein patient neither can pass feces nor flatus.**
- **Constipation can occur due to many causes—habitual, congenital cause like congenital megacolon (Hirschsprung's disease), anorectal malformations and acquired causes like colonic carcinoma, stricture.**

Diarrhea

Diarrhea is defined as more than *3 stools* per day, containing *300 mL* or more of fluid per day. It is usually soft, often foul smelling. Often it may be associated with incontinence. It is *graded* as frequency of 3-4 times/day (1); frequency 4-6/day (2); frequency >7/day or with incontinence or need parenteral nutrition (3); needs intensive care with hemodynamic collapse (4).
- *Surgical causes of diarrhea:* Intestinal tuberculosis, carcinoma colon, amoebic infection, intestinal resection, ulcerative colitis, irritable bowel syndrome.
- *Diarrhea may be acute onset or chronic; it may be watery/bloody/mucus/bloody mucus/dysentery/painful diarrhea/painless/early morning diarrhea.*
- *Steatorrhea* is copious, frothy, pale stool.

■ PHYSICAL EXAMINATION

It should be done in privacy. Female patients should be examined in presence of a female/nurse. Examination should be done with limited clothing to elicit proper findings. Broad day light is ideal for examination. Usage of other lights may mislead or mimic some clinical findings like jaundice **(Figs. 1-6 to 1-9).**

General Examination

This part of the examination is essential preliminary step in all patients. Patient's intelligence level should be assessed while taking history. Uneducated people can still be intelligent.

General examination is done for proper diagnosis and differential diagnosis; for selecting the patient for anesthesia; to decide type of surgery to be done (mesh hernioplasty is done in inguinal hernia if patient is having chronic respiratory disease or if there is poor abdominal muscle tone); to predict the prognosis (patients with gastrointestinal cancer showing palpable supraclavicular lymph node means poor prognosis). It usually includes—looking for pallor, pulse, respiration, edema feet, clubbing, cyanosis, jaundice, blood pressure. Each will be discussed in detail.

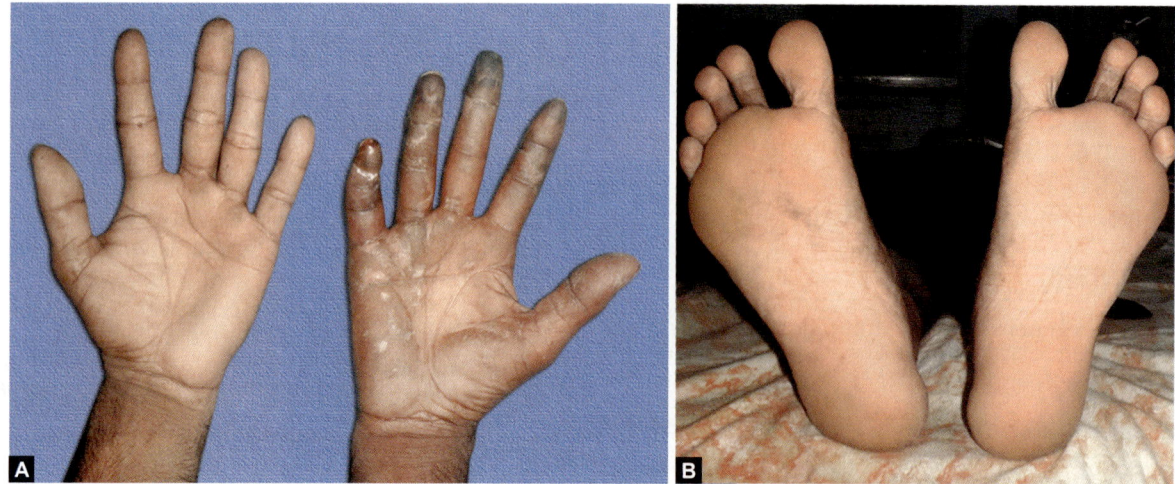

Figs. 1-6A and B Both sides should be examined and compared like—in limbs (hands, feet, forearms, arms, joints), eye, ears, face in bilateral anatomical areas.

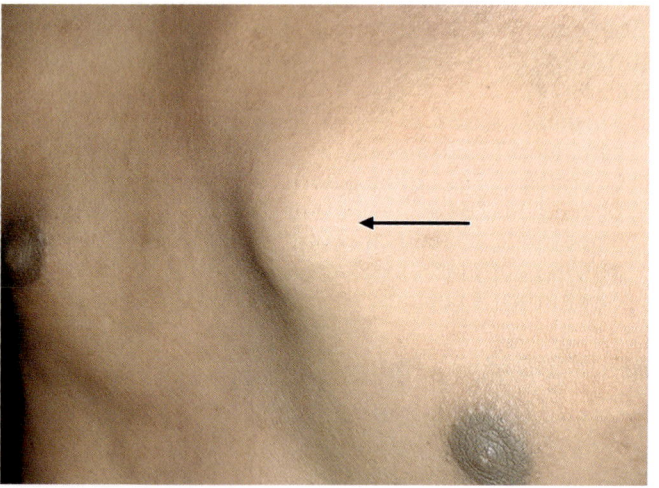

Fig. 1-7 Systemic examination is a must. Note the chest wall swelling in this patient. Clothings should be removed properly while examining the patient. This swelling may be due to secondary in the rib or primary tumor.

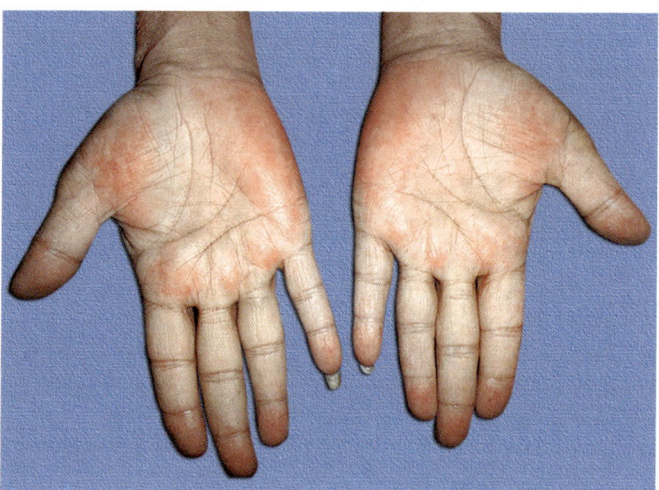

Fig. 1-9 Both hands should be examined. Palmar erythema of both hands is seen in this patient.

Mental Status

Mental status and level of consciousness should be assessed in general but in particular in specific clinical situations like head injury, hepatic encephalopathy, septic shock, etc.

Grading of the mental status	
Grade I	Properly oriented in time, space and person
Grade II	Conscious but without orientation of time, space and person
Grade III	Drowsy and semiconscious
Grade IV	Unconscious but responding to painful stimuli
Grade V	Unconscious and comatose and not responding to painful stimuli

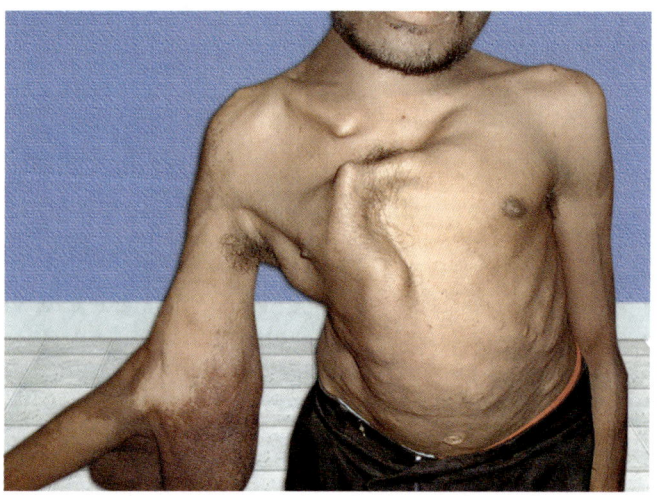

Fig. 1-8 Chest wall deformity.

Built and Nutritional Status

Built and nutritional status of the patient is important to assess.

Built is structural organization of underlying skeleton. It is related to age and sex of the patient. Gigantism is height to that age is in excess than normal (in adult more than 6.5 feet). It may be due to racial; familial; endocrine (hyperpituitarism, hypogonadism); genetic (Klinefelter's syndrome); metabolic (Marfan's syndrome, homocystinuria); overeating; cerebral causes. Dwarfism is height to that age and sex is far less than normal (below 4.5 feet). It can be due to hereditary, chromosomal (Turner's syndrome, Down's syndrome); delayed growth; nutritional (Rickets); endocrine (hypopituitarism, hypothyroidism, excess androgens, congenital adrenal hyperplasia, insulin insufficiency); skeletal (achondroplasia, spinal deformities); systemic diseases (uremia, cyanotic heart diseases, cirrhosis).

In *normal adult*, height of the person is equal to length of arm span. Upper segment from vertex to pubic symphysis is equal to lower segment from pubic symphysis to heel.

In infants upper segment is more than lower segment and height is more than arm span. This *infantile body frame* persists in achondroplasia, cretinism, and juvenile myxedema.

Greater arm span than height and greater lower segment is observed in Marfan's syndrome, homocystinuria, Klinefelter's syndrome, Frohlich's syndrome.

Nutrition is the proportion of soft tissue structures (muscles, soft tissues, fat) in relation to the bony structure. In gastrointestinal malignancy or in other malignancy with metastases patient will be cachexic. Protein deficiency causes rough skin, brittle hair, and edema feet. Fat deficiency causes cachexia, hollow cheeks, and loss of fat in hips, abdomen and subcutaneous tissues of elbow. Deficiency of minerals and vitamins has got specific features.

Severe malnutrition causes wasting of muscles, ill skeletonized look. Reduced weight, loss of subcutaneous fat, edema (generalized), alopecia, decreased hand grip and respiratory muscle power are features.

Assessment of nutrition body mass index (BMI) which is weight in kilogram divided by height in meters square. BMI less than 18.5 suggests malnutrition. Triceps skin fold thickness, mid arm muscle circumference are other tools used to assess malnutrition. Biochemical estimation of serum albumin, prealbumin, transferrin and retinol binding proteins are useful (Figs. 1-10A and B).

$$\text{Body mass index (BMI)} = \frac{\text{Body weight in kilogram}}{(\text{Height in meters})^2}$$

Example: If body weight is 80 kg and height is 1.8 meter; then BMI is $80/1.8^2 = 80/3.24 = 24.69$.

Obesity may be due to idiopathic cause (more intake), mental retardation, alcohol intake, genetic, hypothalamic causes, endocrine (thyroid/parathyroid/adrenal disorders), testicular atrophy, drugs like insulin, oral antidiabetics, steroids, estrogens.

Body Weight

Body weight is controlled by rate of energy expenditure; it is regulated by energy-related hormones. Neuropeptide Y present in the nervous system promotes anabolism by stimulating the secretion of the insulin. Corticotropin-releasing hormone has got catabolic activity. Hypothalamus controls the energy reserve in body.

Nutritional status	BMI (kg/m²)
Underweight	<18.5
Normal	18.5–24.9
Overweight (Preobesity)	25.0–29.9
Obesity	>30
• Class I	• 30.0–34.9
• Class II (Moderate)	• 35.0–39.9
• Class III (Severe/Morbid)	• 40.0
Superobesity	>50
Super superobesity	>60

Weight Gain

It is increase in weight. It is graded as <5% (0); 5–10% (1); 10–20% (2); >20% (3). It is seen in obesity, pregnancy, myxedema, water retention, Cushing's syndrome. Weight gain

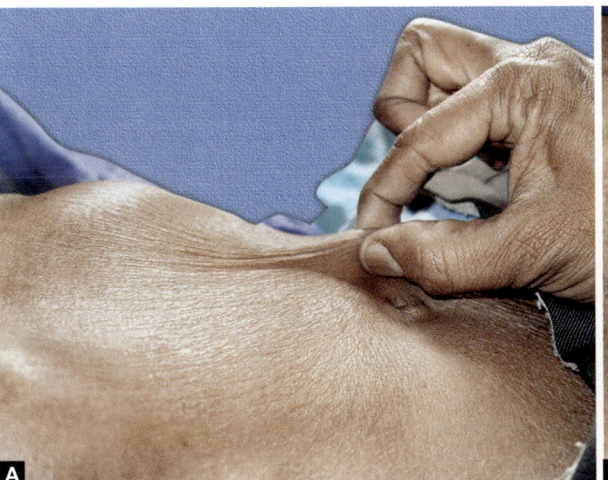
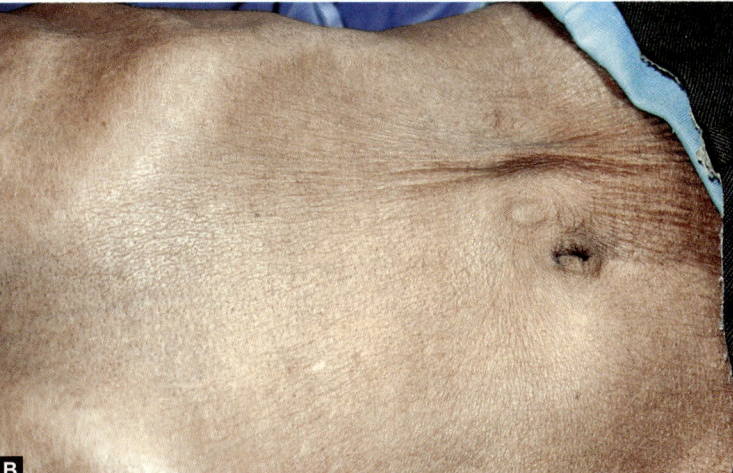

Figs. 1-10A and B Assessment of subcutaneous fat and dehydration.

also occurs in liver/kidney/cardiac failures, hypoproteinemia, lymphedema, increased muscle mass by anabolic steroids, hormone-related causes; ovarian cyst, etc.

Weight Loss

- *Weight loss* is graded as <5% (0); 5–10% (1); 10–20% (2); > 20% (3). But time duration of weight loss is also important.
- **Definition of significant weight loss** *(2009):* Weight loss more than 5% (up to 7.5%) in 30 days; weight loss more than 7.5% (up to 10%) in 60 days; weight loss more than 10% in 180 days.
- Weight loss can occur **with adequate** food intake or **with diminished** food intake.
- Weight loss is assessed by loosening of clothes; clothes mainly trousers at waist will be too commodious.
- It can be **due to increased utilization**—like thyrotoxicosis, anxiousness, drug induced; **decreased absorption**—like chronic pancreatitis, carcinoid disease, hypermotility of bowel, short bowel syndrome; abnormal calorie loss—like gastrointestinal fistula, worm infestations, diabetes.

Causes are—anorexia nervosa, depression, psychosis, gastric ulcer, colitis, worm infestations, liver/biliary/pancreatic diseases, gastrointestinal malignancies, surface malignancies with visceral spread, leukemia, lymphoma, sarcoma with spread, chronic bacterial infections, tuberculosis (pulmonary or erxtrapulmonary like abdominal, urinary), autoimmune diseases like rheumatoid arthritis, systemic lupus erythematosus, alcohol intake, smoking, Addison's disease, chronic lung and cardiac diseases, acquired immune deficiency syndrome (AIDS), chronic renal failure [CRF/CKD (chronic kidney disease)].

Wasting

It is obvious on the upper half of the body as there is often edema due to hypoproteinemia in lower half of body. It is observed in starvation, severe gastroenteritis, tuberculosis, anorexia nervosa, diabetes mellitus, advanced carcinomas, gastrointestinal malignancies, and old age.

Severity of wasting can be assessed by looking at shoulder girdle, loose skin of arms, trunk and buttocks (Fig. 1-11).

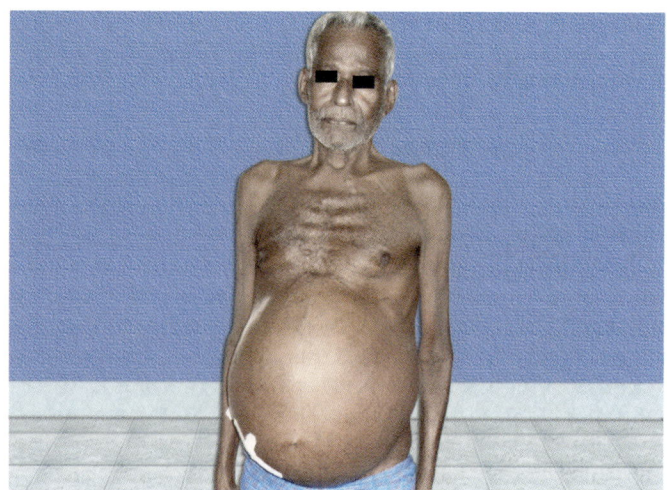

Fig. 1-11 Ascites with wasting of proximal part probably due to malignancy.

Nutritional deficiency is assessed by skin texture, arm circumference, muscle mass, body weight, BMI (Figs. 1-12A and B).

Malignant Cachexia

Here the patient looks *emaciated, languid, sallow, with pale face, loose wrinkled skin, loss of fat, dry skin, with lost appetite/weight/energy* and with oral infection—candida and stomatitis. **Profound loss of weight is typical**. Usually *they do not experience* any pain **(Figs. 1-13A and B)**.

Attitude of the Patient

It is typical changed position of the body or part of the body like limbs. In posterior dislocation of hip, limb is shortened and internally rotated. Comatose patient/paraplegic or quadriplegic patient is silent and immobile. Patient in shock or with peritonitis may not move due to pain. Patient with ureteric stone may be restless and rolling in the bed due to severe colicky pain. Different attitudes in different fractures of the limbs are typical and useful in diagnosing the site of fractures.

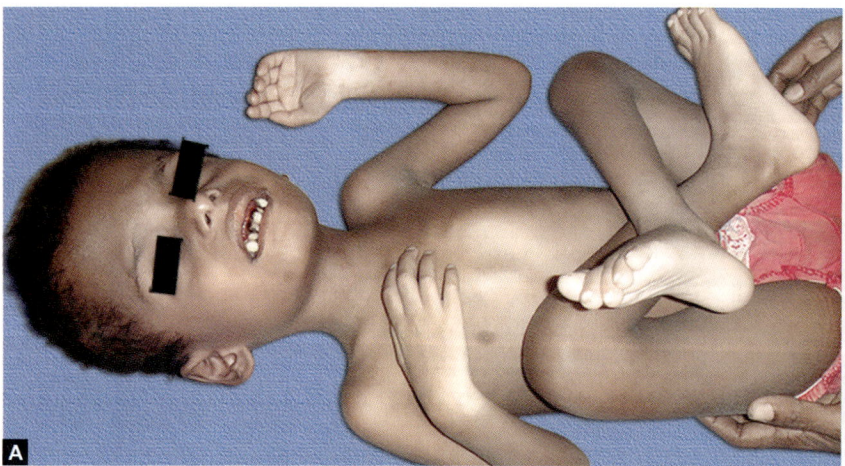 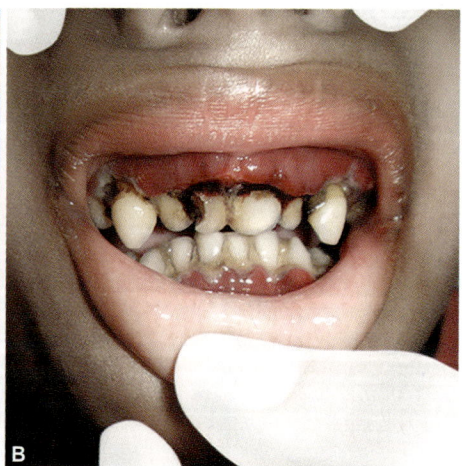

Figs. 1-12A and B Malnourished child with features of protein-energy malnutrition.

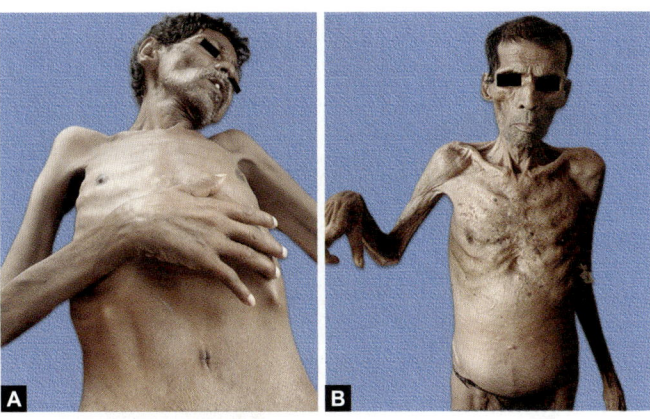

Figs. 1-13A and B Typical malignant cachexia—emaciated, languish, sallow and pale look with dry wrinkled skin.

Decubitus of the Patient

Position of the patient in the bed is called as decubitus. Decubitus is derived from the Latin word ***decumbere*** means '***to lie down***'. First part of the body on which patient is rested is followed by the word decubitus; hence *right **lateral decubitus*** means the patient is lying on his right side (left side up) and *left lateral decubitus* means patient is lying on his left side (right side up) **(Figs. 1-14 and 1-15)**.

- It is often typical in certain diseases like cerebral irritation, cerebral palsy, etc. In hemiplegia patient lies with one side immobile, with affected arm flexed and legs externally rotated and extended. In tetanus patient develops stiff neck. In ureteric colic, patient is restless with rolling and tossing over the bed. In acute peritonitis patient lies in the bed still and motionless. In cardiac diseases, patient is comfortable in sitting up position. In pneumonia, patient lies on the affected side to make that side immobile and restricted so as to reduce the pain.
- Rigid dorsal decubitus is seen as patient lying on back immobile with flexion of both hips.
- Decubitus in tetanus are opisthotonus (spine arching backwards with body resting on head and feet—common); *orthotonus* (straight); *pleurosthotonus* (lateral bending); *emprosthotonus* (forward bending). *Opisthotonus* is also seen in meningitis, strychnine poisoning, uremia, rabies.
- In cardiac diseases patient attains left lateral position to allow expansion of the liver capsule.
- Lateral decubitus with curled up body is called as '*coiled up decubitus*'. It is observed in colicky abdomen of any cause and cerebral irritations.
- Decubitus in thromboangiitis obliterans (TAO)—is sitting on the bed with flexion of hip, knee and holding foot in both palms.
- Kneeling prayer's decubitus in orthopnea is typical as patient kneels forward in the bed holding a pillow. It kinks the iliac veins to reduce the venous return to the heart. *Squatting decubitus* is seen in cyanotic heart disease (Fallot's tetralogy).

Stature of the Patient

It is the total height from vertex to sole. Stature may be short or tall.

- Turner's syndrome is seen in females with only one X chromosome (it is XO instead XX) having short stature, narrow pelvis and wide shoulder with webbing; widened neck with prominently running skin fold from neck to shoulder.
- Achondroplasia is often called as circus dwarf with large head, flat nasal bridge, stunted trunk, hand and fingers with waddling gait.
- Rickets shows bow legs, scoliosis, rickety rosary, Harrison's transverse sulcus across rib cage.
- Tall stature is seen in *Klinefelter's syndrome* [(extra X chromosome as XXY instead XY) in males with low testosterone levels, presents with female distribution of fat in pelvis and breasts but normal hairs in face and pubis with small testes and azoospermia (low sperm count)]; *Marfan's syndrome* (mucopolysaccharides abnormality); hypogonadism; thyrotoxicosis; adrenal disorders; hypothalamus diseases; familial and nutritional.

Posture of the Patient

It is positional relationships of different parts of the body. Posture of the body is observed in standing, sitting as well as in recumbent position. **Normal posture is**—moderate lordosis of cervical and lumbar spine; kyphosis of thoracic and sacrococcygeal region; forward pelvic inclination 30°; normal rotation of femur; line from the mastoid down passes through the middle of the shoulder and hip, anterior to knee and lateral malleolus.

Gait of the Patient

Gait is the typical way which the patient walks. He is made to walk in a straight line for at least 8–9 meters. While walking,

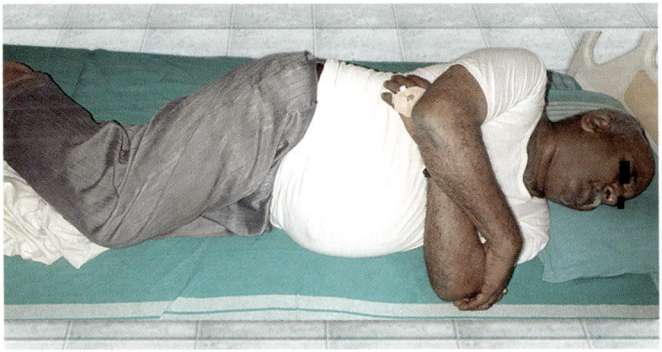

Fig. 1-14 Left lateral decubitus.

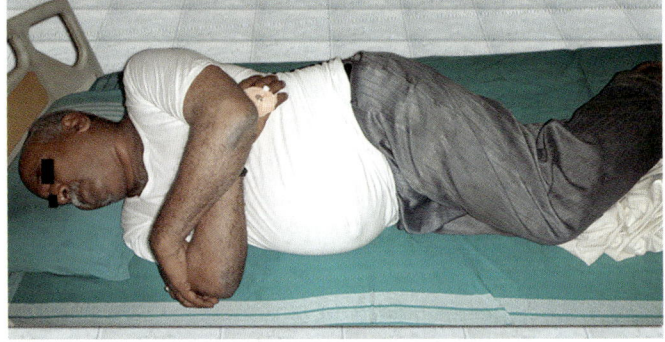

Fig. 1-15 Right lateral decubitus.

positions of the body, upper and lower limb movements, regularity and smoothness of movements, distance between the feet are all observed.
- Abnormal gait may be due to mechanical or structural abnormality [congenital dislocation of hip (CDH) or poliomyelitis]; pain (osteoarthritis); altered muscle tone (hemiplegia, foot drop with high stepping gait); psychological.
- Waddling gait is seen in bilateral congenital dislocation of the hip and bilateral coxa vara; Trendelenburg gait is seen in Legg Calve Perthes' disease, arthritis of hip, poliomyelitis, unilateral coxa vara; high stepping gait in foot drop; circumduction in hemiplegia; festinating gait in Parkinson's disease. Other gaits are—spastic gait, ataxic gait, stuttering gait, antalgic gait in avoiding pain.
- Limp is dragging of the limb during walking.

Face Look/Facies

Face reveals the inner emotions of the mind and body going through. It is the mirror of mind. Typical face is diagnostic of some diseases. Deformity of face as congenital is often obvious **(Fig. 1-16)**.

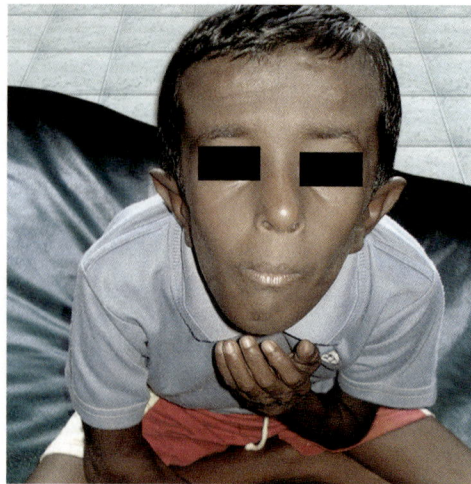

Fig. 1-16 Deformity of face.

Different facies (Face/gum look)

Hippocratic facies: It is seen in patients with acute severe peritonitis with terminal illness. Features are sunken bright eyes, pinched nose, dry, shrivelled tongue, crusted lips, cold clammy forehead, distended abdomen with features of peritonitis.
Adenoid facies: High vaulted palate, narrow dental arch, protruding incisor teeth, earlier was considered as feature of enlarged adenoid is now not accepted. In fact, these features are familial anomaly; nasal obstruction, oral breathing leading into wide opened mouth in a child.
Risus sardonicus: Face of tetanus with trismus—painful smiling. It is due to contraction of zygomaticus major muscle in face leading to sardonic smiling face (*Sardinia plant* when eaten is supposed to produce convulsive laughter ending in death; sardonic means mockery).
Facies of cretinism: Cretin is a neonate with deficient thyroid hormone (cured by thyroid hormone supplement); pale, puffy, wrinkled face; dry cold skin; protruded tongue; open anterior fontanelle; palpable (in endemic type) or impalpable (in sporadic type gland is atrophic) thyroid gland; diagnosed at birth; with broad flat face and nose, wide apart eyes with thick eyelids, protruded tongue with widely open mouth, with dull facial expression.
Face of myasthenia gravis: Unilateral or bilateral intermittent ptosis; drooping jaw; sneering smile face due to reduced action of risorius and zygomatic muscles; here weakness of all muscles is found; in particular of eyelids showing drooping of eyelids with weakness of the face muscles and jaw; lagging of eye lids due to fatigue and 'myasthenia smile' due to weakness of risorius and zygomatic muscles—are typical.
Facies of congenital syphilis: Bossing of frontal bones; interstitial keratitis; Hutchinson's teeth; saddle nose.
Facies of hepatic cirrhosis: Sunken eyes; jaundiced sclera; watery conjunctiva; dull diffusely pigmented sallow face.
Moon face of Cushing's syndrome: Rubicund (red) round face like of full moon; pursed lips; with hirsuitism.
Virile facies: In a woman suffering from adrenocortical hyperplasia or tumor is typical (face looks like that of men).
Carcinoid facies: Typical facial flushing seen in metastatic carcinoid tumor.
Face with typical pale look with half bloated and partially closed eyes is seen in **chronic renal failure**.
Mask face is seen in Parkinsonism; it is due to muscular rigidity of skeletal muscles including of face; but ocular muscles are not involved and so eye movements are normal but with stare.
Acromegaly (due to increased growth hormone in pituitary acidophilic adenoma) shows large face due to overgrowth of soft tissues in face, nose, tongue, air sinuses; large hands (due to enlargement of bones of distal phalanges)—facies of 'Punch and Judy' or an 'Ape man'. Skin is greasy; mental acumen is normal (in myxedema, skin is dry with decreased mental acumen). Lower teeth project in front of the upper; the tongue is enlarged and so mouth is kept open.
Down's syndrome/Mongolism is a congenital abnormality with extrachromosome 21 and total chromosomes 47 (instead of 46); males and females and all races are equally affected. Features are—mental retardation, floppiness, short stature, upward slanting of outer ends of the palpebral fissures slant upwards with prominent epicanthic folds, flat face, protruded tongue and squint.
Face of myxedema shows dull face, rose purple flush over the cheek, eyelid puffiness, with loss of hairs over the lateral 1/3rd of the eyebrow (lateral madarosis), swollen lips and enlarged tongue.
In scleroderma, progressively thickened, pale, waxy skin with reduced facial expressions, microstomia, telangiectases on cheeks, mouth and nose, with fine white horizontal scars in the neck in transverse skin creases (with esophageal stenosis and vasculitis) are seen.
Tabetic facies—drooping of upper eyelid; wrinkling of the forehead; sad expression.
Face in Wilson's disease (hepatolenticular degeneration)—face of fixed emotion.
Face in lupus erythematosus—butterfly erythema over bridge of nose and cheek.
Face in Addison's disease—generalized darkening of the skin of face along with the pigmentation of the mucous membrane of mouth.
Face in Addisonian pernicious anemia—'Lemon yellow' face.
Face in primary polycythemia—red discoloration of the nose, lips, ears and palpebral conjunctiva.
Facial look are typical in chronic alcoholic, drug addict, depressed or anxious individuals.
Scars, discoloration, discrepancies, swellings in the face should be observed and examined.
Discoloration may be due to underlying hemangiomas **(Fig. 1-17)**.
Gums and teeth should be examined for redness, carious teeth, gum hypertrophy, loosened tooth, etc. **(Fig. 1-18)**.

Chapter 1: Introduction to Clinical Approach and Examination

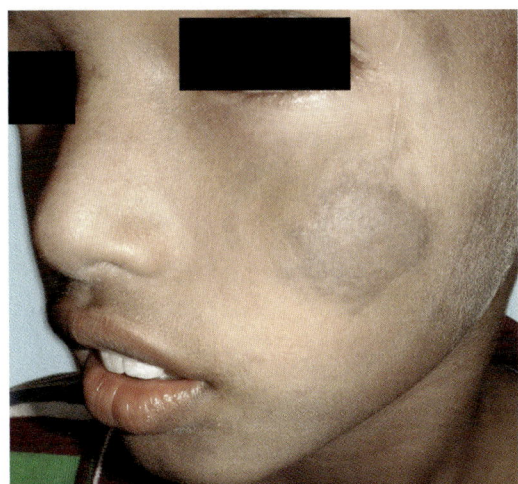

Fig. 1-17 Hemangioma face; note the surface discoloration/pigmentation.

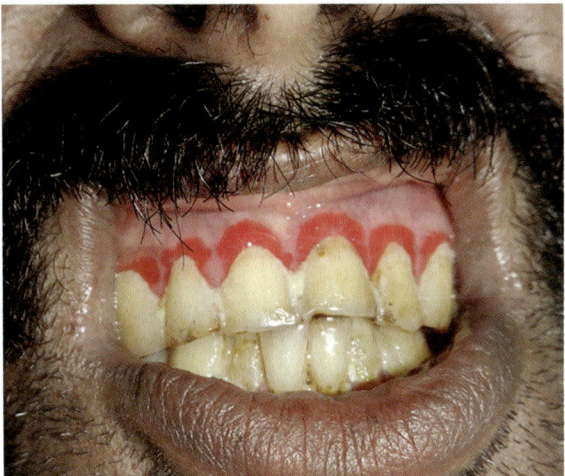

Fig. 1-18 Examination of gums and teeth is a must.

EXAMINATION OF SKIN AND MUCOUS MEMBRANE

It is the largest organ of the human body with surface area of 2 m² and weight of 4 kg. Many of underlying diseases reflect on the skin with different features. It is assessed by changes in color, texture and surface. Common color changes are pallor, cyanosis and jaundice. Color of the skin (brown/black) is determined by pigment—melanin. Generalized pigmentation is seen in Addison's disease. Localized pigmentation can occur in varicose vein disease, hematological diseases, naevus and malignant melanoma.

Pallor

- Causes for pallor are—anemia, massive bleeding, shock and anxiety status.
- Pallor is common in tuberculosis, malignancy, renal failure, myxedema, sepsis, malaria, malnutrition.
- It is checked in lower palpebral conjunctiva, mucous membrane of lips and cheeks, nail beds and palmar creases (Figs. 1-19A and B).

Causes of anemia:
- Nutritional deficiency causing reduced marrow production—deficiency of iron, folate and vitamin B_{12} [diet (cereal rich diet), achlorhydria, pernicious anemia, gastrectomy, Crohn's disease, ileal resection, tropical sprue, celiac disease]; inadequate zinc, cobalt
- Bone marrow hypoplasia—aplastic anemia, Fanconi's anemia, leukemia's, myeloproliferative diseases
- Malignancies—lymphomas, advanced carcinomas, GI malignancies
- Pregnancy, irradiation
- Drug induced—chemotherapy agents, some antibiotics and anticonvulsants
- Chronic blood loss—menorrhagia, bleeding piles, bleeding peptic ulcers, carcinoma stomach, hematuria
- Hemolytic anemia—congenital and acquired
- Hypersplenism
- Other causes—chronic kidney diseases (CKD)

Pigmentation of Skin

It is usually an increase in natural brown pigmentation of the skin. It is determined by the pigment melanin the amount of which is under the influence of hereditary or environmental factors. Often pigmentation by other colors like blue/red also can occur.

Pigmentation can be generalized or localized.
- *Generalized:* It occurs in Addison's disease (seen in skin and buccal mucosa); scleroderma, porphyria cutanea tarda, arsenic/silver poisoning; hemochromatosis; Gaucher's disease; sunburn; irradiation.
- *Localized:* It occurs in pregnancy (around areola, midline abdomen); venous diseases of lower limb (medial third of leg and ankle); *erythema eb agne* (in the exposed part of leg); ultraviolet and high voltage irradiation; *café au lait*

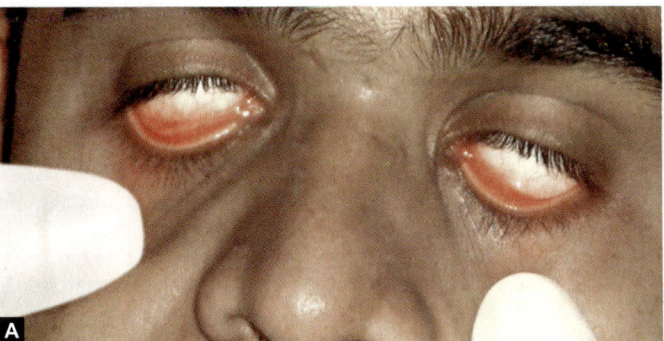
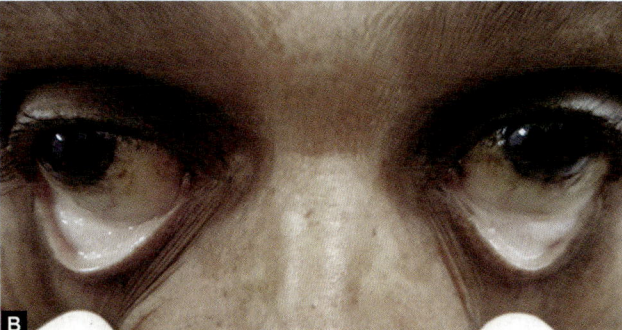

Figs. 1-19A and B Lower eyelid is retracted to see the conjunctiva for pallor. Note the normal conjunctiva and conjunctiva with pallor.

18 Section 1: Examination in General Surgery

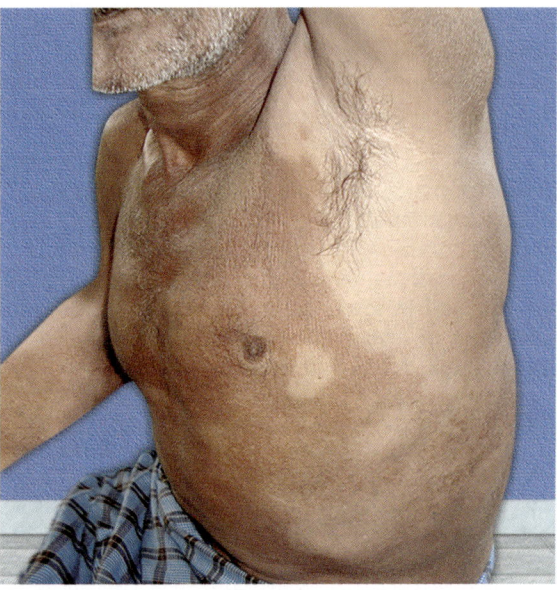

Fig. 1-20 Borderline leprosy with depigmented anesthetic patches.

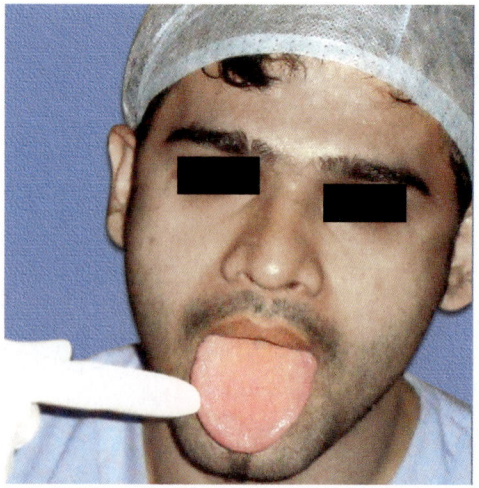

Fig. 1-21 Central cyanosis is checked in the tongue—dorsum.

spots of neurofibromatosis; naevi; melanomas; pellagra (nicotinic acid deficiency); hyperthyroidism (bronzing of eyelids); rheumatoid arthritis.
- *Depigmented patches* are seen in leprosy. There may be loss of sensation, deformities also (Fig. 1-20).

Cyanosis

It is due to increased reduced hemoglobin in the blood causing blue/purple discoloration of the skin and mucous membrane. A minimum of 5 g/dL of reduced hemoglobin should be present in the circulation to cause cyanosis. So in severe anemia (Hb% below 5 g%), cyanosis is not seen.

Two types of cyanosis are observed—*peripheral and central*.

- *Peripheral cyanosis* is due to poor perfusion of peripheral vessels causing reduction in oxyhemoglobin in the capillaries. It is seen in peripheral vasoconstriction due to any cause like exposure to cold temperature, reduced cardiac output, profound shock where blood is diverted from periphery to vital organs like brain, liver, and kidney. Peripheral cyanosis is checked in nail bed, palm and toes, tip of the nose. Here limb is cold and inhaling pure oxygen may not reduce it. *Tongue is not involved in peripheral cyanosis*.
- *Central cyanosis* occurs due to reduced oxygen saturation of arterial blood as a result of poor oxygenation in the lungs. It may be due to congenital heart disease with left to right shunt (cyanotic heart disease), congestive cardiac failure, lung diseases, and low oxygen partial pressure in high altitude. Limb temperature is normal in this type. Clubbing and polycythemia is common here and pure oxygen inhalation reduces the central cyanosis. It is confirmed by *checking the tongue*, nail bed, palms and toes. Central cyanosis is due to *arterial hypoxemia* (chronic obstructive pulmonary disease/COPD), pulmonary fibrosis, pulmonary embolism, pulmonary edema or pneumonia); or due to *arterial hypoventilation* due to mechanical chest wall causes, hypoventilation, laryngeal obstruction, malignancy. Congenital cyanotic heart diseases, left sided cardiac failure are *cardiac causes* of central cyanosis.
- *Methemoglobinemia or sulphemoglobinemia* (abnormal pigments) also causes cyanosis but with normal arterial tension.
- *In carbon monoxide poisoning*, carboxyhemoglobin prevents reduction of oxyhemoglobin and so there will not be any features of cyanosis but cherry-red discoloration is seen. Here *mixed (both central and peripheral) cyanosis* develops. Hemoglobin here contains iron in ferric +3 rather +2 ferrous form. It is a pigmentary cyanosis. Mixed cyanosis often is also seen in cor pulmonale. Lung fibrosis and emphysema causes central cyanosis; right-sided failure or congestive cardiac failure causes peripheral cyanosis.
- Local cyanosis develops in peripheral vascular diseases like Raynaud's phenomenon, thromboangiitis obliterans (TAO), venous diseases.
- Differential cyanosis: Patent ductus arteriosus (PDA) with reversal of shunt causes only lower limb cyanosis. PDA with reversal of shunt with transposition of great vessels causes only upper limb cyanosis. PDA with reversal of shunt with preductal coarctation of aorta causes cyanosis of left upper limb and both lower limbs (Fig. 1-21).

Note: Cyanosis is clinically evident when reduced hemoglobin is 5 g% or more or methemoglobin is 1.5 g% or sulphemoglobin is 0.5 g%.

Skin markers:
- *Purplish striae:* It is seen in lower anterior abdominal wall in Cushing's syndrome.
- *Purpura:* It is seen in idiopathic thrombocytopenic purpura (ITP), coagulopathies, leukemias.
- *Surface hemoangiomas* may be present in central nervous system (CNS) diseases.
- *Spider naevi* is seen in cirrhosis of liver.
- *Palmar erythema* is seen in liver diseases, leukemia, polycythemia, thyrotoxicosis, chronic alcohol intake.
- *Multiple neurofibromas:* von Recklinghausen's disease.
- *Erythema nodosum:* It is seen in primary complex, sarcoidosis and with certain drug intake.
- *Xanthomas*—hyperlipidemia.

Chapter 1: Introduction to Clinical Approach and Examination   19

- *Pigmentation of the oral cavity mucous membrane:* It is seen in Addison's disease, Peutz-Jeghers syndrome.
- *Tuft of hair or lipoma over lumbar spine* in the lower back midline suggests spina bifida.
- *Many cutaneous lesions may suggest the presence of internal malignancies:* Acanthosis nigricans suggests adenocarcinoma of gastrointestinal tract (stomach); necrolytic migratory erythema seen in glucagonoma; pityriasis rotunda in hepatocellular carcinoma; sign of Leser Trelat in carcinoma stomach (sudden appearance of intensely pruritic multiple seborrheic keratosis); palmar plantar keratoderma in carcinoma esophagus and bronchus; migratory thrombophlebitis in carcinoma pancreas; skin hamartoma in Cowden's disease with carcinoma breast and thyroid and GI polyposis.

Polycythemia

It is excess of circulating red blood cells giving the patient a purple-red florid appearance; it heightens the color of all the skin, cheeks, neck, backs of hands and feet whereas cyanosis is limited to tips of hands, feet and nose.

Jaundice/icterus

(Icterus is a **purely a clinical** term; jaundice is **biochemical finding** of raised serum bilirubin).

It is yellowish discoloration of skin and mucous membrane. Serum bilirubin level more than 2 mg/dL causes yellowish discoloration. Tissues and body fluids are also discolored yellow. Bilirubin has more affinity to elastic tissue, blood vessels and nervous tissue. So it is better seen in sclera and skin. During recovery, bilirubin takes longer time to get cleared from elastic tissue and so clinical jaundice persists for little longer time than biochemical disappearance of jaundice.

Initially it is pale lemon yellow color, later gets darkened, becomes yellow-orange, olive greenish yellow as seen in obstructive jaundice. Jaundice is due to deposition of bile pigments with excess of it in plasma. Greenish color is due to deposition of *biliverdin.*

It is checked in upper sclera (better seen against white background; by asking the patient to look at his feet and clinician pulls the upper eyelid upwards). It also can be checked in **nail bed, ear lobule, nasal tip, and under surface of the tongue**. It is checked using normal daylight instead of torch light (**Figs. 1-22A to E**).

Scratch marks observed on the dorsum of the body (forearm, neck, back) is due to deposition of bile acids which release excess histamine causing itching.

Jaundice may be due to *prehepatic* cause (excess hemolysis); *hepatic* (liver dysfunction—hepatitis, sepsis, drugs, cirrhosis*); posthepatic* (CBD stones, carcinoma pancreas, drugs—obstructive); *congenital* hyperbilirubinemia (*Gilbert's syndrome* causing altered bilirubin transport and so increase in unconjugated bilirubin; *Criggler-Najjar syndrome* causing disturbance in bilirubin conjugation and so increase in unconjugated bilirubin; *Dubin Johnson syndrome* and *Rotor's syndrome* causing disturbance in excretion of bilirubin and so increase in conjugated bilirubin).

Aged red cells get lysed in the reticuloendothelial cells and breakdown into haem and globin. Haem is divided into

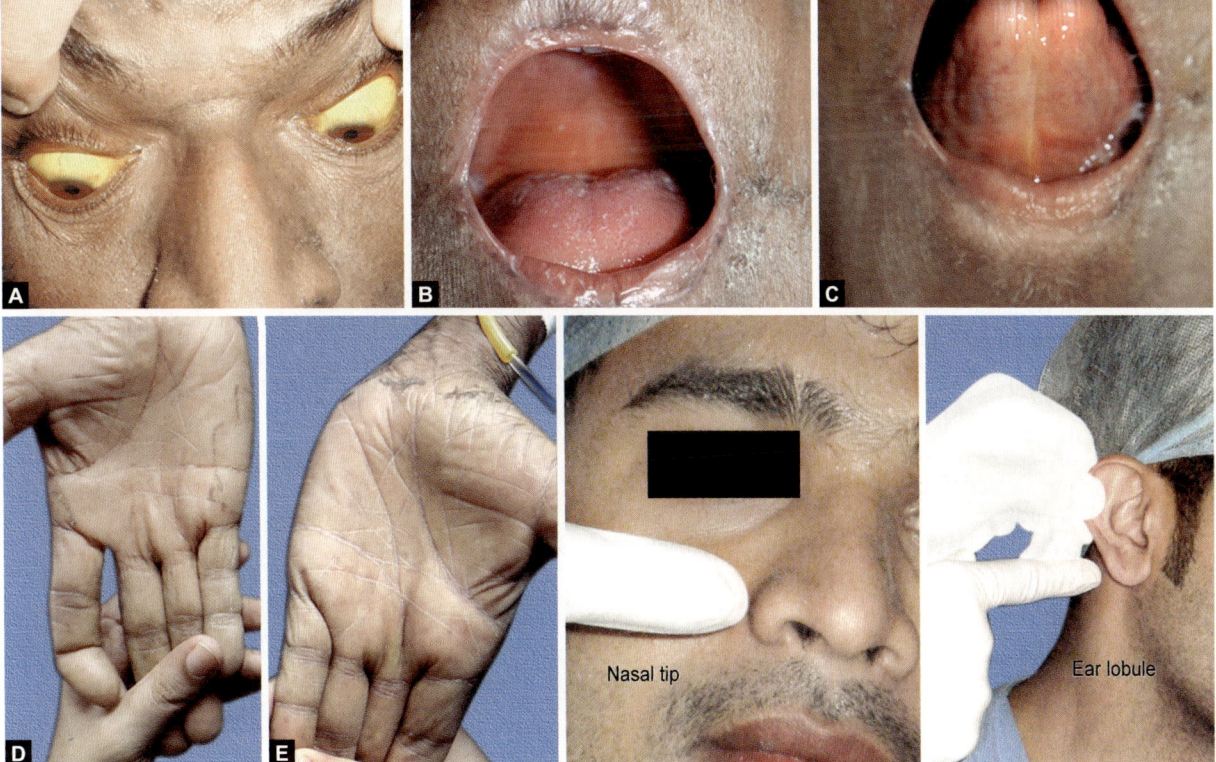

Figs. 1-22A to E Jaundice/icterus is checked in sclera by asking the patient to look on the feet and examiner pulls up the upper eyelids. It is also checked on palate, under surface of the tongue, finger tips, in nasal tip and ear lobule.

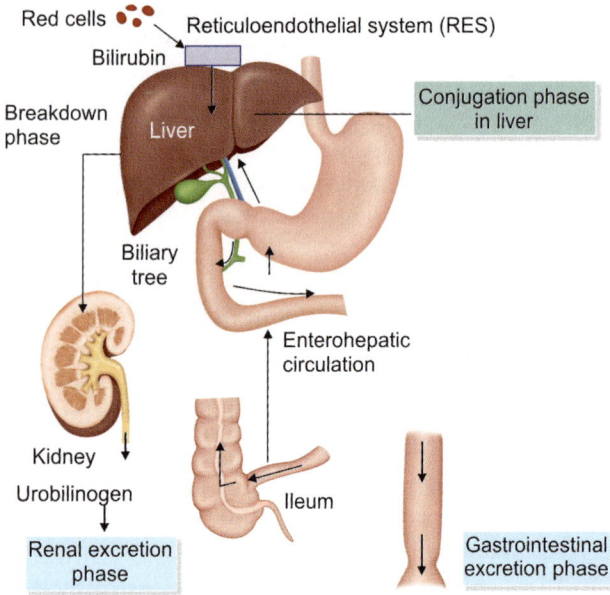

Fig. 1-23 Enterohepatic circulation.

globin and bilirubin. Bilirubin is combined with albumin and transported to liver. In the liver bilirubin get separated from albumin and conjugated to bilirubin glucuronide by glucuronyl transferase. This conjugated bilirubin glucuronide is water soluble and can be excreted in kidney (So in obstructive and hepatic jaundice bile pigment—bilirubin is seen in the urine). This conjugated bilirubin is excreted through biliary canaliculi reaching intestine. In the intestine, it is converted into stercobilinogen and urobilinogen by intestinal bacteria. 70% of this is absorbed in the colon and brought back to liver via enterohepatic circulation. Unabsorbed stercobilinogen colors feces brown. Circulating urobilinogen is taken up by kidneys for excretion. If direct bilirubin in the serum is more than 0.4 mg%, then bilirubin is seen in urine. Normal urinary urobilinogen is 100–200 mg/day. It is absent in obstructive jaundice. Normal fecal stercobilinogen is 300 mg/day. It is also absent in obstructive jaundice (Fig. 1-23).

Hypercarotinemia

It mimics jaundice and is due to increased yellow pigment carotene. It is seen equally on face, palm, sole and skin but **not seen in sclera**. It is common in vegetarians who eat more raw carrot. Mepacrine therapy also causes yellow discoloration.

■ EXAMINATION OF NAILS

Nail is a skin appendage made up of keratin containing nail plate, matrix with bed underneath. **Nail plate** is the main body which is made of layers of flat dead cells, containing keratin; its shape is due to the curvature of distal phalanx underneath. Proximal growing alive part is called as **nail matrix** which produces cells to form eventual nail plate. Whitish crescent shaped base of the nail is called as **lunule. Nail bed** contains epidermis and dermis with capillaries, nerves and lymphatics. Between epidermis and dermis of the nail bed tiny grooves are present which are called as **matrix crests**. Epithelium beneath the tip of the nail plate is called as **hyponychium**; both are attached by a band called as **onychodermal band**. Proximal most part is embedded in the nail sinus and is called as **nail root**. A band of epithelium called as **eponychium** overhangs the nail root in front with cuticle as its distal margin (**Figs. 1-24A and B**).

Skin fold overlapping the lateral margins of the nail is called as nail wall. Tissue around the margins of the nail is called as **paronychium** which is the site of paronychia infection. Rate of growth of nail is 3 mm/month. Nails of fingers regrow completely after removal in 6 months; nails of toes take 12–18 months to regrow completely. Fingernails grow 4 times faster than toenails. Nail of index finger grows faster.

Deformities of the Nail

- A transverse groove (transverse lines/*Beau's lines*) at same levels of each nail is suggestive of systemic disease/general debilitating illness. It is due to temporary alteration in nail plate growth.

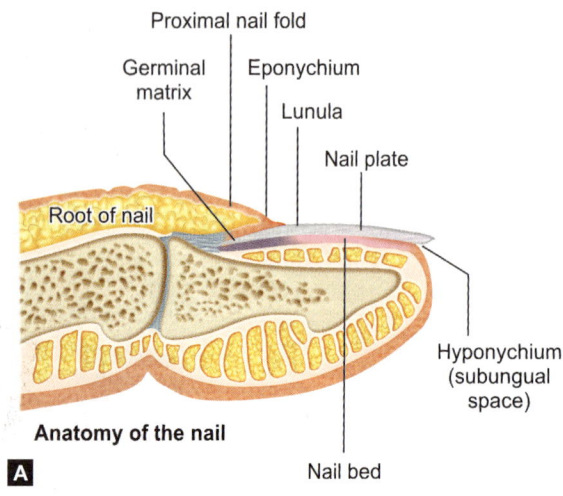
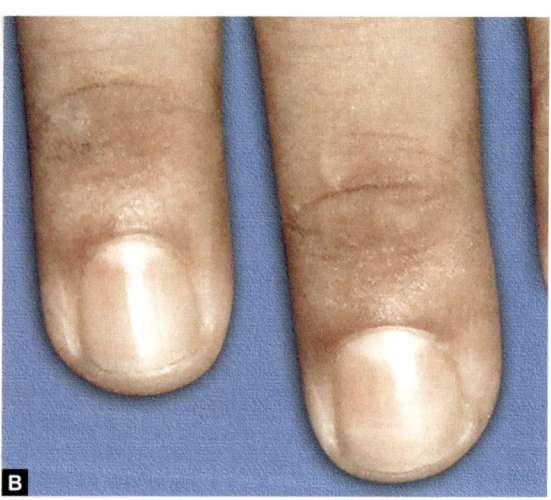

Figs. 1-24A and B Anatomy of the nail.

- **Pallor** can be seen in nail bed. In iron efficiency anemia (*Plummer Vinson syndrome*) nails may be brittle/flat (*platynychia*)/spoon shaped (*kolionychia*) (Figs. 1-25 and 1-26).
- **Splinter hemorrhages** are seen in nail bed in bacterial endocarditis, bleeding disorders.
- Discolored, deformed, **pitted nails** are seen in psoariasis.
- Hypoalbuminemia causes whitening of the nail bed—**Terry's sign**.
- Specific discolorations are seen in Raynaud's disease, silver and mercury poisoning.
- Ribbing, brittleness, falling of nails are seen in syringomyelia, leprosy and tabes dorsalis.
- **Nail bed infarcts** are seen in vasculitis due to SLE or polyarteritis.
- **Onychogryphosis** (in toe) is heaping up of nail and curling over the end of the toe due to failure of normal sliding mechanism of the nail and is due to trauma or old age (Figs. 1-27A and B).
- **Ingrowing toenail** is common in margins of the nail of great toe where irregular edge of the nail grow beneath the lateral nail fold due to improper trimming of the nail causing repeated pain and infection.
- **Dry, brittle, fragile dark** nails are seen in vitamin A, B (B_{12}), D and calcium deficiency. Deficiency of protein, folic acid, and vitamin C causes hangnails. Linoleic acid deficiency causes splitting and flaking of the nails.
- In uremia, nails become dull white proximally with distal brown portion with a well-demarcated transverse line of separation—**Lindsay line**.

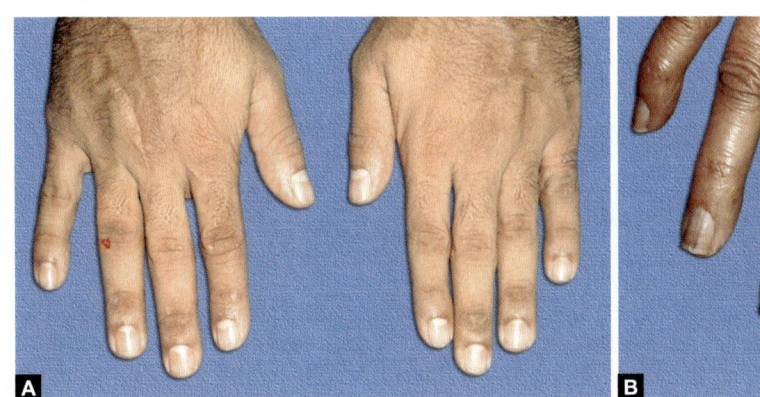
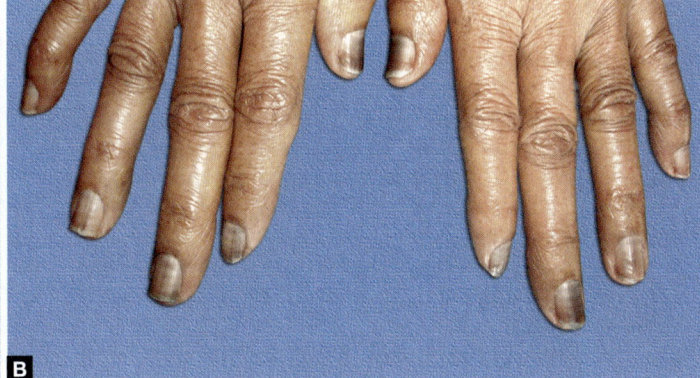

Figs. 1-25A and B Nails should be examined both in hands and feet (fingers and toes) for change in color, splinter hemorrhage, clubbing, pallor, koilonychia and other features.

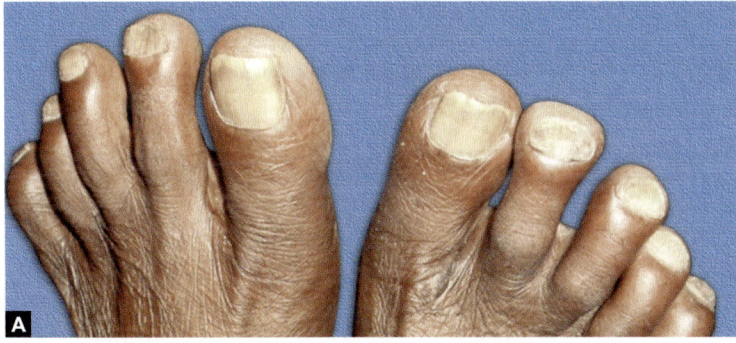
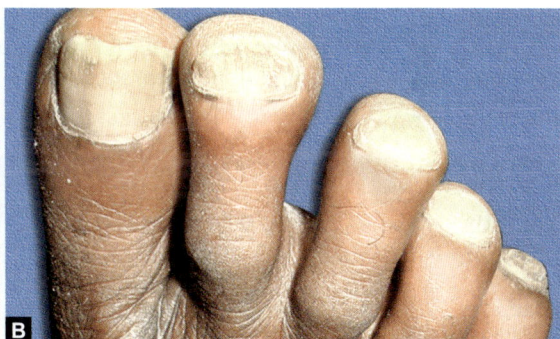

Figs. 1-26A and B Changes in the toenail also should be observed. Note the pallor and koilonychia in the toenails.

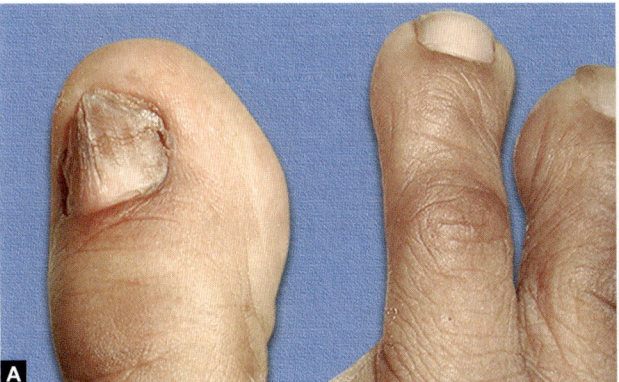
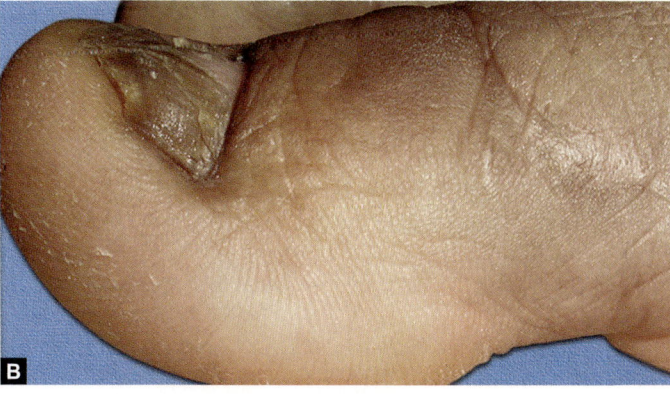

Figs. 1-27A and B Note the change in the great toenail. It could be onychogryphosis.

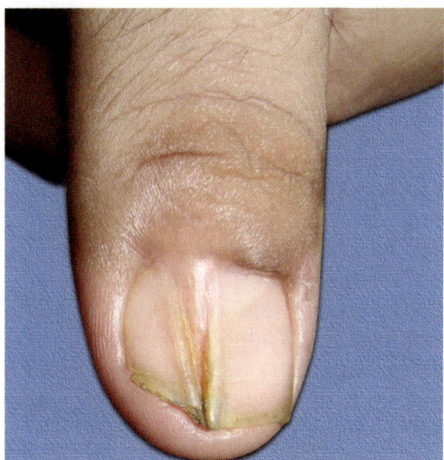

Fig. 1-28 Nail pterygium.

- *White nail* is seen in hypoalbuminemia (leuconychia of cirrhosis); *red nail* (red half moons) in congestive cardiac failure; *blue nail* is in Wilson's disease; *black nail* in Peutz-Jeghers/Cushing's syndrome or Addison's disease. *Leukonychia striata* is white patches in nail and *leukonychia punctata* is white dots in nail—are of no pathological significance. *Yellow nail syndrome* has got slowly growing curved yellowish or yellowish green nails in association with lymphedema, bronchiectasis or pleural effusion.
- *Nails are absent* or hypoplastic since birth in ectodermal dysplasia, a familial condition. Scarring and loss of nails occurs due to repeated blistering of fingertips in epidermolysis bullosa, a genetic disorder.
- Scarring and destruction of the nailbed is called as *pterygium of nail* which is seen in lichen planus (Fig. 1-28).
- *Onycholysis* is whitening of the distal nail, seen in psoriasis, thyrotoxicosis due to separation of the distal nail plate.

- *Onychorrhexis* is softening or brittleness of nailbeds, commonly seen in females due to constant wetting of nails.
- *Onychauxis* is hypertrophy of nails.
- *Onychia* is deformity of the nail—seen in fungal infection or tuberculosis. It is due to inflammation of nails.

Clubbing (Hippocratic Fingers)

It is bulbous enlargement of soft parts of the terminal phalanges with both transverse and longitudinal curving of the nails. It is due to interstitial edema and dilatation of the arterioles and capillaries. There is loss of normal angle between surface of the nail and the skin covering the nail bed.

When a normal nail is viewed from side, plane of the nail and the plane of the skin covering the base of the nail bed form an angle of 130–170° (*Lovibond angle*). In clubbing tissue hypertrophy beneath the nail bed makes the base of the nail bulge upwards distorting the nail growth causing nail to be curved in both directions. So in clubbing plane of the nail and plane of the skin covering the nail bed form an angle which is greater than 180°.

Causes of Clubbing

- *Causes*: It can be pulmonary (Carcinoma bronchus, lung abscess, bronchiectasis, tuberculosis with secondary infection); cardiac (cyanotic congenital heart disease, infective endocarditis); gastrointestinal (ulcerative colitis, Crohn's disease, cirrhosis); endocrinal (myxedema, acromegaly, exophthalmic ophthalmoplegia—*thyroid acropachy*); other causes (hereditary, idiopathic), *unilateral* in Pancoast tumor, subclavian/innominate artery aneurysm: *unidigital* in trauma or tophi deposition in Gout, only in upper limbs in heroin addicts due to chronic obstructive phlebitis.

Causes of Clubbing					
Respiratory	**Cardiac**	**Abdominal**	**Mediastinal**	**Extrathoracic**	**Others**
• Bronchogenic carcinoma • Bronchiectasis • Empyema • Idiopathic pulmonary fibrosis • Mesothelioma • Cystic fibrosis • Lung abscess • Fibrotic pulmonary tuberculosis • Arteriovenous malformations • Secondaries	• Congenital cyanotic heart disease • Infective endocarditis	• Cirrhosis of liver • Ulcerative colitis • Crohn's disease	• Lymphoma • Thymoma • Carcinoma esophagus • Achalasia cardia • Esophagitis	• Nasopharyngeal carcinoma • Thyroid carcinoma • Thyrotoxicosis	• Idiopathic • Familial • Congenital

Grading of clubbing:

Grade I: Softening and fluctuation of nail bed;

Grade II: Obliteration of angle of the nail bed with loss of longitudinal ridges and formation of convexity from above downwards and side to side;

Grade III: Swelling of the subcutaneous tissue over the base of the nail causing overlying skin tense, shiny and wet increasing the nail curvature;

Grade IV: Swelling of the fingers occurs in all dimensions associated with hypertrophic pulmonary osteoarthropathy causing pain and swelling of the hand and radiographic features of subperiosteal new bone formation.

In clubbing: Angle between the base of the nailfold and nailbed is more than 180° (normal is 160°).

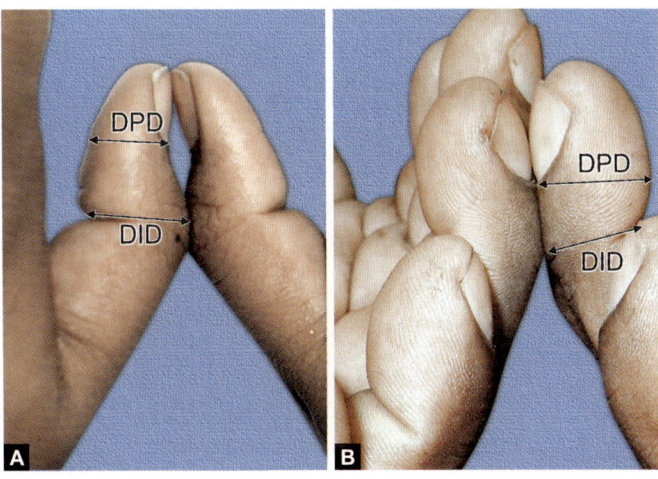

Figs. 1-29A and B *Schamroth's sign*. When distal phalanges of the two index fingers (or opposing fingers) are held in apposition, a closed triangular space (diamond-shaped gap) will form in normal individual, but will be absent in clubbing; it is due to widened distal phalangeal depth (DPD) than distal interphalangeal depth (DID).

- Disappearance of diamond-shaped gap between nails when fingers are apposed is called as *Schamroth's sign* (Figs. 1-29A and B).
- *Pathogenesis:* Hypoxia leads to opening up of deep arteriovenous fistulas which increase the perfusion of the fingers and toes causing its hypertrophy. It may be due to reduced venous blood ferritin which escapes oxygenation in the lungs, which after entering the systemic circulation stimulates dilatation of arteriovenous anastomosis leading to hypertrophy and clubbing of terminal phalanx (Figs. 1-30A to E).
- *Hypertrophic pulmonary osteoarthropathy* is severe clubbing with subperiosteal bone thickening and thickening of the synovium which is often associated with lung cancer.
- *Pseudoclubbing* is seen in hyperparathyroidism and is due to undue bone resorption resulting in disappearance of terminal phalanges causing telescoping of soft tissues into the terminal phalanges which appears like clubbing. Nail is not having curvatures here.

SKIN CHANGES AND ERUPTIONS

Nonpalpable Eruptions

- *Macule:* It is not raised above the skin; there is alteration in color of skin; it is seen but not felt (nonpalpable); capillary naevi or erythema blanch on pressure, purpuric macules do not blanch on pressure. Macule is <1 cm nonpalpable lesion. Macules can be generalized as seen in typhoid, syphilis, purpura or localized type which is called as *roseolar*.
- *Patch:* Circumscribed flat nonpalpable colored area in the skin with diameter >1 cm. Patches are seen in vitiligo, bruises. Macule and patch are nonpalpable lesions.

Palpable Eruptions

- *Papule:* It is raised tiny nodule; usually of few mm in size; it may be epidermal or dermal; seen in measles, chickenpox, smallpox, drugs like sulfonamides, occasionally in

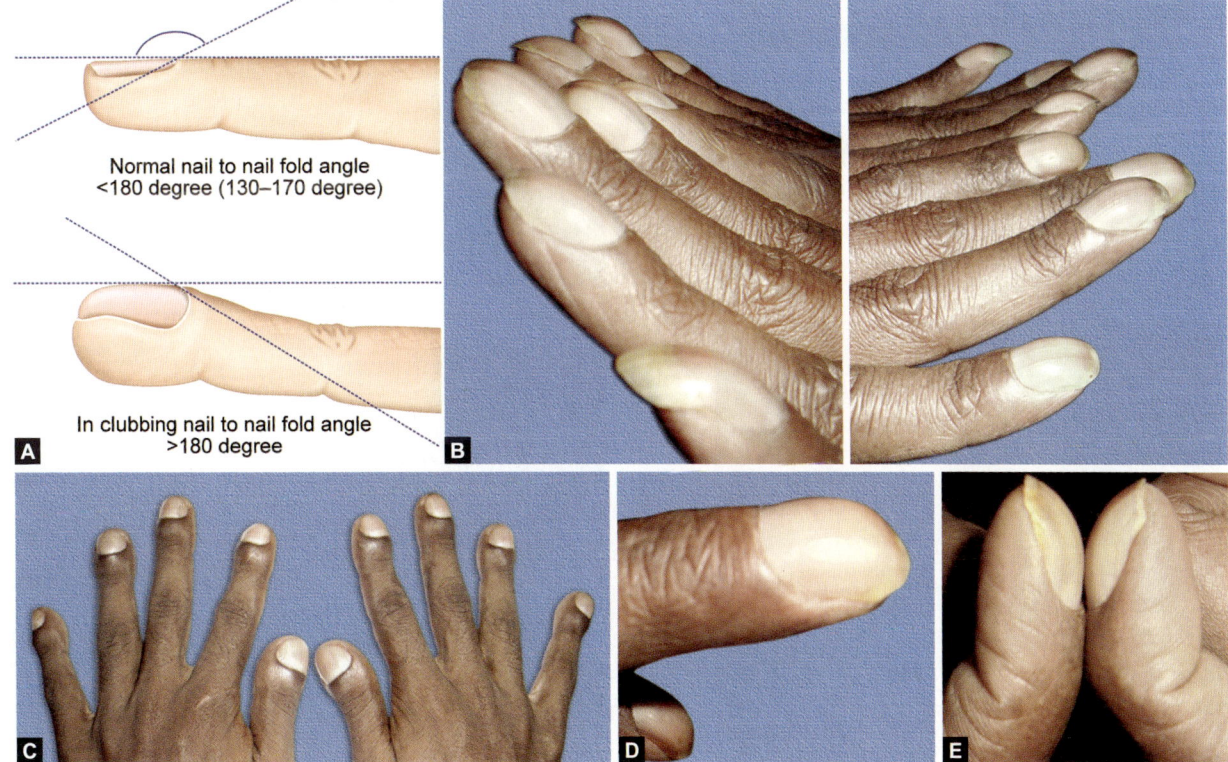

Figs. 1-30A to E Typical clubbing. In normal individual angle from skin to nail fold is 130 to 170 degree (*Lovibond angle*). In clubbing it is more than 180°. In clubbing both longitudinal and transverse curvatures are increased.

tuberculosis, sarcoidosis. It is < 5 mm sized palpable lesion.
- *Granule and nodule:* Large papule >5 mm diameter up to 2 cm is called as granule; size more than 2 cm size is called as nodule. It may be cutaneous/subcutaneous origin; hard (rheumatoid arthritis)/soft (lipoma).
- *Plaque: Confluence of papule/nodule*; flat topped, raised/sunken seen in psoriasis. Papule, nodule and plaque develops due to proliferation of dermal cells which may be inflammatory or neoplastic in origin (Figs. 1-31 and 1-32).

Note:

Different eruptions occur in different conditions. Drug reactions commonly observed in the skin can involve systemically causing renal failure, respiratory distress or cardiac problems. Viral, bacterial, parasitic infections, radiation and chemotherapeutic agents can cause different skin eruptions, like vesicles, pigmentation, dermatitis, alopecia, thrombophlebitis, etc. **(Figs. 1-33 to 1-42).**

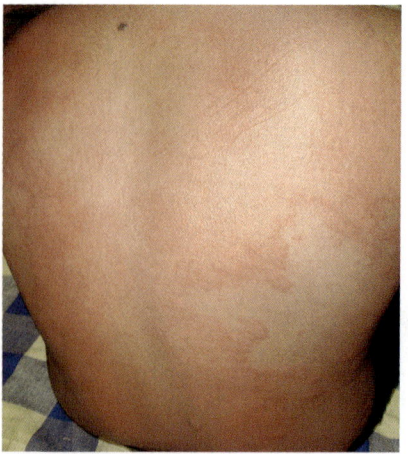

Fig. 1-33 Drug-induced allergic rashes on the back extensively involved.

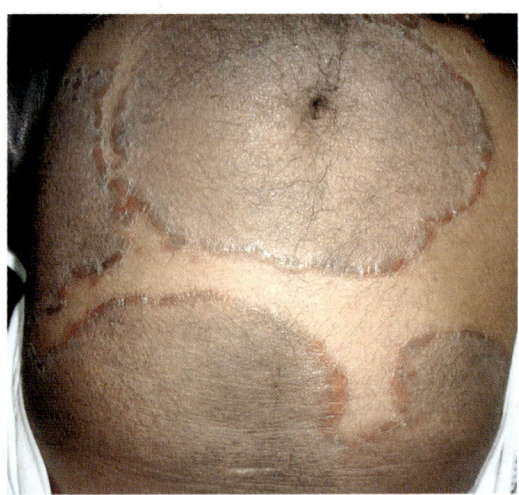

Fig. 1-31 Psoriasis; it can involve nails also. It is red, scaly, patches or papules or plaques. Plaque psoriasis is commonest type. Pitting of nails is common. Immune system mistakes a normal skin cell for a pathogen causing overproduction of new skin cells; it is probably genetically related but stress and environmental factors also responsible.

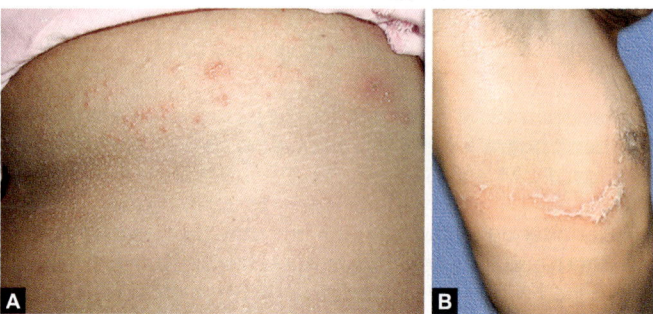

Figs. 1-34A and B Herpes zoster infection.

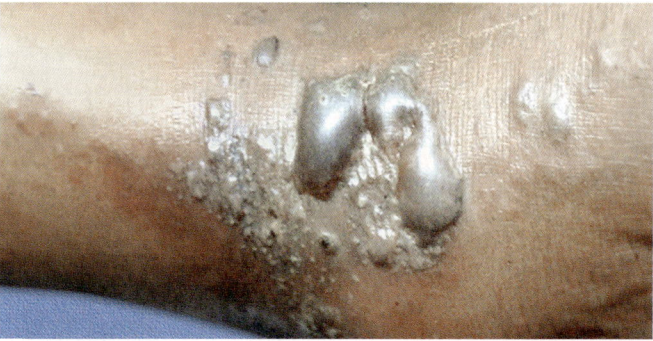

Fig. 1-35 Skin vesicles.

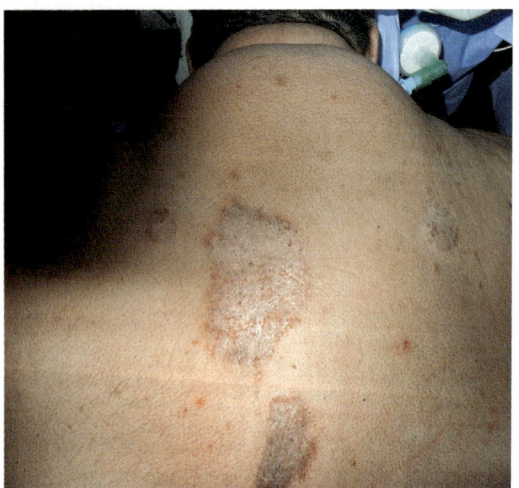

Fig. 1-32 Psoriasis—back area.

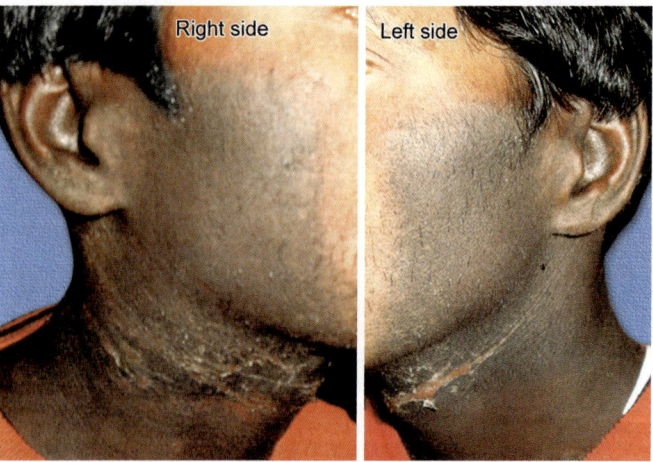

Fig. 1-36 Radiation dermatitis on both sides of neck and face.

Chapter 1: Introduction to Clinical Approach and Examination 25

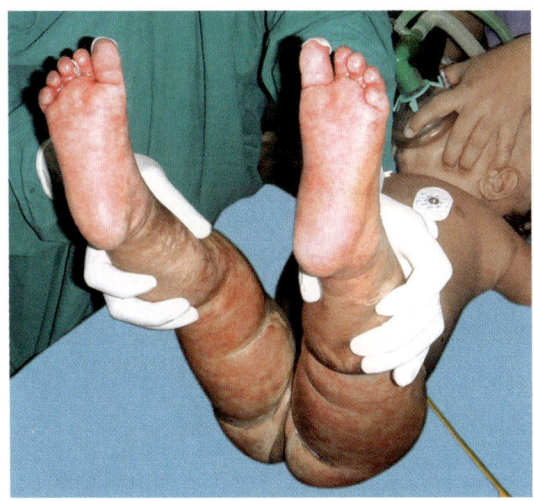

Fig. 1-37 Acute drug reaction in a child causing burn like injury of the entire skin of the body. It could be TEN (toxic epidermal necrolysis).

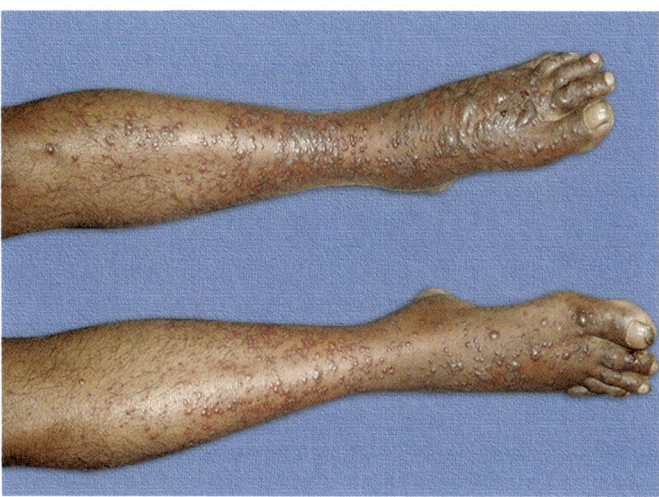

Fig. 1-40 Vasculitis—multiple vesicles and bullae in the skin.

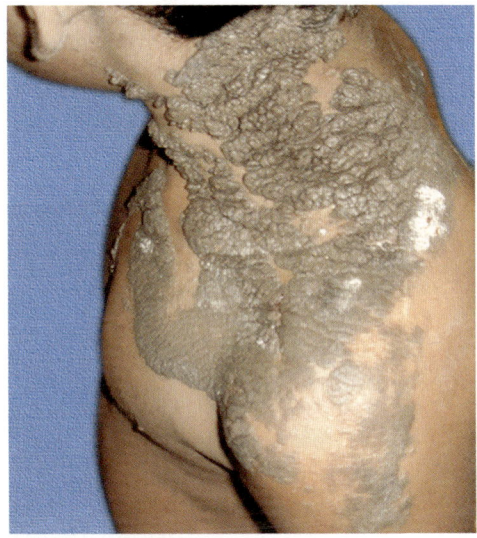

Fig. 1-38 Verrucous epidermal naevus.

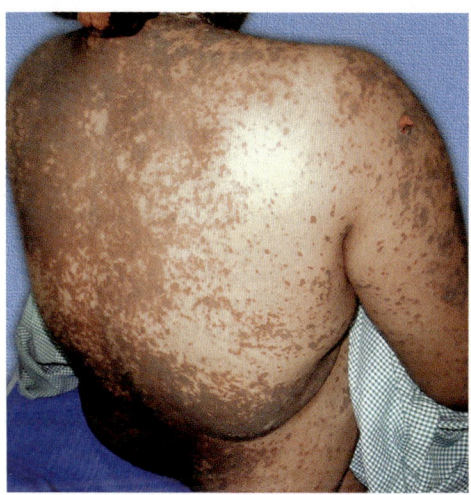

Fig. 1-41 Toxic epidermal necrolysis TEN, Lyell's syndrome (Alan Lyell, 1956). It is severe drug reaction often life-threatening; mimics Steven Johnson syndrome.

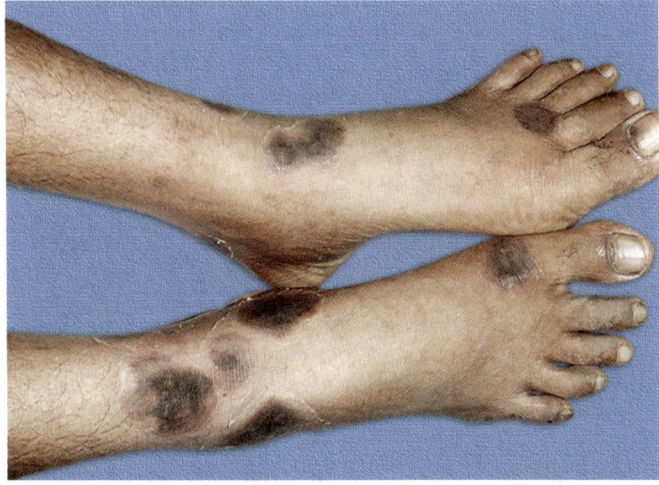

Fig. 1-39 Drug-induced skin reaction—fixed drug reaction.

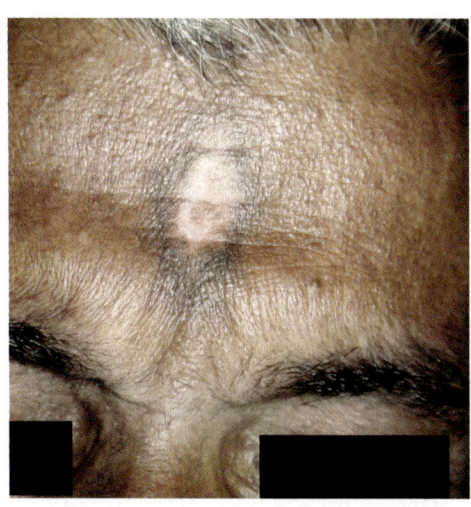

Fig. 1-42 Allergy on the forehead due to traditional kumkum application.

Fluid Collections in the Skin

- **Vesicles:** They are small blisters (<5 mm in size); elevations from epidermis containing clear or milk like fluid within; seen in chickenpox, smallpox, herpes. There is cleavage in the layers of the epidermis causing intraepidermal vesicles or cleavage can occur at epidermo-dermal interface causing subepidermal vesicles.
- **Bulla:** Large blister (>5 mm diameter); unilocular/multilocular; may contain serous/seropurulent/hemorrhagic fluid within (Fig. 1-43).
- **Pustules:** They are circumscribed epidermal elevations containing purulent exudate (white/yellow/greenish yellow); due to bacterial (like streptococcal) infection. It may develop in hair follicle or independently.
- **Wheal:** It is elevated patches on the skin with pallor at the center than the periphery; it is edematous elevation with itching; it is seen in allergic conditions (urticaria). Fluid accumulation occurs in diffuse pattern in wheal. Urticaria is elevated round lesion with white center and pale red periphery.

Others

- **Scales:** It is formed by desquamating layer of skin; occurring due to imperfect keratinization; small (dandruff), large (psoriasis).
- **Crusts:** It is dried exudation of serum, blood or pus over the skin, may be thin/thick; adherent/friable; colored yellow (serum)/dark red (blood)/green (pus).
- **Café au lait spots:** They are coffee brown colored patches in the skin; if more than 5 in number and with each more than 1.5 cm in size is significant; seen in von Recklinghausen's disease of neurofibromatosis with regular outline and deep indentations; occasionally also seen in Albright's syndrome where the outline is irregular.
- **Petechiae:** Tiny hemorrhagic spots less than 1 mm in size.
- **Purpura:** Hemorrhagic spots of 2–5 mm in size (Fig. 1-44).
- **Ecchymosis:** Hemorrhagic spots more than 5 mm in size.
- **Hematoma:** Hemorrhage causing elevation of skin (Fig. 1-45).

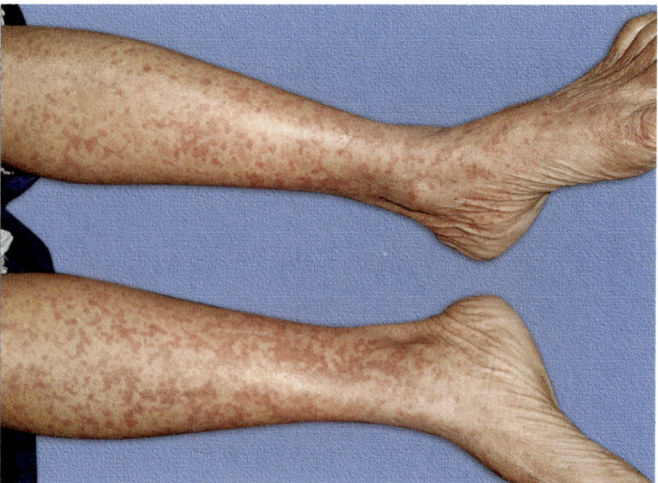

Fig. 1-44 Henoch-Schönlein purpura. It is purplish rash involving legs and buttocks due to inflammation and bleeding of small vessels in the skin, bowel, kidney and joints. Purpuric rashes are reddish purple spots; joint swellings mainly in knee and elbow due to hemarthrosis; abdominal pain, bloody stools, intussusception as gastrointestinal features; hematuria and proteinuria due to involvement of kidneys. It is common in children (boys) after an attack of upper respiratory tract (viral) infections; common in seasons other than summer; may also be due to insect bite, exposure to cold, and drugs.

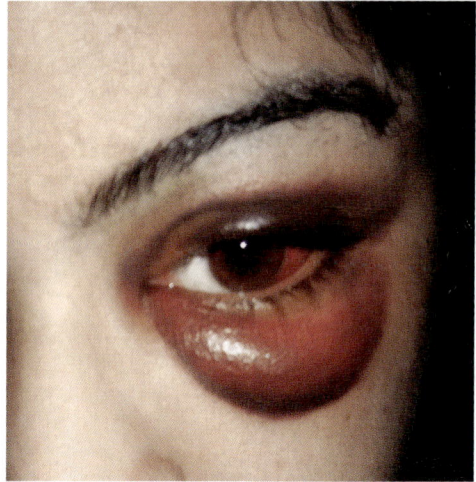

Fig. 1-45 Hematoma lower eyelid.

- *Scar over the skin* may be present; it may be due to old trauma, earlier surgery, healed infected area or childhood branding as a tradition (Fig. 1-46).

TEXTURE OF THE SKIN

Texture of the skin gives idea about different conditions and often severity. It should be seen as well as felt.
- **Dry skin:** Seen in dehydration and myxedema.
- **Moist skin:** Seen in myocardial infarction, shock of sudden onset (hemorrhage), toxic thyroid.
- **Thick skin:** Seen in myxedema, acromegaly, and scleroderma.
- **Thin skin:** Seen in old people, and wasting diseases.
- **Pinched skin** a feature of dehydration, malnutrition.

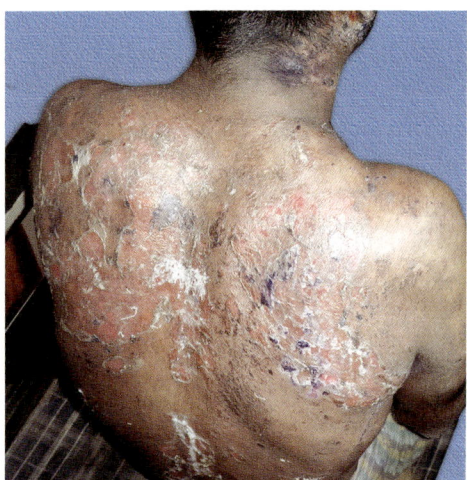

Fig. 1-43 Pemphigus is bullous lesions in the skin due to development of antibodies against desmoglein of skin. It can be erythematous lesions also.

Chapter 1: Introduction to Clinical Approach and Examination

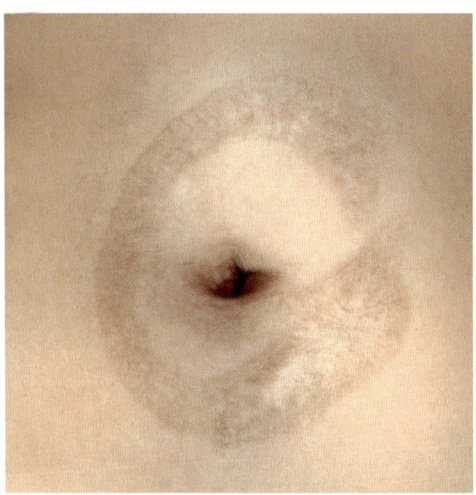

Fig. 1-46 *Branding* using heated iron rod at various parts of the body during childhood to prevent evil effect is an old belief which was practiced in many parts of the world. One of the common sites is around the umbilicus. It forms a circumferential burn scar.

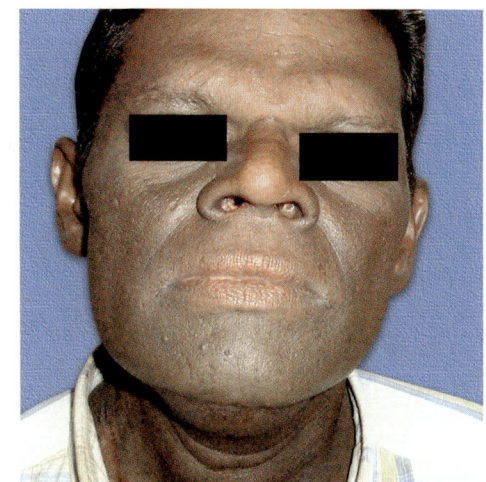

Fig. 1-47 Pigmentation of skin over the face.

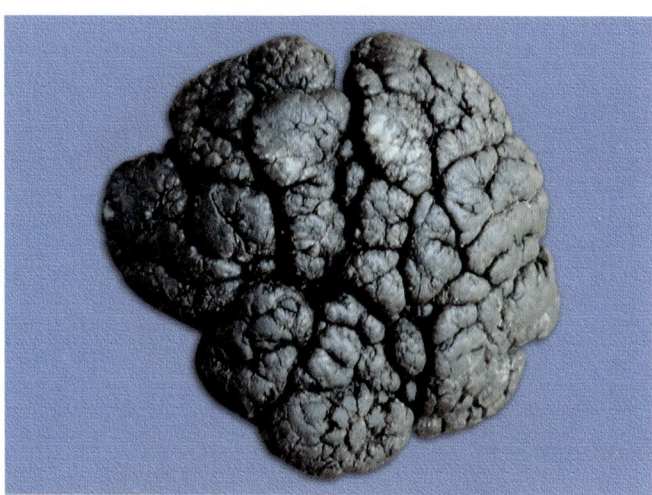

Fig. 1-48 Seborrheic keratosis (basal cell papilloma, senile wart, verruca senilis). Note the sulci and gyri appearance; it is often better evident using a dermoscopy. It is brown/black/tan colored waxy, scaly slightly elevated single or multiple lesions. They are not precancerous; but mimic carcinoma. It is benign cutaneous basal layer overgrowth with oily look. It is common in old age; may run in families. It can be removed by scraping, cryosurgery, cautery or laser. Excision is done if diagnosis is not certain.

PIGMENTED LESIONS IN THE SKIN

It may be due to Naevus of different types, malignant melanoma, pigmented carcinoma (basal cell or squamous cell type), seborrheic keratosis, *café au lait spots,* cutaneous hemangiomas, spider naevus (an acquired condition with single dilated feeding skin arteriole with many small radial branches, which is compressible as it fades on pressure and is common on the upper trunk, face and arms), *Campbell de Morgan spot* (bright uniform deep red, painless noncompressible spot of 1-3 mm in size with collection of dilated capillaries fed by one or cluster of arterioles, seen in upper parts of the trunk of individual after the age of 45), *Vin rose patch* (congenital dilatation of the subpapillary dermal vascular plexus with pale pink skin), systemic diseases like liver cell dysfunction, adrenal diseases, drug induced, solar keratosis, etc. **(Figs. 1-47 and 1-48).**

HAIR

Hair is skin appendage with flat stratified multilayered keratinized squamous epithelium. Hair growth cycle shows three phases—anagen; catagen; telogen. Hair grows at a rate of 1.25 cm per month. *Anagen* is the initial growth phase of the hair; next *catagen* phase shows shrinkage of the hair follicle with diminished blood supply and nutrition to the hair follicle and this phase lasts for 2 weeks; eventual *telogen* phase lasts for 2-4 months where static hair lasts with resting phase. Once again new anagen phase begins at its hair follicle with shedding out the earlier hair.

Fetal entire skin is covered by fine, silky, *Lanugo hairs* which are shed by 8th month of intrauterine life. Fine, nonpigmented childhood hair (both male and female) is called as *vellus*. Long, pigmented, soft silky hair called *intermediate hair* is common in shoulder region (often is also seen along with vellus hair in Cushing's syndrome). *Terminal hair* is coarse, pigmented; nonsexual terminal hair present in scalp, eyebrows, arms and legs. *Ambosexual hair* is present in axillae, lower pubic triangle and limbs; *sexual hair* is present in upper pubic triangle, face, nose, ears, trunk and limbs in males (in females if present it is abnormal—*hirsutism*).

Hair can overgrow or curl on its own. *Plica polonica* is a condition where long hairs of the scalp gets thickened, rough and curl on its own causing difficulty in combing and poor cosmesis. It is matted, filthy condition of hair which is sticky and moist; hairs cannot be disentangled; often mimics bird's nest. It may be due to poor hygiene. A condition called plica polanica which is first observed in Poland wherein long hairs in young females suddenly curl and twist on its own to create tough rough hairs. It is difficult to treat **(Fig. 1-49).**

Falling of Hair

Normally 50–100 hairs fall daily. Excessive hair fall is seen in infectious fevers like typhoid, chemotherapy for

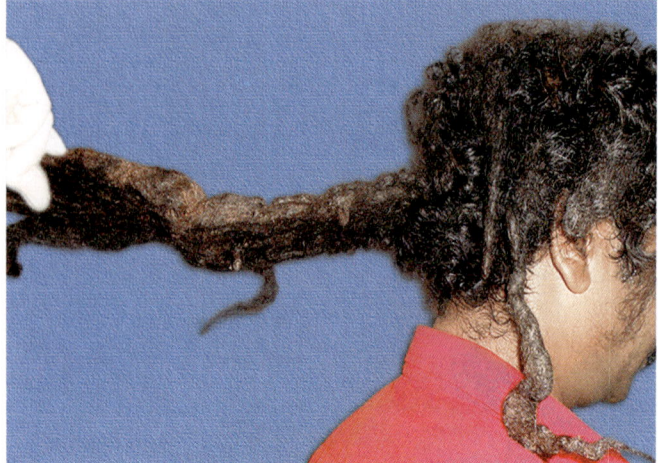

Fig. 1-49 Plica polonica.

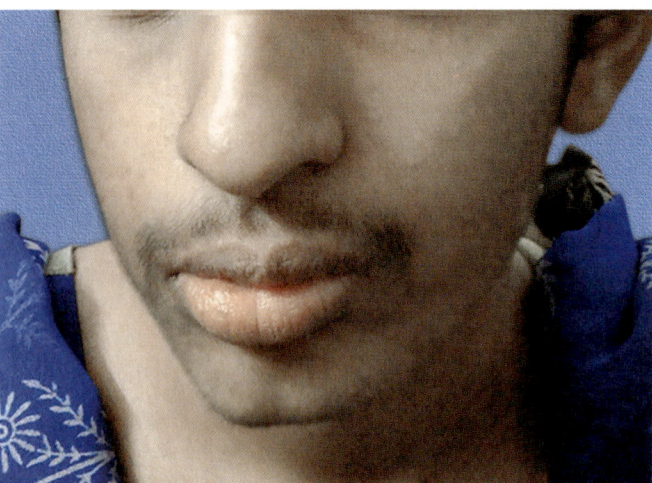

Fig. 1-51 Hirsutism in a young female.

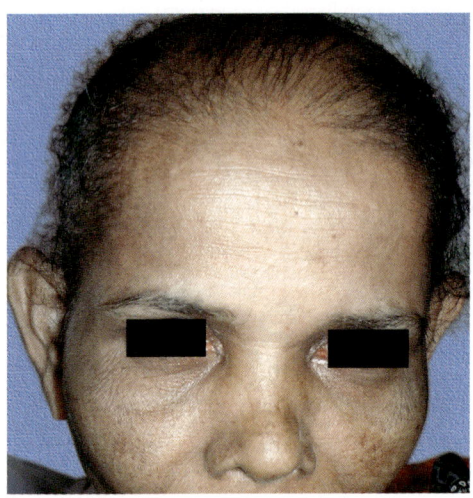

Fig. 1-50 Alopecia scalp developed after chemotherapy.

malignancies, drugs (heparin, allopurinol, bismuth, vitamin A, amphetamine) and hereditary. As hair follicle cells divide very quickly, chemotherapeutic agents inhibit hair growth and cause hair fall; after chemotherapy hair growth resumes in 3–10 months. Other causes of hair fall—SLE (systemic lupus erythematosus), myxedema, hyperthyroidism (Fig. 1-50).

Patchy hair loss is seen in fungal infections, alopecia areata, syphilis.

Loss of hair in outer third of eyebrow is seen in leprosy, myxedema. Absence of axillary, pubic and facial hairs is seen in hypopituitarism, hypogonadism.

Alopecia

Alopecia is often an autoimmune disease. Alopecia can occur with *normal or abnormal* scalp skin. Abnormal scalp skin in alopecia is observed due to scarring as in SLE, lichen planus, radiotherapy, scleroderma, dermatitis, tinea capitis, folliculitis. Normal scalp skin in alopecia is observed in alopecia areata, secondary syphilis, traction alopecia, alopecia totalis, endocrine causes, telogen effluvium (here hair bulbs of anagen phase shrinks entering into telogen phase and hair falls later; 300–400 hairs fall daily in this condition). Alopecia can be—*localized; generalized; male pattern*.

Alopecia areata: It may be due to noninflammatory, autoimmune condition, may be associated with SLE, thyroid disorders, where there is single or multiple patches of hair loss. It can be familial (30%); it is patchy hair loss with normal scalp skin.

Alopecia totalis—when whole scalp is involved.

Alopecia universalis—when whole body is involved.

Androgenic alopecia: Male pattern of baldness with frontal recession of hairline.

Excessive Hair Growth

It is seen in women in Cushing's syndrome, adrenocortical syndrome, myxedema, ovarian tumors, drugs (androgen, minoxidil, diazoxide, anabolic steroids, phenytoin).

Hirsutism is exaggeration of hair growth (excessive) in females in androgen sensitive area where normal hair growth is absent. It may present as alone (due to polycystic ovarian disease) or may be accompanied with virilization (enlargement of clitoris, amenorrhea, temporal balding, reduction in size of breasts, loss female body contour) (Fig. 1-51).

Hirsutism is either due to excessive secretion of androgens from ovary (raise in levels of serum testosterone) or from adrenal glands [secretes proandrogen-dehydroepiandrosterone (DHEA) and dehydroepiandrosterone sulphate (DHEAS); causes raise in serum DHEAS]. Hirsutism can be seen as idiopathic, familial; seen in anorexia nervosa; epilepsy, pulmonary tuberculosis; spina bifida, poliomyelitis. Hirsutism can be physiological as in pregnancy.

■ EDEMA

It is the collection of fluid in the interstitial spaces or soft tissues. Edema will be clinically evident only when fluid accumulates more than 5 liters. Pitting on pressure occurs only when circumference of the limb is increased by 10% **(Figs. 1-52A and B).**

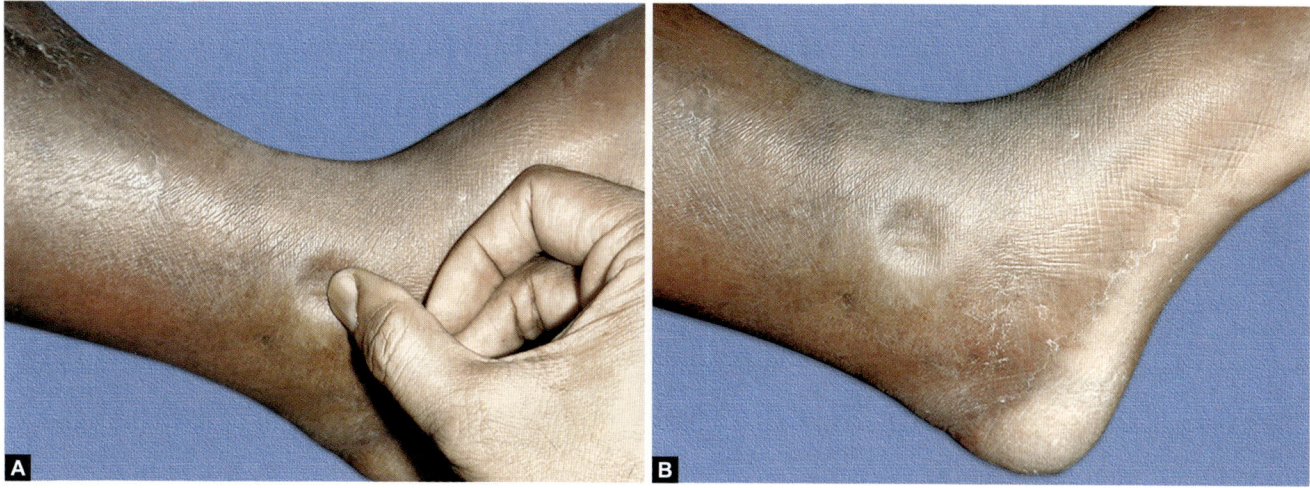

Figs. 1-52A and B Pitting edema leg. Pitting is elicited over the ankle (malleolus) or lower leg on medial aspect on a bony point using pulp of the thumb (ideally) or other fingers; deep continuous pressure for 30 seconds is applied and released to observe the pitting.

Mechanism

Normal hydrostatic pressure at the arteriolar end of the capillary bed is 35 mm Hg; at the venular end it is 12–15 mm Hg. *Oncotic pressure* of plasma is chiefly maintained by plasma proteins and is 20–25 mm Hg. Fluid volume in different compartment of the body is maintained by hydrostatic pressure at the arteriolar end that tend to push the fluid into the interstitium; oncotic pressure at the venous end which tend to push the fluid from the interstitium to intravascular space. The normal lymphatic flow helps to recirculate the albumin extruded from intravascular compartment into the interstitium.

Fluid accumulates in the interstitial space following—increased capillary permeability like in acute inflammation (cellulitis); increased capillary pressure (cardiac failure); decreased osmotic pressure (hypoproteinemia); lymphatic block (filariasis).

Pitting on pressure is the cardinal sign of edema. Firm pressure is applied using pulp of the finger/thumb for few seconds on the skin over a bone surface like lower part of medial aspect of leg just above the malleoli. Indentation or pitting is seen on releasing the finger. Slow reaccumulation of fluid in few minutes is observed.

Nonpitting edema is observed in late stage of lymphedema.

Edema is commonly observed in *most dependent part*—lower limbs. In bedridden patient, it may be seen on sacral region. Often limb edema may also be associated with ascites or pleural effusion. Upper limb edema can also occur. Edema can be unilateral or bilateral (**Fig. 1-53**).

Edema can be generalized or localized.

==Generalized edema== is called as *anasarca*. It is due to cardiac, renal, hepatic or nutritional (Figs. 1-54 and 1-55).

==Localized edema== is due to cellulitis, lymphatic causes (filariasis, radiotherapy, lymph node block dissection, Milroy's disease), venous diseases (DVT, thrombophlebitis, varicose veins), pretibial myxedema of thyrotoxicosis.

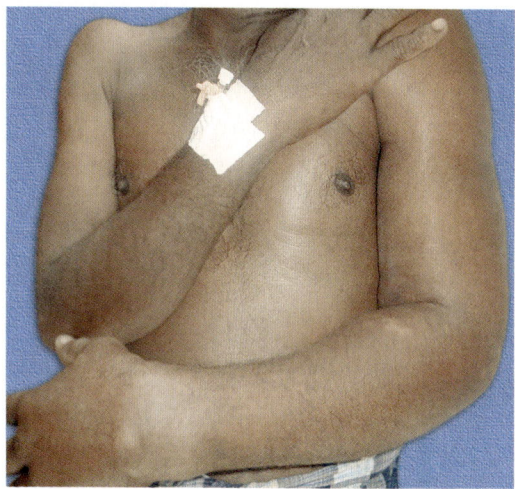

Fig. 1-53 Upper limb edema can occur as unilateral or bilateral. It can be due to axillary vein thrombosis, as a part of generalized edema, lymphedema (filarial), or due infection (cellulitis)

Allergic edema can occur on face or other parts of the body also (Fig. 1-56).

Causes may be classified as bilateral (cardiac, renal, hepatic, IVC obstruction, allergic, nutritional, toxic) or unilateral (lymphatic, traumatic, infection, metabolic like gout, DVT/varicose veins, hereditary) (Figs. 1-57A and B).

In CCF (congestive cardiac failure) edema is in most dependent position—in lower limbs and is more in evening.

In LVF (left ventricular failure) pulmonary edema develops early and so dyspnea, basal crepitations, and cough are typical. In pericardial effusion, lower limb edema, ascites, hepatomegaly (soft smooth liver), raised JVP without pulmonary edema is observed.

Edema due to renal cause develops first in eyelids and face, and then it becomes generalized into legs and ascites.

In edema due to hepatic cause like portal hypertension, ascites develops first due to increased portal pressure and hypoproteinemia, and then lower limb edema develops.

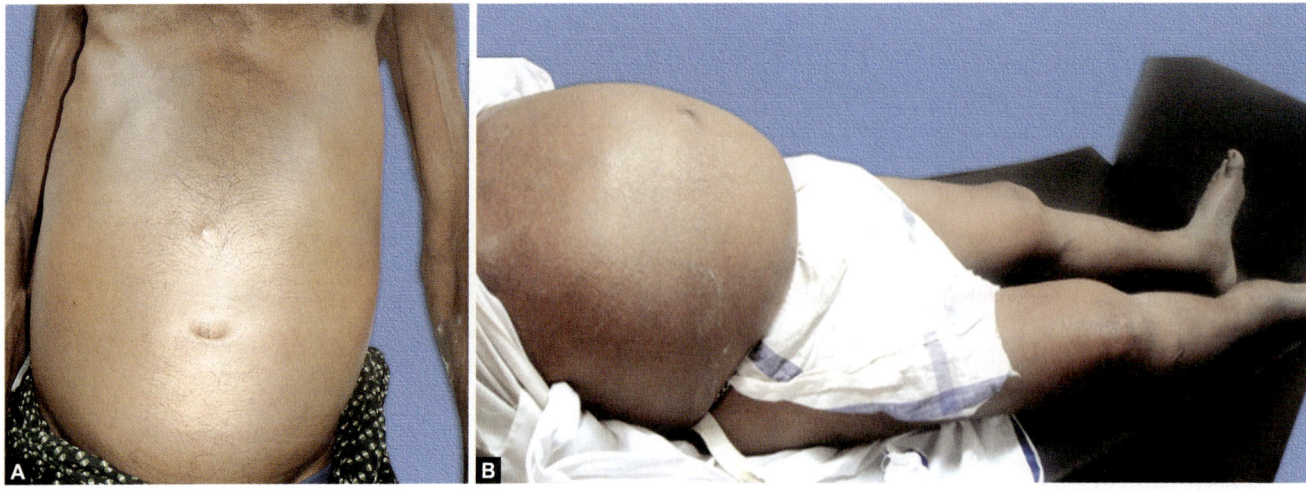

Figs. 1-54A and B Severe ascites with everted umbilicus (*smiling umbilicus*); ascites with edema limbs and face as generalized is called as *anasarca*.

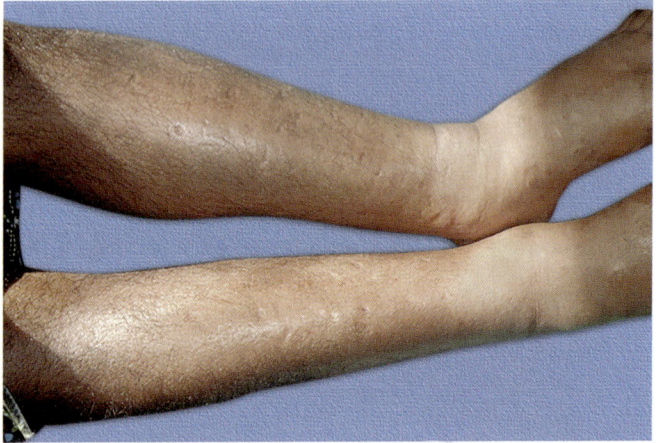

Fig. 1-55 Bilateral edema is due to cardiac/renal/liver diseases. It could be due to myxedema, pretibial myxedema (in primary thyrotoxicosis) or other metabolic causes. Anemia and hypoproteinemia also cause bilateral edema.

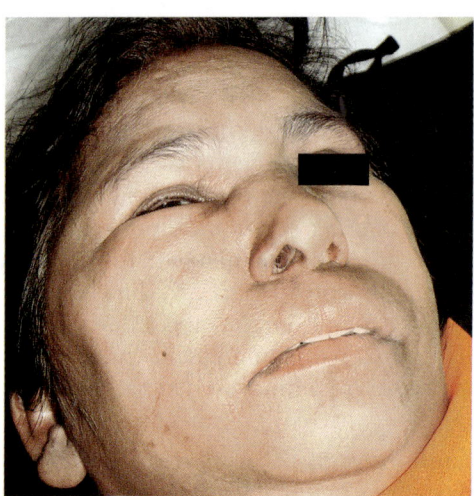

Fig. 1-56 Edema face due to allergy.

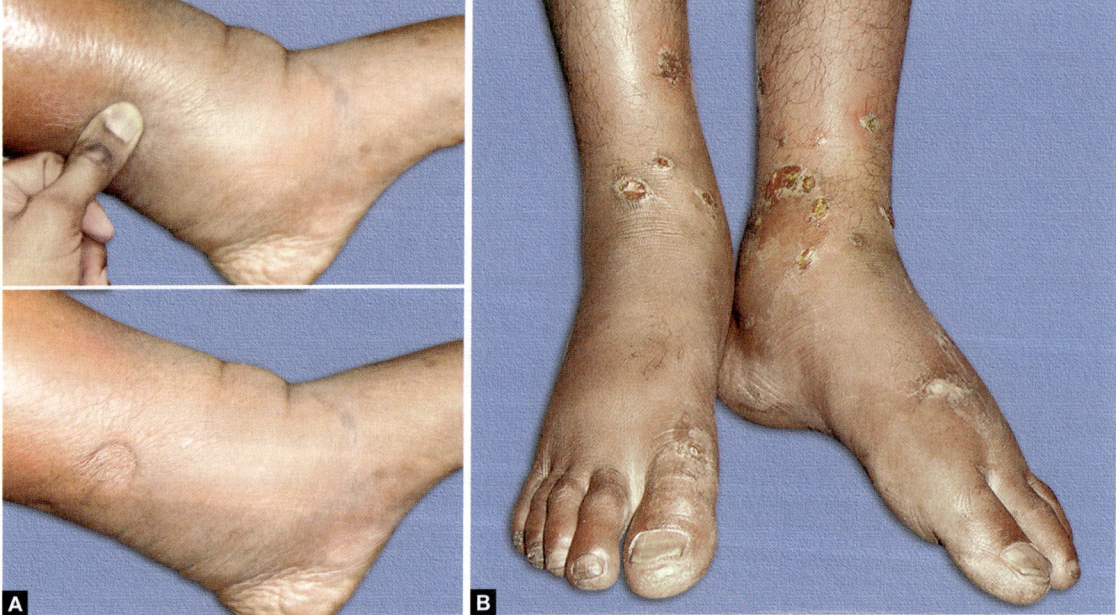

Figs. 1-57A and B Pitting edema in the leg. Note edema with multiple ulcers in another photo.

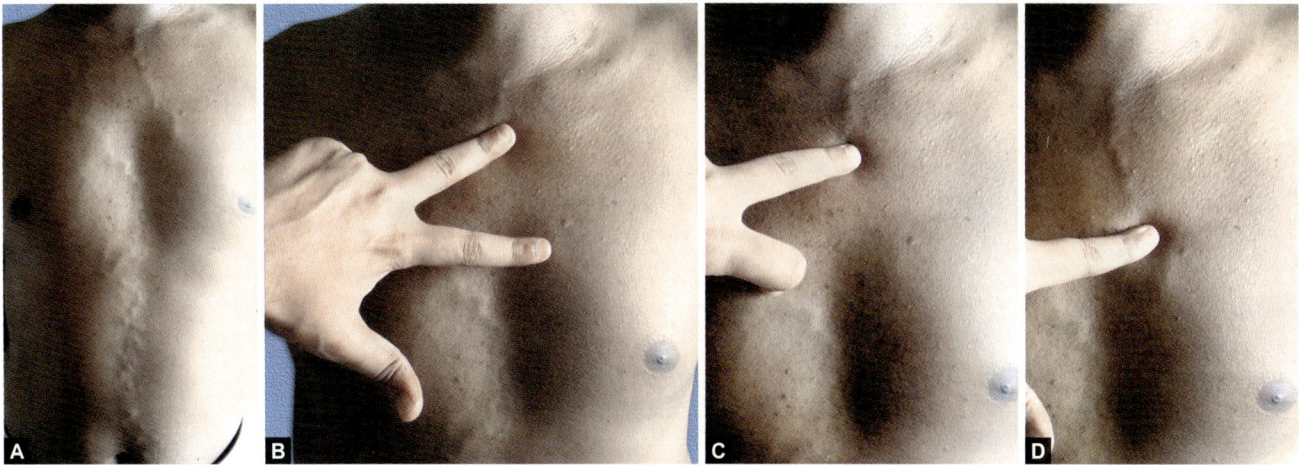

Figs. 1-58A to D Superior vena caval obstruction causing dilated veins in the chest wall. Note the direction of flow from above downwards towards lower abdomen and to inferior vena cava.

In myxedema, edema is nonpitting. Here edema over the lateral aspects of the eyelids is typical.

> **Grading of edema:**
> None (0); asymptomatic, does not require drug therapy (1); symptomatic requires drug therapy (2); symptomatic, with limited function, not responding to therapy (3); anasarca (4).

■ VISIBLE VEINS

Patient should be examined for visible veins over limbs (usually lower), abdomen, trunk and neck. With normal venous pressure external jugular vein is invisible or just visible for short distance. Raised venous pressure causes engorgement of external jugular vein. Bilateral engorgement of external jugular vein/neck veins may be due to myocardial infarction or intravenous fluid infusion or retrosternal goiter/thoracic outlet obstruction. Unilateral engorgement of vein is due to compression by lymph nodes, tumor.

In toxic goiter neck veins may be prominent due to increased vascularity.

In SVC (superior vena cava) obstruction, inguino-axillary veins, chest wall veins, neck veins may be prominent with flow of blood from above downwards and through groin veins (across watershed area) to IVC (inferior vena cava) (Figs. 1-58 and 1-59).

In IVC obstruction, veins in the flanks (both sides) will be prominent, with direction of flow from below upwards towards axillary vein along inguinoaxillary vein. Such unilateral flow is observed in unilateral blockage of common or external iliac vein. *Caput medusae* **is visible dilated veins radiating from umbilicus, seen in portal hypertension (Figs. 1-60A and B).**

Varicose veins in the leg suggest valvular incompetence in the saphenous system, either congenital nor acquired.

Jugular Venous Pressure/pulse (JVP)

JVP is superficial, wave like pulsation with 3 waves per beat; better visible than felt; alters with position and during phases of respiration. JVP decreases during inspiration but becomes prominent during expiration. Normal jugular venous pressure is **3–4 cm of water** (H_2O) **(Figs. 1-61 to 1-63)**.

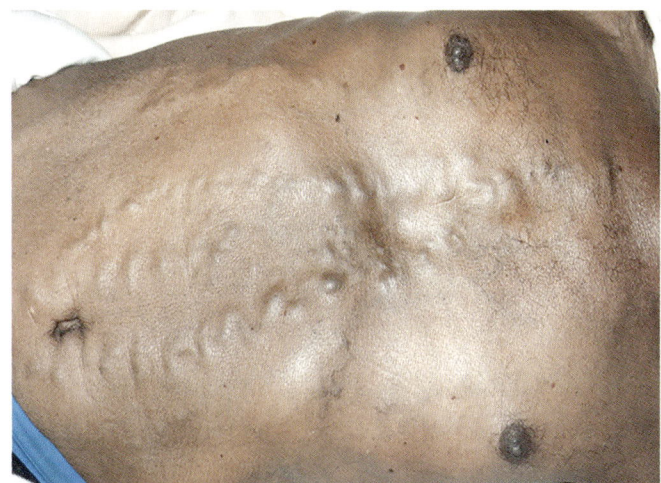

Fig. 1-59 Visible chest wall veins—SVC (superior vena caval) obstruction.

JVP is assessed by observing internal jugular vein on right side with 45° semirecumbent position, with neck turned towards opposite side. Right side is chosen because vein on right side is in direct communication with the atrium. Distance (vertical) from sternal angle to the top of blood column in the internal jugular vein is measured to get the JVP. IJV runs from the medial end of the clavicle up to the level of ear lobule under the sternocleidomastoid muscle. Normal JVP is less than 4 cm. Raised JVP suggests increase in central venous pressure (CVP)—as an indirect evidence. External jugular vein also will be distended in these patients.

Moodley's sign: Radial pulse is felt and simultaneously JVP waveform is observed; the waveform that is seen immediately after the felt arterial pulsation is the 'v wave' of the JVP. This sign is used to determine which waveform is viewed.

Internal jugular vein (IJV) if distended with visible jugular pulsation in sitting position also suggests raised JVP.

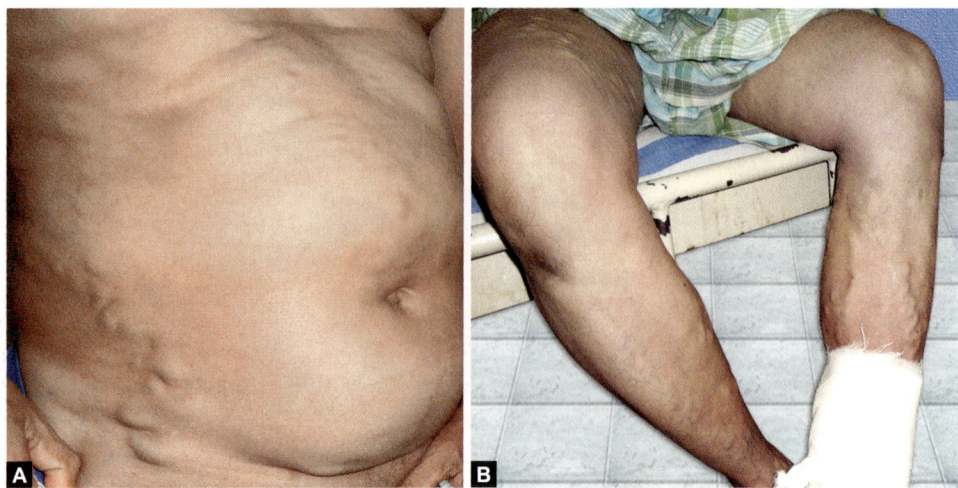

Figs. 1-60A and B Dilatation of abdominal veins including inguino-axillary vein and bilateral varicose veins in IVC (inferior vena cava) obstruction in a patient.

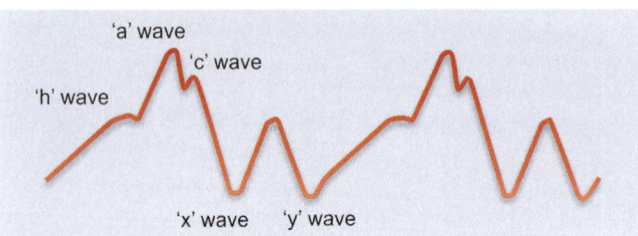

Fig. 1-61 Normal jugular venous pulse—waves (Mackenzie's polygraph)

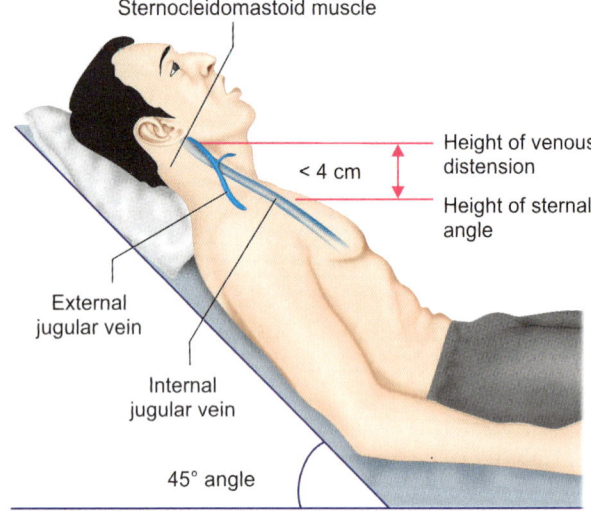

Fig. 1-62 Position and anatomical location of jugular veins to assess JVP.

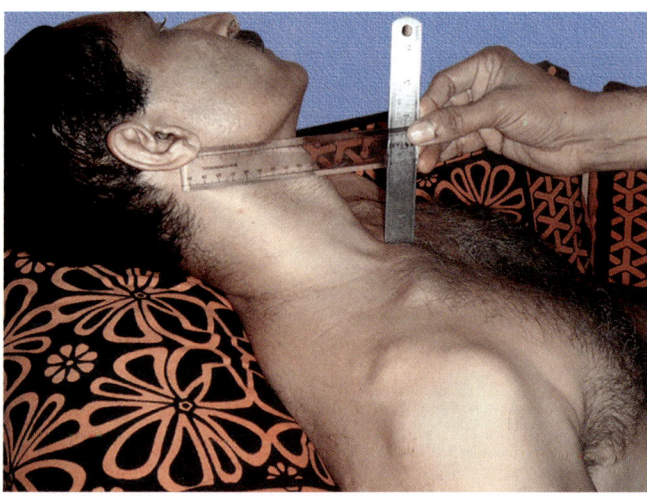

Fig. 1-63 Measuring the JVP using two scales. Position of the patient is 45° semirecumbent position with neck turned towards opposite side.

Elevated jugular venous pressure is seen in cardiac tamponade, right ventricular failure, tricuspid stenosis, increased blood volume, asthma, emphysema, superior vena caval (SVC) obstruction.

JVP is reduced in shock, dehydration. During normal inspiration, intrathoracic pressure falls and venous blood flow to thorax increases causing inspiratory collapse of jugular venous pressure. In constrictive pericarditis when intrapericardial pressure rises, there will be paradoxical increase in jugular venous pressure during inspiration—*Kussmaul's sign*.

Nonpulsatile elevation of JVP occurs in obstruction of SVC/brachiocephalic or jugular veins—mediastinal tumors, bronchial tumors, thrombosis of these veins.

Pulsatile elevation of JVP is common; it is seen in congestive cardiac failure (CCF), fluid overload like renal cause or pregnancy, right sided failure, tricuspid regurgitation/stenosis, pericardial effusion, constrictive pericarditis, massive pulmonary embolism, thyrotoxicosis, anemia, high fever.

Prominent antecubital vein or superficial veins of the hand (Gaertner's) or veins under surface of the tongue (May's) are all suggestive of raised JVP.

Hepatojugular reflux can be elicited by compression of liver causing raised right atrial pressure and so the distended jugular vein; it is also called as abdominojugular test. Positive abdominojugular test suggests that pulmonary capillary wedge pressure is 15 mm Hg or more.

Normal JVP has 3 positive waves a, c and v and 2 negative waves x and y.

'a' wave is due to right atrial contraction. It is absent in atrial fibrillation; prominent in tricuspid/pulmonary stenosis/atrial septal defect/pulmonary hypertension. *Cannon a wave* is seen in complete heart block, ventricular tachycardia, premature atrial rhythm and atrial flutter.

'c' wave is due to carotid artery impact into jugular vein and right ventricular systole. It corresponds to right ventricular contraction causing the tricuspid valve to bulge towards the right atrium.

'x' wave is due to fall in right atrial pressure and atrial relaxation. It is absent in tricuspid regurgitation. It is prominent in constrictive pericarditis.

'v' wave is due to right atrial filling. Giant v wave is seen in tricuspid regurgitation.

'y' wave is due to opening of tricuspid valve causing rapid inflow of blood from right atrium into the right ventricle. Rapid y descent occurs in constrictive pericarditis, heart failure and tricuspid regurgitation.

EXAMINATION OF PULSE

Pulse means-arterial pulse. It is a waveform felt by the palpating finger over an artery produced by cardiac systole. It gives the overall idea about the status of the heart, circulation, arrhythmias, systolic pressure and condition of the vessel wall. Pulse is an ideal indicator of severity of many diseases. It is increased in sepsis, severe pain, shock, fever, toxic thyroid. It is also altered in all cardiac conditions **(Fig. 1-64)**.

Assessment of Pulse

Pulse is assessed by rate (count the pulse); rhythm (regularity); tension and force; volume; character; condition of arterial wall; radiofemoral delay.

Pulse felt usually is radial pulse (against head of the radius) but when indicated, other pulses in the body also should be examined (dorsalis pedis, posterior tibial, popliteal, femoral, brachial, carotid, superficial temporal; bilateral pulses are compared for rate, rhythm and volume). It is felt using three fingers—index, middle and ring. Ring finger is kept distally to obliterate the retrograde pressure transmission; middle finger is used to feel the pulse; index finger is kept proximally to control and fix the artery to reduce the blood flow while checking the vessel wall thickness. **Pulse is counted for full one minute.** *Counting for few seconds and then multiplying is wrong.*

Force of a pulse is the minimum pressure required to obliterate the pulse; which reflects on systolic pressure of the patient.

Pulse volume is the uplift created towards the palpating finger; reflects on the stroke volume. ***Pulsus parvus*** is small volume pulse seen in shock and valvular stenosis. ***Pulsus magnus*** is large volume pulse seen in heart block, anemia, thyrotoxicosis, high fever. It is the amplitude of the pulse; it can be normal/low/high volume.

Amount of pressure required by the palpating finger to feel the pulse is called as *pulse tension*; it reflects on diastolic pressure.

Normal pulse rate is 60–100/minute. Tachycardia means increased pulse rate more than 100/minute. ***Bradycardia*** (Greek—slow) is decreased pulse rate less than 60/minute. ***Relative bradycardia (Faget's sign)***—Every degree rise in temperature pulse rate will increase by 10 usually (**Liebermiester rule**); in condition like ***typhoid fever*** this rise in pulse rate per degree of rise in fever is less than 10 (less than expected rise, but still having increased pulse rate); it is called as relative bradycardia. It is often also observed in *yellow fever, Legionella pneumoniae, Mycoplasma pneumoniae, Brucellosis, drug fever (beta blockers)*.

Normal Pulse Wave

Normal pulse has got a small anacrotic wave (limb) in the upstroke (which is not felt), a big tidal percussion wave which is felt. During down stroke (*catacrotic* limb), there is a dicrotic notch with a dicrotic wave (both are not felt) (Fig. 1-65).

Anacrotic wave pulse is felt in severe aortic stenosis.

Pulsus bisferiens is rapid rising, twice beating waves in the systole of the pulse; felt in idiopathic hypertrophic subaortic stenosis, severe aortic incompetence with mitral stenosis.

Dicrotic pulse is twice beating pulse with initial normal percussion wave of systole and eventual abnormal prominent dicrotic wave in diastole. It is seen in reduced peripheral resistance like CCF, cardiac tamponade, typhoid fever.

Pulsus alterans is strong and weak beats alternatively; due to alternate contractions of the cardiac muscle; seen in left ventricular failure, toxic myocarditis.

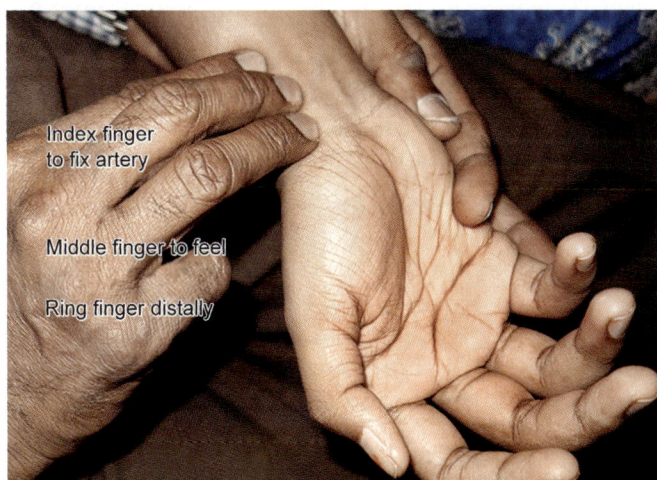

Fig. 1-64 Palpation of the radial pulse. Ring finger is kept distally to block retrograde pressure feel; middle finger is used to feel the pulse and index finger to fix the artery proximally.

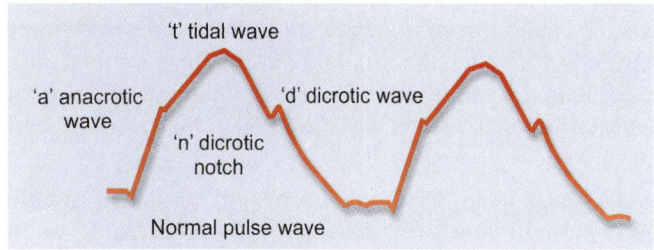

Fig. 1-65 Normal arterial pulse wave.

Pulsus paradoxus—During inspiration there is increased venous return to right atrium; lung expansion causes pooling of blood in the pulmonary vessels causing decreased venous return to left atrium and ventricle. It causes decreased left ventricular output and arterial pressure during inspiration by 3–10 mm Hg. When this fall in systolic pressure is exaggerated more than 10 mm Hg, it is called as pulsus paradoxus. It is seen in SVC obstruction, airway obstruction, asthma, pericardial effusion. In immobile thoracic cage pulsus paradoxus does not exists.

Pulsus bigeminus with coupling occurs in atrio-ventricular block.

Thready pulse is rapid, small waved pulse is seen in shock, cardiac diseases.

Waterhammer pulse (*collapsing/Corrigan's*) is large bounding pulse with a forcible jerk and disappearing quickly. It is due to sudden fall in peripheral resistance; seen in thyrotoxicosis, AV fistula, beriberi, aortic regurgitation, PDA.

■ BLOOD PRESSURE (BP)

BP is essential part of the general examination in all cases. It gives the idea about the general condition of the patient along with other parameters. BP is lateral pressure exerted by the column of blood on the walls of the arteries. Systolic pressure is due to stroke volume of the heart and stiffness of vessels. It is the maximum pressure produced during (cardiac cycle) systole. Diastolic pressure is due to peripheral resistance. BP varies in phases of respiration. It is the minimum pressure exerted during cardiac cycle (diastole). It is related to emotion, exercise, smoking, alcohol, tobacco, relation to meals, temperature, anxiousness, circadian rhythm, age, race, obesity, etc.

Recording the Blood Pressure

BP is recorded by indirect method. ***Riva Rocci* invented *sphygmomanometer***. It contains mercury manometer, cuff and air pump. Russian surgeon ***Korotkoff*** (1905) originated the method of placing of stethoscope over cubital fossa to hear sounds (***Korotkoff's sounds***) of brachial artery.

Types of devices available are—*mercury, aneroid and digital* (Figs. 1-66 to 1-68).

Aneroid sphygmomanometer is manual sphygmomanometer with a manometer gauge for measuring blood pressure. It is widely used and is safer than mercury type. ***Mercury blood pressure apparatus*** is a desktop model capable of determining blood pressure up to 300 mm of Hg. The complete inflation system is enclosed in an aluminium case.

It is measured by ***palpatory or auscultatory or oscillatory*** methods. Usually palpatory and auscultatory methods are used. Palpatory method is done first; then auscultatory; it avoids missing the ***silent gap*** observed in hypertension and aortic stenosis.

Procedure of taking BP should be meticulous. Patient should be explained about the procedure. Patient should be in rest for 5 minutes prior to checking of BP. Patient should avoid exertion or meals 30 minutes prior to checking of BP. Clothing of the arm should be removed or kept as it is without folding (folding may cause constriction band). Width of the inflatable bladder cuff should be about 40% of the upper arm circumference (12–14 cm width in average adult); length of the inflatable bladder should be 80% of upper

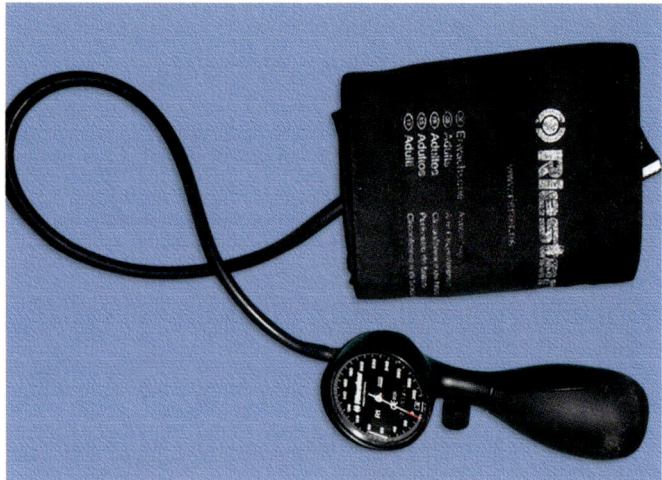

Fig. 1-66 Aneroid type of blood pressure apparatus.

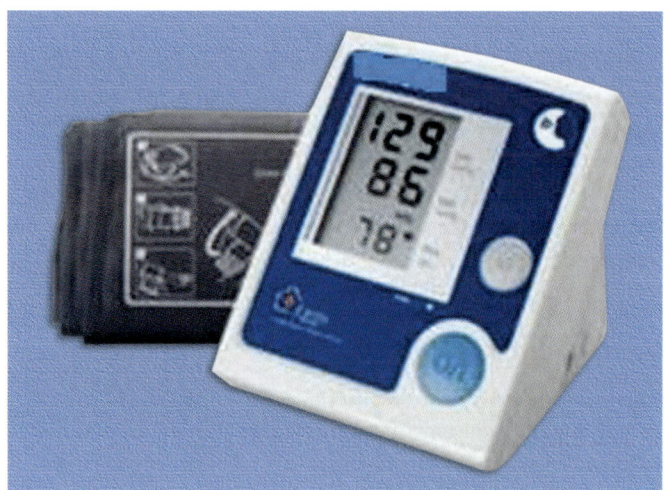

Fig. 1-67 Digital type of blood pressure apparatus.

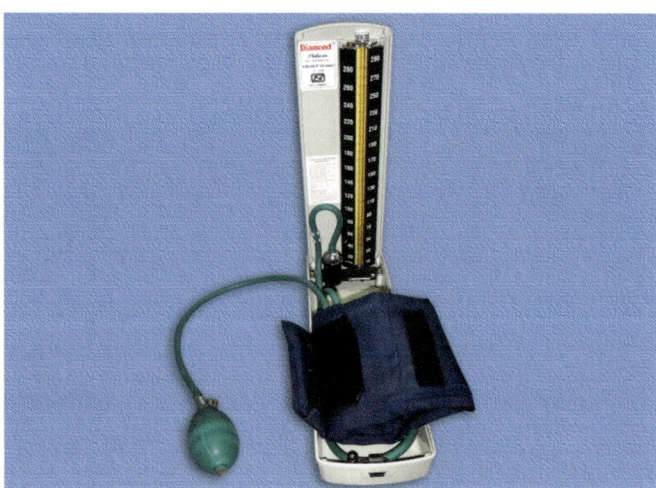

Fig. 1-68 Mercury type of blood pressure apparatus.

arm circumference, almost long enough to encircle the arm. Standard cuff commonly used is 12 × 23 cm size. In the thigh cuff of 18 × 24 cm is used. In obese, 12 × 35 cm sized cuff is used. In children smaller sized cuff (width 3 cm in infants; 8 cm in children) is used. Bladder of the BP cuff should encircle the arm completely; center of the bladder cuff should be over brachial artery; ideally rubber tubes should be placed on the inferior aspect in the line of the brachial artery (even though tubes are commonly placed superiorly to make stethoscope placement over cubital fossa easier); bell of stethoscope gives better sound; but diaphragm of the stethoscope is commonly used as its ability to cover wider area and easier to secure it. Usual position is supine lying down with arm supported to heart level. In sitting/standing position arm should be horizontal at 4th intercostal space of the sternum. If arm is not supported, arm with isometric contraction will elevate the diastolic BP by 10%. In normal individual, there is not much difference in BP in standing, sitting or lying down positions. BP in right arm is higher by up to 10 mm Hg; if BP is more than 10 mm Hg then it should be analyzed carefully. Repeat inflations of cuff will raise the systolic and diastolic BP and give false readings. So cuff should be inflated rapidly and deflated early and completely; further repeat readings are taken with a 15 seconds gap.

==Hypertension== is persistent raised systolic (above 140 mm Hg) or diastolic (above 90 mm Hg) BP. It is sustained elevation of systemic arterial pressure. It could be due to—essential HT; renal; vascular; endocrinal; neurological; hematological.

==Hypotension== is diminished BP (systolic pressure less than 90 mm Hg). It could be due to—postural, cardiac, endocrinal like Addison's disease, tuberculosis, malignancy, dehydration, shock, hemorrhage, hypovolemia, anemia, anorexia nervosa.

Phases in BP measurement:

Phase I: Faint clear tapping sound appearance which gradually increases in intensity;
Phase II: Softening or swishing sounds;
Phase III: Return of sharper crisper sounds;
Phase IV: Soft, blowing, muffling of sounds;
Phase V: Disappearance of sounds completely.

Phase I is systolic BP; Phase V is diastolic BP.

Note about blood pressure:

While checking the BP, *apparatus* should be properly functioning; mercury column should be at zero prior to inflation; size of the cuff should be proper; cuff should not be too tight or too loose (but should have *snug fit*).

Cuff should be inflated 30 mm Hg more (super systolic) than the point at which radial pulse disappears; cuff should later be deflated at a rate of 2 mm Hg per second; mercury level should be carefully observed; rapid inflation and deflation should be avoided which may result in wrong recording of BP. Width of the cuff should be 20% larger than the diameter of the limb at the point; it is to compress soft tissue effectively.

BP should be checked on *both arms* while checking it first time to confirm equality on both sides.

BP should be checked at least on *3 occasions* prior to labeling individual as hypertensive.

Normal systolic BP in adult is 120 mm Hg (90–150); *normal adult diastolic pressure* is 80 mm Hg (60–90); normal pulse pressure is 40 (30–60). BP at birth is 55/35; early childhood it is 90/60; adolescence it is 105/65.

Femoral artery is in direct line with that of aorta and so *femoral pressure* is 10 mm Hg more than that of brachial; but in aortic incompetence this difference is more than 15 mm Hg (Hill's sign). It is also seen in coarctation of Aorta, tumors pressing subclavian artery, dissecting aneurysm of aorta, cervical rib.

Diastolic BP is more relevant as it is not influenced by external factors; it reflects the constant load subjected towards arterial tree.

Hypertension (sustained elevation of BP systolic >140 mm Hg; diastolic >90 mm Hg) can be essential or secondary. Secondary can be renal [renovascular; renal parenchymal (nephritis, chronic kidney disease); renin secreting tumors; polycystic kidney disease], endocrine (adrenal causes), others (pregnancy related, aortic causes).

Malignant hypertension is BP >200/140 mm Hg; it is associated with papilledema, grade 3 or 4 retinopathy, blurring vision, hematuria, hematospermia, mental impairment.

Hypotension is fall of BP below 90 mm Hg systolic and 60 mm Hg diastolic. It may be due to familial, postural, vasovagal, shock of any cause, myocardial infarction, cardiac failure, Addison's disease, Simmond's disease (pituitary), anemia, hypothyroidism, aortic regurgitation, malignancy.

Wide pulse pressure (systolic BP is high; diastolic BP is low) is seen essential hypertension, high fever, thyrotoxicosis, complete heart block, aortic regurgitation, severe anemia, hyperdynamic circulation of any cause [AV fistula, patent ductus arteriosus (PDA), Paget's disease of bone, beriberi].

Decreased pulse pressure (less than 20 mm Hg) is seen in mitral stenosis with pulmonary hypertension, aortic stenosis, shock, cardiac tamponade, high venous pressure in severe congestive cardiac failure (CCF).

Ankle pressure is checked with knee in semiflexed (45°) position and foot kept flat on the floor, by placing the cuff around the calf with its lower edge is 2.5 cm above the ankle (malleoli); anterior tibial or dorsalis pedis artery pulsation is checked; cuff is inflated 30 mm Hg above the disappearance of pulse; slowly deflated at a rate 2 mm Hg per second; both systolic and diastolic pressures are checked. Hand held Doppler is better to check/hear the pulse/pulse waves.

Ankle brachial pressure index (ABPI) is noninvasive method used to identify the severity of peripheral vascular disease. Patient should be supine with all 4 limbs at same level (to avoid orthostatic pressure which will give false high BP); vascular cuffs with long bladder that wrap the entire circumference of the limb is ideal (all 4 cuffs are placed and pressures are checked one by one); continuous waveform bidirectional Doppler should be used in all 4 limbs [even though hand held Doppler is often (commonly) practiced]; both brachial pressures are checked and highest of two are taken as value; both ankle pressures are checked and highest of two is taken as value (please note—not average); (usually ipsilateral brachial pressure, ipsilateral ankle pressure; contralateral brachial and ankle pressures are checked) highest of the two ankle pressure divided by highest of the two brachial pressure is ABPI. Normal value is 1; if less than 0.9 it suggests ischemia; if less than 0.3 it suggests critical ischemia. In arteriosclerosis with calcification ABPI may be more than 1.3 as falsely high (drawback of test) **(Figs. 1-69A and B)**.

If ABPI is more than 1.3 then *toe brachial pressure index* is evaluated (TBPI/TBI). Both brachial cuffs and both great toe cuffs are placed; using Doppler brachial, and same side toe pressure, then similarly opposite side brachial and toe pressures are checked. For toe pressure photoplethysmograph (ppg) should be placed on the pad of the great toe to achieve waveform graph; this pad should not touch the toe cuff placed proximally in the great toe. Waveform in the chart recorder is observed; cuff is inflated through aneroid/mercury sphygmomanometer; when waveform in the chart disappears pressure is noted; pressure is raised by inflation for another 30 mm Hg; pressure is slowly released at a rate of 2 mm Hg per second until waveform in ppg reappears and this toe pressure is noted. Highest toe pressure divided by highest of brachial pressure is TBPI. Normal value is 0.65 or above. Normal toe pressure is less than ankle or brachial pressure. A toe systolic pressure greater than 30 mm Hg is normal. TBPI less than 0.64 suggests poor blood supply; less than 0.52 suggests claudication; less than 0.23 suggests critical limb ischemia.

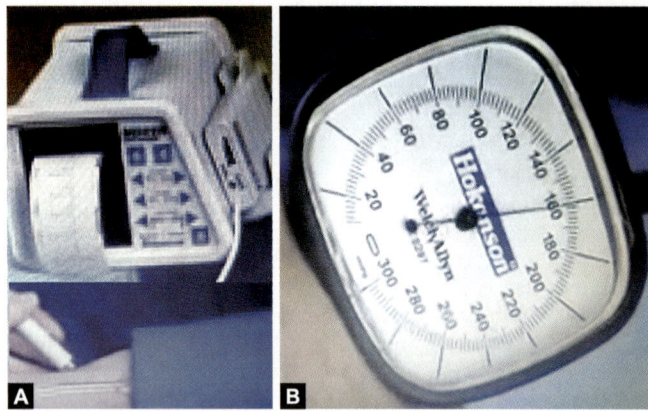

Figs. 1-69A and B To check ankle brachial pressure index aneroid manometer is used; along with wave form Doppler; all four limbs are cuffed with separate BP bladder cuffs.

RESPIRATION

Normal respiratory rate is 16–20/minute; in children it is more. It is usually 1/4th of the pulse rate. In male it is abdominothoracic; in females it is thoracoabdominal. Tachypnea is rapid breathing seen in fever, shock, hypoxia, acidosis, tetany, hysteria. Bradypnea is decreased breathing—seen in narcotic poisoning, diabetic coma, uremia and raised intracranial tension.

Irregular respiration often seen in meningitis, coma and shock. Gradual deepening of respiration alternating with short periods of apnea is called as *Cheyne-Stokes respiration* (John Cheyenne and William Stokes, 1846). It is a periodic breathing; with alternate apnea and hyperventilation; apnea lasts for 30 seconds; hyperapnea lasts for 3 minutes with 30 or more breaths; amplitude of breathing will increase and decrease. **It is common in deep sleep, narcotics, left ventricular failure, pneumonia, respiratory infections, uremia, cerebrovascular diseases, severe head injuries, cerebral tumors.**

EYES

Eyes are evidence of many diseases. Observation of eyes is very important. Normally eyes blink 3–5 times a minute; infrequent blinking is observed in thyrotoxicosis and parkinsonism.

Orbital margin appears sunken in dehydration/malnutrition; puffiness seen in nephrotic syndrome; sclera looks yellow in icterus/jaundice; red in conjunctivitis, iritis, keratitis. Sclera and conjunctiva looks pale in anemia; grayish white color is seen in limbus (Figs. 1-70 and 1-71).

Arcus senilis is seen in elderly due to atherosclerosis, hypertension; there is deposition of cholesterol in the eyelids. It can also occur in old age commonly. It is asymptomatic common entity seen in 60% of old people. *Arcus cornealis* is deposition of lipid droplets and cholesterol in superficial and deep layers of cornea forming a yellowish white ring about 2 mm wide with clear space between it and sclerocorneal junction at the limbus. It is seen as bilateral peripheral calcification of cornea.

Argyll Robertson pupil: It occurs in neurosyphilis; unequal, irregular miotic pupil; presence of accommodation reflex but absence of miotic and ciliospinal reflex is seen.

Exophthalmos is bilateral outward protrusion of eyeballs from their normal positions, seen in primary thyrotoxicosis. Proptosis is unilateral/bilateral outward protrusion of eyeball due to condition other than thyrotoxicosis (Fig. 1-72).

Enlargement of lacrimal glands is seen in *Sjögren's syndrome.*

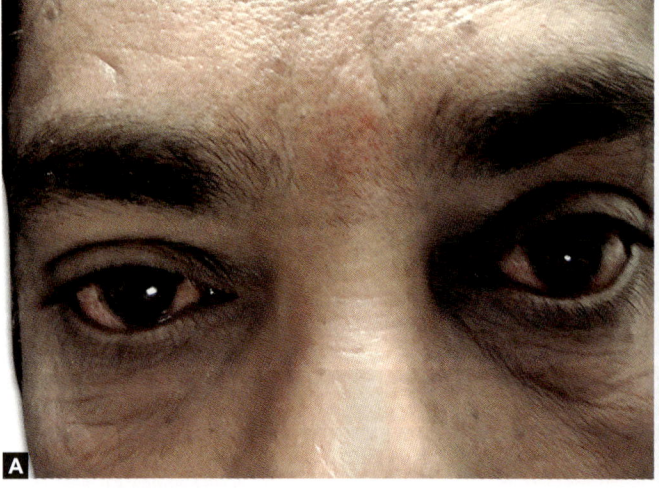
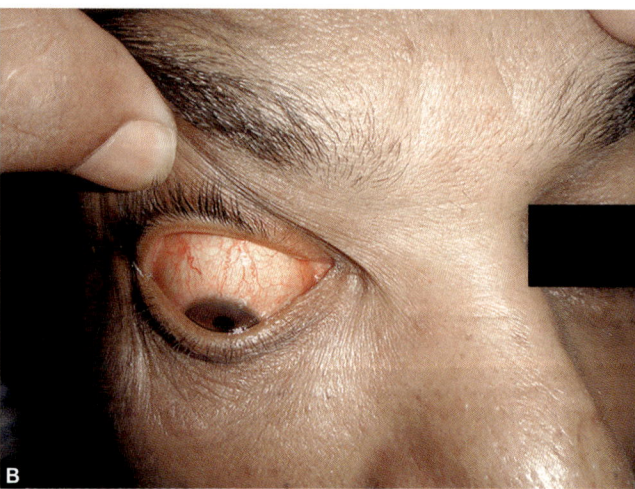

Figs. 1-70A and B Sclera should be examined for congestion, redness, discoloration (jaundice); in this patient there is redness and congestion in sclera due to leptospirosis.

Chapter 1: Introduction to Clinical Approach and Examination 37

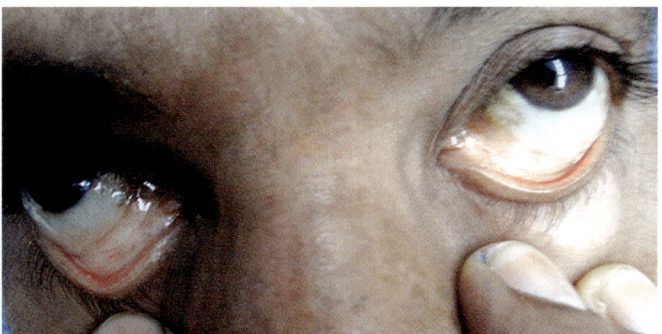

Fig. 1-71 Examination of conjunctiva.

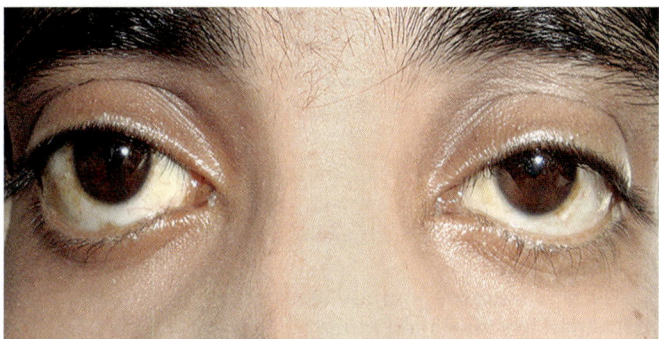

Fig. 1-72 Eyes and face should be examined carefully as part of general examination. Note the visible lower sclera—could be due to exophthalmos.

Ptosis: It is inability of upper eyelid to achieve elevation causing drooping (of the upper eyelid). *Causes*: Congenital is due to weak levator palpebrae muscle. Acquired is due to Horner's syndrome, paralysis of 3rd cranial nerve, myasthenia gravis, multiple sclerosis, edema/trachoma/tumor of the eyelid and trauma. Tabes dorsalis (neurosyphilis) causes pseudoptosis. 3rd cranial nerve (oculomotor) palsy may be due to trauma, ischemia, tumor, aneurysm. It causes unilateral complete ptosis with squint and large pupil. Myasthenia causes bilateral transitory ptosis which is more towards evening due to muscle fatigue.

Horner's syndrome: Enophthalmos due to Müller's muscle weakness; drooping of upper eyelid [partial ptosis (in 3rd nerve palsy ptosis is complete)]; anhidrosis; miosis due to paralysis of dilator papillae; absence of ciliospinal reflex; flushing of face and nasal congestion. Reasons for Horner's syndrome: It is due to interruption of sympathetic nerve supply to head and neck. Preganglionic fibers arise from 1st and 2nd thoracic segments of the spinal cord synapses with three cervical sympathetic ganglia. Any disruption of preganglionic fibers or cervical ganglia or their fibers will cause Horner's syndrome. Causes are: Posterior inferior cerebellar artery thrombosis; often cervical sympathectomy; Pancoast's tumor; secondaries in the neck; advanced thyroid malignancy; carotid artery aneurysm; spinal cord lesions; injuries to lower root of brachial plexus. Unilateral diseases, cervical sympathectomy causes unilateral Horner's syndrome (Fig. 1-73).

Edema of the eyelids: It can be unilateral or bilateral. It is due to drug allergy, physiological (crying, sleeplessness), nephrotic syndrome, part of anasarca, cardiac/liver failure, protein deficiency, etc.

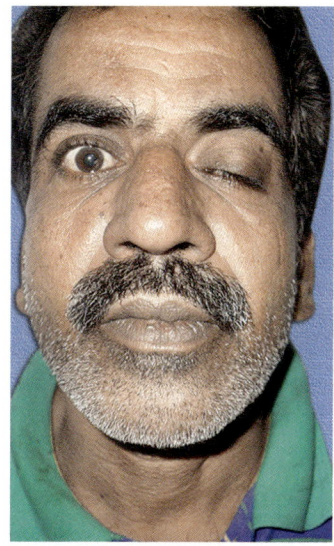

Fig. 1-73 Unilateral left sided ptosis due to Horner's syndrome/3rd nerve palsy (oculomotor).

Xanthelasma: It occurs in eyelids as yellow/orange plaques or nodules. It may be single or multiple; unilateral or bilateral. It is seen in old age, diabetes mellitus and ischemic heart disease. Pain, itching or inflammation will not be present.

Other conditions like cataract, eyelid swelling (chalazion), eyelid edema, retinal tumors can occur; conditions should be identified and proper ophthalmic opinion should be sought for (Figs. 1-74 to 1-76).

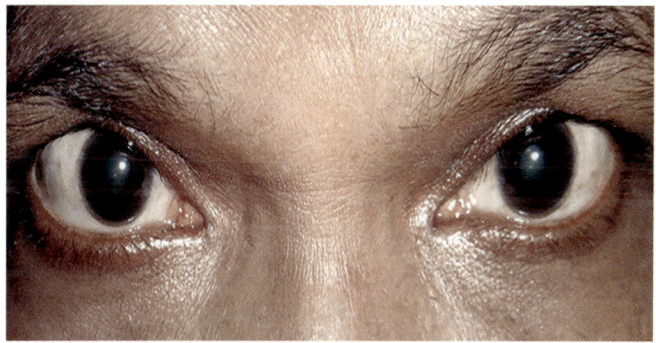

Fig. 1-74 Cataract both eyes; note the opaque lens.

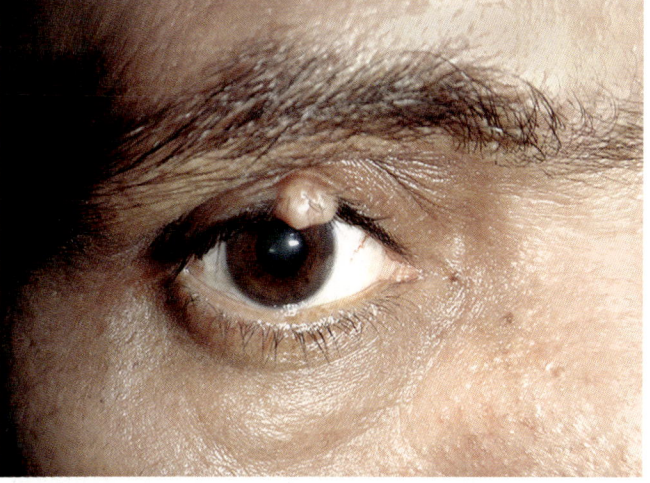

Fig. 1-75 Eyelid swelling; chalazion.

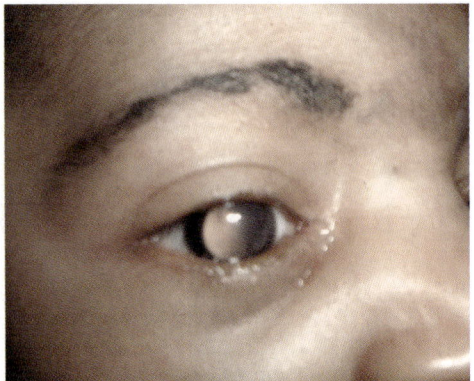

Fig. 1-76 Retinoblastoma eye in an infant.

■ NOSE

Depressed bridge of the nose is called as **saddle nose**. It is due to destruction of the nasal cartilage; seen in Hansen's (leprosy) disease, congenital syphilis, cutaneous Leishmaniasis. It can be congenital also. Hypertrophy and adenomatous changes in the sebaceous glands in the tip of nose causing thickened, widened nasal tip is called as **rhinophyma**.

■ EARS

Ear is made up of 6 ear tubercles. So **dermoid cyst** can occur due to sequestration. **Bat ear** is congenital one which protrudes out from the side of the head. Multiple subperichondrial hematoma in the ear can cause **cauliflower ear** deformity. **Keloid** can occur in the ear at the site of ear prick; shows soft or firm nodule hanging down often pedunculated. **Accessory auricle** may be present in front of the tragus. **Hansen's disease (leprosy)** can cause ear deformity (**Figs. 1-77 and 1-78**).

■ FEVER/RISE IN TEMPERATURE

Normal body temperature is balance between heat gain and loss maintained by hypothalamus. It is the temperature of

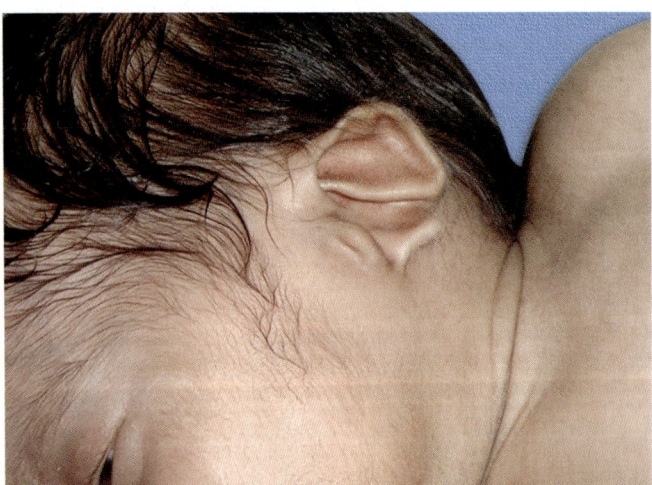

Fig. 1-77 Congenital deformity in the ear is not uncommon; it requires reconstructive surgery for correction.

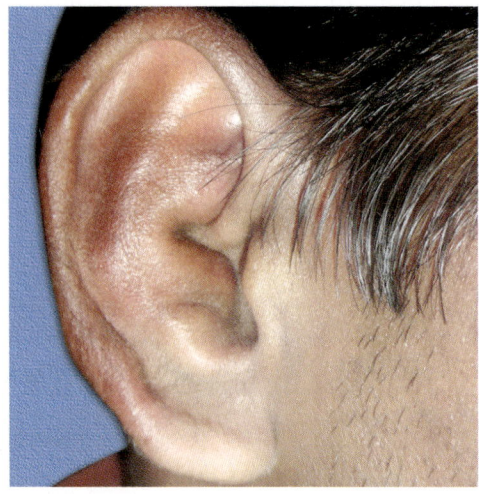

Fig. 1-78 Diffuse swelling in the ear—cauliflower ear.

viscera and body tissues. Normal temperature is 36.7°C–37.5°C (98 to 99°F – 98.6°F). A diurnal variation of 1°C is normal; lowest temperature is during morning 2–4 AM, highest being in afternoon.

Fever is increase in body temperature more than 1°C or more than the maximum range.

Types of Fever (Fig. 1-79)

Continuous fever: Fever persists throughout the day and temperature does not fluctuate more than 1°C in 24 hours. It is seen in pneumonia, urinary infection, endocarditis.

Remittent fever: Temperature is above normal throughout the day but there is fluctuation of more than 1°C in 24 hours.

Intermittent fever: Fever is present for only few hours a day and reaches to normal. It is observed in malaria, kala-azar. When fever develops daily, it is called as *quotidian*; when fever develops on alternate days it is called as *tertian*; when it occurs every third day it is called as *quartan*.

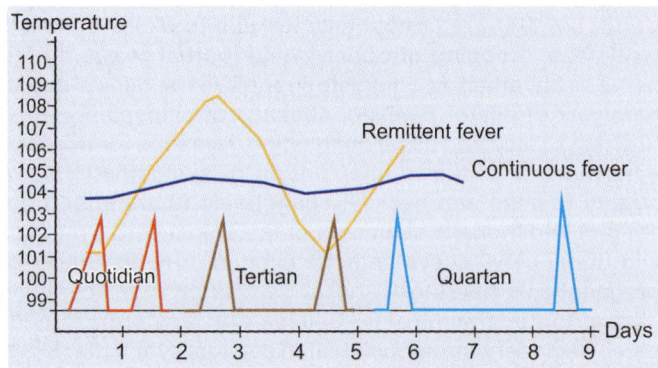

Fig. 1-79 Different types of fever.

Hypothermia is 35°C/95°F or below;
Subnormal temperature is 35°–36.7°C/95°–97°F;
Normal is 36.7°C–37.5°C/98° to 99°F (98.6°F);
Mild fever is 37.2°–37.8°C/99°–100°F;
Moderate fever is 37.8°–39.4°C/100°–103°F;
High fever is 39.4°–40.5°C/103°–105°F;
Hyperpyrexia is more than 40.5°C/106°F.

Chapter 1: Introduction to Clinical Approach and Examination 39

Note about fever:

Fever with exanthematous rashes are seen in chickenpox (1st day); measles (3–4th day); typhoid (7–8th day).

Febrile convulsions—convulsion occurring in infants and children at temperature more than 40°C.

Thermoregulatory center is located in *hypothalamus*.

Morning 6 AM body temperature is 98.6°F; evening 6 PM it is 99.6°F—as 1°F *diurnal variation*.

Axillary temperature is 1°F less than oral; *oral temperature* is 1°F less than *rectal temperature*. Rectal 1°F > Oral 1°F > axilla. 1°F is 0.6°C.

In females, during ovulation, temperature rises by 1°F and persists till menstruation due to progesterone effect; later till ovulation temperature will be subnormal.

Temperature raise of 1°F after 100°F causes raise in pulse rate by 10; raise in respiratory rate by 4; raise in BMR by 7; raise in oxygen consumption by 13%.

Elevation of body core temperature more than 106°F (41°C) with inadequate heat dissipation is called as *hyperthermia*. It may be due to cerebral malaria, meningococcal meningitis, septicemia, rheumatic fever, pontine hemorrhage. *Malignant hyperthermia* is an inherent abnormality of skeletal muscle cell sarcoplasmic reticulum which is unable to store calcium with raise in intracellular myoplasmic calcium activating myosin ATPase converting ATP to ADP, PO_4 and high heat. Hyperthermia also occurs in heat stroke, inhalation of the anesthetics like halothane and cyclopropane or muscle relaxant like succinylcholine.

Pel Ebstein fever: Recurrent bouts of fever and afebrile periods occur at regular alternations. Temperature rises for 3 days, remains high for 3 days, remits in 3 days and goes for an afebrile period of 9 days to develop fever again in the same manner. It is observed in brucellosis; earlier also thought to be due to Hodgkin's lymphoma. It is a cyclical/relapsing fever with a pyrexial period of one or two weeks and then an apyrexial fever period of again one or two weeks.

Relapsing fever: Here febrile episodes are separated by normal temperature for more than one day; like in Borrelia fever; ratbite fever.

Drug fever: It is prolonged fever starts 1–3 weeks after drug intake; persists 2–3 weeks after withdrawal of drug. Drugs which cause fever usually are—sulphonamides, penicillins, iodides, propylthiouracil, methyldopa, anticonvulsants and antitubercular drugs. This fever is associated with rashes, pruritus, arthralgia, eosinophilia, relative bradycardia and hypotension.

Fever with chills and rigors: Fever with chills is sensation of cold with fever. *Rigor* is profound chill with piloerection (*gooseflesh*) with teeth shattering and shivering.

Causes for Fever:
- Infective (bacterial, viral, fungal, parasitic);
- Neoplastic (lymphoma, leukemia, hepatoma, renal cell carcinoma, carcinoma colon);
- Cardiovascular (myocardial infarction, pulmonary embolism, pontine/subarachnoid hemorrhage);
- Traumatic;
- Collagen diseases; endocrinal;
- Metabolic (Gout, acidosis); hemolytic.

Grading of Fever:
- None (0); 38–39°C (1); 39.1–40 (2); >40 for 24 hours (3).

Pyrexia unknown origin (PUO): It is defined as—fever with temperature more than 101°F; more than 3 weeks of duration; failure to reach a diagnosis even after one week of inpatient investigation.

■ TONGUE

It is muscular organ of mastication often red in color, with prominent fungiform papillae at the edge and tip of the tongue; filiform papillae at the dorsum; circumvallate papillae at the junction of anterior 2/3rd and posterior 1/3rd; which help in appreciating various tastes. The color, size, surface, shape, coating, mobility, and any other lesions are to be noted.

Mouth dryness is graded as:

Normal (0);
Mild (1);
Moderate (2).

Tongue may be large called as *macroglossia*. It is seen in lymphangioma, hemangioma, acromegaly, myxedema, critinism, amylodosis.

Tongue tremor is observed in thyrotoxicosis (primary). It is checked with tongue kept inside the oral cavity. If tongue is protruded out tongue twitchings may mimic tremor.

Tongue is bright red in color normally—due to rich blood supply through capillary network. Pallor is seen in anemia, hemorrhage. Discoloration can occur after colored food intake, tobacco chewing, Addison's disease, iron tablets intake. *Black* discoloration is *melanoglossia* due to iron and bismuth intake; *brown* discoloration is seen in uremia; scarlet red discoloration—niacin deficiency; *white centrally coated* tongue is seen in enteric fever and leukoplakia. In central cyanosis, tongue appears *blue*.

Tongue is *moist* normally; dry tongue suggests dehydration, shock. *Dry brown tongue* is a feature of uremia, Sjögren's syndrome, intestinal obstruction.

Furring of tongue is seen in smokers, stomatitis, and poor oral hygiene.

Black hairy tongue is seen in fungal infection.

Bald tongue is due to atrophy of papillae. It is seen in iron deficiency anemia, vitamin B_{12} deficiency.

Curdy coating is seen in candidiasis infection (Refer chapter 11).

Leukoplakia is a whitish opaque thickened epithelium; it is often associated with superficial glossitis.

Congenital *fissuring* can occur with irregular folds. Fissuring may also be a presentation of carcinoma of tongue. Lozenge shaped loss of papillae and fissuring is seen in midline in front of the foramen cecum.

Lingual thyroid may be seen posteriorly in midline.

Inability to protrude tongue is seen (*ankyloglossia*) in tongue tie, advanced carcinoma tongue infiltrating the genioglossus muscle.

While protruding, tongue may deviate *towards same side* in hypoglossal nerve palsy.

Ulcers in the Tongue

Single	Multiple	Recurrent
Tuberculosis	Aphthous ulcers	Aphthous
Carcinoma	Herpes	SLE
Syphilis	Secondary syphilis	Lichen planus
Dental irritation	Vitamin B deficiency	

Note: One should look for carious tooth, dentition, any artificial dentures, sharp tooth; should observe for the mucous membrane of cheek, palate, floor of the mouth for any ulcers, leukoplakia and pigmentation; should observe for lip pallor, cracks, fissuring, ulcer, and angle of the mouth for cheliosis.

Causes for abnormal pigmentation in tongue:
- Addison's disease
- Peutz-Jegher's syndrome
- Malnutrition
- Nelson's syndrome

CREPITUS

It is crackling or grating sensation felt on palpation of subcutaneous tissue or joint or bone. Crackling sensation is felt when air is under the palpating fingers. Pockets of air moves in between separated subcutaneous or soft tissues causing crackling feel. Grating sensation is felt in bone or joint as crepitus.

Types

Various types of crepitus is seen depending on the contents (gas/liquid/solid) in the mass felt.

Crepitus in subcutaneous (surgical) emphysema: It is crackling sensation felt under examining fingers with gentle pressure similar like a palpating horse hair mattress. It can often be heard by placing a stethoscope over the surface. Subcutaneous emphysema is better felt (often seen as bull neck) in neck, shoulder and chest wall. Causes of subcutaneous emphysema are—traumatic (injury to lung and pleura following fracture ribs, bronchial/tracheal/laryngeal injury, tracheostomy, fracture skull with air sinus like frontal sinus injury); after surgery (air may get trapped in the subcutaneous plane) prior to closure of skin, after laparoscopic surgery; infective (in gas gangrene); after esophageal rupture (Boerhaave's syndrome—here mediastinal emphysema, subcutaneous emphysema, shock, toxicity occurs).

Crepitus of tenosynovitis: It is seen in de Quervain's tenosynovitis. Here hand is laid upon arm above the wrist, and the patient is asked to close and open the hand. Crepitus is felt at the junction of extensor pollicis brevis and abductor pollicis longus crossing the extensor carpi radialis longus and brevis.

Crepitus of bursitis: It is felt when lining of bursa is rough or contains loose fibrinous particles.

Joint crepitus: It is felt when affected joint passively moved by one hand, and by placing other hand over the suspected joint.

It can be—*fine*, even crepitations of chronic and subacute joint diseases; *coarse*, irregular crepitations of osteoarthritis, Charcot's joints; *a click* due to loose body or displaced cartilage.

Bone crepitus: It is elicited over the fracture segments of the bone when two fragments are moved against each other. A grating sensation is typical. But this should be elicited with utmost gentleness; only when radiological doubt exists. Crepitus is an unmistakable, diagnostic sign of fracture.

LOCAL EXAMINATION

Following rules should always be followed:
- It should be done in the presence of a nurse/ attendant.
- It should be done under good light preferably day light otherwise signs like jaundice may be missed.
- Proper positioning of the patient in relaxed and comfortable manner is a must for a successful examination.
  Various positions are:
  » *Supine* for abdomen, extremities, chest, and head and neck.
  » *Prone* for back.
  » *Sitting position* for face, eyes mouth, thyroid swellings, neck swellings, back and breast.
  » *Standing position* for hernia, varicosities of lower limb, inguinoscrotal swelling, spine.
  » *Lateral position* for rectal examination.
  » *Lithotomy* for vaginal examination.
- Examination should be carried by the examiner, standing or sitting comfortably on the right side or front of the patient.
- Various parts have to be exposed adequately for proper examination, for example:
  » *For neck lesion*—from chin to nipple.
  » *For chest lesion*—from chin to umbilicus.
  » *For abdomen*—from nipple to thigh.
  » *For hand*—finger to axilla.
  » *For foot*—toes to inguinal region.
- Bilateral examination should be done to compare the disease with normal part.

Local Examination should be Done in a Systematic Way by Observing the Following Steps

Inspection (Look): It is observing the diseased area carefully for clinical features. It should be done with proper complete exposure of the part; compared with normal side.

Palpation (Feel): It is done by feeling of affected part using hand and fingers.

Percussion (Move/Tap): It is tapping of the affected area directly using flexed finger (direct method) or using pleximeter finger and percussion finger (indirect method). Percussion is used over sternum, abdomen (ascites, over mass to find out note, liver dullness,), respiratory system (in pleural effusion, pneumothorax).

Auscultation (Hear): Stethoscope is used to hear abnormal sounds like adventitious breath sounds, altered bowel or absence bowel sounds or loud intestinal sounds (*Borboygmi*) or *succussion splash* in pyloric stenosis; bruit over vessel or organ.

Examination of regional lymph nodes: It is essential as many diseases like inflammation and malignancy may spread to regional nodes. Involvement of regional nodes gives idea about the severity of the disease and staging in case of malignancies.

Movements: Active and passive movements of the joints related are tested to note the abnormal movements; movements are compared to opposite side.

Measurements: Circumferential girth of abdomen is taken for ascites, intestinal obstruction; circumferential girth of upper and lower limb is taken for soft tissue growth/edema; length of limb in case of fracture of long bones.

SYSTEMIC EXAMINATION

Systemic examination is essential in all patients. It includes examination of respiratory and cardiac systems, abdominal examination, central nervous system examination and skeletal system examination.

Respiratory system: Chest wall movements; breath sounds, vocal fremitus, presence of pleural effusion, vocal resonance, tracheal shift, etc.

Cardiac system: Apex beat location, heart sounds, alerted sounds, muffled sounds, murmurs, etc.

Abdominal examination: Inspection of the abdomen for movements, fullness, umbilicus, hernial orifices, visible mass/pulsation, any scars of previous surgeries; palpation for mass and palpable organs like liver or spleen; percussion for the liver dullness (right 5th intercostal space in the midclavicular line), percussion over the mass, percussion for free fluid (ascites); auscultation for bruit around umbilicus; digital examination of the rectum for sphincter tone, rectal ulcers/lesions, prostate enlargement in males, rectal stricture, secondaries in rectovesical or rectouterine pouch.

Skeletal system: Spine should be examined for deformity, tenderness, paraspinal spasm and movements. Rotation movement of the spine should be checked by making the patient to sit in a stool.

> **Other examinations to be done according to the need:**
>
> *Head and neck region:* Cranial nerve functions; eyes (visual field, pupils for equality and reaction, accommodation reflux, conjunctiva, eye ball movements, fundus examination); mouth and pharynx (teeth, gums, soft palate movement, tongue, tonsils, lip); neck (movements of neck, neck veins, neck nodes, carotid pulse, trachea, thyroid).
>
> *Upper limbs:* General look of hands, forearm, arm (muscle wasting); vascular system (pulsation); nervous system (sensation, muscle power, muscle tone, reflexes); axillary nodes; joints and movements; fingers and nails. Both hands, forearms, arms and joints should be inspected.
>
> *Thorax:* Examination of chest for deformity; dilated veins; swelling; pulsations; breasts; apex beat; lungs and heart.
>
> *Abdomen:* Abdominal wall (umbilicus, scar, dilated veins); reflexes of abdomen; visible peristalsis; visible pulsation; hernial orifices; palpation; percussion; auscultation; rectal digital examination; per vaginal examination if needed in females; examination after catheterization if needed.
>
> *Lower limbs:* Examination of feet, legs, thighs; feeling of peripheral pulsation; nervous system in the lower limbs; edema feet; varicose veins; examination in standing; joints; inguinal nodes.
>
> *Examination of genitalia:* Testis (its size, texture, presence of hydrocele); epididymis; vas deferens, skin over the scrotum; penis for phimosis, balanoposthitis, chordee, hypospadias.
>
> *Skeletal system:* Spine and skull.
>
> *Note:* In bilateral anatomical areas: Both sides should be examined and compared like—in limbs, eye, ears, face, etc.

FINAL DIAGNOSIS

- It is identification/determination of proper anatomical, pathological and etiological (cause) nature of the disease with its extent, severity based on which proper investigations and treatment can be planned. It is purely analytical. Analysis is based on detailed history, clinical findings and their application towards a disease correlating anatomy, pathology, etc.
- As it happens in many occasions if it is not possible to conclude towards a single disease and features correlate to more than one disease then differential diagnosis is put forward. Each diagnosis listed out in differential diagnosis are analyzed and assessed.
- All positive features in history, **symptoms and signs** are put together to analyze the anatomical location (tissue of origin), extent and pathological nature of the disease. Sometimes negative features are also important to consider or rule out certain diseases.

> **Diseases are also classified as congenital, traumatic, inflammatory, neoplastic or others:**
>
> **Congenital**
> - It can present at birth or at a later period
> - At birth—cleft lip/palate; spina bifida, microstomia, exomphalos, ectopia vesicae, hypo or epispadias, anorectal malformations, tracheoesophageal fistula, biliary or intestinal atresia, limb anomalies.
> - Presentation at a later age group—hemangiomas, branchial cyst, dermoid cyst, thyroglossal cyst, indirect inguinal hernia, congenital pelviureteric junction (PUJ) obstruction causing hydronephrosis
>
> **Traumatic**—mechanical, electrical, chemical, thermal, radiation induced
>
> **Inflammatory**—viral; fungal; protozoal; parasitic; bacterial (specific like tuberculosis, syphilis, leprosy; nonspecific bacterial)
>
> **Neoplastic conditions:** Benign—neurofibroma, lipoma; Malignant—primary like carcinoma, sarcoma; secondary as metastases
>
> **Others**
> - Occlusions—of blood vessels; lymphatics; intestine; biliary duct, salivary duct, urinary tract, Fallopian tube, of cerebrospinal flow (CSF causing hydrocephalous)
> - Metabolic diseases
> - Degenerative diseases
> - Deficiencies of vitamins, minerals
> - Endocrine diseases—diabetes mellitus, thyrotoxicosis
> - Collagen diseases like rheumatic disease, autoimmune diseases
> - Foreign body impaction in various structures like esophagus, trachea, etc.
> - Functional diseases like inflammatory bowel disease
> - Poisoning conditions

- Iatrogenic diseases: It is occurrence of disease due to some act of the clinician during therapy period; urethral stricture after catheterization or instrumentation; drug-induced hematemesis

Based on the tissue of origin diagnosis can be considered as arising from—skin, fat, fascia, muscles, blood vessels, lymphatics, nerves, bones, joints, lymph nodes, organs like liver/spleen/lungs, etc.

Tissue contents will help to identify anatomical and pathological nature of the disease—*solid cellular* swelling (firm/hard, nonfluctuant, nontransilluminating); soft/cystic/tensely cystic *liquid swelling* (soft/firm), fluctuant may be transilluminating (if fluid is clear one) containing serous/purulent (pus)/bloody/lymph fluid; content may be *gas* (air/hydrogen sulphide/toxic gas) like in surgical emphysema or laryngocele or gas gangrene; or combination of more than one of the above.

Diseases are classified as congenital (begins at birth); acquired which develops at a later period or idiopathic when cause is not identified.

Note: Detailed history taking is essential. First history should be taken with suitable questions; one should wait patiently for right answers; one neither should nor force the answer of our need; leading questions are asked only at the end after complete history is taken. First complaint is noted down; detail of that complaint is elicited; system relevant to that complaint is explored by asking simple direct questions; then history in relation to other systems are asked.

In differential diagnosis most common possible diagnosis should be mentioned first; then in descending order as per correlation of findings.

Investigations are planned depending on the clinical diagnosis; only relevant investigations are to be done. Investigations are done for tissue diagnosis; for system involvement by the disease; relevant for preparation for anesthesia and surgery.

LEVELS OF EVIDENCES

Different levels of evidences are used in clinical practice. It is important to know so that recommendations or strength of evidence is assessed. High quality RCT, systemic reviews, high quality synthesized evidence are evidences beyond reasonable doubt. High quality review of literature is best practice evidence.

Levels of evidences

Evidence	Level description
I a I b	Evidence from meta-analysis from randomized controlled studies (RCT) Evidence from at least one RCT
II a II b	Evidence from at least one controlled study without randomization Evidence from at least one other type of quasi-experimental study
III	Evidence from nonexperimental descriptive studies, such as comparative studies and case control studies
IV	Evidence from expert committee reports or opinions or clinical experience of respected authorities or both

ECOG PERFORMANCE STATUS (Eastern Cooperative Oncology Group)

This performance status is used as a guide to plan the therapy. It is also important in clinical trials to select the patient.

ECOG (Zubroad) scale	Performance
0	Fully active and able to carry out work without restriction
1	Symptoms restrict strenuous physical activity but ambulatory and able to carry light sedentary work
2	Ambulatory but unable carry out work; up and about >50% waking hours
3	Only limited self-care; confined to bed or chair for more than 50% of waking hours
4	Completely disabled; confined to bed or chair
5	Dead

KARNOFSKY PERFORMANCE STATUS (KPS)

In 1948 *David A Karno*fsky devised the scale as a uniform objective assessment of functional status. The KPS is a method of measuring co-morbidity mainly in solid tumors especially in head and neck malignancies as an independent reliable predictor of the outcome.

Karnofsky performance status (KPS)	
100	Normal; no complaints; no diseases
90	Able to carry on with normal activity; few symptoms and signs of the disease
80	Able to carry on with work with effort; some symptoms and signs of the disease
70	Inability to do normal activity or active work;' but can care for self without assistance
60	Able to carry out most of basic needs; but occasional assistance is needed
50	Frequent medical care and considerable assistance is needed
40	Needs special care and assistance—disabled
30	Hospitalization is needed with severe disability; but death is not imminent
20	Hospitalization, active supports are needed; very sick
10	Moribund, rapidly deteriorating
0	Dead

Knows in clinical practice

- Know the patient
- Know the anatomy
- Know the disease
- Know the time of intervention
- Know the machines
- Know the right and wrongs both
- Know – "The Team"
- Know what you don't know
- Know the technique
- Know when "NO' or 'NOT REQUIRED"
- Know yourself
- Know what patient wants
  - Relief
  - Resumption of work
  - No complications
  - No recurrence
  - Cost feasibility
- Know the risks and complications
  - Know how to avoid them
  - Know how to recognize them
  - Know how to treat them

2 | Investigations

Competency: AS3.1; AS3.2; AS3.4; AS3.5; IM12.9; SU1.3; SU9.1; SU9.2; SU9.3.

■ INTRODUCTION

Even though clinical diagnosis is finalized, it is essential to do further investigations to:

- *Confirm the diagnosis:* It is done using different biochemical methods, imaging and tissue diagnosis. Biochemical methods may be done by analysis of fluid (pus, discharge, urine, bile, etc.), blood/serum, tumor markers, culture, cytology, etc. For cellular diagnosis, fine needle aspiration cytology (FNAC) is done. For tissue diagnosis, various biopsies are done. Gastroscopy, colonoscopy, bronchoscopy, laparoscopy, thoracoscopy, mediastinoscopy are other things used. Immunohistochemistry (tissue and receptor marker study) needs tissue for assessment and is useful in various malignancies like sarcomas, lymphomas, carcinoma breast; it gives the idea about the needed chemotherapy agents including number of cycles and prognosis as well.
- *Assess the severity of the disease:* It is done by various imaging methods like ultrasound, CT scan, MRI scan, angiogram. It is used to stage the disease in case of malignancy (local or systemic spread) or to find out the severity/extent like in case of tuberculosis (to assess location, size of the lesion), fungal/parasitic (hydatid cyst), congenital (arteriovenous malformations).
- *Often to know the exact etiology of the disease:* Estimation of serum calcitonin in patient with medullary carcinoma of thyroid and in his/her family members; estimating alpha-fetoprotein (AFP) in hepatocellular carcinoma (HCC); estimating serum parathormone (PTH), calcium levels in hyperparathyroidism.
- *Plan and implement the treatment strategy and to predict the prognosis:* Many investigations are analyzed properly like histopathology report, imaging, markers, biochemical studies. They should be correlated to clinical diagnosis. It is often better to discuss with radiologists and pathologists regarding your suspicion of the condition to have a proper conclusion prior to surgery or other therapeutic modalities. Often during surgery, on-table investigations are needed to have an additional information like on-table ultrasound, C-arm imaging, etc. Frozen section biopsy may be needed while operating on malignancy to confirm resection clearance is adequate or not.
- *Identify associated illness, if any:* Often patient may suffer from more than one disease; if such doubt arises, patient should be evaluated for additional associated illness, as that particular disease may alter the treatment and prognosis of this specific disease.
- *As a preoperative preparation* in case patient needs surgery. It is done with complete hemogram, blood sugar, cardiac and respiratory assessment; it is better to have fitness opinion from a physician especially if patient is above 40 years of age. It is essential to evaluate in detail if patient is having comorbid conditions like diabetes, cardiac/respiratory/renal/liver diseases or coagulopathies. Patient should be made acceptable (*optimized*) for anesthesia prior to surgery in these patients. If patient is on any anticoagulant therapy, it should be stopped 3–5 days prior to surgery. Prothrombin time (PT, INR) and ideally activated partial thromboplastin time (APTT) should be assessed; these patients may require injection vitamin K or fresh frozen plasma (FFP) prior to and during the surgery. In trauma, and in critically ill patients, preoperative preparation is done later after initial adequate resuscitation.

■ TYPES OF INVESTIGATION

Investigations may be

- *Noninvasive:* It is preferred one at initial period of assessment—ultrasound, Doppler, X-rays, echocardiography, etc. are noninvasive methods.
- *Invasive:* It is done by some means of invasive methods wherein it creates some level of inconvenience to the patient. Biopsy, endoscopies, intravenous contrast studies are some examples.

Needed investigations are decided by the intelligent clinician as a supportive tool to his clinical diagnosis. Without clinical examination, ordering the investigations does not make any sense. Often first imaging like ultrasound done prior to clinical examination is also entirely wrong. Clinician should keep his discretion to decide which investigations are essential and which are not necessary based on individual case/patient study. However, present trend is changed towards more and more investigations due to more legal litigation against practitioners. Clinician is becoming defensive in the fear of negligence. Change in the social system and loss of trust towards clinicians should only be blamed for this.

Investigations done often as

- **Negative confirmative evidence:** In gallbladder stone disease, CT abdomen is done to confirm that common bile duct (CBD) is normal so that laparoscopic cholecystectomy can be undertaken safely. Ultrasound abdomen is done to rule out right ureteric stone or ovarian pathology (in females) to confirm severe pain in right iliac fossa is due to acute appendicitis. Normal orthopantomogram (OPG) of the mandible confirms that there is no mandibular infiltration in oral cancers. It is the method of exclusion (Fig. 2-1).
- **Positive confirmative evidence:** Presence of stones in gall bladder in an ultrasound is positive confirmative. Showing fracture in an X-ray is positive confirmative evidence (Fig. 2-2).

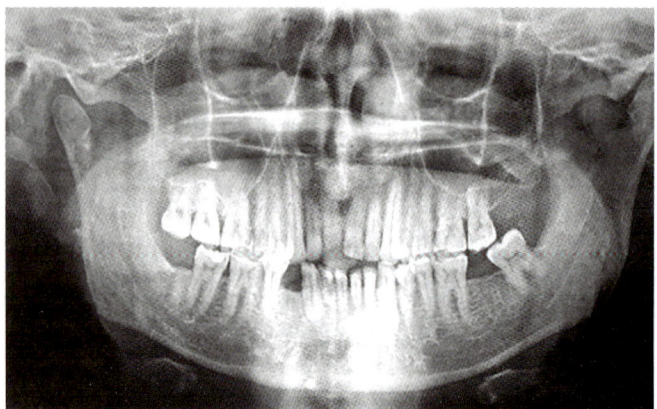

Fig. 2-1 X-ray orthopantomogram (mandible) which is normal; taken in a patient with carcinoma oral cavity; it confirms that mandibular infiltration by tumor is not present.

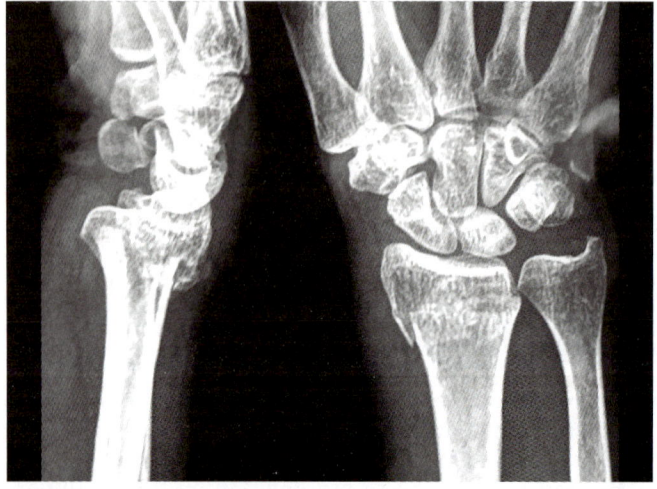

Fig. 2-2 Fracture in X-ray bone is positive confirmative evidence (here fracture is just above wrist, Colles' fracture).

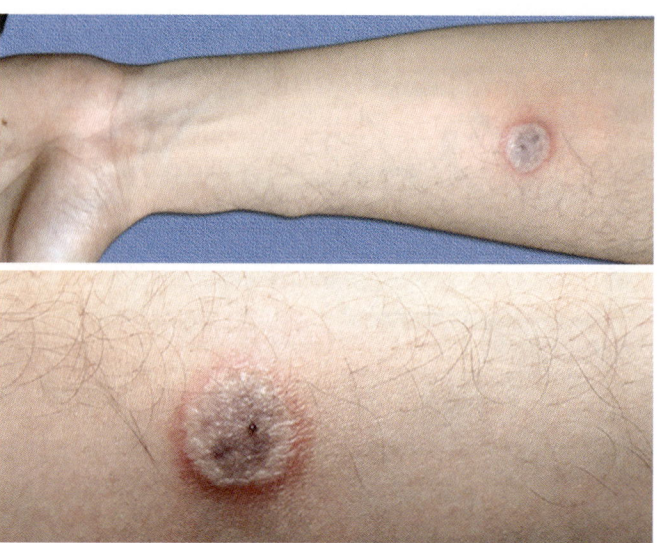

Fig. 2-3 Mantoux skin test done for tuberculosis (positive in this patient).

Skin tests are often used to assess allergy, antigen reactions, etc. Casoni's skin test for hydatid, *Mantoux skin test* for tuberculosis are few of them. Antigen is injected intradermally, area is marked, extent of redness and *induration* is observed in 48–72 hours (Fig. 2-3).

CELLULAR STUDY

It is the study of cells (*cytology*) for diagnosing mainly malignancy (tumor cells) and often tuberculosis (epithelioid cells). It is done either by **FNAC** (Fine needle aspiration cytology), **exfoliate cytology** (secretions from the hollow viscera may contain tumor cells which are shed from the tumors in the particular lining; these secretions are collected for cellular study to confirm malignancies, for example: Cytological study of sputum for carcinoma lung; of stomach fluid for carcinoma stomach; of urine for carcinoma urinary bladder; vaginal secretions of female genital tract; nipple discharge for carcinoma breast, etc.), **imprint cytology** (here excised specimen is transected and cut surface is pressed firmly over a slide without any movement and slide is immediately fixed with ethylalcohol and stained with Papanicolaou stain), **brush cytology** in respiratory system during bronchoscopy or from biliary tree during ERCP [endoscopic retrograde cholangiopancreatography] or from urinary system; **sponge cytology** using sponge over the surface lining.

BIOPSY

- '**Bio**' means life or tissue; '**opsis**' means vision or microscopy. **Biopsy** means study of tissues using microscopy. It is the removal and examination of a sample of tissue taken from usually a living individual for diagnostic purpose to have histological examination using different staining and microscope study; tissue so obtained is called as biopsy specimen (biopsy specimen is dead one).
- Biopsy can be incision, excision, trucut, Pap smear, FNAC, frozen section, punch, US/CT guided, laparoscopic/thoracoscopic/endoscopic/proctoscopic/open by

laparotomy/thoracotomy/craniotomy, etc. Biopsy is sent in 10% formalin. To assess receptors and histochemistry, it is sent often in low temperature in normal saline or special ingredients. Tissue blocks are made. It is cut using microtome up to 5 μ thickness. It is studied after staining with hematoxylin and eosin. Bone specimens are *decalcified* for 7–21 days using HCl.
- *Cautery use* should be *minimized* while taking biopsy. *Specimen* in the lab is kept for 6 weeks; *blocks* for 30 years; *slides* are kept for 10 years. Risk of false positivity in malignancy should be remembered. Repeat biopsy/repeat sectioning/second opinion should be done in such doubtful situations. Special stains, histochemistries are very useful.

Types

Biopsy can be Closed or Open Type

Closed type: Needle biopsies, punch biopsy, drill biopsy, Crosby capsule biopsy are different closed method biopsies. *Vim Silverman, Menghini, Travenol needles* are used to do biopsies of liver, kidney, prostate and muscle. Bone marrow biopsy is also done using specialized needle with guard.
- *Drill biopsy* is done under local anesthesia; a stab incision is made and the drill introduced into the tissue; the drill rotates at a speed of 15,000 rpm and cores out a cylinder of tissue (1–2 cm long) which is then dislodged with a syringe into the preservative fluid; bleeding and infection rates are very minimal; possible drawback is tumor dissemination; but studies proved that such chances are uncommon (Burn et al) **(Fig. 2-4)**.

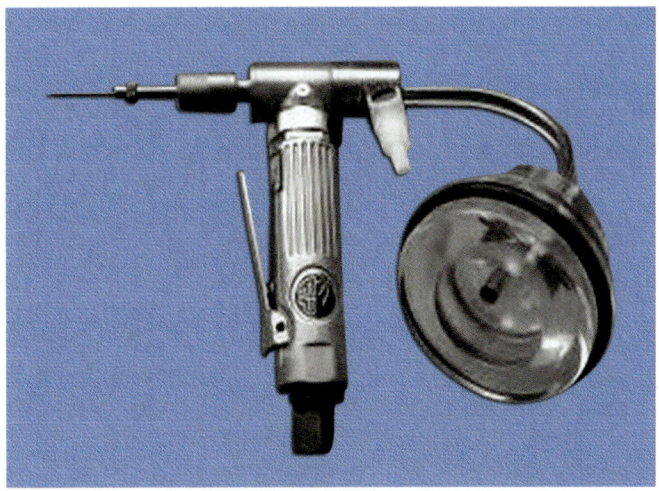

Fig. 2-4 Drill biopsy device.

- The *Crosby-Kugler capsule (Crosby capsule; Dr William H Crosby)* is a device used to take biopsy from small intestine mucosa in small bowel diseases (mainly in children to diagnose Sprue). The capsule with attached long tube is swallowed; other end of the tube remains outside the patient's mouth. Once the capsule has reached the desired part of the small intestine, suction is applied to the tube to cause a spring-loaded knife to sweep across an aperture in the capsule by trigger mechanism, cutting away the mucosa protruding into the aperture. The capsule is then pulled out by the tube to retrieve the biopsy specimen from capsule chamber. Capsule can be used along with gastroduodenoscopy. Crosby capsule biopsy is done under image guidance (C arm) **(Figs. 2-5A to C)**.

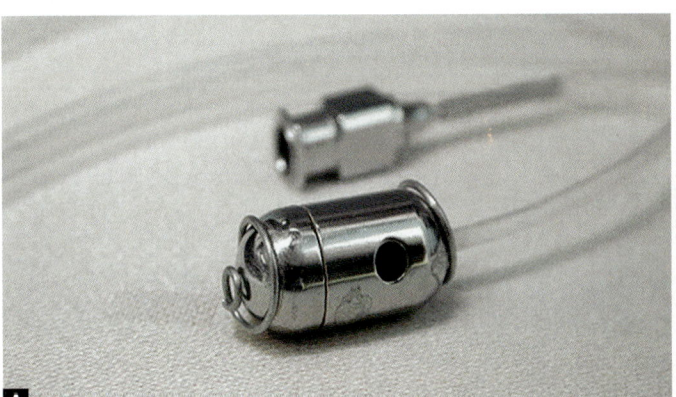
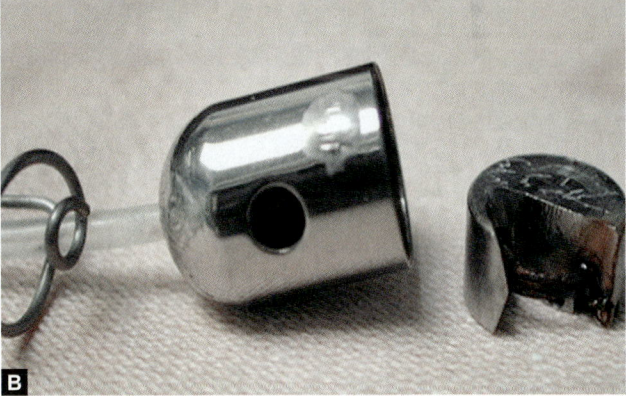
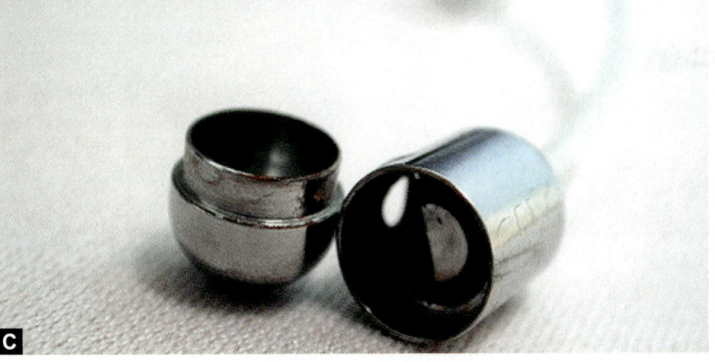

Figs. 2-5A to C Crosby-Kugler capsule biopsy device.

Open type: Here biopsy is taken under vision by open method. *Incision biopsy* to take wedge biopsy from an ulcer or incision biopsy of soft tissue sarcoma; *excision biopsy* of a swelling or melanomas or small skin lesions are examples.

- **Incision biopsy** is taken from the *edge of ulcer* along with the normal tissue; usually two wedge biopsies should be taken; it is contraindicated in melanoma and lymph node secondaries. There is not much difference between wedge (*wedge biopsy* means removal of a cuneiform shaped tissue with part of the normal tissue adjacent) and edge biopsy which is actually wedge biopsy from the edge in case of an ulcer. So better terminology could be *wedge biopsy or incision biopsy from the edge*. Wedge biopsy can also be taken from solid organ like liver, kidney or lungs.
- *In post-radiotherapy recurrent cancers and syphilitic ulcers,* biopsy is done from center as the center contains actively multiplying cells with blood supply and there is no actively multiplying tissue in the edge due to radiotherapy (radiotherapy reduces the blood supply at the edge and tumor proliferates at the center).
- **Excision biopsy** is useful in lymphoma (lymph node), melanoma (incision/wedge biopsy is not advisable in melanoma), and doubtful lesions wherein FNAC is not clear. It does not have chance of spreading the tumor.
- **Needle biopsy** is done by passing a needle through the tissue. *Vim Silverman needle* is used for liver biopsy. Kidney biopsy is done using needle under ultrasound guidance.
- **Fine needle aspiration cytology (FNAC)** is aspiration of fluid and cell content of the tissue of interest to have cytological study using a device with 24 G needle. It is useful in thyroid, breast, parotid, lymph node and other surface lesions. US/CT guided FNAC is commonly advocated. It is contraindicated in testicular tumor for the fear of spread of malignant cells along the needle track. Negative FNAC may require repeat FNAC or open biopsy. Often positive FNAC should be also reconfirmed by repeat FNAC or second opinion (occasional false positive may create problem in managing conditions like carcinoma breast) **(Fig. 2-6)**.
- **Trucut biopsy** is done using a specialized device with a gun to fire the needle to decore the tissue of interest. It is done in prostate, breast and surface tumors **(Fig. 2-7)**.
- **Punch biopsy** is used in hollow organ and skin. Punch biopsy is also taken from cervix. It takes a cylindrical biopsy with adequate depth. Miniature punch biopsy is done using endoscopes; bronchoscopic punch biopsy of bronchial tree/gastroscopic punch biopsy of gastric ulcer/cystoscopic punch biopsy of urinary bladder/**ERCP** (endoscopic retrograde cholangiopancreaticography) guided punch biopsy of biliary tree are different examples. It is taken from the edge and base of the lesion like in four quadrant biopsy from gastric ulcer. It should include abnormal along with adjacent normal tissue *with base* but avoiding sloughed part **(Fig. 2-8)**.

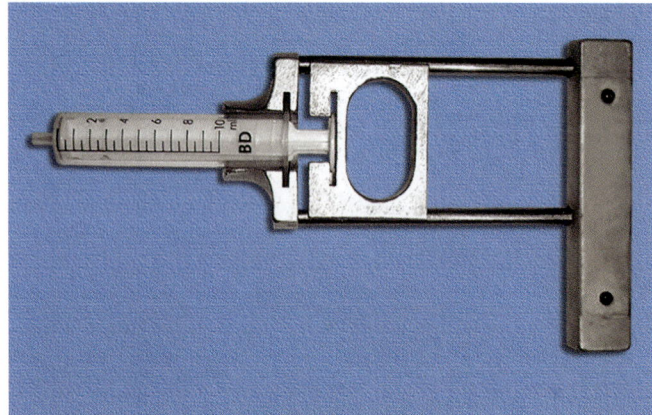

Fig. 2-6 Device used for FNAC (Fine needle aspiration cytology).

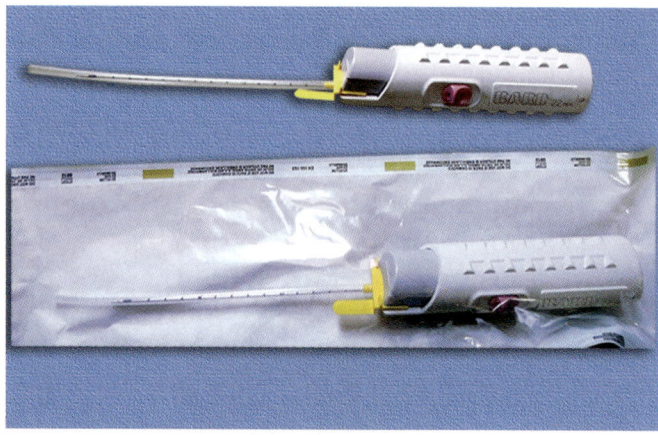

Fig. 2-7 Trucut biopsy device.

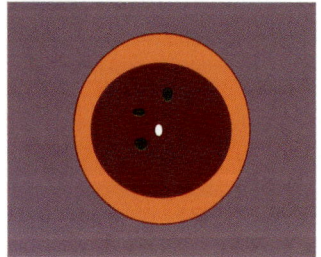

'Punch biopsy' of the cervix

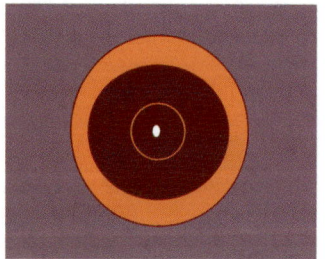

'Cold cone biopsy'—a large area of cervix mucosa is removed circumferentially using no. 15 blade

In lithotomy position, cervix is visualized using speculum

Fig. 2-8 With patient in lithotomy position punch biopsy is taken from cervix using punch biopsy forceps following per speculum visualization; much wider cone biopsy can also be taken.

ENDOSCOPIC EXAMINATION

- It is the visualization of the inner lining of the hollow viscera or cavities and their contents using specialized devices called endoscopes. It is named depending on structure which is examined—proctoscopy (anorectum), sigmoidoscopy, colonoscopy, esophagoscopy, gastroduodenoscopy, enteroscopy, cystoscopy, ureteroscopy, nephroscopy, culdoscopy, hysteroscopy, thoracoscopy, mediastinoscopy, laparoscopy, choledochoscopy, arthroscopy, bronchoscopy and laryngoscopy.
- **Endoscopy can be rigid, fiberoptic or video endoscope. Rigid is sturdy and strong and is used for therapeutic purpose like foreign body removal; it needs general anesthesia; complications are more. Fiberoptic is one where light is transmitted through optical glass fibers with an opaque coating and scope tube is flexible; direct visualization is possible. Biopsy, irrigation, suction, sclerotherapy can be done under direct vision. Presently video endoscopes are available which are ideal with images of good clarity and magnification. Virtual images including virtual histology can be assessed in present generation scopes. Endoscopic ultrasonography (EUS) is done by placing/attaching a specialized device to the end of the endoscope through which ultrasound pictures and images of the layers of the wall of the gastrointestinal tract can be assessed including taking EUS needle aspiration/biopsy of bowel wall and adjacent lymph nodes. EUS is useful in esophagus, stomach, duodenum and rectum.**

X-RAY AND IMAGING

Plain X-ray

Plain X-ray is useful to identify radiopaque pathology, fractures, mass lesions, fluid levels, erosions/rarefactions of the bone, etc. Usually two films are taken—anteroposterior and lateral; as X-ray is two dimensional, two films give better idea about the visualization of the needed area. Chest X-ray

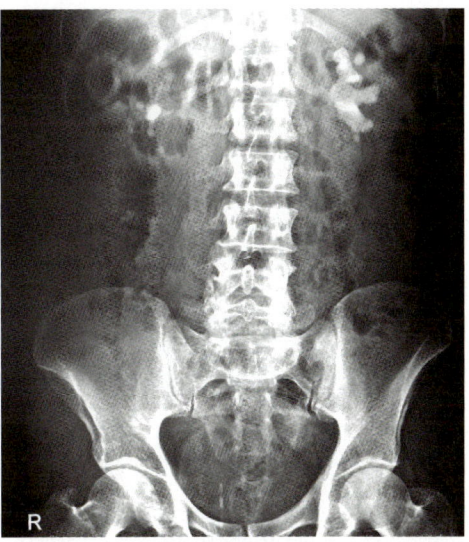

Fig. 2-9 X-ray KUB (kidney, ureter and bladder) showing left sided staghorn calculus.

is done usually in posteroanterior view; when needed lateral X-ray chest is taken. X-ray may be taken at different areas like chest, abdomen, urinary region [KUB (kidney, ureter, bladder)], pelvis, skull, paranasal sinuses (PNS) **(Fig. 2-9)**.

Chest X-ray is useful in identifying pleural effusion, mass lesion, tuberculosis, consolidation; but if lesion is in posterior lobe, chest X-ray may look normal; and in such situation, CT chest is ideal (Figs. 2-10 to 2-13).

Plain X-ray abdomen is useful to visualize gas under diaphragm, multiple air fluid levels of intestinal obstruction, to see pancreatic stones/calcification in chronic pancreatitis (Fig. 2-14).

Contrast X-ray

Clarity of the visualization in X-ray can be augmented by introducing contrast into the cavities or into the vessels. Barium meal, barium meal follow through X-ray, barium

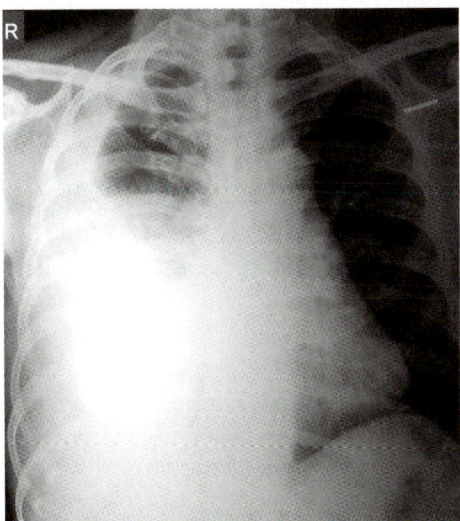

Fig. 2-10 Chest X-ray showing right sided pleural effusion—could be due to tuberculosis.

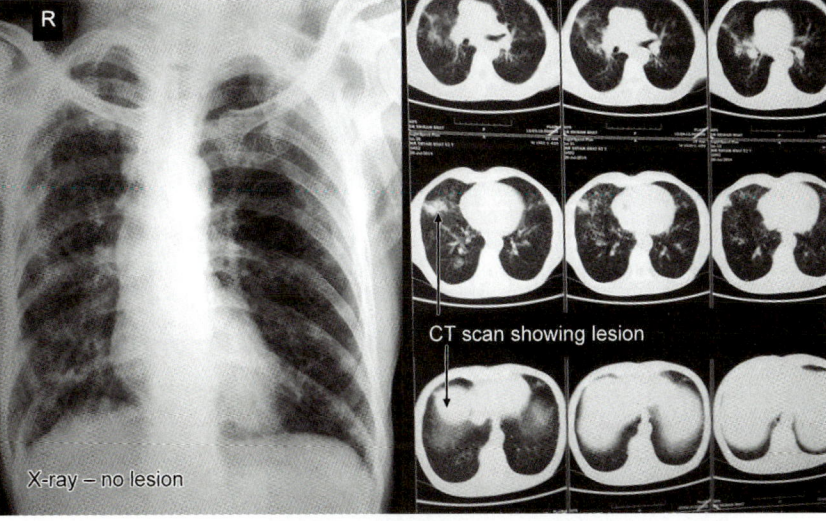

Fig. 2-11 Chest X-ray is commonly taken; often chest X-ray may be normal but CT chest may show a lesion. 30% cases of X-ray chest may miss a lesion especially in posterior lower lobe.

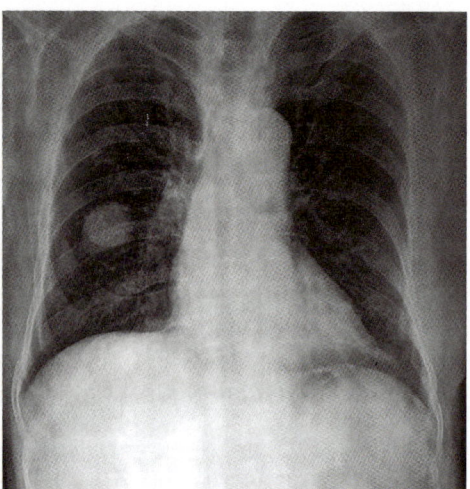

Fig. 2-12 Chest X-ray PA view showing solitary homogenous opacity—coin lesion. It could be carcinoma lung or solitary secondary in the lung.

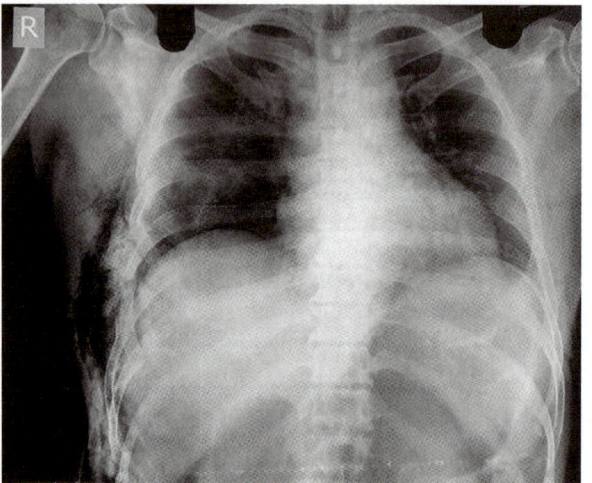

Fig. 2-13 Chest X-ray showing surgical emphysema right chest wall.

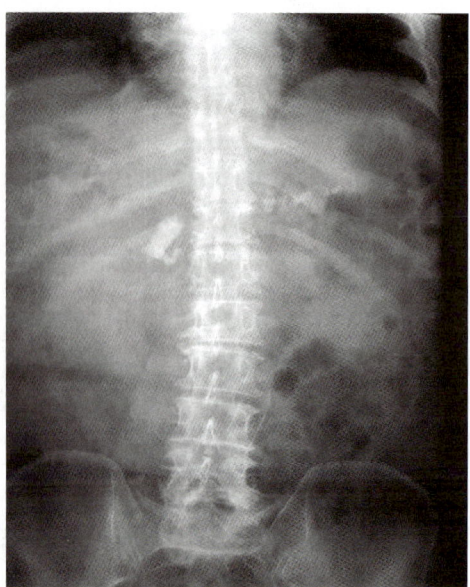

Fig. 2-14 Plain X-ray abdomen showing pancreatic duct stones due to chronic pancreatitis.

enema, cholecystogram, cholangiogram, percutaneous transhepatic cholangiogram (PTC), myelography, endoscopic retrograde cholangiopancreatography (ERCP), lymphangiography, intravenous urography (IVU), angiography are different contrast X-rays.

Double Contrast X-ray

Here X-ray augmentation is done by two contrast agents. Air and barium or air and water soluble iodine dyes are different examples. Double contrast barium enema is a good example. Double contrast cystography using air and water soluble iodine dyes within with additional air insufflation in presacral area is called as triple contrast X-ray.

Ultrasound Examination (Ultrasonography/USG)

Ultrasound contains waves with a frequency of more than 20,000 cycles/second which the human ears cannot hear. It is modified and developed from SONAR (sound navigation and ranging) and RADAR (radio detecting and ranging) system used in First World War.

In medical sonography, frequencies used are commonly 2–10 MHz. The transducer or the probe works as both transmitter of *sound waves* and receiver of *echoes*. The piezoelectric crystal is the producer of ultrasound waves. Received signals from the patient are fed into the computer which forms the image. Sound waves of high frequency reflect at the junction of different tissues of the body; tissue absorption of sound waves vary from tissue to tissue and when sound waves strike they interfere with two media of differing acoustic impedance; energy which is reflected towards first media is called as ultrasonic echo. A detector records it as ultrasonic beam and is displayed using an oscilloscope as unidimensional wave—amplitude modulated wave (A mode). When two dimensional waves are used, it is called as B mode (brightness modulated).

There are three types of ultrasound image display:

1. **A (amplitude) mode**: Only one dimensional static display as spikes is obtained. It is used only in eye scan.

2. **B (brightness) mode**: Two dimensional real time images in the form of grains. It is most widely used type. Using this mode, *transverse, longitudinal or oblique* sections can be taken **(Fig. 2-15)**.

Gray scale USG machine produces varying shades of gray pictures called as gray scan ultrasound. It is B-mode ultrasonography in which the strength of echoes is indicated by a proportional brightness of the displayed dots. The display of the ultrasound echo amplitude or signal intensity as different shades of gray, improving image quality compared with the obsolete black-and-white presentation **(Fig. 2-16)**.

Real-time ultrasonography is B-mode ultrasonography using an array of detectors so that scans can be made electronically at a rate of 30 frames per second, thus giving a true display of motion, such as that of the heart.

3. **M (motion) mode**: Here images are recorded as dots. It is mainly used in moving parts like echocardiography. M-mode is also called as TM mode, i.e. *Time Motion Mode*.

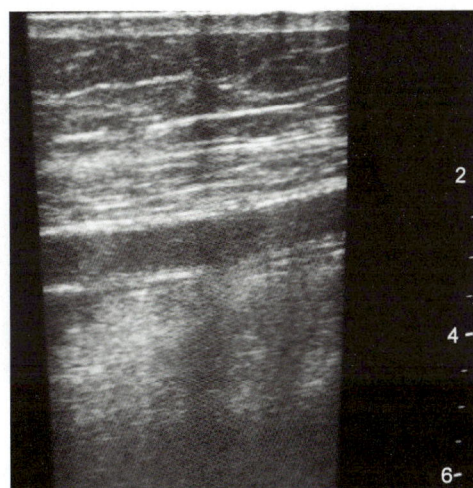

Fig. 2-15 B-mode ultrasound. It is without color.

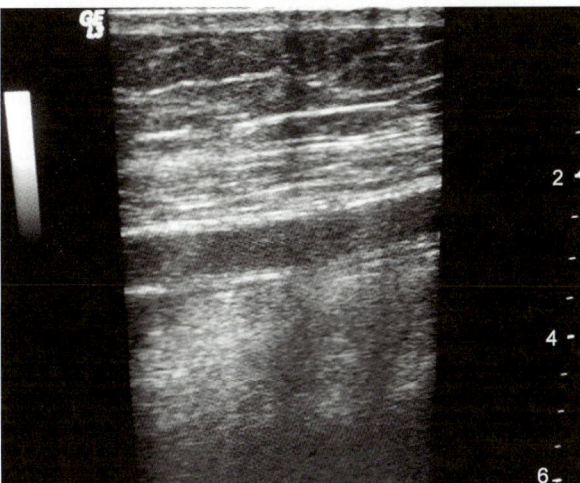

Fig. 2-16 Ultrasound B-mode gray scale.

Uses

- Ultrasonography is used in all abdominal and pelvic conditions and often in thoracic conditions.
- *Ultrasound of thyroid* is very useful method to differentiate between solid and cystic lesions. Ultrasound is used in testicular tumors, epididymo-orchitis, trauma to testis, erectile dysfunction, etc.
- *Ultrasound breast* is used to differentiate solid from cystic tumors; soft tissue and musculoskeletal ultrasound helps in identifying the pathology.
- Ocular ultrasound is ideal method to image eye and intraocular structures.
- *Interpretation* is based on echogenicity, either *hyperechogenic* or *hypoechogenic*. Fluids in the body are echofree and sonolucent, solid tissues are echogenic, better tool to identify the lesion as solid and cystic or mixed one. In pregnancy fetal movements, development, sex, growth, anomalies can be picked up using good USG. Stones are well-visualized as echogenic with *acoustic shadow*. Inferior vena cava, portal vein, liver lesions, cysts in the abdomen, renal diseases like stones, hydronephrosis and neoplasms are well-detected.
- *Therapeutic uses*: Examples are ultrasound guided aspiration, USG guided biopsy of deeper organs, USG guided drainage of abscess and insertion of pigtail catheter into the cavity; during laparoscopy or laparotomy, on-table assessment of the tissues or organ or lymph node status by placing USG probe directly on the site so that extent of the disease or operability or extent of resection can be planned well.

Advantages

There is no radiation, noninvasive, simple, effective with efficiency, painless, low cost, available even as portable machines, dye is not needed, harmless in pregnant women and radiology work persons, reasonably reliable, very useful as an outpatient and bedside (in critically ill) procedure, can be done in all age groups.

Disadvantages

Interpretation can be inadequate; bowel shadow may prevent proper visualization; in obese patient, image will be inadequate.

Advanced Ultrasound Techniques

(1) Endosonography (EUS) is used in visualization of walls of esophagus or stomach through gastroscopy; biopsy using a needle through EUS can be taken from adjacent lymph nodes; (2) Transvaginal ultrasound; (3) Transrectal ultrasound to see prostate; (4) Doppler ultrasound to study arterial and venous diseases.

Doppler Study

- A Doppler *(Christian Johann Doppler, Austrian physicist)* ultrasound uses reflected sound waves to see blood flow through a blood vessel; so that arteries/veins in neck, limbs, abdomen and umbilical cord can be assessed. It assesses the blocked or reduced flow of blood through the vessel like in stroke, deep vein thrombosis, pulmonary embolism, pregnancy (fetal blood flow). A hand held Doppler instrument (transducer) is placed on the skin over the vessel area to send and receive sound waves on the vessel which are amplified through a microphone.
- The sound waves bounce off from solid objects, including blood cells. The movement of blood cells causes a change in pitch of the reflected sound waves (called the Doppler effect); if there is no blood flow, the pitch does not change. These reflected sound waves can be processed by a computer to provide graphs or pictures that represent the flow of blood through the blood vessels. These graphs or pictures can be saved for future review or evaluation.
- *Doppler effect* is a change in the perceived frequency of sound emitted by a *moving source*. So it measures blood flow. Spectral Doppler wave form and ultrasound image with color are combined in *Duplex scanning* (**Figs. 2-17 and 2-18**).

Types: (1) **Continuous waves:** This type uses the change in pitch of the sound waves to provide information about blood flow through a blood vessel; the clinician listens to the sounds produced by the transducer to evaluate the blood flow; this type of Doppler ultrasound can be done at the bedside with

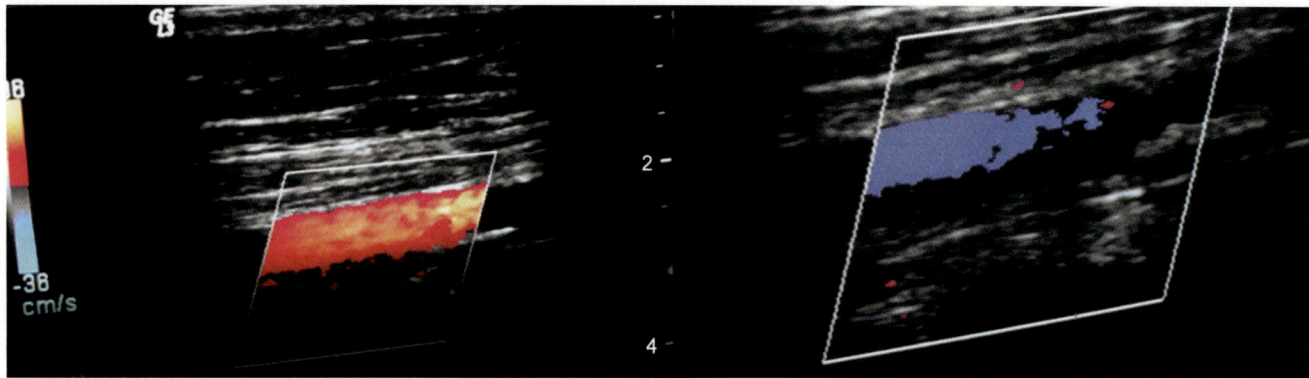

Fig. 2-17 Colored ultrasound with Doppler with gray scale.

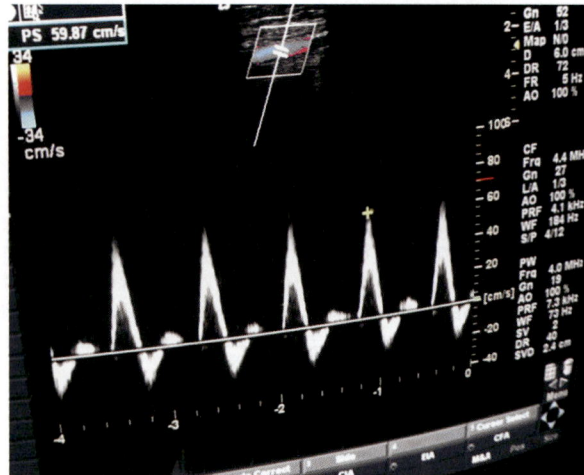

Fig. 2-18 Ultrasound (colored) image with Doppler wave form (Triplex).

a portable machine to provide a fast estimate of the extent of blood vessel damage or disease. (2) **Pulsed waves:** Doppler will provide both audio and video signals. Here picture of a blood vessel and the surrounding organs with a computer converted Doppler sounds into a graph is created that gives information about the speed and direction of blood flow through the blood vessel.

Color Doppler imaging displays flowing blood as ***red*** when direction of flow is towards the transducer. Image will be ***blue*** if flow is away from the transducer. Computer converts the Doppler sounds into colors that are overlaid on the image of the blood vessel and that represent the speed and direction of blood flow through the vessel. ***Power Doppler*** is a special type of color Doppler. Power Doppler, a special type can get images that are impossible to get using standard color Doppler; commonly used to evaluate blood flow through vessels within solid organs.

Uses: **To study cardiovascular system; to study vascularity of tumors; to study blood flow and velocity in arterial diseases so as to assess stenosis (its extent, cause, etc.) like in atherosclerosis, thromboangiitis obliterans (TAO), cervical rib, aneurysm, A-V fistulas; to find out deep venous thrombosis (DVT), varicose veins, perforator incompetence; to study grade of varicocele in males.**

Advantages: **It has replaced venogram and angiogram in many places as a diagnostic tool. It is reliable and noninvasive.**

> Density of tissues is numbered as *Hounsfield Number (HN):*
> Water—Zero HN;
> Air—Minus 1,000
> Bone—Plus 1,000
> The density of other tissues come in between air and bone with different HNs

CT Scan Imaging

- Computerized tomography scan (earlier computerized axial tomography scan—CAT scan) was invented by ***Godfrey Hounsfield*** in 1963. He was a physicist. He received ***Nobel Prize*** (1972) for the same. The first CAT scan is in London museum.
- Narrow X-ray beams are passed from a rotating X-ray generator through *the gantry* where patient is placed. When X-rays pass through the tissues, some of the X-rays get absorbed and some pass through, depending on the tissue density. The different grades of absorption in different tissues are detected through sensitive detectors which are translated to a Gray scale image by a computer.
- Attenuated X-ray beam passes through the part of the body as a thin cross-section (salami slice); highly sensitive scintillation detector placed diagonally on opposite side measures the amount of X-ray photons transmitted through the patient. Very fine resolution can be detected; further contrast enhancement can be achieved by injecting iodine contrast agents intravenously.
- *Presently spiral CT scan* has become popular. They are faster and in a single breath holding time, whole CT scan can be taken. Both plain and contrast CTs are done whenever required (Fig. 2-19).
- *Contrast agents:* (a) **Ionic**: Water soluble iodide dyes like ***sodium diatrizoate, meglumine iothalamate (conray, urografin, angiograffin)***. They are cheaper but often toxic and cause anaphylaxis. (b) **Non-ionic:** Safer but expensive, like ***iohexol (omnipaque), iopamiro***. In abdominal CT, contrast agents can be given orally to delineate bowel properly.

Indications

- **Trauma like head injury, chest injury, abdomen trauma. In trauma, *only plain CT scan* is taken.**

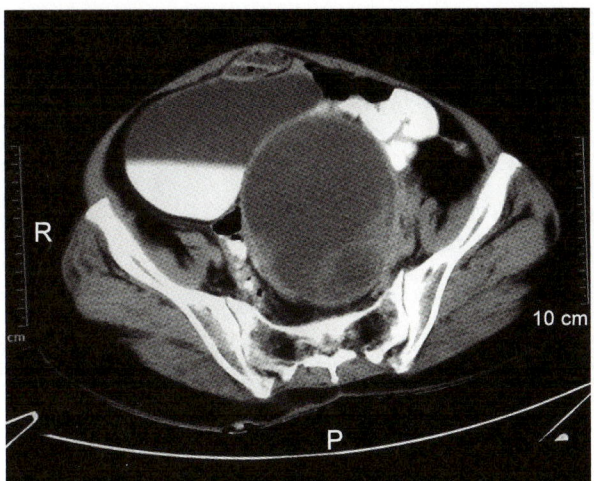

Fig. 2-19 CT scan abdomen showing retroperitoneal tumor.

- **Neoplasms:** To see the exact location, size, vascularity, extent and operability. For example, brain, abdominal, retroperitoneal, thoracic tumors.
- **Inflammatory conditions** in various sites; for example, psoas abscess, pseudocyst of pancreas.

Findings: For example, extradural hematoma—*biconvex lesion;* subdural hematoma—*concavoconvex lesion;* smooth margin in benign condition; irregular margin in malignant condition.

Advantages of CT scan:
- One to 2 mm sized sections are possible
- Proper cross-sectional images—transverse and longitudinal
- More accurate, sensitive, and specific
- Small lesions are also detected
- CT guided biopsies are done at present, safely

Advantages of spiral CT scan:
- It reduces scan time; useful in children and critically ill-patients
- Imaging in both arterial and venous phases is possible
- Improved lesion detection. Missing a lesion is uncommon

Multiplanar and 3-dimensional analysis like CT angiography, complex joint imaging, facial bone imaging is possible

High resolution CT *(HRCT)* is a CT technique used in chest scan where thin sections are taken to have better quality images

Disadvantages:
- *Interpretation* by an experienced radiologist is important
- *Artefacts* can be present
- Cost factor and availability

Magnetic Resonance Imaging (MRI)

Earlier, named as *nuclear magnetic resonance (NMR) imaging,* the term is not used now.

Principle

When patient is placed in an *external high magnetic field,* protons of hydrogen atoms rotate in phase with each other and gradually return to their original position releasing small amounts of energy which is detected by sensitive coils. Proton density and relaxation time are assessed by radiofrequency pulse and the computer generates a Gray scale image from this data. Strong magnetic field and emitted radiowaves by nuclei due to this magnetic field influence the protons and neutrons; when body is placed in gantry containing this super conducting magnetic field, nuclei align their direction against the magnetic field.

T1 relaxation time is the time taken to return to original axis. *T1 images* are used to find out *normal anatomical details.* It has got high soft tissue discrimination. Here fluid (CSF) looks black. *T2 relaxation time* is the time taken by the proton to diphase. It is used to assess *pathological processes.* In *T2 images,* fluid looks white. *In proton density images,* fluid looks in between black and white.

It can be *plain MRI or contrast MRI.* Contrast agent is *gadolinium,* given intravenously.

Advantages of MRI:
Artefacts are not common
More sensitive and specific than CT scan

Disadvantages:
Availability and *cost factor*
It is time consuming
Patient compliance is poor
It is not feasible in patients suffering from *claustrophobia*
It is not ideal in emergencies and critically ill patients
It is not useful in lung pathology and subarachnoid hemorrhage

Precaution:
Before entering the MRI room, the patient and other personnel should remove all magnetically attractive materials

Contraindications:
Patients with **prosthesis in the body, metallic foreign bodies, pacemakers, cochlear implants, cranial aneurysm clips should *never* undergo MRI**

Uses of MRI

It is very useful in intracranial, spinal and musculoskeletal lesions including *joint pathologies.* It gives direct anatomical sections of the area, with lesions at a high resolution. *MR angiogram* is done without injecting IV contrast agents. *Cardiac MRI* is very useful. *Breast MRI* is used in multifocal recurrent cancers. *Magnetic resonance cholangiopancreatography (MRCP)* is a very useful noncontrast diagnostic tool which may replace diagnostic ERCP. *MR spectroscopy* is chemical analysis of elements in a tissue to differentiate between tumor, inflammation, and degeneration. MRI is very useful to identify soft tissues in pelvis and pelvic tumors. MRI identifies pathological anatomy of fistula-in-ano also clearly (Fig. 2-20).

Radionuclide Imaging (Scintiscan)

- It represents function of an organ than morphology. Isotope of an element is a nuclide with the same atomic number but different mass number. Isotopes while disintegrating emits radiation. γ-rays emitted can penetrate many centimeters in the body tissues. Geiger Muller γ-ray counter detects γ-rays as scintillating light. These isotope emissions can be either printed using a mechanical dotter or displayed in a oscilloscope screen as scintillations.
- Isotope to be used in medical field should have short half-life; should get excreted rapidly; should have ability to concentrate selectively in the specific organ of interest. Isotope is given either orally (I_{123}) or intravenously

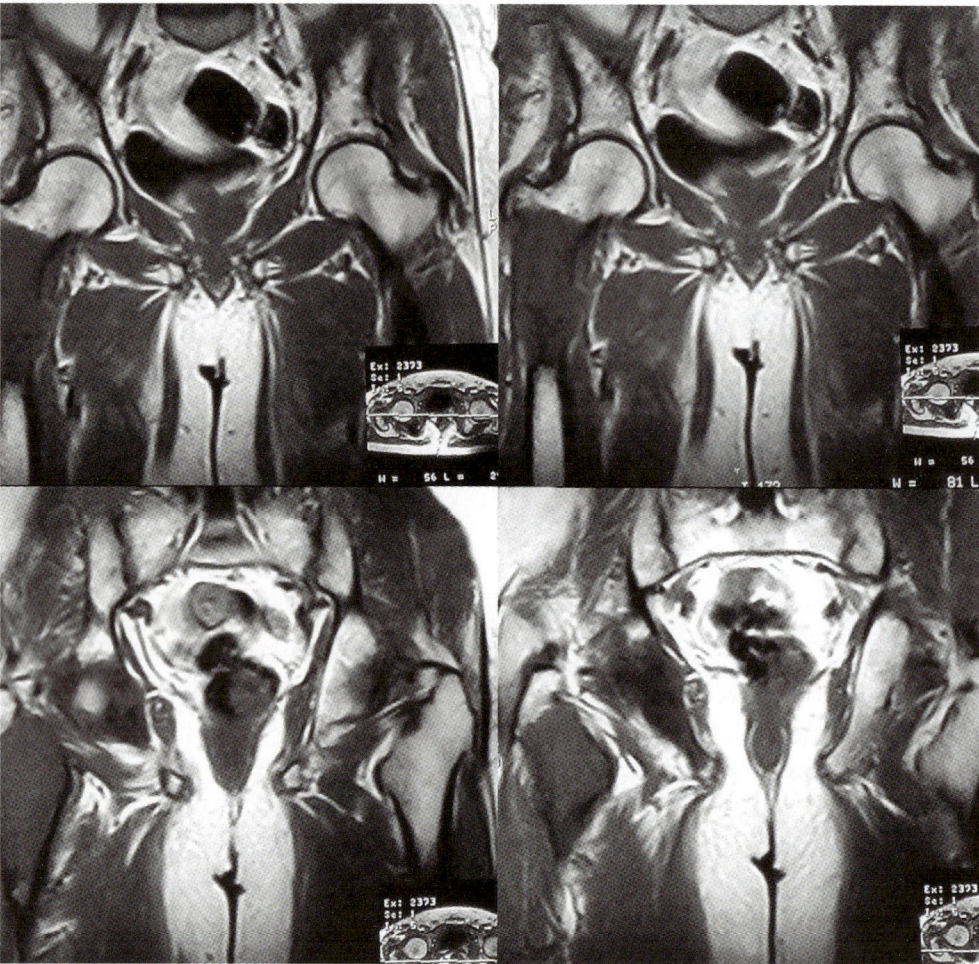

Fig. 2-20 MRI of pelvis and perineum is very useful investigation.

(technetium). Organ is scanned using a gamma camera to assess uptake, either low or high. Isotope scintiscan is used to study circulation of the organ; structure and function of an organ like liver/thyroid/bones/lungs, etc. *Rays*: α-particles are emitted by the natural radionuclides like radium, which are no longer used in medicine. β-particles are useful for therapy but not for diagnosis. γ-rays pass out of the body and so used for the diagnostic purpose. Mapping is done using sophisticated gamma camera

- *Technetium 99m:* It is commonest radionuclide used (99 is mass number; m–metastable.); it is administered intravenously; it is pure γ-rays emitter with short half-life; widely used gamma ray detectors are specified to Tc99m.

Uses

- ^{99m}Tc labeled serum albumin is used to detect pulmonary emboli.
- ^{99m}Tc labeled phosphate is used to image bone.
- ^{99m}Tc labeled sulfur colloid is used to detect the functions of liver, spleen, bone marrow.
- ^{99m}Tc labeled HIDA (Hippuric immunodiacetic acid) or PIPIDA is used to study the functions of hepatocytes and biliary tract.
- ^{99m}Tc labeled DMSA (Dimercaptosuccinic acid) which is taken up by the renal cortical cells, is used in renal function tests.
- ^{99m}Tc labeled DTPA (Diphenyl triamine penta acetic acid) measures glomerular filtration rate (GFR).
- ^{99m}Tc labeled HMPAO (Hydroxy methyl propylamine oxime) is used in Alzheimer's disease and schizophrenia as it crosses the blood brain barrier.

Other radionuclides used: Thallium 201 chloride for cardiac imaging; Gallium 67 nitrate to detect tumors and inflammation; I_{123} radioisotope.

Advantages: Safer, easier, no side effects/no biological ill effects.

Disadvantages: Availability problem, cost factor, not specific, fast half life. It gives only abnormal imaging and will not give any idea about the cause. Examples: It is difficult to differentiate between fracture and osteomyelitis or liver secondaries and cirrhosis. It is interpreter dependent; false positive or false negative results may appear.

Positron Emission Tomography (PET Scan)

It is a noninvasive diagnostic method to assess the biochemical and physiological status of a tissue. It is used in complimentary with CT scan and MRI. Two protons are used, they are positive electrons (***positrons***). Most clinically used positron emitting radionuclide is fluorodeoxyglucose (FDG), others are ^{82}Rb, ^{15}O, ^{13}N, ^{18}F, ^{11}C. Detectors used are bismuth germanate (BGO) crystals or sodium iodide crystals.

Principle of ***electronic collimation*** is used to produce images from the radiation emitted from positron emitting tracers.

Uses: **To assess myocardial perfusion (^{82}Rb) and viability (FDG) study; in epilepsy—to localize temporal lobe epilepsy (FDG); in cancer imaging like lung cancer (detection and staging), colorectal cancer, melanoma, head and neck cancer and breast cancer, musculoskeletal tumors, thyroid cancer (I_{131}). It is very specific but very expensive with limited availability. It gives idea about the physiological status, metabolic processes of the tissue or the pathological status of the diseases.**

EXAMINATION BY EXPLORATION

When all evaluation methods fail, cavity is/cavities are opened to find out what pathology is existing and decision of the procedure to be done as a therapy is taken on-table and is called explorative procedure. When abdomen is opened it is called explorative laparotomy, similarly explorative thoracotomy/craniotomy, etc.

Diagnostic laparoscopy/thoracoscopy/mediastinoscopy are good alternatives for exploration. If it shows any positive finding or operability of the tumor/disease then opening can be done. It will avoid unnecessary opening of the abdomen/thorax in inoperable cases.

PREANESTHETIC ASSESSMENT (CHECK UP FOR FITNESS FOR SURGERY)

- It is the detail evaluation of the patient prior to surgery to achieve safe anesthesia, recovery and to avoid post-surgery anesthetic complications. It helps in determining and minimizing the risk factors, optimizing the patient, plan the technique of perioperative care in anesthesia, taking proper consent for anesthesia.
- It is done by operating surgeon, physician and mainly by involved anesthetist; but in reality, it is team work and decision of surgeon, physician, anesthetist and often cardiologist, neurologist so on depending on the need

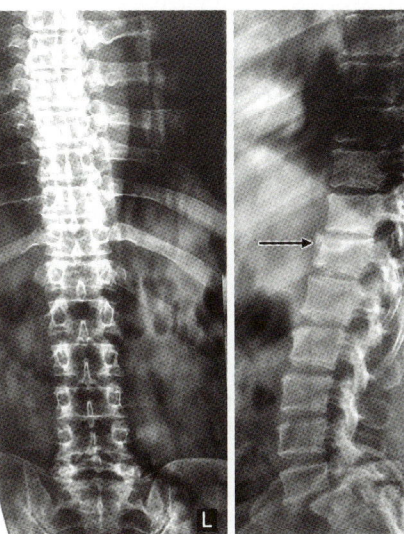

Fig. 2-21 X-ray spine showing fracture spine.

in individual patient (case) basis. Final assessment and decision should be done by the anesthetist. It is better to have preanesthetic assessment far early (a day or before) so that there will be enough time to prepare the patient.
- Detail history present/past/drug/allergy/old records/old surgery/old anesthesia are needed.
- Anesthetist should go through all the reports (especially laboratory) and should ask for any additional investigations which may be useful during anesthesia.
- Which anesthesia should be given is decided by anesthetist with opinions by surgeon and physician. In spine trauma and disc prolapse spinal anesthesia may be avoided. In lower limb and groin procedures, spinal anesthesia is preferred (Fig. 2-21).

In high-risk patients, benefit—risk ratio should be assessed and decision is taken; and high-risk explanation and consent should be taken. In such situations minimal needed procedure should be done—like drainage of pus, colostomy only instead of colectomy, ileostomy, etc. More aggressive radical surgery should be postponed for later period after patient recovers and becomes fit by proper resuscitation and optimization.

Anesthetists should discuss with the surgeon about the type of procedure, time needed, need for blood transfusions and should plan for it during preoperative assessment only.

LABORATORY INVESTIGATIONS

Blood examination

Hemogram

Red cell count; white cell count (total count and differential count—TC/DC); hemoglobin (Hb%); packed cell volume (PCV); platelet count; reticulocyte count; blood indices; erythrocyte sedimentation rate (ESR)

Biochemical estimation

Serum electrolytes (sodium, potassium, bicarbonate, chloride, calcium, phosphorus, magnesium)

Nutritional assay—Blood sugar, lipid profile (serum cholesterol, triglyceride [TG], high density lipoprotein [HDL], low density lipoprotein [LDL], very low density lipoprotein [VLDL], chylomicrons); serum proteins (total, albumin, globulin, A:G ratio).

Functional assessment of the organs: liver [(LFT)—Serum bilirubin direct and indirect, serum proteins, serum alanine phosphatase, serum glutamic pyruvate transaminase (SGPT), serum glutamate oxaloacetic transaminase (SGOT)]; kidney [blood urea, serum creatinine, serum electrolytes, serum nonprotein nitrogenous substances (NPN)]

Hormone assay: Pituitary—TSH [thyroid stimulating hormone]; Thyroid—Serum T3, serum T4; Pancreas—plasma insulin; Adrenal—serum cortisol, serum catecholamine, serum vanillylmandelic acid (VMA); Others—serum prolactin, follicular stimulating hormone (FSH), serum luteinizing hormone (LH), serum testosterone, estrogen estimation.

Enzymes—serum lipase, amylase, acid phosphatase, etc.
Coagulation profile and assessment of abnormal hemoglobins—bleeding time, clotting time, prothrombin time, platelet count, estimation of clotting factors, activated partial thromboplastin time (APTT); Hb spectroscopy; fetal hemoglobin estimation, osmotic fragility test of blood
Arterial blood gas analysis (ABG)—pCO_2, pO_2, pH of the blood

Immunological evaluation:
Receptor study by immunohistochemistry: ER (estrogen receptor) and PR (progesterone receptor) study in carcinomas of breast.
Enzyme linked immune sorbent assay (ELISA) is used in conditions like HIV
Radio immune assay (RIA) to assess the specific antibodies that bind to the hormones. *VDRL, WIDAL, Weil–Felix tests; Australia antigen*, rheumatoid arthritis factor, immunoglobulins like IgA, IgG, IgM, IgE, IgD
Assessment of tumor markers like carcinoembryonic antigen (CEA), alpha-feto protein (AFP), calcitonin, human chorionic gonadotropin (β-hCG)

Others:
Blood grouping and cross-matching
Blood culture for growth of bacteria and checking for bacterial sensitivity
Peripheral smear for malaria, filarial, cellular component observation, etc.

Examination of secretions:
Gastrointestinal tract secretions
Gastric: Fractional test meal, gastric secretion analysis during fasting and postprandial for bile/blood/acid/alkali/pH, insulin/Hollander's test, augmented histamine test, tubeless gastric analysis [quinine resin indicator test (1950)]
Pancreatic: Analysis of biliary and pancreatic secretions, bile culture, Lundh test (1965, after a liquid test meal to assess trypsin concentration in the duodenum), secretin-pancreozymin test, etc.

Cerebrospinal fluid (CSF) analysis:
CSF is collected by lumbar or cistern puncture. It is examined physically for color, turbidity, cobweb formation, specific gravity; chemically for glucose, proteins; microscopically for cytology, cell count, bacteria; culture for bacteria and antibiotic sensitivity

Serosal fluid examination:
Peritoneal fluid analysis for culture, specific gravity, AFB, proteins, sugar, bacteria, cytology for malignant cells, etc.
Pleural tapping for pleural fluid analysis; pericardial fluid tap; synovial fluid tap
Amniotic fluid aspiration for determination of sex in legal cases only

Other secretions:
Semen analysis in case of infertility, etc.

Examination of excretions:
Urine
Color, odor, pH, specific gravity; chemical examination for sugar, proteins, Bence Jones proteins, bile salts, bile pigments, acetone, occult blood; 24 hour urine sample to assess creatinine (creatinine clearance in renal failure); vanillylmandelic acid (VMA for pheochromocytoma); 11 hydroxycorticosteroids and 17 oxysteroids for adrenocortical hyperfunction; 5 hydroxy indole acetic acid (5 HIAA) for carcinoid syndrome; calcium in hyperparathyroidism; porphyrins in porphyrias; hydroxyproline and calcium in secondaries in bone
Urine microscopy for bacteria, casts, pus cells, red cells (trauma, tumors, glomerulonephritis, transplant rejection), epithelial cells, crystals
Urine examination for cytology, AFB, culture and sensitivity

Stool:
Gross: Color, stickiness, froth, odor; bloody in (carcinoma, infection), slimy (inflammation or inflammatory bowel disease/IBS), bulky frothy undigested in malabsorption, clay colored in obstructive jaundice
Chemical: For occult blood, fat, stercobilinogen
Microscopy for bacteria, ova, cyst; Entamoeba histolytica cysts and trophozoites
Stool culture for bacteria like vibrio cholera, bacterial dysentery and antibiotic sensitivity

Sputum:
For color, odor, quantity
Culture and sensitivity, AFB staining and culture, cytology

Other excretions:
Pus, excretions from ear, nose, pharynx, urethra, vagina for gross/microscopy, culture and cytology

Patients' *current medications* like insulin, antihypertensives, antidiabetics, anticonvulsants, anticoagulants should be assessed. Anticoagulants [warfarin, clopidogrel (aspirin intake is presently not a contraindication; but better to stop 3 days prior to surgery is practiced by many anesthetists)] should be stopped 5 days prior to surgery to avoid bleeding/oozing. In emergency cases, adequate fresh frozen plasma (FFP) and packed cells should kept ready in operation theater.

Preanesthetic note should be written by the anesthetist with detail history, comorbid status, all laboratory values, chest X-ray, imaging, ECG, echocardiography finding of the patient and need for additional evaluation. These are routine investigations required in most of the patients of course based on type of surgery, age and status of the patient. Specific investigations like thyroid function tests, respiratory function assessment like arterial blood gas analysis, spirometry, 2D echocardiography and TMT (Treadmill test) with fitness from cardiologist, etc. are required often.

Hepatitis B and C tests, ELISA for HIV are usually done. It allows surgical team to take adequate precautions, and add additional treatment to the patients whenever needed.

Preoperative medications by sedatives are usually given to the patients as advised by anesthetist.

> **American Society of Anesthesiologist (ASA) physical status classification provides a predictive value for anesthesia**
> Class 1 – Normal patient—healthy as for anesthesia
> Class 2 – Mild systemic disease
> Class 3 – Severe systemic disease
> Class 4 – Severe systemic disease with a constant threat to life
> Class 5 – Moribund patient who will not survive without surgery
> Class 6 – Declared brain dead patient whose organ can be removed for donation
>
> In case of emergency, designation 'E' is added. 1E, 2E, 3E, 4E, 5E, 6. 6E does not exist as it is brain dead.
> *An emergency* is defined as a situation existing when delay in (surgical) treatment would significantly increase the threat to patient's life or body part. By this definition, fracture bone, ureteric stone, fissure-in-ano and similar conditions are not emergencies.

Recommended Preanesthetic Investigations

Hematocrit—full blood count	*Blood sugar estimation*
• Age >40 years • Anemia clinically • Hematological disease • Renal disease • Patients on hemotherapy • Possible blood loss >15%	• Age >40 years • Diabetes mellitus—fasting and post prandial; glycosylated hemoglobin • Liver and pancreatic diseases
Renal parameters (profile)	*Electrocardiogram (ECG)*
• Age >40 years • Renal and liver diseases • Diabetes mellitus • Cardiac illnesses • Possible blood loss >15%	• Age >40 years • Cardiovascular diseases • Diabetes mellitus • Liver disease • History of smoking
Serum electrolytes estimation In vomiting, dehydration, shock patients, peritonitis, renal failure, acute conditions, major procedures	*Chest X-ray* • Age >40 years • History of smoking • Any past or present history of respiratory diseases like bronchial asthma, tuberculosis, chronic obstructive pulmonary disease (COPD)
Urine examination • Renal failure • If urinary catheterization is needed	*Coagulation profile* • Blood disorders • Liver diseases • Patients on anticoagulant drugs • Thoracic or cranial or major surgical procedures • Liver/biliary/pancreatic diseases or surgeries • Chronic alcohol intake

■ EXAMINATION OF FECES

- It gives indirect evidence of different pathologies in the gastrointestinal tract.
- The quantity—copious/scanty; consistency—liquid/semisolid/semiformed/formed/hard.
- Color—black—in upper GI bleed, iron or bismuth intake/pale colored stool is seen in obstructive jaundice (absence of bile in the bowel). Rapid transit of stool is seen in diarrhea, malabsorption, chronic pancreatitis. Blood from small bowel is dark red; from large bowel it is red jelly like; from anorectum, it is bright red and fresh.

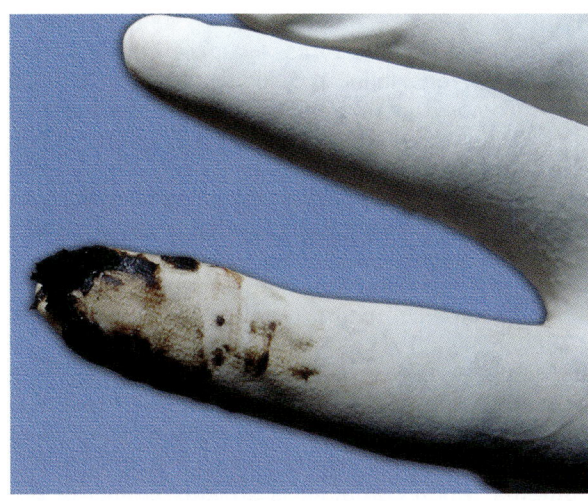

Fig. 2-22 Typical black, foul smelling tarry colored stool seen in upper gastrointestinal bleeding.

- Odor: Offensive in jaundice, semen like odor in acute amebic dysentery, odorless in acute bacillary dysentery.
- Type: Slimy stool in carcinoma colon, colitis of different causes; purulent stool in bacterial dysentery.
- Blood in stool is seen in different conditions. They are *melena,* that is, black, tarry, foul smelling stool seen in upper gastrointestrinal bleed; red pigmented clots (maroon colored) in Meckel's diverticulum; red currant jelly in intussusception; bright red colored in rectal and anal diseases.
- *Steatorrhea* is large quantity, pale, porridge like stool that sticks to lavatory and is difficult to flush. It is due to severe degree of pancreatic insufficiency causing malodorous, voluminous stool which floats on the water. Patient passes large quantity of fat that separates from the nonfatty part of the fecal matter that resembles melted butter that becomes solid again.
- *Spurious diarrhea* is seen in carcinoma colon.
- *Pipe stem stool* occurs in rectal stenosis usually due to malignant rectal stricture.
- *Toothpaste stool* is seen in Hirschsprung's disease.
- *Meconium (Greek—a poppy):* It is seen in neonates for first 2–3 days of birth. It is greenish black, odorless, sticky, scanty semisolid feces. It disappears gradually in a week to form thin golden yellow pasty or pale putty like feces.
- *Melena/melaena* is passage of black/tarry, sticky, semisolid, often foul smelling stool due to presence of altered blood; black color is due to hematin. It suggests upper GI bleed; *50 mL of blood* in the stomach can cause melena; *one liter of blood* in the stomach can produce melena for 5 days (Fig. 2-22).

■ EXAMINATION OF URINE

- Random *fresh urine sample* is usually taken for routine urine examination. *Early morning sample* of urine is better in many occasions like for tuberculosis due to its lower pH and so preserves contents.
- *24 hours urine sample* is needed in assessing chronic renal failure and many biochemical evaluation. It is collected from morning of one day after discarding early morning sample till the next day morning which

includes next day early morning sample. 24 hour urine sample is done to assess creatinine (creatinine clearance in renal failure), vanillylmandelic acid (VMA for pheochromocytoma), 11 hydroxycorticosteroids and 17 oxysteroids for adrenocortical hyperfunction, 5 hydroxy indole acetic acid (5 HIAA) for carcinoid syndrome, calcium in hyperparathyroidism, porphyrins in *porphyrias*, hydroxyproline and calcium in secondaries in bone.

- *Mid urine sample* is needed for bacterial culture.
- *Sediment* in the urine may be due to phosphate or pus; phosphate sediments disappear after adding few drops of acetic acid.
- *Color:* Normal is pale yellow due to urobilin. Blood, bile, lymph and drugs alter the color. Cloudy urine occurs when there is pus, phosphates, urates, chyle, and fungus. Urine appears *greenish brown* color when it contains bile pigments; when container is shaken, yellow or brown foam appears. Urine will become greenish if it is kept like that for sometime due to oxidation of bilirubin to biliverdin. *Porphyria* makes urine orange colored, which on exposure to air for few hours turns amber colored. *Drugs:* Salicylic acid, pyridium, rifampicin make urine reddish yellow; sulfonyl makes urine pink; cascara, senna, rhubarb make urine brown. *Beeturia:* Urine becomes light red or like cherry brandy after intake of beetroot due to betacyanin (betacynuria). *Chyluria:* Milky white urine is seen in chyluria and is due to fat glubules of chyle. It may be due to rupture of dilated lymphatics due to thoracic duct obstruction. It may be due to filarial infection, tuberculosis or tumors.
- *Odor:* Normally odor is aromatic. Once allowed like that after voiding, urea releases ammonia causing distressing ammoniacal smell.
- *pH of urine* is 4.5–7.0 (6.0) due to weak organic acids. Blue litmus turns red in acid urine; red litmus turns blue in alkaline urine.
- *Specific gravity* of urine is normally 1.003 to 1.030. Sodium, urea, chlorides, phosphates, albumin and sugar alter the specific gravity. Fixed specific gravity of 1.010 is observed in end stage renal disease with inability to concentrate urine. Urine is collected in a conical flask; urinometer is floated into it; reading (from 1.001 to 1.030) is checked. Specific gravity is adjusted to 20°C; correction should be done by adding or deducting 0.001 for each raise or fall in temperature of 3°C.
- *24 hours urine protein* is normally less than 50 mg% which is undetectable by conventional methods, if it is detectable it is abnormal and called proteinuria. It is checked by *heat test*—by heating the upper part of the urine taken in a test tube after filtering (and rendering it acidic by adding 3% acetic acid if needed). Lower part of tube is not heated as it will take longer time to show the precipitate and unlike upper part comparison will not be achieved as entire column gets precipitated if lower part is heated. Three drops of 3% acetic acid are added to cloudy precipitate, if it persists means it is due to proteins; three drops of HNO_3 (nitric acid) is added to that again; if cloudy precipitate persists means it is due to albumin/globulin; if it disappears it is due to nucleoproteins and mucin. If more acetic acid is added or urine is alkaline, false negative results appear. *Other tests for proteinuria* are: (1) Adding 3% sulfosalicylic acid to 2 mL urine may show precipitation after 10 minutes. (2) Adding drop by drop urine to a test tube containing nitric acid will show white ring if there is proteinuria—*Heller's test*. (3) An indicator tetrabromophenol blue which is yellow at pH 3.0 becomes blue if more pH due to presence of proteins—*Clinistix*. (4) *Esbach's reagent* containing picric acid and citric acid is added to dilute urine taken in *Esbach's albuminometer*; closed tube is kept undisturbed to allow proteins to settle down; reading is multiplied by dilution factor; it is multiplied by 24 hours urine volume to get 24 hours protein excretion; if it is multiplied by 10, it states presence of proteins in gram%. (5) 2.5 mL of urine and 7.5 mL of sulfosalicylic acid is taken in a test tube, mixed and kept for 5 minutes to get turbidity if proteins are present—*Kingsbury test*.
- *Sugar* in the urine is assessed by *Benedict's quantitative test* using eight drops of urine and 5 mL of reagent which is boiled to get different colors based on quantity of sugar in the urine like blue, green (+), yellow <1%: ++), orange (1–2% - +++), brick red)>2%: - ++++).
- *Ketone bodies* are checked by *Rothera's test* (5 mL of urine + saturated ammonium sulfate + one crystal of sodium nitroprusside + ammonia liquid from side → permanganate ring develops. *Gerhardt's test* is also positive.
- *Specific tests* are done for blood (*Benzidine*), bile pigments, bile salts (*Hay's test*), Ehrlich's aldehyde test for urobilinogen.
- *Microscopic examination* of urine is done by centrifuging 10 mL of urine at 3000 rpm for 5 minutes. Centrifuged deposit is collected in a slide for analysis. It is looked for crystals, casts, red cells, pus cells, epithelial cells and bacteria. Casts are found in renal tubules by coagulation of albuminous material with cylindrical shape. Granular casts are seen in renal disease; blood casts are in acute glomerulonephritis; waxy casts in end stage renal disease; hyaline and epithelial casts are nonspecific.

3 CHAPTER

Examination and Clinical Approach of an Ulcer

Competency: SU6.1; SU6.2.

DEFINITION

An ulcer is a break in the continuity of the covering epithelium, either skin or mucous membrane due to molecular/cell death.

Wound is simply a *disruption* of any tissues—soft tissue or bone or internal organs, i.e. *structurally and functionally* whereas ulcer is a disruption or break in the continuity of *any lining tissue*—may be skin, mucous membrane. Ulcer is one of the types of wounds (Fig. 3-1).

PARTS OF AN ULCER (FIGS. 3-2 AND 3-3)

1. **Margin:** It may be regular or irregular. It may be rounded or oval in shape. It may be well defined or ill defined. Margin is peripheral limit of an ulcer. It is connected to floor through edge of an ulcer.
2. **Edge:** Edge is the one which connects floor of the ulcer to the margin.

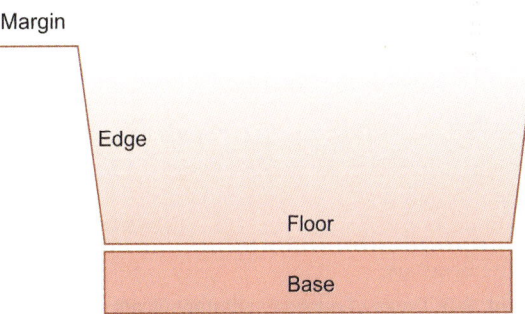

Fig. 3-2 Parts of an ulcer (diagrammatic).

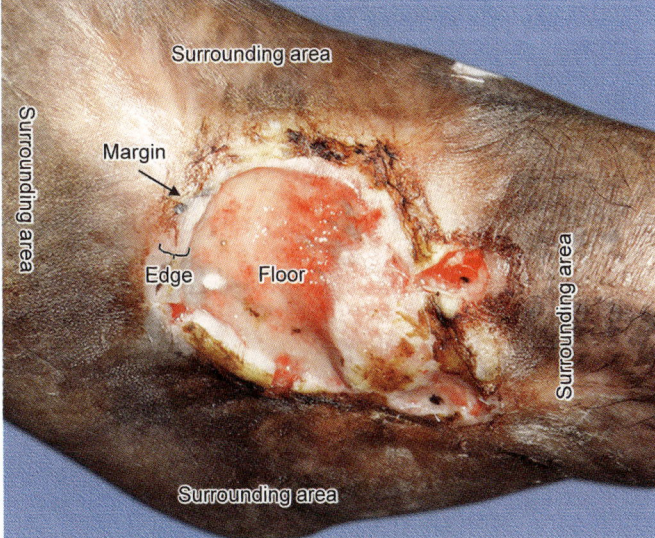

Fig. 3-3 Parts of an ulcer (Photograph).

Different edges are (Figs. 3-4 to 3-9):

Sloping edge: It is seen in healing ulcer. Its inner part is red is due to healthy granulation tissue; middle part is blue due to epithelial proliferation; outer part is white due to scar/fibrous tissue.

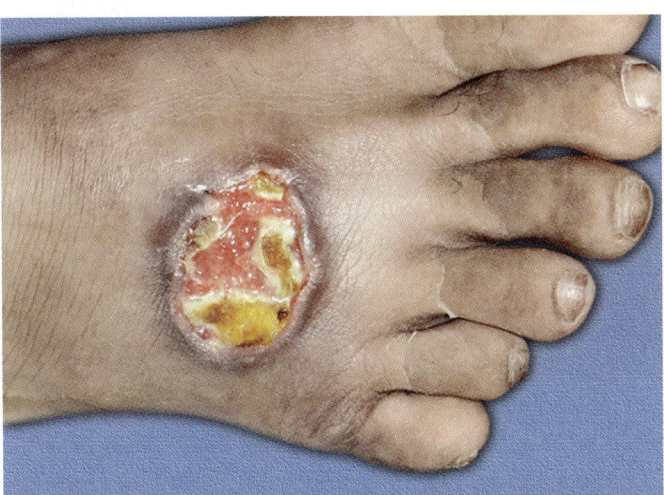

Fig. 3-1 *Typical ulcer* with margin, edge, floor with slough, and surrounding area. *Slough* is dead soft tissue in situ. *Crust or scab* is dried up discharge on the surface.

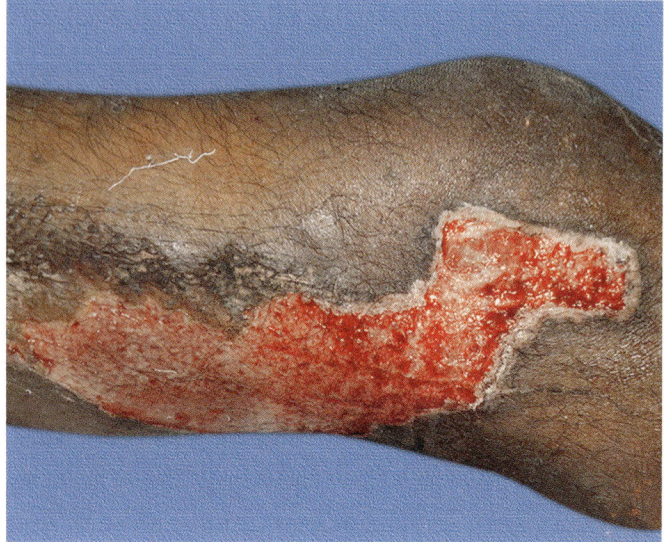

Fig. 3-4 *Sloping edge* in a healing ulcer.

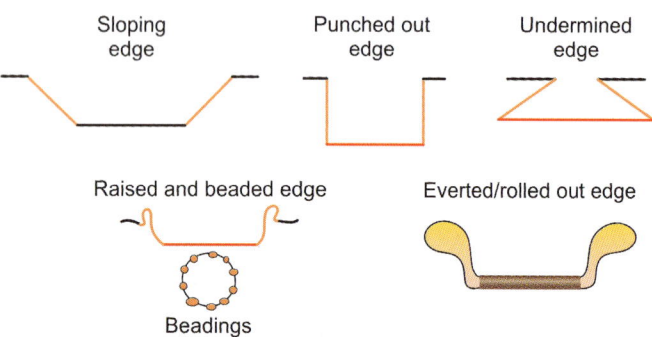

Fig. 3-5 Types of edges in different ulcers.

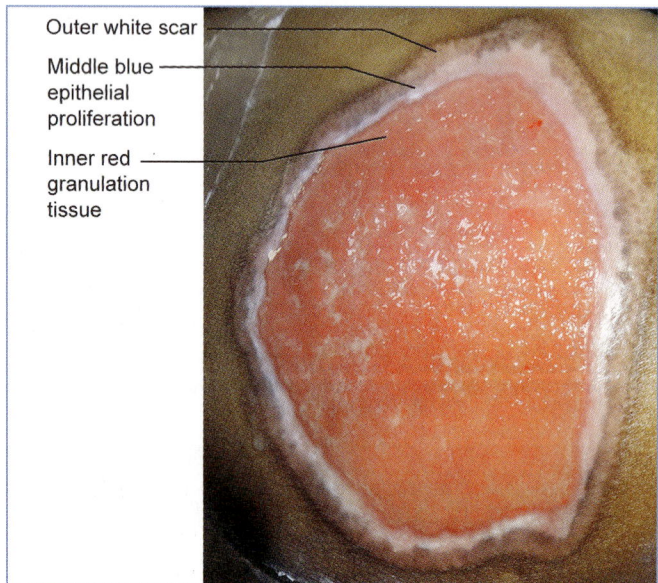

Fig. 3-6 Typical look of an edge in a healing ulcer.

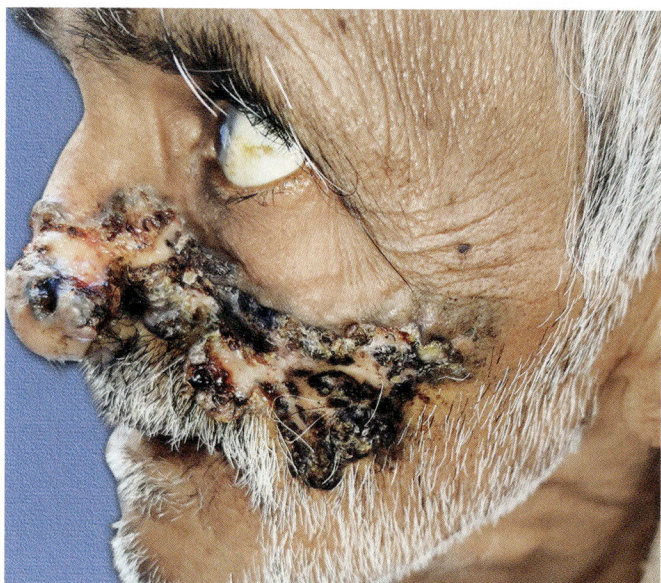

Fig. 3-7 Typical basal cell carcinoma (BCC) with *beaded edge*.

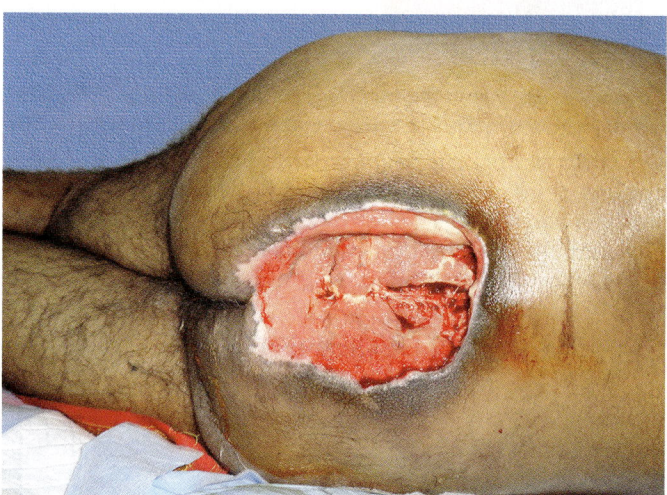

Fig. 3-8 Bed sore is a typical trophic ulcer.

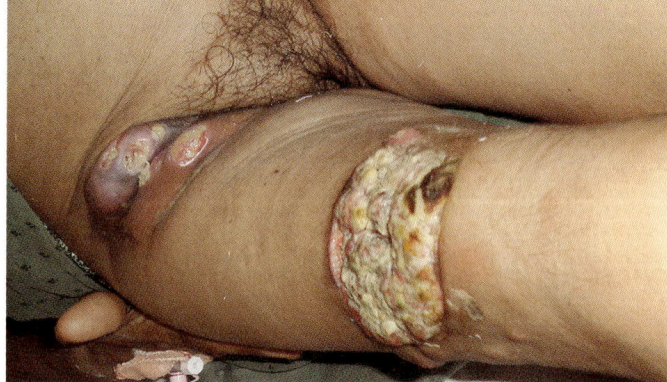

Fig. 3-9 Typical squamous cell carcinoma (SCC/epithelioma).

Undermined edge is seen in tuberculous ulcer. Disease process advances in deeper plane (in subcutaneous tissue) whereas epidermis (skin) proliferates inwards. Overhanging skin is blue and unhealthy.

Punched out edge is seen in gummatous (syphilitic) ulcer and trophic ulcer. It is due to end arteritis. It is due to rapid destruction of full thickness skin. It is deep with bone as base (Fig. 3-10).

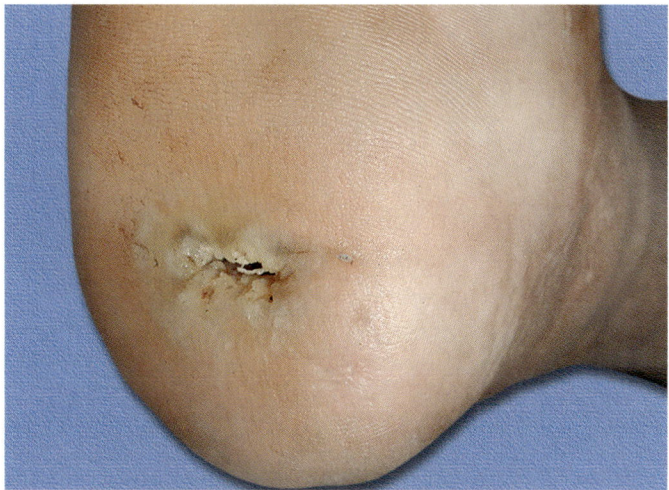

Fig. 3-10 *Trophic ulcer*—punched out edge.

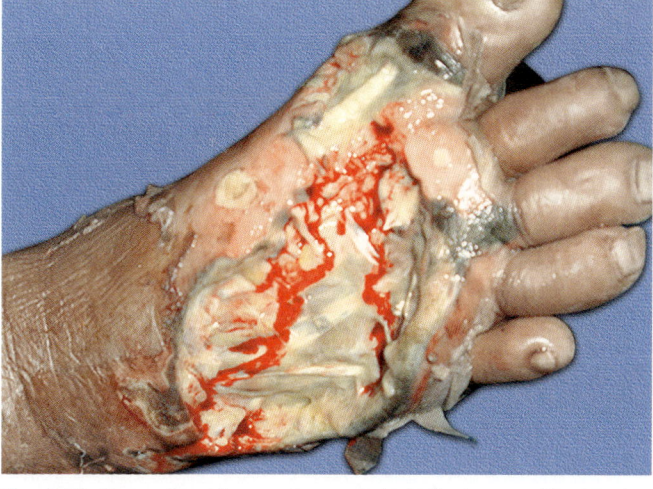

Fig. 3-12 *Spreading ulcer* copious purulent discharge with slough.

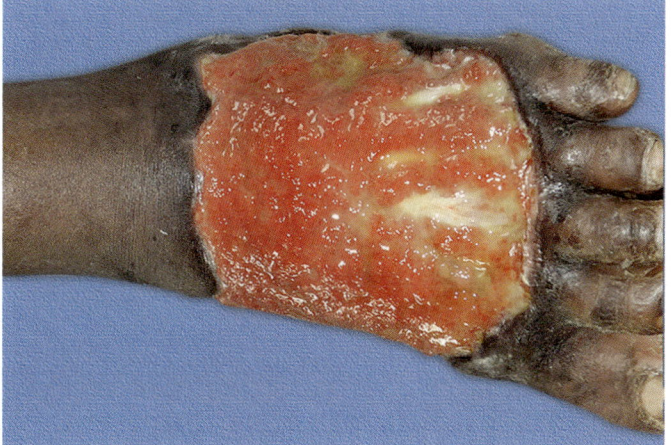

Fig. 3-11 *Active ulcer* with discharge, slough.

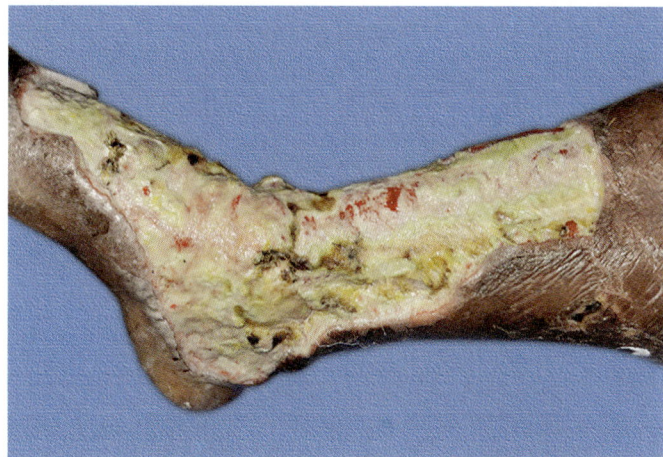

Fig. 3-13 Typical *spreading ulcer* with purulent discharge.

Raised and beaded edge (pearly white) is seen in rodent ulcer (BCC). Beads are due to proliferating active cells.
Everted edge (rolled out edge): It is seen in carcinomatous ulcer due to spill of the proliferating malignant tissues over the normal skin.
3. *Floor*: It is the one which is seen. Floor may contain discharge, granulation tissue or slough (Fig. 3-11).
4. *Base*: Base is the one where ulcer rests. It may be bone or soft tissues. Base is felt; not seen.

LIFE HISTORY OF AN ULCER

Stage of extension: Ulcer with inflammation spreads along subcutaneous and fascial planes and becoming bigger.
Stage of transition: Appearance of granulation tissue and serous discharge in the floor.
Stage of repair: Formation of healthy granulation tissue, neoepithelialization, fibrosis and scarring.

Classifications

Classification I (Clinical)

1. *Spreading ulcer*: Here edge is inflamed, irregular and edematous. It is an *acute* painful ulcer; floor does not contain healthy granulation tissue (or granulation tissue is absent), with profuse purulent discharge and slough; surrounding area is red and edematous. Regional (draining) lymph nodes are enlarged and tender due to inflammation. There will be associated fever, pain, impairment of functions with local tissue destruction and with little evidence of regeneration (Figs. 3-12 and 3-13).
2. *Healing ulcer*: Edge is sloping with healthy pink/red healthy granulation tissue with *scanty/minimal serous discharge* in the floor; slough is absent; regional lymph nodes may or may not be enlarged but when enlarged always nontender. Surrounding area does not show any signs of inflammation or induration; base is not indurated. *Three zones* are observed in healing ulcer. *Inner most red zone* of healthy granulation tissue; *middle bluish zone* of growing epithelium; *outer whitish zone* of fibrosis and scar formation (Figs. 3-14 and 3-15).
3. *Nonhealing ulcer*: It may be a *chronic* ulcer depending on the cause of the ulcer; here edge depending on the cause may be—punched out (trophic), undermined (tuberculous), rolled out (carcinomatous ulcer), beaded (rodent ulcer); floor contains unhealthy granulation tissue and slough, and serosanguinous/purulent/bloody discharge; regional draining lymph nodes may be enlarged but non tender (Fig. 3-16).

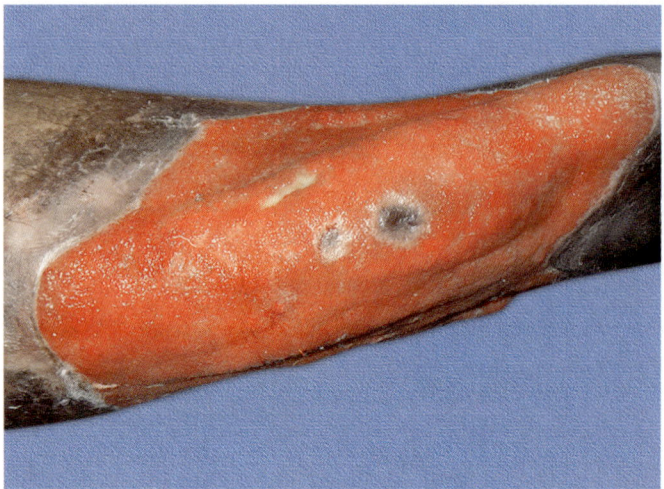

Fig. 3-14 Typical *healing ulcer*.

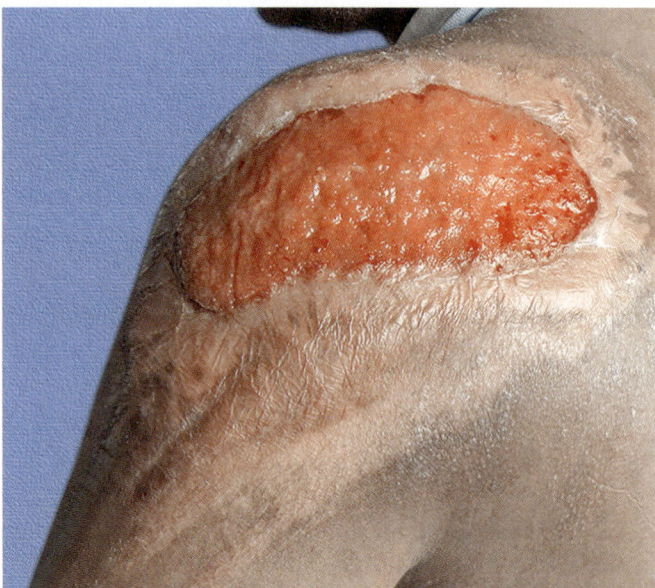

Fig. 3-15 *Healing ulcer* with healthy granulation tissue in the floor; it is ready for split skin grafting.

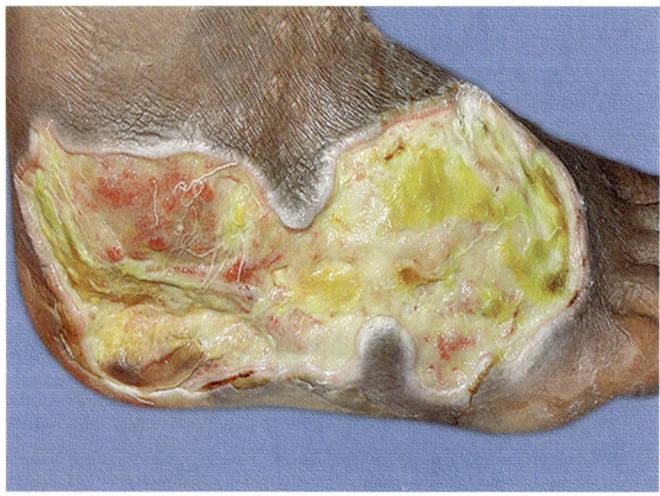

Fig. 3-16 *Nonhealing ulcer* with pale unhealthy granulation tissue and slough.

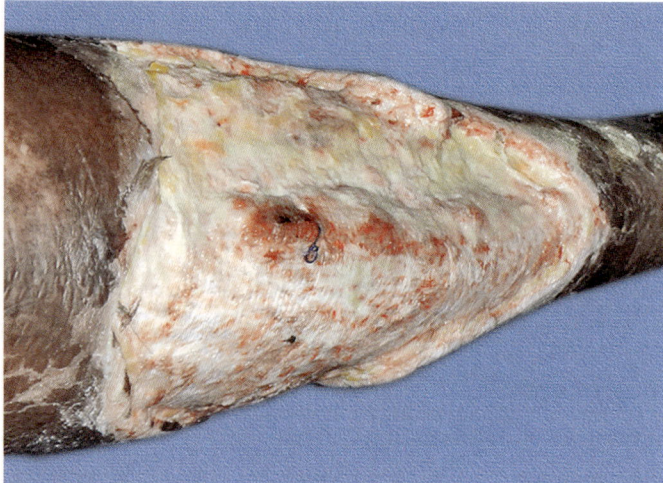

Fig. 3-17 *Callous ulcer* without any sign of healing and, without any granulation tissue.

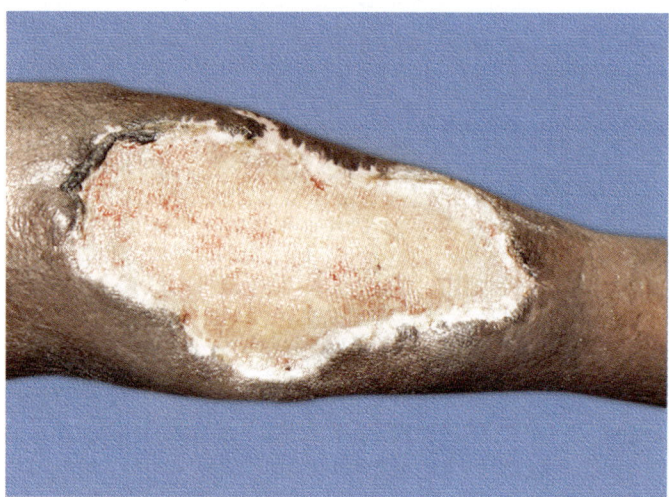

Fig. 3-18 *Callous ulcer*. It is stationary ulcer without any sign of healing. There is no healthy granulation tissue at all in the floor.

4. **Callous (stationary) ulcer:** It is also a *chronic* ulcer; floor contains pale unhealthy, flabby, whitish yellow granulation tissue and thin scanty serous discharge with indurated non tender edge; base is indurated, nontender and often fixed; and the *ulcer has no tendency to heal*. It lasts for many months to years. Tissue destruction is more with absence of or only minimal regeneration. Induration and pigmentation may be seen in the surrounding area. There is no/less discharge. Regional lymph nodes may be enlarged; are firm/hard and nontender (Figs. 3-17 and 3-18).

Classification II (Pathological)

1. *Specific ulcers:*
   » Tuberculous ulcer.
   » Syphilitic ulcer: It is punched out, deep, with 'wash-leather' slough in the floor and indurated base.
   » Actinomycosis.
   » Soft sore (Ducrey's ulcer).
   » Herpes simplex ulcer, fungal ulcer, etc.

Note: Specific ulcers may be *acute*—amoebic, typhoid; or *chronic*—tuberculous, syphilis, fungal, peptic ulcer.

2. *Malignant ulcers:*
   » Carcinomatous ulcer.
   » Rodent ulcer.
   » Melanotic ulcer.
3. *Nonspecific ulcers:*
   » *Traumatic ulcer:* It may be due to mechanical injury (dental ulcers in the tongue), physical (electrical burn), and chemical (alkali injury). Any trauma leading into denudation of epithelium can cause traumatic ulcer. *Footballer's ulcer* is a traumatic, chronic, deep ulcer in the shin.
   » *Arterial ulcer:* Atherosclerosis, thromboangiitis obliterans (TAO), Raynaud's disease.
   » *Venous ulcer:* Gravitational ulcer, post-phlebitic ulcer.
   » *Neuropathic ulcer:* It is also called as neurotrophic ulcer. It is due to loss of sensation and often motor power. It (often) causes trophic ulcer. Main cause of neuropathic ulcer is loss of sensation in the skin and tissues. Ulcer with surrounding area is typically painless; surrounding tissue usually has normal blood supply. It indirectly causes local ischemia causing deep penetrating punched out ulcers. *Commonest site* is over the heads of 1st and 2nd metatarsals. It is due to both components of peripheral neuropathy—*motor neuropathy* → paralyses of small muscles of the foot → unopposed actions of long flexor tendons in the foot → shortening of the longitudinal arch of the foot → increased load on the metatarsal heads during walking; *sensory neuropathy* → loss of pain sensation → repeated unnoticed trauma → neuropathic ulcer. Neuropathic ulcer occurs as a part of peripheral neuropathy (Hansen's disease, nerve injuries, diabetes mellitus) or as a part of the spinal cord disease (spina bifida, spinal injury, tabes dorsalis, syringomyelia).
   » *Trophic ulcer:* Bed sore; perforating ulcers in the sole.
   » *Infective ulcers:* Pyogenic ulcer.
   » *Tropical ulcers:* It occurs in tropical countries. It is callous type of ulcer, e.g. Vincent's ulcer.
   » Ulcers due to chilblains and frostbite (*cryopathic ulcer*).
   » *Martorell's hypertensive* ulcer.
   » *Bazin's ulcer:* Ulcers occur in young females due to development of mild ischemia in lower leg and around ankle; it is due to significantly smaller than normal perforating arteries arising from deeper arteries in this region, causing superficial, small, multiple nodules with ulcers which are hypersensitive for temperature (blue, cold skin in cold weather; hot, edematous, painful ankle in hot weather due to reactive hyperemia). Subcutaneous fat around ankle is thick and abnormal.
   » *Diabetic ulcer:* It is often progressive spreading ulcer as infection is rapid and associated ischemia worsens the ulcer early (Figs. 3-19A and B).
   » *Ulcers* due to leukemia, polycythemia, jaundice, collagen diseases, lymphedema, anemia, rheumatoid arthritis, gout, vitamin deficiency.
   » *Cortisol ulcers* are due to long time application of cortisol (steroid) creams to certain skin diseases. These ulcers are callous ulcers, last for long time and require excision and skin grafting.
   » *Factitious ulcer (artifact ulcer/man made ulcer):* Factitious disorders are defined as acts of self harm that directly or indirectly result in clinically relevant injury. They are typically performed in secret; small

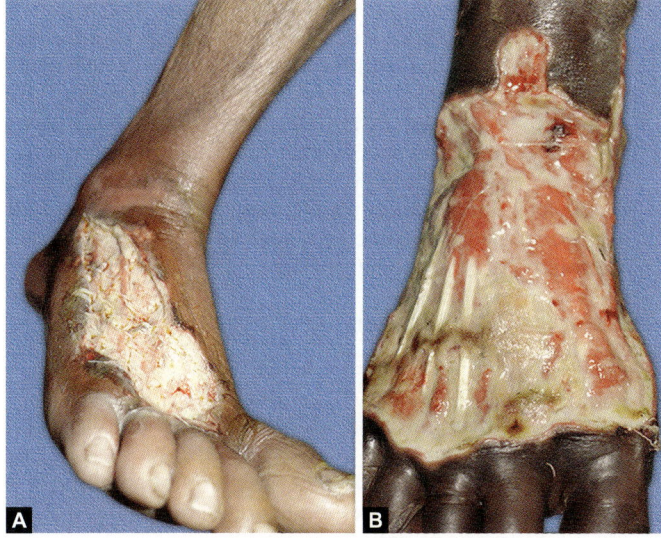

Figs. 3-19A and B Diabetic ulcer foot with exposed tendons, discharge and is spreading with features of ischemia.

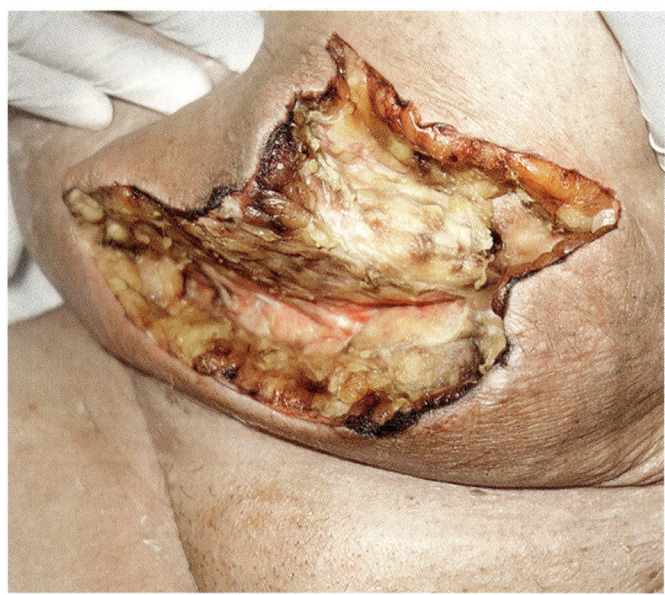

Fig. 3-20 Meleney's gangrene/ulcer.

objects like blade, coins, corrosives are used to inflict; but without direct intention of suicide. Such trauma induced ulcers are called as factitious ulcers; they are multiple, recurrent and superficial; evaluation for all causes of ulcer will be negative; these ulcers heal with usual ulcer treatment rapidly. It is a psychosomatic disorder; so psychiatric counseling and treatment is needed. These automutilation ulcers may be part of the Munchausen's syndrome.
» *Meleney's ulcer:* It is postoperative infection and ulcer formation in lower abdomen, perineum and often in chest wall in an immunosuppressed individuals (Fig. 3-20).
» *Other ulcers:* Ulcers can occur in vitamin deficiency, erythrocyanosis frigida, gout (increased uric acid deposition in small joints like of great toe as deposit called *tophi* which may ulcerate to form gouty ulcer), rheumatoid arthritis (nodules can break down to form

ulcer), Paget's disease of bone, sickle cell anemia, Felty's syndrome, ulcer poliomyelitis leg, diphtheritic ulcer (*Vela sore*/cutaneous diphtheria), decubitous ulcer, iatrogenic ulcer (over intravenous cannula site, over injection site), etc. Infection in *diphtheritic cutaneous ulcer* occurs due to skin breach; initially begins as straw colored vesicles which ruptures to form a tender shallow acute ulcer to begin with; later becomes chronic. Diphtheria bacteria multiply releasing exotoxins causing dangerous carditis or peripheral neuropathy.

Classification III (Wagner's Grading)

Grade 0—preulcerative lesion/healed ulcer.
Grade 1—superficial ulcer.
Grade 2—ulcer deeper to subcutaneous tissue exposing soft tissues or bone.
Grade 3—abscess formation underneath/osteomyelitis.
Grade 4—gangrene of part of the tissues/limb/foot.
Grade 5—gangrene of entire one area/foot.

Classification IV (Based on Duration)

- *Acute ulcer:* Duration less than 6 weeks.
- *Chronic ulcer:* Duration more than 6 weeks.

■ HISTORY

Name: **Sex:**
Age: Certain ulcer types may be more common in certain age groups.
Occupation: Venous ulcers are more common in individuals whose occupation requires long hours of standing like nurses, surgeons, traffic policemen, watchmen and bus conductors.
Place: Tropical ulcers are common in tropical regions of Africa, India, South America whereas ulcers due to chilblains and frost bite in cold countries.
Chief complaints: History of ulcer and its duration should be mentioned. Asking duration is important as it determines the chronicity of ulcer. History of specific condition related also should be mentioned.

History of Present Illness

Mode of Onset and Progression

It is the initial way of formation of an ulcer. It may be after an attack of cellulitis of the part which causes skin necrosis and later sloughs off, or after trauma which breaks the continuity of the epithelium or spontaneously due to any cause. Common cause of ulcer is trauma. Even minor trauma can cause extensive necrotizing fasciitis and ulcer later. Traumatic ulcer may heal fast or may progress into chronicity if it is on a joint or due to improper rest to the part or if patient is diabetic or due to recurrent infection, poor blood supply.

Often patient will be having the idea of the cause of ulcer. Tuberculous lymphadenitis leading into collar stud abscess eventually may form a fistula or an ulcer. Ulcerative lesion may be rodent ulcer **(Fig. 3-21)** carcinomatous ulcer or melanotic ulcer originating spontaneously. Syphilis may lead into gummatous ulcer. Ulcer may occur as a result

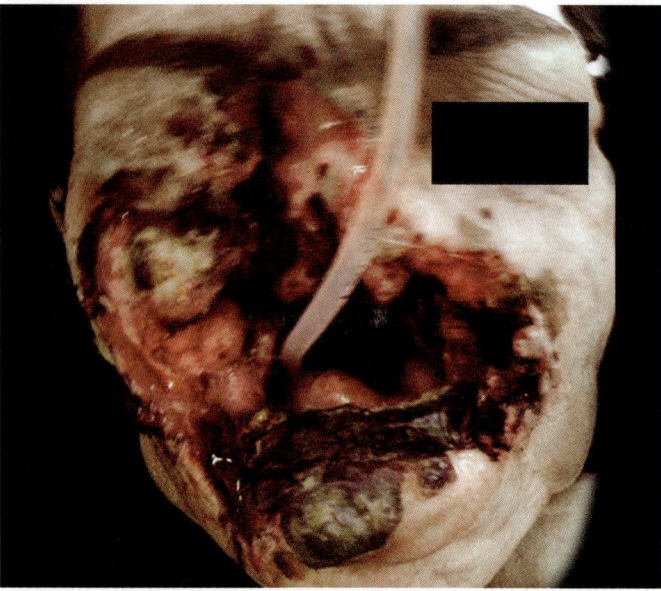

Fig. 3-21 *Rodent ulcer* with destruction into bone and cartilage. It is basal cell carcinoma which is locally malignant. It erodes deeply hence the name (gnaws/eats like a rat).

of varicose veins due to chronic venous hypertension or arterial insufficiency as in ischemic ulcer or over pre-existing scars like of burn scar.

Regressing or progressing of an ulcer formed in specific method is important. Acute ulcers are fast spreading in nature; chronic ulcers are slow to progress (tuberculous, gummatous, varicose ulcers, perforating ulcers). Ulcer may often heal spontaneously and reform later repeatedly in the same site, e.g. formation of an ulcer in a pre-existing burn scar or formation of venous ulcer repetitively around ankle. Here ulcer heals by rest and reforms by trauma or other precipitating causes. Such unstable long standing scar (of burns or venous ulcer) can turn into squamous cell carcinoma called as **Marjolin's ulcer (Fig. 3-22)**.

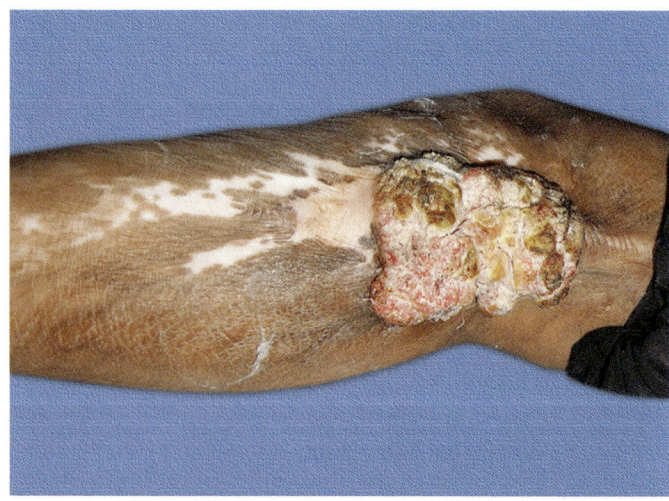

Fig. 3-22 Typical *Marjolin's ulcer* occurring in a chronic scar. It occurs in an unstable scar of long duration; usually chronic venous ulcer, burn scar or scar after snake bite.

If it is progressing then method of progressing is also noted. Change in size, shape, depth, discharge during progression period should be asked.

Duration

Ulcer may be of long duration like in chronic venous ulcer or of short duration like in acute ulcer after trauma or cellulitis. Incubation period may be longer (3–4 weeks) for syphilitic Hunterian chancre; 3–4 days for chancroid. Venous ulcers usually show more than a year duration; malignant ulcers show few months duration.

Pain

Ulcer may be painful or painless. Often malignant ulcer is painless to begin with but may eventually become painful due to secondary bacterial infection or infiltration to deeper plane or nerve ending. Some ulcers are painful to begin like *acute ulcer* (**Fig. 3-23**), but becomes painless once it turns to chronicity. Its time of onset, progress, and severity should be asked. Trophic ulcers, syphilitic ulcer, ulcers of neurological diseases like spinal injury/spina bifida/peripheral neuropathy/tabes dorsalis, leprosy are painless. Pain may interfere with patient's daily routine activities like walking, eating, bathing, defecation, etc. Tuberculous ulcer is usually *painless* except on the tongue. Superficial ulcers are *more painful* than deep ulcers. Ulcers in the ventral aspect of the body are *more painful* than ulcers in the dorsal aspect of the body.

Claudication pain in leg/thigh or rest pain with formation of ulcer suggests ischemic ulcer may be due to atherosclerosis in elderly or thromboangiitis obliterans (TAO) in young age. Varicose vein with venous ulcer patients have evening time crampy pain in calf.

History of Fever

Presence of fever signifies existing acute inflammation in an ulcer or in surrounding area.

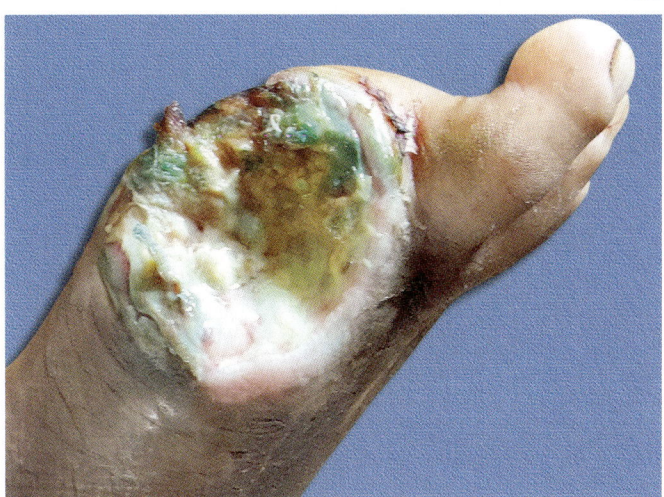

Fig. 3-24 Green discharge in ulcer suggests *Pseudomonas* infection.

Discharge from Ulcer

Whether ulcer is having discharge or not is asked and also its duration. Discharge can be also assessed by looking at the dressing pads. The quantity of discharge is enquired. Discharge may be profuse, scanty or absent. Patient often gives history of the quantity of dressing pads soaked and its color. Color and smell of the discharge is important. Whether discharge is serous or purulent which often indicates the type of bacterial infection involved is also important to be noted; like in Pseudomonas infection the discharge is greenish in color (**Fig. 3-24**).

Number of Ulcers

Often ulcers can be *multiple* (**Figs. 3-25 and 3-26**). If it is so, which ulcer developed first and which one later should be asked.

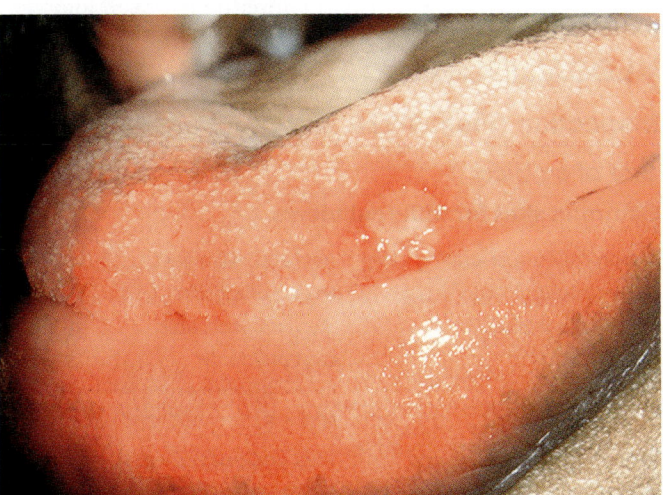

Fig. 3-23 Ulcer over lateral margin of the tongue due to dental injury. It is an *acute ulcer*.

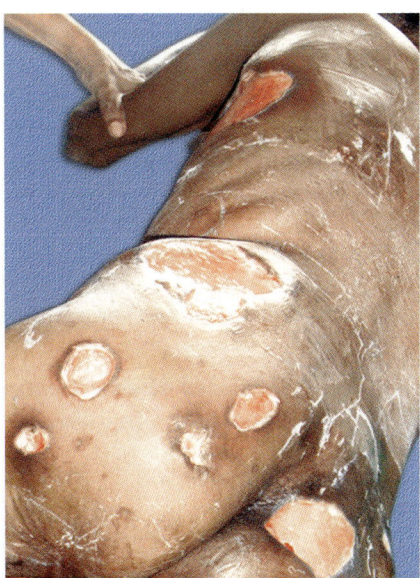

Fig. 3-25 Multiple ulcers all over the body in a malnourished immunosuppressed individual.

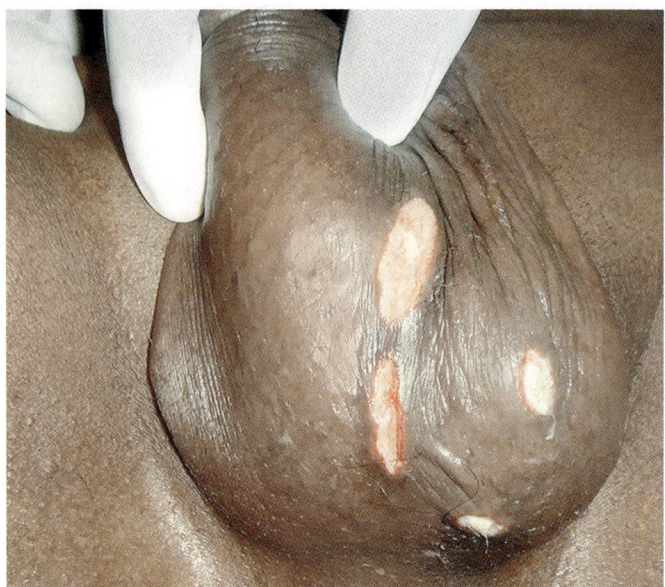

Fig. 3-26 Multiple ulcers in the scrotum.

Associated Symptoms

History of presence of varicose veins; claudication, rest pain of arterial insufficiency should be asked for. Features suggestive of chronic renal failure [CRF/CKD (chronic kidney disease)], tuberculosis, diabetes mellitus, spinal trauma/diseases (transverse myelitis, syringomyelia), Hansen's (leprosy) disease, AIDS, systemic malignancies should be asked. History of edema, deformity and loss of function of the part/limb should be asked for.

History of loss of sensation in feet from distal to proximal is typical of neuropathy which may be caused by diabetes mellitus (commonest cause), leprosy and peripheral neuropathy of other causes like vitamin deficiency. In sickle cell disease, there will be jaundice with recurrent ulcers in leg (over the shin). *Recurrent ulcerations* often multiple may be due to drug induced (reactions) or may be related to certain dermatological conditions.

Past History

Past history of ulcer treated by dressing/drugs/skin grafting/hospital stay should be asked in detail. Number of days hospitalized, time taken up for healing of the ulcer should be noted. Previous history of treatment for tuberculosis, syphilis, diabetes, hypertension, leprosy, neurological diseases, sickle cell disease (anemia) or any other illness is important.

History suggestive of associated disease/treatment history like for tuberculosis, tabes dorsalis, spinal diseases or diabetes mellitus has to be asked. If patient is on treatment for any of such ailment, type of drugs taken, dose and method of intake should be asked.

Whether the patient was on any steroid cream for long duration has to be asked as callous ulcer are common in these patients.

Past history of surgery like tumor wide excision (removal of tumor), its detail, which year and which hospital, result/outcome, biopsy report if any; any further treatment taken like radiotherapy or chemotherapy or antituberculous drug therapy or treatment for leprosy; name of drugs, doses, side effects; recovery should be asked for in detail. Past history of toe(s) amputation(s) on one or both feet and if so details of it; it is common in diabetic foot.

Personal History

History of alcohol consumption/smoking/tobacco chewing/history of sexual contact/dietary habits are also important. Duration of such habits, quantity should be asked for. It has got direct relation to ulcer formation or ulcer healing or treatment strategy. *Altered appetite or weight loss* can also be mentioned under personal history—may be due to advanced malignancy or tuberculosis.

Family History

Family history of any specific disease (tuberculosis, leprosy, hypertension, diabetes mellitus, varicose veins) should be asked.

GENERAL EXAMINATION

Doing a detailed general examination is very essential. Presence of anemia/edema/jaundice/clubbing/lymphadenopathy/raise in temperature/attitude of the patient/nutritional assessment by skin texture, subcutaneous fat, weight, body mass index/any other relevant findings should be mentioned. Rate and volume of radial pulse/palpation of all peripheral pulses/blood pressure should be noted. Malignant tumor infiltrating nerves or ulcer with a chronic scar or large chronic ulcer or painful acute ulcer can alter the attitude of the limb. Increased pulse rate and temperature suggests ulcer with acute inflammation. Features suggestive of tuberculosis, vascular disease, spinal disease, syphilis or neurological diseases should be looked for.

LOCAL EXAMINATION OF AN ULCER

Inspection (Figs. 3-27A and B)

Site of an Ulcer

Common sites for different ulcers

Trophic ulcer (perforating ulcer)	Heel and ball of feet
Tuberculous ulcer	Neck, axilla, groin
Gummatous ulcer	Sternum, skull, tibia
Traumatic ulcer	Leg commonly
Rodent ulcer	Face—Above the line joining the angle of the mouth and ear lobule
Arterial ulcer	Toes, fingers, feet, legs
Venous ulcer	Around ankle (gaiter's area)
Neuropathic ulcer	Heads of 1st and 2nd metatarsals

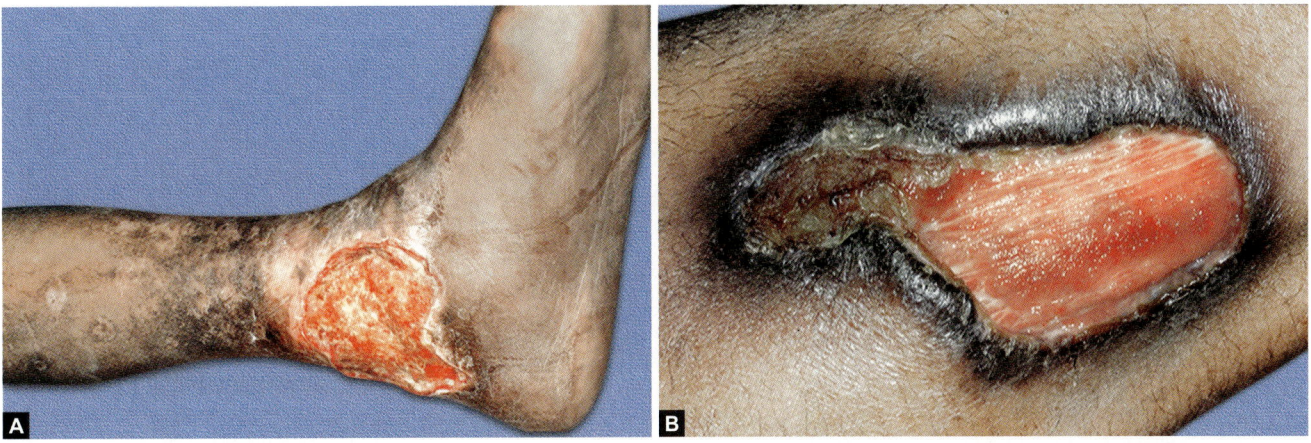

Figs. 3-27A and B Inspection of ulcer for its site, size, shape, margin, edge, floor and surrounding area.

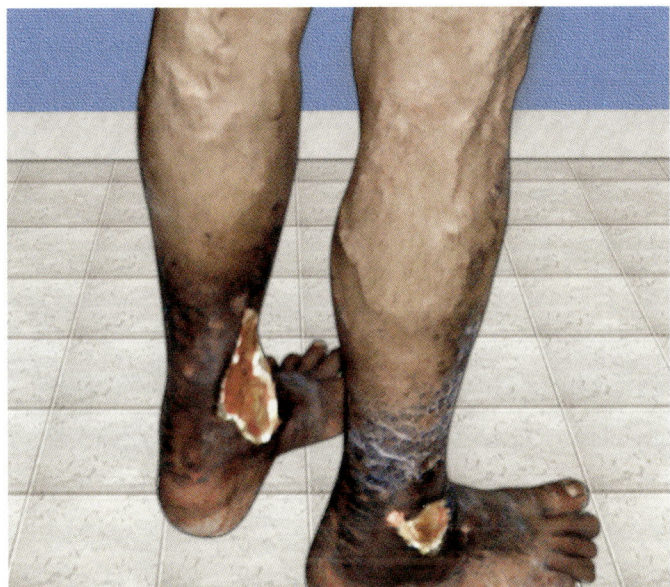

Fig. 3-28 *Inspect the limb in standing position* for evidence of varicose veins in case of suspected venous ulcer. This area around ankle and lower leg is called as *gaiters area* (gaiter is leather or cloth or polyester used as protective covering around ankle used in military or during horse ride).

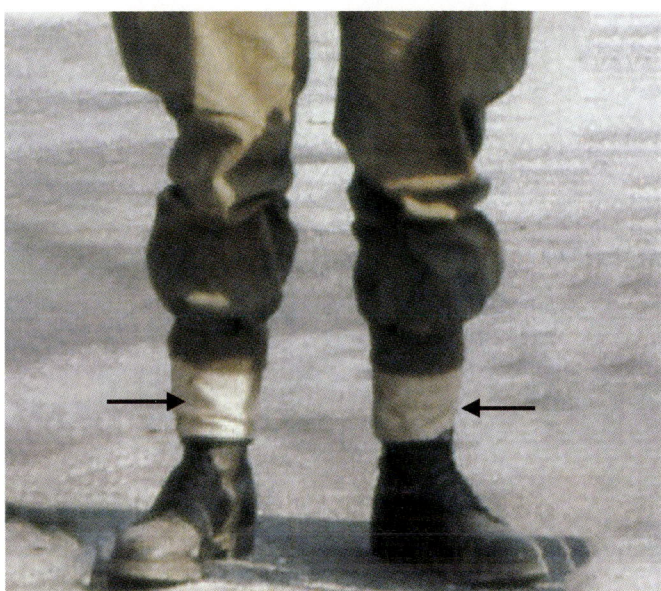

Fig. 3-29 *Typical gaiters* used by military infantry men in olden days.

Exact anatomical location of the ulcer is noted. It is mentioned in relation to particular anatomical point usually bony point. **Venous ulcers** occur over malleoli around ankle **(Figs. 3-28 and 3-29)**. **Basal cell carcinomatous ulcer/rodent ulcer** occurs in the face commonly above the line joining angle of the mouth to the ear lobule (common site is inner canthus of eye) **(Fig. 3-30)**. **Tuberculous ulcer** occurs commonly in the neck, axilla, chest wall or groin. It can occur anywhere in the body. **Syphilitic gummatous ulcer** occurs over subcutaneous bones like tibia, sternum, palate or skull. **Trophic ulcer** occurs in the sole of the foot (heel, over the heads of the metatarsals). **Malignant ulcers** can occur anywhere in the skin. **Meleney's ulcer** occurs over the perineum, groin and lower abdominal wall; **syphilitic** and **chancroid ulcers** over the external genitalia; **melanoma** over the sole.

Size of an Ulcer

Ulcer size should be assessed approximately both *vertically and horizontally* in centimeters.

Shape of an Ulcer

Ulcers of different causes may have different shapes. Venous ulcer is vertically *oval* in shape. Tuberculous ulcer is *circular/oval/crescentic* in shape. Malignant ulcer is *irregular* in shape. *Serpiginous* ulcer looks like a serpent (in chronic ulcers). Here healing occurs in one place; while disease extends in another/adjacent place.

Number

Malignant ulcer is usually solitary. Venous ulcers can be multiple. Tuberculous ulcers can be multiple.

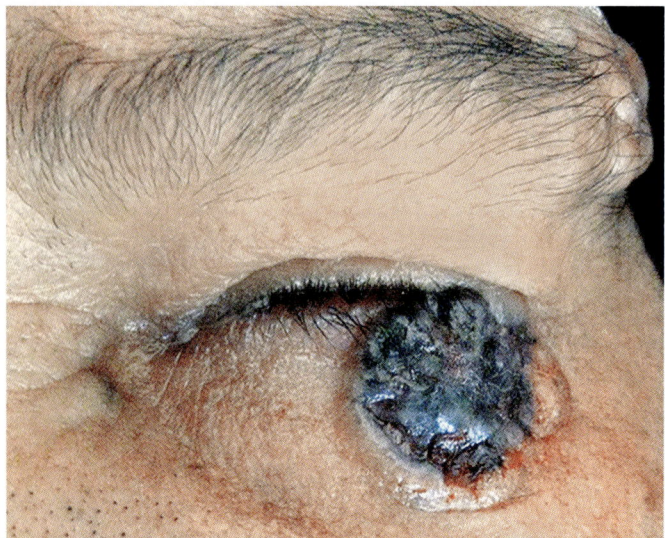

Fig. 3-30 BCC (rodent ulcer) which is pigmented involving lower eyelid—a common site.

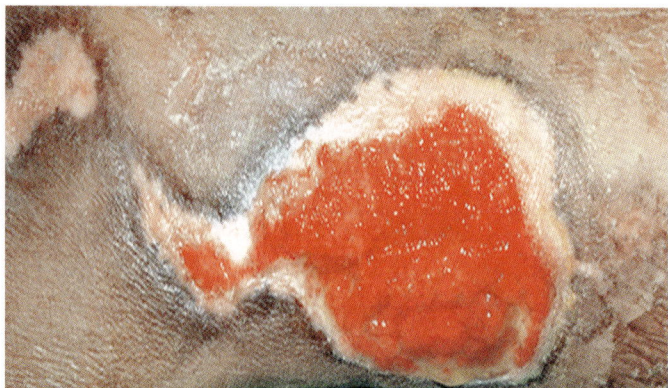

Fig. 3-32 Healing ulcer with healthy granulation tissue. Note the sloping edge.

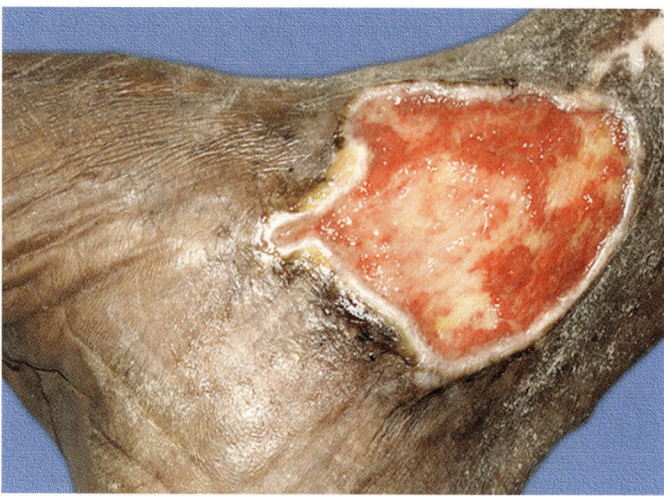

Fig. 3-33 Healing ulcer with healthy granulation tissue in the floor with sloping edge.

When **multiple**, which ulcer started first, its progress and about other ulcers should be asked; most prominent and large ulcer should be examined first **(Fig. 3-31)**.

Margin of an Ulcer

Margin, whether regular/irregular/well-defined/ill-defined should be observed. Margin is the junction of the normal skin around to the outermost end of the edge. **Margin** is the boundary of an ulcer. Part beyond margin is called as **surrounding area**.

Edge of an Ulcer

Edge of an ulcer is *a part from floor to margin*; destruction, proliferation, regeneration is maximum at the edge. Different edges occur in different conditions:

Sloping edge occurs in healing ulcer. It shows three zones from inside out. First is **red zone** due to central healthy red granulation tissue; second is middle **blue zone** consisting of active growing epithelium; third is outermost **white zone** consisting of fibrous tissue and scar. It is seen in **healing ulcer** **(Figs. 3-32 and 3-33)**.

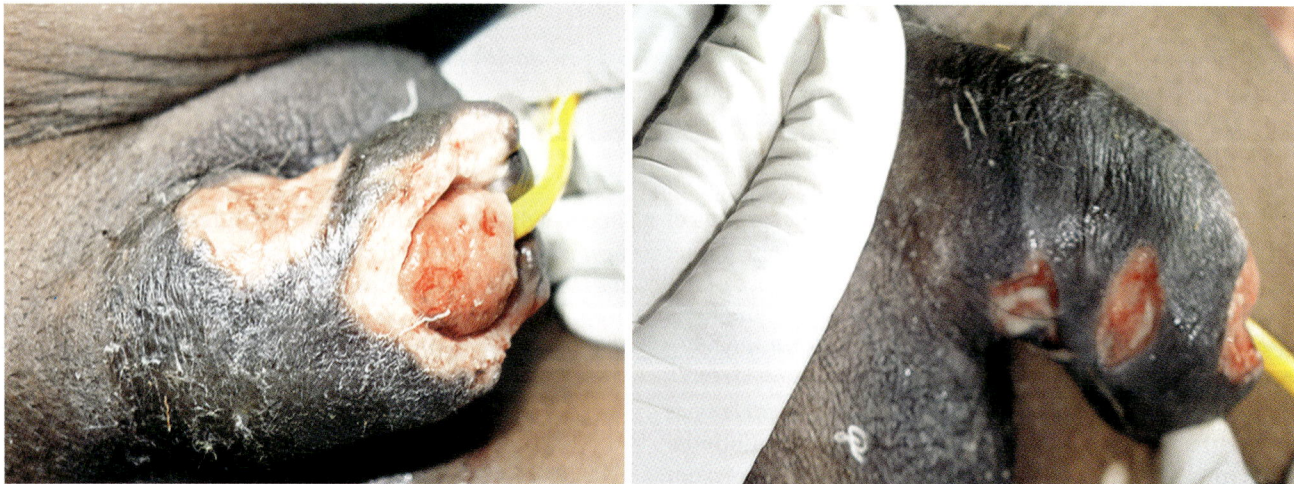

Fig. 3-31 Multiple ulcers in the penis with phagedena. **Phagedena** (eating away) is deep, destructive necrotizing infection of skin and tissues (destruction without proliferation).

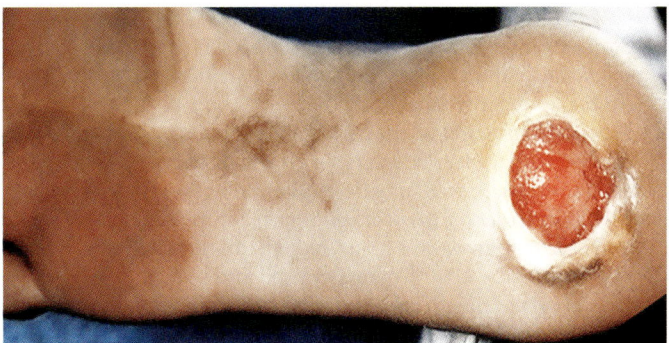

Fig. 3-34 Trophic ulcer heel—typical punched out edge.

Punched out edge is edge that run deeply perpendicular to the skin margin. It is commonly seen in **trophic ulcer** (due to localized deep inflammation) and gummatous ulcer (due to end arteritis obliterans). Disease is localized to ulcer area and does not spread to surrounding structures **(Fig. 3-34)**.

Undermined edge is one where edge is burrowed deep and lateral to the skin margin. *Edge in tuberculous ulcer* is typically undermined. It is due to faster spread of tuberculosis in subcutaneous plane than skin. Overlying skin which is pointing towards the center of the ulcer is bluish, thin, and friable **(Figs. 3-35A and B)**. *Undermined edge* may be also seen in Bazin's disease, Meleney's ulcer, amebic ulcer, soft sore, bed sore, tropical ulcer.

Aphorism—*syphilis bites; tuberculosis nibbles.*

Raised and beaded edge is seen in **rodent ulcer** (BCC ulcer). Beads are pearly white in color and are due to actively multiplying malignant cells. Probably in between these beads are predominantly the dormant inactive cells **(Fig. 3-36)**.

Everted edge/rolled out edge is one which fills, heaps and spills outward from the edge towards margin. It is typical of **epitheliomatous ulcer** (squamous cell carcinoma/malignant ulcer). It signifies rapidly growing tissues **(Fig. 3-37)**. Ulcer showing proliferation (usually in the edge) is proliferative ulcer. Growth showing ulceration is ulcerative growth.

Spreading ulcer shows edematous, inflamed edge.

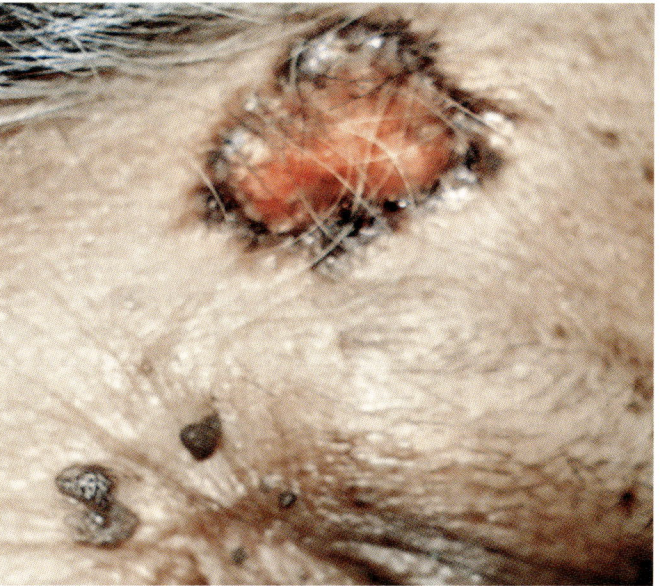

Fig. 3-36 Basal cell carcinomatous ulcer (rodent ulcer) with beaded edge.

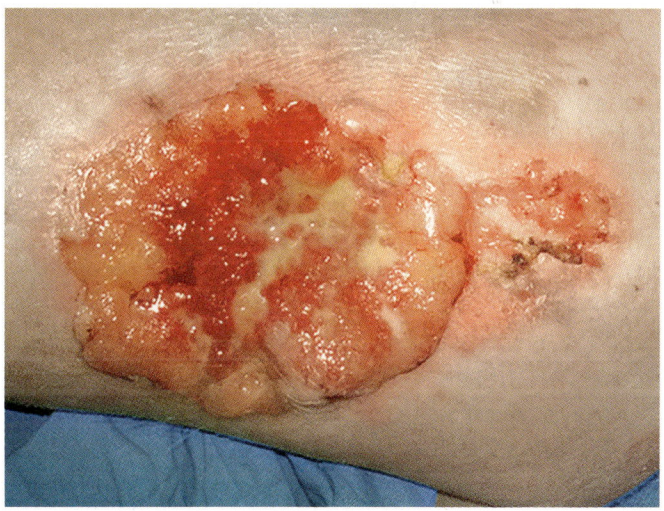

Fig. 3-37 Squamous cell carcinoma shoulder region. Note the everted edge of SCC (carcinomatous ulcer/epithelioma).

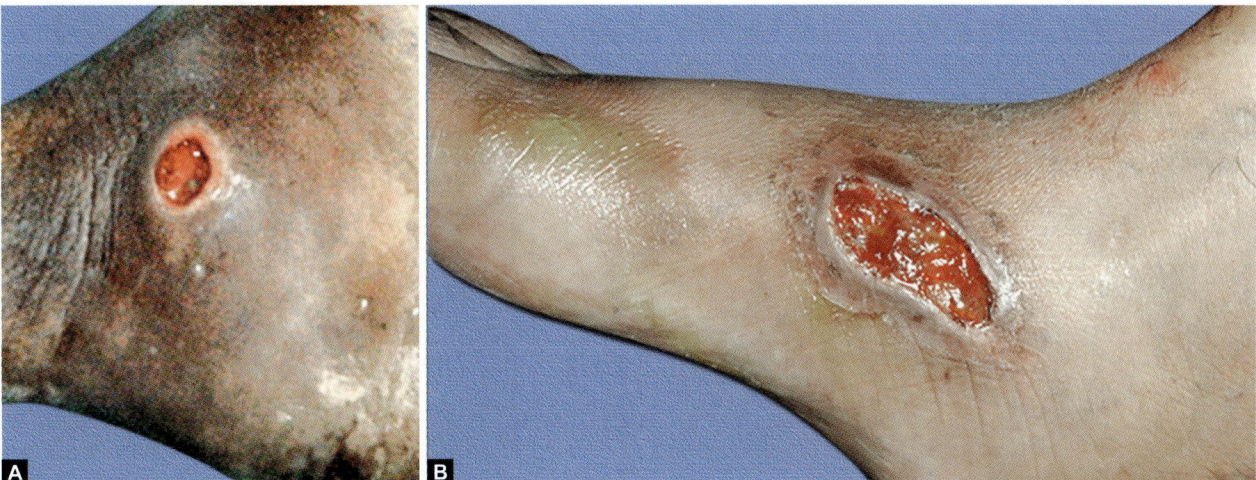

Figs. 3-35A and B Tuberculous ulcer foot with undermined edge.

Floor of the Ulcer (Figs. 3-38 to 3-42)

Floor is the one what is seen. It rests on the base (base is not seen; it is only felt). Floor may contain red granulation tissue in healing ulcer; pale, unhealthy granulation tissue in non-healing ulcer; thick slough without any granulation tissue in chronic callous ulcer; pigmented tissue in melanoma or pigmented BCC or pigmented SCC (**Fig. 3-38**). Floor may be covered with ***crust/scab/ slough.*** ***Wash leather slough/wet chamois leather slough*** is seen in gummatous ulcer. Wash—leather slough is also seen in post-radiation necrosis. Often moving maggots may be present in the floor. They eat necrotic dead tissue only. Cultivated maggots are used as therapeutic desloughing agent. In melanoma, black pigmented mass of tissue is observed in the floor.

Note:
- ***Slough*** is insensitive mass (yellowish/brownish) formed by *dead soft tissue in situ*; it is often foul smelling. ***Scab*** *is dried up discharge* (in the floor of the ulcer).
- ***Floor is depressed*** in specific and nonspecific ulcer; raised in carcinomatous ulcer due to rapid growth of tissue. Floor may also contain exposed fascia, muscle, tendon, bone, nerve (trophic ulcer).
- ***Floor is visible on inspection;*** it is examined for the presence and type of granulation tissue, slough, discharge, nodules, level of floor (depressed and deep or raised and outer).
- ***Red granulation tissue*** in the floor suggests healing (also indicates good blood supply); *bluish granulation* or *apple jelly* granulation suggests tuberculosis; *wash leather slough* suggests gummatous ulcer or post-radiation necrosis; *yellow slough* suggests gram-positive bacterial infection; *greenish slough* may suggest pseudomonas infection; *black mass* in the floor may suggest malignant melanoma. Ischemic ulcer shows *minimum or no granulation tissue* (indicates poor blood supply). Non healing, callous ulcers show *unhealthy pale granulation tissue.*

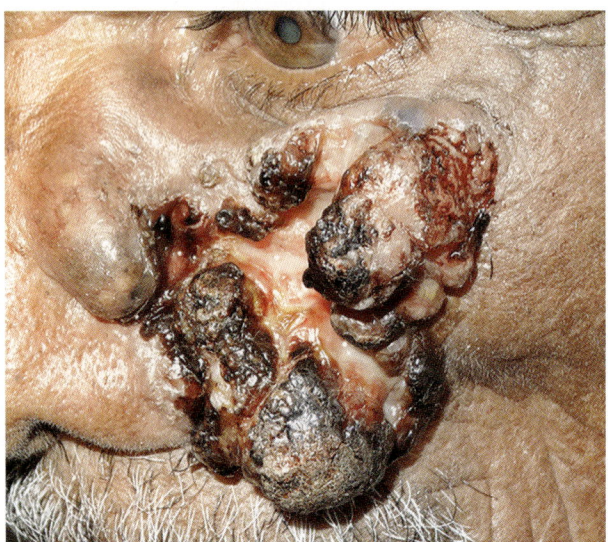

Fig. 3-38 Pigmented ulcer. It could be pigmented BCC or pigmented SCC.

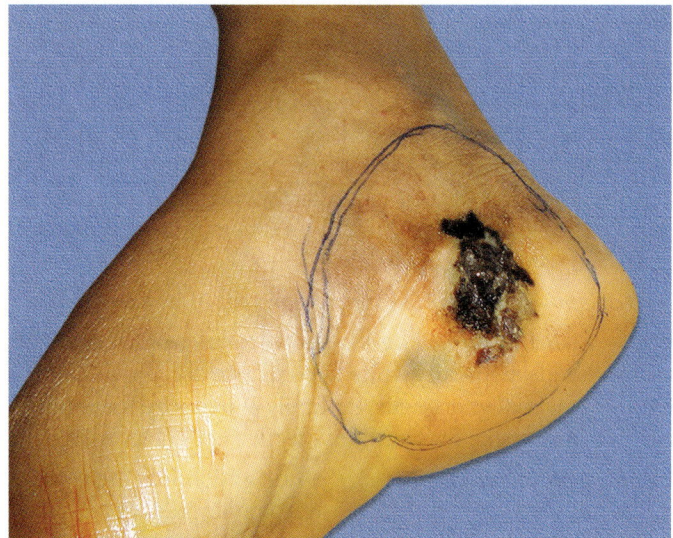

Fig. 3-40 Pigmented tissue mass in the floor of melanoma.

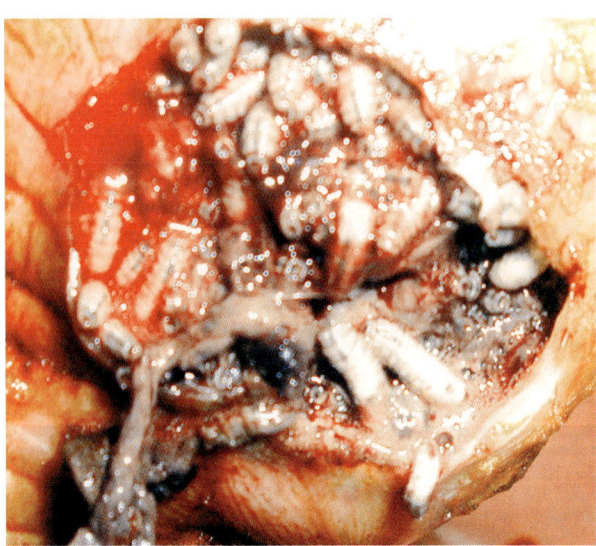

Fig. 3-39 Maggots in an ulcer.

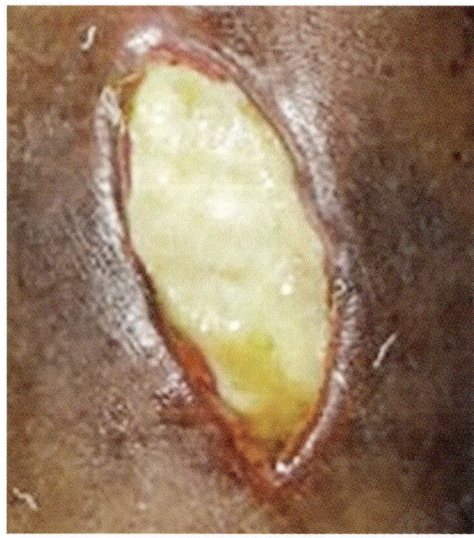

Fig. 3-41 Typical floor of an ulcer with slough.

Chapter 3: Examination and Clinical Approach of an Ulcer

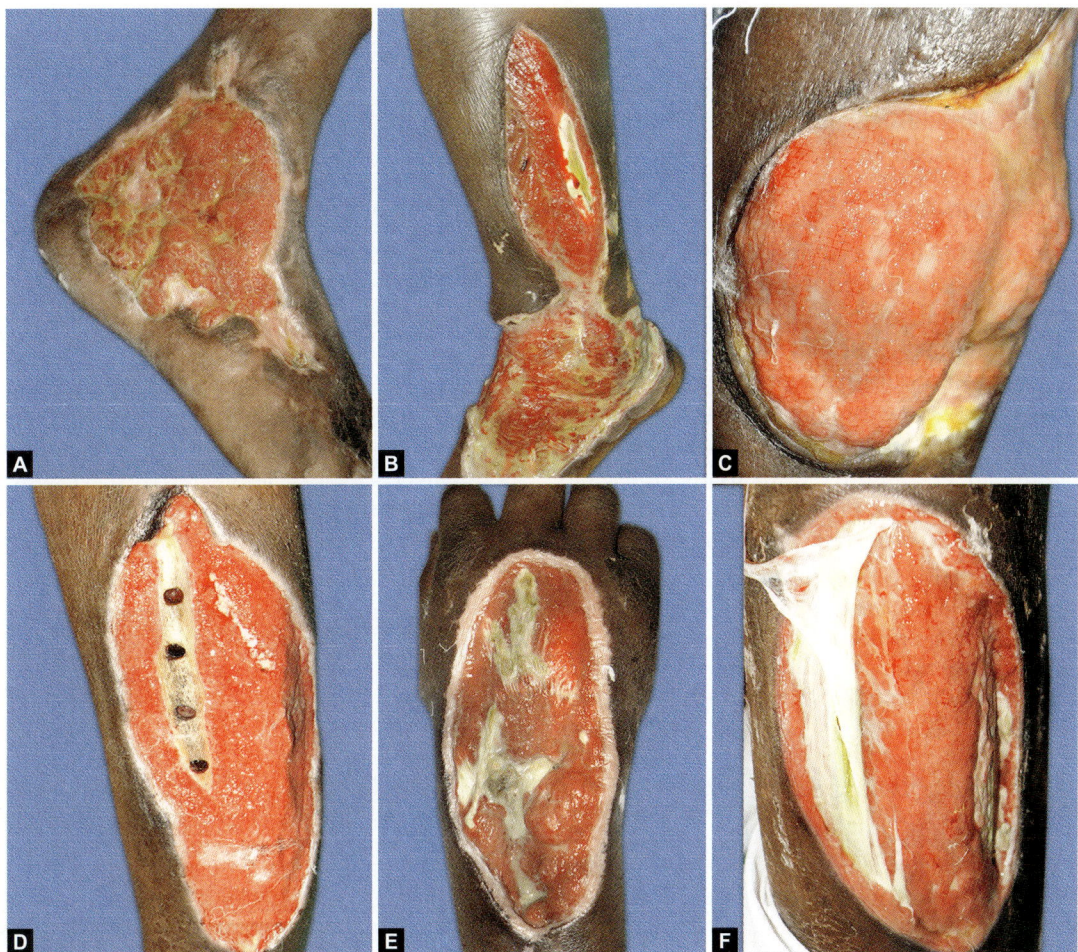

Figs. 3-42A to F *Different contents of floor.* (A) Floor with healthy granulation tissue; (B) Floor with slough, granulation tissue, and tendon; (C) Floor with exuberant granulation tissue; (D) Floor with exposed bone (tibia which is drilled to promote formation of granulation tissue); (E) Floor with granulation tissue, slough, exposed bone; (F) Ulcer with slough on the surface getting separated from the floor.

Discharge from Ulcer Bed

It can be serous (healing ulcer), serosanguinous, bloody (malignant ulcer), purulent (infective ulcer); color of discharge—greenish in *Pseudomonas* infection (**Fig. 3-43**).

Quantity, quality, color and smell of discharge should be assessed.

Quantity: Discharge may be scanty or profuse. Spreading ulcer may have profuse thick discharge; venous, arterial, trophic ulcers have scanty discharge; in Hunterian (syphilitic) hard chancre, gummatous ulcer, carcinomatous ulcers discharge will be absent unless it is secondarily infected. Dried up discharge looks like scab in the ulcer floor [*scab/crust* is a dried up *discharge* (and it is seen often with slough); *slough* is yellowish/brownish mass of dead soft tissue in situ].

Quality: Spreading ulcer will have purulent discharge; healing ulcer shows serous discharge; tuberculous ulcer shows serosanguinous and malignant ulcer shows bloody or serosanguinous discharge. Discharge with bony spicules is typical of underlying chronic osteomyelitis.

Color: *Yellowish* or *dark* brown colored discharge in spreading ulcer; reddish or *pinkish* in healing ulcer; greenish discharge

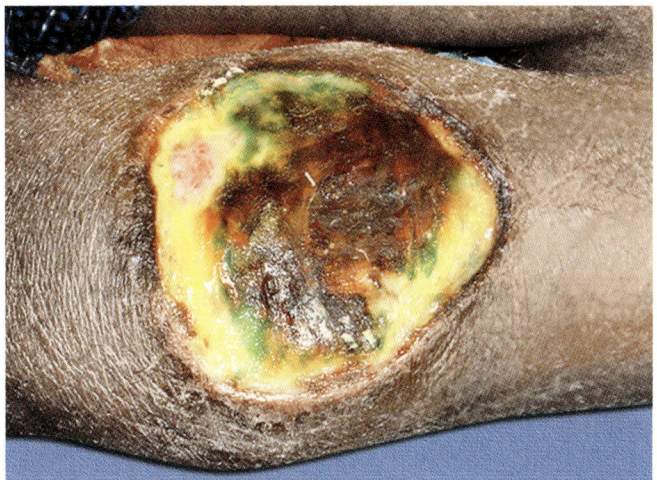

Fig. 3-43 Nonhealing ulcer leg in a diabetic patient with *Pseudomonas* infection. Note the greenish discharge in the wound. *Pseudomonas* infection is commonly hospital acquired.

with typical smell is characteristic of pseudomonas infection (**Fig. 3-43**); yellowish colored caseation in tuberculous ulcer (often looks like apple jelly in face, lupus vulgaris); yellowish sulphur granules in actinomycosis infection; black color in malignant melanoma.

Smell: Healing ulcer is odorless (no smell); foul smell is seen in spreading ulcer with bacterial infection. In anerobic infection, smell is bad which is nauseating.

Surrounding Skin and Area

Surrounding skin/area has to be examined for inflammation, edema, pigmentation, pallor, eczema, color, texture, scar, presence or absence of hair, visible veins. **Multiple scars** of healed ulcers or sinuses may be present in recurrent diseases like venous ulcers or ulcers due to osteomyelitis **(Fig. 3-44)**.

Swollen limb of deep venous thrombosis or chronic venous disease, equines deformity (venous ulcer), claw toes, muscle wasting of ischemic ulcers, multiple discharging sinuses in surrounding area of Madura foot, previously amputated toe(s) in diabetic foot—should be observed **(Figs. 3-45 and 3-46)**.

Note: Inspection of the entire part or limb should be done for varicose veins, features of deep vein thrombosis, arterial diseases and neurological cases. Examination (inspection) of the limb for muscle wasting, joint movement is also important. Area proximal to the ulcer; area distal to the ulcer for wasting, edema, deformity also should be examined.

Opposite Side and Neighboring Structures

Opposite side or limb should also be inspected. **Neighboring structures** should be inspected like inspection of groin in limb ulcers for possible enlarged lymph nodes; inspection of the abdomen, etc.

Palpation

Tenderness

Tenderness should be elicited over the edge, base and surrounding area. Acute ulcers are tender. Chronic ulcer is usually nontender but can be tender if there is secondary infection, involvement of deeper structures like periostitis in venous ulcer. Tuberculous ulcers are painless unless over the tongue. Neurotrophic ulcers are painless. Malignant ulcer is nontender to begin with. It may only become tender in later period when it infiltrates into deeper plane.

Temperature

Warmness over **surrounding area** signifies acute inflammation **(Figs. 3-47A and B)**.

Palpation of Edge for Tenderness and Induration

Induration is feeling of hardness. It often suggests carcinoma. In chronic ulcer hardness can be felt because of thick fibrosis **(Fig. 3-48)**.

Varying degree of induration (hardness) is common in chronic ulcers; **marked induration** is seen in carcinomatous ulcer. Induration extends well beyond the edge into the surrounding area in carcinoma, but in chronic ulcer it usually confines to ulcer area, however, sometimes induration can be felt even in chronic ulcer well beyond the ulcer in the surrounding area.

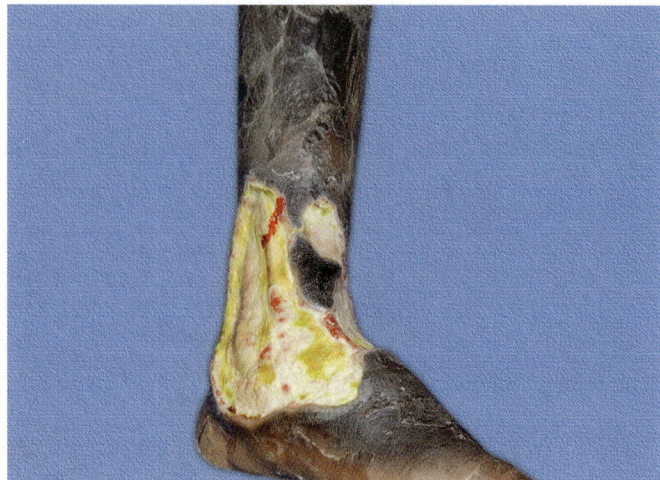

Fig. 3-44 *Surrounding area* of the ulcer should be examined; note the chronic nonhealing/callous ulcer with pigmented unhealthy surrounding area.

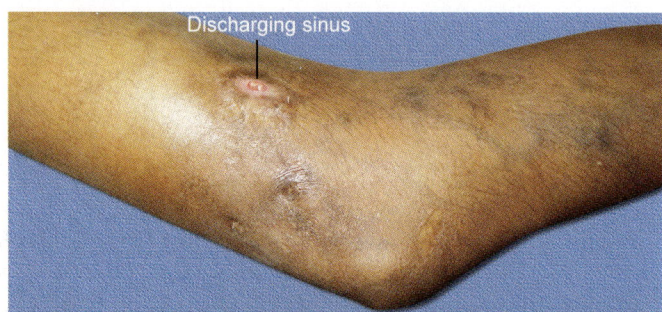
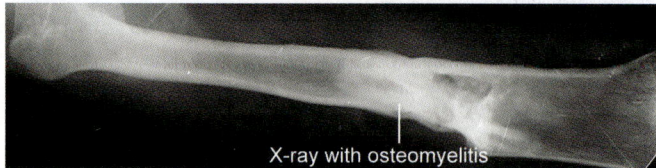

Fig. 3-45 Ulcer with great toe amputated. Note the slough in the floor.

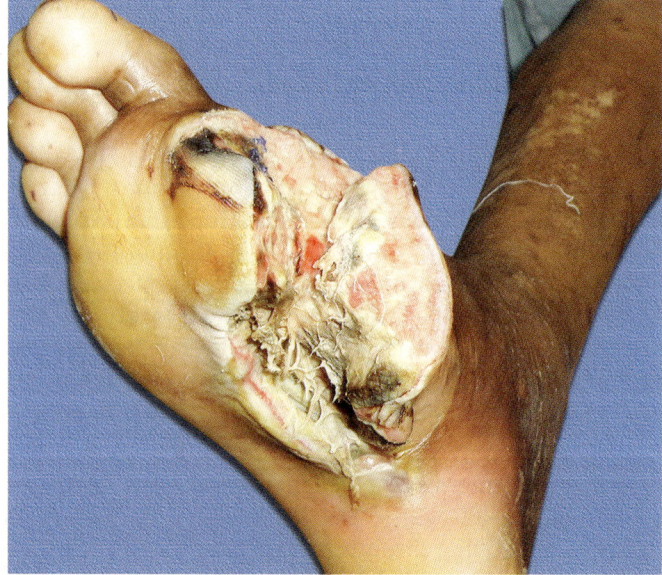

Fig. 3-46 Discharging sinus with bony spicules with X-ray showing chronic osteomyelitis.

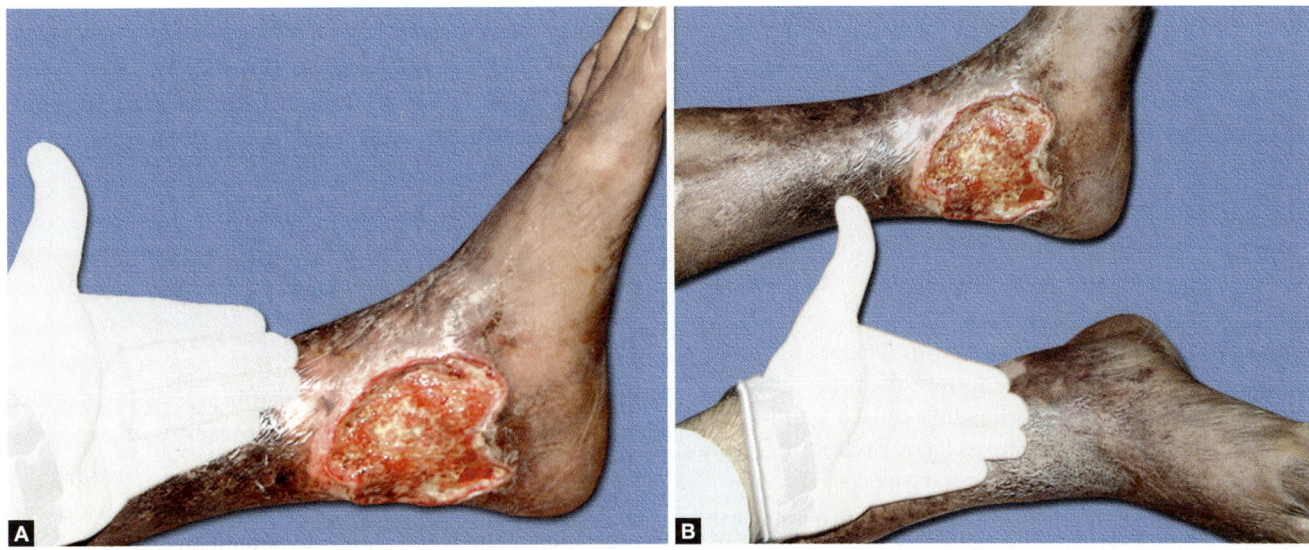

Figs. 3-47A and B Checking the temperature in surrounding area and comparing with opposite/normal area.

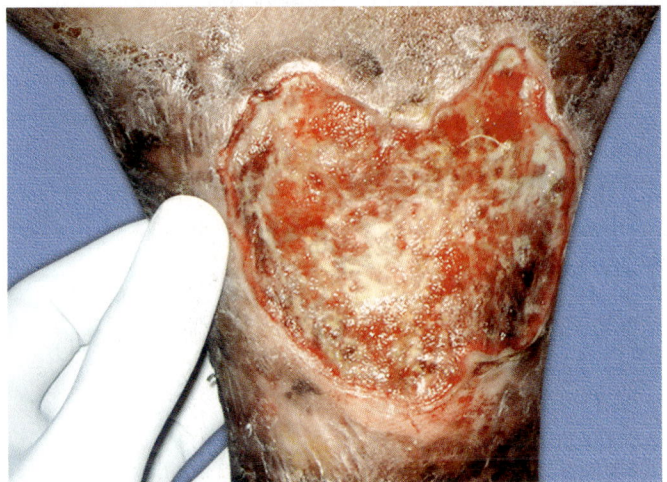

Fig. 3-48 Palpating the edge for tenderness and induration.

Palpation of Base for Induration/Fixity

Base is the one on which ulcer lies. Base may be fascia, soft tissues or bone. If base is formed by bone then ulcer is fixed and non-mobile. Mobility should be checked in two planes, perpendicular to each other by holding the ulcer firmly using thumb and fingers. Induration of base and fixity of ulcer is important in carcinoma and is due to infiltration. Base is wider than floor in carcinomatous ulcer. Hunterian chancre also shows induration. In tuberculous ulcer induration is less/absent; benign chronic ulcer may show induration due to fibrosis. Base may be soft and supple or indurated and hard; tender or nontender; mobile or fixed **(Figs. 3-49A and B)**.

Note:

Induration is a clinical palpatory sign; it is observed in well differentiated squamous cell carcinoma and adenocarcinoma. It is absent or less in poorly differentiated carcinoma or malignant melanoma. Induration is felt at edge, base and surrounding area. Induration at surrounding area signifies extent of the disease; outermost part of the indurated area is taken as the point where clearance margin for wide excision has to be planned. Brawny

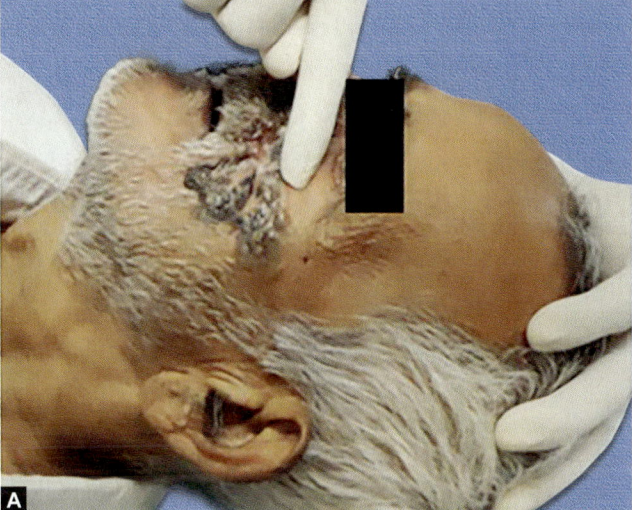

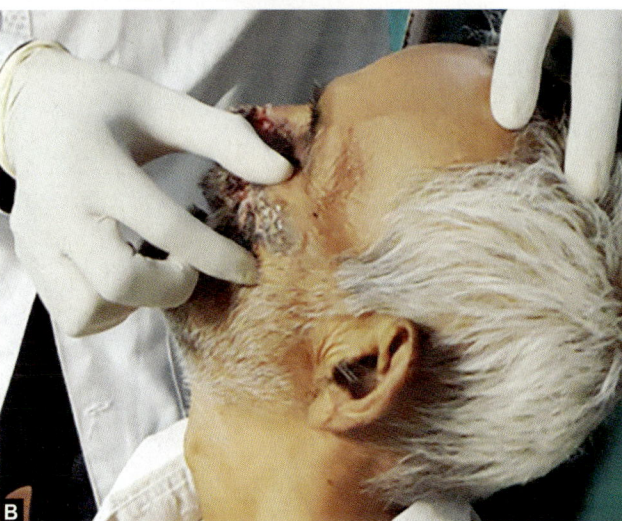

Figs. 3-49A and B Palpation of base for induration and fixity.

induration is a feature of an abscess. Specific indurations are observed in venous diseases (cyanotic induration of chronic venous congestion) and deep vein thrombosis.

- **Base** is felt; not seen (*base is palpated, not inspected*). Base may be soft and supple or indurated or hard; base may be tender or nontender. Ulcer may be fixed or free. Base often can be held between fingers. If ulcer is mobile that means it is not fixed to bone underneath; in such situation muscle underneath is made to contract against resistance and mobility of ulcer is checked; then if ulcer is not mobile means it is fixed to the underlying muscle.
- **Edge** is *both inspected and palpated*; **Base** is *only palpated*; **Margin** can only be inspected.

Depth and Size of the Ulcer

Depth of the ulcer is measured in mm. Venous ulcer is not deep but shallow; will not penetrate deep fascia usually. Ischemic ulcer is deep extending into muscles and tendon; trophic ulcer is deep with bone as base; carcinomatous and rodent ulcers may penetrate deeper tissues.

Size of the ulcer is measured using a measuring tape in centimeters; ulcer floor is covered with a sterile gauze or disposable transparent plastic sheet to place the measuring tape over it; first vertical measurement is taken, then horizontal. *Caliper (Vernier)* can be used to measure the size **(Figs. 3-50 to 3-52)**.

Bleeding on Palpation and Touching

Floor and edge should be palpated gently for this sign after wearing a sterile glove. Malignant ulcer is vascular and friable hence bleeds on touch. Healthy and exuberant granulation tissues in the floor can bleed on touch **(Figs. 3-53A and B)**.

Palpation of Deeper Structures and its Relation to Ulcer (Mobility)

Bone and soft tissues should be palpated. Bone thickening signifies periostitis or osteomyelitis due to ulcer penetration. It is felt by running thumb firmly over the surface of the bone. It is commonly elicited over lower tibia and malleoli

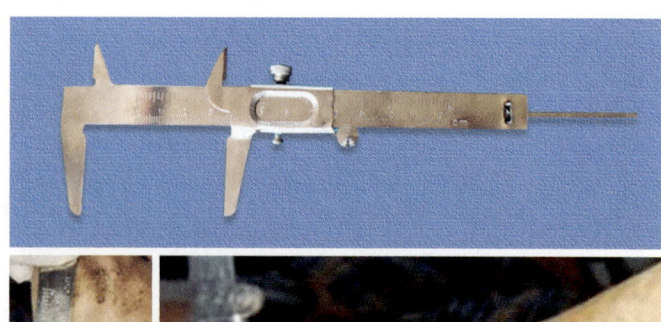

Fig. 3-51 Ulcer can also be measured using Vernier calliper.

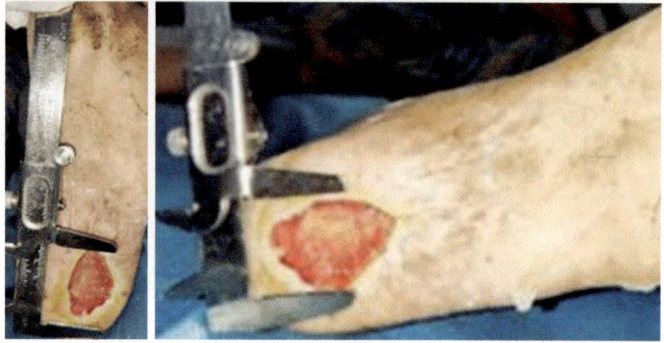

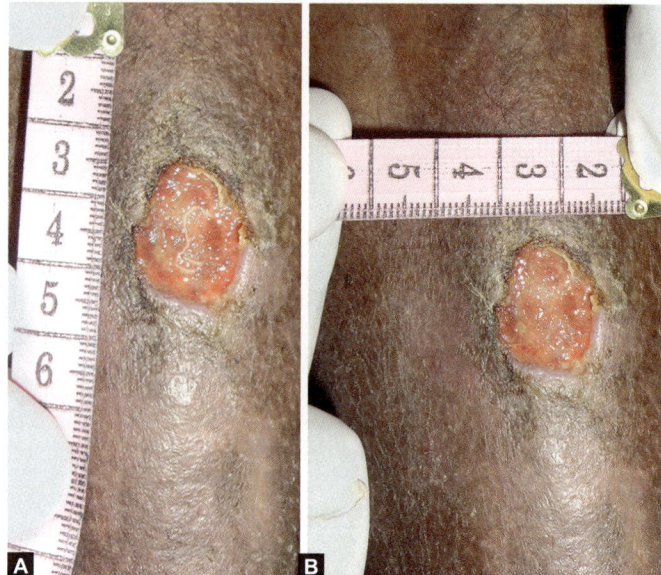

Figs. 3-52A and B Measuring an ulcer using measuring tape in centimetres—vertical and horizontal dimensions.

in case of venous ulcer; on calcaneum in trophic ulcer. Mobility also of an ulcer should be checked by wearing a glove. Ulcer is held firmly at two opposite points over the margin and tried to move over the base. It should be checked in two perpendicular directions **(Figs. 3-54A and B)**. Ulcer may be mobile (benign) or fixed (locally advanced malignancy).

Surrounding Area

Surrounding skin should be palpated for warmness (is seen in inflammatory ulcers), tenderness, induration, extension, infiltration, fixity in case of carcinoma, sensation, underlying ***bone thickening*** (suggest periostitis or osteomyelitis) **(Figs. 3-55 and 3-56)**.

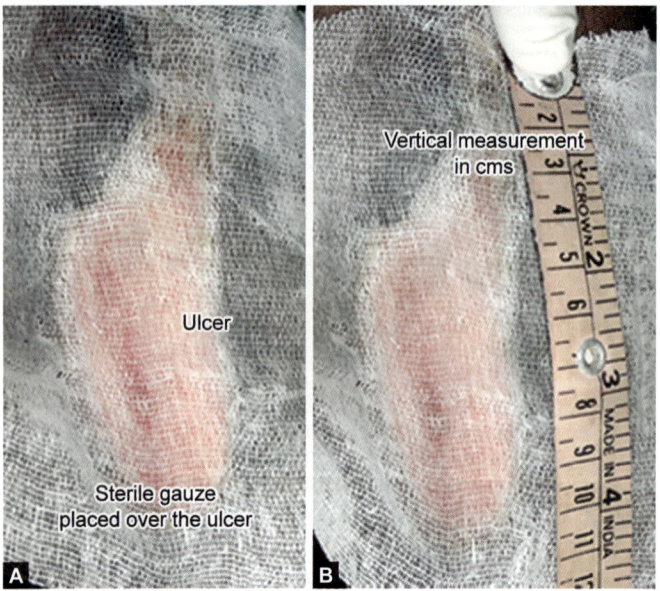

Figs. 3-50A and B Measurement of an ulcer—vertical and horizontal in centimeters; after placing sterile gauze.

Chapter 3: Examination and Clinical Approach of an Ulcer

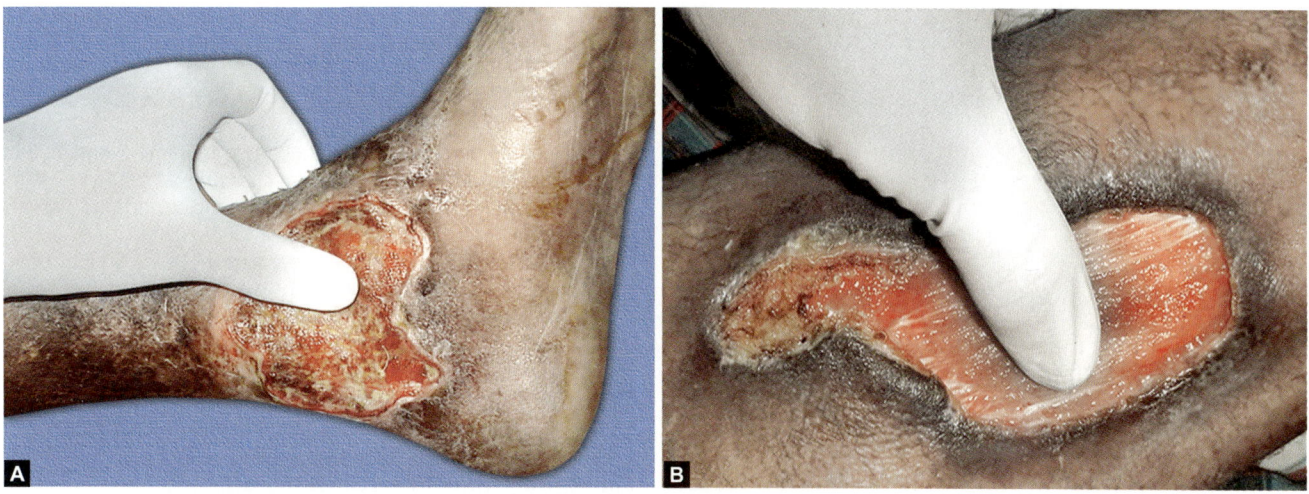

Figs. 3-53A and B Palpation may cause bleeding on touch in healthy granulation tissue or carcinoma. Base of an ulcer also should be palpated for tenderness and induration.

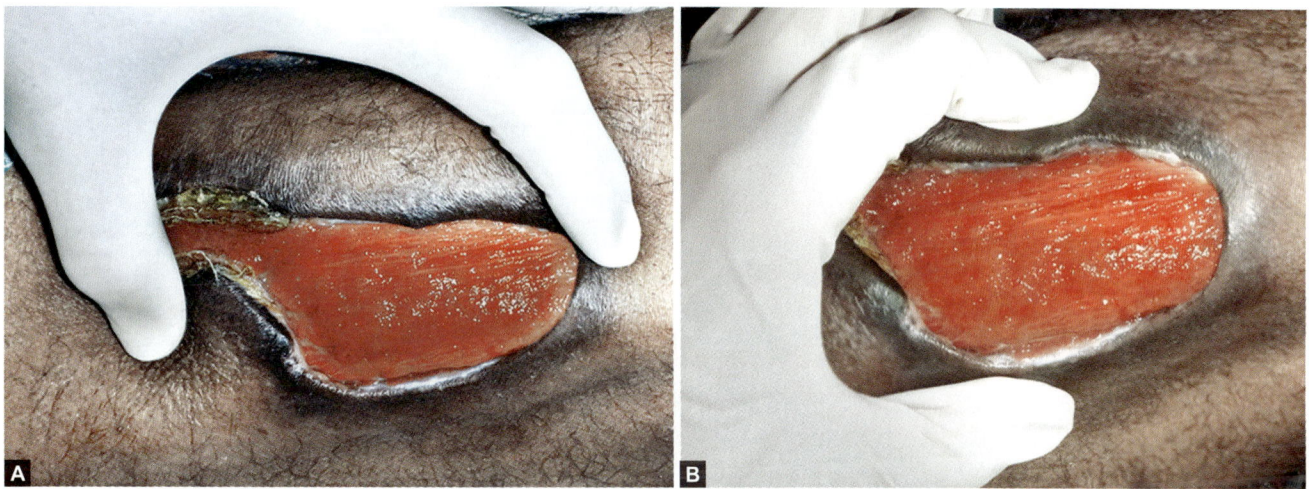

Figs. 3-54A and B Mobility of an ulcer should be checked. If there is free mobility it means it is not fixed to bone. If mobility is absent then it could be fixed to bone.

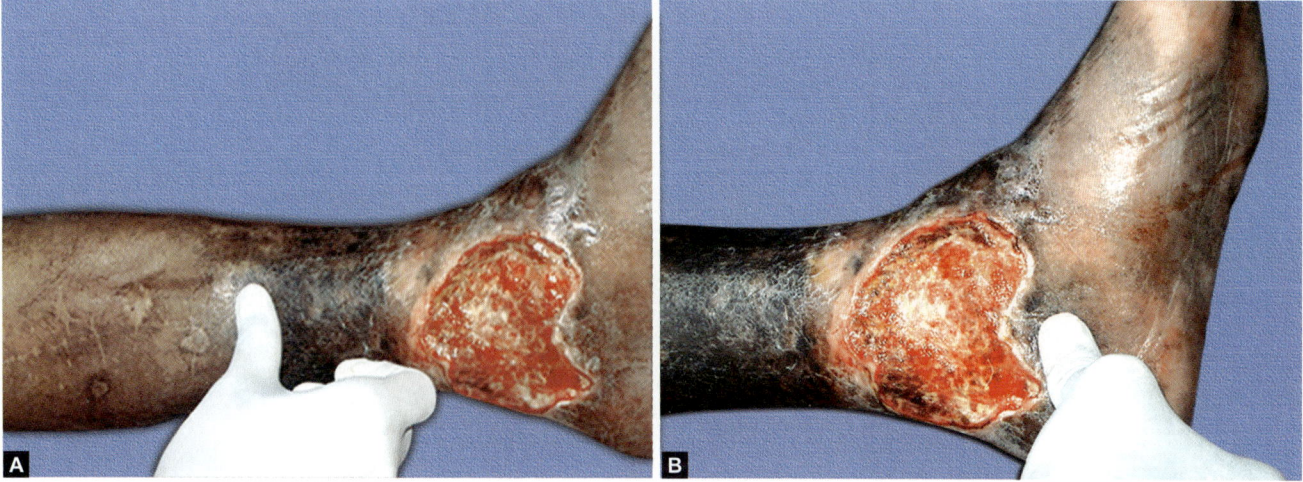

Figs. 3-55 and B Bone thickening should be felt by palpation over proximal and distal part of the ulcer. Here ulcer is in ankle region and so thickening of tibia and calcaneum should be checked.

Section 1: Examination in General Surgery

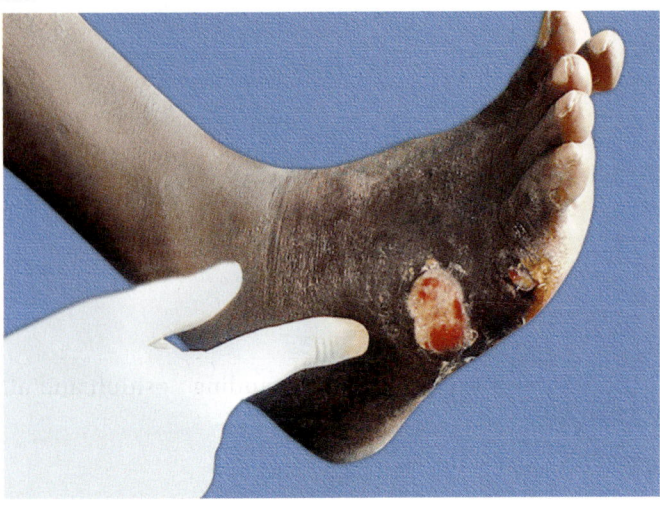

Fig. 3-56 Surrounding area should be palpated for relevant findings.

Girth of the limb adjacent to ulcer should be checked for wasting and should be compared to opposite side.

CLINICAL PEARLS

- 95% of the ulcers can be diagnosed on clinical examination.
- Typical look is the most relevant clinical examination.
- Always examine regional nodes, neurological, arterial, venous systems depending on the location of the ulcer.
- Effects of chronic ulcer (>6 weeks) are—pain, itching, odor, discharge, infection, chronicity (>6 weeks), nonhealing, social factor, inability to work, psychological impact.

Examination of Adjacent Joint (Figs. 3-57A and B)

Joints are examined for both ***active and passive movements***. Active movements are done by the patient. Passive movements are elicited by the clinician.

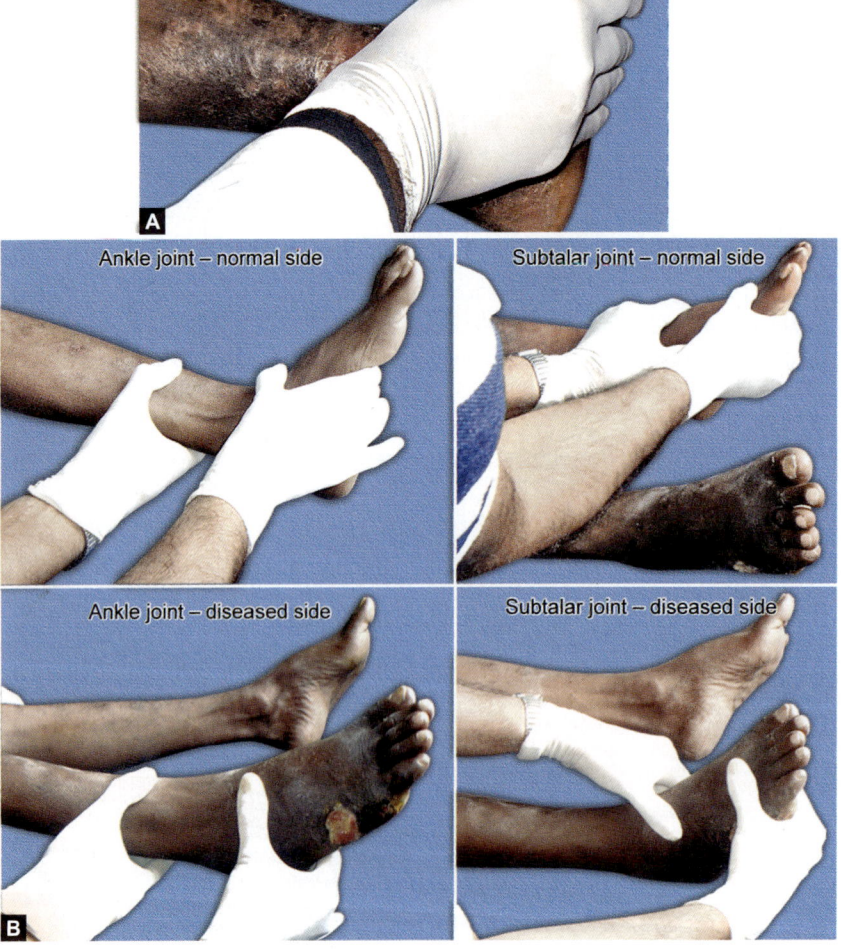

Figs. 3-57A and B Joint proximal to the ulcer area should be checked for any change in movement. Fibrous ankylosis and total loss of joint movement can occur. Ankle joint should be examined by holding lower leg flexed with left hand and right hand placed just distal to ankle joint (with heel off the ground) to check for dorsiflexion (normal is 25°) and plantar flexion (normal 35°). Inversion (20°) and eversion (20°) is checked by holding the calcaneum with one hand and foot distally with other hand.

Examination of Regional Lymph Nodes (Figs. 3-58A and B)

Examination of regional lymph nodes is essential. Number, size, surface, consistency, tenderness, mobility, fixity—superficially (skin) or to deeper structures are to be examined.
- *Tender,* palpable regional lymph nodes are found in acute infective conditions.
- *Shotty, firm, discrete* lymph nodes are felt in Hunterian chancre.
- Lymph nodes are not enlarged in BCC/rodent ulcer as malignant cells block the lymphatics early. In actinomycosis and gummatous ulcers lymph nodes are not enlarged.
- *Stony hard,* initially discrete and mobile lymph nodes, but later when advanced fixed to deeper structures are features of secondaries from carcinoma. Initially regional lymph nodes may get enlarged due to infection as such, and not due to primary existing carcinoma. Such nodes are usually firm, not hard and may regress by trial antibiotic therapy.
- Lymph nodes enlarged due to sepsis may get suppurated and may form an abscess as *soft, tender swelling*.
- Lymph nodes involved by tuberculosis are *matted, firm,* often may lead to cold abscess or collar stud abscess.

In leg ulcers, vertical group of lymph nodes are examined; further above *external iliac nodes* are also examined (**Figs. 3-59A and B**). Number, size, tenderness, surface, consistency, mobility or fixity (skin and deeper) should be checked. External iliac nodes are located above and medial part of the inguinal ligaments; palpable external iliac nodes suggest severity of the disease whether inflammatory or neoplastic. In malignancy (of leg) iliac node involvement alters the stage of the disease and outcome of the therapy.

Examination for Varicose Veins

Varicose veins are examined in standing position and all relevant tests should be done in case of venous ulcers.

Examination of Peripheral Pulses

Examination of peripheral pulses should be done to confirm if there is any ischemia (**Fig. 3-60**).

Examination of Spine and Neurological System

Examination of spine and neurological system like sensation and muscle power in the region and specific segments (**Figs. 3-61A to C**).

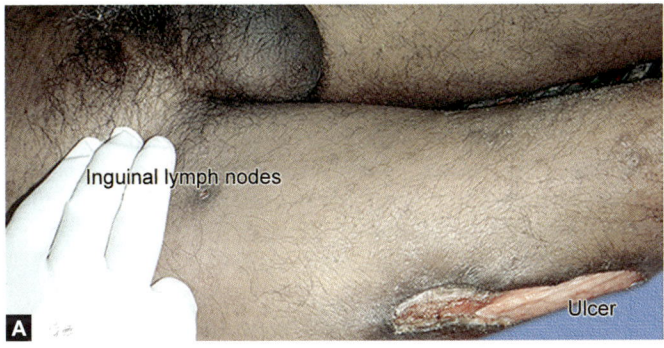
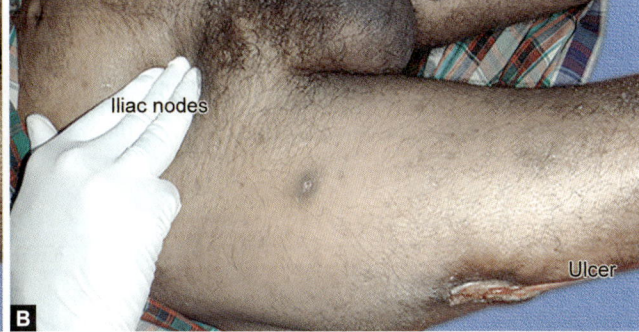

Figs. 3-58A and B Regional lymph nodes should be palpated for enlargement. In lower limb ulcer, vertical superficial group of inguinal nodes are palpated. External iliac nodes are also checked above and on medial aspect of the inguinal ligament. Its enlargement signifies severity of the disease.

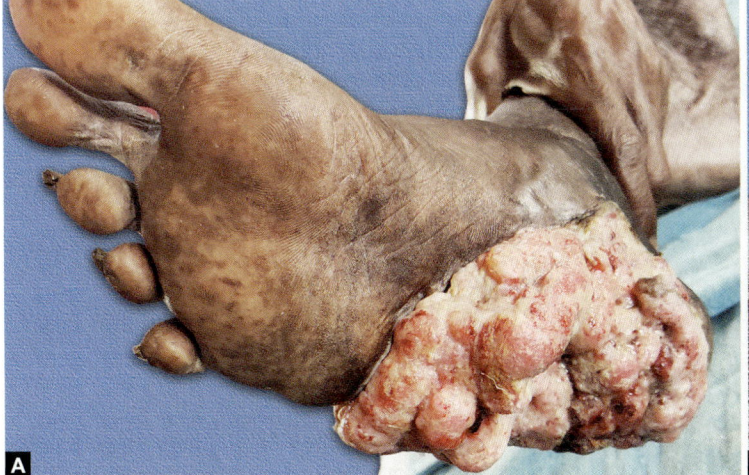
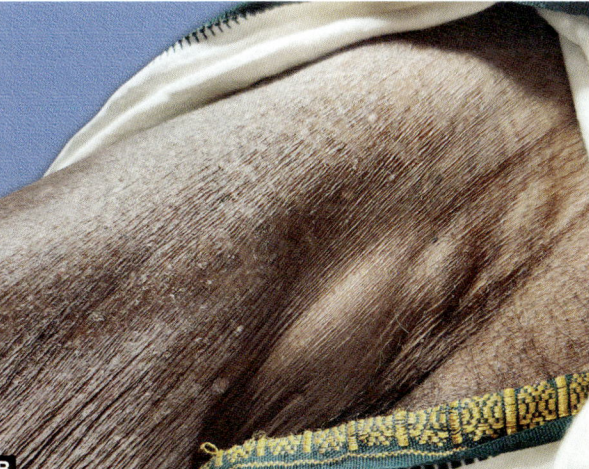

Figs. 3-59A and B Typical squamous cell carcinoma heel (epithelioma) with inguinal and external iliac nodes palpation.

Section 1: Examination in General Surgery

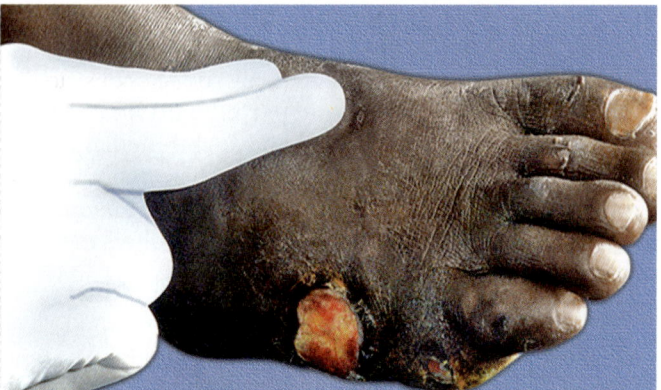

Fig. 3-60 Palpation of peripheral pulses to find out ischemia in ulcer foot is important.

It is significant in leprosy, peripheral neuritis, spinal diseases or trauma. In suspected case of Hansen's disease, one should look for hypopigmentation, nerve thickening, etc. Spinal tuberculosis is not uncommon; may present with gibbus, neurological deficits, psoas abscess, etc.

Gait of the Patient

Gait of the patient should be checked to find out the severity of loss of function due to ulcer (**Fig. 3-62**).

Systemic Examinations

Systemic examinations like of abdomen, respiratory and cardiovascular system should be done properly (**Figs. 3-63A and B**). Hepatosplenomegaly in case of blood dyscrasias; altered breath sounds or pleural effusion in tuberculous ulcer (may be present but not necessary always).

Investigations of an Ulcer

Study of Discharge (Fig. 3-64)

Discharge is examined for specific bacteria—*Streptococcus/ Staphylococcus/Gonococcus*. Sensitivity of antibiotics is

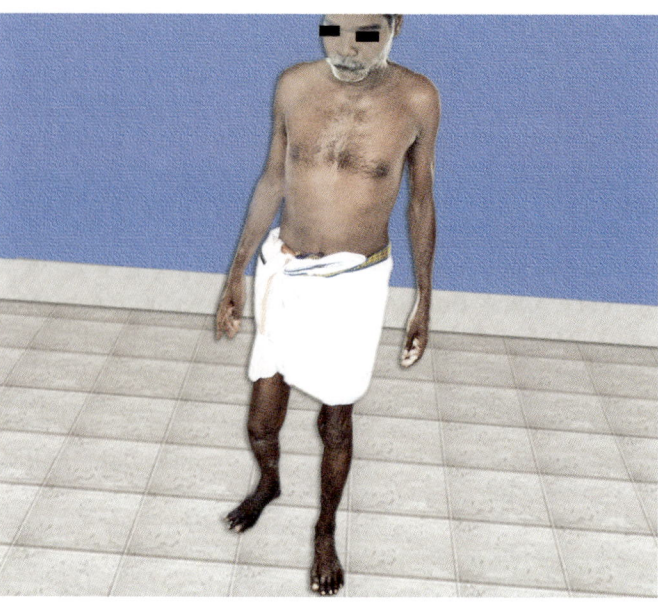

Fig. 3-62 Checking the gait in an ulcer patient.

also checked. Tuberculous bacteria are detected by AFB study. Cytology of discharge is done when malignancy is suspected. Discharge is useful to identify actinomycosis (sun ray appearance), Madura infection and fungal infection.

Wedge Biopsy

Wedge shaped biopsy is taken from the edge because edge contains multiplying cells. Usually two biopsies are taken. Because of central necrosis, biopsy may be inadequate if taken from the center. But in recurrent post-radiation malignant ulcer biopsy is taken from center, as active proliferating cells are present in the center not in periphery due to vascular fibrosis in the edge by radiotherapy.

Imaging

X-ray of the part (underlying bone) to see periostitis or osteomyelitis (Fig. 3-65); to check infiltration in malignancy; to

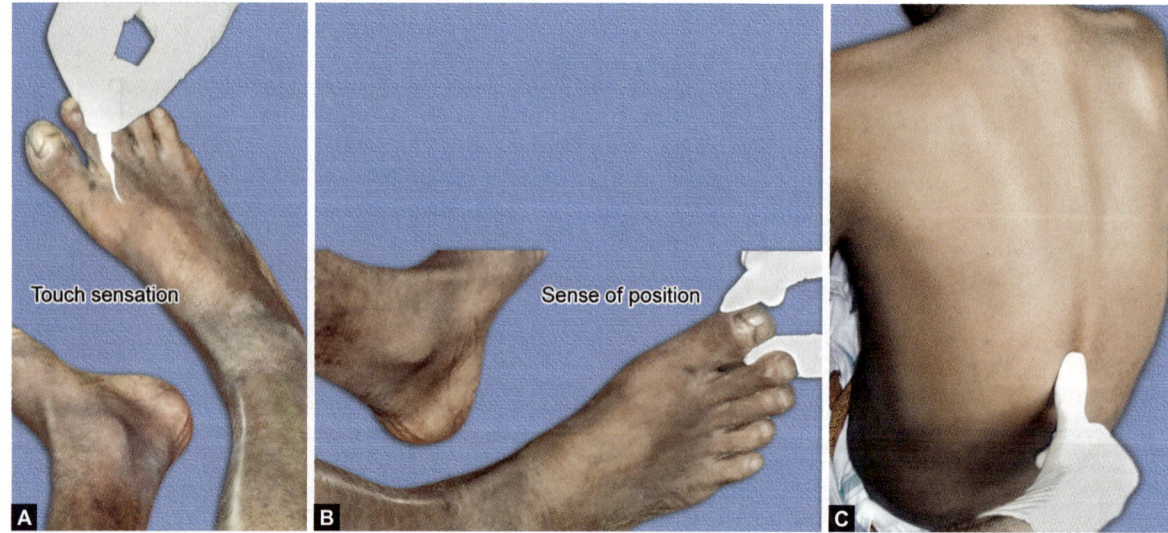

Figs. 3-61A to C Examination of neurological system is a must. Touch sensation and sense of positions are commonly tested. Checking the muscle power and grading should also be done. Spine should be examined for tenderness/deformity.

Chapter 3: Examination and Clinical Approach of an Ulcer

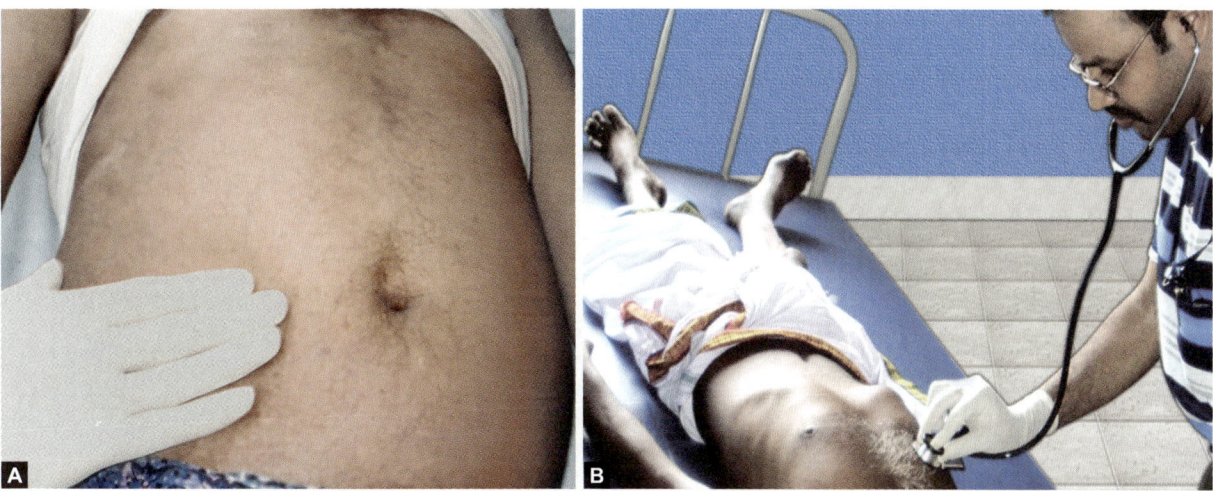

Figs. 3-63A and B Systemic examination like of abdomen, respiratory, cardiovascular system, spine, neurological examination is a must.

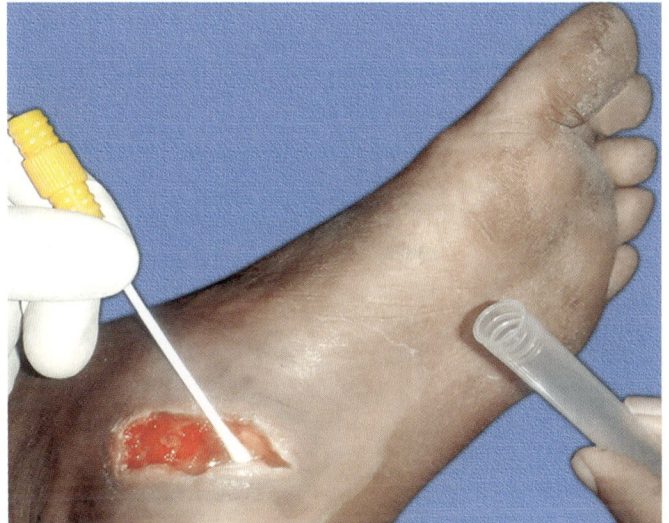

Fig. 3-64 Discharge is taken in a sterile swab to study culture and sensitivity and AFB.

find out involvement of bone in case of syphilis (gummatous ulcer) and in trophic ulcer.

MRI imaging is often better to identify bone, joint adjacent and soft tissue problems. MRI of spine if spinal pathology like tuberculosis/bifida/tumor is suspected.

Imaging for specific disease like for tuberculosis elsewhere in the body are to be assessed. Chest X-ray/CT chest in case of tuberculosis, angiogram in case of vascular cases.

Doppler imaging of the limb either arterial (in diabetic/ischemic ulcer) or venous (in venous ulcer). Plethysmography may be useful but not used routinely.

MRI spine in case of spinal diseases causing trophic ulcer.

Other Tests

FNAC of the regional lymph node is done in case of malignancy.

Blood tests: Hemoglobin and albumin levels in blood are important. Granulation tissue will not develop if Hb% is

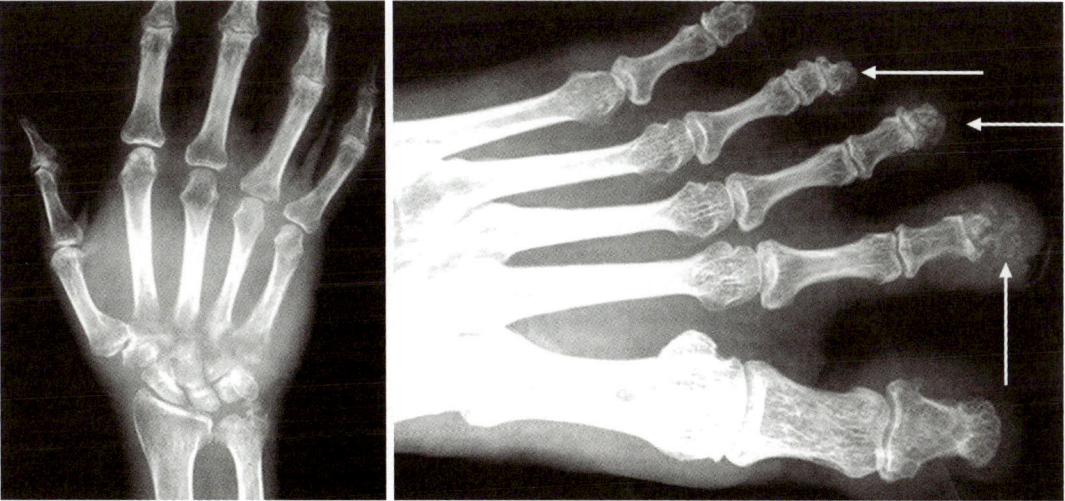

Fig. 3-65 X-ray showing osteomyelitis of the carpal bones in a diabetic patient with osteomyelitis of the terminal phalanges of the 2nd and 3rd toes. Clinically it is suspected by bone thickening.

below 10 g%; and if albumin is less than 3 g%. TC, DC, ESR (increased in tuberculosis), blood sugar/glycosylated hemoglobin (diabetic ulcer), VDRL (syphilitic), tests for HIV are done as needed.

Mantoux test in suspected case of tuberculous ulcer.

> Investigations are usually classified for clinician's easiness as:
> - *Routine investigations* like hemogram, ESR, blood sugar, serum creatinine, fasting lipid profile, ECG which is done in general in most of the surgical cases [it helps in identifying anemia, tuberculosis (indirectly), arthritis, diabetes].
> - *Specific/relevant investigations* are done in specific and relevant to that particular clinical condition in that particular patient like biopsy, X-ray of part, FNAC, discharge study, Doppler study etc. It is the clinician's discretion to identify which is routine and which is specific in that particular condition in that particular patient. It is standard practice to mention routine investigations first then specific investigations; however, specific investigations are *more important* in evaluation of the patient at that point of time.

> **Assessment of an Ulcer**
> Cause of an ulcer should be found—diabetes/venous/arterial/infective. Clinical type should be assessed. Assessment of wound is important—anatomical site; size and depth of the wound; edge of the wound; mobility; fixity; induration; surrounding area; local blood supply. Wound perimeter may be useful in assessing this. Wound imaging is done by tracing it on a transparent acetate sheet at regular intervals. Presence of systemic features; regional nodal status; function of the limb/part; joint movements; distal pulses; sensations should be assessed. Severity of infection should be assessed—culture of discharge. Specific investigations like edge biopsy; X-ray of part; blood sugar; arterial/venous Doppler; angiogram are done.

Granulation Tissue

It is seen on the floor of an ulcer consisting of proliferating new capillaries and fibroblasts intermingled with RBCs and WBCs with thin fibrin cover over it. It contains fine capillary loops, fibroblasts with thin fibrin and plasma covering. It is a reparative tissue preceding to epithelialization.

Types:

Healthy granulation tissue: It is seen in a healing ulcer. It has got sloping edge. It bleeds on touch. It has got serous discharge. Skin grafting takes up well in an ulcer with healthy granulation tissue (Fig. 3-66). Streptococci growth in discharge culture should be less than 10^5/gram of tissue before skin grafting.
Note: Healthy granulation tissue is—pink, pinpoint, painless, without pus, bleeds on pressure.

Unhealthy granulation tissue: It is pale with purulent discharge. Its floor is covered with slough. Its edge is inflamed and edematous. It is seen in spreading ulcer.

Unhealthy, pale, flat granulation tissue: It is seen in chronic nonhealing ulcer (callous ulcer).

Exuberant granulation tissue (proud flesh/hypergranulation/overgranulation): It is friable, soft, red overgrowth of granulation tissue protruding outwards from the floor of the ulcer which is due to prolonged stimulation of fibroblasts

> **Case sheet writing in an ulcer patient**
> **History**
> Name: Age:
> Occupation: Sex: Place/residence:
> **Chief complaints**
> *History of present illness*
> - Site and number
> - Mode of onset and progression
> - Duration
> - Pain in detail and fever
> - Discharge from ulcer
> - Associated symptoms
>
> *Past history*
> - Past history of ulcer
> - Tuberculosis, spinal diseases, diabetes, leprosy, malignancies
> - Past history of treatment and surgery
>
> *Family history*
> - Family tree; history of tuberculosis, ulcer, malignancies; treatment history
>
> **General examination**
> **Local examination**
> *Inspection*
> - Site and number
> - Size
> - Shape
> - Extent
> - Margin
> - Edge
> - Floor
> - Surrounding skin
> - Opposite side and neighboring structures
>
> *Palpation*
> - Tenderness
> - Temperature
> - Palpation of edge
> - Palpation of base
> - Depth and size of ulcer
> - Bleeding on palpation and touching
> - Palpation of deeper structures and its relation to ulcer
> - Palpation of surrounding area
>
> **Examination of adjacent joint(s)**
> **Examination of regional lymph nodes**
> **Examination of varicose veins**
> **Examination of peripheral pulses**
> **Examination of spine and neurological system**
> **Gait of the patient**
> **Systemic examinations**
> **Clinical diagnosis**
> **Investigations of an ulcer**
> *Routine investigations*—Blood tests
> *Specific investigations:* Study of discharge; wedge biopsy; imaging; FNAC
> **Final diagnosis**

and angiogenesis during the phase of secondary intention of healing process. It prevents the epithelial tissue/cells migration and so arresting the ulcer healing and contraction. Sprouting granulation tissue usually occurs in a sinus opening often with a retained foreign body in the sinus cavity or bone piece of dead tissue in the cavity underneath (Figs. 3-67 and 3-68).

Chapter 3: Examination and Clinical Approach of an Ulcer

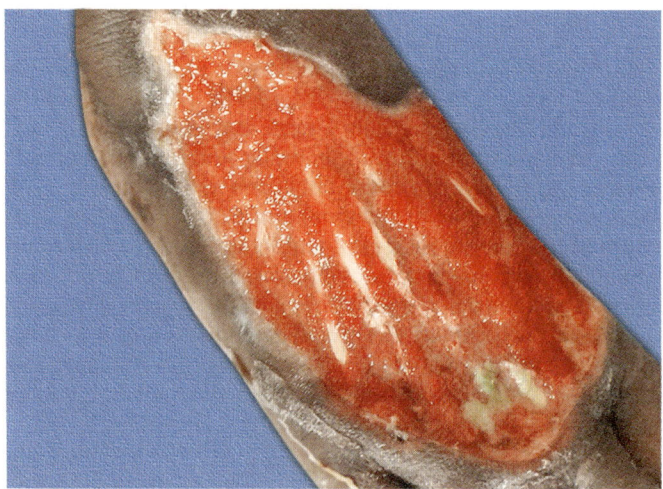

Fig. 3-66 Ulcer with healthy granulation tissue ready for split skin grafting.

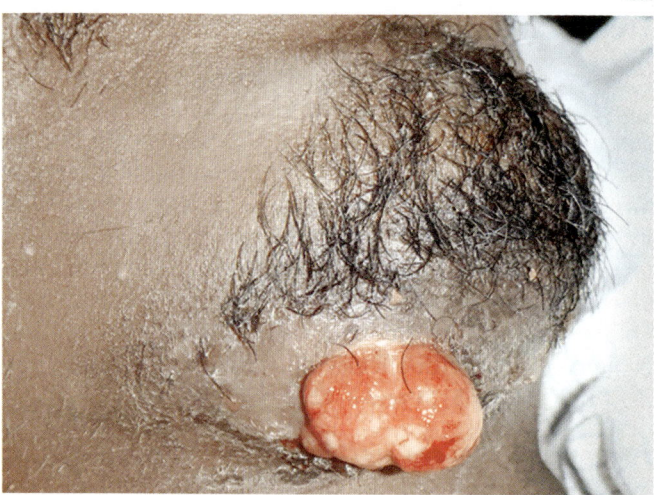

Fig. 3-69 Pyogenic granuloma.

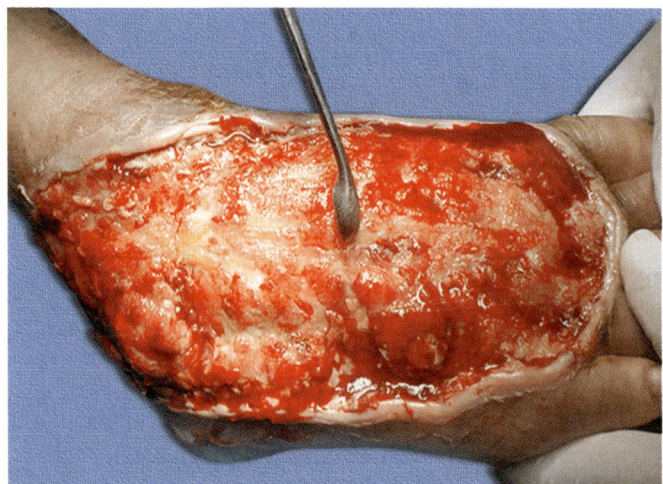

Fig. 3-67 Exuberant granulation (*proud flesh*) in an ulcer. It should be scooped out using Volkmann's scoop prior to skin grafting.

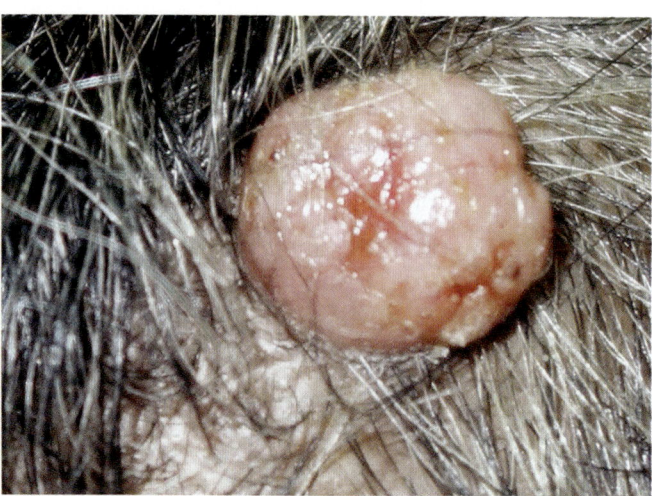

Fig. 3-70 Pyogenic granuloma scalp.

Causes of Nonhealing/Delayed Healing of an Ulcer

Local causes	General causes
• Lack of rest and immobilization • Repeated trauma, scratching and infection • Osteomyelitis of the underlying bone • Presence of edema, pus, fibrous tissue • When situated over the joints and bones • Presence of foreign body, sequestrum in the ulcer wound • Very large ulcer, immobile ulcer • Underlying arterial, venous, lymphatic diseases • Neurological causes	• Old age, anemia and hypoproteinemia • Vitamin deficiency—C, B, A • Diabetes mellitus • Debilitating diseases • Tuberculosis, syphilis, malignancy • Hypertension • Chronic liver and kidney diseases • Steroid therapy, HIV infection • Malignancy, radiotherapy, chemotherapy

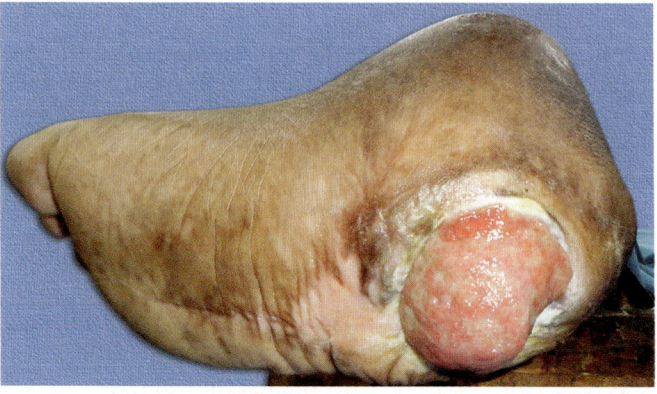

Fig. 3-68 Exuberant granulation in a heel ulcer.

Pyogenic granuloma: It is a type of exuberant granulation tissue. Here granulation tissue protrudes out from an infected wound or ulcer bed presenting as well localized, red swelling which bleeds on touch (Figs. 3-69 and 3-70).

Trophic Ulcer (Neurogenic/Neuropathic Ulcer)

It occurs due to impaired nutrition may be defective blood supply or more commonly due to neurological deficit. It is common in heel, heads of metatarsals, buttocks, over ischial tuberosity, over the shoulder or occiput. Initially callosity forms which extends deep as a central cavity due to repeated trauma, pressure, suppuration involving deeper muscles, tendons and bone causing typical perforating or penetrating ulcer. It is painless ulcer, with punched out edge; like a deep hole or burrow which is nonmobile with bone as base; its floor is often covered with offensive slough. Surrounding skin is anesthetic (**Figs. 3-71 and 3-72**).

> *Neurological causes are:* Diabetic neuropathy, peripheral neuritis, tabes dorsalis, spina bifida, leprosy, spinal injury, paraplegia, peripheral nerve injuries, syringomyelia, meningomyelocele.
> *Factors are:* Pressure, repeated trauma, moisture, anemia, malnutrition, bedridden patient, urinary incontinence and soiling.

Pressure sore/bed sore: It is the classical example of trophic ulcer. Once external pressure to skin increases more than 30 mm Hg (capillary occlusive pressure) blood flow to skin decreases causing tissue hypoxia, necrosis, and ulceration. It occurs over the bony prominences.

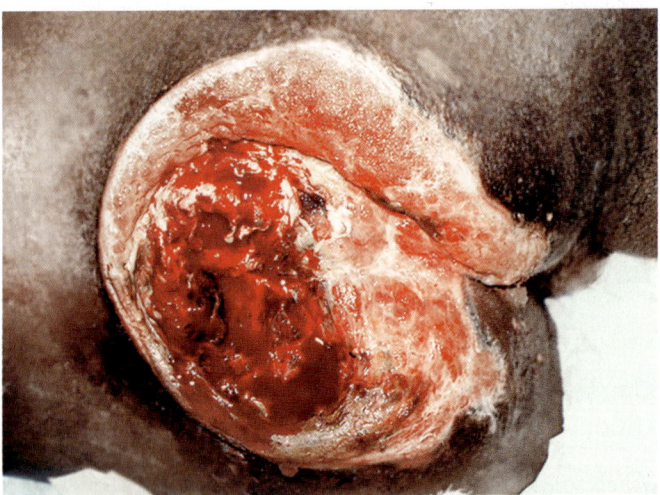

Fig. 3-71 Bedsore (decubitus ulcer) in sacral region—it is a trophic ulcer. It is usually with punched out edge.

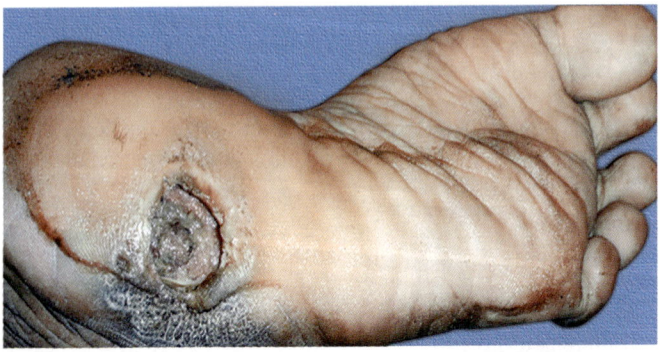

Fig. 3-72 Trophic ulcer heel. It is a punched out deep ulcer.

Tropical Ulcer

It is an acute ulcerative lesion of the skin in the legs and feet following trauma or insect bite observed in tropical regions like Africa, India and South America. It is associated with lower socioeconomic group, anemia, and malnutrition and vitamin deficiency. It is commonly caused by *Fusobacterium fusiformis* (Vincent's organisms) and *Borrelia vincenti*. They begin as abrasions, redness, papule and pustule formation, with acute regional lymphadenitis and severe pain, copious, serosanguinous discharge in floor with often undermined and raised edge is common. Eventually, it forms a chronic indolent large ulcer. After long time when it heals, it forms a pigmented, parchment paper like scar. Squamous cell carcinoma may be a occasional late complication in such disease.

> Tropical ulcer:
> - Caused by Vincent's organisms
> - Common in monsoon ridden tropics
> - Occurs in lower leg and foot in bare foot walkers
> - Unremitting constant pain
> - Slight constitutional symptoms
> - Copious seropurulent discharge
> - Overpowering vile (unpleasant) odor
> - Undermined edge
> - *Phagedena*, destruction of soft tissues widely and rapidly can occur
> - Chronic indolent ulcer may form lasting for many months or years
> - On healing, permanent parchment like faint pigmented scar
> - Squamous cell carcinoma can occur occasionally
>
> *Note:* Phagedena – Greek – to eat; it is rapid destruction without proliferation unlike in malignancy there is destruction with proliferation. Phagedena also occurs in chancroid and cancrum oris (Noma).

Diabetic Ulcer

Causes: Increased glucose in the tissue precipitates infection; diabetic microangiopathy affects microcirculation; increased glycosylated hemoglobin decreases the oxygen dissociation; increased glycosylated tissue protein decreases the oxygen dissociation; diabetic neuropathy involves all sensory, motor and autonomic components; associated atherosclerosis affects the circulation.

Sites: Foot-plantar aspect—is the commonest site; leg; upper limb; back; scrotum; perineum, etc. Diabetic ulcer may be associated with ischemia. Ulcer is spreading and deep (Figs. 3-73 and 3-74).

Painless ulcer to begin with, becomes deep penetrating, chronic type due to constant infection, varying in size and shape with inflamed edges, slough and seropurulent discharge in floor, with base fixed and surrounding skin relatively healthy. There may be loss of underlying muscle reflexes and limb deformity in chronic ulcer. Diabetic ulcer can be trophic type when there is neuropathy.

Problems with diabetic ulcer: Neuropathy, in foot—clawing of toes, hammer toe (due to intrinsic muscle paralysis); multiple deeper abscesses; osteomyelitis of deeper bones are common; reduced leucocyte function; resistant infection; spreading cellulitis; arterial insufficiency; septicemia; diabetic ketoacidosis; associated cardiac diseases like ischemic heart disease.

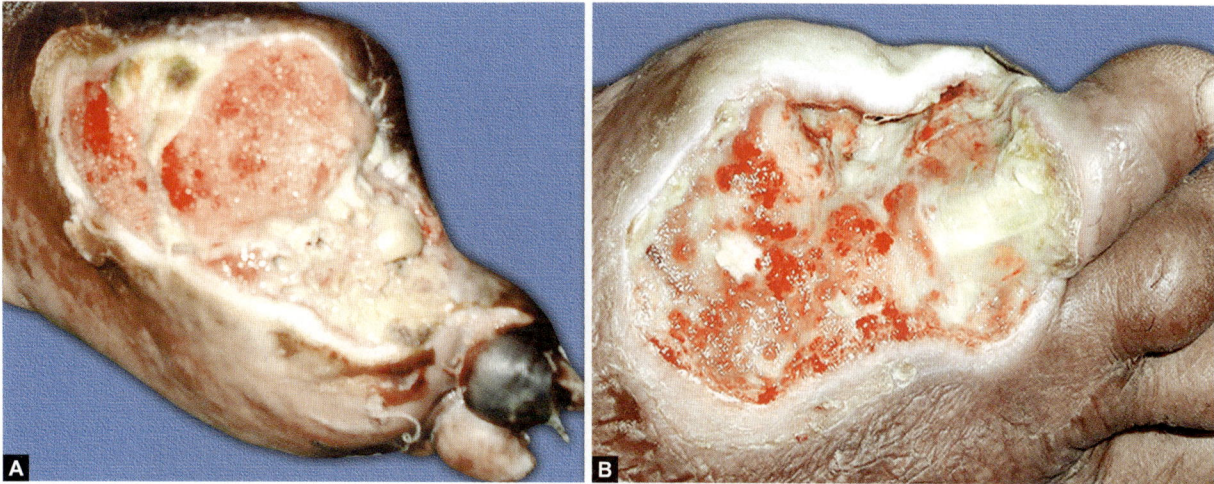

Figs. 3-73A and B Foot is the commonest area for diabetic infective problems. It can cause abscess, ulcer, osteomyelitis, gangrene, septicemia. Initially patient undergoes toe amputation but later eventually may require below knee or above knee amputation.

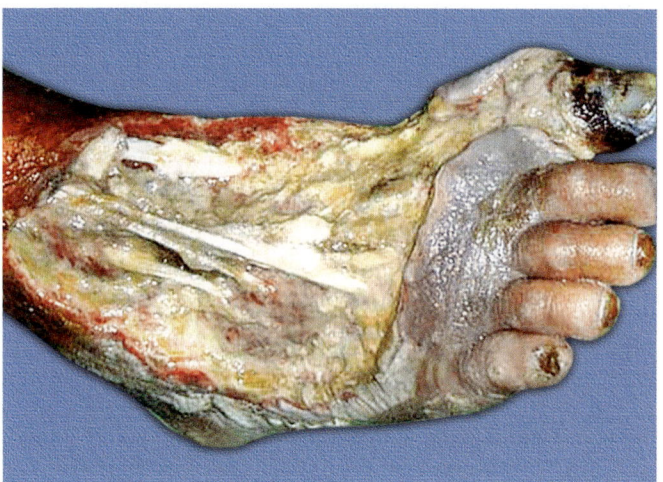

Fig. 3-74 Infective ulcer in the foot. Note the quantity of slough, exposed tendon and gangrenous great toe. Patient might require below knee/above knee amputation.

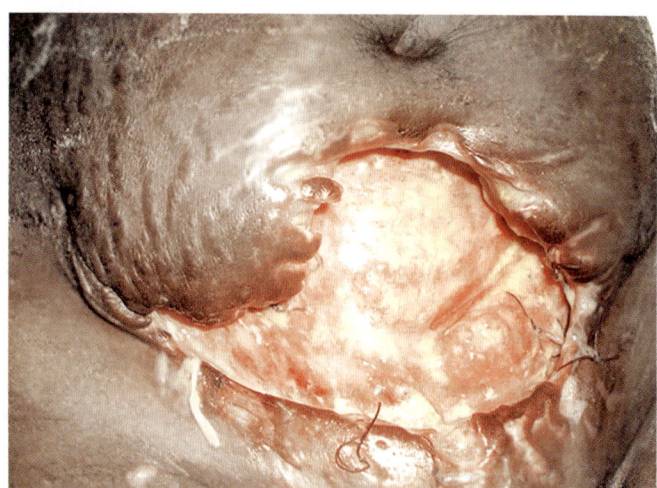

Fig. 3-75 Meleney's postoperative synergistic gangrene.

Meleney's Ulcer (Postoperative Synergistic Gangrene, Pyoderma Gangrenosum)

It is commonly seen in postoperative wounds in abdomen and chest wall like in drainage of empyema or surgery for peritonitis. It is an acute rapidly spreading ulcer with gangrene of skin and subcutaneous tissues. It is common in old age, immunosuppressed people and when surgery is done in infected conditions. It is caused by *symbiotic effect* of microaerophilic nonhemolytic streptococci and hemolytic *Staphylococcus aureus*. It occurs commonly in lower abdomen after surgical treatment for perforated bowel or in the thorax after surgical treatment of the drainage of empyema thoracis. It can occur in other areas of skin also. Very rarely it can occur in leg or back of hand when patient is suffering from ulcerative colitis. Clinically, patient is toxic. Ulcer is rapidly spreading painful and tender with large quantity of foul smelling serosanguinous discharge, showing undermined deep edge with surrounding area having immediate deep purple zone and outer red zone. Floor is covered with abundant unhealthy granulation tissue. Infection is severe with endarteritis of the skin leading to ulcer and destruction. It needs an emergency critical care therapy. Condition has got high mortality (Fig. 3-75).

Tuberculous Ulcer

It is due to breaking of the underlying cold abscess and collar stud abscess or tuberculous lesion of bones and joints onto the surface of skin. It is common in neck, axilla and groin. But it can occur anywhere in the skin. Primary cutaneous tuberculosis with single or multiple ulcers (usually) also can occur. Tuberculous ulcer are usually painless presents with thin, *bluish and undermined edge* (Figs. 3-76A and B). Disease spreads more in the deeper subcutaneous plane than in the skin. Hence, skin overhangs directing towards centre. It *is rounded or oval* in shape. Floor contains pale, blue granulation tissue (apple *jelly appearance*). Yellowish discharge which is caseating material is common. Base is not indurated, surrounding skin may be pigmented. Regional lymph nodes may get enlarged which are *matted, firm* and nontender. Ulcer may form after burst open/rupture of the *caseating tuberculous lymphadenitis*. Mantoux test; study of

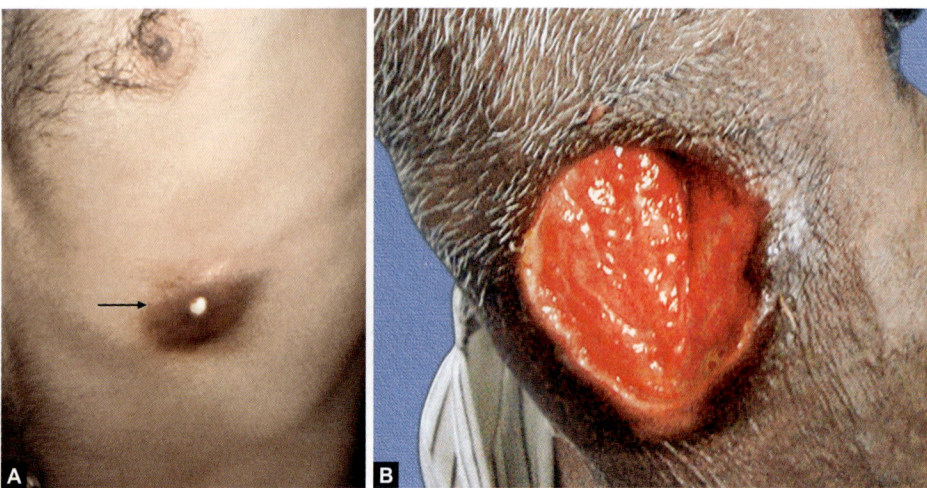

Figs. 3-76A and B Tuberculous ulcer over chest wall and neck. Neck is the common site and is from tuberculous lymphadenitis. Note the undermined edge. Discharge study, biopsy and later antituberculous drugs are the treatment.

discharge; AFB staining (Ziehl Neelsen), AFB culture using Lowenstein Jenson media; wedge biopsy from the edge to look for epithelioid cells; ESR, chest X-ray are needed investigations. *Epithelioid cells* (modified histiocytes) are typical of tuberculosis.

Lupus Vulgaris

Lupus means 'wolf'. It indicates the *spreading destructive* lesion. It is cutaneous *tuberculosis* which occurs in young age group. Commonly it is seen in face, hands and forearm; starts as *typical apple-jelly nodule* with congestion of face around. It is confirmed by preparing the area using a glass slide which removes the surrounding hyperemia temporarily. Biopsy of the lesion for AFB (acid fast bacilli) and tissue histology confirms tuberculosis. It begins as superficial single or multiple nodules in skin which eventually forms multiple superficial ulcers with scarring, necrosis and *undermined edge*. Center area gradually heals apparently; periphery shows active spreading disease. Often lesion extends into nose and oral cavity involving mucosa. Due to lymphatic obstruction edema of face can occur. Long standing lupus vulgaris can turn into *squamous cell carcinoma (Marjolin's)*.

Traumatic Ulcer

Such ulcer occurs after trauma. It may be mechanical—dental ulcer in the margin of the tongue due to tooth injury; physical like in electrical burn; chemical like in alkali injury. Such ulcer is acute, superficial, painful and tender. Secondary infection or poor blood supply of the area make it chronic and deep.

Arterial/Ischemic Ulcer

It is common in toes, feet or legs; often can occur in upper limb digits. It is due to poor blood supply following blockage of the digital or medium sized arteries. Atherosclerosis and thromboangiitis obliterans (TAO) are common causes in lower limb. Cervical rib, Raynaud's phenomenon and vasculitis are common causes in upper limb. Ulcer initially occurs after

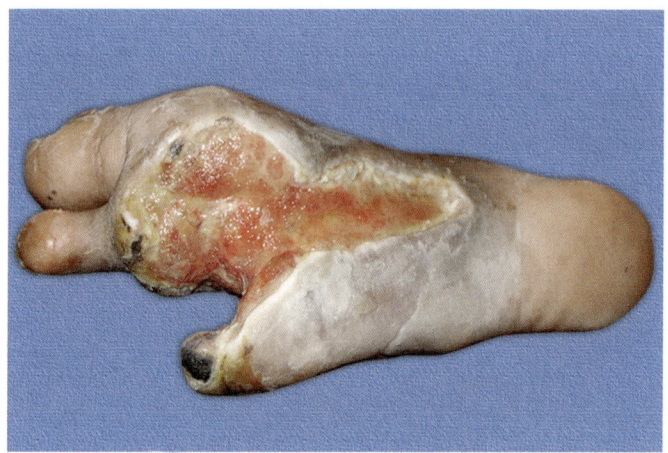

Fig. 3-77 Ischemic ulcer foot. Note little toe is blackish.

trauma, soon becomes nonhealing, spreading with scanty granulation tissue. Ulcer is very painful, tender and often hyperesthetic. Digits may often be gangrenous. Intermittent claudication, rest pains are common. Other features of ischemia are obvious in the adjacent area. They are—pallor, dry skin, brittle nail, patchy ulcerations, and loss of hair. Peripheral pulses may be weak/absent. Ulcer is usually deep, destructs the deep fascia, exposing tendons, muscles and underlying bone. Dead tendons look pale/greenish with pus over it. Arteriography, Doppler, plethysmography are done for diagnosis (Fig. 3-77).

Venous Ulcer (Gravitational Ulcer)

It is common around ankle *(gaiter's zone)* due to chronic venous hypertension. It is due to *varicose veins* (long saphenous vein/short saphenous vein/perforators) or *post-phlebitic* limb. Post-phlebitic limb is partially recanalized deep venous thrombosis which causes increased venous pressure around ankle through perforators. Varicose veins are common in *females*. 50% of venous ulcers are due to varicose veins; 50% is due to post-phlebitic limb (previous DVT). Pain, discomfort, pigmentation, dermatitis, lipodermatosclerosis, ulceration, periostitis, ankle joint ankylosis, talipes equinovarus deformity and Marjolin's ulcer are the problems of varicose veins and later venous ulcer. Ulcer is initially painful; but once chronicity develops it becomes painless. Ulcer is often vertically *oval*; commonly located on the *medial side*; occasionally on lateral side; often on both sides of the ankle; but *never* above the middle third of the leg. *Varicose ulcer* is *superficial*, *painless* and usually *will not* penetrate deep fascia; base is indurated and usually free and mobile. *Post-thrombotic/post phlebitic ulcer* is due to previous deep vein thrombosis; it is *painful* and *always* penetrates the deep fascia; hence base is fixed to deeper structures. Floor is covered with pale or often without any granulation tissue when well granulated edge is sloping. Induration and tenderness is seen often in the base of an ulcer. Ulcer heals on rest and treatment; but reforms again. Inguinal lymph nodes (*vertical* group) are often enlarged whenever there is active or recurrent infection and inflammation. Ulcer often attains very large size which is nonhealing, indolent and callous. Scarring is common due to repeated healing and recurrent ulcer formation (Fig. 3-78). This *unstable scar* of long duration may lead into squamous cell carcinoma (*Marjolin's ulcer*) (Fig. 3-79).

Venous Doppler, venography, study of ulcer discharge, wedge biopsy, X-ray part are done as investigations.

Carcinomatous Ulcer (Epithelioma, Squamous Cell Carcinoma, SCC)

It arises from prickle cell layer of skin. It may initially begin as a nodule or ulcer; but later forms an ulcerative lesion with rolled out/everted edge (Fig. 3-80). Floor of this *nonhealing ulcer* contains unhealthy tumor tissue which is friable, with blood and necrotic yellowish material. Ulcer bleeds on touch and is vascular and friable. *Induration* is felt at the base and edge. It is usually circular or irregular in shape. Initially, ulcer is mobile but becomes nonmobile once it infiltrates into deeper tissues. Hard, discrete, initially mobile but later fixed regional lymph nodes are often palpable. Lymph nodes can fungate eventually. Ulcer and lymph nodes are initially painless; but becomes painful and tender once there is deeper infiltration or secondary infection. Systemic spread is rare. It is a *locoregional malignant* disease.

Verrucous carcinoma is exophytic, locally malignant well differentiated squamous cell carcinoma without lymphatic spread.

Epithelioma (*SCC*) occurs due to chronic irritation, exposure to sunlight, Bowen's disease (Fig. 3.81), leukoplakia, chronic venous ulcer, radiation dermatitis, lupus vulgaris, papilloma, immunosuppressed individual, and senile keratosis. It is common in skin, oral cavity, esophagus, larynx, respiratory tract, penis, anus, vulva; it can occur as squamous metaplasia from columnar cells and then squamous cell carcinoma in esophagogastric junction, stomach, gallbladder, and bronchus; as metaplasia from transitional cells in urinary bladder. It can be ulcerative, nodular, proliferative (cauliflower like), ulceroproliferative (Fig. 3.82). It may begin as nodule or crack or fissure or ulcer. Histologically malignant cells with epithelial pearls are diagnostic. Based on epithelial pearls it is graded (*Broder's*) as—(1) more than 75% pearls; (2) 50–75% pearls; (3) 25–50% pearls; (4) less than 25%. (For details refer Chapter 4: Examination and Clinical Approach of a Swelling/Lump).

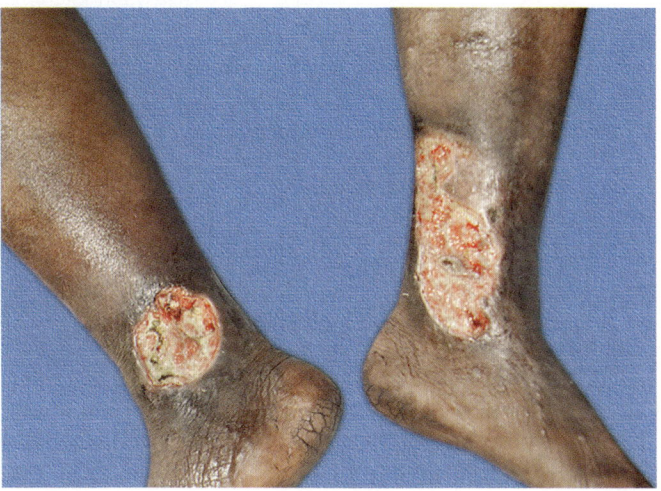

Fig. 3-78 Venous ulcer both legs (gaiter's zone). Ulcer once granulates needs split skin grafting; also needs definitive therapy for varicose veins.

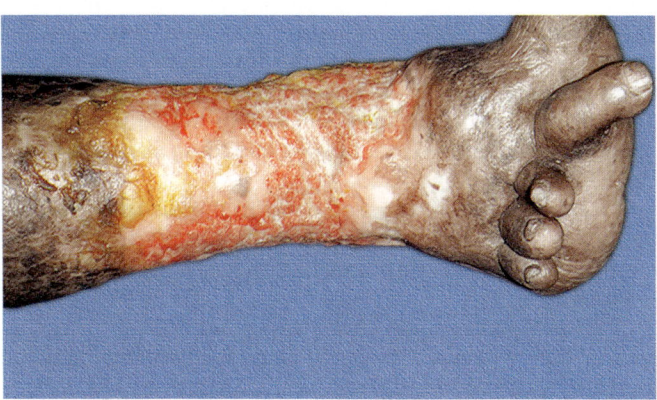

Fig. 3-79 Marjolin's ulcer occurring in an old scar (burn scar or scar of venous ulcer).

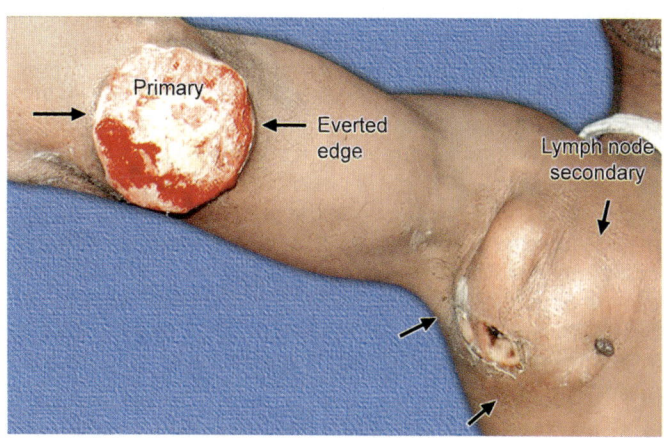

Fig. 3-80 Squamous cell carcinoma in the arm with secondaries in the axillary lymph node. Friable tumor tissues in the floor causing bleeding after trauma. Secondaries are fixed with ulceration. It is advanced disease.

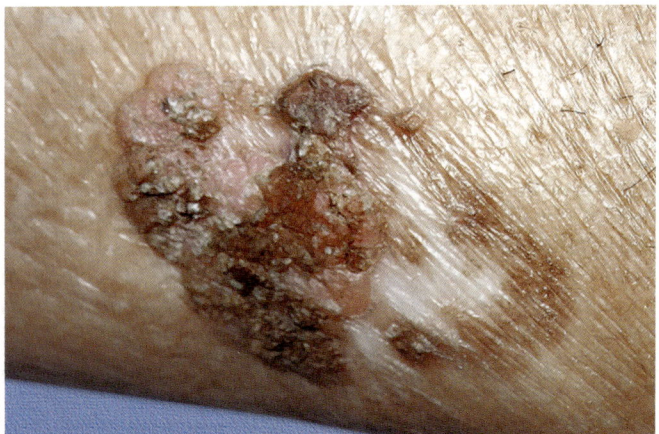

Fig. 3-81 Bowen's disease over the shoulder region. It is erythematous plaque with irregular border with crusts and scales; it is squamous cell carcinoma in situ. It is common in women, in sun exposed areas. Erythroplasia Queyrat is a type of squamous cell carcinoma in situ which occurs in the glans or prepuce in males; vulva in females; it may be caused by human papilloma virus (HPV).

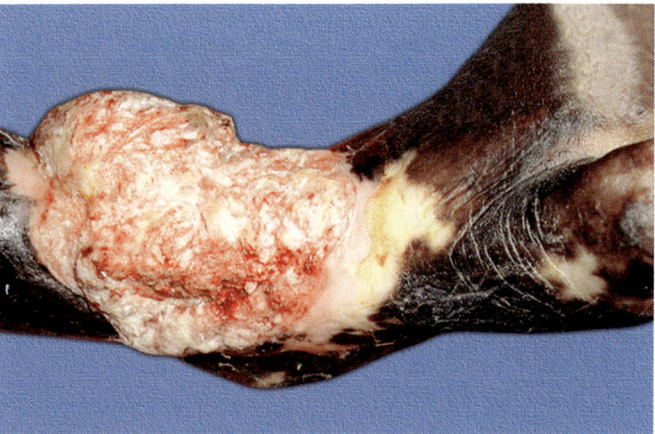

Fig. 3-83 Marjolin's ulcer in the leg. It occurs in an unstable scar of long duration. It does not spread through lymphatics.

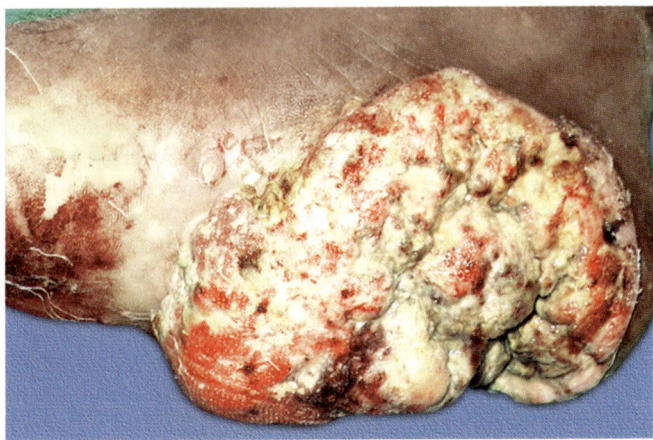

Fig. 3-82 Proliferative squamous cell carcinoma heel. Note the rolled out (everted) edge.

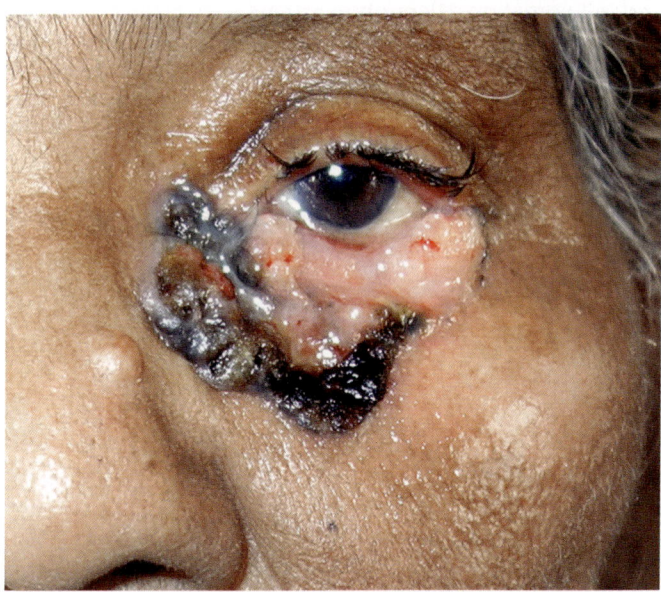

Fig. 3-84 Typical basal cell carcinoma (BCC) with beaded look. Typical site above the line joining the angle of the mouth to ear lobule (*Onghren's line*) is observed.

Marjolin's Ulcer (1828) [Rene Marjolin (1812–1895, Surgeon, Paris) Identified it in Scar of Burns]

It is *slow* growing *locally* involved malignant lesion—a very well differentiated squamous cell carcinoma occurring in *unstable scar of long duration*. It is commonly seen in chronic venous ulcer scar. Often it is observed in burns scar and scar of previous snake bite. Lesion is ulcerative/proliferative. Edge may be everted or may not be. It is painless as scar does not contain nerve fibrils. It *does not* spread into lymphatics as scar is devoid of lymphatics. Induration is felt at edge and base. There is marked fibrosis also. Once lesion spreads into adjacent normal skin, it can spread into regional lymph nodes (Fig. 3-83).

Rodent Ulcer

It is ulcerative form of basal cell carcinoma which is common in face (*tear cancer*, occurs at the site where tears roll down) (Fig. 3-84). Ulcer shows central area of dry scab with peripheral active raised and *beaded (pearly white)* edge. Ulcer is circular in outline; edge is not everted but raised, heaped up with tiny nodules with a peculiar pearl like luster with a minute venules. Edge is raised or rolled but *never everted*. Often floor is pigmented, and covered with scab containing dried serum and epithelial cells. It erodes into deeper plane like soft tissues, cartilages and bones hence the name— *rodent ulcer* (it gnaws/eats tissues including bone like a rat). Base is indurated and fixed.

As lymphatics are blocked early in the disease by large tumor cells (*tumor emboli*), it does not spread to regional lymph nodes. Blood spread is absent. It is only *locally malignant*.

It is common in area where bright sunlight (UV light) is present like Australia; it is rare in dark skinned; it is common in old age; common in males; very slow growing in months or years. It is common in face; rarely it can occur over tibia, external genitalia, mucocutaneous junction. It does not occur in mucosa (For details refer Chapter 4: Examination and Clinical Approach of a Swelling/Lump).

Melanotic Ulcer

It is ulcerative form of melanoma. It can occur in skin as de novo or in a pre-existing mole. Ulcer is pigmented often with a halo around (Fig. 3-85). Ulcer is rapidly growing, often with satellite nodules and 'in-transit' lesions. It is very aggressive skin tumor arising from melanocytes. It spreads rapidly to regional lymph nodes which are pigmented (Figs. 3-86A and B). Blood spread is common to liver, lungs, brain, and bones. It can occur in mucosa, genitalia, and eye. It is a systemic malignant disease (For details refer Chapter 4: Examination and Clinical Approach of a Swelling/Lump).

Syphilitic Ulcer

It is caused by *Treponema pallidum;* nowadays it is rare. It is sexually transmitted disease.

Primary syphilis occurs 4 weeks after infection. Typical genital chancre (hard/Hunterian chancre) is painless, hard, indurated nonbleeding ulcer. Chancre can occur in lips, breasts and anal region. Shotty painless, firm, discrete groin nodes are common. Healing occurs spontaneously.

Secondary syphilis features are—snail track ulcers in mouth; condyloma lata at mucocutaneous junction; shotty, discrete painless epitrochlear and suboccipital nodes; iritis, hepatitis (hepar lobatum, massive hepatomegaly); meningitis, osteitis with ivory sequestrum; moth eaten alopecia.

Tertiary syphilis features are—deep, punched out, painless, nontender gummatous ulcer with wash leather slough, indurated base, silvery tissue paper scar seen in subcutaneous bones like tibia, palate, skull. It can occur in tongue, scrotum (in front). Clutton's joint, sabre tibia, neurosyphilis, aneurysm of arch of aorta are other features. Lymph nodes are not enlarged in secondary syphilis. Tabes dorsalis with generalized paralysis of insane is called as later tertiary or quaternary syphilis.

Syphilitic stigmatas are—bossing of skull, nasal bridge depression, interstitial keratitis, otitis interna, perforation of nasal septum/palate, chronic superficial glossitis, Hutchinson's teeth, alopecia, mucosal patches, condyloma lata, enlarged epitrochlear and suboccipital lymph nodes, gumma testis, Clutton's joint, sabre tibia.

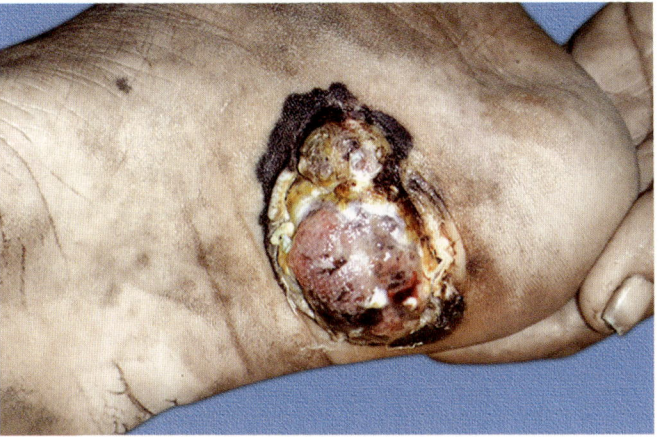

Fig. 3-85 Melanoma may present as pigmented ulcer.

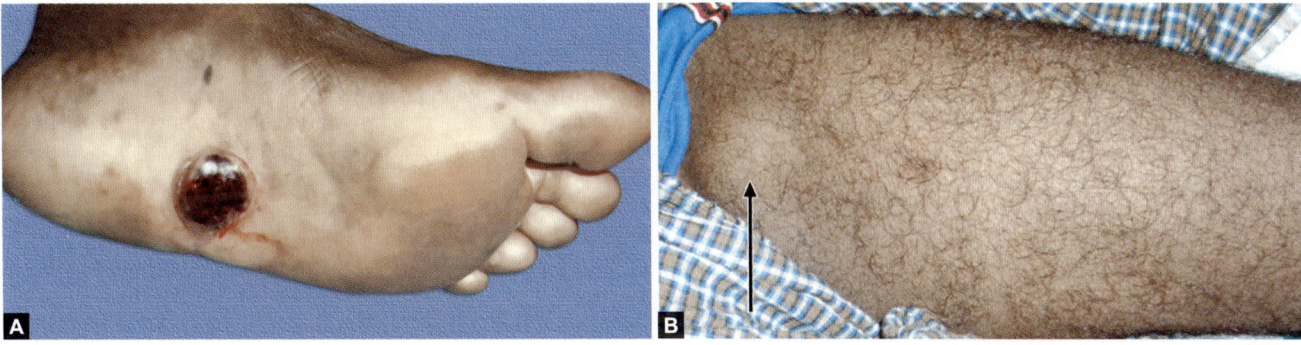

Figs. 3-86A and B Melanoma in the sole (foot) with secondaries in the inguinal lymph node.

■ OTHER ULCERS

Type	Causative factors	Features
Ulcer due to chilblains 'perniosis'	Due to exposure to intense cold causing cutaneous vasoconstriction	Blisters and superficial ulcers in the feet; common in women and children; common in winter
Ulcer due to frostbite	Due to exposure to wet cold below the freezing point causing intense arteriolar spasm	Gangrene of feet with deep ulcers
Martorell's ulcer	Seen in hypertensive patients often with atherosclerosis; common in females	Seen in calf, bilateral, painful, deep punched out ulcers extending into the deep fascia; all peripheral pulses are present and normal
Bairnsdale ulcer (Buruli ulcer)	Due to *Mycobacterium ulcerans*	Chronic, irregular, deep ulcer with undermined edges, with extensive dermal necrosis

Contd...

Contd...

Type	Causative factors	Features
Bazin's disease (erythema induratum/erythrocyanosis frigida)	May be due to *Mycobacterium tuberculosis*. Seen in adolescent girls with thick subcutaneous fat around ankle	Symmetrical, purple nodules develop in ankle and lower leg which later break down forming multiple, small, painful superficial ulcers with ankle edema and pigment scars. In cold season, ankle becomes cold, bluish and tender; in warm season ankle becomes warm, red, edematous, painful and tender due to hyperemia
Soft chancre or bubo	Venereal disease—*Haemophilus Ducreyi*	Acute, painful tender, nonindurated ulcers in genital region with acute regional lymphadenitis causing soft fluctuant inguinal swelling 'bubo'
Climatic bubo or tropical bubo	• Venereal disease—*Lymphogranuloma inguinale* (LGV)—L 1,2,3 • Lymphatic blockage and scarring can cause rectal stricture and vulval elephantiasis (esthiomene) in females	• Small, painless ulcers in the genitals in primary stage • Inguinal nodes enlarge suppurate with discharging sinuses in 2 weeks in males—second stage (intrapelvic/pararectal nodes in females) • In tertiary stage, eye, joint, meninges many involve after many years
Yaws (Frambesia)	*Treponema pertenue*	Multiple painless ulcers in leg and feet which spontaneously heel leaving tissue paper like scar
Oriental sore (Delhi boil/Baghdad sore)	*Leishmania tropica*	Indurated papule on face and exposed parts of body causing chronic indolent ulcer
Diphtheria desert sore	*Corynebacterium diphtheriae*	Initially forming as pustules in legs later bursting into an ulcer
Staphylococcal ulcer	Poor hygiene, trauma	Poor hygiene can cause typical multiple, small, red, recurrent, disturbing *Staphylococcus aureus* ulcers in leg and feet. **Footballer's ulcer** is traumatic staphylococcal ulcer seen in footballers; presents as chronic, deep ulcer in the shin

Leg ulcers:
Commonest site of an ulcer in the human body is lower limb (*foot and lower leg*).
Causes of leg ulcers:
Venous (varicose and postphlebitic/post-thrombotic), arterial, both venous and arterial; neuropathic/trophic; gummatous; diabetes mellitus; hemolytic anemia, polycythemia, ulcerative colitis, rheumatoid arthritis, Paget's disease of bone, traumatic; ulcers due to sickle cell anemia, Felty's syndrome, carcinomatous ulcer (malignant), melanoma; Marjolin's ulcer; tropical ulcer; Bazin's disease, tuberculous ulcer, hypertensive Martorell's ulcer; Meleney's ulcer; factitious ulcer.

Foot ulcers:
Foot ulcer may be isolated or often associated with leg ulcers. It can be one side or both sides.
Causes of foot ulcers:
Ischemic—diabetes mellitus, atherosclerosis.
Neuropathic—diabetes mellitus, Hansen's disease, peripheral neuropathy, chronic alcohol intake, poliomyelitis, spinal cord diseases or trauma.
Vascular diseases—autoimmune diseases like systemic lupus erythematosus (SLE), scleroderma, and hereditary spherocytosis.
Infections—Madura foot—fungal; Meleney's ulcer; tuberculous, syphilitic, other bacterial.
Malignancy—carcinoma, melanoma, Marjolin's ulcer, sarcoma (Kaposi's).

CASE DISCUSSION

A 40-year-old white complexion female finds a pigmented ulcerative lesion on her right waist which is increasing in color and size gradually for 3 months. Lesion is black, painless but with itching. No lesions are present elsewhere in the body. Size of the lesion is 1.5 cm. Lesion on examination showed slight bleeding on touch; induration is absent; 1.5 cm rounded ulcer with pigmentation; edge is spreading and irregular. Ulcer is mobile; not fixed to deeper structures. Surrounding area is normal.

What other clinical examination you will do?
Regional lymph nodes should be examined; here it is inguinal and external iliac lymph nodes—horizontal superficial inguinal nodes are examined; external iliac nodes are palpated above and medial to the inguinal ligament. Number, tenderness, size, surface, consistency, mobility, fixity, adherent to each other and to skin or deeper structures should be checked. If lesion is above the level of the umbilical region, axillary lymph nodes of same side should be examined. If it is at the level of the umbilicus both groin and inguinal nodes should

be examined. Abdomen should be examined for palpable liver often it may be massive hepatomegaly; its surface, consistency should be checked. Respiratory system, spine, other bones, central nervous system should be examined for metastases as melanoma can have systemic spread to lungs, liver, brain or bones.

How will you confirm the base of the ulcer?
Initially ulcer is checked for mobility; if it is freely mobile or mobility is restricted in one direction then muscle underneath should be contracted against resistance (*see Chapter 4: Examination of Swelling*) and mobility of the ulcer should be checked, if now there is no mobility then ulcer base is muscle underneath. If ulcer still shows mobility then base may be subcutaneous tissue or deep fascia. of base is formed by bone then there will be absent of mobility to begin with and ulcer will be deep.

What is your diagnosis and why and possible differential diagnoses?
Most probable diagnosis is malignant melanoma; reasons are—pigmented ulcerative lesion which is of short duration, progressive with itching and bleeding touch, there is absence of induration. Pigmented squamous cell carcinoma should be a differential diagnosis. But carcinomatous ulcer usually is ulcerative or ulceroproliferative with everted edge with induration of edge, base and often surrounding area. Foul smelling serosanguinous discharge is common. Regional nodes may be enlarged but systemic spread is uncommon in carcinomatous ulcer but can occur very rarely.

What you will do?
First routine and relevant (specific) investigations should be done. Specific investigations for melanoma are—excision biopsy, ultrasound abdomen, liver function test, chest X-ray or ideally CT chest; in suspected cases CT brain and radioisotope bone scan. If it is carcinomatous ulcer, wedge biopsy from the edge is done. In melanoma wedge biopsy is contraindicated as it will cause early spread of tumor cells systemically through opened vessels.

What is the staging and treatment?
TNM staging is done in melanoma only after excision biopsy report as 'T' part is based on the depth in mm of the lesion. Treatment is Handley's wide local excision with 2 cm clearance but depends on the depth of invasion of the tumor (Breslow's grading). Staging for squamous cell carcinoma is different.

(Please refer Chapter 3 and Chapter 4 of SRB's Clinical Methods in Surgery and melanoma topic of SRB's Manual of Surgery, current editions for discussion).

CHAPTER 4

Examination and Clinical Approach of a Swelling/Lump

Competency: SU6.1; SU18.1; SU18.2; SU18.3.

Swelling is a gross terminology which means protrusion from the body part usually considered as abnormal. It may be due to various causes like neoplasm, trauma, inflammation, familial, congenital, etc. which will be discussed in detail in later part of this chapter. In different places different terminologies are commonly used. In breast, 'breast *lump*' term is used; in abdomen '*mass* abdomen' term is used; they are rather a preferential usages of terms in clinical surgical practice.

'*Swelling*' denotes clear protrusion without affecting the gross nature of the part or organ, like swelling in the leg/thigh/arm/neck, etc., whereas '*lump*' is defined as lesion within the organ or causing the alteration in the gross nature/shape of the part or organ, like—lump in the breast; '*mass*' means lesion with difficulty to define its extent like —'mass abdomen' **(Figs. 4-1A and B)**.

■ HISTORY

Age: Cystic hygroma, a swelling in the neck commonly seen in infants and children. Benign swelling can occur at any age; sarcomas usually occur in younger age group **(Fig. 4-2)**.

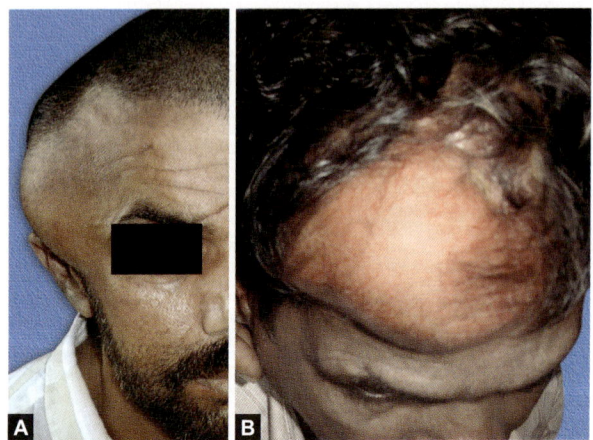

Figs. 4-1A and B Scalp swellings. It could be dermoid or skull secondaries (vascular) or intracranial tumor extending outward.

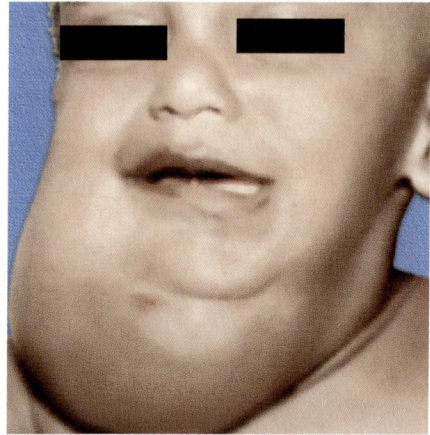

Fig. 4-2 Cystic hygroma—typical site.

Sex: Hypogastric swelling may be related to uterus or ovaries in females.

Occupation: Bursa, housemaid's knee or clergyman's knee, are swellings around the knee joint specific to certain occupation.

History of Present Illness

Swelling

Duration: It is important to note the duration of all swellings. Swelling which has been present since birth could be **congenital** like meningocele. Swelling of short duration associated with pain may be of **inflammatory** origin. Acute inflammatory swelling will be of short duration with severe pain. Chronic inflammatory swellings often have long duration with mild pain. **Benign tumors** are usually painless swelling of long duration. **Malignant tumors** present as swellings of short duration, rapidly enlarging, initially painless (but can be painful later). Patient may not be aware of the existence of a painless swelling for a long time. Often patient will not give much importance to a painless swelling **(Figs. 4-3 to 4-12)**.

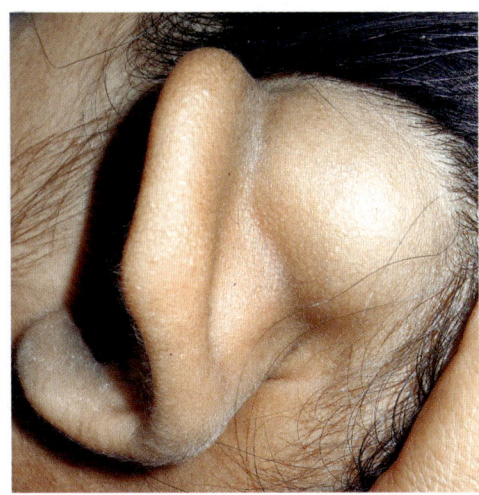

Fig. 4-3 *Post-auricular* dermoid; it is a sequestration dermoid.

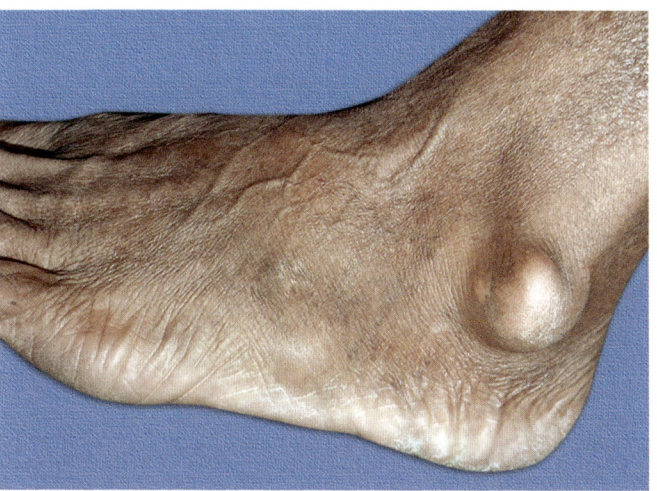

Fig. 4-6 *Adventitious bursa* over the lateral malleolus.

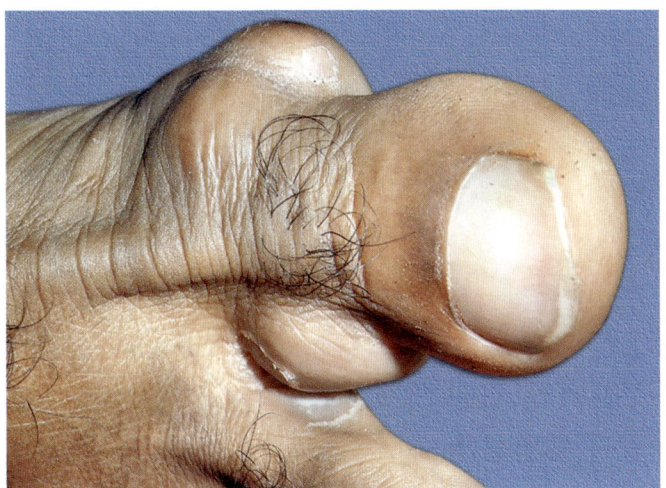

Fig. 4-4 *Implantation dermoid* foot around great toe.

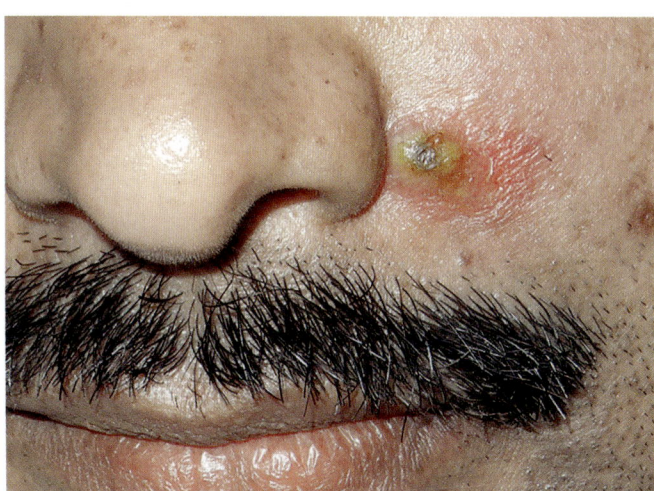

Fig. 4-7 *Inflammatory swelling* face; note the pus, redness–feature of a formed abscess.

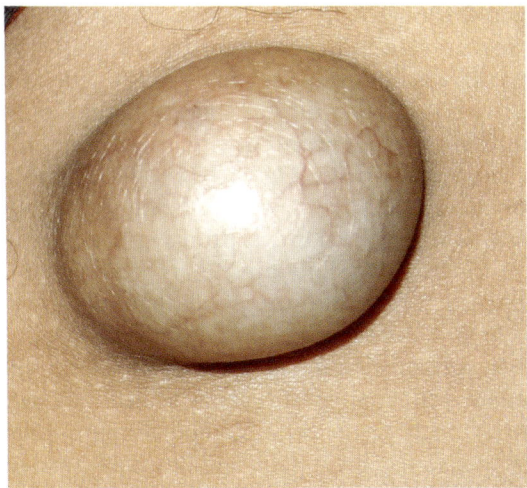

Fig. 4-5 Cyst in the thigh; it is subcutaneous; could be *sebaceous cyst*.

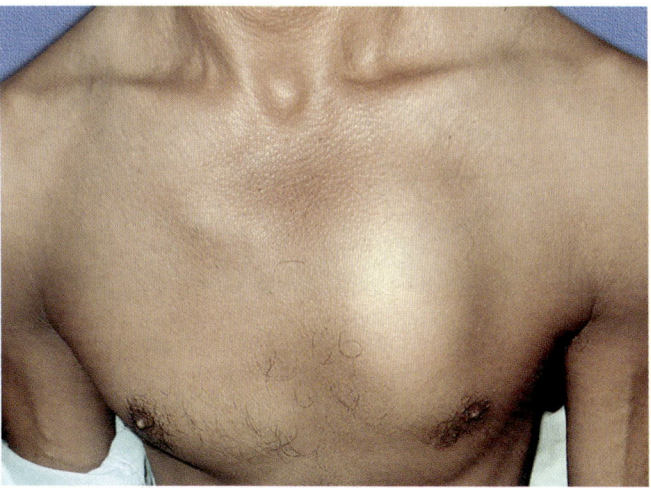

Fig. 4-8 Left sided *chest wall swelling*—it could be soft tissue tumor or cold abscess chest wall.

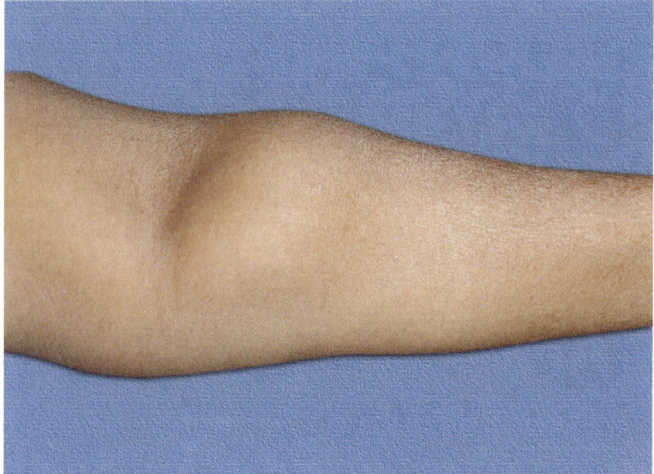

Fig. 4-9 *Benign swelling* forearm; it could be intramuscular lipoma.

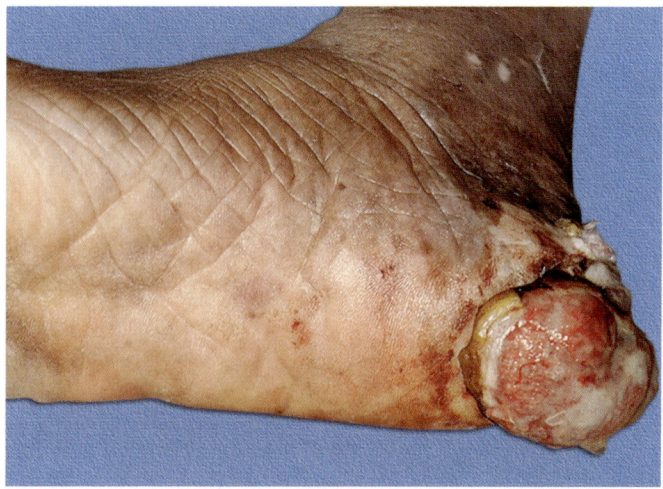

Fig. 4-10 *Malignant swelling* in the heel; it could be soft tissue sarcoma or amelanotic melanoma or aggressive squamous cell carcinoma.

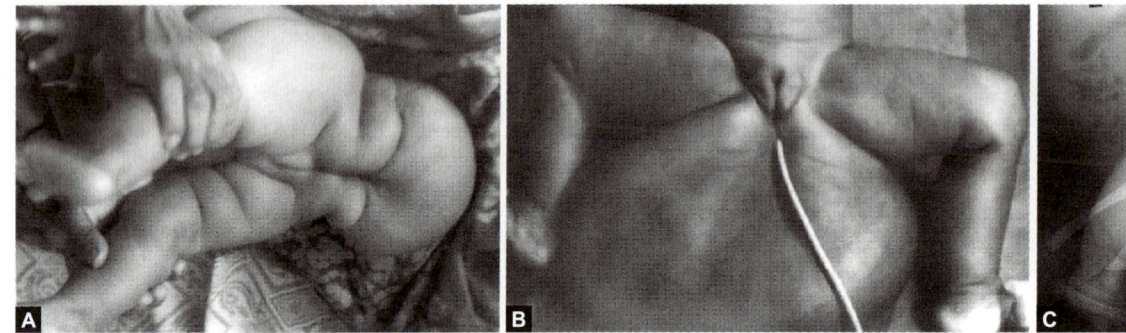

Figs. 4-11A to C *Sacrococcygeal teratoma* in newborn infants and also X-ray of the same condition.

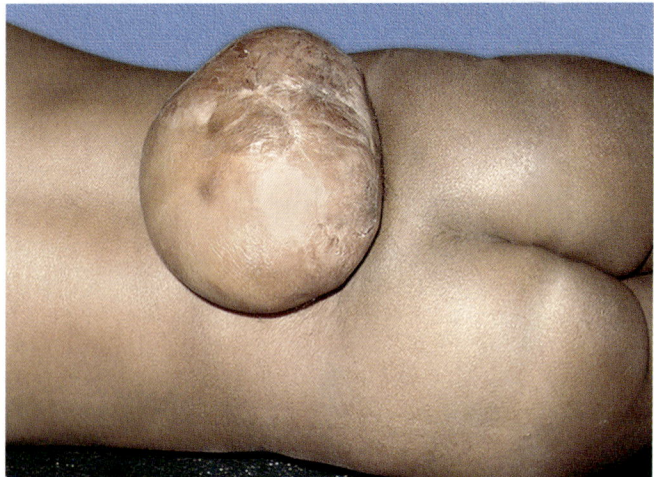

Fig. 4-12 *Spina bifida*—a congenital anomaly of spine presenting as swelling. Failure of fusion of posterior part of the spine is called as spinal dysraphism. It can be spina bifida occulta or spina bifida aperta. Meningocele, meningomyelocele, syringomyelocele, myelocele are different types of spina bifida aperta.

Mode of onset and progress: It is very important to take the history regarding the mode of onset of the swelling. Swelling whether occurred after trauma (example—hematoma) or spontaneously. It is important to note the rate of progress, whether rapid or slow; malignant swellings progresses rapidly whereas benign swellings progress slowly (lipoma, dermoid cyst). Sudden hemorrhage in a swelling can increase in size rapidly in minutes to hours. Sarcomas may progress rapidly in weeks. Swelling that shows recent rapid progress in size means probably benign lesion is turning into malignancy (naevus turning into melanoma; neurofibroma into neurofibrosarcoma). Swelling which eventually shows reduction in size is probably of inflammatory origin. Certain swellings may be stationary—status quo, i.e. neither progressive nor regressive. Pain and appearance of swelling after intramuscular injection into deltoid or gluteal region could be *injection abscess* (**Figs. 4-13A and B**); proper asepsis while giving injection will prevent formation of injection abscess. **Keloid** may develop over a previous scar over sternum or ear prick site or vaccination site in the shoulder. Keloid may increase in size continuously independent of the size of the scar and progress onto the adjacent skin (**Figs. 4-14A and B**). **Hypertrophic scar** can occur on a previous burn scar or traumatic scar wherein wound has healed with secondary intention; it progresses for certain period of time (6–12 months) and is limited to scar area; will not progress onto the adjacent normal skin. Thorn prick or needle prick (in tailors) can cause **implantation dermoid** due to forcible implantation of few cutaneous cells into deeper plane which causes reaction and localized adherent swelling (**Figs. 4-15A and B**).

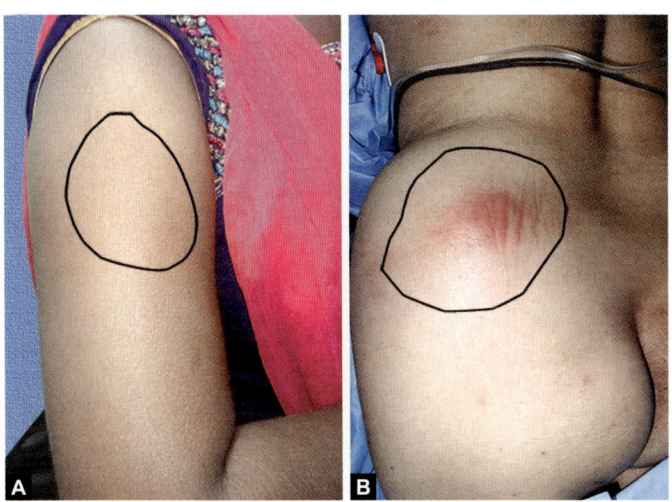

Figs. 4-13A and B *Injection abscess* in deltoid (A) and gluteal (B) region; it is often diffuse, red and warm with brawny induration; fever and difficulty in moving the arm will be common.

Site of beginning of the swelling: Site of beginning of the swelling and eventual progression is also often an important history to find out the anatomical origin of the swelling **(Figs. 4-16 to 4-18)**. Side and exact site should be asked. Size and shape of the swelling at the time of initial observation should be asked.

> **Recent increase in size of swelling, one should think of:**
> - Hemorrhage/hematoma
> - Infection/suppuration/abscess formation
> - Malignant change in a preexisting benign swelling
> - Hormonal changes–breast lump—ANDI
> - Luminal obstruction—increase in size of the submandibular salivary gland while eating due to obstruction of the duct by a salivary calculus

Number of swellings: Number of swellings patient has observed and which swelling has appeared first and next in order should be asked. Progression of each should be clarified **(Figs. 4-19 to 4-21)**.

Behavior of swelling: It may appear on standing and disappear on lying down as in case of hernia and saphena varix.

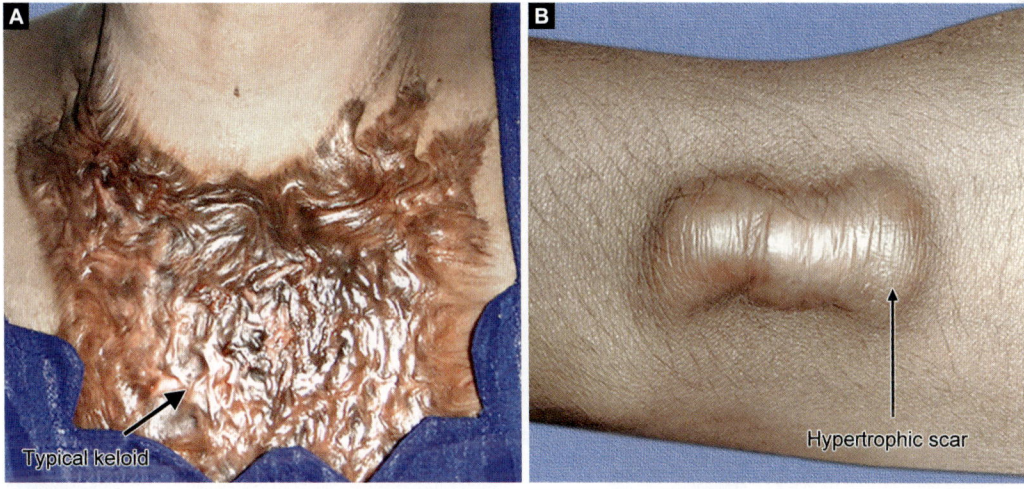

Figs. 4-14A and B (A) Typical look and site of the *keloid* over the sternum; (B) *Hypertrophic scar* is different from keloid.

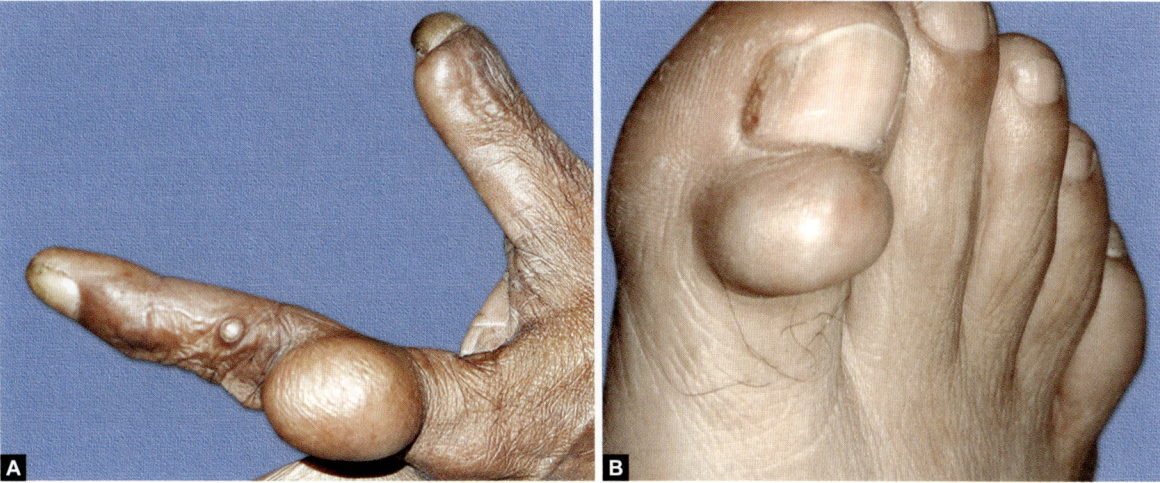

Figs. 4-15A and B Typical *implantation dermoid*—finger and the foot are the common sites.

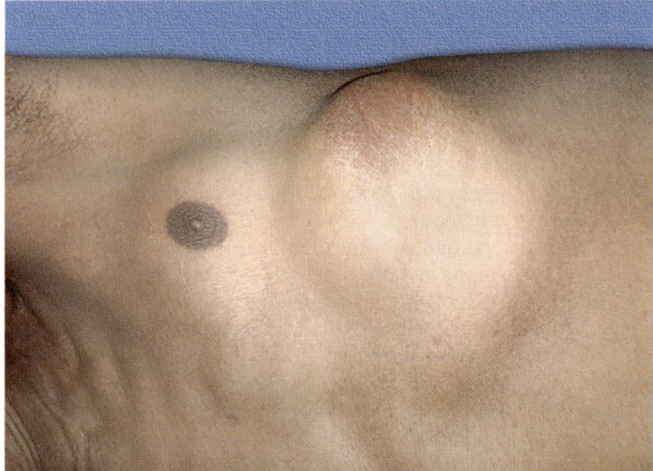

Fig. 4-16 *Abscess on chest wall.* Patient presented with swelling of acute onset and short duration with pain, redness, fever, swelling and tenderness.

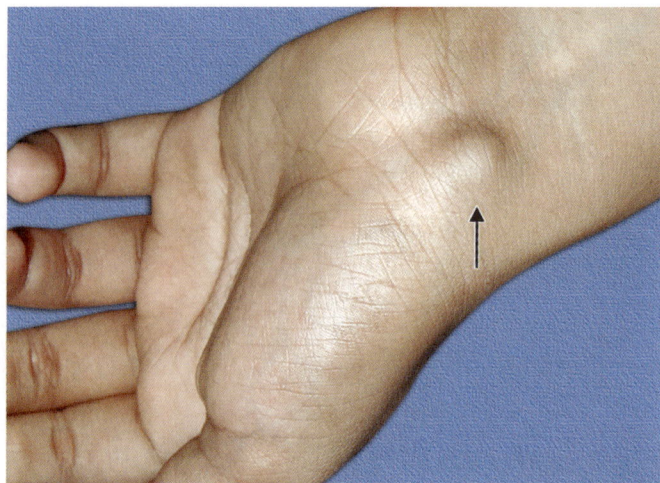

Fig. 4-18 Ganglion wrist—typical location. It is arising from the synovial sheath of the joint or tendon.

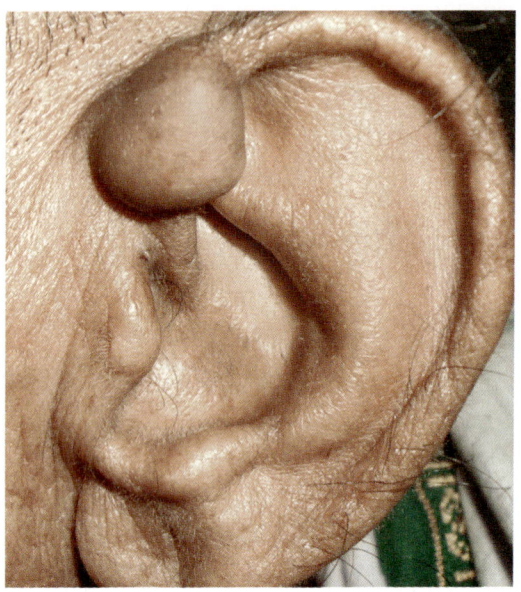

Fig. 4-17 Hematoma ear. It is subperichondrial hematoma, which usually occurs in boxers, wrestlers and rugby players, can also occasionally occur spontaneously. It presents as discoursed, doughy soft swelling with feeling of heaviness and discomfort. Fluctuation may be absent as there may be complete clotting of extravasated blood. It resolves very slowly. Often there is edema of adjacent part of the ear. Pain is usually absent. Repeated multiple subperichondrial hematomas of ear leads to cauliflower ear which is unsightly, deforming and often may lead into cartilage necrosis and destruction. Bleeding disorders should be thought of if hematoma is of spontaneous onset.

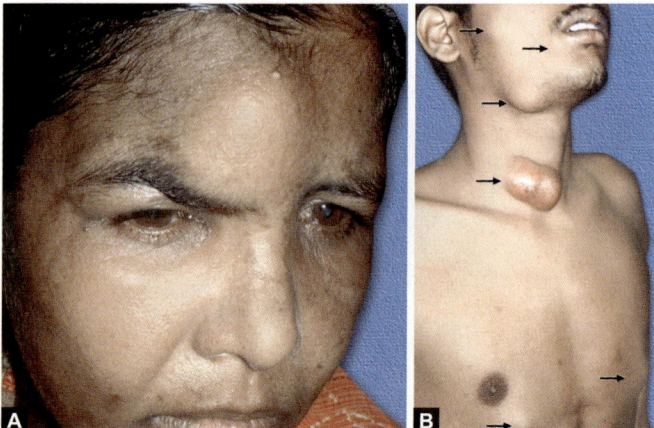

Figs. 4-19A and B (A) *Single (solitary) swelling* forehead region; it could be dermoid cyst, lipoma, osteoma or bony secondary; (B) *Multiple swellings (abscesses)* in different places; it could be pyemic abscess or multiple pyogenic abscess in immunosuppressed individual.

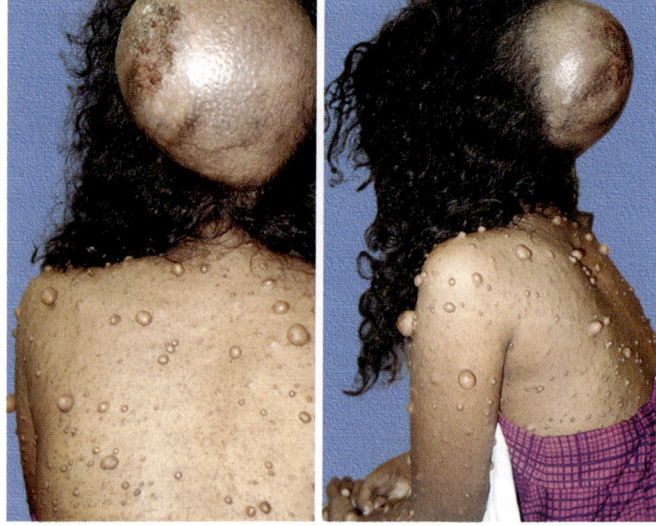

Fig. 4-20 Multiple neurofibromatosis—Von Recklinghausen's disease of neurofibromatosis. Note the multiple swellings all over the body. One of the swellings in the scalp has gone for malignant transformation—neurofibrosarcoma.

Pain

When did the pain start? Detailed history of location of pain/type of pain/severity/whether it interferes with work or not, is to be noted. Inflammatory conditions are painful, whereas malignant conditions are painless to begin with but later become painful. Infiltration into the nerves, soft tissues; ulceration; necrosis or inflammation may be cause of the pain

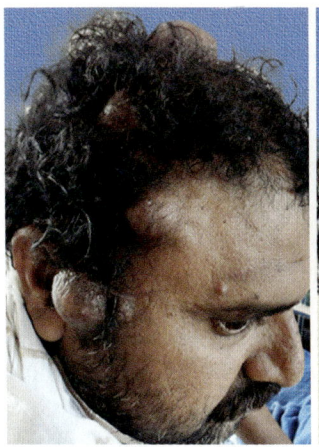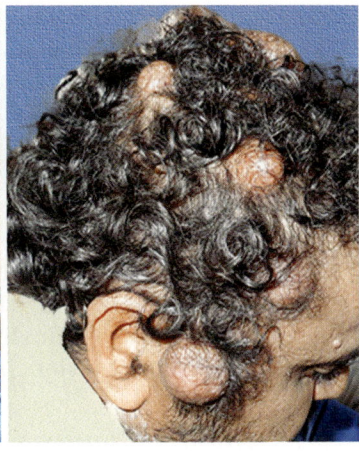

Fig. 4-21 Multiple scalp swellings—Turban tumor.

in malignancy eventually. Rapid enlargement of malignant tumor or hemorrhage also can cause pain in malignancy. Pain is usually over the swelling but often it can be deep seated pain or **referred pain** towards different place away from the swelling. In a large swelling, pain may be only over certain part of the swelling.

Nature of the pain is important to be noted. Pain may be **throbbing** in acute inflammation or suppuration; **burning** in inflammatory or neurological like herpes zoster infection, *aching, stretching, distending, deep seated, sharp, vague, stabbing,* etc.

Character of pain: Whether pain is mild/moderate/severe/ unbearable; continuous or intermittent; dull aching or throbbing (like in abscess or hematoma).

Pain is absent in benign swellings; present and is severe in acute inflammation; mild to moderate in chronic inflammation; pain is absent to begin with and later becomes painful in malignancy; dull ache pain may be a feature of few sarcoma to begin with prior to appearance of the swelling (osteosarcoma). Pain appears first in acute inflammatory conditions later swelling. Gastrointestinal malignancies, renal cell carcinoma, carcinoma breast, etc. are painless to begin with and becomes painful if there is deeper infiltration (nerves), infection, ulceration, etc.

Duration and specific features of pain in the swelling should be asked in detail.

Presence of Fever

Fever may be present in inflammatory conditions. Pyogenic abscess, acute lymphadenitis is associated with fever, often of high grade. Certain malignancies also can present with fever at later stage like in Hodgkin's lymphoma or renal cell carcinoma.

Presence of Other Lumps

Multiple neurofibromatosis, lipomatosis (Dercum's disease), multiple abscesses in the body generalized lymphadenopathy of any cause (Lymphomas) are the examples of multiple swellings in the body.

Secondary Changes

Secondary changes in the swelling like ulceration/fungation/ bleeding has to be noted.

Loss of Function

History of loss of function of a part or as a whole should be asked. Patient with cold abscess may show spinal pathology with alteration in limb movements, sensation, etc. Swellings adjacent or from the joint will show impaired joint function.

Loss of Weight

Loss of weight and decreased appetite may signify that swelling is related to malignant condition, probably advanced or tuberculosis.

Pressure Symptoms

Swelling may exert pressure on the adjoining structures producing symptoms, e.g. pressure on the larynx and trachea—hoarseness of voice and difficulty in breathing; on the esophagus—difficulty in swallowing.

Past History

History of previous surgery for similar swelling at the same site or different site or biopsy taken has to be asked for. Neurofibroma even though once excised often may occur at some other place in the body. Incomplete removal of an earlier benign lesion, either cyst or tumor or if the lesion is a malignant one, then recurrence can occur at the same site. Past history of diabetes mellitus, hypertension, tuberculosis, syphilis, gonorrhea often may be useful and should be asked for.

Previous treatment history, type of treatment—surgical or not, and if surgical—nature of surgery and its details like scar, drain, etc., hospitalization, outcome of the treatment, name of the hospital and treating doctor and whether patient is cured of the earlier illness or not, details of the earlier illness, whether earlier illness is related or similar like present one should be asked for.

Reappearance/recurrence of the swelling after the earlier surgical removal at the same site may indicate as recurrence of the disease, e.g. excision of the malignant swelling without clearance margin or sebaceous cyst excision with retained cyst wall enucleation in pleomorphic adenoma of salivary gland, excision of keloid may cause recurrence. Perianal abscess or pilonidal abscess (sinus) abscess may recur after drainage. How long before surgery was done, its details, any biopsy reports available should be asked in detail. Recurrence may be *true* recurrence like after adequate wide excision of the tumor; *perceived* as recurrence like appearance of similar swelling elsewhere (fibroadenoma appearing in different quadrant of breast after removal; neurofibroma occurring in different place close to the site of removal), *persistence recurrence* (residual disease) due to incomplete removal of the tumor.

Personal History

Personal history of alcohol consumption/smoking/tobacco chewing/history of sexual contact/dietary habits are also important. Altered appetite or weight loss can also be mentioned under personal history.

Family History

Family history suggestive of similar swellings is important. Neurofibromatosis is often familial. History of tuberculosis among the family members may be relevant in cold abscess. Certain malignancies can run in families.

■ GENERAL EXAMINATION

Detailed general examination is very essential. Anemia/edema/jaundice/clubbing/lymphadenopathy/radial pulse/blood pressure/raise in temperature/attitude of the patient/nutritional assessment by skin texture, subcutaneous fat, weight, body mass index/any other relevant findings should be mentioned. *Cachexia* signifies advanced malignancy or tuberculosis. Bone tumors, malignant tumor infiltrating nerves can alter the attitude of the limb. Increased pulse rate and fever suggests swelling with inflammatory pathology.

■ LOCAL EXAMINATION

One should never hurry to touch unless properly inspected.

Inspection

It should be carried out under a good light with proper exposure in the presence of a nurse, in proper position of the patient. *Opposite side also should be inspected and compared*. Often condition may be *bilateral* **(Figs. 4-22A and B)**.

Location, Size, Shape and Extent of the Swelling

Exact anatomical *location (site/position)* of the swelling is noted. Site of the swelling is mentioned as how far swelling is [in distance (in cm)] from a fixed bony prominence like tibial tubercle, sternal angle, angle of the mandible, etc. Some swellings have got typical locations, for examples, postauricular dermoid behind the ear, external angular dermoid at lateral end of the eyebrow, internal angular dermoid occurs near root of the nose but is rare, meningocele over the midline back, thyroglossal cyst in front of the neck near thyroid cartilage, adventitious bursa is common in angle due to constant friction over the malleoli or foot bones, it is an acquired condition.

Dermoid cysts occur in midline/outer canthus of eye/or any embryonic line of fusion. Lipoma can occur anywhere in the body.

Size as vertical and horizontal dimension in centimeters should be assessed approximately (should be measured using a measuring tape or Vernier caliper during palpation) **(Figs. 4-23 to 4-27)**.

Its *shape*—globular or hemispherical or oval or pear-shaped or pyriform or irregular or kidney-shaped or butterfly-shaped, diffused or well localized is noted. As deeper part of the swelling is not seen, it is not possible to say that a swelling is 'circular' but can be told as spherical.

Extent of the swelling should be observed both vertically and horizontally.

Skin Over the Swelling

Skin over the swelling should be inspected. It may be tense, glossy with prominent veins as in sarcoma and malignancy. Dilatation and engorgement of subcutaneous veins is also seen in hemangioma. Skin is *red* and edematous in inflammatory swellings. Pigmentation (common after radiotherapy), ulceration/fungation/discharge from ulcer/bleeding from the fungation should be inspected. ***Bluish*** color over the skin is seen in hemangioma, black in melanoma. ***Black punctum*** over the summit of the swelling suggests sebaceous cyst. In sarcoma, skin will be tense with ***dilated veins*** over the surface. ***Peau d'orange*** over the swelling is due to cutaneous lymphedema following blockage of cutaneous lymphatics usually by malignant cells. It is commonly seen in carcinoma breast.

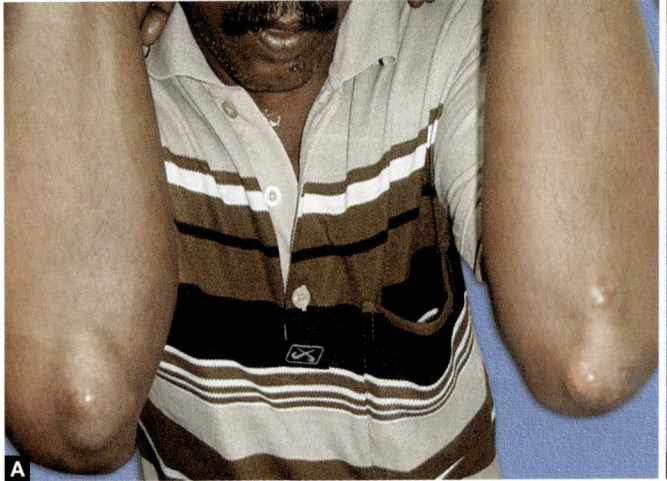
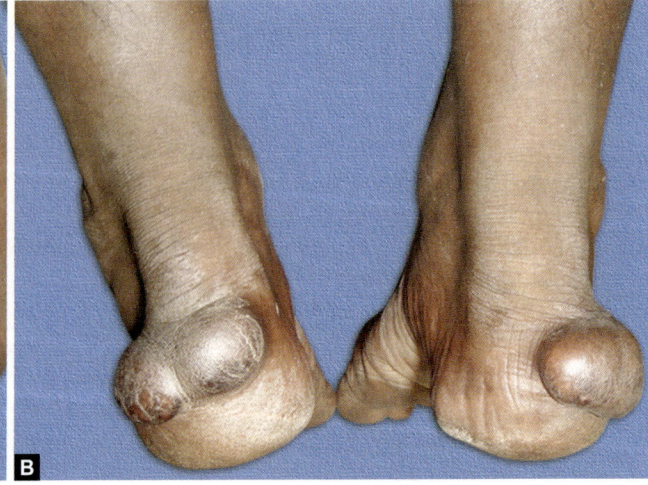

Figs. 4-22A and B Bilateral elbow and heel swellings. Corresponding opposite side should be examined.

Chapter 4: Examination and Clinical Approach of a Swelling/Lump

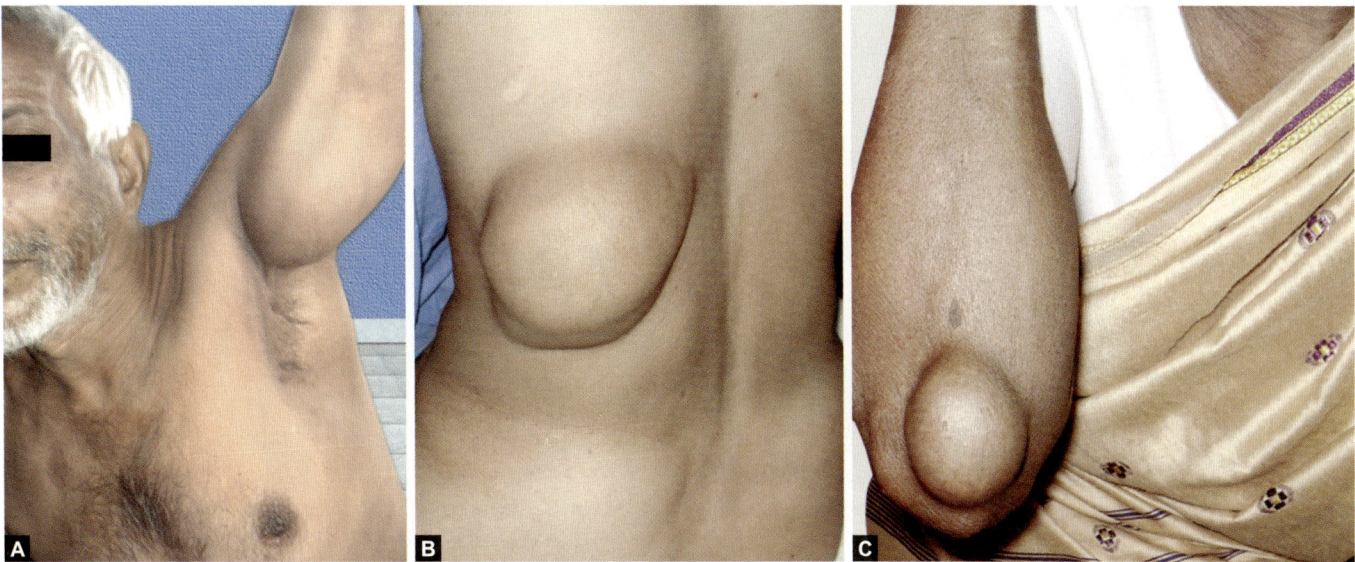

Figs. 4-23A to C Swelling should be inspected properly for its exact anatomical location, shape, size and extent.

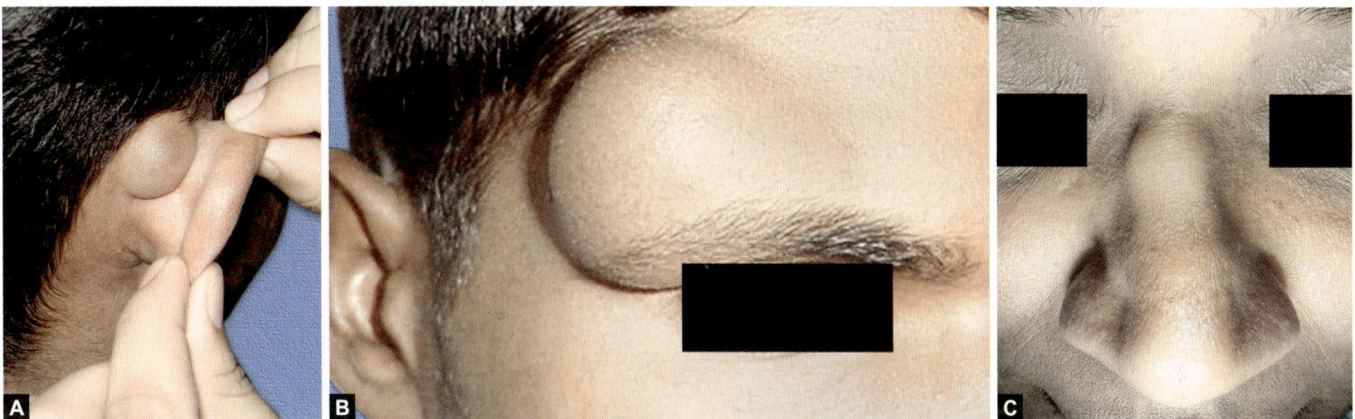

Figs. 4-24A to C Typical sites of *sequestration dermoid*—postauricular and external angular. Dermoid is usually single. Internal angular dermoid is a rare type of dermoid.

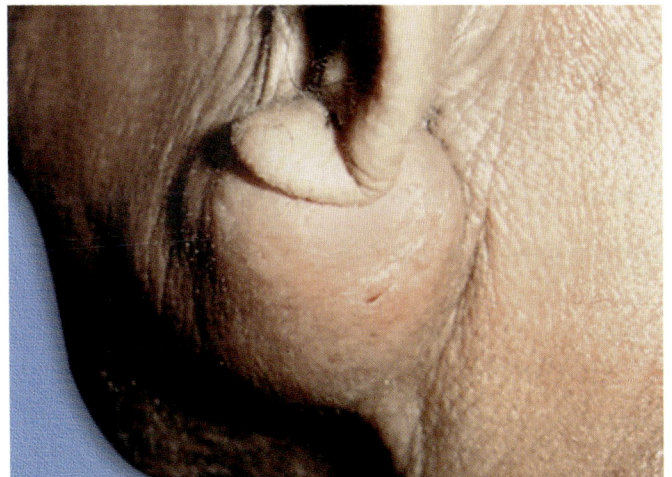

Fig. 4-25 In a parotid swelling, *rise of ear lobule* is an important finding which should be observed during inspection.

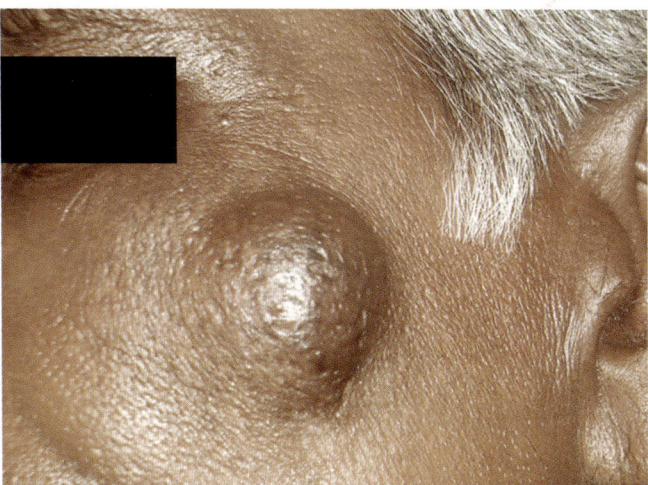

Fig. 4-26 Sebaceous cyst face—face (*most common*), scalp and scrotum are common sites.

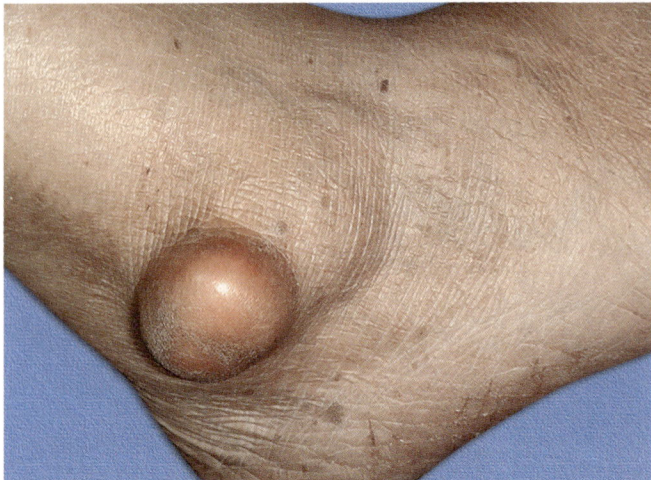

Fig. 4-27 *Adventitious bursa* in ankle region on lateral aspect of the foot. It is infected.

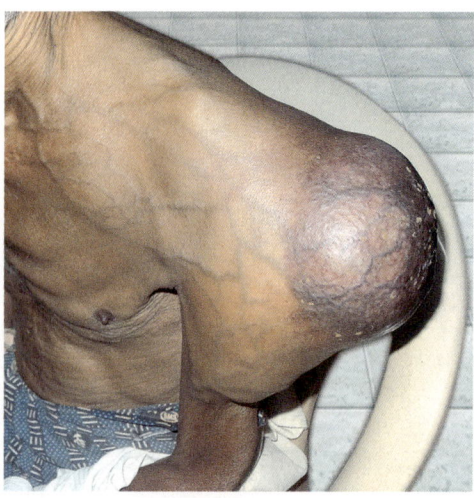

Fig. 4-29 Sarcoma over the shoulder. Note the *large swelling with dilated visible* veins.

Scar, if present—its size, features whether healed by primary intention or secondary intention should be mentioned. Scar may be linear and regular/broad, puckered and irregular has to be noted. Scar may be hypertrophied or **keloid**.

The skin may show **loss of hair** over the swelling, e.g. sebaceous cyst.

Skin over surrounding area of the swelling should be inspected for edema, color changes, texture, scar, visible veins and hair loss **(Figs. 4-28 to 4-30)**.

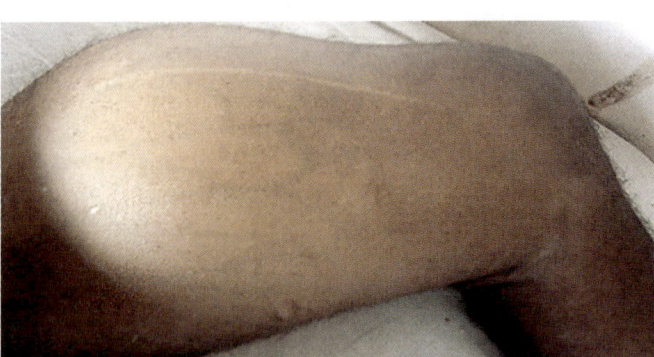

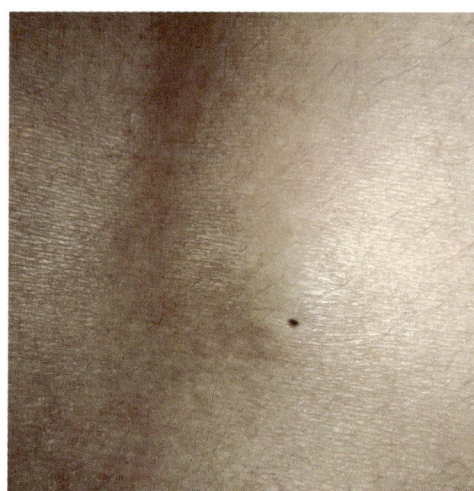

Fig. 4-30 Sebaceous cyst surface—*punctum like a black spot* is clearly visible.

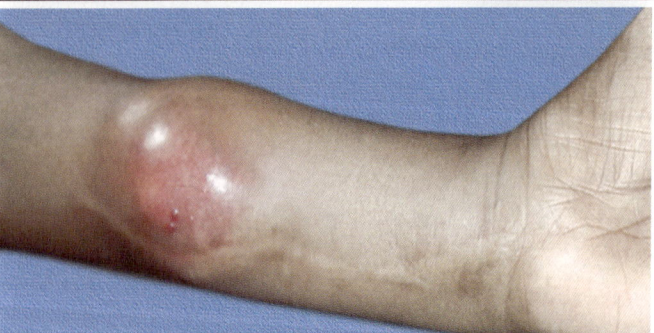

Fig. 4-28 Recurrent soft tissue tumor (sarcoma) thigh and forearm. Note the *scar of previous surgery in thigh*. This scar has healed by primary intention. It is a linear, smooth and supple scar. Scar of forearm surgery is wide, irregular which has healed by secondary intention.

Color of the Swelling

Blue color of venous hemangioma, red color in arterial hemangiomas, black color in nevus or melanoma, blue color of ranula are often typical. Pigmentation is also seen after radiotherapy, local application of some ointments or solutions or medicinal leaves (in Ayurveda or traditional methods), birth marks, plaster of Paris cast, etc. **(Figs. 4-31 to 4-36)**.

Surface Over Swelling

The surface may be smooth (cyst)/irregular (papilloma)/nodular/cauliflower-like (squamous cell carcinoma)/lobular (lipoma) **(Figs. 4-37 and 4-38)**.

Number of the Swellings

Multiple swellings can be neurofibromas, sebaceous cysts, lipomatoses (Dercum's disease), multiple exostosis (diaphyseal aclasis), multiple abscesses and often secondaries in skin. Generalized lymphadenopathy is multiple lymph

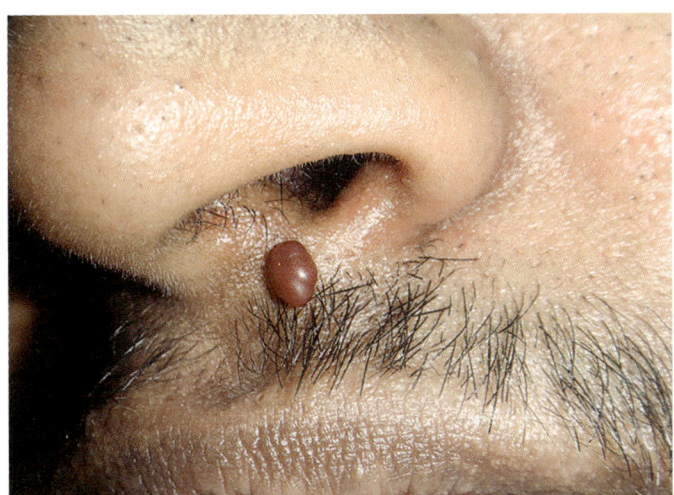

Fig. 4-31 *Color of the swelling* should be noted. It could be hemangioma or granuloma.

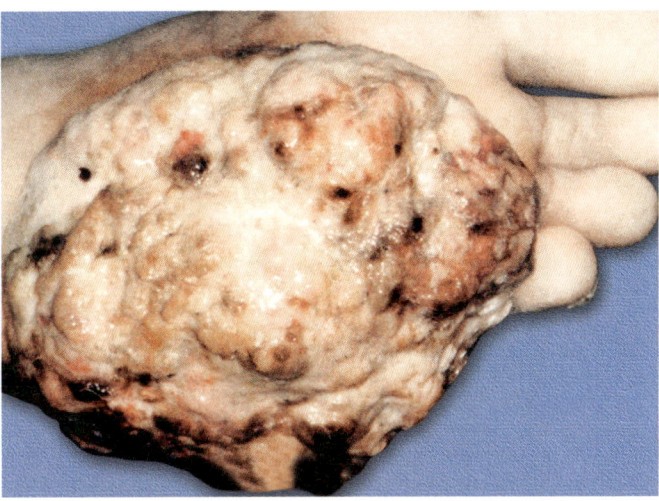

Fig. 4-34 Proliferative cauliflower-like *epithelioma* (squamous cell carcinoma); *note* the *cauliflower-like* surface.

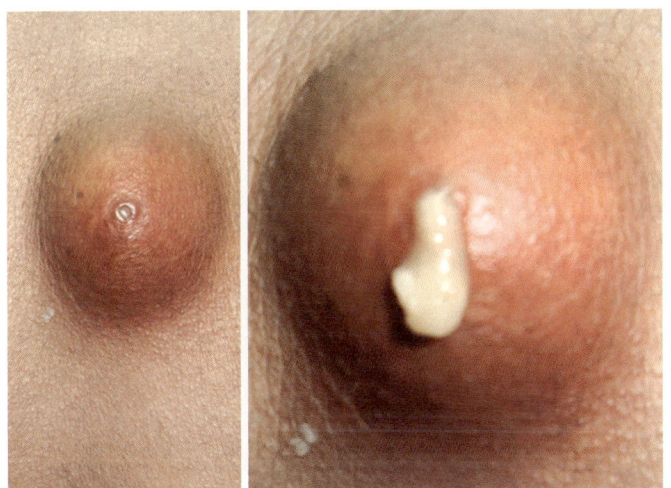

Fig. 4-32 Note the surface of the swelling in sebaceous cyst showing infection and extrusion of the *pultaceous material* after burst.

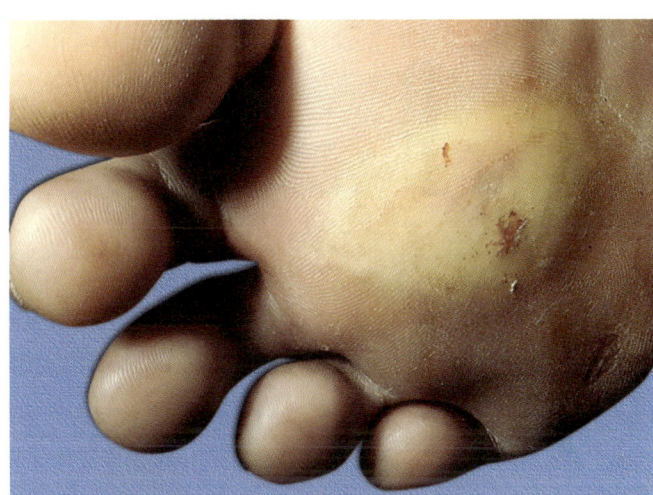

Fig. 4-35 *Abscess foot*—plantar aspect. Note the *color of the surface*.

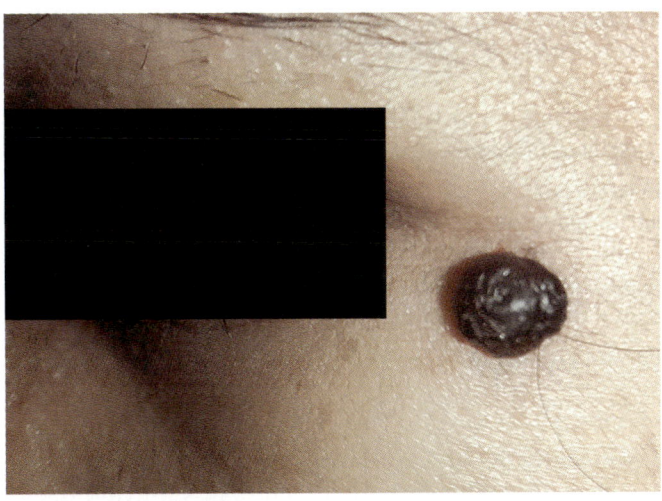

Fig. 4-33 *Papilloma face*. Note the color and surface.

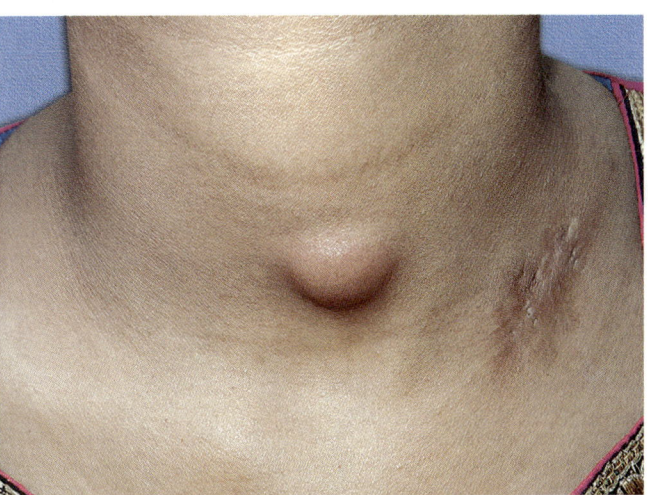

Fig. 4-36 *Cold abscess* neck and scar adjacent below. It could be a collar stud abscess (*tuberculous origin*).

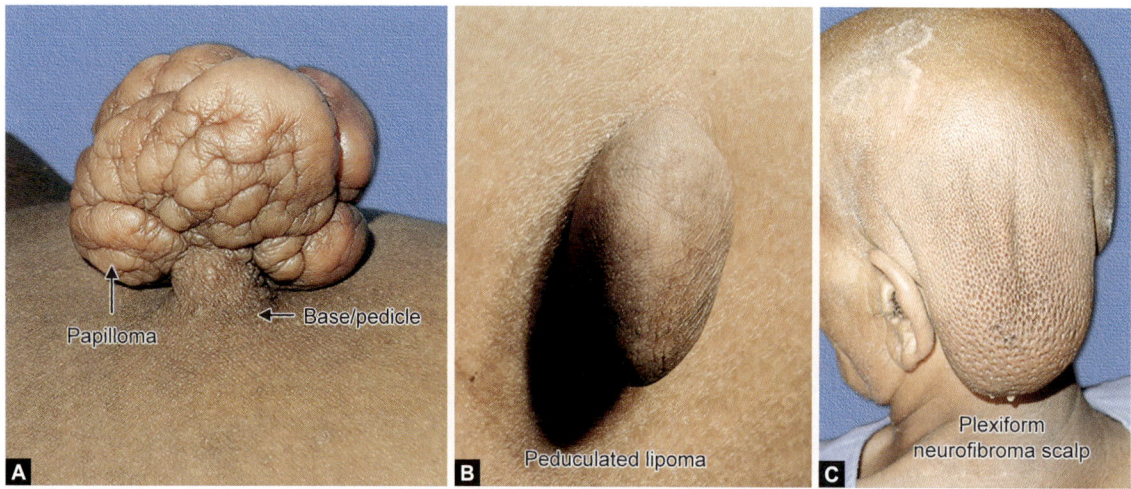

Figs. 4-37A to C *Surfaces look differently in different swellings*: (A) Papilloma (pedunculated); (B) Pedunculated lipoma; (C) Plexiform neurofibroma of scalp.

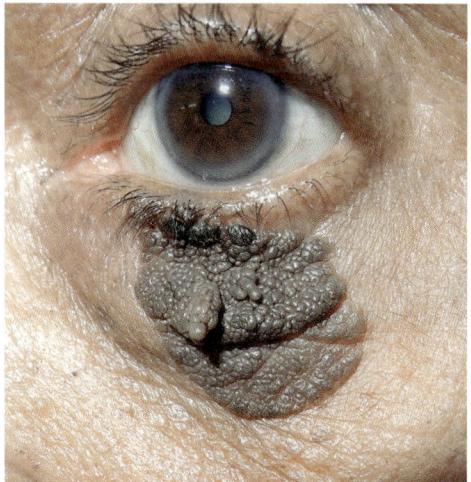

Fig. 4-38 Seborrhoeic keratosis.

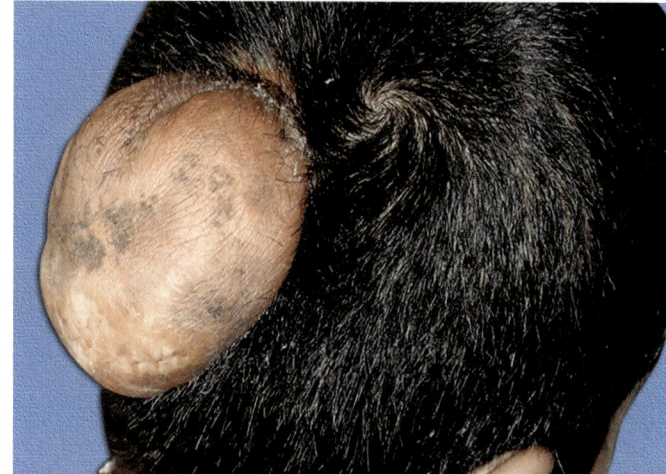

Fig. 4-39 Dermoid in occipital region. Dermoid is usually a single swelling.

node enlargements. Dermoid cyst is usually single (**Figs. 4-39 and 4-40**).

Edge or Margin of the Swelling

In a swelling, edge and margin are considered as same. Margin may be well-defined or ill-defined, pedunculated or sessile. Lipoma, sebaceous cysts are well-defined; acute inflammatory conditions are ill-defined; papilloma is often pedunculated; malignant swelling is well-defined and irregular; deep seated mass has vaguely defined edge (**Figs. 4-41 to 4-43**).

Movements of the Swelling

It may be an *active movement* of the lump itself due to intrinsic force within, which may be vascular (*pulsatile*)/intestinal (*peristaltic*); or *passive movement* when external force is transmitted to the swelling—*transmitted impulse* is observed when patient coughs, cries, strains as seen in hernia. If the swelling is attached (directly/indirectly) to any structure that moves, the swelling will also exhibit its movement. For example, thyroid swellings as attached to cricoid cartilage moves up with deglutition; thyroglossal cyst moves up as the tongue is protruded out due to its attachment to foramen cecum.

Respiratory movements make the mass arising from upper abdomen organs to move up and down along the phases of respiration, e.g. gallbladder, liver, spleen, kidney, stomach, hepatic splenic flexure of colon as these organs are in close contact with diaphragm.

Peristaltic movement is seen in intestinal mass due to gastric/intestinal obstruction. It is checked by the side of the bed keeping eyes at the level of the patient's abdomen.

Movement of the swelling during certain specialized action, e.g. thyroid swelling, thyroglossal cyst, subhyoid bursa, pretracheal lymph nodes move upwards **during deglutition**

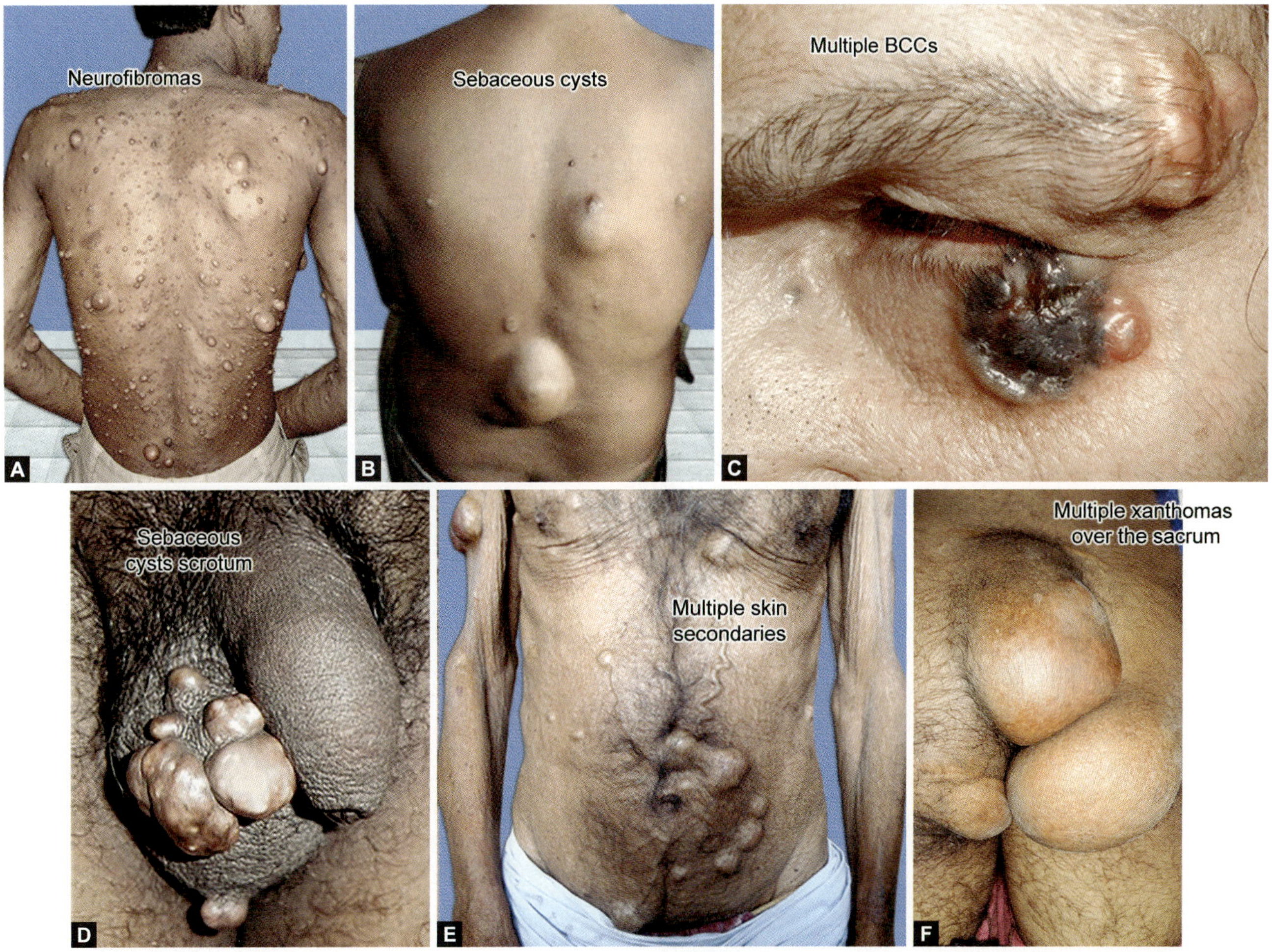

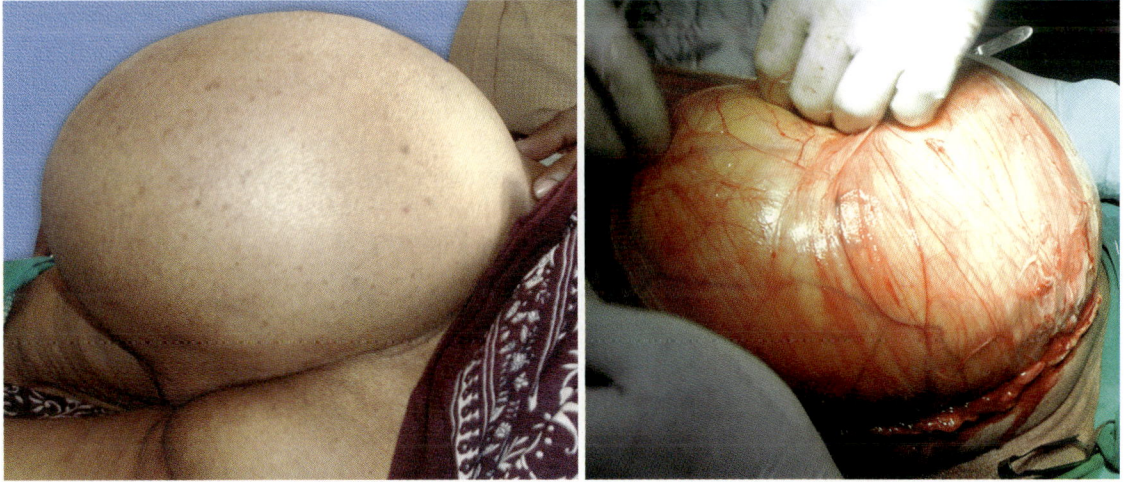

Figs. 4-40A to F Neurofibromas, sebaceous cysts, basal cell carcinomas (rodent ulcer), cutaneous secondaries (metastases) can be multiple. In the scrotum, multiple sebaceous cysts are common. Multiple xanthomas in sacral region.

Fig. 4-41 *Well-defined* swelling on back—lipoma. Lipoma is usually well-defined; but in the sole and back it can be diffused.

because of the attachment to larynx or trachea; thyroglossal cyst moves upwards with a tug while ***protruding the tongue*** out as thyroglossal tract/duct is attached to the base of the tongue through foramen cecum.

Falling forward of the lump should be checked for like in breast lump.

Pulsation over the swelling: Arterial swelling has got *expansile pulsation* (It is checked by keeping two fingers over the swelling during palpation). Swelling which is very close to artery or adherent to it also can show pulsation but it is *transmitted pulsation*. On inspection, it is possible only to tell whether swelling is pulsatile or not.

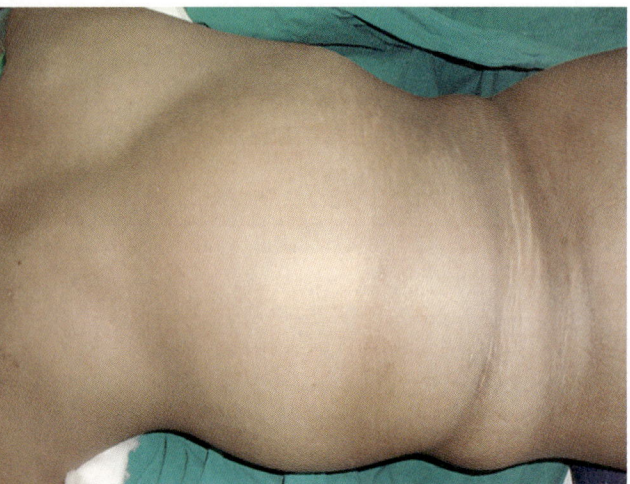

Fig. 4-42 *Diffuse* large lipoma on back.

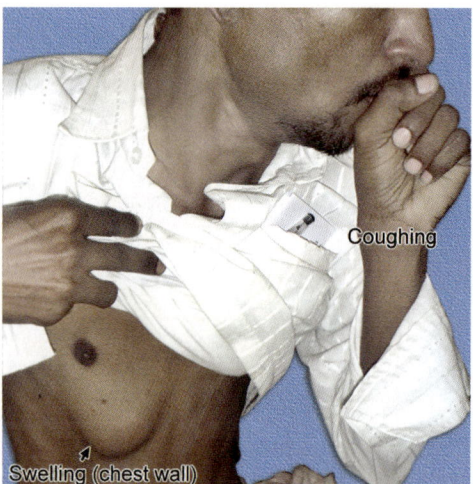

Fig. 4-44 In a swelling related to cavities like thorax, abdomen or cranium, *expansile impulse on coughing should be checked* for to identify the possible intracavity extension.

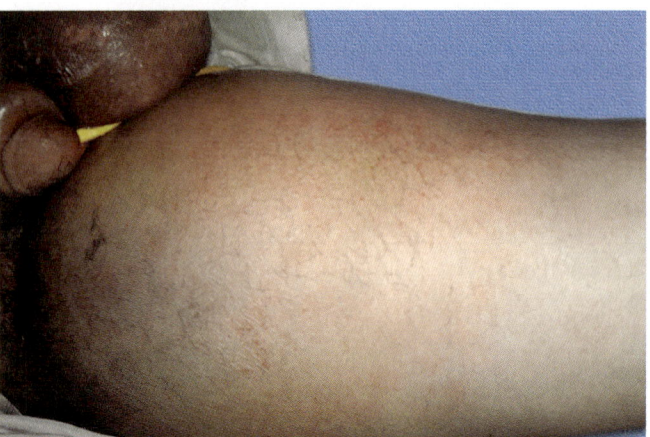

Fig. 4-43 Cellulitis thigh; it is *ill-defined*; redness and diffused swelling is noted.

Presence of expansile impulse: Presence of expansile impulse on coughing signifies hernia or communication into the deeper cavity like abdomen or thorax or pharynx or spinal canal or cranium. Raise in pressure in these cavities during coughing or straining causes *momentary increase in the size of the swelling* if swelling is communicating to these cavities underneath. For example, abdomen (hernia, iliopsoas abscess), chest (empyema necessitans), in pharynx (pharyngeal pouch), spine (meningocele), cranium (occipital meningo-encephalocele). In children coughing/crying will show expansile impulse, e.g. cranial/spinal meningocele (communication with cranial/spinal cavity), empyema necessitans (thorax) **(Fig. 4-44)**.

Pressure Effects

Pressure effect in the limb distal to the swelling and in the neck proximal to the swelling is (inspected) looked for *edema* (block in the venous or lymphatic drainage), *dilated veins, muscle wasting, deformity, paralysis. Wasting* may be due to trauma, disuse atrophy, nerve injury or ischemia (wasting should be confirmed by proper measurement of the part from equal distance from a bony point during palpation). Axillary or groin swelling (enlarged lymph node mass) may cause edema (lymphedema or venous edema) distally (upper or lower limb) due to infiltration or compression or blockage of the lymphatics or veins underneath.

Palpation

It is done to define the swelling properly anatomically and also to find out the nature of the content and its pathology. *It gives the definitive clue to the clinical diagnosis.*

Local Raise of Temperature

Local raise of temperature is checked using **back of the fingers** which is more sensitive than palmar aspect, as dorsum of the fingers is thin and has got rich nerve supply. The temperature should be checked in the beginning of palpation as in later part of palpation, swelling may apparently feel warmer due to manipulation. It should be compared with surrounding unaffected skin or opposite corresponding part. Warmness may be due to inflammation (infection) or due to tumors with increased vascularity. Sarcoma is warmer; cellulites, pyogenic abscess are warm. Cold abscess (due to tuberculosis) is not warm as there are no signs of acute inflammation. But secondary infection in a cold abscess can make it warm **(Fig. 4-45)**.

Tenderness

While palpating the swelling, tenderness is checked by observing the face of the patient. Palpation is started from normal to diseased area. Patient expresses the tenderness on his face; often he cries. Inflammatory conditions are tender. Neoplastic conditions are initially non-tender but later can become tender. Tenderness should be elicited gently.

Size, Shape and Extent of the Swelling

The swelling may be bigger than it appeared on inspection. Size is measured using tape (vertical dimension in cm × horizontal dimension in cm; *or* longitudinal × transverse dimension in cm in a lengthy oval swelling); shape is confirmed and extent of the entire swelling and its anatomical location should be mentioned properly. Tape is placed on the outer margin of the swelling on both sides; if tape placed over the surface of the swelling across its summit then half diameter/circumference of the swelling only will be assessed. Length and breadth of the swelling ideally can be measured using *Vernier caliper* but it is not practicable in a given patient **(Fig. 4-46)**.

Edge or Margin

Edge of the swelling can be ***well-defined (distinct)*** or ***ill-defined (indistinct***, i.e. merges into the surrounding structures). It is ill-defined in acute conditions and deep swellings. It is well-defined in superficial swellings. Margin may be irregular in malignancy and is regular in benign swellings.

Edge of the swelling is examined using ***pulp of the index finger. Erosion of the margin into the deeper plane*** like bone is also checked. Dermoid cyst commonly shows ***erosion into the bone*** **(Fig. 4-47A)**. Entire margin is palpated as it may be well-defined at one place and ill-defined at other region. In

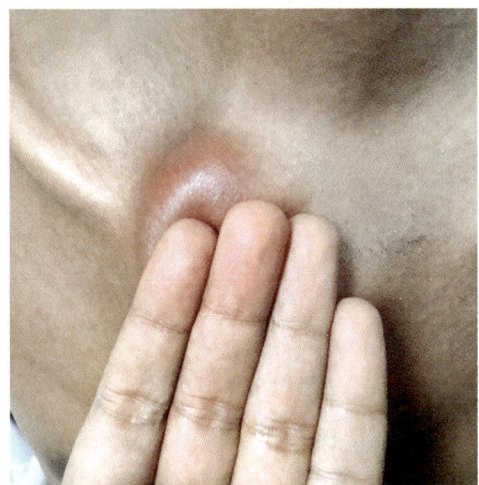

Fig. 4-45 *Back of the fingers* is used to check the local raise of temperature.

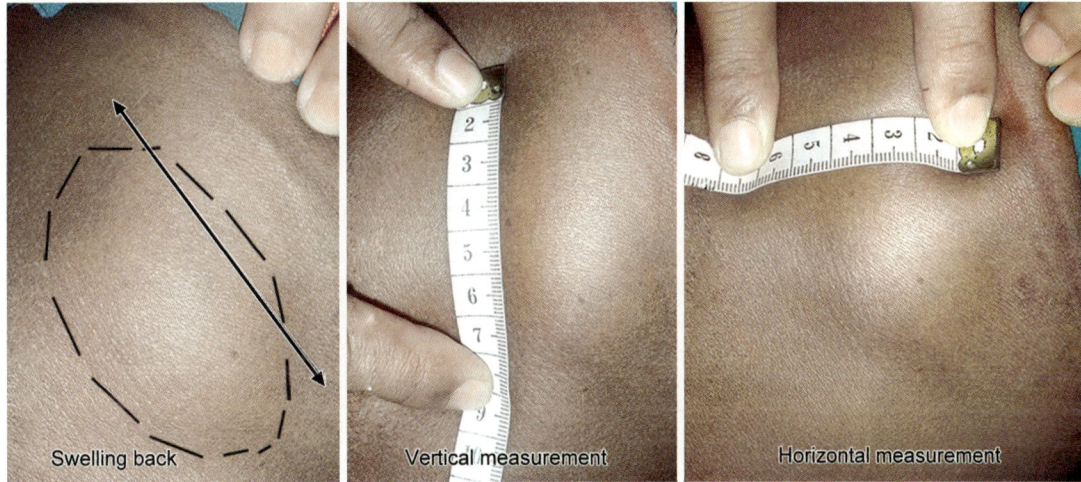

Fig. 4-46 Swelling should be measured using a measuring tape or scale. Usually the measurement is described in centimeter. Firstly, vertical measurement is mentioned and later, horizontal measurement.

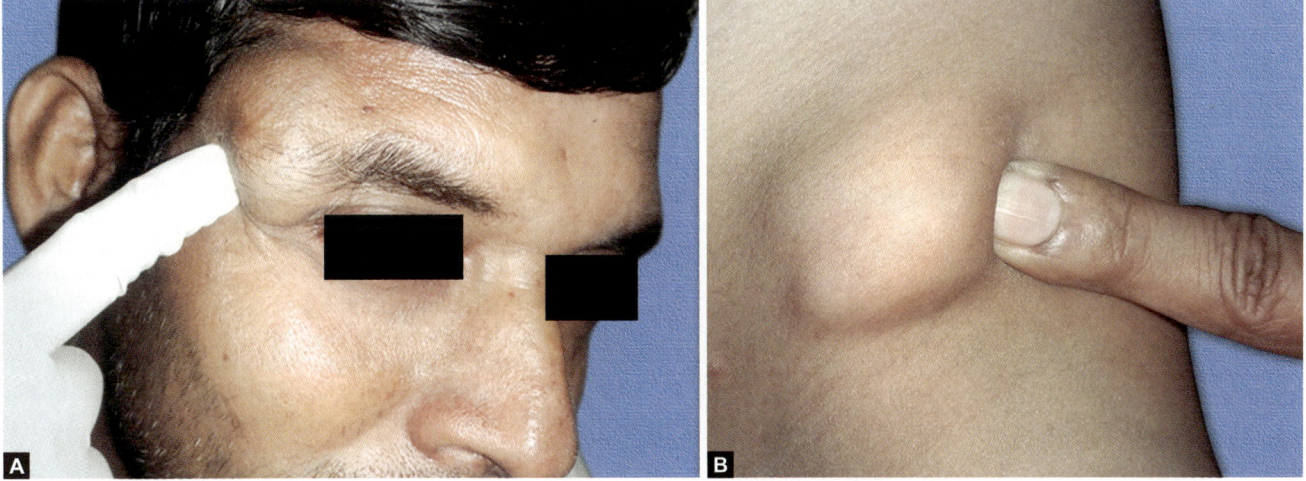

Figs. 4-47A and B (A) External angular dermoid. *Erosion of the bone at the edge should be checked* by feeling the edge using index finger; (B) *Typical slip sign* is positive in lipoma (*Lipoma slips; cyst yields*).

lipoma, margin does not yield to the pressure of the palpating finger and slips away from the finger—*slip sign* (Fig. 4-47B). It is tested by pressing the fingertip at the edge of the swelling. In sebaceous cyst, margin gets *yielded* by the finger.

Surface of the Swelling

It is felt with the palmar surface of the fingers. It may be smooth like in a cyst/nodular in lymph nodes/lobular in lipoma/matted in tuberculous nodes/irregular in carcinoma. Surface may be variable and if so should be mentioned which part is smooth and which is nodular (Fig. 4-48).

Consistency

It is one of the important characteristic features of the swelling which denotes its density and type/nature of contents of the swelling. Contents may be solid, liquid, gas, or mixture of these. *Solid* content has got cell mass having fixed volume and shape; *liquid* has got fixed volume but variable shape; *gas* has got variable volume and shape.

Consistency may be termed as *very soft* (like jelly)/*soft* (like consistency of lip/relaxed muscle)/may be *firm* (like consistency of nose/contracted muscle)/may be *hard* (like consistency of forehead). Myxoma is very soft; lipoma is soft; branchial cyst is cystic (soft and fluctuant); fibroma is hard; osteoma is bony hard; carcinoma is stony hard. Solid cellular swelling but having noncohesive cells makes the swelling often cystic (Figs. 4-49 and 4-50).

Uniform consistency in a swelling is observed/felt when swelling is of acute onset (abscess) or benign in nature or often in malignancy of shorter duration. *Variable consistency* may be observed in one swelling. In such occasion, which area is soft, and which area is firm or hard should be confirmed properly. Variability may be due to tumor necrosis/inflammation/hemorrhage in the swelling.

Often based on the contents, consistency of a swelling may be classified as—*hard* means it do not change its shape on application of pressure; *firm* means it may slightly change

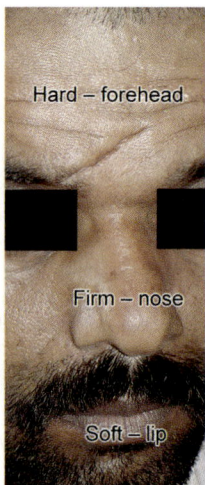

Fig. 4-49 Consistency can be very soft, soft (like lip), firm (like nose) or hard (like forehead).

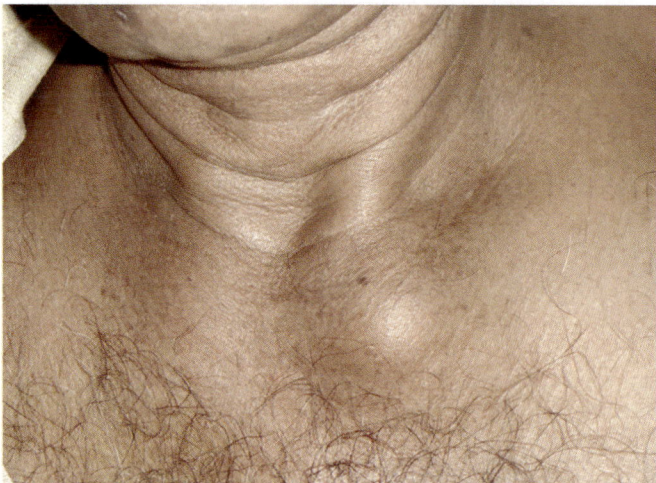

Fig. 4-50 Bony swelling arising from clavicle.

its shape with application of pressure; *elastic* means it changes its shape with application of pressure but there is immediate recoiling once the pressure is removed (Hodgkin's lymphoma); *soft* means it yields easily by pressure. Cystic swelling denotes the typical feel of fluid which changes their shape by pressure, e.g. cyst, abscess.

Note: *Cystic nature* or cystic in consistency is mentioned only when swelling is confirmed to have fluid clinically by doing fluctuation test; without getting positive fluctuation, swelling cannot be called as cystic and in such situation it is better to say that swelling is soft in consistency. Swelling containing fluid need not be always cystic in consistency; it may be firm due to increased tension of fluid in the swelling, e.g. thyroglossal/thyroid cyst. Occasionally solid swelling may feel cystic due to tumor/cell necrosis within or undifferentiated rapidly multiplying cells [*paradox in consistency (cystic swelling can be firm and solid swelling can be cystic)* for example, thyroid paradox]. If surface of the swelling while palpating for consistency, pits on pressure it may be due to inflammatory cause or venous/lymphatic block by tumor.

Lipoma, cystic swellings, abscess are soft; neurofibromas, certain nodal enlargements are firm; chondroma, osteomas

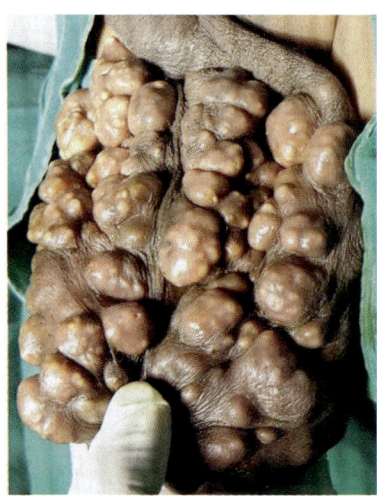

Fig. 4-48 Multiple (calcified) sebaceous cysts scrotum (*Strawberry scrotum*).

are *bony hard*; malignant swellings (carcinomas) are *stony hard*; fibroma, chondromas are *woody hard*. Fibroma often can be firm also. Swelling like sebaceous cyst or dermoid cyst which contains pultaceous (porridge-like) material or putty-like material gets *moulded (sign of indentation)* **(Figs. 4-51 to 4-53)**.

Following are the features to be observed or clinical methods to be elicited to know the contents of the swelling (cell mass/fluid/gas). *Pitting on pressure:* With fingertip, firm pressure is applied over the swelling and removed after few seconds. One may see or feel the depression on removal of the finger which is due to displacement of fluid from the edematous tissue on pressure. It is often seen in brawny edema in a deeply situated abscess. *Indentation/moulding:* Obvious depression is seen when swelling like sebaceous cyst (often dermoid cyst) is pressed with tip of finger for 15–30 sec; which is due to putty-like material within which gets moulded on pressure. Moulding can also be elicited in colon loaded with fecal matter. *Crepitus* in subcutaneous emphysema suggests presence of gas/air in the subcutaneous plane. Crepitus is felt as sensation of palpating a horse hair mattress (on auscultation it is heard as crackling sound). Crepitus is felt in chest trauma along with bloated look of face, neck, thorax and abdomen. It is also felt in injury to nasal sinuses, trachea, bronchus, esophageal rupture, after tracheostomy, in gas gangrene. Crepitus can be localized or generalized. Crepitus also often seen in bone (fracture), joint, tenosynovitis.

Fluctuation

Fluctuation test is most commonly used and better method to evaluate the content of the swelling.

Principle: When a swelling is compressed at one spot, the increased pressure within the swelling is transmitted equally at right angle to all parts of the wall. This test helps to confirm the presence of liquid/gas within the swelling. It is a sense of movement/expansion/wave/impulse felt or perceived by the fingers due to displacement of the contents of the swelling on pressure over a *soft swelling* having a *nonrigid wall*. ***Fluctuation implies transmitted impulse in two planes at right angles to each other (by Marsh).*** *Pascal's law:* Pressure exerted to a fluid is transmitted *equally* in all directions.

Technique of standard fluctuation (Marsh, London): Swelling is fixed by holding it with thumb and middle finger of both hands (fixing the mobile swelling is important prior to eliciting the fluctuation test, otherwise swelling itself may get pushed away significantly giving wrong result of positive fluctuation). With the index finger of one hand, one side of the swelling is pressed and index finger of the other hand placed diagonally on the opposite side feels the fluid movement and also a rise/elevation/sense of movement underneath. Procedure is repeated in perpendicular direction to confirm fluctuation (two right angle planes) (*Note:* Often muscle gives fluctuation-like feeling when elicited in one direction (muscle feels fluctuant like in horizontal direction; *pseudofluctuation*) but not in two perpendicular directions). Alternatively finger used to press the swelling is called as *displacing finger* and finger that is used to feel (which is kept as passive) is called as *feeling/perceiving/watching finger*. Watching finger should be *kept motionless* throughout the procedure. This is *standard fluctuation*. Positive fluctuation signifies presence of fluid. Examples are hydrocele, cysts, etc. Alternatively thumb and forefingers of one hand can be used to fix the swelling, and

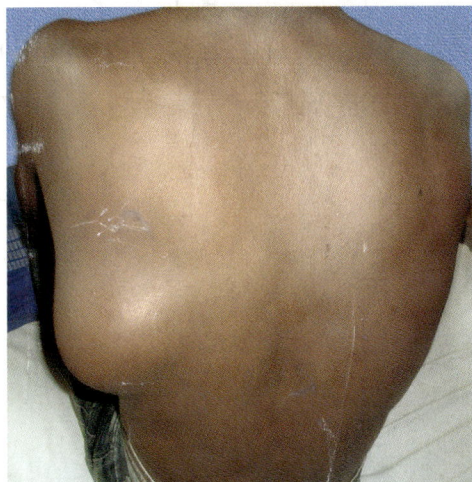

Fig. 4-51 Large lipoma over back which is *well localized, smooth, soft and lobulated*.

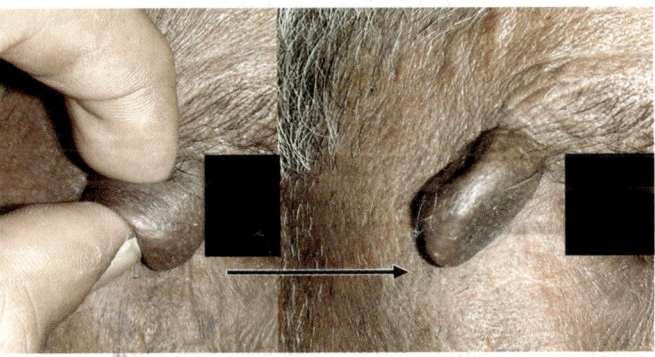

Fig. 4-52 *Moulding* is seen in a cyst where content is pultaceous (porridge-like) material; commonly seen in sebaceous cyst; can occasionally occur in dermoid cyst also.

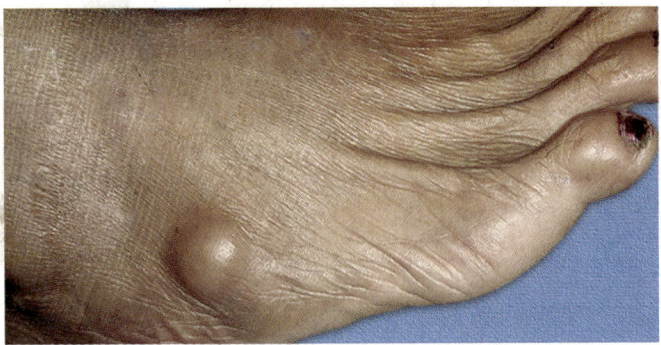

Fig. 4-53 Ganglion foot. It is tensely cystic swelling. *Paget's test will be positive.*

104 Section 1: Examination in General Surgery

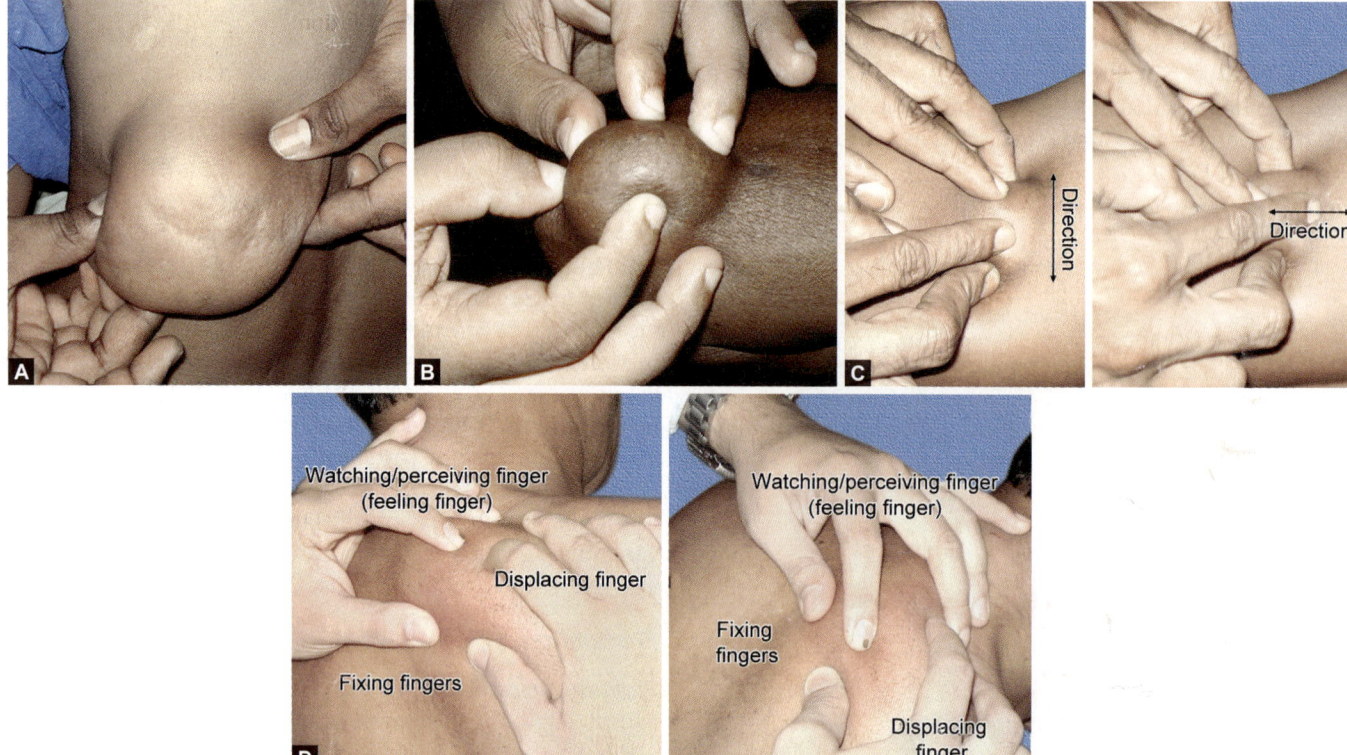

Figs. 4-54A to D Swelling should be fixed before eliciting the fluctuation. Fluctuation cannot be elicited in intra-abdominal swelling as it cannot be fixed. It should be done in two perpendicular directions. With one finger (displacing finger) swelling is pressed to displace the fluid content and its movement is felt with other finger (watching/perceiving/feeling finger) placed.

fingers of the other hand can be used to displace and feel the fluid **(Figs. 4-54A to D)**.

In a *small swelling* which cannot accommodate two fingers to do standard fluctuation test, margin of the swelling is fixed using two fingers (index and ring as perceiving fingers) and using middle finger summit/center of the swelling is pressed/indented to feel displacement of the fluid/*yielding sensation*. This test is called as **Paget's test** of fluctuation (done for a small swelling of 1–2 cm in size)**(Figs. 4-55 and 4-56)**. In a swelling smaller than 1 cm in size, it is difficult to elicit even Paget's method; here fluctuation can be elicited using two matchsticks—*matchstick test* **(Fig. 4-57)**. But one has to remember that it is often difficult to elicit fluctuation in a small swelling. ***Note: Cystic swellings are softer at center than periphery; solid swellings are firmer at the center than periphery.***

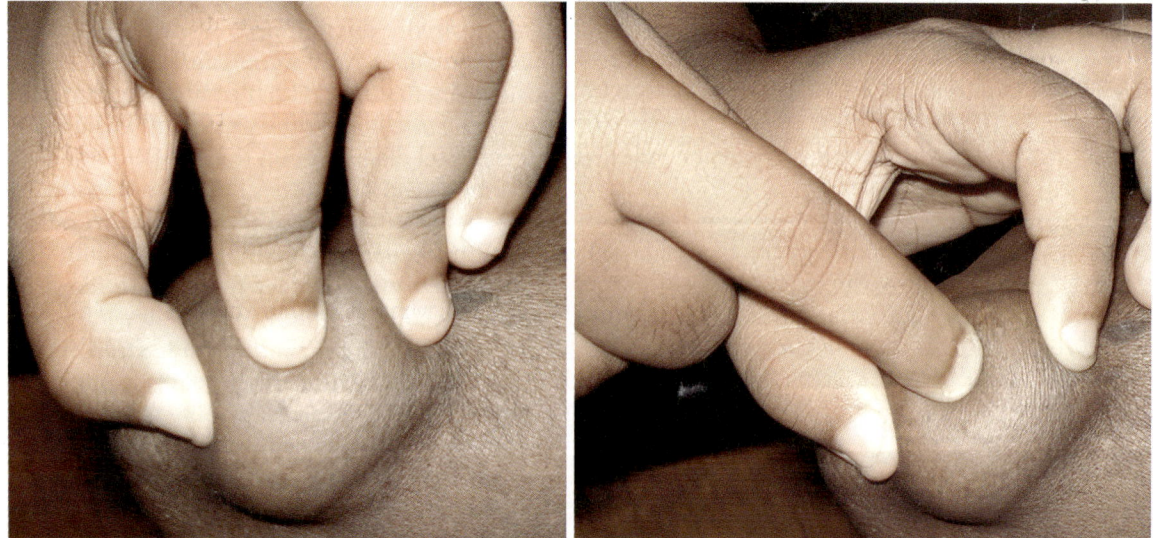

Fig. 4-55 *Paget's test* is done for a small swelling to elicit fluctuation. Swelling is fixed with index and ring fingers; middle finger while pressing/indenting over the summit of the swelling displaces the fluid, movement of which is perceived by ring and index fingers (perceiving fingers).

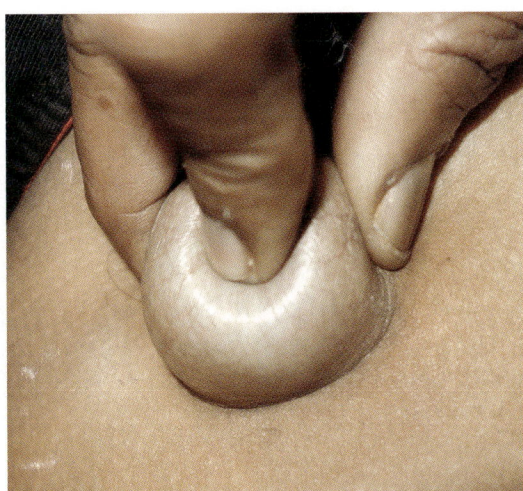

Fig. 4-56 Typical positive Paget's test.

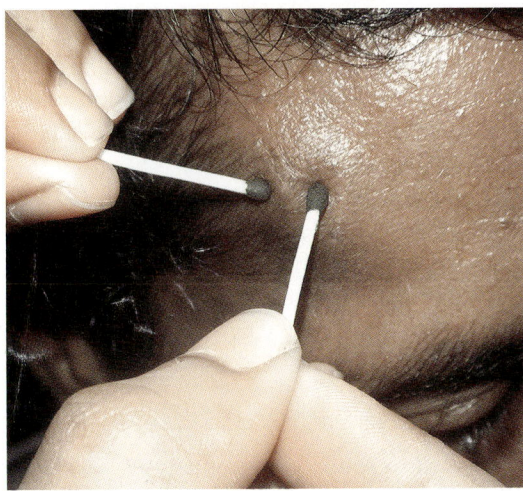

Fig. 4-57 In a very small swelling (<1 cm) match-sticks can be used to feel the displacement; here swelling is difficult to fix. This test is not used commonly.

In *very large swelling*, an assistant will fix the swelling and the swelling is pressed with two fingers (index and middle) instead of standard one finger, as the pressure generated by single finger will not be adequate to be perceived.

It is often difficult to differentiate the content as fluid (cystic) or cell mass *in soft small swelling*. With the displacing finger summit is compressed steadily; perceiving finger kept at the periphery of the swelling will feel a projection (outward) wave in case of cystic swelling but not in case of soft cellular swelling. Very soft swellings are lipoma, myxoma, vascular swellings and soft fibroma. These swellings may show false positive fluctuation *(false sense of fluctuation)*. Pseudofluctuation is a false sense of fluctuation in a soft, often large swelling but not containing fluid.

False negative fluctuation can occur occasionally in a swelling which actually contains fluid. This happens when swelling is very soft with low tension fluid which prevents wave to reach its opposite wall. Very large, very tense, and swelling with multiple septae, thick-walled (calcification of wall) swelling show false negative fluctuation.

> **Remember about the fluctuation:**
> - Both hands should be used
> - Mobile swelling should be fixed
> - Should be done in two planes perpendicular to each other
> - Wall of the swelling should be nonrigid
> - Displacing and perceiving fingers should be kept adequately apart each other
> - Assistant should fix the larger swelling to elicit the fluctuation
> - Watching finger should be kept motionless throughout the procedure

Fluctuation by 'three finger test' is used in hydatid cyst of the liver and is called as **hydatid thrill**. Index, middle and ring fingers of the left hand is placed over the mass with each finger being few millimeters apart; tapping/percussion over the middle phalanx of the left middle finger using right index finger displaces the scolices creating a wave under the index and middle fingers of the left hand.

> **Special tests for soft swellings:**
> - Fluctuation test
> - Transillumination test
> - Expansile impulse on coughing
> - Reducibility
> - Compressibility

Cross fluctuation: Fluctuation may be present in a cystic swelling which contains fluid in two components on either sides of an anatomical barrier (*across an anatomical barrier*). It is called *cross fluctuation*. Plunging ranula (across mylohyoid muscle), iliopsoas abscess (across inguinal ligament), compound palmar ganglion (across flexor retinaculum), bilocular hydrocele (across a band or superficial inguinal ring) are cross-fluctuant.

Transillumination Test

Demonstration of transmission of light through a swelling is called as *transillumination*. Positive transillumination test means fluid content is clear with a thin transparent wall. Translucency or transilluminant swelling can transmit light through it. This test is only contributory, never confirmatory. Cyst containing clear fluid will be brilliantly transilluminant. It is negative when it contains blood, pus, pultaceous material or thick-walled. This test is preferably done in a dark room. Torch light is placed on one side of the swelling and illumination is observed on the diagonally opposite side using a rolled paper or rolled X-ray sheet/*transilluminoscope*. *Transillumination test* should be done across full thickness of the swelling to avoid surface translucency except in hydrocele where it is done from side to avoid false negativity by the posteriorly situated testis. Lymph cyst, cystic hygroma, ranula, meningocele, hydrocele are transilluminant swellings.

> **Swellings which are brilliantly transilluminant:**
> - Ranula
> - Cystic hygroma and lymph cyst
> - Hydrocele
> - Epididymal cyst (Chinese-lantern pattern)
> - Meningocele
> - Hydrocele of the canal of Nuck

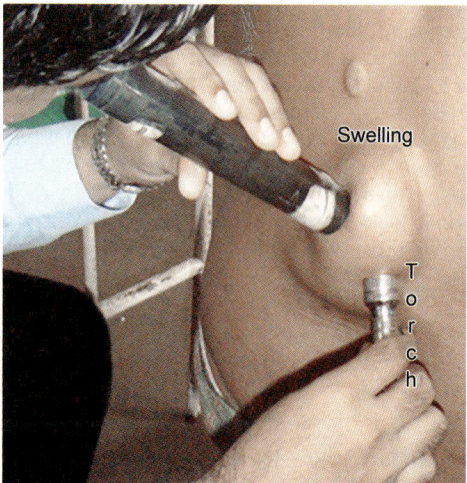

Fig. 4-58 *Transillumination* should be elicited using pen torch and dark visualization tube (folded X-ray tube/transilluminoscope). All fluctuant swelling should be checked for transillumination.

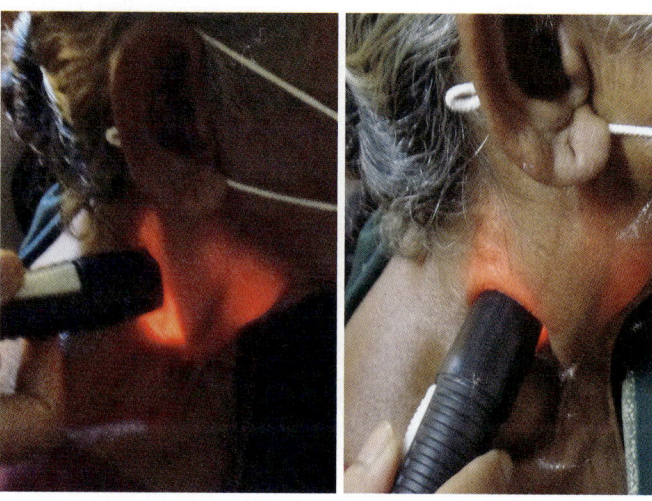

Fig. 4-61 Lymph cyst in the neck which is brilliantly transilluminant; transillumination is checked in dark room.

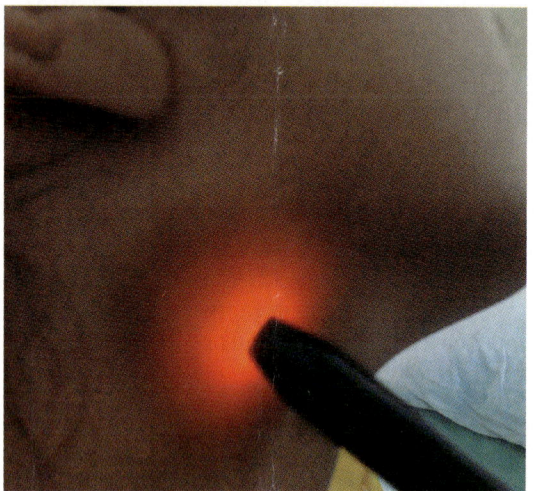

Fig. 4-59 *Brilliantly transilluminating swelling.* Here it is branchial cyst. While checking transillumination, transillumination of normal skin should be carefully eliminated.

Negative test is seen in dermoid cyst, sebaceous cyst, hematocele, chylocele, pyocele, chronic hydrocele as fluid here is not clear but opaque. Calcified or thick walled cyst will show false negative result.

False positive (transillumination is present but no fluid inside) transillumination is seen across skin folds, finger webs and congenital inguinal enterocele. *False negative* (means clear fluid is present but transillumination cannot be elicited) results are seen in thick-walled cyst, calcified cyst (**Figs. 4-58 to 4-60**).

Reducibility

Patient is asked to relax; swelling is pressed/compressed from all sides with a sustained, uniform, gentle pressure; swelling which gets reduced in size, content (viscera) moves completely into the adjoining cavity and disappears, is said to be a reducible swelling. Uncomplicated inguinal hernia, saphena varix, varicocele, meningocele are reducible. On

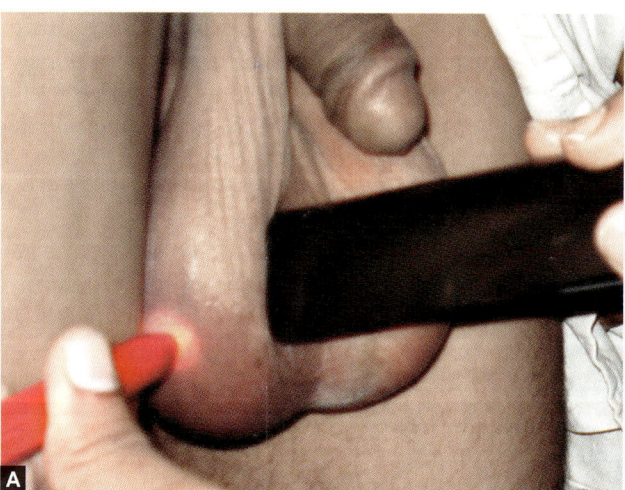 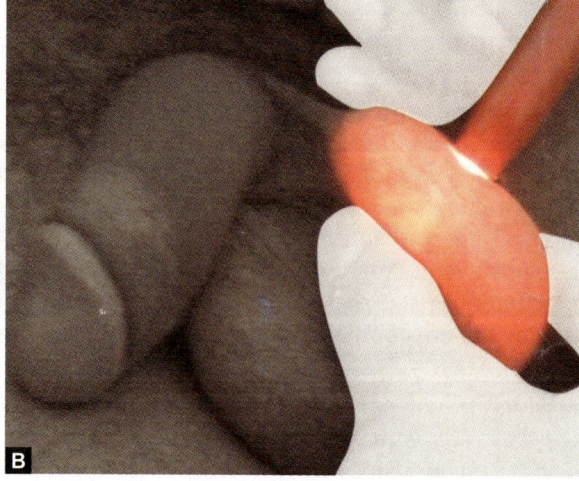

Figs. 4-60A and B *In hydrocele*, transillumination should be checked by placing torch and tube in opposite directions (side to side) in the front aspect of the swelling. It should not be from front to back as testis will prevent light to pass and makes transillumination test improper.

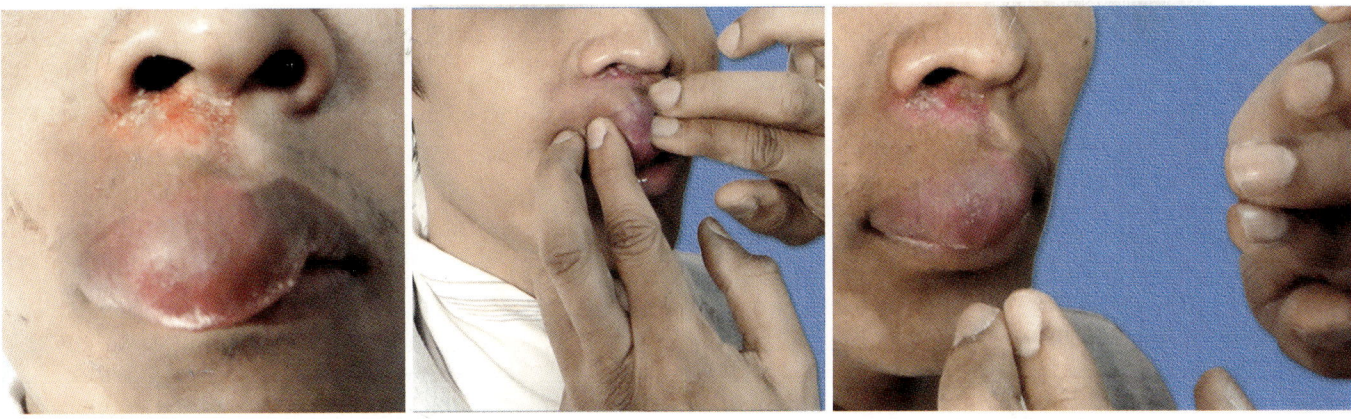

Fig. 4-62 *Checking compressibility.* By applying pressure swelling disappears partially; by releasing it swelling comes back to its original shape and size.

standing or under gravity, only this reduced swelling may reappear spontaneously or by coughing or straining. Often swelling may get reduced only partially like in some inguinal hernias (indirect/irreducible).

Expansile Impulse on Coughing

It is visible momentary increase in size of the swelling synchronous with the coughing or crying (in children). Swellings which are reducible, can have an impulse which is seen as well as felt on straining, coughing, sneezing. These swelling are in continuity with abdominal cavity (hernia, psoas and lumbar abscess); pleural cavity (empyema necessitans), spinal and cranium (meningocele). It is also present in saphena varix, laryngocele, lymph varix and varicocele.

Expansile impulse on coughing also should be confirmed by palpation. Swelling is held with one hand firmly and patient is asked to cough to elicit impulse. Expansile impulse is better seen than felt; but should also be confirmed by palpation.

Compressibility

Swelling on applying pressure decreases in size *only partially and will not disappear completely* and on releasing the pressure, swelling again *comes back to its original size and shape immediately* without any external factors like straining or coughing **(Fig. 4-62)**. Compressible swellings do not have communication with the body cavities. Usually vascular and lymphatic swellings are compressible. Example—hemangioma, lymphangioma.

Pulsatility

When a finger is placed firmly over the swelling if it raises *synchronously* with each heartbeat of the patient, then swelling is called as pulsatile. **Examining the pulsatile swelling:** Two fingers are placed over the swelling with adequate gap between the two fingers. If fingers over the swelling are *raised, separated and moved apart* with each beat of the artery it means pulsation is *expansile*. Here with pulsation, the swelling initially increases in size denoting expansion in all direction. If fingers are only *raised (only lifted up) but not separated* from each other, then pulsation of the swelling is *transmitted*. Pure arterial swelling like aneurysm shows *expansile pulsation* **(Figs. 4-63A and B)** (swelling arising from artery). Swelling which is close to the artery may show pulsation because

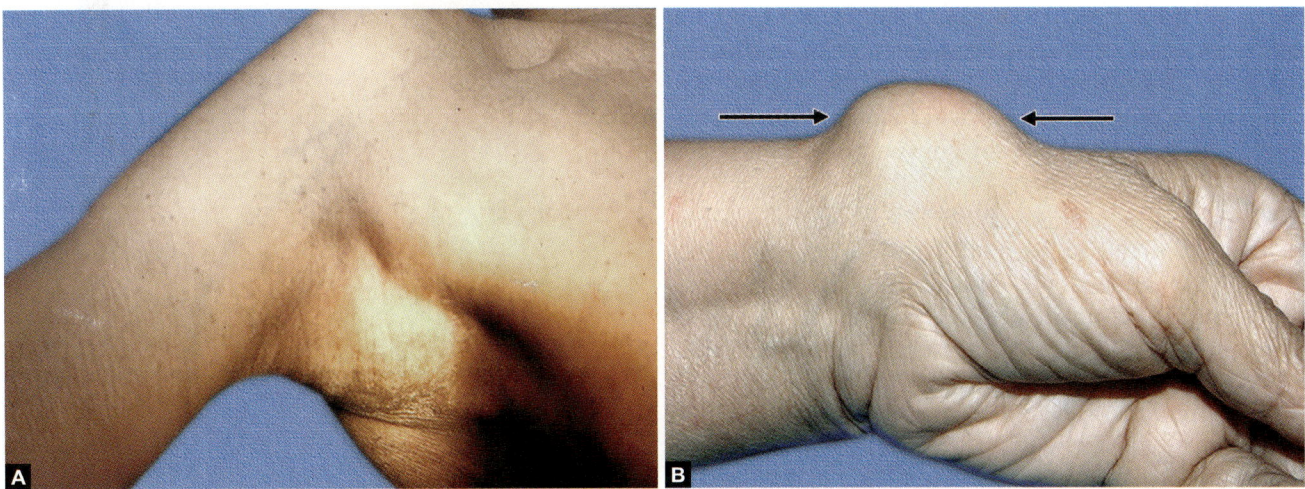

Figs. 4-63A and B Aneurysm of the axillary artery and radial artery. Aneurysm shows *expansile pulsation*.

of its proximity to the vessel and it is only transmitted pulsation. In transmitted pulsation, the swelling is merely raised with pulsation. Swelling which is very vascular also can be pulsatile.

Pseudocyst in the abdomen shows transmitted pulsation because of its close proximity to aorta. Pulsatile tumors may lie along the course of the artery except highly vascular tumors. Follicular carcinoma of thyroid causes localized, highly vascular, warm, often pulsatile secondaries in skull bone (commonly frontal bone). Telangiectatic osteogenic sarcoma is also often pulsatile due to its high vascularity.

Thrill

It is the feeling of the movement of the fluid underneath the palpating finger. It can be felt as a flow of fluid abnormally in natural structures like altered (rapid flow through a normal caliber vessel like in thyrotoxic goiter or turbulent blood flow through a narrowed arteries like stenosed vessel) arteries where thrill felt is systolic or arteriovenous fistula where thrill felt is machinery (both systolic and diastolic); or collected fluid is made to move/flow by external tapping to feel the thrill like in eliciting fluid thrill of ascites. In A-V, communication/malformation thrill can also be felt for some distance along the course of the vessel.

Plane of the Swelling

Plane of the swelling is checked to confirm whether the swelling is adherent to the superficial or deeper structures. Skin and mucous membrane are usually mobile. But skin in the palm, sole, ear, nose and mucous membrane of the hard palate and gums are adherent to deeper structures. **Gliding** (**gliding test**, rolling, moving) of the skin outer to the swelling or **pinching** (pinching test) of the skin from the underlying swelling is done to confirm the whether swelling is fixed to the skin or not. **Dimpling** of the skin can be demonstrated by pulling the underlying swelling away; it implies the attachment of fibrous septa or duct to the skin which may be due to infiltration of the tumor or fibrosis.

Swellings arising from the skin will move along with the skin over subcutaneous tissue if the said swelling is not adherent to subcutaneous or deeper plane **(Figs. 4-64 and 4-65)**. Examples are—skin papilloma, melanoma, squamous cell carcinoma, skin adnexal tumors. Malignant skin tumors if adherent to deep structures will be nonmobile. Fixity to deeper plane is checked by contracting the muscles underneath or by its mobility.

Fixity to the skin: Mobility of the skin over the swelling is checked by rolling or pinching skin over the swelling to confirm whether skin is free or attached to the swelling underneath. In sebaceous cyst, skin over it is adherent to the cyst over the summit often with a punctum (70%). In dermoid cyst, skin is always free. In lipoma skin is usually free. In neurofibromas skin may be adherent, but depends on from which nerves neurofibroma arises, whether from deeper plane or from cutaneous nerves. When skin is fixed to swelling it cannot be pinched out. For example, carcinoma,

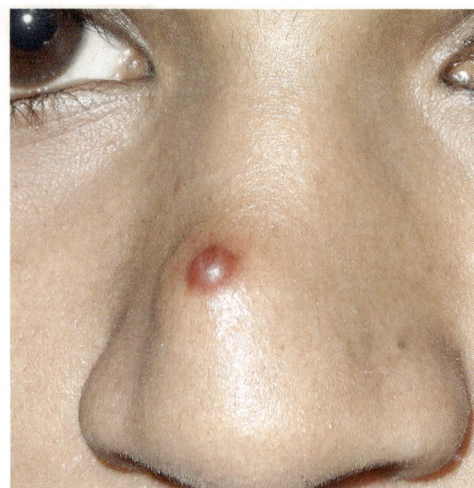

Fig. 4-64 *Swelling which is attached to skin*; it is arising from skin and is pigmented.

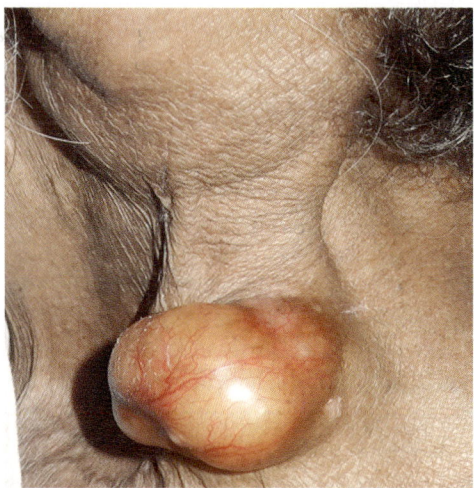

Fig. 4-65 *Swelling neck which is adherent/fixed* to the sternocleidomastoid muscle.

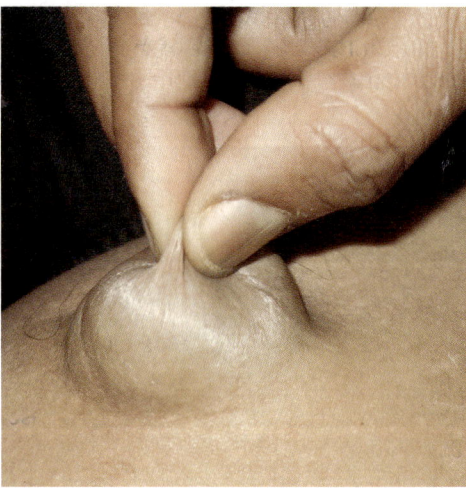

Fig. 4-66 Skin over the swelling should be *pinched/held* to check swelling is adherent to skin or not. *Gliding the skin* over the swelling is also another method.

inflammatory condition. In sarcoma skin may be stretched and still not adherent to tumor **(Fig. 4-66)**.

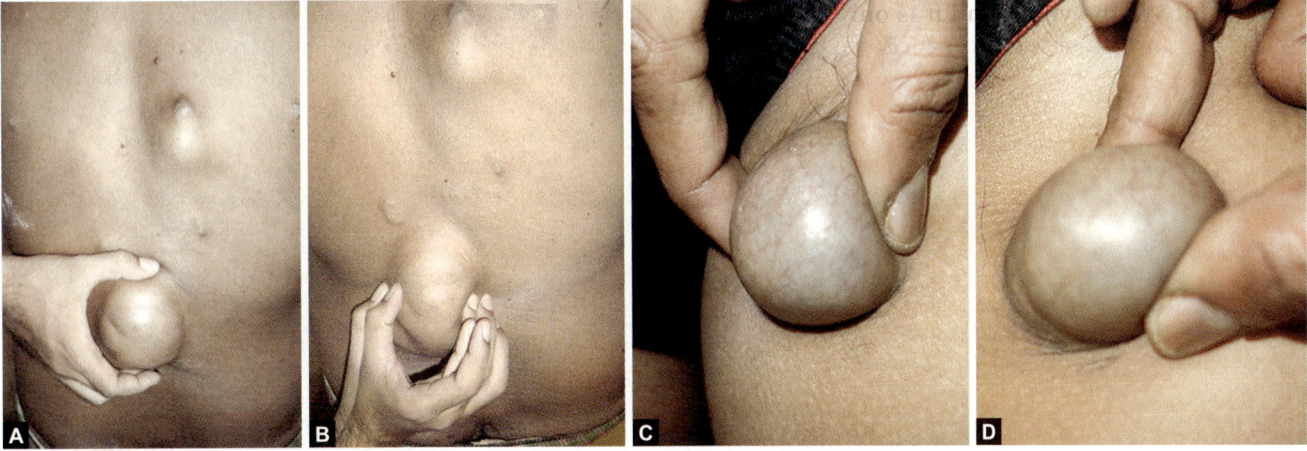

Figs. 4-67A to D Mobility of the swelling should be checked in *two perpendicular planes (both directions)* perpendicular to each other to find out the plane of the swelling.

Fixity to deeper structures: *Relation of swelling to underlying structures:* **Movements of the swelling in relation to the muscle underneath is checked before and after the muscle contraction** (Figs. 4.67A to D). This is an essential clinical method for any swelling to confirm whether it is outer or inside or deeper to the underlying muscle. Swelling arising from the muscle tissue moves with the muscle, becomes less mobile and decreases in size when muscle contracts. In abdominal swelling, swelling becomes less prominent if arising beneath the rectus muscle or remains unaltered or becomes more prominent if arising in front of the muscle. In breast lump, if it is adherent to pectoralis major muscle, mobility of swelling will be restricted. Clinician should know the names and surgical anatomy of the muscles underneath and their movements properly.

Swelling in subcutaneous plane: If swelling is freely mobile in all directions, it could be in subcutaneous plane. Lipoma, sebaceous cyst, often neurofibroma are subcutaneous swelling. Neurofibroma in subcutaneous plane will be mobile only transversely not along the line of the nerve. Swelling in subcutaneous plane which is not adherent to the muscle underneath will still be mobile freely after contraction of the muscle.

Adherent to deep fascia: A swelling being underneath is difficult to assess even though there may be some restrictions of all mobility (but not necessarily always). Tumors arising from the fascia like fibroma are relatively less mobile compared to that of subcutaneous fascia. Deep fascia cannot be put into contraction (exception: tensor fascia lata).

Swelling adherent to a tendon underneath will be mobile in the direction perpendicular to the line of the muscle fibers; but when the tendon of the specific muscle is taut (against resistance) mobility will be restricted. **Example:** Ganglion around the wrist adherent to the tendon; its mobility will be restricted on contracting the tendon underneath.

If swelling is adherent to muscle underneath, then when muscle is contracted against resistance mobility of the swelling is restricted and it becomes more prominent. While muscle is relaxed, swelling will be mobile. So mobility of the swelling should be checked in both directions before and after contracting the muscle underneath *against resistance.*

If swelling is arising from the muscle **(myoma)** or *deep to muscle,* then size of the swelling decreases (becomes less prominent) when muscle is contracted. Swelling arising from the muscle, mainly in the middle of the muscle will be transversely mobile. Again mobility, which was present initially will disappear completely during contraction of the muscle. Disappearance occurs much more significantly in swelling which is deeper to the muscle. Active movements of the muscle occur by isometric contraction wherein only few muscle fibers are involved; in muscle contraction against resistance, isometric contraction of all muscle fibers occurs.

Swellings arising from vessels or nerves will move only in horizontal direction/perpendicular to the line of nerve but will

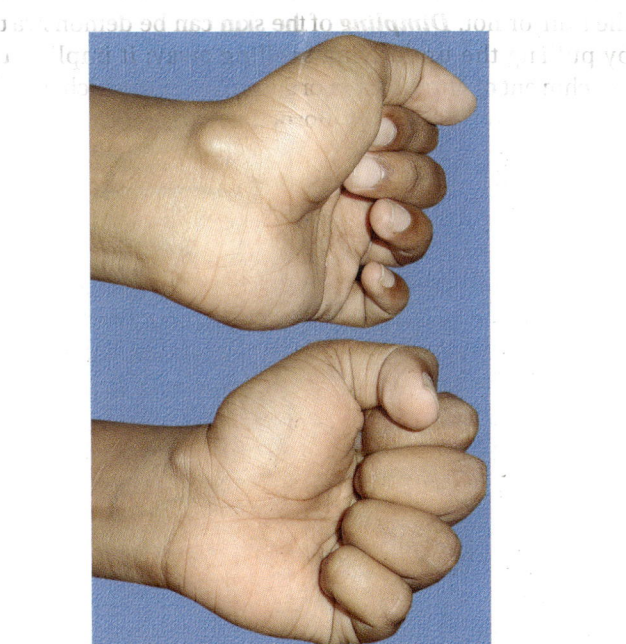

Fig. 4-68 Ganglion around the wrist adherent to the tendon; its mobility will be restricted on contracting the tendon underneath.

not show any mobility in longitudinal direction. Examples—neurofibroma, aneurysm.

> **Mobility of the swelling (Figs. 4-69A to C):**
> **Extrinsic mobility**
> - *Movement on deglutition*—thyroid swelling, thyroglossal cyst, subhyoid bursa
> - *Movement on protrusion of the tongue*—thyroglossal cyst moves on protrusion of the tongue–creates 'tug' with upward movement
> - *Movement with respiration*—it is seen in upper abdominal masses—like from liver, stomach, spleen, gallbladder, flexures of colon (often)
>
> ***Intrinsic mobility of the swelling***—it is checked in any swelling; but especially useful and essential in abdomen mass. Mobility in all directions should be checked. Intrinsic mobility is also checked in breast lump. Fibroadenoma is freely mobile and having intrinsic mobility within her breast tissue. Swelling may be freely mobile; nonmobile (fixed); restricted mobility (often difficult to say–clinician's feel, it is minimum mobility may be felt); mobility in one direction only.

Swelling arising from the bone is hard and absolutely fixed and cannot be moved separately from the bone (**Figs. 4-70 and 4-71**).

Methods of Contractions of Different Muscles Against Resistance

Figures 4-72 to 4-88 show the clinical methods of contracting the different muscles which is useful while examining the swelling in relation to these muscles. Clinician should aware of the attachments of each muscle.

Examination of Part at Distal and Proximal to the Swelling

Examination distally and proximally is essential to see *pressure effects* and wasting. Pressure effects may be on adjacent artery (absence/feeble pulse; ischemic changes). Distal pulses should be checked. Any thrill/murmur should be looked for. Nerves (wasting; paresis; altered sensation; deformities, etc.); bone (pressure erosion of the adjacent bone like in aneurysm, dermoid cyst, malignancy, etc.) are examined for pressure effects.

Examination of the Neurological (Sensory/Motor) System

Touch, sense of position, pain sensation should be checked for if any possible neurological deficits. Wasting and power of the muscles in relation to the joints distally should be

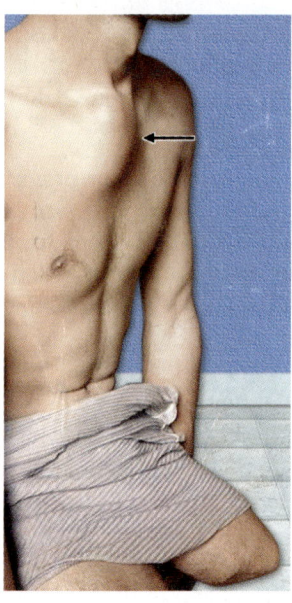

Fig. 4-70 Bony swelling in sternum which is *nonmobile*. In this patient, it is the secondaries from osteosarcoma of lower femur (thigh amputated).

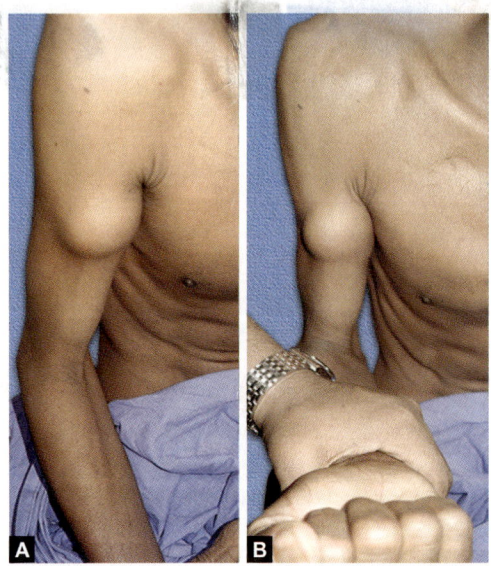

Figs. 4-69A and B Mobility of the swelling is checked initially; then *muscle underneath should be contracted against resistance*; mobility of the swelling is checked again to check fixity to muscle underneath. Clinician should have clear knowledge of the attachments of the muscle underneath.

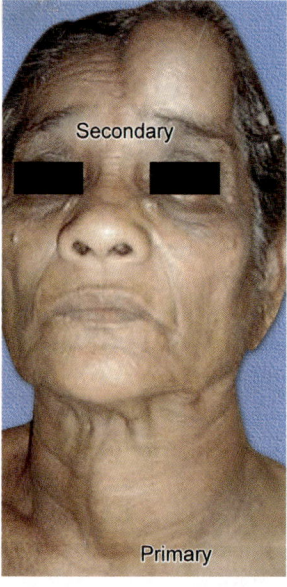

Fig. 4-71 Secondaries in the skull in a patient with primary in the thyroid (follicular carcinoma). Follicular carcinoma of thyroid causes *localized, warm, vascular, pulsatile, smooth, hard/soft (nonmobile)*, secondaries in the skull.

Chapter 4: Examination and Clinical Approach of a Swelling/Lump 111

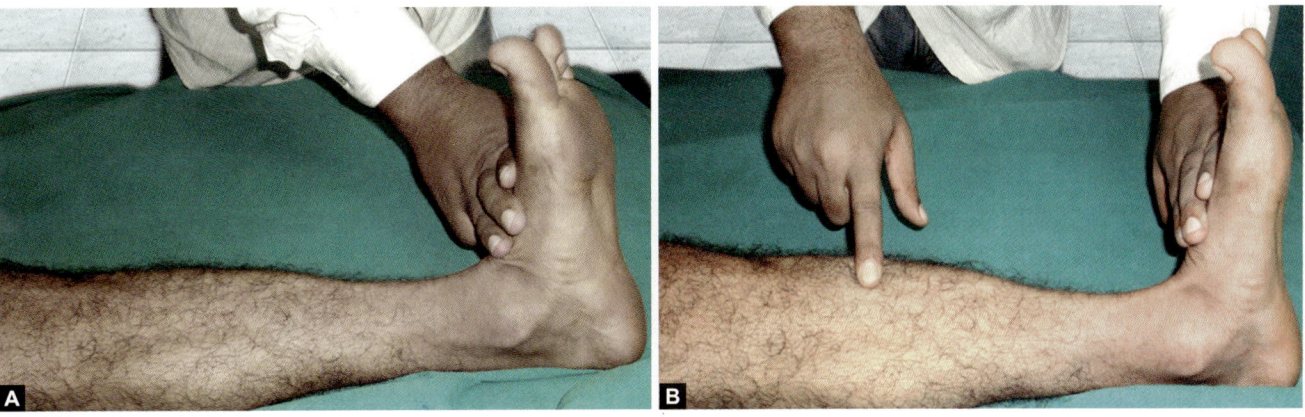

Figs. 4-72A and B Contraction of extensors of ankle.

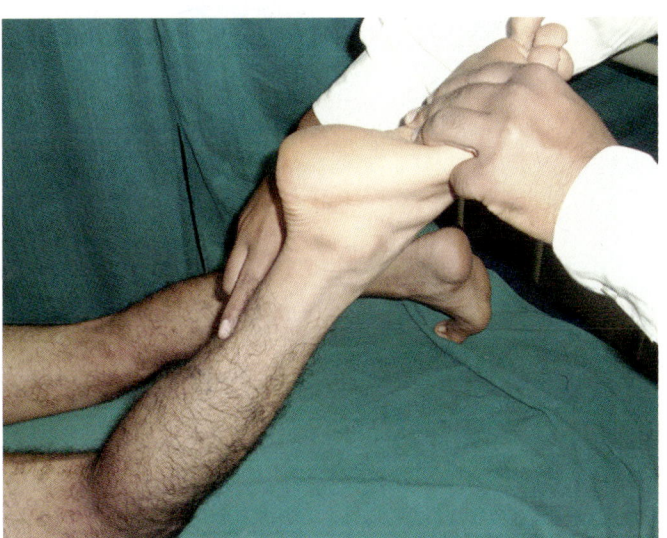

Fig. 4-73 Contraction of flexors of the ankle.

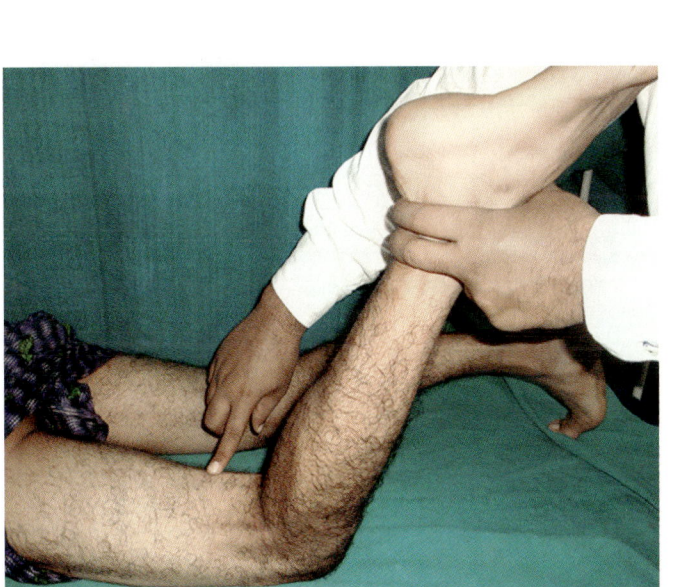

Fig. 4-74 Contraction of hamstring muscles.

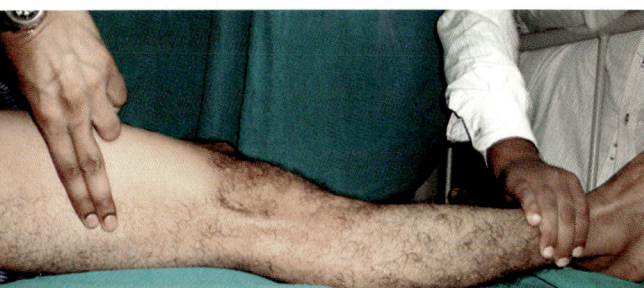

Fig. 4-75 Contraction of gluteus medius muscle.

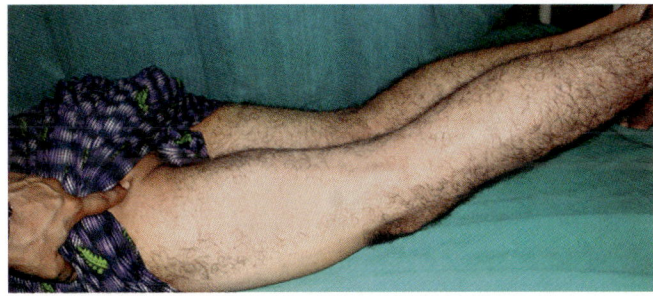

Fig. 4-76 Contraction of gluteus maximus muscle.

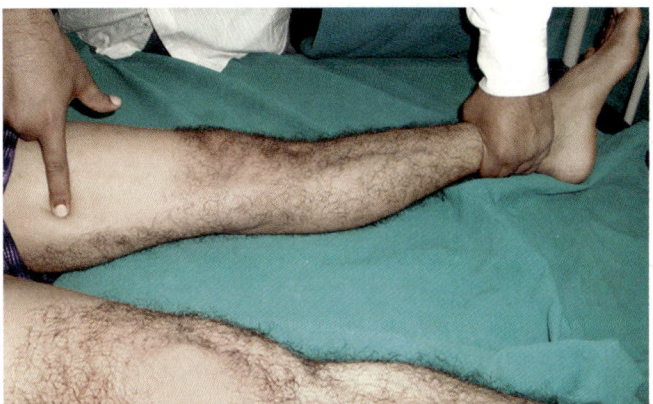

Fig. 4-77 Contraction of adductors of thigh.

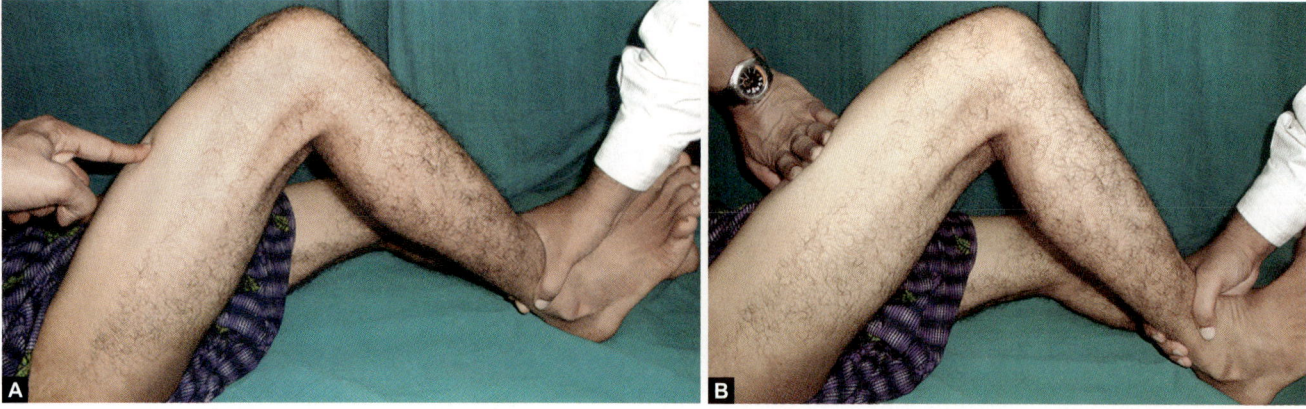

Figs. 4-78A and B Contraction of quadriceps femoris.

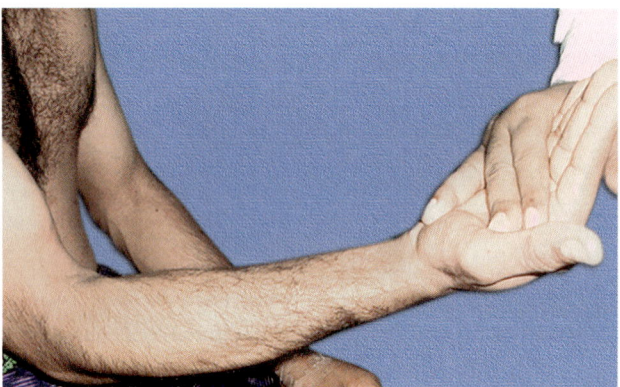

Fig. 4-79 Contraction of wrist flexors.

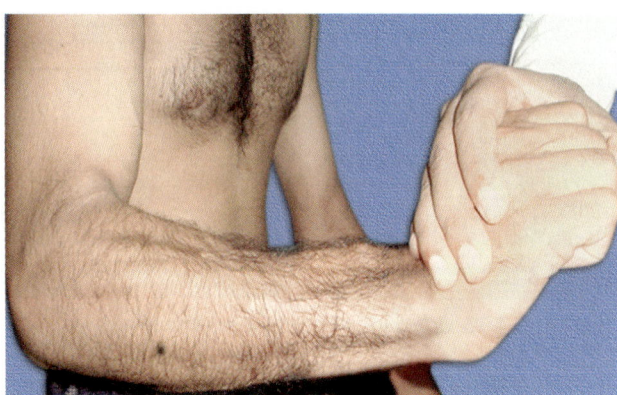

Fig. 4-80 Contraction of wrist extensors.

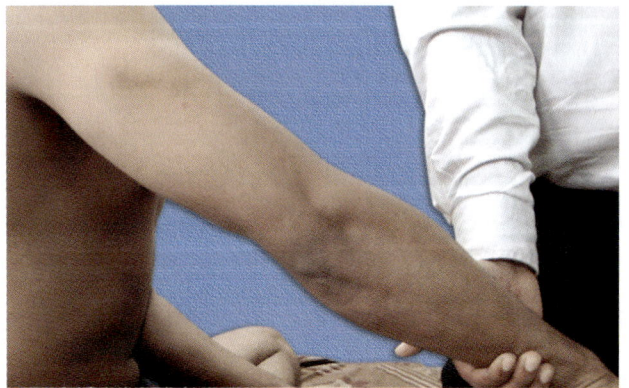

Fig. 4-81 Contraction of triceps brachii muscle.

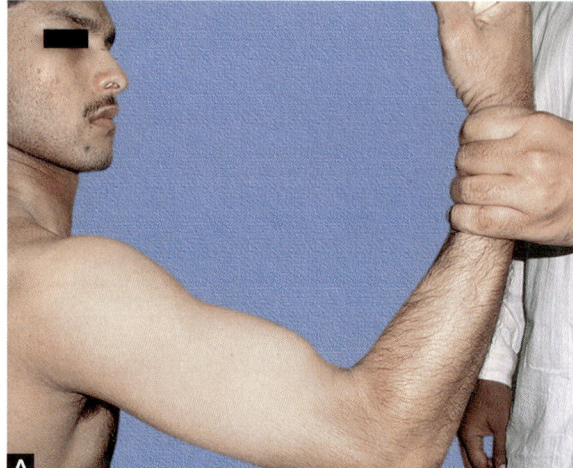

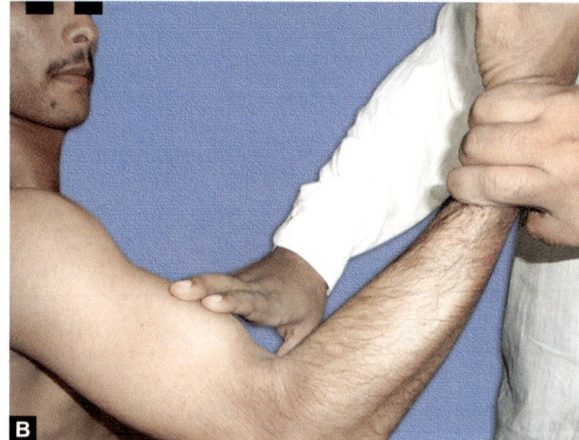

Figs. 4-82A and B Contraction of biceps brachii muscle.

checked and graded (paralysis can occur). In spinal tumors and spina bifida, distal sensations and muscle power may be altered.

Percussion

Percussion over the swelling in relevant area like hernia should be done. ***Laryngocele** in the neck is resonant*. Abdominal mass should always be percussed. Often tenderness may be elicited by percussion.

Chapter 4: Examination and Clinical Approach of a Swelling/Lump 113

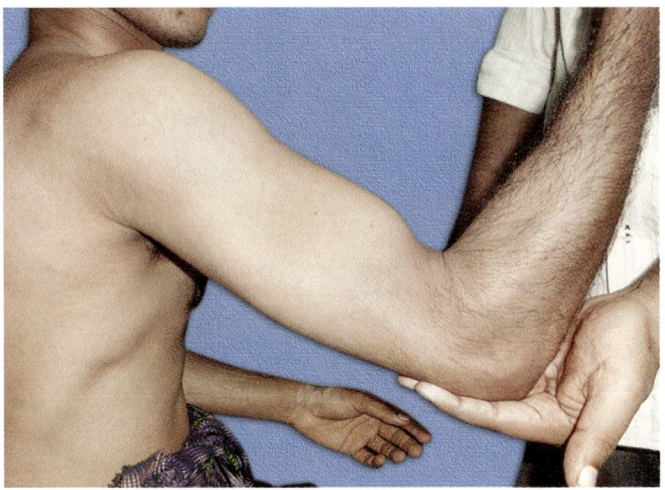

Fig. 4-83 Contraction of latissimus dorsi muscle.

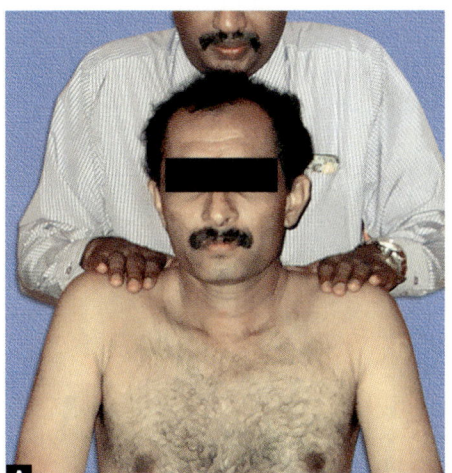

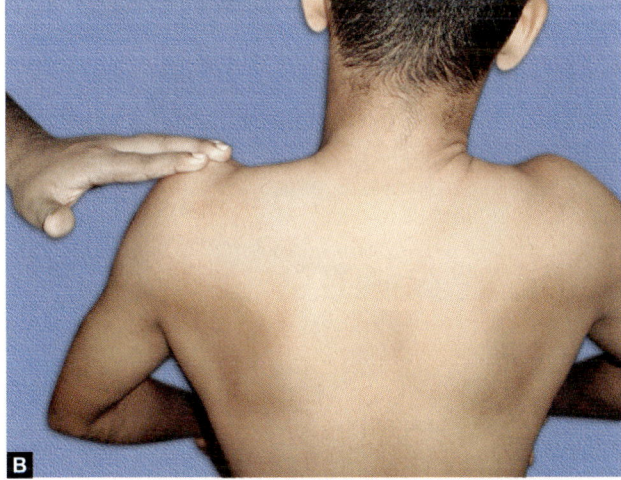

Figs. 4-84A and B Contraction of trapezius muscle.

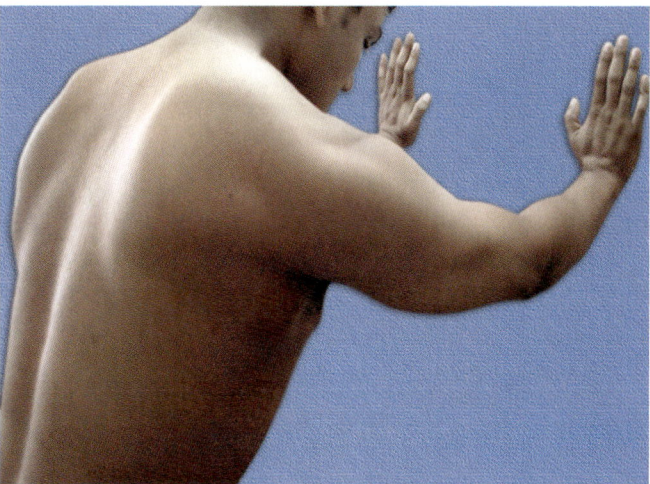

Fig. 4-85 Contraction of serratus anterior muscle.

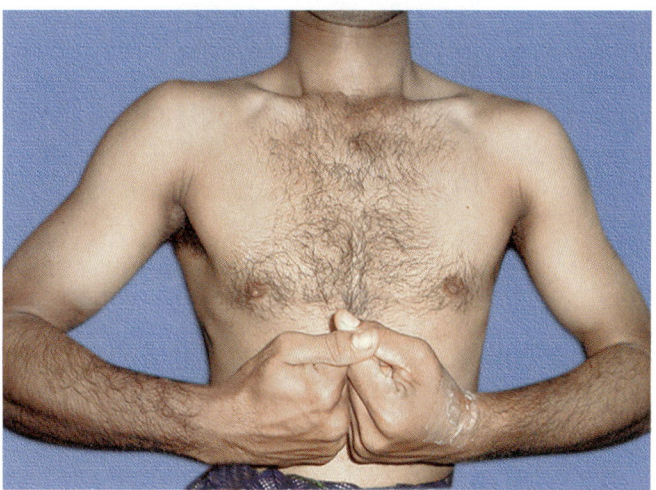

Fig. 4-86 Contraction of pectoralis major muscle.

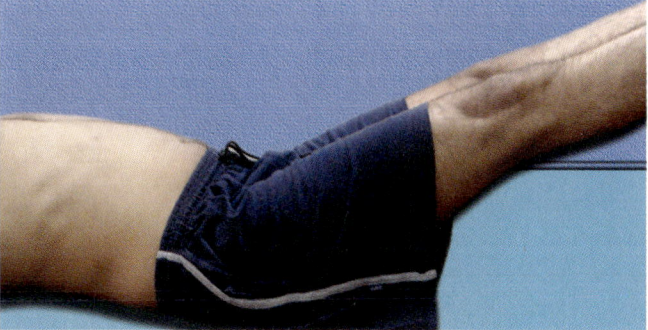

Fig. 4-87 Contraction of abdominal wall muscles.

Auscultation

It is done to look for bruit over the swelling like in A-V malformation, arterial stenosis, aneurysms. **Machinery murmur** is heard in AV fistulas. **Bruit** is short, medium pitched murmur heard over the swelling with each pulse wave/heartbeat **(Fig. 4-89)**.

Movements

Joints above and below the swelling should be examined both for active and passive movements. If the swelling is close to the joint, it should be evaluated clinically to see that whether swelling is communicating with the joint or not. For example Morrant Baker'cyst and semimembranosus bursa are in close relation to the dorsal aspect of the knee joint in popliteal fossa. Baker's cyst lies in the midline, deep and lower; it disappears on flexing the knee joint as

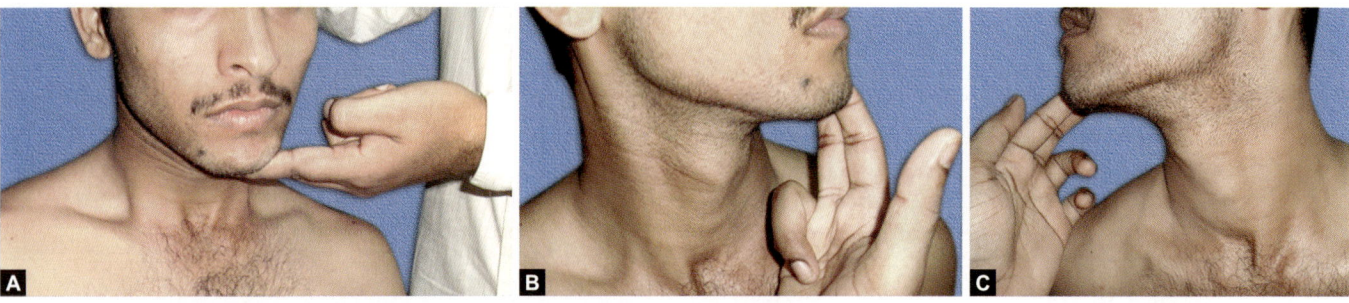

Figs. 4-88A to C *Contraction of sternomastoid muscles* both side together and each side independently.

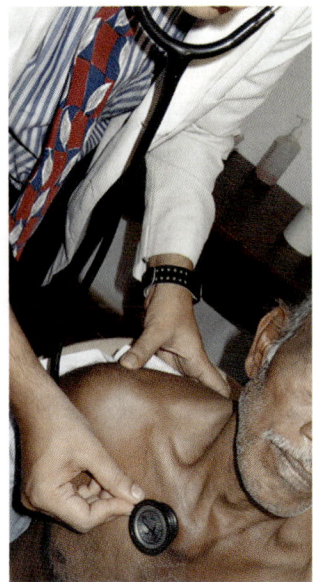

Fig. 4-89 Swelling *should be auscultated for any bruit.*

it communicates with the knee joint through a hiatus in the joint capsule; osteoarthritis of the knee joint is found. Swelling is nontransilluminant but often compressible. Semimembranosus bursa is located in the medial and upper part of the popliteal fossa between semimembranosus muscle and medial head of the gastrocnemius muscle; it becomes flaccid on flexion of the knee joint but will not disappear on flexion of the knee joint; it is commonly transilluminant. Joint is normal in semimembranosus bursa **(Figs. 4-90A to C).**

Measurements

Size of the swelling is measured using measuring tape vertically and horizontally in centimeters. ***Length of limb and girth of the limb*** distally is measured for increase or decrease in size.

Length and girth of the limb is increased in congenital AV malformations (congenital AV fistula). In wasting of the limb muscles, girth only will be reduced.

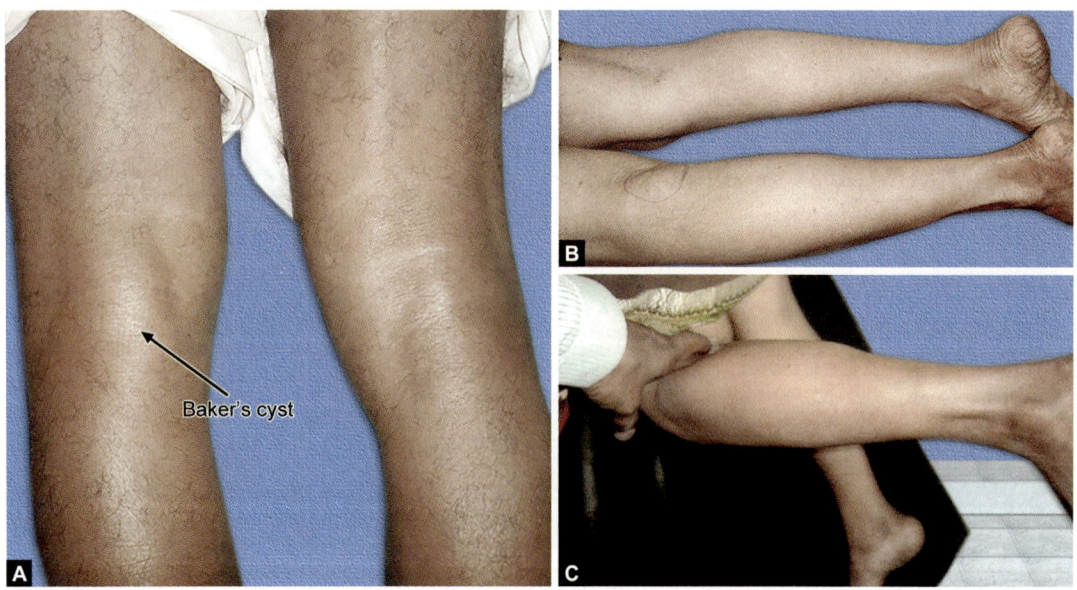

Figs. 4-90A to C (A) Morrant Baker' cyst is located in the popliteal fossa lower midline part; deeply placed swelling is *fluctuant, nontransilluminating, communicates with the joint cavity, disappears on flexion of knee joint*, often compressible on palpation; (B and C): Semimembranosus bursa which is located in the medial and upper part of the popliteal fossa between semimembranosus muscle and medial head of the gastrocnemius muscle; it becomes *only flaccid on flexion of the knee joint but will not disappear on flexion of the knee joint; joint is normal.*

Examination of Regional Lymph Nodes

Regional lymph nodes should be examined for significant enlargement. Other groups/proximal groups should be examined in relevant/systemic clinical indications (**Figs. 4-91 and 4-92**).

RELEVANT SYSTEMIC EXAMINATION

Systemic examination is a very essential like respiratory (pleural effusion, consolidation, cavity), cardiac, skeletal (bones and joints for osteomyelitis, gibbus, kyphosis, scoliosis, deformities) and abdomen (mass, fluid), neurological system (**Figs. 4-93 and 4-94**).

PROPER CLINICAL DIAGNOSIS

Clinical diagnosis of the swelling should be given based on history, clinical findings; it needs proper analysis, correlation of different findings to give a valid conclusion. Three points should be assessed: (1) *Exact anatomical origin*, i.e. from which structure swelling originates; (2) *Its pathological nature*; (3) *Its extent and spread*, i.e. whether swelling is confined to area of the structure or organ or occupied/spread/invaded beyond the organ or structure of origin. In malignancy, whether disease is local or locally advanced or metastatic, i.e. staging of the tumor should be assessed (predicted) clinically.

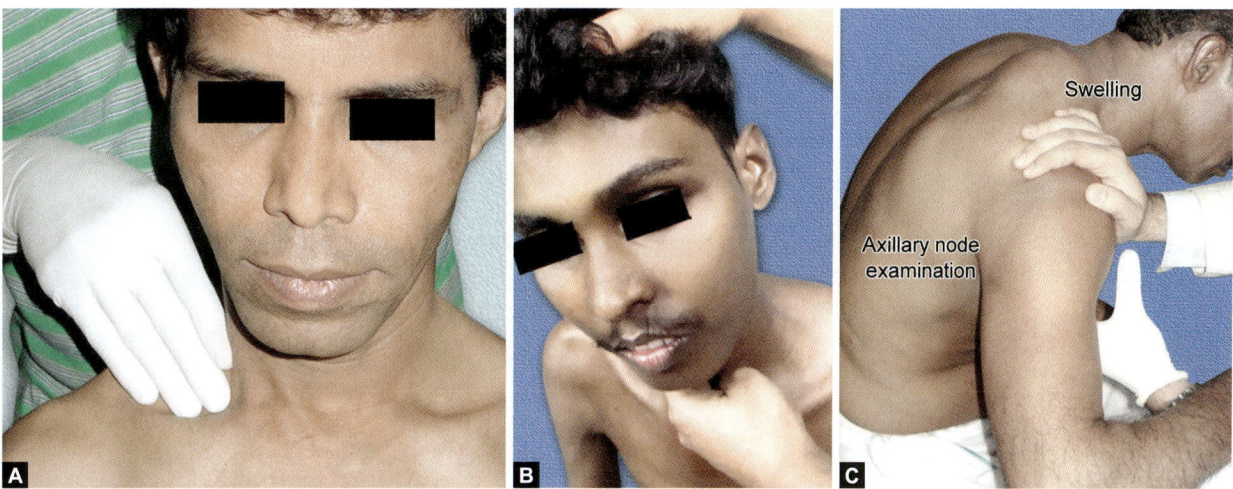

Figs. 4-91A to C *Relevant regional lymph node examination* should be done to look for palpable significant nodes.

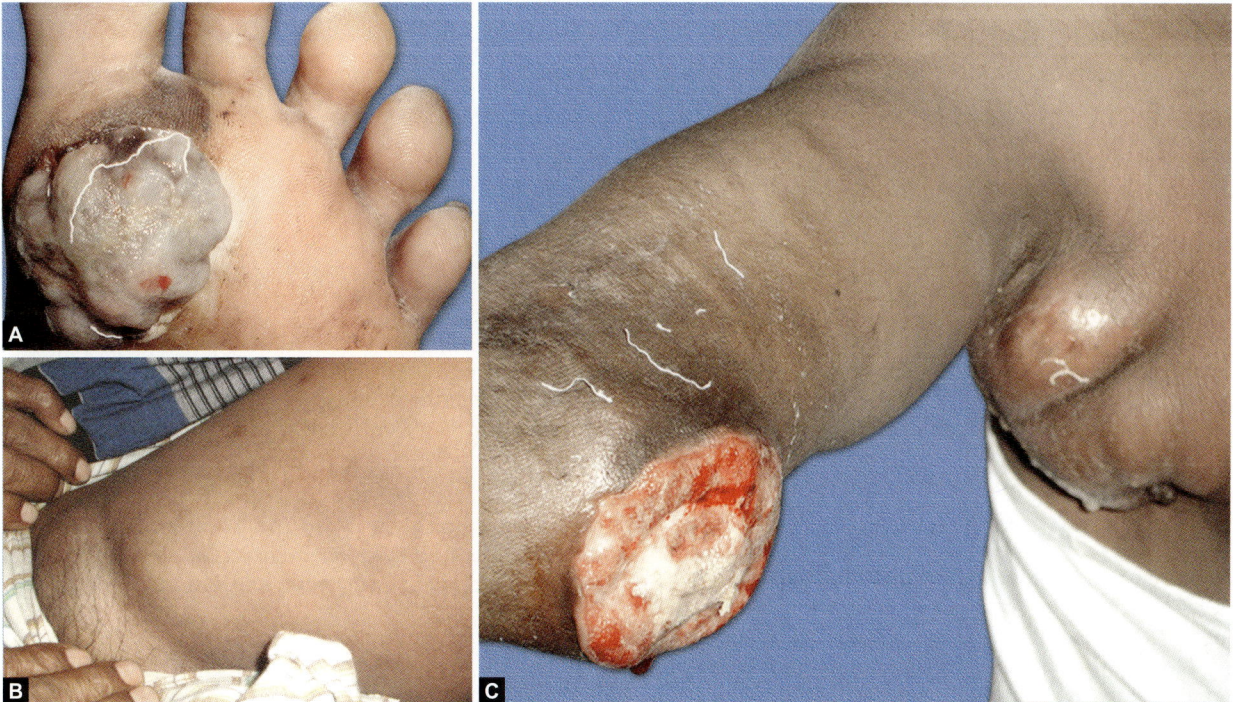

Figs. 4-92A to C (A and B) Melanoma toe causing *inguinal lymph node secondaries*; (C) Squamous cell carcinoma (epithelioma) of the skin over the right elbow with fungating *axillary lymph node secondaries*.

Case sheet writing in a patient with swelling

History
Name: Age:
Occupation: Sex: Place/residence:

Chief complaints

History of present illness
- Swelling – duration, mode of onset and progress, site of origin, number, disappearing or reducing in size
- Pain – origin, nature, character, duration, time of starting of pain, specific features, severity, aggravating or relieving factors
- Fever – type, severity, duration
- Other lumps – when started, progress
- Secondary changes like ulceration, fungation
- Loss of function
- Loss of weight
- Pressure symptoms

Past history
- Past history of swelling and treatment for that
- Tuberculosis, spinal diseases, diabetes, leprosy, malignancies
- Past history of treatment and surgery

Family history
- Family tree; history of tuberculosis, diabetes, malignancies; treatment history

General examination
Anemia, edema, jaundice, clubbing, lymphadenopathy, pulse, blood pressure, temperature, attitude, nutrition, body weight

Local examination
Inspection
- Swelling – location, size, shape, extent, color, surface of the swelling, skin over the swelling, number, edge/margin/border of the swelling, movement of the swelling, pulsation, impulse on coughing
- Pressure effects – edema, dilated veins, paralysis, deformity, wasting

Palpation
- Local raise of temperature, tenderness
- Size, shape and extent of the swelling, edge of the swelling, surface of the swelling, consistency
- Fluctuation, transillumination test
- Reducibility, expansile impulse on coughing, compressibility, pulsatility, thrill
- Plane of the selling, mobility, fixity to skin or deeper structures
- Examination proximal and distal to swelling
- Examination of regional neurological and vascular systems

Percussion
Auscultation
Movements of adjacent joints
Measurements of limb girth and length
Gait
Examination of regional lymph nodes
Systemic examination – abdomen, respiratory, cardiac and central nervous systems

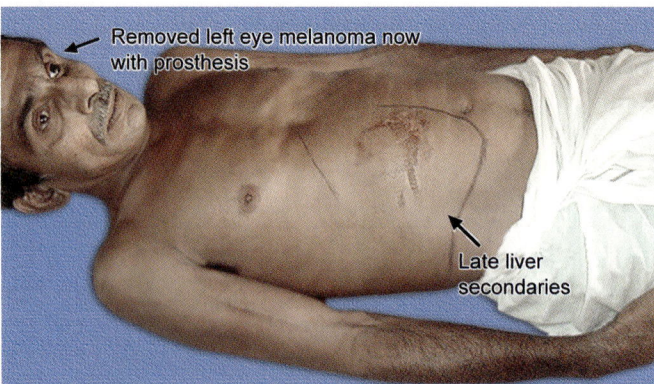

Fig. 4-93 Secondaries in liver—here large enlarged liver is present (massive hepatomegaly); *primary lesion was in the eye* which was removed surgically many years back and prosthesis was kept. Melanoma from the eye is known to cause *late liver secondaries*.

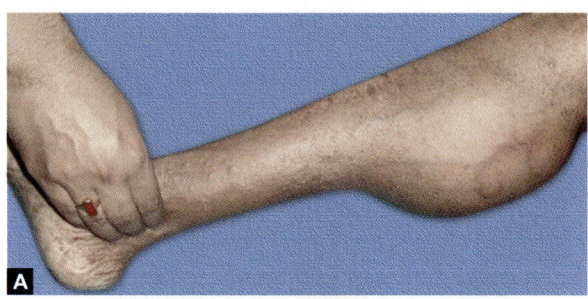

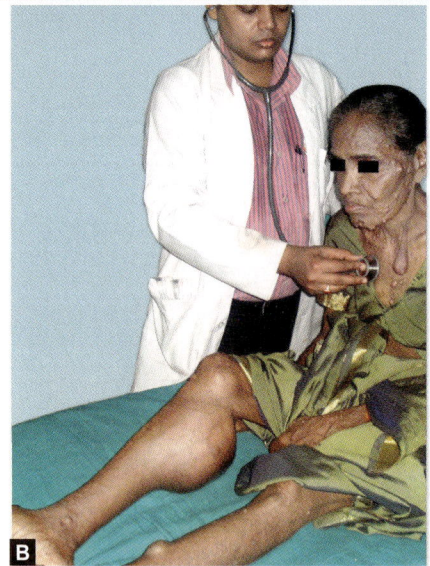

Figs. 4-94A and B Neurofibrosarcoma leg. Distal pulse should be examined for *pressure effect*. Respiratory system (chest) should be examined in this patient for *lung secondaries*.

■ RELEVANT INVESTIGATIONS

HB% (anemia in chronic infection, tuberculosis, malignancies); Total WBC count (raised in acute inflammatory condition), DC, ESR (raised in tuberculosis and malignancy), random blood sugar (raised in carbuncles), blood urea and serum creatinine (to assess the renal function).

Fine needle aspiration cytology (FNAC), ultrasound (US) of part, computed tomography (CT) scan (Fig. 4-95), magnetic resonance imaging (MRI) for bony and joint swellings, angiography and Doppler in vascular swellings, incision or excision biopsy in soft tissue sarcomas.

■ DIFFERENTIAL DIAGNOSIS

Swellings may be *congenital/traumatic/inflammatory (acute/subacute/chronic)/neoplastic*. Neoplastic swelling may be benign or malignant. In malignancy, it may be early or

Chapter 4: Examination and Clinical Approach of a Swelling/Lump

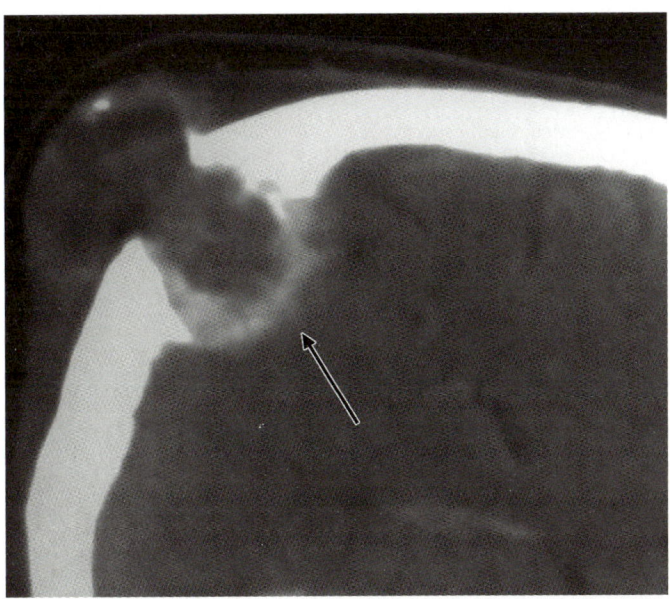

Fig. 4-95 CT head showing *swelling eroding into the cranium*; it is also possible that intracranial swelling can erode skull to present as swelling scalp.

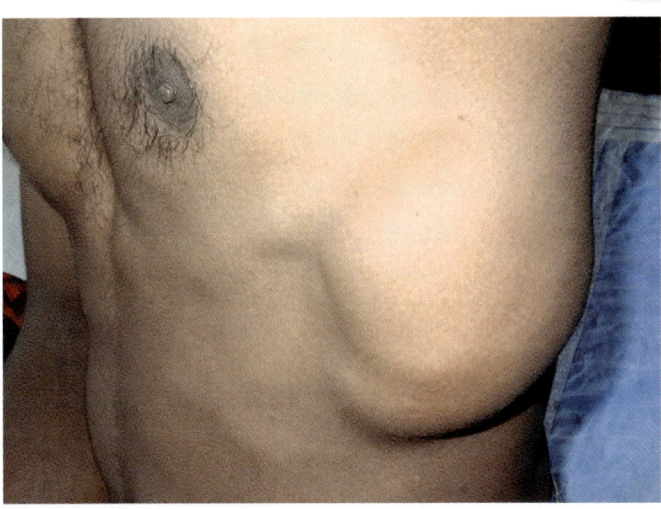

Fig. 4-97 Chest wall swelling. Note that *swelling is well localized*.

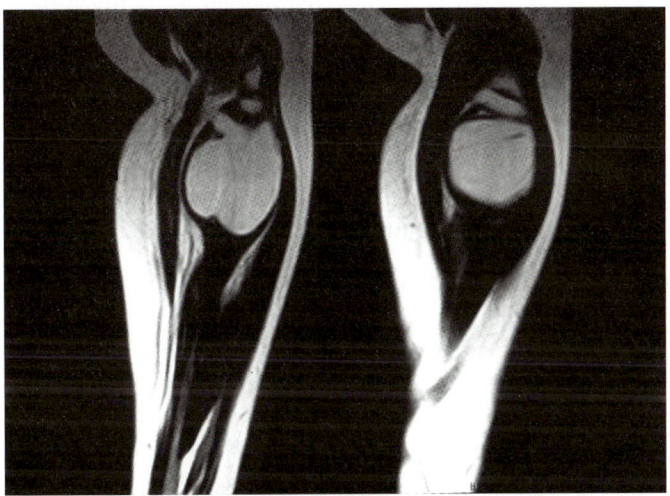

Fig. 4-96 MRI showing intramuscular lipoma.

advanced. First *anatomical diagnosis* of the swelling should be made by clinical methods and proper analysis. It means from which anatomical structure the swelling is arising from. Anatomical diagnosis can be by various clinical methods like movements, relation to muscle, plane of the swelling (Fig. 4-97). Then *pathological diagnosis* is made out by examining the surface, consistency, fluctuation, transillumination, tenderness, warmness. When features elicited are not suitable for one diagnosis, it is not possible to give a single diagnosis. Then differential diagnoses should be given. While giving differential diagnosis, clinical features which correlate to most possible condition should be given as first possible diagnosis; like that second, third, so on. *It is not necessary to give every condition as differential diagnosis*. Only conditions that is relevant to those clinical features should be given as differential diagnosis. Congenital conditions are—hemangiomas, dermoid cyst, etc. Cellulitis, abscess, boil, carbuncle are inflammatory conditions. Neoplasms can be benign or malignant. Lipoma, papilloma, neurofibromas are examples of benign swellings. Tumors like carcinoma, melanoma, skin tumors, sarcomas are malignant tumors. Other swellings like sebaceous cyst, keloid, pyogenic granuloma are also important.

Classification of Swellings

	Cutaneous swellings	*Subcutaneous swellings*	*Soft tissue swellings: Deep to deep fascia*	*Bony swellings*
Congenital	Mole, hemangioma, lymphangioma	Sequestration and tubulodermoids, sebaceous cyst, lymph cyst	Branchial cyst, thyroglossal cyst	Bony deformities
Traumatic	Vesicles, bulla, keloid, corn	Hematoma, implantation dermoid, bursa	Soft tissue hematoma, ruptured tendon	Fractures
Inflammatory	Acute—boil, erysipelas, impetigo, carbuncle, keratoacanthoma Chronic—pyogenic granuloma, hidradenitis suppurativa, lupus vulgaris, condyloma lata	Acute—cellulitis, abscess, lymphadenitis Chronic—lymphadenopathy, antibioma	Myositis ossificans, lymphadenitis, deep abscess	Osteomyelitis
Neoplastic	Benign—wart, nevus, dermatofibroma, skin adnexal tumor	Benign—lipoma, fibroma, neurofibroma, neurilemmoma	Soft tissue tumors—benign—myxoma, rhabdomyoma	Bony tumors—benign (osteoma, osteochondroma, chondroma);

Contd...

	Cutaneous swellings	Subcutaneous swellings	Soft tissue swellings: Deep to deep fascia	Bony swellings
	Malignant—epithelioma, basal cell carcinoma, melanoma, dermatofibrosarcoma, malignant skin adnexal tumor	Malignant—fibrosarcoma, neurofibrosarcoma	Malignant—soft tissue tumors arising deeper to deep fascia—synovial sarcoma, liposarcoma, rhabdomyosarcoma, nerve sheath tumors, etc.	Malignant (secondaries in bone, osteosarcoma, Ewing's tumor, osteoclastoma, chondrosarcoma)
Others *Swellings arising from cavity like cranial, thoracic or abdominal can be included here with specifications*	Seborrheic keratosis, cutaneous horns	Ganglion, sebaceous cyst, lymph cyst, rheumatic nodule		
Features	From epidermis; projects outside from skin surface; color changes are common; skin is adherent–pinching or gliding is not possible; shiny and stretched; superficial plane; mobile all round	Freely mobile; not adherent to skin or deeper plane; does not project out from skin; skin texture is normal; pinching or gliding of skin is possible; plane is deeper to skin; mobile even after contracting the muscle underneath	Deeper plane; mobility restricts while contracting the deeper muscle and swelling may reduce in size; without contracting the muscle it will be mobile; not adherent to bone underneath	Very deep swelling; totally nonmobile; bony hard; usually superficial structures are free (skin, subcutaneous tissue, soft tissues); but may come out of all these tissues towards skin causing sinus or fungation in either chronic osteomyelitis or malignant tumors of bone

Cystic Swellings

Cystic swellings are common surgical clinical entity. Common cystic swellings are discussed in the table. They are usually nontender unless infected, smooth, soft, fluctuant well localized swellings. They are transilluminant if they contain clear fluid as content. They are usually single; some may be multiple. Dermoids, sebaceous cyst, ganglions, bursae are common cystic swellings.

Cysts

Cyst is a collection of fluid in a sac lined by epithelium or endothelium. Word meaning of cyst is '*bladder*' (Greek). In true cyst, cyst wall is lined by epithelium or endothelium. If infection occurs cyst wall will also be lined by granulation tissue. Fluid is usually serous or mucoid derived from the secretion of the lining. In false cyst, cyst does not have epithelial lining. Fluid collection occurs as a result of exudation or degeneration. *Examples:* Pseudocyst of pancreas, wall of cystic swelling in tuberculous peritonitis, cystic degeneration of tumor, after hemorrhage in a hematoma red cells are lysed, get absorbed and fluid remains as a false cyst. '*Apoplectic cyst*' is formed in brain as a result of ischemia causing collection of fluid.

Classification of Cysts

1. **Congenital cyst:** *Dermoids*: Sequestration dermoid; *Tubulodermoids*: Thyroglossal cyst, postanal dermoid, ependymal cyst, urachal cyst; *Cysts of embryonic remnants*: Cysts from paramesonephric duct and mesonephric duct; Cysts of urachus and vitellointestinal duct.
2. **Acquired cysts:** *Retention cysts*: They are accumulation of secretion of a gland due to obstruction of a duct. Examples: Sebaceous cyst, bartholin cyst, cyst of pancreas, cyst of parotid, breast, epididymis. *Distention cyst*: Lymph cyst, ovarian cyst, colloid goiter. *Exudation cyst*: Bursa, hydrocele.
3. **Cystic tumors:** Dermoid cyst of ovary, cystadenomas.
4. **Traumatic cyst:** Due to trauma, hematoma occurs usually in thigh, loin, and shin. It eventually gets lined by endothelium containing brown colored fluid with cholesterol crystals.
5. **Degenerative cyst:** Due to cystic degeneration of a solid tumor (due to necrosis of tumor).
6. **Parasitic cyst:** Hydatid cyst, trichiniasis, cysticercosis.

Clinical features of a cyst: Hemispherical swelling which is smooth, fluctuant, nontender, well-localized. Some cysts are transilluminant. Presentation varies depending on its anatomical location.

Effects of a cyst: *Compression* to adjacent structures: Choledochal cyst compressing over the CBD; *infection*; sinus formation; *hemorrhage*; *torsion* like in ovarian cyst; *calcification*; cachexia: in malignant ovarian cyst patient goes for severe cachexia.

Dermoids

1. Congenital dermoid (formed in intrauterine life and manifest later in life)—sequestration, tubulodermoid.
2. Acquired—implantation dermoid.

Types

1. **Sequestration dermoids:** It occurs at the line of embryonic fusion due to inclusion of epithelium beneath the surface which later gets sequestered forming a cystic swelling in the deeper plane.

Common sites are: Forehead; external angular dermoid; root of nose; post-auricular dermoid; sublingual dermoid; in the ear; anywhere in midline or in the line of fusion. Dermoids occurring in the skull may extend into the cranial cavity.

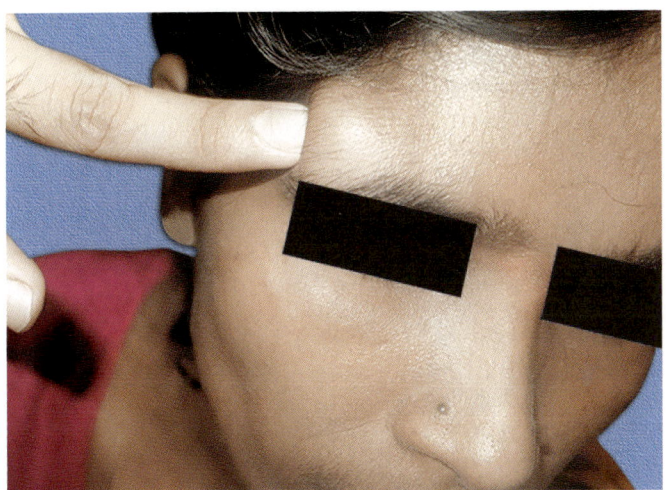

Fig. 4-98 External angular dermoid; bone resorption should be checked by *indenting the finger on the edge*/margin of the swelling.

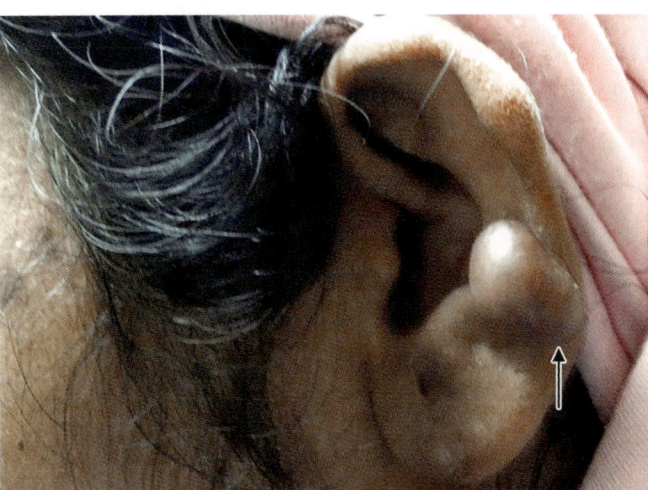

Fig. 4-99 Dermoid in the ear. It arises due to sequestration *at the fusion line of one of the six developmental ear tubercles* (Each ear develops from six ear tubercles).

When it occurs as external angular dermoid, it extends into the orbital cavity. Or it can extend into any cavity underneath in relation to its anatomical location (e.g., thorax, abdomen). Dermoid cyst contains putty-like desquamated material along with hair, hair follicles, sweat and sebaceous gland. It is lined by both dermal and epidermal components.

External angular dermoid: It is a sequestration dermoid situated over the external angular process of the frontal bone (frontozygomatic suture). Outer extremity of the eyebrow extends over some part of the swelling. This typical feature differentiates it from the swelling arising from the lacrimal gland. It may extend into the orbital cavity also (Fig. 4-98).

Internal angular dermoid: It is a sequestration dermoid cyst in central position at the root of the nose. Dermoid cyst in scalp may lie purely in the scalp or may cause a defect in the skull with attachment to dura, or may be partly intracranial and partly extracranial with a stalk between the two parts, or very rarely purely intracranial lying deep into the skull and outer to dura but attached to it.

Clinical features: Painless swelling in the line of fusion, presents in the second or third decade onwards, which is smooth, soft, nontender, fluctuant (*Paget's test positive,* i.e. swelling is fixed with two fingers and summit is indented to get yielding sensation due to fluid), nontransilluminating, with free skin often adherent to the deeper plane (Fig. 4.99). There will be resorption *and indentation* of the bone beneath . Impulse on coughing may be evident if there is intracranial extension. It should be differentiated from lipoma and sebaceous cyst. Slip sign and free mobility are features of lipoma. Skin is adherent in sebaceous cyst often with a punctum. X-ray part or CT scan is often needed to evaluate its deeper extent.

Submental dermoid: It is a congenital sequestration dermoid occurring during fusion of 1st and 2nd branchial arches. It is deep to deep fascia of neck. It presents as soft, cystic, fluctuant, nontransilluminating, swelling in midline in submental region which does not move with deglutition nor moves while protruding the tongue out. It should be differentiated from thyroglossal cyst, cold abscess from submental lymph nodes or sebaceous cyst.

2. **Tubulodermoids:** It arises due to fluid collection in a nonobliterated portion of embryonic ectodermal tubular structure. Examples include—thyroglossal cyst, ependymal cyst, and postanal dermoid.

3. **Teratomatous dermoid:** It is cystic structure arising from totipotent cell, i.e. from all germinal layers ecto, meso and endoderms but with the preponderance of ectoderm. It occurs in ovary, testis, retroperitoneum, superior mediastinum, presacral region. It contains hairs, teeth, cartilage, and muscle. It can be benign or malignant.

4. **Implantation dermoid:** Due to minor pricks or trauma, epidermis gets buried into the deeper subcutaneous tissue which causes reaction and acquired cyst formation (trauma is often forgotten). It is common in fingers (common in tailors), toes and feet (Figs. 4-100A and B). It is slowly progressive swelling after a trauma which is smooth, soft, mobile, tensely cystic, nontransilluminating and adherent to skin. It contains cheesy-like material lined by squamous epithelium, without hair follicle/sweat glands/sebaceous glands. It can cause infection, rupture or pressure effects on digital nerves.

Sebaceous Cyst (Wen)

It is a *retention cyst*. It is due to obstruction at the mouth of a sebaceous duct, causing a cystic swelling due to collection of its own secretion. It is common in face, scalp, and scrotum. *It is not seen in palms and plantar aspect of foot (sole)* as there are no sebaceous glands. Sebaceous cyst contains yellowish white material with fat, desquamated epithelium (forming thick porridge like) which is having putty-like cheesy consistency, with a parasite in the wall of the cyst—*demodex folliculorum*. Its lining is only epidermal layer of squamous epithelium.

Clinical features: Painless swelling which is *smooth, soft, nontender, freely mobile, adherent to skin especially over the summit, fluctuant (positive Paget's test), nontransilluminating with punctum over the summit. It moulds on finger indentation. Punctum* is present over the summit in 70% of cases because here sebaceous duct directly opens into the skin which gets blocked. Punctum is depressed black colored spot over the summit of the sebaceous cyst. Because of the denuded

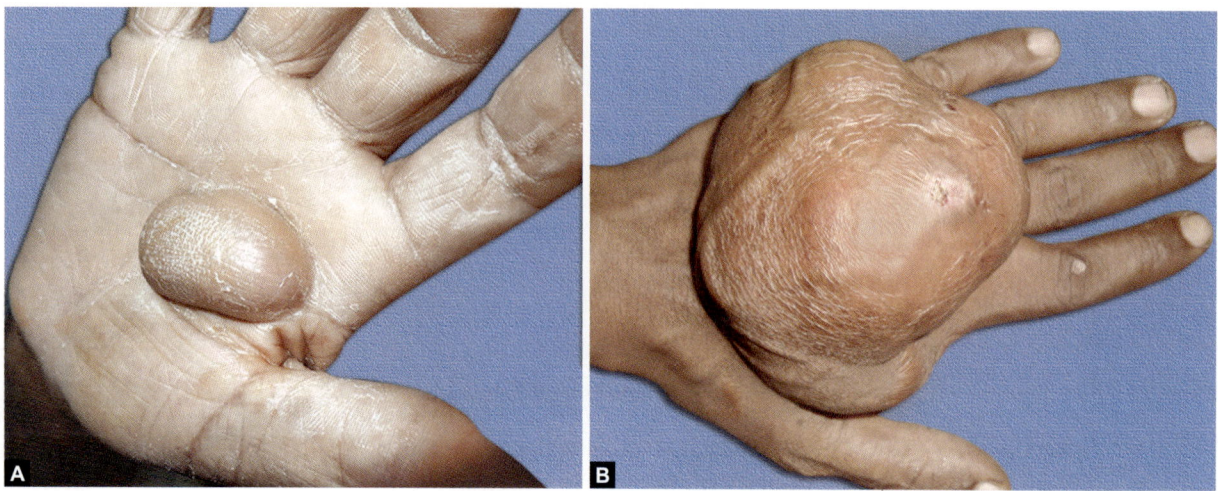

Figs. 4-100A and B *Implantation dermoids* in the hand-palmar and dorsal aspect.

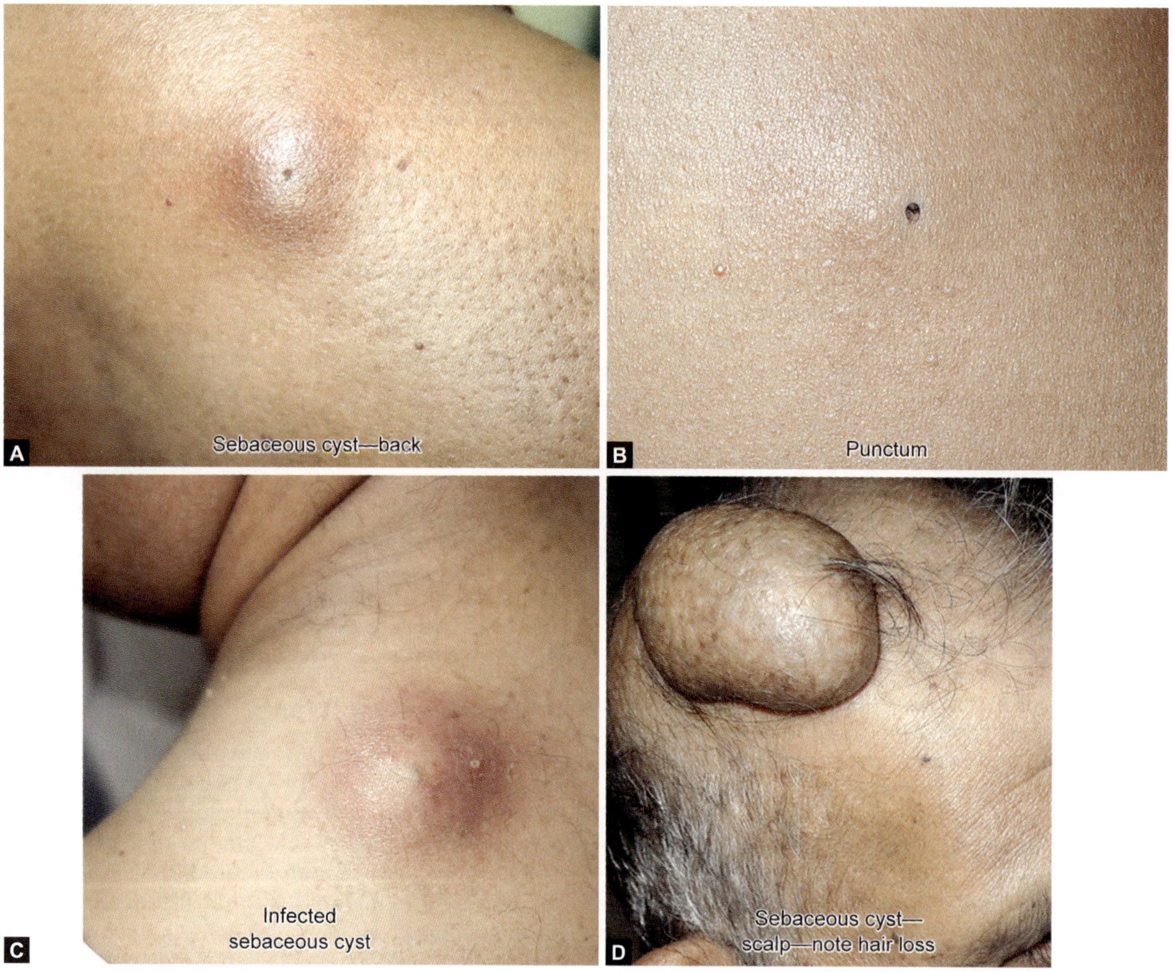

Figs. 4-101A to D (A) Typical sebaceous cyst back; (B) Note the punctum; (C) Infected sebaceous cyst; (D) Sebaceous cyst scalp—usually seen with loss of hair.

squamous epithelium (keratin), it is black in color. In 30% cases, punctum is not seen, as sebaceous duct opens into hair follicle. Other view is that it may arise from epidermal rest cell or pleuripotent cells of skin. Sebaceous cysts can be multiple, commonly in face and scrotum. Often hairs are scanty or skin over the summit of the sebaceous cyst is bald (Figs. 4-101A to D).

Complications: The contents may get spontaneously squeezed through the punctum resulting in disappearance of the swelling. *Infection* and abscess formation may occur; Surface may *rupture* and gets *ulcerated* with foul-smelling discharge and chronic inflammation, this discharge often spreads to surrounding tissues and hardens, and is called as—*Cock's peculiar tumor when occurring in the scalp,* which

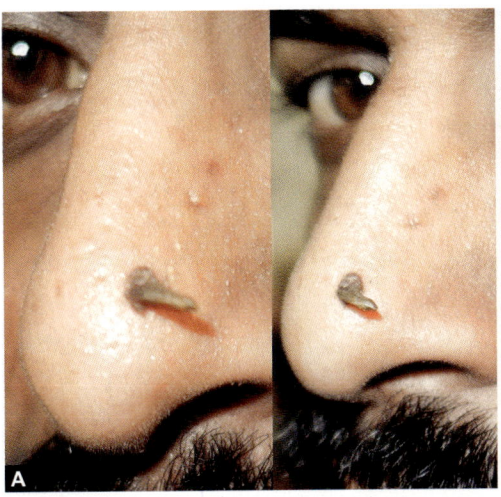
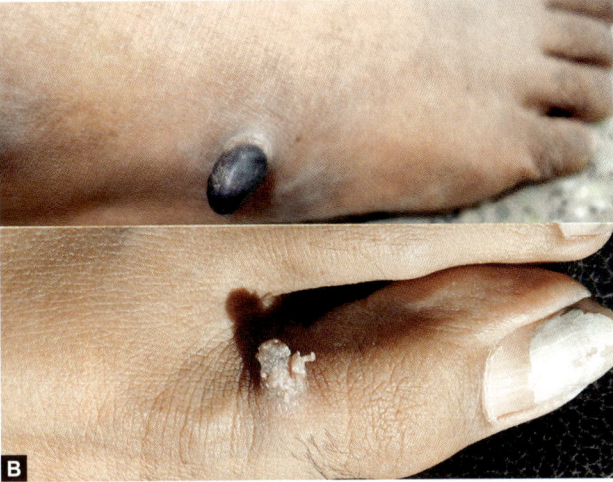

Figs. 4-102A and B Sebaceous horn—nose and feet.

often resembles epithelioma. It is a misnomer. Occasionally, yellowish sebum discharges slowly through a wide punctum and gets hardened. Inspissated dried sebaceous material in layers on the skin is known as *sebaceous horn* (Length greater than its base diameter, is called as horn) (Figs. 4-102A and B). *Calcification* also can occur in sebaceous cyst. *Rupture and sinus formation* can occur. Punctum is usually absent in sebaceous cysts of the scrotum *Fordyce's disease* is heterotopic sebaceous glands in mucosa of lip and oral cavity).

Other cystic swellings	*Etiology and pathology*	*Features*
1. Epidermoid cyst (epidermal/keratin/infundibular cyst/ follicular infundibular cyst) – Benign cyst that originates from follicular infundibulum – Often associated with Gardner's syndrome, basal cell nevus syndrome – Tiny superficial cysts called Milia – common in neonates and younger age	• Exposure to UV light and human papilloma virus infection • Plugging and occlusion of pilosebaceous unit, high testosterone levels are observed	• Common in face, trunk, neck, extremities, scalp • Contains cheese like material often with typical foul smell
2. Trichilemmal cyst/pilar cyst Benign cyst lined by stratified squamous epithelium of isthmus of the hair follicle without granular cell layer	Autosomal dominant, hereditary/acquired	Incidence is 10%; 90% in scalp Multiple, common in females (middle aged); often mistaken for sebaceous cyst but no punctum; can form horn
3. Ganglion Cystic swelling that occur in relation to tendon sheath or synovial sheath or joint capsule **Common sites:** Dorsum of wrist (near scaphoid – lunate articulation); flexor aspect of wrist; around ankle joint	• Cystic degeneration of the tendon sheath; or leakage of synovial fluid through joint capsule; or presence of small islets of microspaces in synovial sheath which often fuse together or one of them enlarges to form ganglion • 30% recurrence rate after excision	• Well-localized, smooth, soft, cystic [tensely cystic]; Paget's test positive; nontender; transilluminant; mobile but mobility restricted when tendon contracts against resistance **(Figs. 4-103A to C)** • Communicates with joint capsule occasionally; contain gel-like fluid • Differential diagnosis: Lipoma, sebaceous cyst, neurofibroma, lymph cyst
4. Lymph cyst (lymphatic cyst) – Acquired type of dissension cyst. – Common site: limbs and neck	Lymphatics form a diffuse encapsulated swelling commonly due to trauma	• Usually occurs in subcutaneous plane, well-defined, smooth, soft, nontender, mobile, non-compressible, fluctuant (positive Paget's test), brilliantly transilluminant **(Fig. 4-104)**; Usually not adherent to skin; can get infected to form abscess • Differential diagnosis: Cold abscess; dermoid cyst

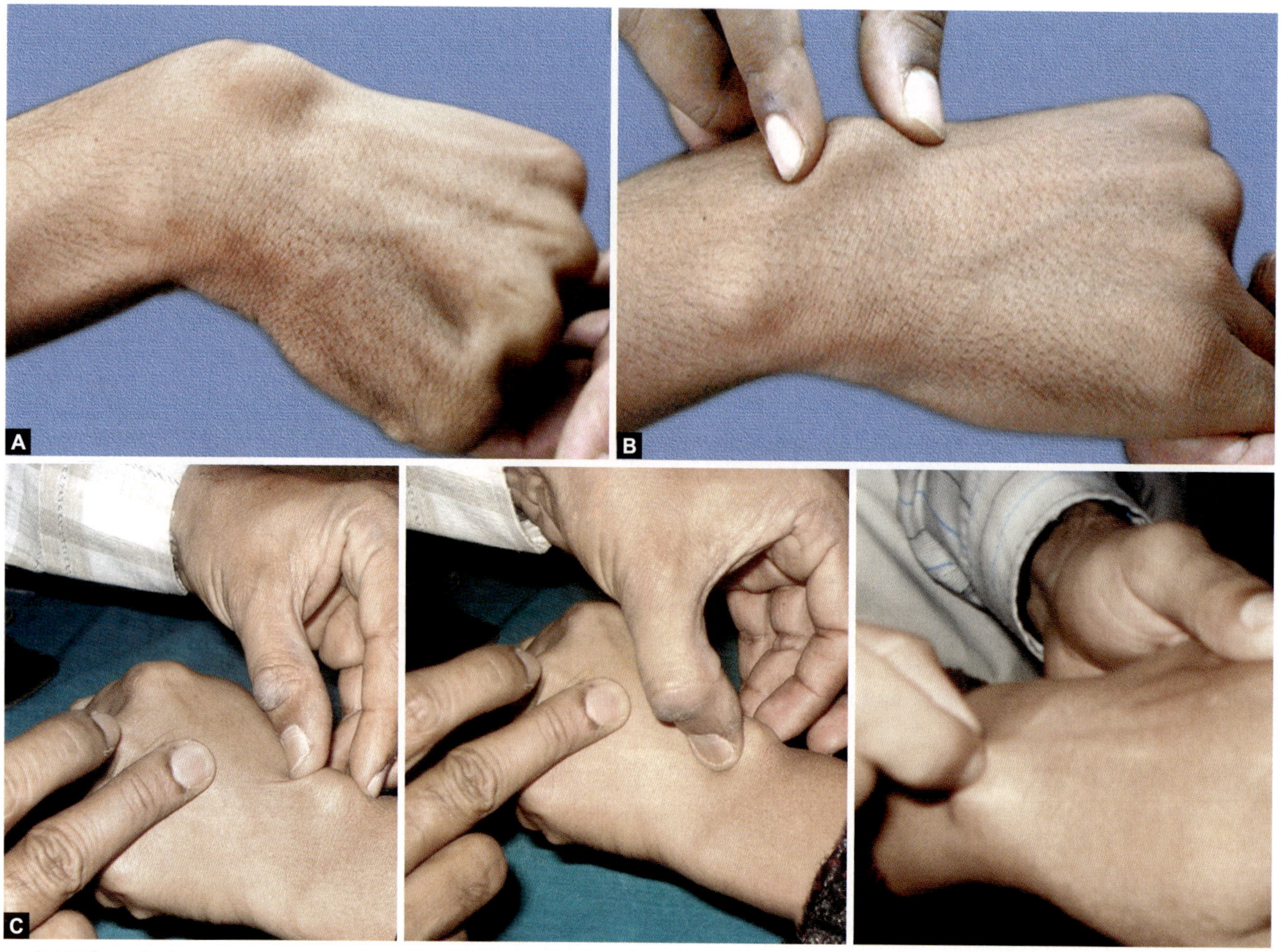

Figs. 4-103A to C Ganglion over the wrist. Its *mobility should be checked both when wrist relaxed as well as extended against resistance*. Skin should be held/pinched to confirm that ganglion is not fixed to skin.

Sequestration dermoid	Sebaceous cyst
Occurs in the line of fusion	Occurs anywhere except palm and sole
Skin is not adherent (free)	Skin is adherent over summit
Extends often into deeper plane or cavities through suture line	Subcutaneous plane—do not extend to deeper plane
Punctum is absent	Punctum is present—70% cases
Bone resorption and indentation is common	Freely mobile without bone resorption
Restricted mobility	Superficial swelling, mobile
Needs proper evaluation with X-ray/CT scan	
Excision is done under general anesthesia	Excision is done under local anesthesia

Bursae

- Bursa is a sac-like cavity lined by endothelium, containing fluid within, which in normal location prevents friction between tendon and bone. It is smooth, soft/firm (tensely cystic), fluctuant, cystic. Skin may be free or often adherent due to chronic inflammation. Sometimes tenderness can occur in bursae due to acute inflammation or abscess

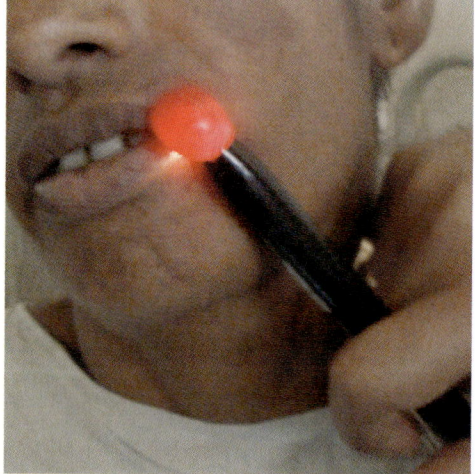

Fig. 4-104 Lymph cyst. It is an *acquired condition and transilluminant swelling*.

formation. Usually, it is mobile but inflammation may restrict the mobility.

- It should be differentiated from sebaceous cyst, soft tissue tumor, lipoma and neurofibroma. Minor injuries and pressure leads into bursitis, which will present as a swelling at the site. Inflammation of this bursa due to friction causes *bursitis*, which commonly presents as swelling, pain, and restricted movements at the joints.

On long standing, when lining becomes rough and fluid contains loose bodies, one may appreciate crepitus on palpation.

- *Different types:* It can be *anatomical or adventitious*.

Anatomical type of bursa	Pathology	Features
1. Subhyoid bursa	A horizontally oval swelling situated below the hyoid bone and in front of the thyrohyoid membrane	Mimics thyroglossal cyst; moves upwards with deglutition
2. Subacromial bursa	Located in front and lateral to humeral head in relation to supraspinatus tendon between acromion and greater tuberosity of humerus	Often presents as painful, tender swelling
3. Olecranon bursa (Student's elbow, Miner's elbow)	Acquired bursa due to friction behind elbow joint (Fig. 4-106)	Soft, cystic, fluctuant localized swelling
4. Psoas bursa	Located over lesser trochanter under the attachment of iliopsoas tendon	A tensely cystic swelling beneath and below the inguinal ligament on the lateral aspect of the femoral triangle. But it will not extend above the inguinal ligament into the iliac region (unlike in psoas abscess, which extends above and is cross fluctuant)
5. Prepatellar bursitis (Housemaid's knee) (Fig. 4-106)	It occurs in bursa located in front of lower part of patella and upper part of patellar tendon due to constant pressure (like kneeling)	
6. Infrapatellar bursitis (Clergyman's knee)	It is inflammation of bursa occurring in relation to lower half of the patellar tendon	
7. Semimembranosus bursa	• Cystic swelling, under the semimembranosus tendon; outer to medial head of gastrocnemius. Common in young individuals	• Soft, smooth, cystic, often transilluminant, nontender, noncompressible swelling; on the upper medial aspect of popliteal fossa • Swelling becomes flaccid on flexion; prominent on extension • Does not communicate with knee joint; joint movement is normal
8. Morrant Baker's cyst Cystic swelling in the lower midline of popliteal fossa Common in middle-aged individuals	Occurs due to herniation of synovial membrane of the knee joint as a result of chronic arthritis.	• Smooth, soft, cystic, often tender swelling that disappears on flexion; becomes prominent on extension • Pain and tenderness in knee joint with effusion • Positive patellar tap; joint movements are painful
9. Bursa anserina	Located under the tendons of Guy ropes (sartorius, gracilis and semitendinosus tendons) *(Goose's foot)*	
10. Retrocalcaneal bursitis	Occurs between calcaneum and tendo-Achilles	

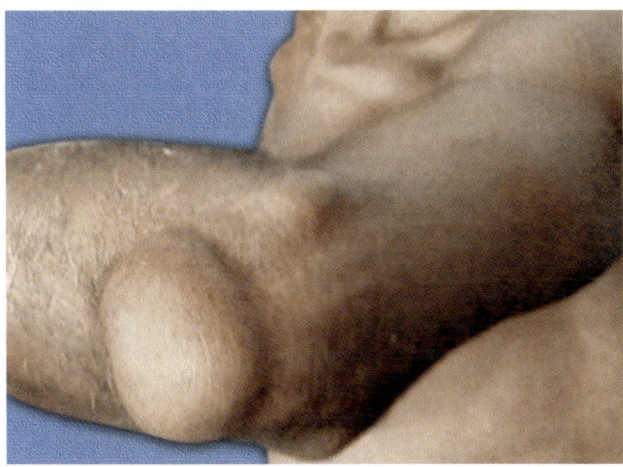

Fig. 4-105 *Bursa* near elbow joint.

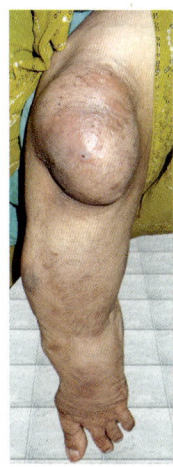

Fig. 4-106 *Housemaid's knee*—prepatellar bursitis.

Adventitious Bursa

Adventitious bursa occurs in an unusual site like in hallux valgus (*bunion*) (Fig. 4-107) over first metatarsal, over lateral malleolus (*tailor's bursa*), between clavicle and skin near shoulder (*porter's bursa*), over C7 vertebra (*Billing's gate hump*), between gluteus maximus muscle and ischial tuberosity (*weaver's bursa*), between tendo-Achilles and skin (*retro-Achilles bursitis*) or over gluteal tuberosity. It occurs due to constant prolonged pressure or friction over bony prominences in persons with particular deformity or occupation, commonly unilateral.

Benign Swellings

Benign swellings are very common. Different types of benign swellings we come across during our surgical practice. Lipoma, neurofibromas are common and often multiple.

Lipoma

It is a benign tumor arising from yellow fat (tumor arising from brown fat is called as *hibernoma*). It is called as *universal tumor/ubiquitous tumor* as it can occur anywhere in the body having fat (except in brain). Areas like eyelids, tip of nose, ear (cartilaginous part), brain that is devoid of fat do not produce lipoma. It is the *most common benign tumor*. It can be superficial and deep seated; deep seated tumors are difficult to diagnose and are hence called 'ambiguous tumor'. It can be *diffuse or localized*. *Diffuse lipomas* are not encapsulated, not well-localized (Fig. 4-108). They are common in palm, sole, head and neck region, difficult to be removed. Diffuse type is often called as *pseudolipoma*. It is usually harmless except with some cosmetic problem. It is more common in alcoholics. Lipoma can be single or multiple. Multiple lipomas (5%) are often associated with many syndromes like *multiple endocrine neoplasia syndrome* (*MEN Syndrome*). Types—Painful lipomas are called as *neurolipomas. Dercum's disease* is tender deposition of fat especially on the trunk, also called as *adiposis dolorosa. It is common in females. It is basically multiple neurolipomatosis.* Fibrolipoma; nevolipoma; lipoma arborigens (pedunculated lipoma); neurolipoma are different histological variants of lipoma. *Localized lipoma* is the most common type. It is encapsulated type. It can occur anywhere but more commonly observed in nape of the neck, back, neck and shoulder. It is most common in subcutaneous plane. It also can be intermuscular; subfascial; intramuscular;

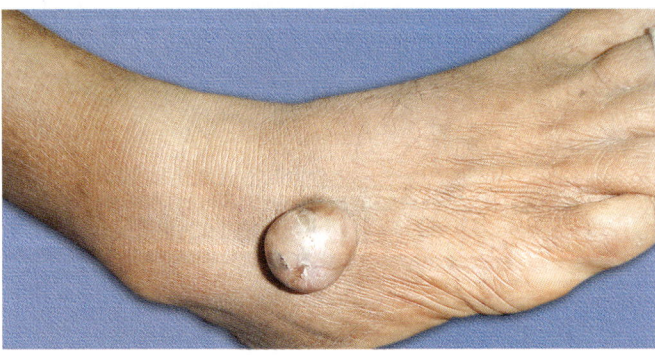

Fig. 4-107 Adventitious bursa over lateral aspect to foot—a *common site*.

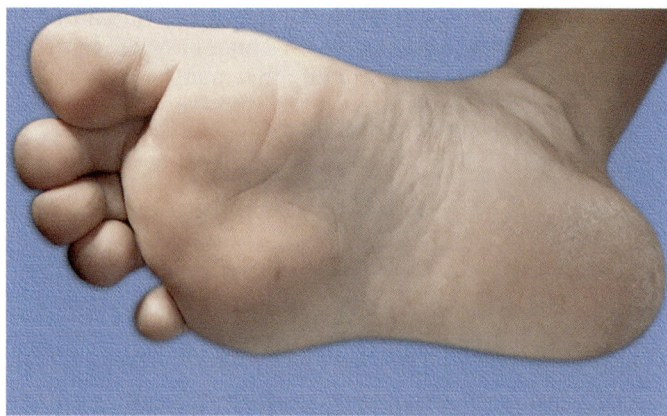

Fig. 4-108 Diffuse lipoma sole. *Diffuse lipoma is common in sole and back.*

parosteal; subserosal; submucosal; extradural; subdural (not intracerebral); subserosal; intra-articular or subsynovial. Lipomas attain large size in thigh, shoulder, retroperitoneum, back which may often turn into sarcoma (Fig. 4-109).

Clinical features: Localized painless swelling, which is lobular, nontender, freely mobile, with edge slipping between the palpating fingers (slip sign), having overlying free skin; often feels like fluctuant but actually not. Using index finger edge of the lipoma when pushed will slip under the palpating finger (*slip sign*) (Fig. 4-110). Nevolipoma shows dilated veins over the surface and so called as lipoma telangiectasis. Fibrolipoma contains more fibrous tissue and so it is firm. Neurolipoma also contains nerve tissue also and so is painful. At times, lipomas may be pedunculated. Lipoma is not transilluminant.

Differential diagnoses: Neurofibroma and other cystic swellings.

Complications: *Note:* Liposarcoma developing from a preexisting lipoma is disproved now. Myxomatous change; saponification; calcification; submucosal lipoma in intestine can cause intussusception and so intestinal obstruction, in respiratory tract causes respiratory obstruction. Repeated

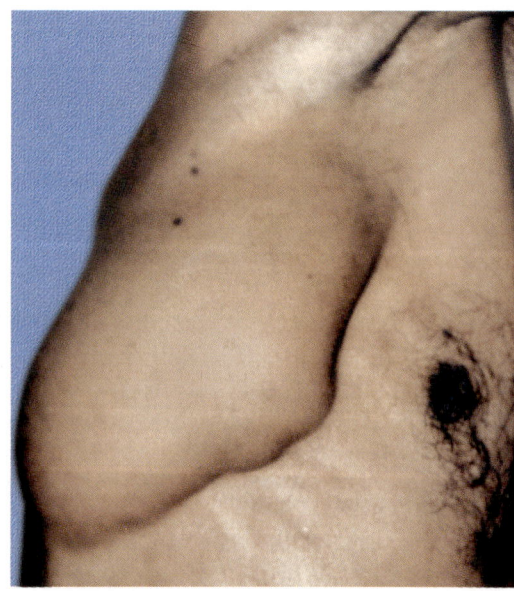

Fig. 4-109 Typical lipoma. Note the *well defined edge*.

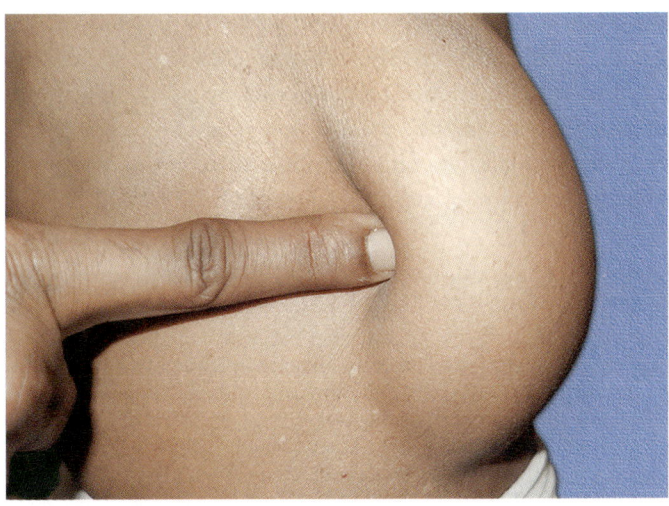

Fig. 4-110 Typical '*slip sign*' in a lipoma.

trauma may cause ulceration over the summit which is more often seen in pedunculated lipoma.

Neurofibroma

It is a benign tumor arising from connective tissue (neural—ectodermal and fibrous—mesodermal) of the nerve sheath. It can be single or multiple. Neurofibromas may be associated with pheochromocytomas, hypertension and few syndromes. Sites—*Cranial, spinal and peripheral.*

Clinical Types

a. Nodular neurofibroma presents as single smooth, firm, tender (often) swelling which moves horizontally (perpendicular to the direction of the nerve), not along the direction of the nerve. Pressure effects of the tumor over the nerve fibers cause pain, tingling sensation and hyperesthesia/paresthesia along the distribution of the nerve. Neurofibroma is the most common intradural extramedullary spinal tumor.
b. Plexiform neurofibroma commonly occurs along the distribution of 5th cranial nerve in the skin of the face. It is more common in ophthalmic division of trigeminal nerve. It often occurs in the cutaneous distribution of the peripheral nerve. It attains enormous size with thickening of the skin which hangs downwards. It causes erosion into the bone, orbit and deeper structures. It may also undergo myxomatous degeneration. It causes cosmetic problem. Rarely, it does occur in upper limb. Development of sarcoma is very rare in this type. *Pachydermatocele* is a variant of plexiform neurofibromatosis observed in the neck. Plexiform type may affect viscera like small intestine known as *visceral neurofibromatosis,* which may or may not be associated with surface tumor.
c. Generalized neurofibromatosis (von Recklinghausen's *disease*): It is an inherited autosomal dominant disease (congenital) wherein there will be multiple neurofibromas in the body (1:4,000 live births; chromosome 17). It commonly involves peripheral nerves; often spinal and cranial nerves. So it is often classified as cranial, spinal or peripheral. It is commonly associated with pigmented spots (coffee colored) in the skin, often seen on the back, abdomen, thigh (*café au lait spots* (Fig. 4-111). It signifies common neuroectodermal origin of nerve sheath cells and melanocytes) (more than 5 in number with each more than 1.5 cm in size are significant) (Fig. 4-112). Axillary or groin freckles with *Lisch nodules* may be present. Familial neurofibroma may be associated with scoliosis or multiple endocrine neoplasia syndrome type II b (MEN II b syndrome)—medullary carcinoma of thyroid; pheochromocytoma; hyperparathyroidism; multiple neurofibromas in eyelids, lips and face.
d. Elephantiatic neurofibromatosis: It is of congenital origin involving limbs. Subcutaneous fat is replaced by thick edematous fibrous tissue often mistaken for filarial elephantiasis. Skin of the limb is greatly thickened, dry and coarse.

Complications: *Sarcomatous changes (5%)*: When it occurs, it shows rapid enlargement, warmness, more vascularity with

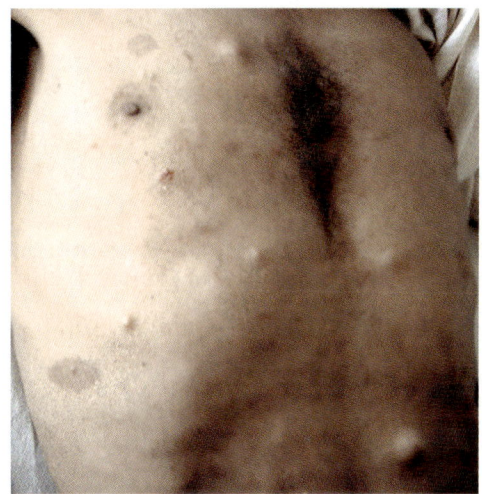

Fig. 4-111 *Café au lait spots*. It is a feature of von Recklinghausen's disease of neurofibromatosis. It is coffee colored pigment spots in the skin. More than 5 in number with each more than 1.5 cm in size is significant.

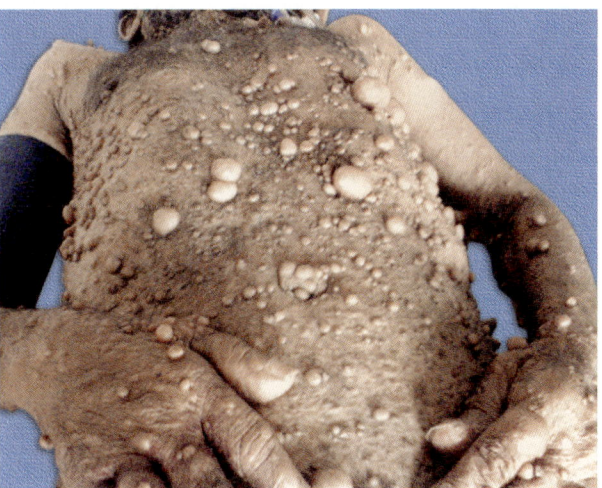

Fig. 4-112 Multiple neurofibromas *(von Recklinghausen's disease).*

dilated veins. Persistent severe pain; fixity and fungation also can occur. Secondaries in lungs can occur through blood spread. *Hemorrhage* can occur into the tissues. Spinal and cranial neurofibromas can cause neurological deficits. *Erosion* can occur into the deeper planes, bone, orbit. *Calcification, cystic degeneration, saponification, disfigurement, myxomatous changes and pressure symptoms* developing as local complication based on the sites of the tumor. Deafness in acoustic neuroma, neurological pressure symptoms, spinal cord compression by dumb-bell tumor arising from spinal root, mediastinal symptoms when tumor is in mediastinum are other complications. Intestinal neurofibroma may precipitate *intussusception*.

Benign swelling types	Etiology and pathology	Features
1. Neurilemmoma (Schwannoma) Common in acoustic nerve but do can occur in any peripheral nerve *Note:* Schwannomas typically grow within a capsule and remain peripherally attached to the parent nerve. Neurofibromas on the other hand contain not only Schwann cells, but also other elements of the peripheral nerve including fibroblasts, perineural cells and axons. Neurofibromas grow diffusely within and along the nerve	Benign, ectodermal tumor arising from Schwann cell of nerve sheath **Types:** Anthoni A (contain *verocay bodies*) Anthoni B (contain amyloid areas)	• Lobulated, encapsulated tumor along the course of nerve; freely mobile, soft, whitish in appearance; displaces the nerve from which it arises • Pain along the distribution of nerve; hyperesthesia and tenderness • Usually single/can be multiple • Rarely can turn into malignancy • Recurrent schwannoma are malignant and very aggressive
2. Neuroma Benign swelling arising in relation to nerve fiber **Types:** 1. *True neuroma*—Develops in relation to sympathetic nervous system 2. *False neuroma*—Occurs due to injury to nerve by trauma or surgery like amputation; arises from connective tissue of the nerve sheath	**True neuroma - types** a. *Ganglioneuroma*—contains ganglion cells and neuron; arises in sympathetic chain b. *Myelinic neuroma*—Contains only nerve fibres without ganglion cells; seen in spinal cord and pia mater **False neuroma – types** a. *End neuroma*—seen in amputation stump b. *Lateral (side) neuroma*—seen after traumatic partial nerve injury	• Mass in the neck, thorax, retroperitoneum or adrenal medulla; benign; attains large size • Tender localized firm, swelling adherent to scar underneath; causes stump neuralgia; proper usage of prosthesis becomes difficult • Present as tender, firm swelling along the line of peripheral nerve
3. Fibroma – Benign tumor arising from fibrous tissue – True fibroma rare; mostly combined with mesodermal tissues Nerve sheath—neurofibroma; Fat—fibrolipoma; Muscle—fibromyoma **Aggressive fibromatosis:** Diffuse firm or hard in nature without capsule **Desmoid tumor:** Variant of aggressive fibromatosis (Desmos = tendon; eidos = appearance)	**Types:** a. *Soft fibroma*—contains immature fibrous tissue b. *Hard fibroma*—contains well formed fibrous tissue • Unencapsulated proliferation of fibrous tissue, common in abdomen and chest wall • Common in females; in rectus sheath of abdominal wall	• Soft brown swelling; common in face • Common in palms and soles • Locally malignant; recurrence common; does not spread through lymphatics and blood • Often associated with *Gardner's syndrome*
4. Glomus tumor (glomangioma) – Often seen in limbs—tips of finger, toes, palmar surfaces of phalanges – Common in nail beds – Not a congenital disease	Arises from the *cutaneous glomus* which is composed of tortuous arteriole that communicate directly with venule (special type of a-v communication) surrounded network of small nerves (medullated and nonmedullated sensory nerves). They regulate temperature of skin	• Blue/reddish color circumscribed swelling, 2–3 mm in size; severe burning sensation and stabbing pain out of proportion to the size of the lesion; more when limb is exposed to sudden changes in temperature • Compressible but slightest pressure will cause excruciating pain • On increasing the pressure in the arm above systolic, pain disappears • Never turn into malignancy
5. Calcinosis cutis (Figs. 4-113A to C) – Type of calcification in/under the skin – Common in females; common in waist	It is due to constant friction leading to degeneration of skin and immediate deeper structure; with increased alkalinity of the tissue causes precipitation of calcium	• Circumscribed swelling in the skin which is solid, hard • Cut section shows hard, yellowish material • Differential diagnosis: calcified lipoma; neurofibroma

Contd...

Chapter 4: Examination and Clinical Approach of a Swelling/Lump

Contd...

Benign swelling types	Etiology and pathology	Features
6. Callosity (Fig. 4-114) Common in hands and feet	Due to excessive wear and tear in relation to occupation	Greyish brown; hyperkeratotic patch of skin; not painful; protrudes outwards; when top layer is removed, shiny, homogenous, translucent dead skin layer exposed
7. Corn (Fig. 4-115) Common in soles; tips of toes; over the dorsal surface of inter-phalangeal joints	• Often due to ill-fitting footwear • It consists of severe keratoses with central degenerated dead cells and cholesterol (yellowish white core)	• Localised, smaller, deeper lesions with palpable painful tender nodule • Hard in the soles; can be soft between 4th and 5th toes • *Complications:* Infection; abscess • *Differential diagnosis:* Plantar wart (soft branching processes)
8. Chordoma (Fig. 4-116) Seen in sacrococcygeal region; sphenoidal sinus; around foramen magnum	Arises from remnants of notochord	Invades into surrounding tissues like nerves; often aggressive

Benign Swelling of the Skin

Many lesions arise from skin itself which is categorized separately as swellings in relation to skin. Benign skin swellings are quiet common. Keloid and hypertrophic scars are common in skin.

Keloid (Fig. 4-119)

- Word meaning keloid is '*like a claw*". It is abnormal proliferation of immature fibroblasts, immature blood vessels and type III thick collagen stroma which occurs due to irritation of mesenchymal cells around the

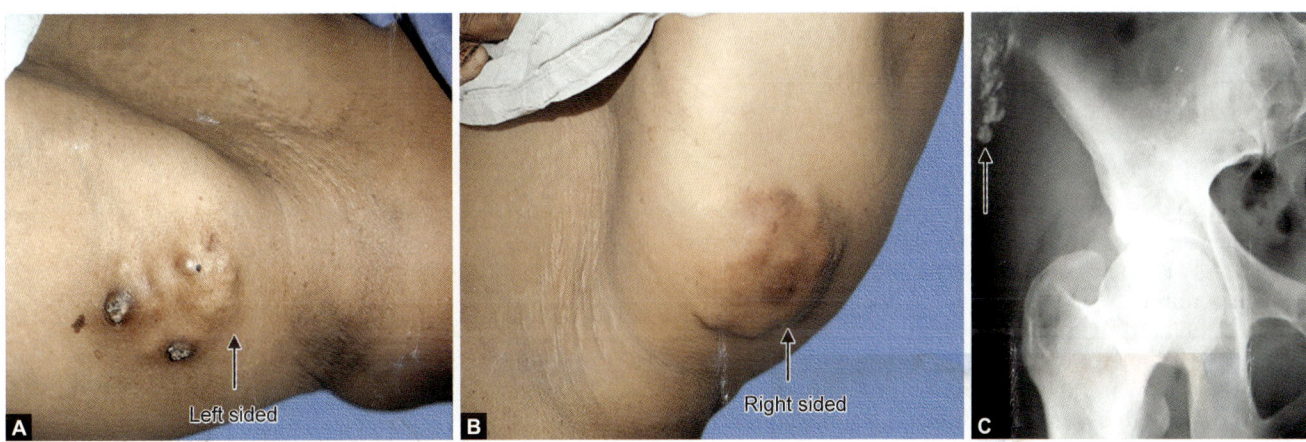

Figs. 4-113A to C Calcinosis cutis—both waists. It is common in females; X-ray shows calcification. It is often bilateral (in this patient). It is *dystrophic calcification*.

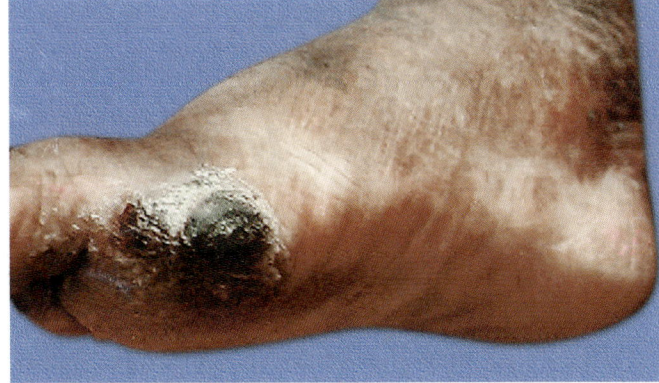

Fig. 4-114 Callosity foot. It is *outward protruding grayish brown hyperkeratotic patch* of skin in the foot/hand. It is *not a painful* condition.

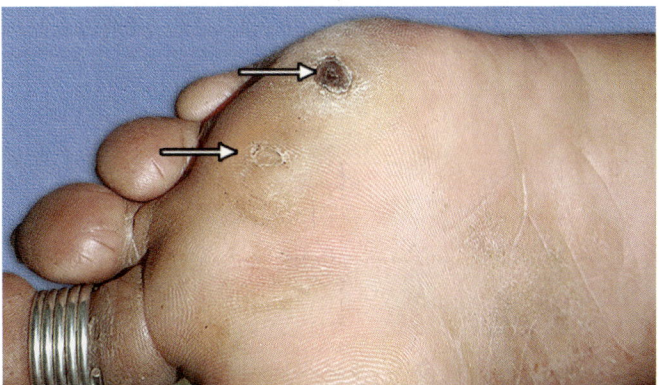

Fig. 4-115 Typical corn in the foot. It is *localized, painful, tender, deep lesion with a deep core* that contains degenerated dead keratotic cells and cholesterol.

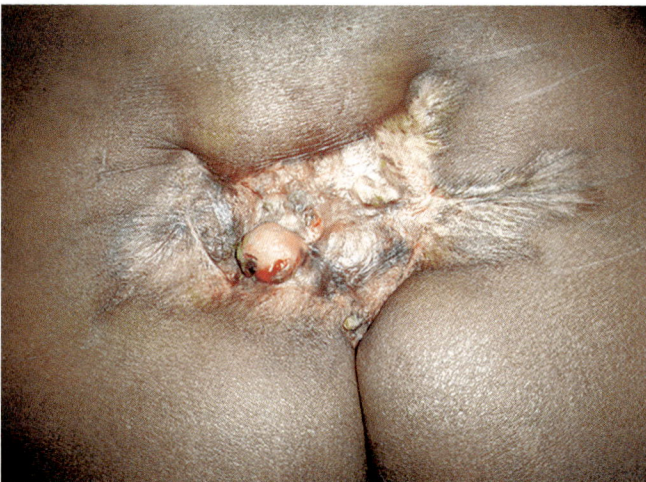

Fig. 4-116 *Chordoma* over the sacrum.

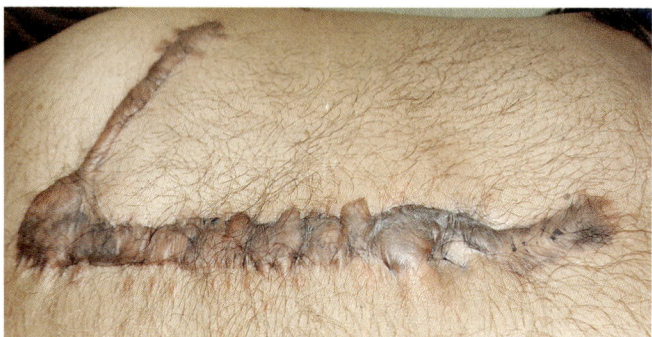

Fig. 4-117 Keloid in laparotomy wound site.

- Scar of minor injury also can form keloid. Fibrous tissue continues to grow even after 6 months to many years. It extends like finger into adjacent normal skin and attains *vascularity*. It forms *pinkish black, painful, hyperesthetic, tender swelling* (not a tumor but tumor-like) which spreads into the surrounding skin and causes itching.
- It can occur as *spontaneous keloid* without a scar after an unnoticed trauma which is common in *Negroes*.
- Recurrence is common if excised.
- *Other complications*: Infection.

Hypertrophic Scar

- It is overgrowth of fibrous tissue (type III *fine* collagen) in any scar and is *limited to scar* area only (Fig. 4-119); which grows up to 6 months; *not* genetically predisposed (unlike keloid); will *never* extend to normal adjacent skin restricting to area of trauma only; occurs *anywhere in the body*; self limiting; *not vascular*.
- It is common on the *flexor* aspect. It is *equal* in both sexes.
- There is *no* racial descrimination.
- *Precipitating factors* are lacerated wounds, infected wounds, scars healed by secondary intention, burns wound, scars which cross the Langer's line.

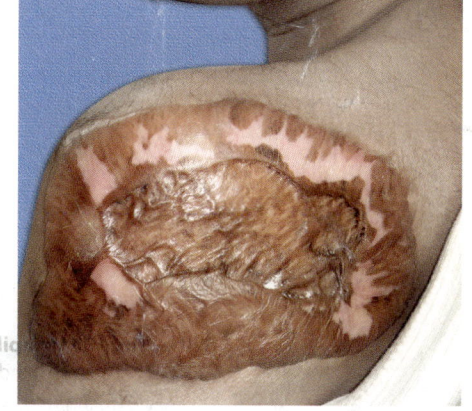

Fig. 4-119 *Hypertrophic scar* shoulder region.

submucus and sweat glands. There is defect in maturation and stabilization of collagen fibrils.
- It is common in blacks (15 times), females, Negroes. It is often familial. It may be associated with *Ehlers-Danlos syndrome* or scleroderma.
- It is common over sternum, upper arm (BCG vaccination scar), upper chest wall, ear, lower neck and abdomen (Figs. 4-118A to C).

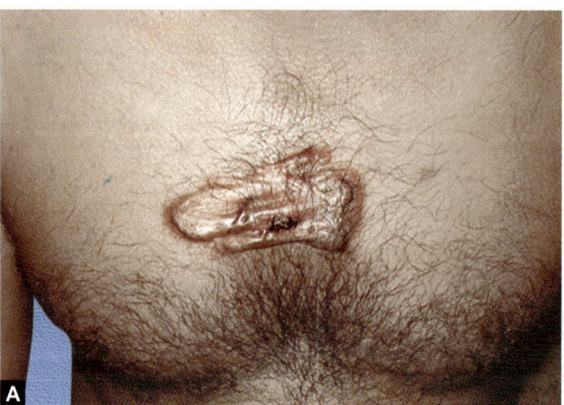
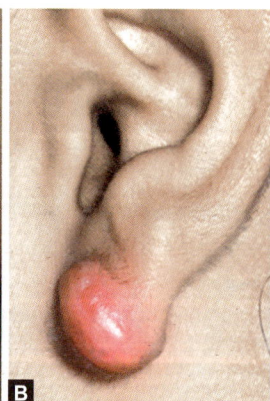
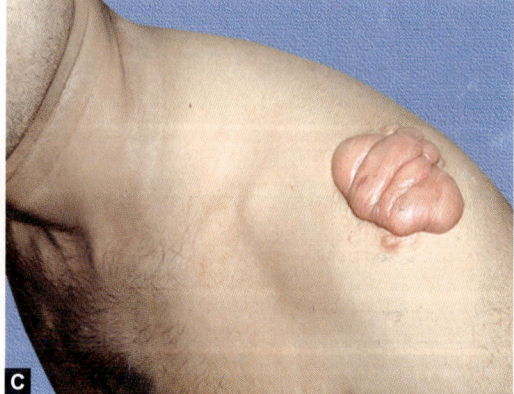

Figs. 4-118A to C *Keloid* over the chest (sternum), ear lobule (ear prick site) and shoulder.

Skin swelling types	Etiology and pathology	Features
1. Seborrheic keratosis (Seborrheic wart; basal cell papilloma) Common in Caucasians; common in elderly. Not pre-malignant	• Benign swelling arising from the overgrowth of basal layer of epidermis • Familial; autosomal dominant • Common sites—back; face; nape of neck	• Protrudes from the surface of the epidermis to give oily appearance—"stuck on" appearance is characteristic; slow growing; pigmented due to melanin; often gets infected; when scabs off leaves a pale pink patch on the skin with visible small capillaries • Lymph nodes not involved
2. Solar keratosis/senile keratosis Common in elderly who were working outdoors for many years. Pre-malignant condition	Seen in sun exposed areas of skin; like face; rim of the ears; dorsum of hands; fingers	• Multiple, hyperkeratotic; dry, scaly, patchy, yellowish gray/brown lesion which soon form ulcers with raised edge • Fixity/tethering; everted edge, recent increase in size and nodal spread –features of malignant transformation
3. Wart Overgrown hyperkeratotic skin; Common in children and youngsters; May disappear spontaneously or remain unchanged **Different types** – **Butcher's wart/pathologist's wart:** Often seen on dorsum of hands of milkmaids – **Plantar wart:** In the sole common in ball or heel of the sole	Often of viral origin. • Types—senile seborrheic warts; common warts, plantar warts; venereal moist wart • Common in finger tips, sole, axilla, face • Due to entry of *Mycobacterium tuberculosis* through broken skin	• Multiple, chronic, painless, asymptomatic, hyperkeratotic, finger- like projections causing disfiguring lesions; can spread to other finger and other part of body (*kiss lesion*). Repeated rubbing causes infection • Bluish red warty lesions with discharges • Pearly white in color with brownish flecks covered by apparently normal skin; gets pushed into the sole of foot • Can be multiple; can be painful and very tender
4. Papilloma Warty swelling from the skin or mucus membrane of viscera (bladder, kidney, breast, intestine)	**Types:** **True papilloma**—Localized overgrowth of all layers of skin or epithelium. Depending on site of occurrence it can be lined by squamous (skin); columnar (intestine; (rectum); cuboidal (gallbladder) transitional (urinary bladder) epithelium. Commonly pedunculated but can be sessile *Pedunculated papilloma is*—villous with central axis containing blood vessels and lymphatics **(Fig. 4-120)** **Infective papilloma**—warty lesion due to infection (condyloma acuminate)	• It is termed as 'skin tag' in skin; contains sweat glands, sebaceous gland, hair follicles. Can be single/multiple • Duct papilloma in breast can cause bloody discharge. Papilloma in vocal cord can cause hoarseness and change of voice • True papilloma can turn into malignancy—sudden change in size, bleeding, ulceration *Differential diagnosis:* Amelanotic melanoma; pedunculated lipoma
5. Keratoacanthoma (Molluscum sebaceum) (Figs. 4-123A and B) It is overgrowth and subsequent spontaneous regression of the sebaceous gland which opens into hair follicle	*Self-limiting benign* neoplasm probably of papilloma virus origin; squamous cells of sebaceous gland proliferate and protrudes out through the sebaceous duct	Solitary lesion; more common in face; hands (abundant sebaceous glands); painless, rapidly growing hard, mobile hemispherical swelling of the skin (grows up to 4–8 weeks); central friable core ulcerates and forms brown crust
More common in males (3:1)		• Spontaneous regression in 4–6 months • Central brown area is hard peripheral rim is firm and rubbery – volcano like • Regional lymph nodes not enlarged • Mimics squamous cell carcinoma (*pseudomalignancy*)
6. Rhinophyma (Potato nose; Bottle nose) (Fig. 4-124) Glandular form of acne rosacea	Due to hypertrophy and adenomatous changes in sebaceous glands	Distal part of the skin of nose is immensely thickened with visible openings of sebaceous follicles. Nose is bluish red in color with dilated capillaries
7. Skin adnexal tumors (Figs. 4-125A and B) Tumors arising from accessory from accessory skin structures like sebaceous glands, sweat glands and hair follicles	Can be benign or malignant	• Painless, well-localized swelling in the skin; skin adherent, ulcerated • Can undergo malignant change—nodular, hard, indurated and often fungation occurs with palpable lymph nodes

Contd...

Section 1: Examination in General Surgery

Contd...

Skin swelling types	Etiology and pathology	Features
8. **Turban tumor** Entire scalp looks like a turban because of multiple scalp swellings	Can be due to multiple cylindromas; multiple hidradenomas; subcutaneous neurofibromas; nodular basal cell carcinoma *Cylindroma*—variant of eccrine spiradenoma *Hidradenoma*—benign sweat gland tumor	Multiple tumors commonly look like a turban in scalp. Painless; disfiguring; cosmetically problematic; soft; boggy; non-fluctuant; noncompressible swellings; commonly observed in middle age
9. **Dermatofibroma (sclerosing angioma; subepithelial benign nodular fibrosis; dermal histiocytoma) (Fig. 4-126)**	Benign tumor containing 'mat like/cartwheel' pattern spindle cells arising from dermal dendritic cells	Red, brownish yellow or bluish black, firm, single, or multiple nodules occurring in limbs

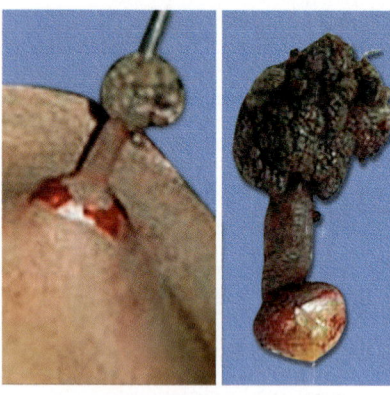

Fig. 4-120 *Papilloma* which is pedunculated. Note its base.

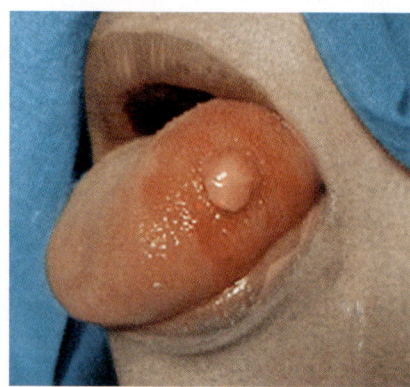

Fig. 4-121 Papilloma tongue. Note: *Papilloma can also occur in mucous membrane* like oral cavity, urinary, gallbladder and rectum.

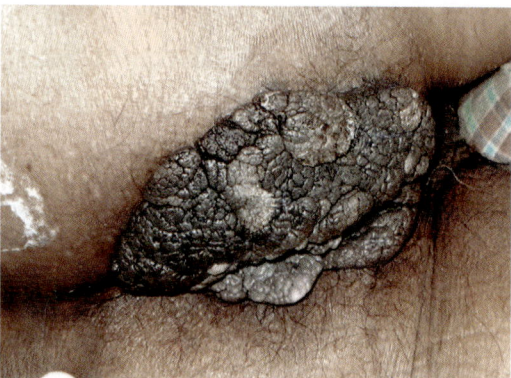

Fig. 4-122 Anal canal papilloma. *It is often called as condyloma*. It is dry, raised lesion in the anal canal. Condyloma lata is seen in secondary syphilis. Condyloma acuminata is of viral origin.

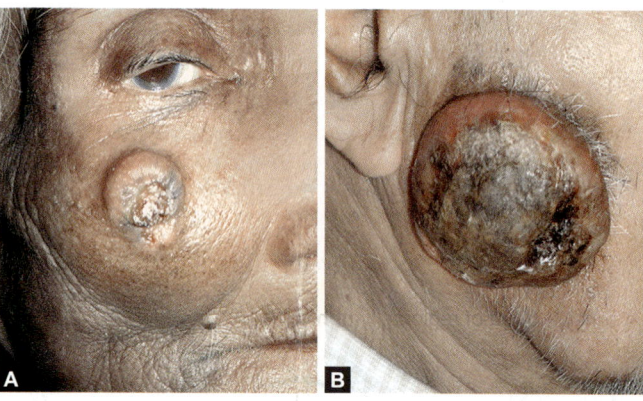

Figs. 4-123A and B: Keratoacanthoma in female and male patients. *Note the central brown area. It mimics epithelioma.*

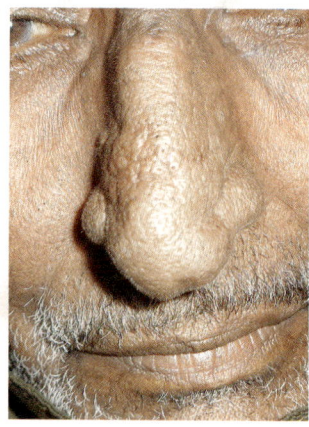

Fig. 4-124 Rhinophyma.

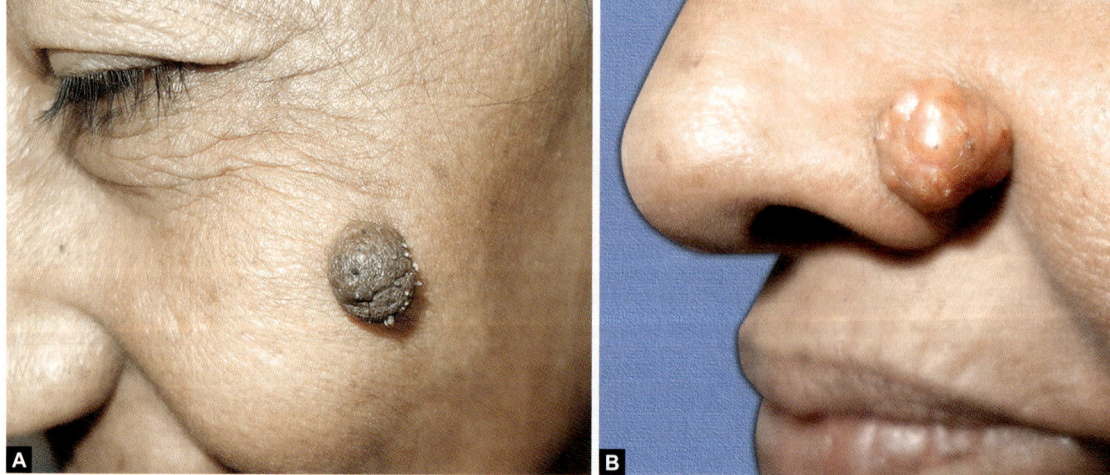

Figs. 4-125A and B *Skin adnexal tumor.*

Chapter 4: Examination and Clinical Approach of a Swelling/Lump

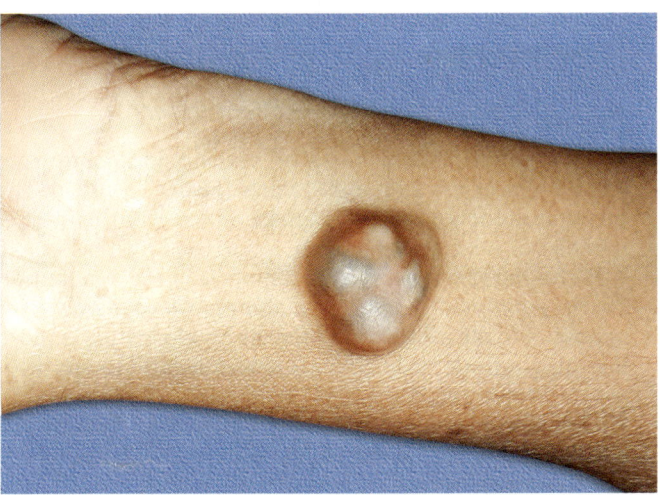

Fig. 4-126 *Dermatofibroma*—forearm.

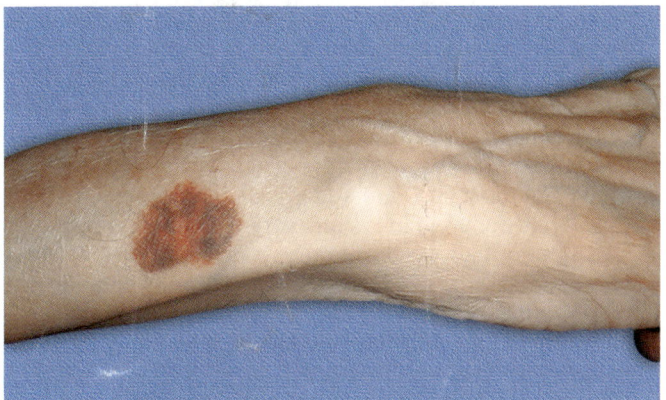

Fig. 4-127 Nevus is a *pigmented lesion*.

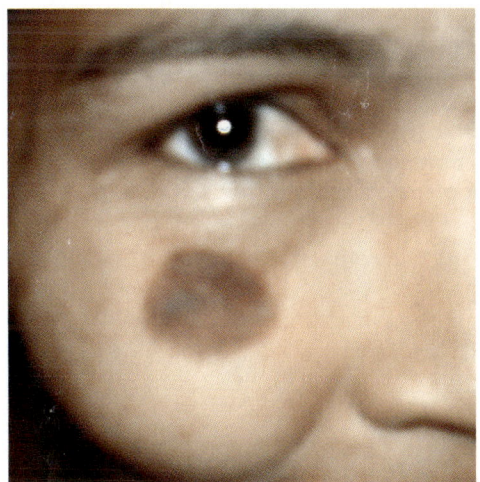

Fig. 4-128 *Congenital nevus*.

Nevus (Mole)

It is excessive or altered stimulation of melanocytes often with hyperplasia or neoplasia (Fig. 4-127). But actually Nevi in general denote neoplastic and non-neoplastic, congenital (Fig. 4-128) and acquired as well as hereditary and nonhereditary skin lesions. Currently considered as—Nevi are visible, circumscribed, long-lasting lesions of the skin

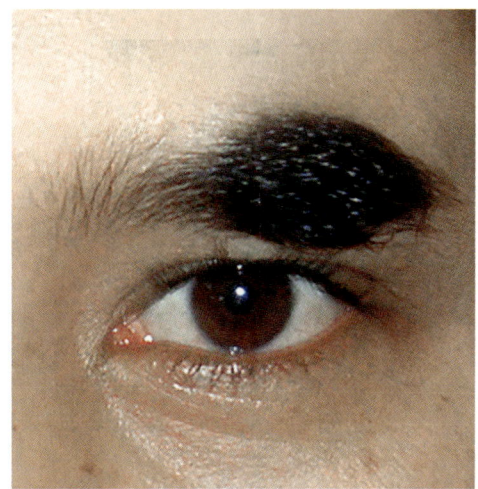

Fig. 4-129 *Hairy nevus* in the left eyebrow.

or the neighboring mucosa, reflecting genetic mosaicism. Few nevi may present at birth. Number increases with age. Adult has got 60-100 moles. It is common in Caucasians and Australians. Moles are not seen in Albinos. Childhood moles may get pigmented more or may get regressed fully. Usually moles at birth do not protrude over the skin surface; but those appear at later age group will not usually protrude over the skin surface. Moles are common in limbs, face and mucocutaneous junction like mouth and anus. Moles can turn into malignancy. In children and African blacks, Moles turning into malignancy is less common. Moles are usually light brown or brown or black in color which does not fade by pressure. Usual size of a mole is 1-3 mm.

Features of malignant change in a mole
- Itching
- Enlargement
- Ooze and bleeding
- Ulceration
- Gets deeply pigmented or develops halo around the mole
- Satellite nodule
- Enlargement of regional lymph node

Nevus–types	Features
Hairy mole Most common type (Fig. 4-129)	Flat/slightly raised with hair growing on surface; also contains sebaceous glands which can get infected
Non-hairy mole Smooth mole	Not elevated from the surface, smooth, brown pigmented lesion without hairs
Blue nevus Uncommon, smooth mole, seen in children	Common in buttock (*Mongolian spots*), hands and feet. Located deep in dermis, so even-though brown pigmented due to overlying dermis color appear faded to blue
Intradermal nevus Flat/raised/hairy/non-hairy	• Consists of clusters of melanocytes in dermis • Common in arms, trunk, face. Hardly becomes malignant
Junctional nevus (Fig. 4-130)	Centred in the junctional layer/basal layer of epidermis. Common in palms, digits, sole and external genitalia. *Commonly turn into malignancy*

Contd...

Contd...

Nevus–types	Features
Compound nevus Combination of intradermal and junctional nevus	Intradermal component is inactive; junctional component is potentially malignant
Juvenile melanoma (Spitz nevus) Junctional appearing before puberty	Seen in face
Hutchinson's freckle Macular and tumor stage	Seen in elderly, common in face, neck and trunk Macular stage—smooth, brown Tumor stage—dark, irregular *Can often turn into malignancy (difficult to identify clinically)*
Halo nevus	Area of depigmentation around pigmented nevus
Spindle cell nevus	• Dense, black pigmented lesion containing spindle cells and atypical melanocytes at junction • Common in females; *high malignant potential*
Nevus spilus	Low malignant potential Hyperpigmented throughout
Nevus of Ota	Dermal melanocytic hemartoma seen in the maxillary/ophthalmic divisions of trigeminal nerve; common in females of Oriental and African race
Nevus of Ito	Similar lesions as above seen in shoulder region

Malignant Lesions of the Skin

Dermatofibrosarcoma Protuberans

It is a low grade slowly growing fibrosarcoma occurring in trunk (common site—50%), back, head and neck and abdominal wall (Fig. 4-131). It is nodular, hard, often multiple swellings with redness and ulcerations over the summit. Regional lymph nodes may get enlarged. Spread to lungs can occur only rarely. It should be differentiated from squamous cell carcinoma or skin adnexal tumor. Often there is melanin pigmentation over the surface (*Bedner's tumor*).

Basal Cell Carcinoma (BCC, Rodent Ulcer)

- It is low grade, locally invasive, carcinoma arising from basal layer of the skin, hair follicle, sweat or sebaceous gland or mucocutaneous junction.
- It does not arise from mucosa.
- It is the *most common* skin tumor. It is more common in *white skinned* people. It is common in places where exposure to ultraviolet rays (causes single lesion) is more like in *Australia*. It is also common in individuals with arsenical dermatitis (multiple lesions).
- It is common in males and older people.
- It is common over the *face.* In the face, it is common above the line drawn between angle of the mouth and ear lobule (90%). As it is common in area where tears roll down, it is called as *tear cancer (Figs. 4-132A to D).*
- It can occur occasionally in other parts of skin (scalp, neck, arms, and hands) or mucocutaneous junction like in anal region, genitalia.
- It is only *locally malignant.* It *does not* spread through blood or lymph nodes. It can *erode* deeply into adjacent deeper tissues even cartilages or bone and hence called as *rodent ulcer.* But most BCC are superficial and confined to skin. Erosion is common in lesions very close to nose or eye.
- It can be nodular, cystic, nodulocystic, ulcerative, multiple (associated with syndromes), pigmented, geographical/ field fire/forest fire (wide area of involvement with central scabbing and peripheral active proliferating edge) or basisquamous type (combination of BCC and SCC. It behaves like SCC with regional nodal spread).
- BCC *never* spreads into regional lymph nodes.
- *Clinicopathologically*—It can be superficial; morphoeic or fibroepithelioma *type of Pinkus.*
- *Histologically*, it contains outer columnar cells arranged in palisading manner with central polyhedral cells *without prickle cells or keratinization.*
- *Clinically,* it is commonly *nodulocystic/noduloulcerative (90%),* nontender, slowly growing; nonmobile if fixed to deeper plane, raised and *beaded edge* (not everted) with

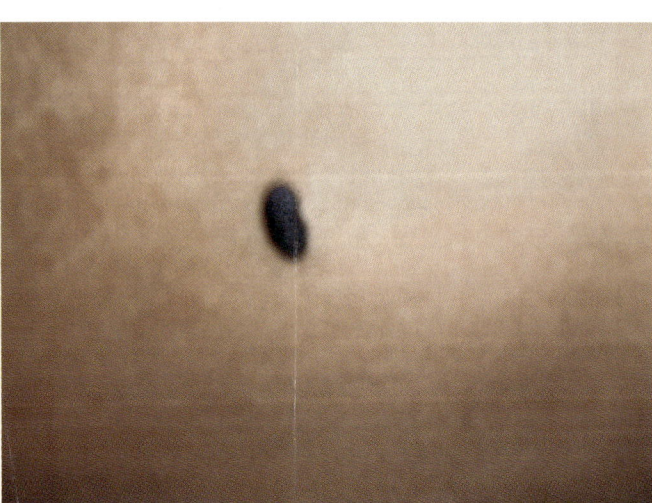

Fig. 4-130 *Junctional nevus.*

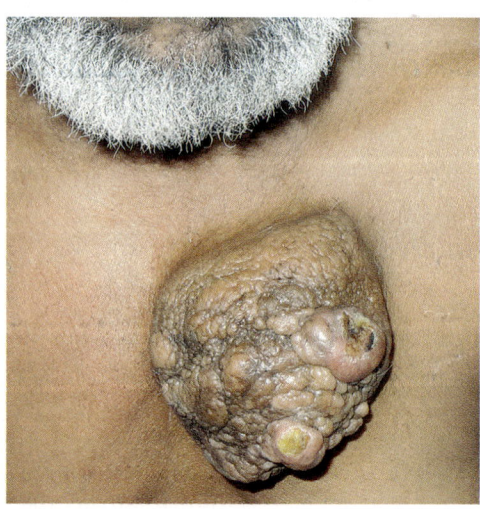

Fig. 4-131 *Dermatofibrosarcoma*— chest wall.

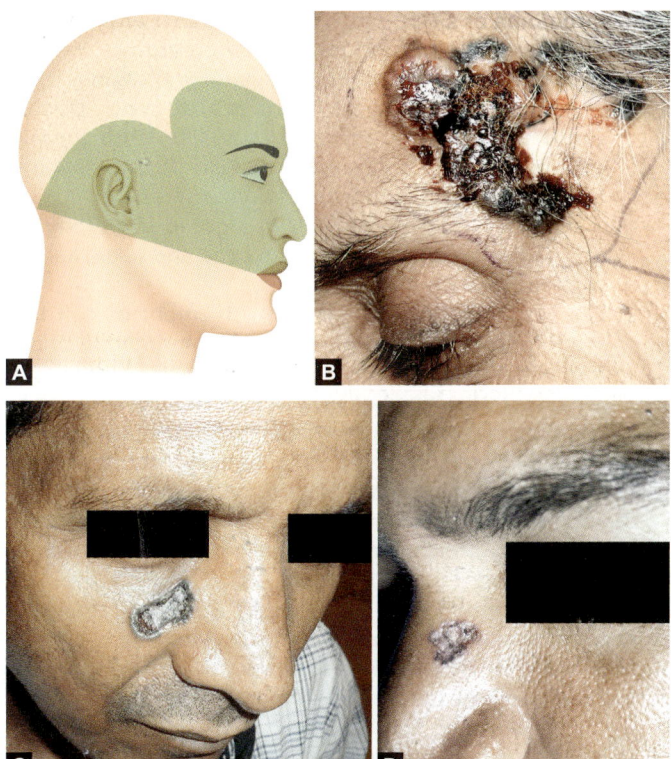

Figs. 4-132A to D Common site of basal cell carcinoma—above the line drawn between angle of mouth and ear lobule. Also picture showing typical location of basal cell carcinoma.

central area of *scabbing*. Scab repeatedly falls off and reforms. Itching over the scab can be present. Often it is disfiguring. It gives a false impression of spontaneous healing to the patient. Beads signify area of active proliferative cells.
- Regional nodes are *not* involved due to early obliteration and destruction of lymphatics by large sized cells.
- It should be differentiated from squamous cell carcinoma, melanoma, keratoacanthoma or seborrheic keratosis. BCC near the eye/nose/ear and BCC more than 2 cm size are called as high-risk BCC. Central polyhedral cells surrounded by perpendicularly arranged darkly stained columnar cell confirm the diagnosis in biopsy.

Squamous Cell Carcinoma (Epithelioma, SCC)

- Squamous cell carcinoma of skin arises from squamous layer (prickle cell layer) of the skin.
- It is the second most common skin cancer.
- Exposures to UV light and chronic irritations are precipitating factors.
- It is common in males.
- It occurs usually in preexisting lesions like Bowen's disease, leukoplakia, chronic scars, chronic chemical irritation, radiodermatitis, senile keratosis, Khangri cancer in Kashmir, chimney scrotal cancer, and Kang cancer of Tibetans, chronic venous ulcer, lupus vulgaris, Paget's disease of nipple.
- It can also occur as de novo.
- Grossly lesion can be proliferative, ulcerative or red plaque-like. It is common in face, cheek, lips, hands, and legs and sole. It can also occur in penis, vulva, buccal cavity, tongue, larynx, esophagus, areas lined by columnar epithelium undergoing metaplasia— bronchus, gallbladder, cardiac end of stomach, anorectum, areas lined by transitional epithelium, underlying metaplasia— renal pelvis and urinary bladder.
- *Clinical features:* Ulcerative or ulceroproliferative lesion with *raised and everted edge*; indurated edge and base (Fig. 4-133). Floor may be containing necrotic slough with serosanguineous discharge or nodular tumor with hard, nodular, nontender; base is indurated and often later gets fixed to underlying structures. As the edge contains actively multiplying cells it is raised above the surrounding area.
- Regional lymph nodes are involved eventually which are nodular, hard and may gets fixed later. Blood spread is not common in SCC.
- *Marjolin's ulcer* is a well-differentiated SCC occurring in *unstable chronic scar* of long duration. It is common in scars of snake bite, venous ulcer and burns. It is only locally malignant without nodal spread. *Verrucous carcinoma* is a variant of well-differentiated SCC occurring in mucous membrane or mucocutaneous junction presenting as dry, exophytic, warty, indurated growth without any nodal spread carrying good prognosis. Verrucous carcinoma of foot is called as *carcinoma cuniculatum. Histologically,* concentrically arranged prickle cells around *epithelial pearls* (malignant squamous) cells with epithelial/keratin pearls are typical. More than 75% keratin pearls are well-differentiated; 50–75% is moderately differentiated; 25–50% poorly differentiated; <25% is undifferentiated.
- *Differential diagnoses:* BCC; melanoma; keratoacanthoma; skin adnexal tumor. A rare variety of multiple self-healing SCC is observed usually in face as familial autosomal dominant (chromosome 9q) disease in western Scotland— *Ferguson-Smith syndrome.*

Melanoma

- It is a malignant tumor arising from melanocyte or melanoblast and is the most aggressive cutaneous malignant tumor. It is of *neural crest* (ectodermal) origin.
- It is 20 times more commonly seen in *whites* than blacks.

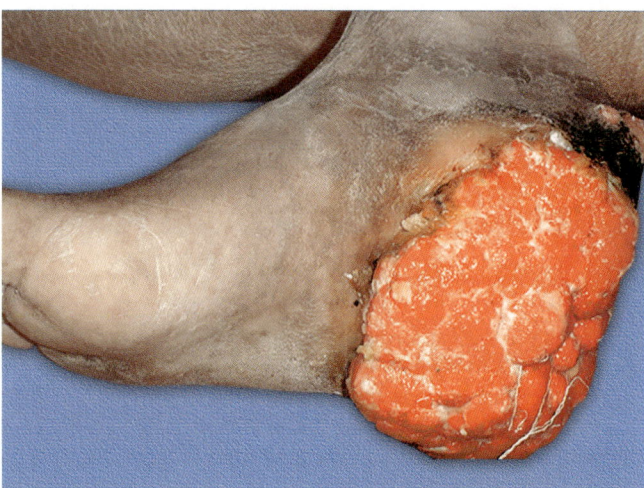

Fig. 4-133 Squamous cell carcinoma heel—it is *proliferative lesion, cauliflower-like.*

- Incidence is equal in both sexes. Incidence increases over years. It is not known to occur before puberty. In females, leg is the most common site. In males trunk is the commonest site. In Bantu tribe sole is the commonest site (Figs. 4-134 and 135).
- It can occur in eyes, mucocutaneous junction, mucosa, head and neck. It is common in *Australia.* It is common in white skinned people. Prolonged exposure to ultraviolet light predisposes to melanoma.
- Risk factors—high society people; albinism; xeroderma pigmentosa; junctional naevus; familial dysplastic naevus syndrome; congenital naevi; family history of melanoma; previously other skin cancer if occurred.
- *Clinical Types:*
  1. Superficial spreading (64%): It is the most common type. It has got more radial growth than vertical. It arises from preexisting nevus. It carries better prognosis.
  2. Nodular melanoma (20%): It shows more vertical growth with invasion; more aggressive; common in mucosa and mucocutaneous junction; it appears as de novo in skin. Nodal spread is common; it is uniform and nodular; carries poor prognosis.
  3. Lentigo maligna melanoma (10%): Less common; least malignant; common in elderly females; common in face, neck, hands. It is slow growing, in situ type.
  4. Acral lentiginous melanoma (5%): Least common; common in palms and soles; common in Japan, Africa and Asia; nodular with vertical growth; attains large size; has poor prognosis; less common in whites; mimics fungal infection or pyogenic granuloma.
  5. Amelanotic melanoma: It is worst type. Due to undifferentiation tumor cells will not synthesize melanin; rapidly progressive pinkish fleshy growth is the presentation; mimics soft tissue sarcoma.
  6. Desmoplastic melanoma: It has got high affinity for perineural invasion; common in head and neck; carries high recurrence rate.
  7. Subungual melanoma: It is involvement of nail fold matrix; progressive widening and pigmentation of nail fold with nail dystrophy is typical—Hutchinson's sign.
- *Clinical features*: It can occur in a preexisting nevus or de novo in normal skin. Pigmentation with irregular surface, irregular margin; ulceration; bleeding; itching; color changes; depigmentation halo around the pigmented area; recent increase in size of the preexisting mole. Melanoma can spread both through regional lymph node as well as through blood (Figs. 4-136 and 4-137).
- *ABCDE of melanoma*: *A*symmetry; *B*order irregularity; *C*olor variation; *D*iameter >6 mm; *E*volving.
- Induration is *not seen* in melanoma.
- Melanoma spreads through lymphatics to *regional nodes* by permeation or embolization; through *blood* to liver (massive pigmented liver); lungs (cough, hemoptysis, pleural effusion, cannon ball secondaries); brain (convulsions, localizing features, raised intracranial pressure); bones (bone pain, pathological fracture, neurological deficits); skin; viscera (melanuria). Secondary skin nodules within 2 cm of primary are called as *satellite nodules* (Figs. 4-138A and B); nodules beyond 2 cm from primary up to the regional nodes are called as *'in-transit' nodules*.
- Melanoma in choroids carries better prognosis as there are *no* lymphatics.
- Late massive liver secondaries even after 20 years is known to occur when primary is specifically in choroid. Presentation initially as secondaries is possible when occult primary exists in anus, scalp, genitalia, eye, nailbed, external auditory canal, adrenal medulla.
- Differential diagnoses are other pigmented lesions of the skin.

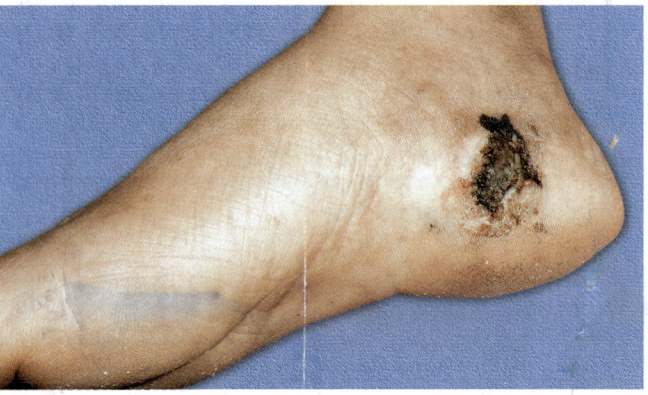

Fig. 4-134 Melanoma sole.

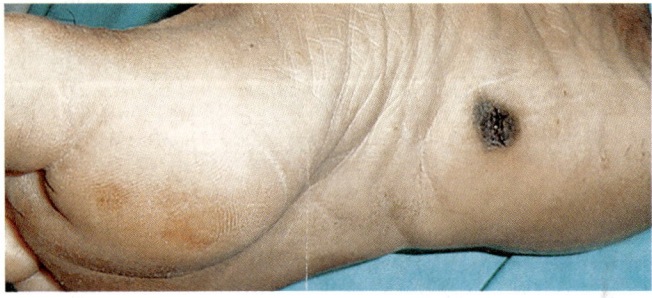

Fig. 4-135 Melanoma on the plantar aspect of the foot. Patient often will not observe this lesion. *Note the deep pigmentation and ulceration over it.*

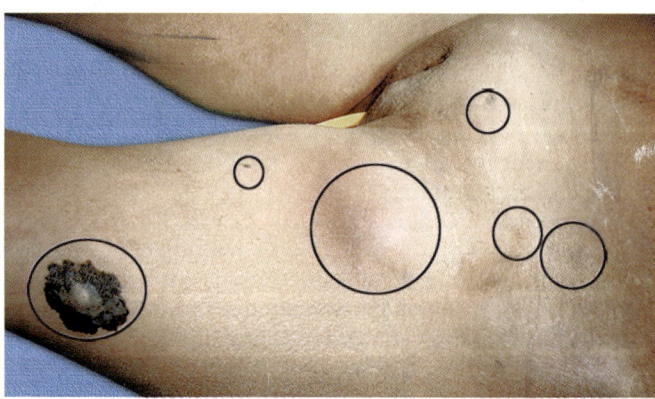

Fig. 4-136 Melanoma thigh with *secondaries in inguinal lymph nodes.*

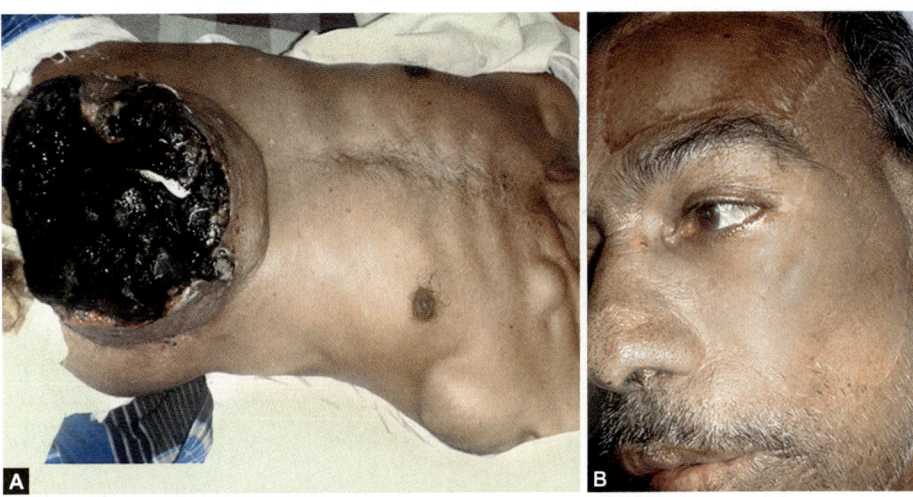

Figs. 4-137A and B Melanoma causing *abdominal wall secondaries*; patient has undergone wide excision with flap reconstruction for melanoma face few years back.

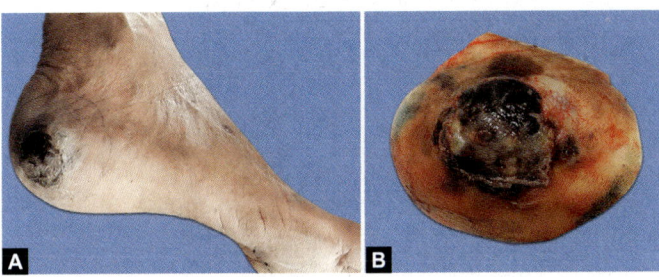

Figs. 4-138A and B Melanoma in sole with *satellite nodules*. Satellite nodules occur within 2 cm of the primary lesion.

Pigmented lesions of the skin
• Seborrheic keratosis
• Dermatofibroma
• Pigmented BCC
• Nevus
• Cutaneous hemangioma
• Melanoma
• Skin adnexal tumors
• Solar keratosis
• Pyogenic granuloma

• Angiosarcoma of skin
• Café au lait patch
• Campbell de Morgan spot
• Venous dermatitis

Sarcomas

Sarcomas arise from soft tissues and bone. They are less common than carcinomas. They are usually rapidly growing nonencapsulated fleshy malignant tumors. It is 1% of adult malignancy. It is common in younger age group. Commonest site is lower limb; common types are liposarcoma and undifferentiated pleomorphic sarcoma (UPS). It spreads mainly through blood to lungs. Few also may spread to lymph nodes like rhabdomyosarcoma, synovial sarcoma, angiosarcoma. It presents clinically as painless, smooth, vascular, progressive swelling of short duration with often infiltration into adjacent structures. Skin over the swelling is stretched, glossy, with dilated veins. It becomes painful and tender once there is nerve infiltration, tumor necrosis, infection. Features lung secondaries like chest, pain, dyspnea and hemoptysis may be seen in metastatic disease. FNAC is not useful; Trucut or Incision biopsy is ideal.

Sarcoma (Swelling) types	Etiology and pathology	Features
1. **Liposarcoma** Most common of all sarcomas	Can occur denovo- or in a pre-existing lipoma. **Types**: Well-differentiated; myxoid; round cell; pleomorphic	Thigh, back, retroperitoneum—most common sites.
2. **Malignant fibrous histiocytoma/ MFH (Now called as Undifferentiated pleomorphic sarcoma/UPS)** Most common type of extremity sarcoma	• It is common in thigh, pelvis, abdomen; it can occur in lungs, head and neck, orbit, naso and oropharynx, CNS. • Often associated with hypoglycaemia, lymphoma, multiple myeloma	Seen in adults and elderly; aggressive rapidly progressive type of sarcoma.
3. **Leiomyosarcoma** Arises from smooth muscles with whorled out appearance	Common in retroperitoneum and viscera	
4. **Rhabdomyosarcoma** – Arises from skeletal muscle – Most common sarcoma in children. Rare in adult	Common in head, neck, thigh, arm **Types**: pleomorphic; embryonal; botryoidal, alveolar	• Grayish pink; soft; fleshy; well-circumscribed tumor • Very aggressive tumor; can spread to lymph nodes

Contd...

Contd...

Sarcoma (Swelling) types	Etiology and pathology	Features
5. **Synovial sarcoma (Fig. 4-140)** Originates from tendon sheath, joint capsule. Occurs in younger age group	Common in shoulder, thigh, leg	High grade aggressive sarcoma; blood spread; 20% cases to regional lymph nodes
6. **Fibrosarcoma** Arises from fibroblasts	Can occur in soft tissue and bone	Slow growing; attains enormous size often
7. **Kaposi's sarcoma** Arises from vascular smooth muscles or pericytes **Types:** *European's Kaposi's sarcoma* *African Kaposi's sarcoma* *Transplant associated Kaposi's sarcoma* *AIDS associated Kaposi's sarcoma*	• Linked to human herpes virus (HHV8) • Common in skin, mucus membrane, lymph nodes or viscera • Common in extremity; rare in viscera; common in old age • Common in children and young; involves skin and lymph nodes • Wide disseminated involvement with spread	Multiple reddish blue nodules in the skin with ulceration over the nodule • Lymph node spread • Very aggressive

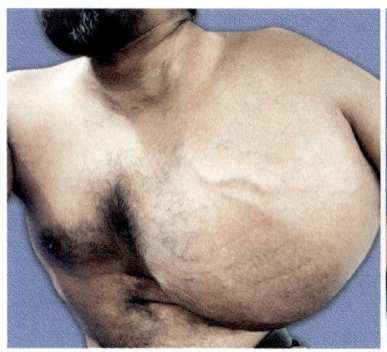
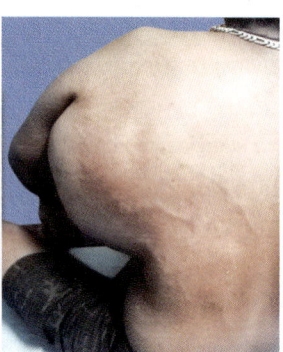

Fig. 4-139 Soft tissue sarcoma over chest wall.

Hamartoma; Hemangioma; Vascular Malformations and Lymphatic Malformations

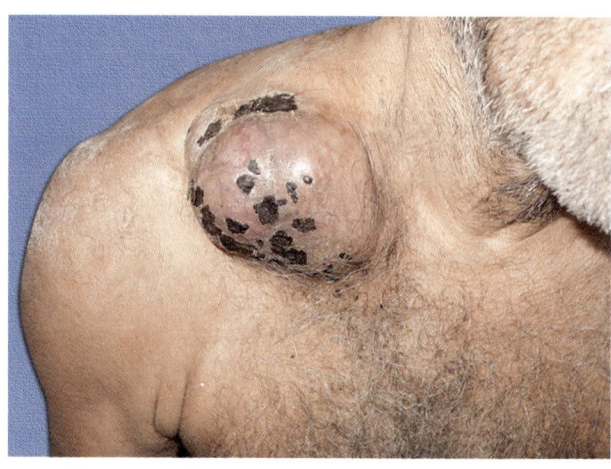

Fig. 4-140 *Synovial sarcoma* over right shoulder.

Hamartomata (Hamartano means – I miss [Greek] or fault or misfire or error) is a benign lesion with aberrant differentiation producing a mass of disorganized but matured tissue or specialized cells indigenous to particular site. It is tumor like overgrowth of tissue proper to that part. Hemangioma, lymphangiomas used be categorized with this; but this terminology is only of academic use as it is no longer used. Currently newer classifications are used.

Vascular malformations and related swelling types	Etiology and pathology	Features
1. **Hemangioma** – Benign vascular endothelial tumor, common in girls – Grows rapidly in first year; involutes in 7 years **Types:** a. **Capillary hemangioma** (Strawberry hemangioma/ Hemangioma simplex): Starts at birth; common in white girls (girl: boy:: 3:1). Most common hemangioma b. **Cavernous hemangioma (Fig. 4-142)** May present at birth	• Commonly seen in skin and subcutaneous tissue but can occur in liver, brain, lungs, other organs • Common in head and neck region **(Fig. 4-141)** Contains immature vaso-formative tissues; involves skin, subcutaneous tissue, often muscle also; Common in head and neck region. *Complications*: Bleeding and ulceration after minor trauma • Consists of multiple venous channels; often contains feeding vessels which is of surgical importance • *Sites*: Head, brain, neck, face, lips, mouth limbs, tongue, liver, kidney and other internal organs • *Complications*: Hemorrhage, thrombosis; infection, ulceration; septicemia; erosion into the adjacent bone; high output cardiac failure • Hemangioma in periorbital region may obstruct the vision in newborn with amblyopia	• Early lesion—bright red, irregular • Deep lesion—bluish colored • On involution color fades, lesion shrinks, leaving behind crepe paper like area It may begin at birth or child may be normal at birth; Begin in first to third week as bright red mark increases in size rapidly in three months; lesion is compressible warm with bluish surface. It slowly begins to disappear after one year of age and completely disappears in 7–8 years • Smooth, soft, well-localized, warm, fluctuant, *compressible*, non-transilluminant, non-pulsatile swelling with *bluish surface* occurring in skin and mucus membrane • Reduces in size partly or completely when pressed attains original size and shape when pressure released - *compressibility* • Non-tender unless infected or undergone thrombosis or in case of hemorrhage

Contd...

Chapter 4: Examination and Clinical Approach of a Swelling/Lump 137

Contd...

Vascular malformations and related swelling types	Etiology and pathology	Features
c. **Cirsoid aneurysm** Rare variant of capillary hemangioma	• Hemangioma in nasal area may obstruct the airway • Occurs beneath skin where an abnormal artery communicates with distended veins • Commonly seen in *superficial temporal artery and its branches*	Pulsatile swelling (*pulsatile bag of worms*) in relation to superficial temporal artery, warm, compressible, arterialization of adjacent veins, thinning of bone due to pressure, systolic bruit and thrill
2. **Capillary vascular malformation** a. **Salmon patch (stork bite)** Resent at birth	Caused by an area of persistent fetal dermal circulation	• Involves wide area of skin; occurs commonly in nape of neck, face, scalp and limbs. Goes for spontaneous regression and disappears completely in one year
b. **Port-Wine stain (Nevus flammeus) (Fig. 4-143)** Present at birth and persist throughout life without any change.	• Results from defect in maturation of sympathetic innervation of skin causing localized vasodilatation of intradermal capillaries • Often associated with syndromes like - Sturge Weber; Klippel–Trenaunay; Proteus, etc.	• Common in head, neck, face; often involving the skin of maxillary/mandibular dermatomes of 5th cranial nerve • Present as smooth, flat, reddish blue/intensely purple area; eventually surface become nodular and keratotic; blanch on pressure; do not increase in size
3. **Other vascular conditions:** a. **Vin rose patch:** Congenital intradermal pale pink vascular malformation with dilatation of vessels in subpapillary dermal plexus		• Associated with hemangiomas; AV malformations in limbs; congenital lymphedema
b. **Campbell de Morgan spots (cherry angiomas)**		• Usually smaller (2–6 mm), circular bright red swelling; common in trunk, common in elderly
c. **Spider nevus:** Acquired solitary lesion. Commonly associated with alcoholic cirrhosis		• Contains *a single dilated central arteriole* (bright red, 1 mm diameter) which acts a feeding vessel to multiple small branches in radial manner • Multiple spider nevi are common in face, upper arm proximal chest; compressible on pressure or slide which refills on release of pressure
4. **Lymphangioma** Congenital condition where there is localized clusters of dilated lymph sacs in skin and subcutaneous tissue that has failed to join the normal lymph system during developmental period a. **Capillary lymphangioma** Can be present at birth or lesions may appear within few years	Common at the junction of body to limb—near shoulder, axilla, groin, buttock involving an area of 5–20 cm area **Types**: a. Lymphangioma circumscriptum—<5 cm in size b. Lymphangioma diffusum—> 5 cm in size c. Lymphangioma ab agne—if it is with reticulated ridges	• Multiple, white colored, skin vesicles, 0.5–4 mm size containing clear watery/yellowish-fluid may turn into brown or black due to bleeding within vesicles. Vesicles will not fade on pressure • Area is soft spongy, often fluctuant, with fluid thrill and translucency, not compressible • Lesion can be painful and tender if infected • Regional lymph nodes not enlarged • Condition does not block normal lymph drainage so there is no skin edema
b. **Cavernous lymphangioma**	Common in neck, pectoral region, face mouth lips (*macrocheilia*); tongue (macroglossia)	• Soft, lobulated, fluctuant, compressible, brilliantly transilluminant large swelling with multiple communicating lymphatic cysts
c. **Cystic hygroma** Collection of clustered, sequestered, lymph sacs in subcutaneous tissue (occurs during developmental period of fetus in utero) seen in newborn	Common in posterior triangle of neck (75%); axilla (20%); rarely in cheek, tongue, retroperitoneum, groin, mediastinum When occurs in neck—*hydrocele of the neck* Complications: Big sized cyst can cause obstructed labor, respiratory obstruction in newborn, may rupture leading to lymphorrhea, infection septicemia	• Large painless swelling which is soft, sessile, smooth, fluctuant, *brilliantly transilluminant, compressible*, having *ill-defined margin* • Contains aggregation of *soap-bubble like multiple cysts*, larger ones on surface smaller ones in deeper plane. Cysts are intercommunicating, so compressible • Lined by endothelium, contains clear/straw colored fluid which does not coagulate

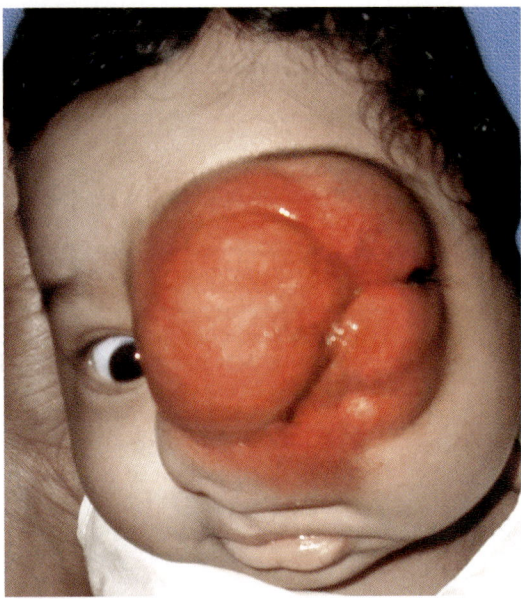

Fig. 4-141 Hemangioma in a child involving face extensively. *Hemangioma is usually compressible*. On applying continuous pressure swelling partially gets reduced and on releasing swelling comes back to original size. Cystic hygroma, aneurysms are compressible. Thrombosed aneurysm is not compressible (*Courtesy:* Professor Ganesh Pai, MCh).

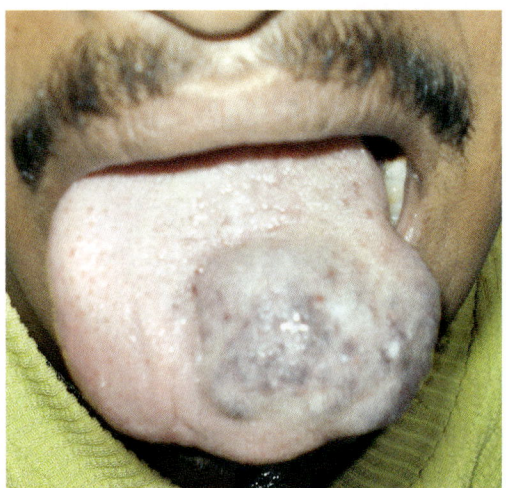

Fig. 4-142 Cavernous hemangioma—tongue.

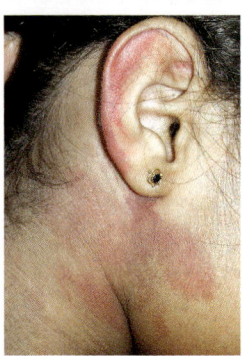

Fig. 4-143 Portwine stain (Nevus flammeus).

Infective Swellings

Cellulitis: It is *spreading inflammation of subcutaneous and fascial planes*. Infection may follow a small scratch or wound or incision. Common causative agents are *Streptococcus pyogenes* organisms and other gram-positive organisms. Often gram-negative organisms like *Klebsiella, Pseudomonas, E. coli* are also involved. Cellulitis can be superficial or deep, can occur anywhere in the body but spreads rapidly in loose connective tissue of forearm, abdominal wall, face. *Sequelae of cellulites*—Infection can get localized to form *pyogenic abscess;* Infection can spread to cause *bacteremia, septicemia, pyemia;* Often infection can lead to *local gangrene. Clinical features* are fever, toxicity (tachycardia, hypotension); diffuse swelling which is spreading in nature; pain and tenderness, red, shiny, boggy area with stretched warm skin. Brawny look of the area with pitting edema without any edge are the typical features (*Absence of edge; absence of fluctuation; absence of pus; absence of limit*). Cellulitis will progress rapidly in diabetic and immunosuppressed individuals like patients with HIV infection. Associated lymphangitis is often seen as raised red streaks which blanch on pressure. Tender palpable regional lymph nodes are common due to associated lymphadenitis. Often these lymph nodes get suppurated forming an abscess eventually (Figs. 4-144 to 4-146).

Orbital cellulitis: Cellulitis in orbit causes proptosis, leading to impairment of ocular movements and blindness. It can spread through ophthalmic veins into cavernous sinus causing *cavernous sinus thrombosis*. It requires admission and immediate aggressive treatment with higher generation antibiotics.

Cellulitis face: Inflammatory condition in dangerous area of face like boils, furuncle, if not treated, can spread to

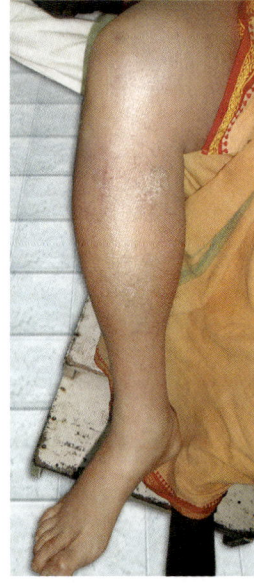

Fig. 4-144 Cellulitis leg with lymphangitis. Note the *edema and redness*.

cavernous sinus leading to life-threatening condition. Patient may present with high grade fever, vomiting, headache, may become delirious or semiconscious. As there will be involvement of 3rd, 4th, 6th cranial nerves, movement of eyeball will be absent with edema of conjunctiva, eyelids, and sluggish pupils.

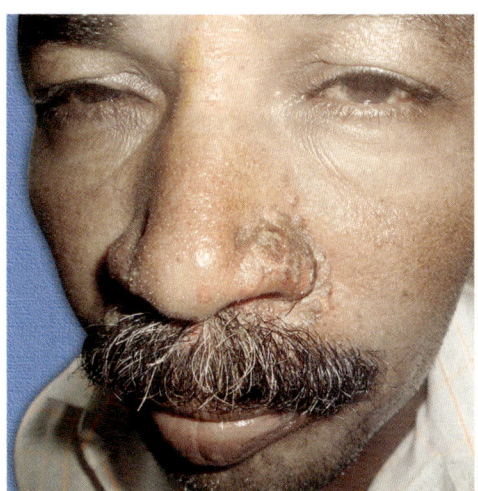

Fig. 4-145 Cellulitis face. *Dangerous area of face— area of upper lip and lower part of nose.* Infection from this area spreads through deep facial vein → pterygoid plexus → communicating vein → cavernous sinus causing its life-threatening thrombosis.

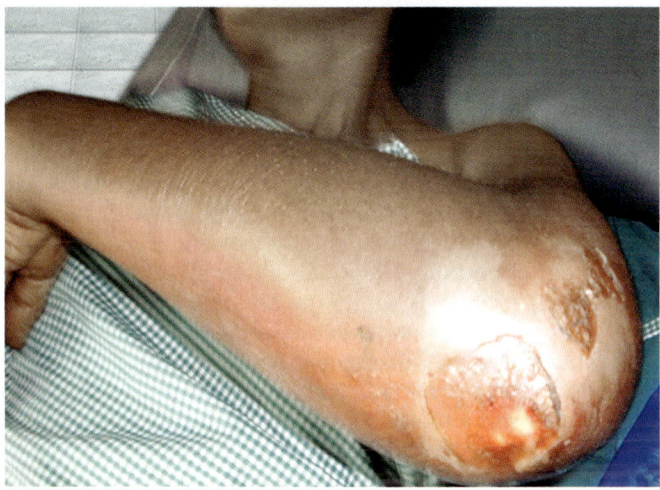

Fig. 4-146 *Extensive cellulitis* of arm and forearm with abscess formation.

Ludwig's angina: It is cellulitis of upper part of the neck involving submandibular region and floor of the mouth along the fascial planes; develop deep to deep fascia of submandibular and submental region. *Clinical features:* Diffuse swelling, redness, tenderness and induration in the floor of the mouth and submandibular region; difficulty in opening the mouth *(Trismus);* toxic features like fever, tachycardia and tachypnea; *severe laryngeal edema* (presents with respiratory distress, stridor and cyanosis). *Complications:* Septicemia; mediastinitis; spread of infection into the parapharyngeal space leads to *thrombosis* of internal jugular vein which may extend above into the sigmoid sinus which may be fatal.

Erysipelas (Greek–red skin): It is a spreading inflammation of the skin and subcutaneous tissues due to infection caused by *Streptococcus pyogenes*. There will be always cutaneous lymphangitis with development of rose pink rash with cutaneous lymphatic edema. Eruptions → erythema → livid hue → brown → yellow → vesicles → pustule. Vesicles which form eventually will rupture to cause serous discharge. Common sites are—orbit, face and scrotum. In face and orbit, it causes severe edema. Eyelid may get closed completely. Hands, genitalia, umbilicus of infants, around decubitus ulcer of lower limb are other rare site. *Clinical features* are toxemia; rash which is fast spreading and blanches on pressure; rash is raised with sharp margin; discharge is serous (In cellulitis discharge is purulent); *Milian's ear sign* is a clinical sign used to differentiate erysipelas from cellulitis wherein ear lobule is spared. Skin of ear lobule is adherent to the subcutaneous tissue and so cellulitis cannot occur. Erysipelas being a cutaneous condition can spread into the ear lobule. Disease is common in poorly hygienic, debilitated individuals. Tender regional lymph nodes may be palpable.

Erysipeloid disease is also called as '*Fish handler's disease*'. It is a self-limiting disease with mild features of both cellulitis and erysipelas. It occurs following minor trauma in fish and meat handlers. It is common in hands.

Pyogenic abscess: It is a *localized collection* of pus in a cavity lined by granulation tissue, covered by pyogenic membrane. It contains pus in loculi. Pus is an inflammatory exudate that contains dead WBCs, multiplying bacteria, toxins and necrotic material. Spread may be direct, hematogenous, lymphatics from adjacent tissues. *Staphylococcus aureus* and *Streptococcus pyogenes* are common organisms. It is often an effect of cellulitis or lymphangitis. Abscess is more common in malnourished people, people with anemia, diabetes mellitus, HIV, immunosuppression or old age. Trauma, hematoma, virulence of the organisms are other factors (Fig. 4-147).

Clinical features: Throbbing pain; fever with chills and rigors; soft, smooth, tender, fluctuant swelling with often visible pus and pointing tenderness. Brawny induration is common in surrounding area. Redness, warmth with restricted movements of the part or adjacent joint are observed. *Visible (pointing) pus, tenderness, fluctuation* are the features of *formed abscess* (Commonly cellulitis occurs first which eventually gets localized to form an abscess). *Sites of an abscess:* It can be *external or internal*, depending on whether the abscess is on the surface or in the deeper cavities like abdomen. *Examples of external sites* are: fingers and hand; neck; axilla; breast; foot; thigh—here it is deeply situated

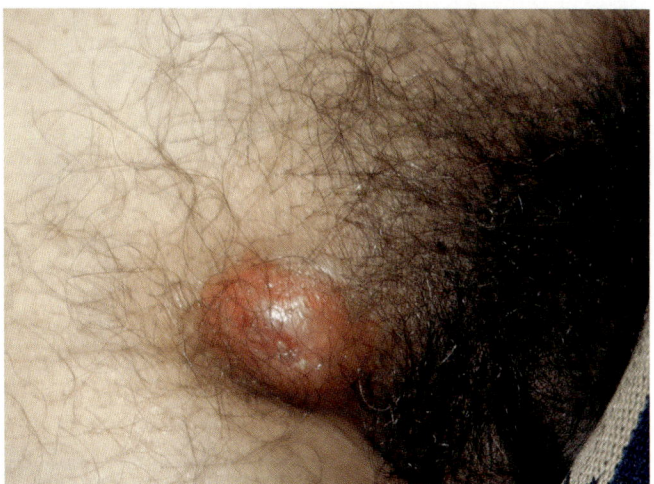

Fig. 4-147 *Abscess groin* showing signs of inflammation.

with brawny edema and deep tenderness; ischiorectal and perianal region; abdominal wall; dental abscess; tonsillar abscess and other abscesses in the oral cavity. *Examples of internal abscess are*: *abdominal*—subphrenic, pelvic, paracolic, amoebic liver abscess, pyogenic abscess of liver, splenic abscess, pancreatic abscess; perinephrenic abscess; retroperitoneal abscess; lung abscess; brain abscess.

Complications of an abscess: Bacteremia, septicemia, and pyemia; multiple abscess formation; metastatic abscess; destruction of tissues due to necrosis; antibioma formation due to antibiotic therapy without drainage (common in breast abscess); sinus and fistula formation; large abscess may erode into adjacent vessels and can cause life-threatening torrential hemorrhage (examples: Pancreatic abscess causing splenic vessel hemorrhage, psoas abscess causing iliac vessel hemorrhage); abscess in head and neck region can cause laryngeal edema, stridor and dysphagia. *Specific complications of internal abscess*: Brain abscess can cause intracranial hypertension, epilepsy, neurological deficit; liver abscess can cause hepatic failure, rupture, jaundice; lung abscess can lead on to bronchopleural fistula or septicemia or respiratory failure or ARDS. *Abscess should be formed before draining. Exceptions for this rule are*: Parotid abscess; breast abscess; axillary abscess; thigh abscess; ischiorectal abscess. Differential diagnoses to be remembered before draining an abscess are—*Aneurysm*, especially in popliteal, femoral and axillary regions. So using a needle always aspirate and confirm the pus; *Soft tissue tumors*—Sarcomas may be smooth, soft/firm and warm with dilated vessels on the surface.

Cold abscess: It means there are no signs of acute inflammation like redness, warmth, tenderness. It is painless, smooth, soft, fluctuant, nontransilluminating. Edema, brawny indurations are absent. Cold abscess is due to caseative necrosis of tuberculous disease. It is commonly observed in caseating tuberculous lymphadenitis; tuberculosis of spine; joint tuberculosis; tuberculosis of ribs, mediastinum, etc. Cold abscess can occur at the site of the disease like in the neck (neck is the most common site) (Fig. 4-148) or often caseating fluid can travel along the fascial or neurovascular bundle to cause abscess at different sites. Such cold abscess is frequently observed in tuberculosis of spine (T_{10}). Psoas abscess; groin abscess; abscess in paraspinal region; abscess in intercostal space are the examples of such type of cold abscess.

Difference between pyogenic and cold abscess:	
Pyogenic abscess	**Cold abscess**
Red, warm, tender, with signs of acute inflammation	No signs of acute inflammation
Pyogenic bacteria are nonspecific organisms (Streptococci/Staphylococci)	Tuberculous bacteria
For drainage, dependent incision is used	Nondependent incision is used
Suturing of the wound is not done	Cavity is curetted and sutured
Drain is placed	Drain is not placed

Pyemic abscess: These are formation of multiple abscesses in the different parts of the body like subfascial plane, deeper planes, in the organs like liver, lungs, brain, spleen, etc. It is due to lodging of the multiple infective bacterial emboli from the circulating blood at different places which cause suppuration and abscesses formation. *Subfascial pyemic abscesses* often do not show the features of acute abscess like warmness, fluctuation, pointing tenderness.

Boil (Furuncle): It is an acute *Staphylococcus aureus* infection of a hair follicle with perifolliculitis which usually proceeds to suppuration and central necrosis. It is common in neck, back and upper limb. Often boil opens on its own and subsides. Furuncle in external auditory meatus is very painful because of rich cutaneous nerves and firmly adherent skin to perichondrium. Pain, indurated swelling, greenish pustule that eventually rupture to create a deep cavity with green slough, often with tender palpable regional nodes are the features (Fig. 4-149). Once it ruptures, red granulation tissue forms in the surface/floor and spontaneous healing takes place with antibiotic coverage. When a boil subsides without suppuration, it is called 'blind boil'.

> Staphylococcal infection of root of one hair follicle—*folliculitis*.
> Staphylococcal infection of root of one hair follicle with perifolliculitis—*boil/furuncle*.
> Multiple boils with normal tissue in between—*furunculosis*.
> Staphylococcal infective gangrene of skin and subcutaneous tissue presenting as multiple boils with involvement of intervening tissue—*carbuncle*

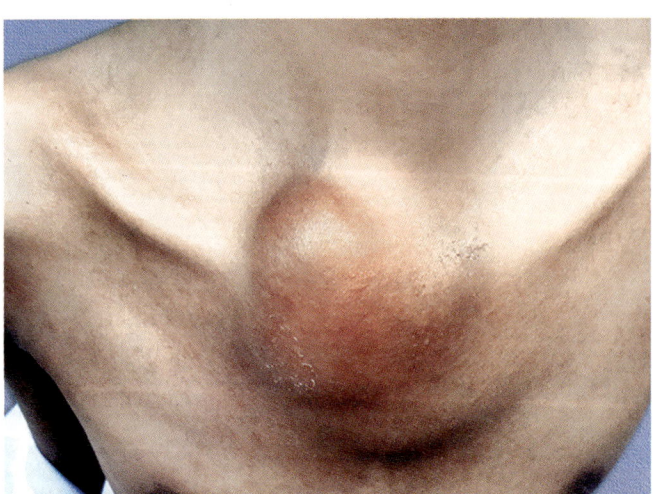

Fig. 4-148 Cold abscess sternal region. *Neck is the common site.*

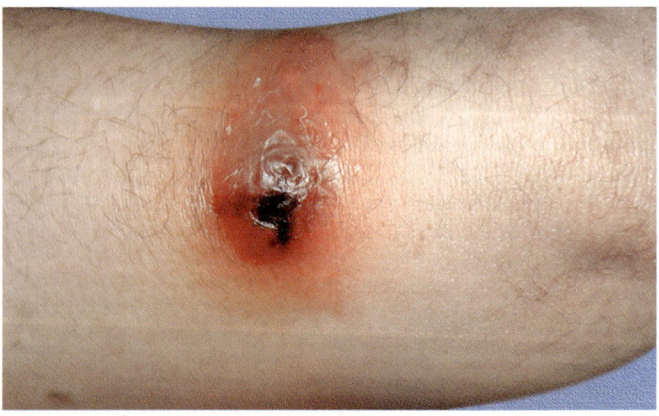

Fig. 4-149 Boil. It is staphylococcal *perifolliculitis* (infection of hair follicle).

Complications: Cellulitis; lymphadenitis; hydradenitis (in axilla—*infection of group of hair follicles*); subcutaneous abscess.

Hidradenitis suppurativa: It is a chronic infective and fibrous disease of the skin which bears apocrine sweat glands. Apocrine sweat glands are coiled sweat glands which open into hair follicle. It is common in axilla, areola, umbilicus, groin and perineum. In the axilla, condition is often bilateral. It is related to obesity, smoking, poor hygiene, diabetes mellitus, steroids. Common bacteria are staphylococci, streptococci and *Propionibacterium acnes*. Keratin blocks the duct of the apocrine sweat glands causing dilatation of the duct leading into infection and suppuration of the glands. Many adjacent glands involve eventually causing fibrosis, scarring and sinus formation. Commonest site is *axilla* (Fig. 4-150). It is common in *females* (4:1). Discharging sinuses, induration, tenderness and edema are common. It often looks like tuberculosis or malignancy.

Carbuncle: *Word meaning carbuncle is charcoal. It is an infective gangrene of skin and subcutaneous tissue.* S*taphylococcus aureus* is the main causative organism (Figs. 4-151A and B). Common site of occurrence is *back and nape of neck*. It is common in *diabetics* and after forty years age. It is common in males. Infection → red, indurated edematous area → small vesicles develop → discharge through multiple openings → sieve-like pattern/cribriform pattern → many fuse together to form a central necrotic ulcer with peripheral fresh vesicle looking like a '*rosette' with ash gray slough* → skin becoming black due to blockage of cutaneous vessels → disease spreads to adjacent skin rapidly. Patient will be *toxic* and in diabetic they are *ketotic*. Renal carbuncle is an entity which occurs in kidney due to infection, forming localized infective mass lesion.

Pott's puffy tumor: It is formation of diffuse external swelling in the scalp due to *subperiosteal pus formation and scalp edema*. It originates commonly in frontal region and may extend into other regions. It is usually due to chronic frontal sinusitis which eventually suppurates and extends into subperiosteal region but trauma also can cause the same. Clinical features: Pain and diffuse swelling in frontal region which is warm, tender. Swelling often extends to face and eyelids. Patient will be toxic and drowsy. Complications: *Osteomyelitis* of frontal bone; spread of infection into intracranial cavity leading to *intracranial abscess* (Extradural or subdural abscess). So it may present with features of raised intracranial tension like headache, coning and convulsions. *Differential diagnosis:* Cellulitis scalp is infection of entire scalp including all layers, where it becomes swollen and boggy.

Pyogenic granuloma (Granuloma pyogenicum): It is a common condition which occurs in face, scalp, nose, fingers and toes (Fig. 4-152). It may be due to minor trauma or minor infection. Infection leads to formation of unhealthy

Fig. 4-150 *Hidradenitis suppurativa*—axilla region.

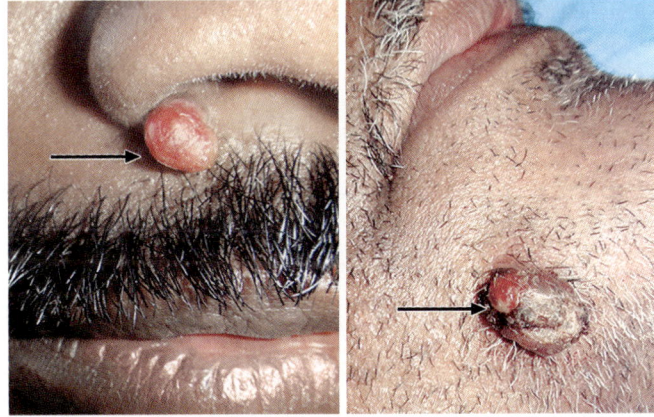

Fig. 4-152 *Pyogenic granuloma* nostril and lower face.

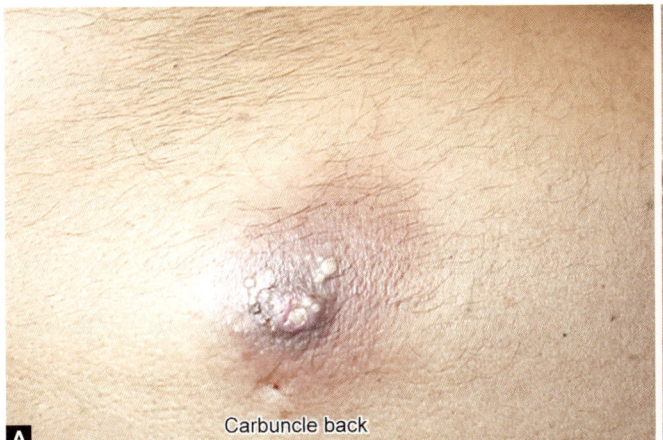

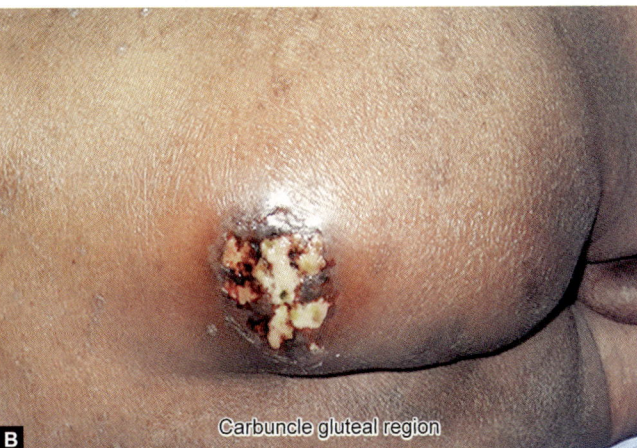

Figs. 4-151A and B *Typical carbuncle.*

granulation tissue which protrudes through the wound. Clinical features: Usually single, well-localized, red, firm, nodule, which bleeds on touch. It is rapidly growing relatively painless and often mimics hemangioma, papilloma, skin adnexal tumor, squamous cell carcinoma and melanoma.

Impetigo: It is highly infectious superficial skin infection caused by staphylococci/streptococci organisms. It is usually seen in children, with formation of multiple blisters that rupture and coalesce, to be covered with honey colored crust. *Scrumpox* is a type of impetigo seen in Rugby players due to staphylococcal infection.

Bacteremia, septicemia, pyemia: These conditions are discussed here as they may cause multiple abscesses in the body or these conditions may occur due to existing abscess itself. *Bacteremia* is presence of bacteria in blood. It causes fever with chills and rigors, tachycardia and leukocytosis. It may get controlled by antibiotics or may lead into septicemia (septic shock). *Septicemia* is presence of overwhelming, multiplying bacteria in the blood with toxins causing *systemic inflammatory response syndrome (SIRS) or multiorgan dysfunction syndrome (MODS)*. Patient presents with fever, oliguria, jaundice, hypotension, feeble pulse, respiratory failure and drowsiness. Fever often may be absent or hypothermia may be evident due to severe sepsis wherein pyogenic response is absent. Septicemia may be due to gram-positive or gram-negative organism. Gram-positive septicemia is due to staphylococci, streptococci, pneumococci, etc. *Overwhelming postsplenectomy infection (OPSI)* is a classical example of gram-positive septicemia. Gram-negative septicemia is commonly observed in urinary infection, biliary sepsis, peritonitis, abdominal infection, sepsis in diabetics and immunosuppressed. It is also called as *endotoxic shock* due to endotoxins released from lysed bacteria. Common gram-negative organisms causing gram-negative septicemia are *E. coli, Klebsiella, Pseudomonas* and *Proteus*. Pyemia is presence of multiplying bacteria in blood as emboli which spreads and lodges in different organs in the body like liver, lungs, kidneys, spleen, brain causing *metastatic abscess*.

CASE DISCUSSION

A 30-year-old man presents with a painless swelling in the left thigh of 3 months duration which is rapidly progressive. But for this swelling he is not having any other symptoms like pain, difficulty in moving the limb, abdominal pain, respiratory symptoms. There is no past history of trauma to the thigh. He is otherwise medically fit. General examination is normal. Swelling on examination is of 6 × 6 cm in size over lower lateral part of the thigh with the skin over it is being normal without dilated veins. On palpation it is nontender, with slight raise in local temperature, smooth surface, firm in consistency, mobile but mobility gets restricted on contracting the lateral muscles; it is not attached to the underlying femur bone. There is no wasting of the thigh muscles. Skin overlying is free. Knee and hip joints are normal. Opposite limb is normal.

What other clinical examination you will do?
Regional nodes (inguinal and external iliac) and *respiratory system (chest)*, abdomen for hepatomegaly, CNS examination should be done for evidence of spread as soft tissue sarcoma is suspected with such findings systemic examination becomes essential.

What is the probable diagnosis and why?
Diagnosis is probably soft tissue sarcoma (STS); as it is of short duration, painless progressive and warm. It is unlikely to be inflammatory conditions like abscess or hematoma which are differential diagnoses for STS. Abscess is warm, tender with fever. Hematoma when develops which is not uncommon will have history of trauma, pain and localization of the swelling with bruises or erythema over the surface.

What is the probable plane of the swelling?
It is probably deep to deep fascia of lower lateral thigh. It is adherent to lateral thigh muscles as mobility gets restricted by contracting those muscles.

How you will evaluate the patient?
Incision biopsy or Trucut biopsy should be done for tissue diagnosis; incision should be longitudinal without raising the flap. MRI of the part is done to assess the extent of the tumor locally. CT chest and abdomen to identify blood spread. FNAC and excision biopsy is usually should be avoided in STS. Core/trucut biopsy may an alternate option accepted.

5

Examination and Clinical Approach of Sinus and Fistula

CHAPTER

Competency: SU6.1.

SINUS

- Sinus is a blind track lined by granulation tissue leading from an epithelial surface into the deeper surrounding tissues (Figs. 5-1 and 5-2).
- Sinus means *'hollow' or 'a bay' (Latin).*
- *Causes: Congenital:* Preauricular sinus. A*cquired:* (1) Traumatic often with presence of foreign body (Fig. 5-3); (2) Inflammatory – Tuberculosis, actinomycosis, chronic osteomyelitis, chronic abscess, median mental sinus; (3) Neoplastic; (4) Other acquired conditions – pilonidal sinus, port site sinus after laparoscopic surgeries.
- *Commonest cause of sinus in the neck is tuberculosis, commonly due to tuberculous lymphadenitis.*

FISTULA (FIG. 5-4)

- Fistula is an abnormal communication lined by epithelium/granulation tissue between two internal hollow viscus or between a hollow viscus and the body surface or between vessels.
- Fistula means *'flute' or 'a pipe or tube'.*
- *Causes: Congenital* like branchial fistula, tracheoesophageal fistula, congenital arteriovenous fistula, umbilical fistula (patent vitellointestinal duct). A*cquired* due to – (1) Trauma (example – abdomen) accidental/operative (post operative) like urinary, biliary, fecal, appendicular, pancreatic, salivary, rectal fistulas; (2) Instrumental (during delivery); (3) Inflammatory (intestinal tuberculosis/actinomycosis); (4) Neoplastic like advanced carcinoma rectum with rectovesical fistula, carcinoma cervix with uterovesical fistula, external fistula with infiltration into abdominal wall, etc.
- Fistula can be *external fistula* like orocutaneous; branchial fistula; thyroglossal fistula; enterocutaneous fistula; appendicular fistula, vesicovaginal fistula or can be *internal fistula* like tracheoesophageal fistula; cholecystoduodenal fistula; colovesical fistula; rectovesical fistula (Figs. 5-5 and 5-6).

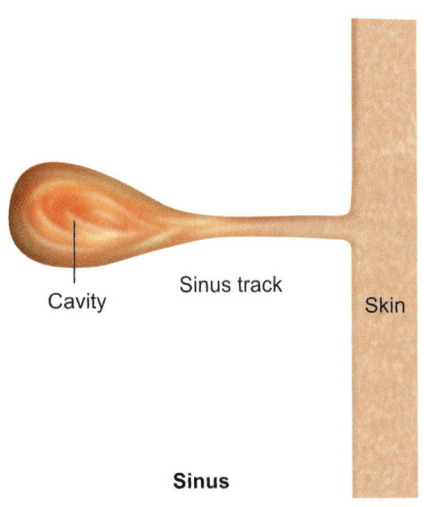

Fig. 5-1 Diagrammatic representation of *sinus.*

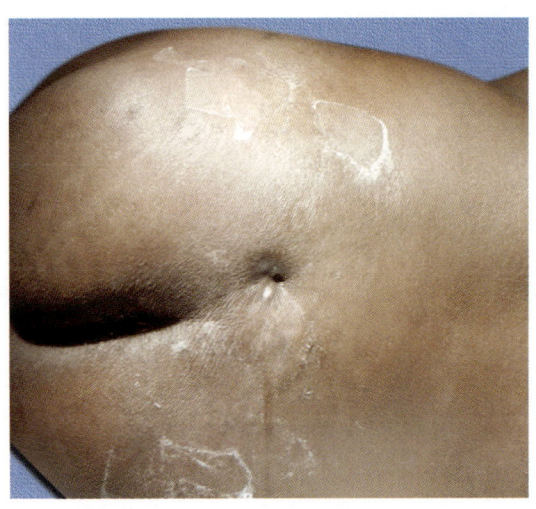

Fig. 5-2 *Sinus* in buttock region.

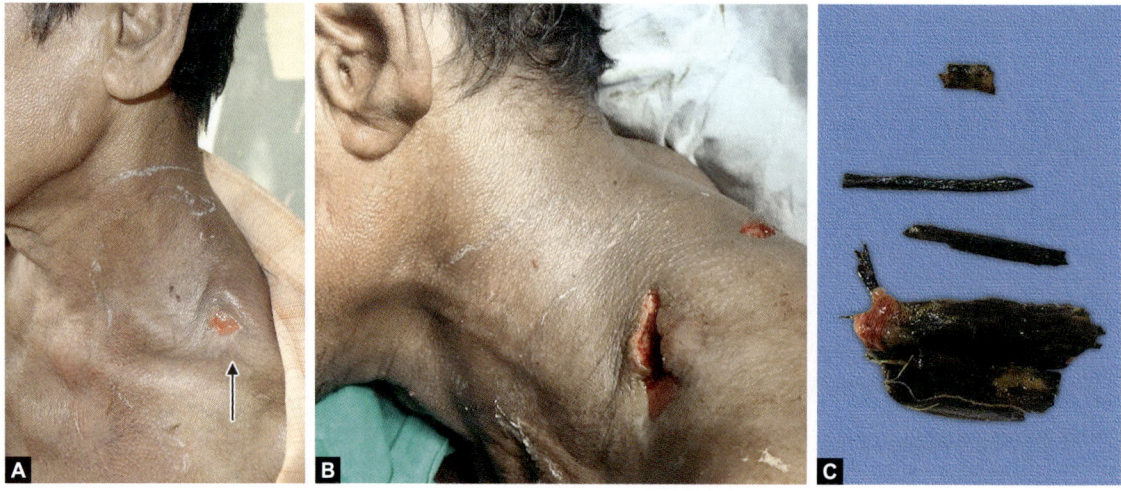

Figs. 5-3A to C *Foreign body neck causing discharging sinus*; after exploration wooden pieces are retrieved from the neck.

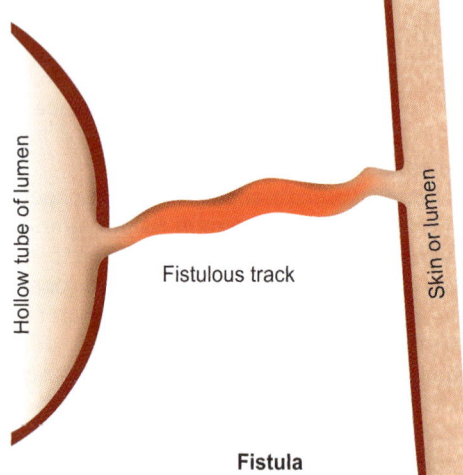

Fig. 5-4 Diagrammatic representation of fistula.

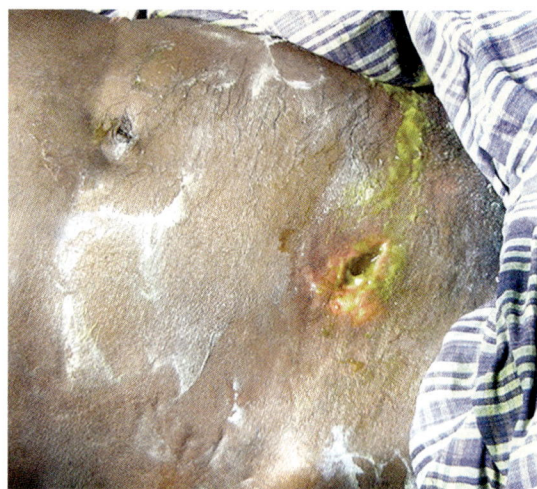

Fig. 5-6 Postoperative gastrointestinal fistula. *Note the skin excoriation.* It can be controlled by local application of zinc oxide cream.

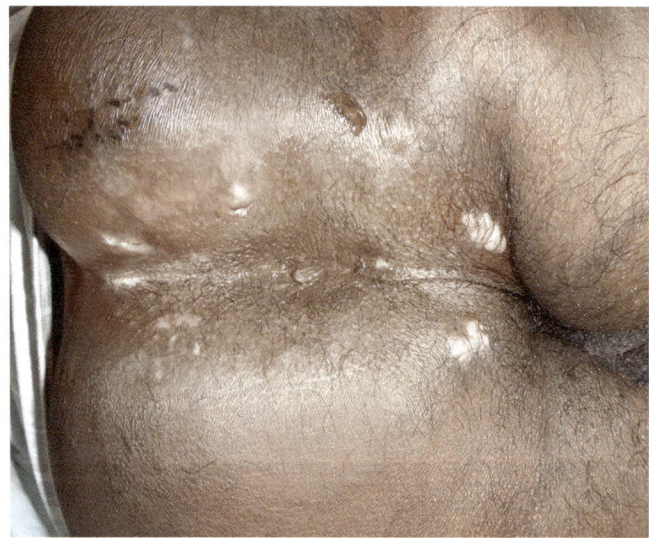

Fig. 5-5 *Fistula-in-ano*—multiple external openings on both sides.

Classification of fistula
- ***Based on number***: It may be single or multiple.
- ***Based on type***: Simple with direct track or complicated with track having variable course.
- ***Based on opening***: Lateral fistula if fistula opening is from lateral aspect of the hollow viscus; end fistula if end of the viscus opens as fistula.
- ***Based on involvement of tissues***: From viscus to skin is external; from viscus to viscus is internal.
- ***Based on output***: High output >500 mL/day; moderate 200–500 mL/day; low output <200 mL/day. In pancreatic fistula high output is >200 mL/day; low output is <200 mL/day.

CLINICAL FEATURES OF SINUS/FISTULA

Discharge from the opening of sinus/fistula—pus, caseating material, bone spicules, sulfur granules depending on the etiology; *no floor*; edge raised and often indurated; indurated base; nonmobile; often *sprouting granulation tissue over the sinus opening* (Fig. 5-7).

Chapter 5: Examination and Clinical Approach of Sinus and Fistula

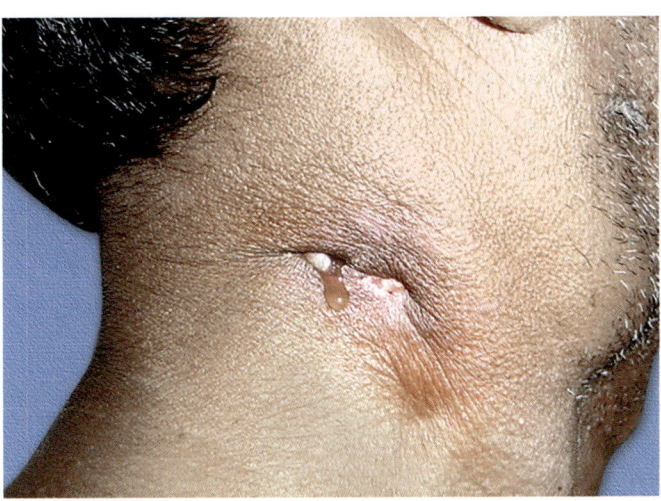

Fig. 5-7 *Secondaries in neck* causing discharging sinus.

Causes of persistence of a sinus or fistula
- Insufficient or nondependent drainage
- Presence of foreign body (wood/metal piece, suture), sequestrum, maggots within the necrotic tissue underneath
- Persistent obstruction in the lumen of viscus or tube distal to fistula, e.g. in fecal fistula, biliary fistulas (distal obstruction)
- Lack of rest
- Walls become lined with epithelium or endothelium
- Dense fibrosis prevents contraction and healing
- Specific infections like tuberculosis, actinomycosis, syphilis
- Presence of malignant disease
- Post surgery due to infected stitch in subcutaneous plane or in deeper plane is not uncommon
- Debilitating diseases like anemia, hypoproteinemia, diabetes mellitus, previous irradiation

HISTORY

Name:

Sex: Pilonidal sinus is common in males.

Age: Certain sinus or fistulas are more common in certain age groups. Pilonidal sinus, branchial fistulas are common in younger age group.

Occupation: Pilonidal sinus in buttock region is common in jeep drivers whereas interdigital pilonidal sinus is common in barbers.

Place:

Chief complaints: History of discharge and its duration should be mentioned. History of specific related condition also should be mentioned.

History of Present Illness

Situation

Exact site where the sinus/fistula has started should be asked. A single sinus in pulp of the finger due to pulp space infection with osteomyelitis of the distal phalanx is called as ***Klap sign***.

Mode of Onset and Progression

- Relevant history regarding how exactly sinus has started and progressed whether present since birth, or it was healing in between and recurring again should be asked for.
- History of trauma should be asked as osteomyelitis can occur after traumatic fracture.
- Detailed history about events happened prior to formation of sinus like swelling, pain, fever, deformity, difficulty in walking, etc. should be asked.
- History of discharging ***bone pieces/spicules*** after an initial episode of fever, pain, swelling in the bone, formation of abscess, localization, giving way through the skin and causing sinus later with bony piece discharge is a feature of ***chronic osteomyelitis***. Bone piece getting discharged is called as sequestrum which is dead bone in situ.
- Often patient gives the history of lymph nodes in the neck which later enlarges forming a soft localized painless swelling called cold abscess; which eventually bursts through the deep fascia to get adherent to the skin forming collar stud abscess; skin gives way causing tuberculous sinus with yellowish caseating material as discharge **(Fig. 5-8)**.
- There may be history suggestive of abdominal surgery like gastrectomy, resections, biliary surgeries followed by discharge from fistula which may progress or regress spontaneously **(Fig. 5-9)**.

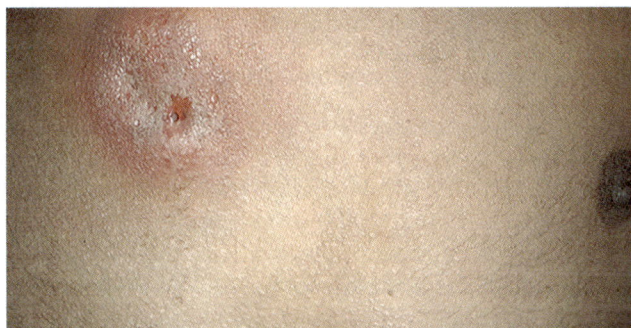

Fig. 5-8 *Tuberculous sinus* over chest wall showing discharge.

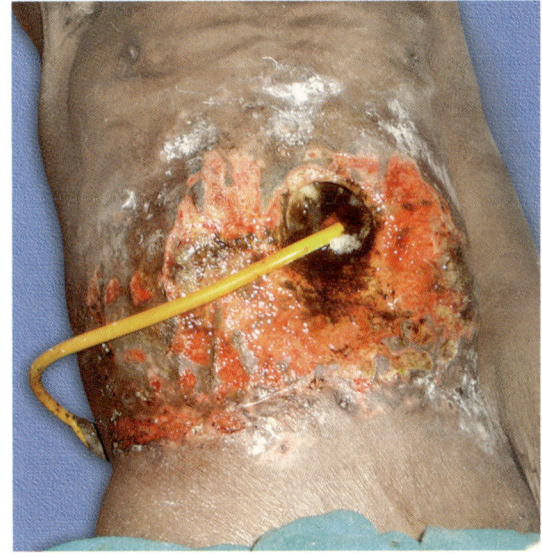

Fig. 5-9 Gastric fistula at gastrostomy site. *One should observe the severe excoriations.*

History of Discharge

- **History of discharge is important** in sinus or fistula. Features of discharge—quantity; quality; duration; color; smell, should be asked. Discharge may be purulent, yellowish/caseous-like in tuberculosis; with bone spicules in chronic osteomyelitis; with necrotic material, bile/feces/saliva/urine in different internal fistulas; sulfur granules in actinomycosis; mucus in branchial fistula, etc. Quantity of discharge, variations at different time, relation to food intake should be clarified. Color may be black, red, yellow green; smell—foul smelling in fecal fistula **(Figs. 5-9 and 5-14)**.
- Discharge may be pus, bile, fecal, urine, serous, cheesy depending on the etiology. Cheesy is seen in tuberculosis; bloody is often seen in malignant sinus or fistula; purulent in bacterial infection and if so its smell, color, quantity should be noted.

History of Pain

History of pain suggests inflammation/blockage/pus formation. Sinus or fistula is usually painless unless it is infected or blocked making pus to accumulate causing throbbing pain or if suffering from malignancy.

History of Fever

History of fever suggests acute/recurrent inflammation.

History Related to Associated Diseases

History related to associated diseases like of bowel disease, tuberculosis, ulcerative colitis, previous surgery, malignancy, etc. should be asked. **Whether patient has earlier undergone surgery** like hysterectomy, bowel resection with details of surgery—when it was done, immediate postoperative problem, sepsis after surgery, recovery, how long after surgery discharge or present symptom appeared. Vesicovaginal fistula may develop after hysterectomy. Fecal fistula may develop due to anastomotic leak after emergency resection and anastomosis for intestinal gangrene.

Past History

- Past history of tuberculosis, Crohn's disease, actinomycosis, diabetes, neurological disorder, surgery for fistula-in-ano, etc. should be asked for.
- Past history of draining perianal abscess may be a cause for fistula-in-ano or treating urethral stricture earlier (urethral stricture may cause urethral fistula). Recurrence of pilonidal sinus or fistula-in-ano is common (30–40%).
- Earlier laparotomy or appendectomy may be the cause for abdominal fistula; type of surgery earlier diagnosis, post operative status should be asked for in detail.
- Previous history of mesh repair and if mesh got infected can cause sinus.

Personal History

History of alcohol consumption/smoking/tobacco chewing/history of sexual contact/dietary habits are also important.

Altered appetite or weight loss can also be mentioned under personal history—may be due to advanced malignancy or tuberculosis.

Family History

Family history of any specific diseases should be asked. Family history of tuberculosis, Crohn's disease, ulcerative colitis, fistula-in-ano can occur in family members.

■ GENERAL EXAMINATION

Detailed general examination is very essential. Anemia/edema/jaundice/clubbing/lymphadenopathy are looked for. Radial pulse/blood pressure/rise in temperature are recorded. Attitude of the patient/nutritional assessment by skin texture, subcutaneous fat, weight, body mass index/any other relevant findings should be mentioned. Increased pulse rate and temperature suggest ulcer with acute inflammation. Features suggestive of tuberculosis, spinal disease, abdominal conditions or chest disease should be looked for.

■ LOCAL EXAMINATION

Inspection

Site of Sinus or Fistula

Preauricular sinus is located in the tragus of ear or root of helix. It is directed upwards and backwards. This occurs due to failure of fusion of ear tubercles. *Branchial fistula* resulting from defective fusion of 1st and 2nd branchial arches occurs in the lower third of the neck along the anterior border of sternomastoid. *Pilonidal sinus* occurs in sacral region. *Tuberculous sinus* is common in neck but can occur in axilla, groin, etc. **(Figs. 5-10 and 5-11)**.

> **Typical sites of sinus/fistula:**
> Preauricular sinus---------------tragus or root of helix.
> Branchial fistula---------------anterior border of sternomastoid in lower 1/3rd
> Thyroglossal fistula---------------midline of neck below hyoid bone
> Mental sinus---------------symphysis menti
> Parotid fistula---------------parotid region
> Pilonidal sinus---------------sacrococcygeal region; interdigital
> Lymphogranuloma venereum---------------groin
> Osteomyelitis---------------over the end of long bone
> Hidradenitis suppurativa---------------axilla often bilateral
> Tuberculous sinus---------------neck, chest wall, limbs and abdomen depends on primary disease
> Appendicular fistula---------------right iliac fossa

Number

- Usually fistulae/sinuses are single (parotid, biliary). Branchial fistula is often on one side of the neck and thyroglossal fistulae are usually single. *Chronic osteomyelitis* of distal phalanx usually causes single discharging sinus *(Klap sign)*; in other bones, it can have single or more often multiple discharging sinuses.
- In actinomycosis, tuberculosis, Madura foot, anal fistula due to Crohn's disease and *watering can perineum* (seen

Chapter 5: Examination and Clinical Approach of Sinus and Fistula

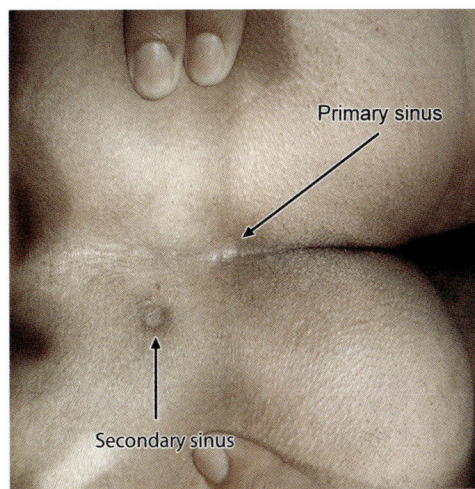

Fig. 5-10 Pilonidal sinus in sacral cleft. *Both primary and secondary sinuses are seen.*

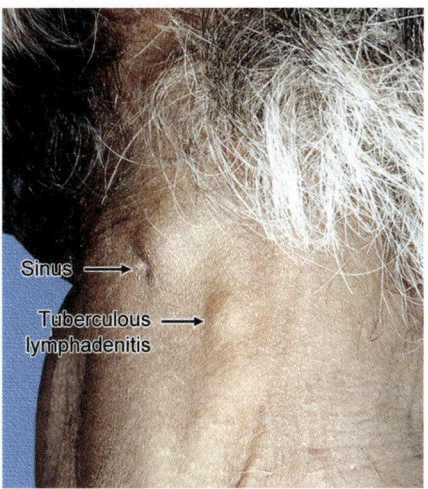

Fig. 5-12 *Tuberculous sinus in the neck with discharge; note enlarged lymph node in the neck due to tuberculosis.*

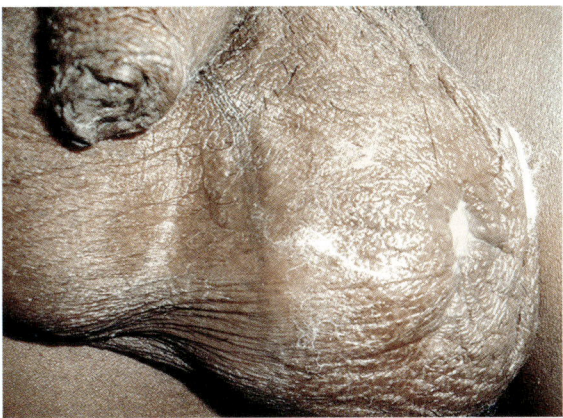

Fig. 5-11 Sinus on the scrotum could be tuberculous or syphilis or other infective focus in the testis or postsurgical cause. *Tuberculosis commonly involves epididymis causing tuberculous epididymitis forming sinus on the posterior aspect. Syphilis involves commonly testis causing syphilitic orchitis forming ulcer/sinus on the anterior aspect.*

in gonococcal urethral stricture with fistula commonly) sinuses, are multiple.
- Hidradenitis suppurativa often is bilateral presents with multiple discharging sinuses which is due to infection of apocrine sweat glands.

Size and Appearance of External Opening

- *Size* of the opening is small with sprouting granulation tissue which indicates the possible presence of foreign body in the depth. *Sequestrum* or foreign body may extrude from the sinus.
- *Margin* is usually raised. In tuberculosis, opening may be wide and its margin is undermined, thin and blue.
- Sinus does not have floor **(Fig. 5-12)**.

Discharge

Discharge should be inspected for color, type (bile, fecal, serous), odor, quantity.

Different discharges in a sinus/fistula: Purulent—bacterial infection; *creamy yellow*—Staphylococcal; *watery opalescent*—Streptococcal; *greenish*—pseudomonas; *caseous*—tuberculous sinus; yellow *sulfur granules*—actinomycosis; red or black granules—Madura foot; *mucus*—branchial fistula; *saliva*—parotid fistula; *feces*—fecal fistula; *bile*—biliary, duodenal fistula; *bone chips*—osteomyelitis sinus; *anchovy sauce*-like pus discharge—amebiasis cutis from amebic liver abscess.

Odor of the discharge is also significant—smell of gas gangrene discharge is sickly-*sweet odor (decayed apple)*; *Bacillus coli* infection in an abdominal wall sinus—objectionable odor; *Escherichia coli* discharge—odorless; *Proteus vulgaris*—proteolytic odor; bacteroides infection in abdominal wall sinus—*over ripe Camembert cheese* odor; fecal odor with bubbles of gas in fecal fistula.

Surrounding Skin

- The surrounding skin may show excoriation in case of biliary fistula due to increased alkalinity of the discharge. Excoriation of skin can also occur in intestinal or fecal fistulas.
- Surrounding skin should be inspected for scar/color/texture/dilated or visible veins/hair loss/pigmentation/dermatitis, etc.
- Surrounding area is red and oedematous in inflammatory conditions; bluish in tuberculous sinus; excoriated in fecal fistula; pigmented in chronic sinuses.

Palpation

Tenderness and local rise in temperature over surrounding area.

Discharge: Apply pressure over the surrounding area to note the type of discharge.

Sinus wall/margin should be palpated for induration or thickening. Chronic long-standing sinuses due to fibrosis will have thick wall.

Mobility of sinus/fistula: Most of the sinuses/fistulae are from deeper plane; Hence, are fixed and nonmobile. Occasionally, superficial sinus when exists, may be mobile.

Palpate for underneath swelling which may be lymph nodes and detailed description of such swelling should be mentioned. Swelling in surrounding area should be looked for. It may be lymph nodal mass as in tuberculosis or malignant mass. Mandibular sinus should be palpated for fixity, mandibular thickening due to osteomyelitis. Tooth/teeth underneath adjacent alveolus should be examined infection of which may be the cause for osteomyelitis (**Figs. 5-13 and 5-15**).

Surrounding skin, tissue and adjacent bone should be palpated for bone thickening (in chronic osteomyelitis), induration, etc. Tuberculous osteomyelitis does not show bone thickening as there is very less new bone formation.

Regional lymph node examination: In tuberculosis, infection and malignancy, regional nodes may be palpable with

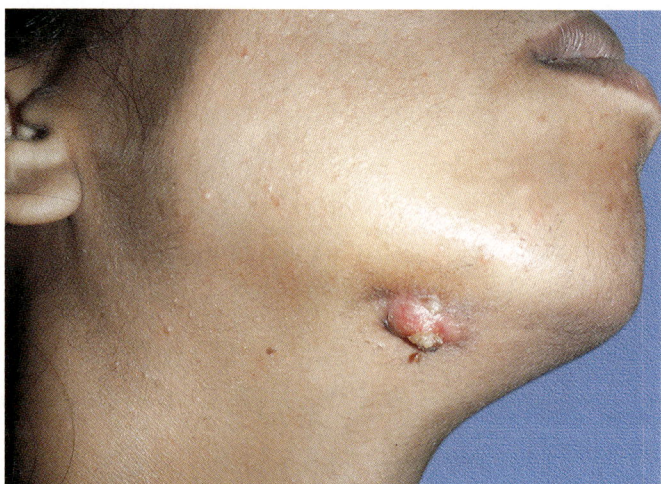

Fig. 5-15 Discharging sinus with granulation tissue. It is due to underlying tooth infection.

different consistency like matted in tuberculosis; hard in malignancy.

Relevant systemic examination should be done: Examination *of respiratory system* is done in case of chest wall sinus. *Thoracic and lumbar spine* examination is done in case of psoas abscess, paraspinal abscess; *urinary system* examination in case of urinary fistula, loin abscess; *Skeletal system* examination in case of osteomyelitis; *Digital examination* of rectum in case of fistula-in-ano; *Vaginal examination* in case vesicovaginal fistula; *adjacent joint* examination like that of hip joint in groin abscess.

Examination using a probe (Probe test): Ideally probe examination of sinus or fistula should be done under general anesthesia with all aseptic precautions and with gentleness. Malleable, blunt metal probe is used for probing the fistula. During probing following points should be looked for—direction, depth and length of the sinus, presence of foreign body, communication to hollow viscus in the depth (free mobility of the passed probe), fresh discharge while removing the probe.

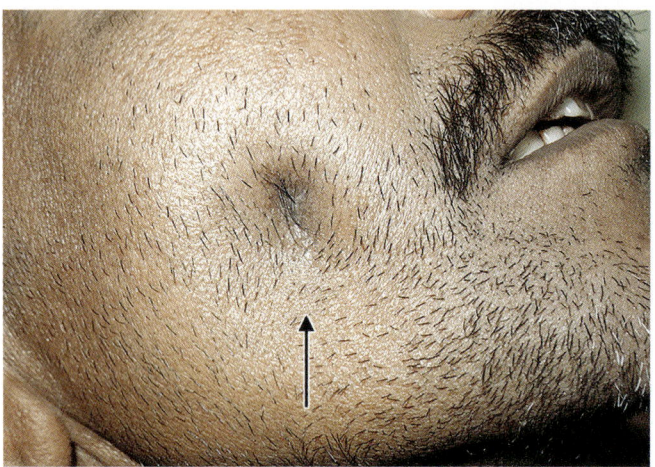

Fig. 5-13 Discharging sinus in the face over the mandible; *could be due to underlying osteomyelitis of the mandible*. It could be due infection of the tooth/trauma/tuberculosis/malignancy or radiation.

▮ INVESTIGATIONS

Fistulogram/sinusogram using ultrafluid lipiodol or water soluble iodine dye injected into the sinus/fistula to know the depth, direction, communication. (lipiodol is poppy seed oil containing 40% iodine);

Very essential and simple is examination of discharge for C/S, AFB, cytology, staining (*gross/physical/chemical/microscopic/staining/culture*);

Biopsy from the edge or entire fistula or sinus tract is excised and sent for biopsy.

Chest X-ray or relevant X-ray of the part like bone/joint to see osteomyelitis or tuberculosis or foreign body (Fig. 5-16). ESR—increases in tuberculosis.

Plain X-ray abdomen or KUB to rule out stone in the urinary tract, foreign body.

CT sinusogram is very useful;

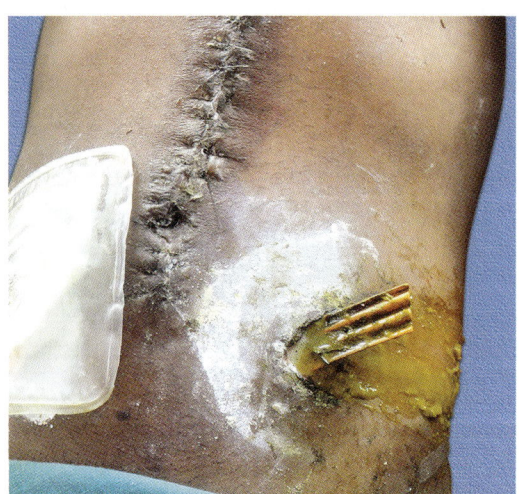

Fig. 5-14 Fecal fistula through drain site after laparotomy; patient has undergone colonic resection and anastomosis.

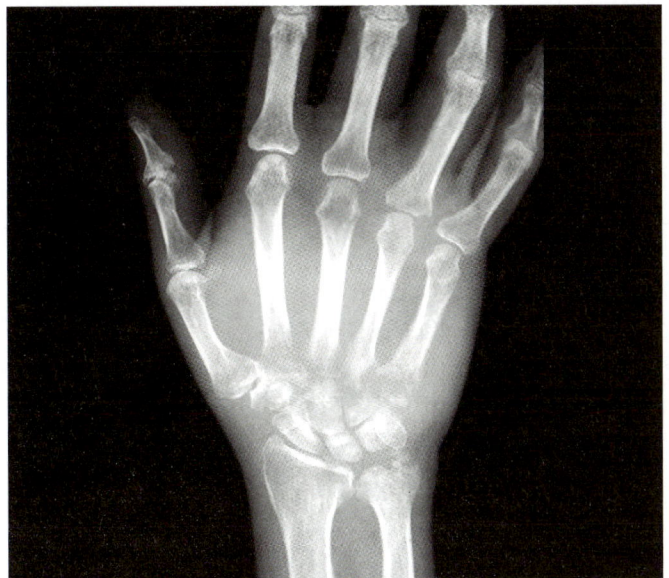

Fig. 5-16 *Osteomyelitis of the carpal bones* presented as discharging sinus.

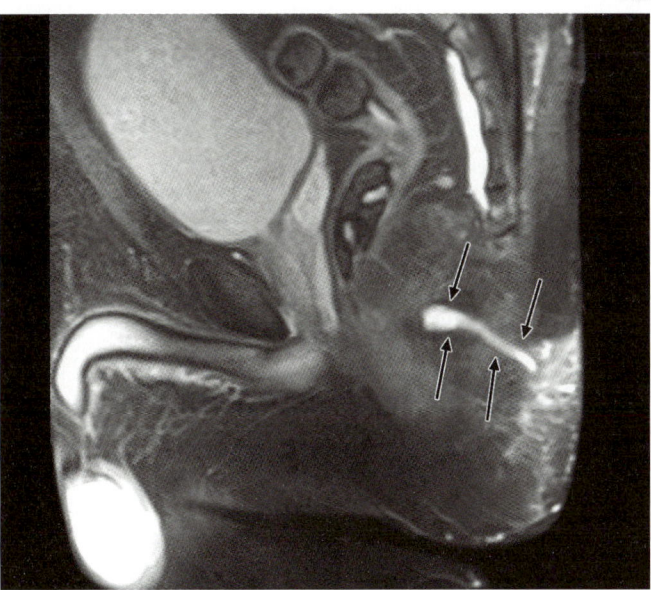

Fig. 5-17 *MR fistulogram* (MRI) showing intersphincteric fistula-in-ano.

MRI is most reliable in assessing *the track anatomy* (Fig. 5-17).

Three swab test in vesicovaginal fistula (vagina is packed with three swab, first swab high up in the anterior fornix, second one at middle of vagina, third one at lower part of vagina and 10 cc sterile methylene blue is infused into the bladder. Patient is asked to walk for 5 minutes and staining of the swab is looked for. Staining of topmost swab suggests vesicovaginal fistula or vesicocervicovaginal fistula, middle one suggests vesicovaginal fistula and lower one urethrovaginal fistula or urethral incontinence. Wetting but no staining of top most swabs suggests ureterovaginal fistula).

Contrast GI study; pyridium intake orally and looking for its excretion as colored urine helps to confirm urinary fistulae.

- Proctoscopy—to visualize the opening of anal fistula
- Cystoscopy—to visualize vesicovaginal fistula (VVF)
- Percutaneous T-tube choledochoscopy—for biliary fistulae
- Barium meal/enema contract CT scan for fecal fistula
- MRI is ideal for fistula-in-ano

Case sheet writing in a patient with Sinus/fistula

History
Name: Age:
Occupation: Sex: Place/residence:

Chief complaints

History of present illness
- Situation/location
- Mode of onset and progression
- Discharge – duration, type of discharge, color of discharge, smell
- Pain – origin, nature, character, duration, time of starting of pain, specific features, severity, aggravating or relieving factors
- Fever – type, severity, duration
- History swelling underneath – when started, progress
- History related to associated diseases like tuberculosis, malignancy
- Loss of weight, reduced appetite
- Pressure symptoms

Past history
- Past history of sinus and treatment for that
- Past history of trauma
- Tuberculosis, spinal diseases, diabetes, leprosy, malignancies
- Past history of surgery like laparotomy and details

Family history
- Family tree; history of tuberculosis, diabetes, malignancies; treatment history

General examination
Anemia, edema, jaundice, clubbing, lymphadenopathy, pulse, blood pressure, temperature, attitude, nutrition, body weight.

Contd...

Contd...

Local examination
Inspection
- Site of sinus or fistula – location, size, shape, extent, color, surface, number, edge/margin/border
- Discharge – type, color, odor, foreign body, bone, etc.
- Surrounding skin

Palpation
- Local raise of temperature, tenderness
- Discharge while palpation
- Sinus wall and margin
- Mobility, fixity of the sinus
- Area underneath the sinus for swelling or palpation of tissues or bone underneath for induration or thickening
- Palpation of surrounding skin for induration, warmness, swelling, edema
- Examination of regional neurological and vascular systems

Percussion if sinus is in chest and abdomen
Auscultation
Movements of adjacent joints if sinus in the limb
Measurements of limb girth and length
Gait
Examination of regional lymph nodes
Examination of sinus using a probe
Systemic examination – abdomen, respiratory, cardiac and central nervous systems

Condition	Pathology and types	Features
Preauricular sinus It is congenital condition occurring in relation to ear, usually in front due to developmental defect of 1st and 2nd branchial arches	• 1st and 2nd branchial arches give rise to 6 tubercles (Hillocks of His; three from each arch). Incomplete fusion of these tubercles leads into preauricular sinus • Sinus connects to the auricular cartilage; but not to the external auditory meatus	Sinus is usually located in front of ear; 25% of patients it is bilateral; sinus, dimple, nodule or cyst in front of the ear may be the presentation; recurrent discharge with scarring is not uncommon
Median mental sinus Chronic infective condition presenting as discharging sinus in the lower jaw in the midline	Root infection of one or more incisor teeth form root abscess that eventually tracks down between two halves of mandible to present as sinus in midline	• Discharging sinus in midline on the point of chin • Incisor infection may or may not be evident • *Differential diagnosis*: Infected sebaceous cyst; tuberculous sinus, osteomyelitis • *Complication*: Osteomyelitis of mandible
Actinomycosis Caused by *Actinomyces Israeli*. • It causes subacute inflammation in the tissues forming induration and nodule formation. This eventually softens, bursts through the skin forming discharging sinus • Pus collected will show yellowish sulphur granules • Pus under microscopy shows branching filaments • Gram staining show gram positive mycelia in center gram negative radiating peripheral filaments – **Ray fungus**	**Clinical types** 1. **Faciocervical**—infection from tonsil or from adjacent infected tooth 2. **Thorax**—lungs and pleura infected by direct spread from pharynx or by aspiration 3. **Abdominal**—ileo-cecal, hepatic	• Diffuse swelling in the lower jaw with multiple sinuses on skin of face and neck discharging pus containing yellowish sulphur granules. Lymph nodes enlarged due to secondary infection • Empyema develops initially, nodules appear later leading to multiple discharging sinuses in the chest wall • Can spread through the diaphragm to liver and subphrenic space • Present as mass abdomen in right iliac fossa with discharging sinuses • Liver infected through portal vein, parenchyma destroyed with multiple abscesses containing sulphur granules
Madura foot (Mycetoma pedis) Chronic granulomatous condition of the foot causing multiple discharging sinuses in the foot **(Figs. 5-18A and B)** Infection in hand—**Madura hand** **Causative organisms**: *Nocardia madurae* (commonest), *Nocardia brasiliensis, Nocardia asteroids, Madurella mycetoma* Common in India, Africa; Common in Tamil Nadu	• Seen in bare foot walkers; Organism enter through a prick in foot evoking chronic granulomatous inflammation, nodule- vesicle formation, burst to form discharging sinuses • Pus contains black, red, yellow granules • Muscles and bones are involved but tendons and nerves are usually spared	• Painless diffuse swelling, of long duration • Multiple-discharging sinuses with serosanguinous purulent granular discharge • Thickening, pigmentation of skin which is fixed to underlying tissues • Lymph nodes enlarge when secondarily infected • Significant limb disability **Investigations**: Discharge study, Gram stain, X-ray foot, and biopsy. MRI is typical
Tuberculous sinus	Tuberculosis in lymph nodes, ribs, spine are the common sites but lungs, other solid organs like kidneys can be foci	• It is common cause of sinus • Yellowish discharge often with cheesy caseation; bluish undermined edge

Contd...

Contd...

Condition	Pathology and types	Features
		without induration is typical; constitutional symptoms with features of underlying involved organ like lymph nodes, ribs or spine or lungs, etc
Chronic osteomyelitis It is one of the common causes of discharging sinus especially in young individuals	It is common in metaphysic of long bones, but other flat bones, jaw bones are also can get involved. Initial bacterial infection leads into acute phase which eventually leads into chronic osteomyelitis with sinus **(Fig. 5-20)**	• History of fever, bone pain; later swelling and sinus formation leading into discharging bony spicules through the sinus with sprouting granulation tissue; thickening is evident due to new bone formation • Sequestrum of different causes has got typical features • Chronic pain, discomfort, deformity are also common

Sequestrum

- A sequestrum is a dead bone that has separated completely from the adjacent normal bone by necrosis (Figs. 5-19A and B).
- Sequestrum is dead bone in situ.
- It can be pyogenic, tubercular (feathery), salmonella (granular), syphilitic (ivory) in origin; tubular and ring (in amputation stump) type.
- It can be *unformed*—means separation between sequestrum and adjacent normal bone has not occurred or *formed*—means there is proper adequate separation between normal bone and sequestrum by forming granulation tissue.
- Radiologically formed sequestrum shows clear lucent area/zone of demarcation. Sequestrum is denser because of the absence of decalcification in the dead bone as there is no blood supply (dead bone is dense bone).
- Sequestrum should be formed prior to surgical intervention—sequestrectomy and saucerization.

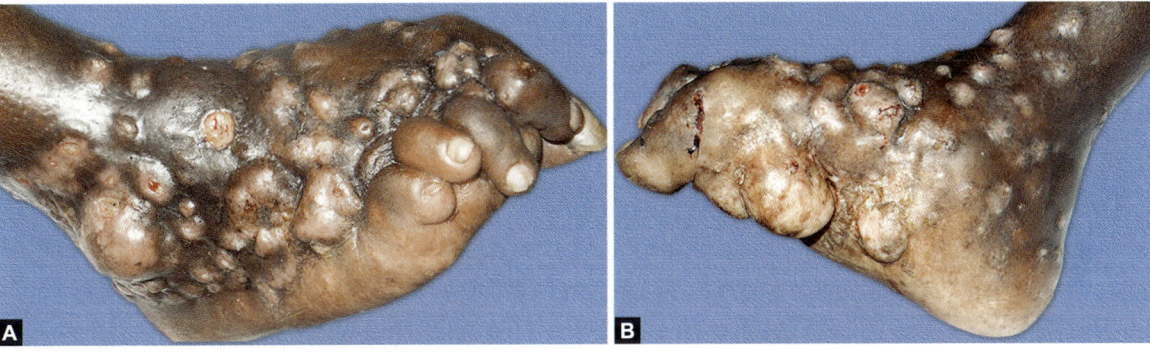

Figs. 5-18A and B Madura foot. Note the *multiple discharging sinuses*

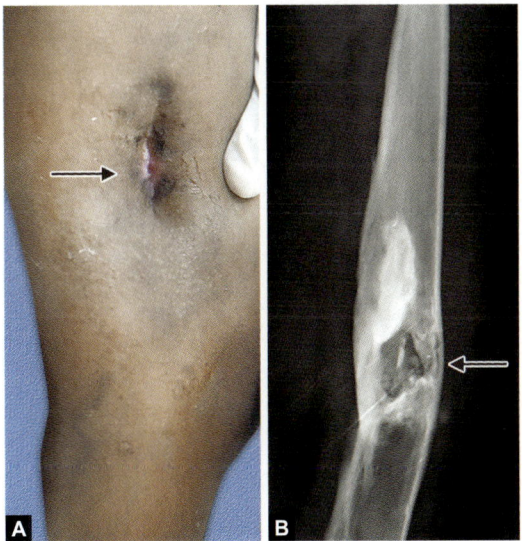

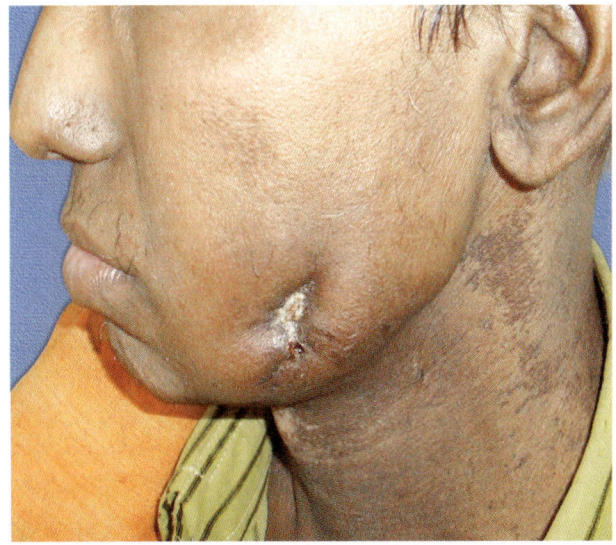

Figs. 5-19A and B Chronic osteomyelitis of femur (thigh); *note the discharging sinus*; X-ray shows *sequestrum* (Latin – to lay aside), new bone formation (*involucrum*).

Fig. 5-20 Discharging sinus from the mandible. It is due to chronic osteomyelitis of the mandible after undergoing radiotherapy for malignancy.

CASE DISCUSSION

A 40-year male comes with history of discharging sinuses in the right foot of one year duration. It started insidiously, slowly progressed. Discharge is purulent and often foul smelled. No history of trauma, no history of cough, hemoptysis, abdominal pain, fever or past history of tuberculosis.

What are your likely differential diagnoses?
Causes are probably tuberculosis, chronic osteomyelitis, Madura mycosis, malignancy (carcinoma).

How will you examine the patient?
After general examination, limb is inspected for number, discharge, location, extent, of the sinuses, size/width of the foot is assessed; foot is compared to opposite side. Warmness, tenderness, surface should be palpated; induration, bone thickening, joint mobility, surrounding area, peripheral pulses (dorsalis pedis, posterior tibial, popliteal) should be checked. Inguinal and external iliac nods should be examined. Gait should be observed. Abdomen for hepatomegaly, respiratory system for tuberculosis should be checked.

How will you analyze the findings?
As there is no visible floor and lesions have restricted mobility with discharge they are sinuses. Type of discharge will give idea about the diagnosis; yellow colored in tuberculosis, bony spicules in chronic osteomyelitis, typical discharge of Madura foot. New bone formation is less in tuberculosis. Inguinal nodes get enlarged in chronic osteomyelitis with recurrent infection, tuberculosis and malignancy. Inguinal nodes are not involved in Madura mycosis unless there is secondary bacterial infection.

How will you evaluate?
X-ray of the part can show bony part and soft tissue shadow and calcification; discharge study (cytology, culture, AFB stain, branching filaments of mycosis); wedge biopsy of the sinus, MRI of the foot, FNAC of the inguinal node; chest X-ray.

6

Examination and Clinical Approach in Arterial Diseases

CHAPTER

Competency: SU27.1; SU27.2; SU27.3; SU27.4; AN20.9.

Arterial diseases are more common in lower limb but occasionally can occur in upper limb. Often both lower and upper limbs may get involved. It is often classified as lower limb ischemia and upper limb ischemia. Irrespective of the locations, detailed examination of both lower and upper limb vessels is required in all patients. Atherosclerosis and thromboangiitis obliterans are two common causes of peripheral arterial occlusive disease which presents with chronic ischemia; both are common causes of limb ischemia and gangrene. Chronic ischemia is a common entity; acute ischemia is a rare one. Acute thrombosis and embolism are common causes of acute ischemia. Raynaud's syndrome, vasculitis of different etiologies, are occasional causes of limb ischemia.

■ HISTORY

Name: **Address:**

Age: Atherosclerosis usually occurs in old age. Diabetes with complications in lower limbs is common in late 5th and 6th decades; mesenteric vascular ischemia occurs in elderly which presents as abdominal angina (pain) with bloody stool; Raynaud's disease is common in 4th decade; TAO is common in 3rd and 4th decades; hereditary cold fingers can occur in children; infants may develop symmetrical digital gangrene. Even though congenital, cervical rib syndrome is seen in middle aged individuals. Vasculitis occurs in younger age group **(Figs. 6-1 and 6-2)**.

Sex: Atherosclerosis can occur in both sexes but more common in males. Thromboangiitis obliterans (Buerger's disease, TAO) occurs in young males. TAO is very rare in females (male to female ratio is 40:1). Cervical rib is more common in females. Raynaud's disease is common in young/middle aged females.

Occupation: People working on vibrating tools/machines are prone to develop Raynaud's syndrome. Thoracic outlet syndrome is more often seen in swimmers, volleyball players, painters and carpenters.

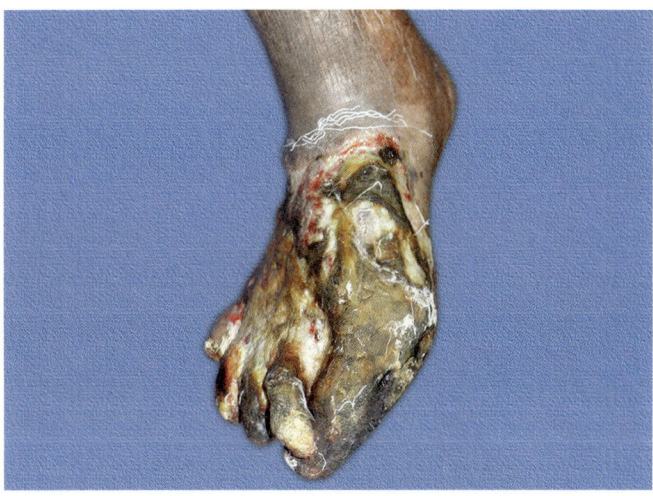

Fig. 6-1 Extensive gangrene foot due to ischemia (*lack of blood supply*). It may be due to atherosclerosis.

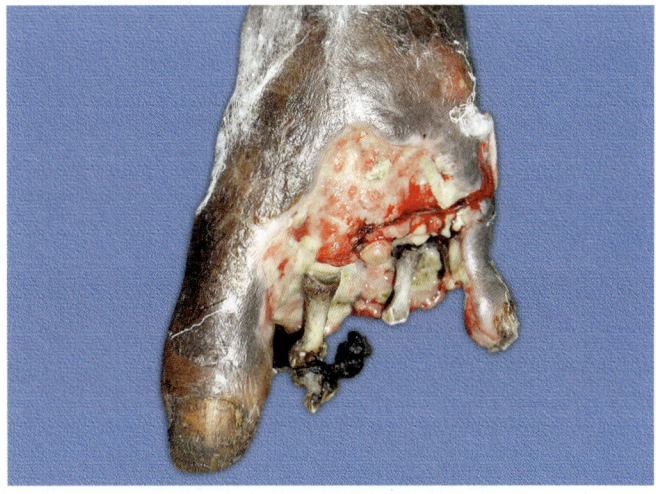

Fig. 6-2 *Severe ischemia* foot with ulceration exposing digital bones.

■CHIEF COMPLAINTS

Pain in the limb right/left/both and its duration.
Intermittent claudication and its duration.
Color change over the skin/ulceration.
Gangrene—blackish discoloration **(Figs. 6-3 and 6-4)**.

History of Present Illness

Pain

- Site of pain, type of pain, whether severe burning, aching or deep persisting type, is asked. History of radiation of pain (along the course of artery) is asked.
- History of **intermittent claudication**, its duration, grade/how much distance patient can walk without pain/whether pain subsides after walking is stopped or after continuous walk/whether patient is able to walk in spite of pain/whether there is any change in the claudication distance/site of claudication—foot/leg/thigh/buttock is asked.
- Presence of **rest pain**—its location/severity/whether the pain gets relieved *slightly* by holding the limb/foot/leg/toes or hanging the leg down or by applying the warmth.

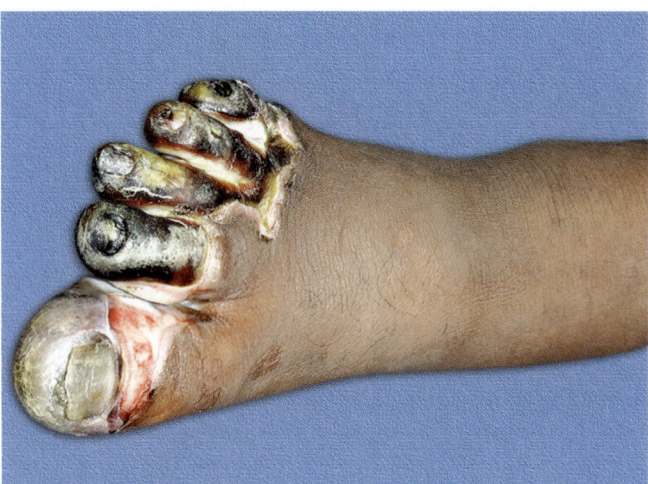

Fig. 6-3 *Gangrene toes* with ischemic changes in the foot.

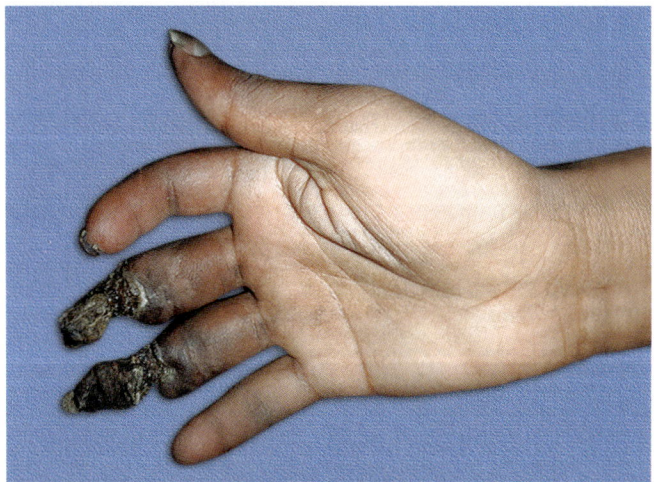

Fig. 6-4 Gangrene of fingers with *ischemic changes in the hand.*

- History of pain, discomfort, color changes when exposed to cold is especially significant in upper limb ischemia. Application of warmth may worsen the arterial occlusion symptoms. Painful part is very sensitive and pain is precipitated/aggravated by any movement/touch or pressure sensation.

Intermittent claudication

- *Claudio means 'I limp' a Latin word*. It is a cramp-like pain in the limb muscles which is ischemic, not felt prior to first step; but develops on exercise or walks and relieved by rest, develops again by similar type of exercise or walk. Due to arterial occlusion, metabolites like lactic acid and substance P accumulate in the muscle and cause pain. It develops only when muscle exercises and subsides by stopping the muscle exercise.

> **Grading of claudicating (Boyd's)**
> **Grade I:** After walk if patient develops claudication pain, which disappears by further walk due to washing of the substance 'P' and other metabolites.
> **Grade II:** Claudication pain persists but patient can still walk with effort.
> **Grade III:** Patient has to take rest compulsorily to relieve claudication pain.
>
> *Note:*
> **Three criteria to diagnose intermittent claudication:**
> 1. *Cramp like pain* in a muscle (e.g. calf muscle)
> 2. Pain develops *only* when muscle is *exercised*
> 3. Pain *disappears* when exercise *stops*

- The site of pain depends on site of arterial occlusion. Commonest site is **calf muscles**.
- It can also occur in the foot, thigh or buttock or forearm or arm. **Claudication distance** is the distance (in meters) walked when cramps develop.
- Pain in foot is due to blockage in lower tibial and plantar vessels. Pain in the calf is due to blockage in femoropopliteal site. Pain in the thigh is due to blockage in the superficial femoral artery. Pain in the buttock is due to blockage in the common iliac or aortoiliac segment often associated with impotence and is called as **Leriche's syndrome**.
- Pain commonly develops when the muscles are exercising. Cause for pain is accumulation of substance 'P' and metabolites. During exercise, increased perfusion and increased opening of collaterals wash away the metabolites. Claudication distance is distance at which claudication appears. It is very essential to assess the distance which is related to the severity of muscle ischemia.
- It is better assessed using a treadmill. Claudication is not so common in upper limb but can occur in muscles of forearm and arm during writing or any upper limb exercise.
- Pain at rest, pain in tissues other than muscles, pain which does not disappear on rest—are not features of intermittent claudication.
- Aortoiliac block causes claudication in buttocks, thighs and calves; absence of femoral and distal pulses bruit over aortoiliac region. Impotence occurs due to defective perfusion through internal iliac arteries and so into the

penis causing erectile dysfunction (Leriche's syndrome). Iliac artery obstruction causes claudication in thigh and calf; bruit over iliac arteries with absence of femoral and distal pulses.
- Femoropopliteal obstruction causes claudication in calf with absence of distal pulses but with palpable femoral. Distal obstruction shows absence of ankle pulses with palpable femoral and popliteal pulses.

Note:
- **Neurogenic claudication** is pain in the leg during walking due to neurological causes. It often mimics vascular claudication but here arterial pulses are normal. It is common in spinal cord stenosis due to narrow canal.
- **Venous claudication** is definitive but a rare entity; and is observed in chronic pelvic venous obstruction as a mechanical high venous pressure probably due to iliac vein thrombosis.

Rest pain
- *Rest pain* is continuous, relentless severe pain even at rest. Patient hangs down his leg to relieve the pain; on elevation of limb, pain increases; pain begins distally first at toes eventually spreads proximally.
- Toes and foot become hypersensitive and elevation, pressure and movements will exacerbate the pain; rest pain worsens at night making the patient sleepless; rest pain may be relieved by hanging the leg down. It is due to ischemic changes in the somatic nerves—*crying of dying nerves*.
- It signifies severe decompensated ischemia.
- Pain is more in the distal part like toes and feet. It gets aggravated with movements and pressure. Hyperesthesia is commonly associated with rest pain.
- Rest pain is more during night time as there is reduced heart rate and blood pressure during night (sleeping time) **(Figs. 6-5 and 6-6)**.

Change in Color

History of change in color of skin on exposure to cold should be asked when Raynaud's syndrome is suspected. Change of color may be in order as blanching and cyanosis producing reddish engorgement.

Raynaud's phenomenon: It has got three stages (1) **Stage of blanching (pallor)** with incapability of finer movements due to vasospasm (local syncope)—part is blanched, white, cold and numb; (2) **Stage of dusky cyanosis** due to accumulation of metabolites in the capillaries causing capillaries to dilate and fill with deoxygenated blood (local asphyxia)—part is cold, blue and numb; (3) **Stage of red engorgement** is due to relaxation of arterioles (relieving of the vasospasm) causing oxygenated blood to return into the dilated capillaries; causing hands to become painful, red with burning sensation; pain is due to increased tissue tension (local recovery). In some patients, occasionally, obliteration of arterioles develop superficial necrosis, ulceration and dry gangrene of digits at their tips (rarely local dry gangrene).

Embolism causes pain, pallor, pulselessness, paresthesia, paralysis, prostration, cold periphery, decreased sweating.

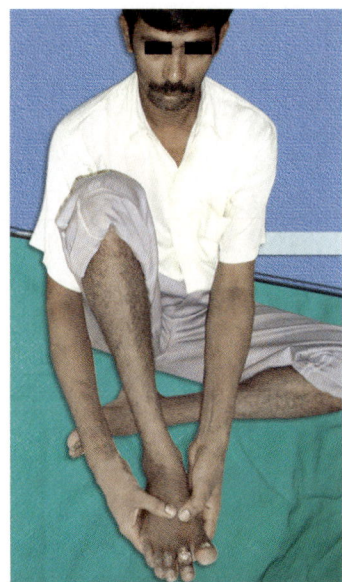

Fig. 6-5 Rest pain in a TAO patient. *Observe the way patient is holding the foot to relieve the pain.*

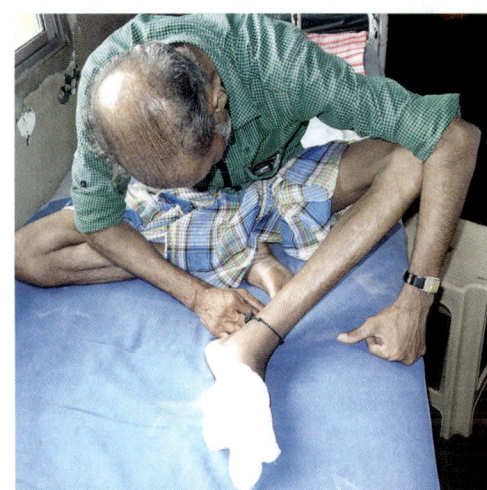

Fig. 6-6 *Typical posture* in a patient with rest pain.

Side of the Symptom or Limb Affected

One should ask which side is the symptom—right or left; one side (unilateral) or both sides (bilateral). If bilateral which side symptoms started first and which side is more severe should be asked. TAO occurs commonly in lower limb. Upper limb is involved following lower limb involvement. Atherosclerosis involves lower limbs. Raynaud's disease occurs in upper limb. TAO and Raynaud's disease are commonly bilateral. Arterial embolism is unilateral causing sudden gangrene. Atherosclerosis is often unilateral to begin with; but eventually becomes bilateral **(Figs. 6-7A and B)**.

Ulceration

Whether spontaneous onset or precipitated by trauma; duration; progression; pain in the ulcer; type; aggravating or relieving factors; type of discharge—serous/purulent/bloody should be asked.

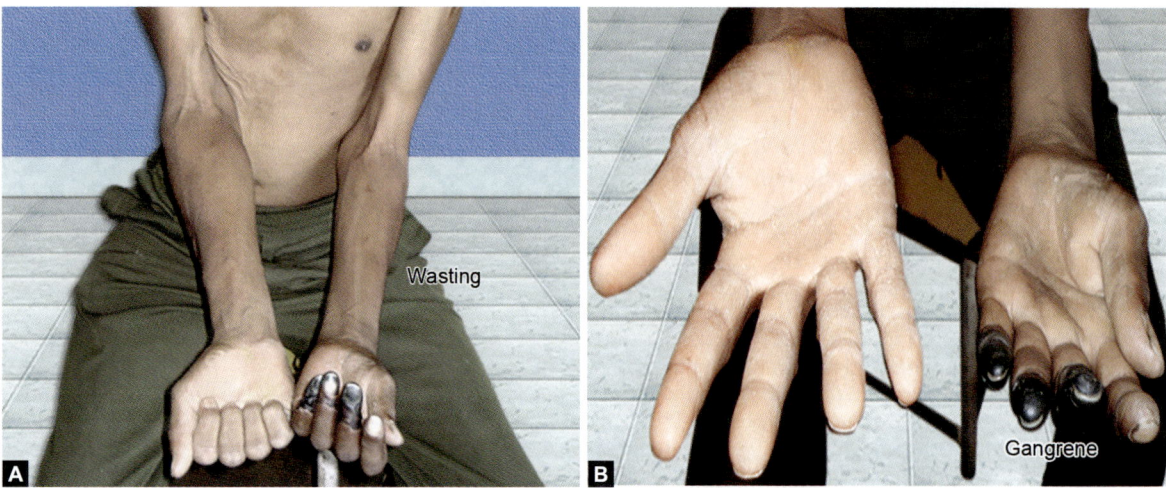

Figs. 6-7A and B Gangrene of left fingers with *ischemic changes* on left side.

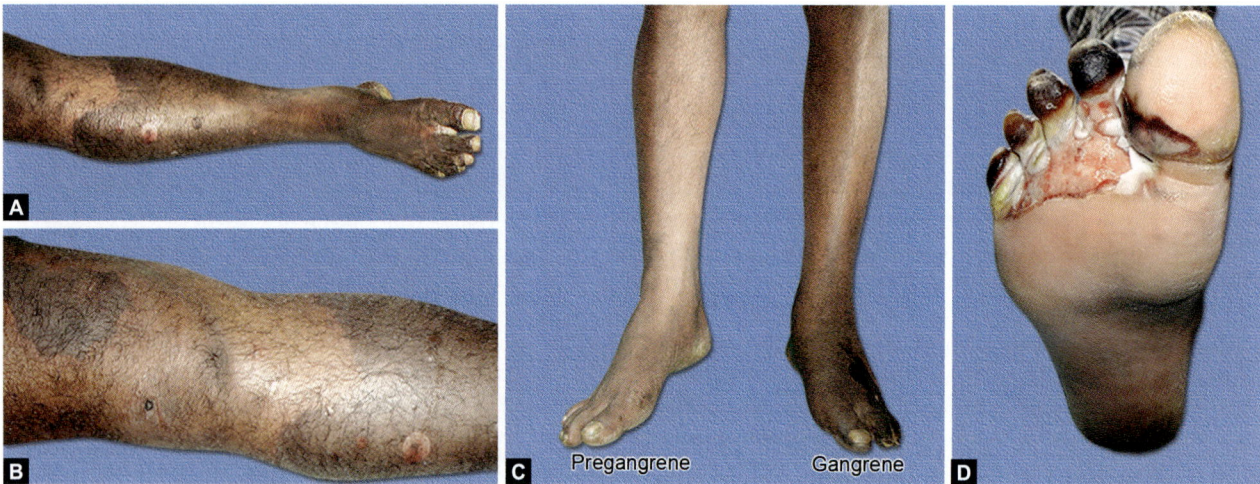

Figs. 6-8A to D Gangrene toes, pregangrenous of some toes, gangrene leg, ischemic changes.
Note: Always inspect the plantar aspect of the foot in all peripheral vascular disease patients.

Gangrene

Site of gangrene; its onset; duration; progression; pain has to be asked. **Gangrene is macroscopic death of tissue *in situ* with putrefaction** (Figs. 6-8A to D).

Mode of Onset

In atherosclerosis/Buerger's disease, process of gangrene is spontaneous and gradual. Gangrene due to embolism is sudden in onset, rapidly progressive with radiating severe pain along the artery.

Duration and Progress

Duration of the disease in the form of pain and ulceration or claudication and duration of appearance of gangrene; whether it is spreading or stationary should be asked for. Time of appearance of the line of demarcation also should be asked. Whether it is progressing rapidly or slowly or intermittently; or disease becomes normal and reappears again like in Raynaud's disease, should be asked. Slow progression means further narrowing of vessels by thrombosis which is important in TAO, intermittent progress is seen in vasospastic conditions, slight remission suggests recanalization of thrombosed arteries as in atherosclerosis. Rapid progression occurs in embolism or sudden narrowing and blockage of the atherosclerotic vessel; remission is also seen in TAO due to opening of the collaterals.

History of Fever

Diabetic gangrene or wet gangrene may be associated with fever due to associated bacteremia or localized suppuration. Often condition may cause septicemia making patients critical mainly in diabetics.

Other Symptoms

History of **cold, paresthesia** in the limb affected.

History of difficulty in walking/altered gait: Duration of such disability and progress; whether it interferes with patient's routine work; whether patient is bedridden due to severe symptoms has to be noted.

History of impotence: Its duration has to be asked [due to bilateral internal iliac artery (aortoiliac) block (*Leriche syndrome*)—pain in buttock, impotence, aortoiliac block]. There is failure of erection.

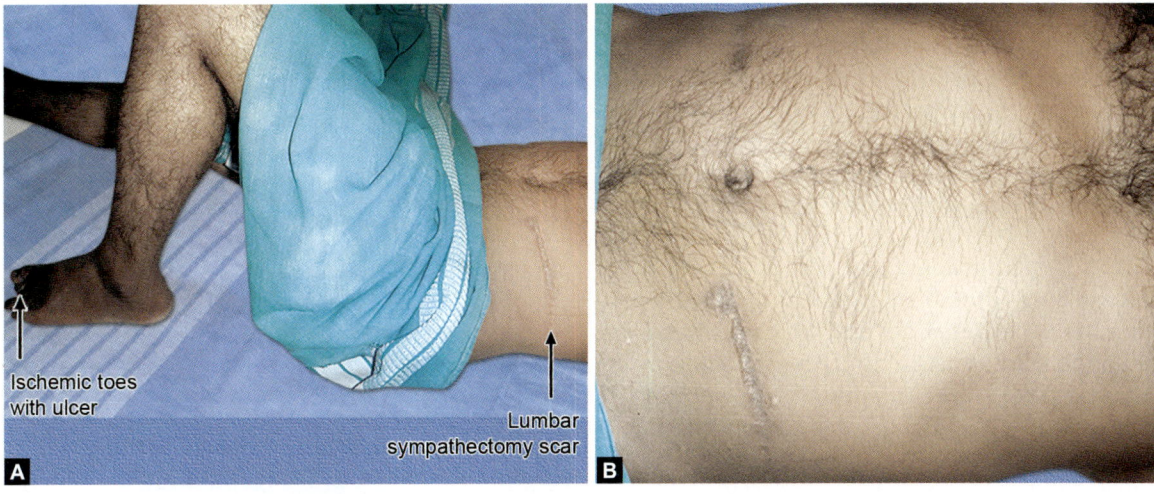

Figs. 6-9A and B *Lumbar sympathectomy scar* with ischemic ulcer foot.

History of tingling/numbness/weakness in the limbs/pins and needles sensation in the skin of foot and leg—*paresthesia* due to shunting of cutaneous blood to deeper muscles.

History suggestive of involvement of other vessels: History of syncope/blackouts/loss of consciousness/blurred vision/transient ischemic attacks/fainting/chest pain/weakness/amaurosis fugax due to *carotid vessel block* (middle cerebral and ophthalmic branches of internal carotid artery); abdominal colic (**post-prandial angina** *due to mesenteric artery block*) with bloody stool or impotence with claudication pain in buttock (**Leriche syndrome**, *involvement of both internal iliac arteries*).

History of chest pain/cough or cardiac related symptoms.

History suggestive of superficial thrombophlebitis like swelling/redness/pain along the line of superficial vein should be asked. It is common in TAO. (There will be cord-like thickening with inflammation and tenderness on the superficial veins).

Past History and Treatment History

History suggestive of similar complaints in the past; history of drug intake earlier for similar conditions like vasodilators/drugs to increase the perfusion; history of surgeries like sympathectomy/omentoplasty in the past; their results or effects are to be noted **(Figs. 6-9 to 6-11)**.

One should enquire about—history of syphilis for endarteritis; history of diabetes for diabetic gangrene along with the nature of treatment for the same; history of repeated superficial phlebitis as in TAO; history of vasospastic attack following exposure to heat or cold; history of exposure to vasospastic drugs (ergot, arsenic, lead, inadvertent injection of thiopentone intra-arterially); history of trauma with injury to vessels; history of rheumatic heart disease in embolism; history of recurrent phlebitis in Buerger's disease; previous history of exposure to corrosives, radiation, electricity, cold, heat; previous history of valve replacement surgeries.

Patient may be taking long acting benzathine penicillin monthly or at regular intervals for mitral stenosis or other

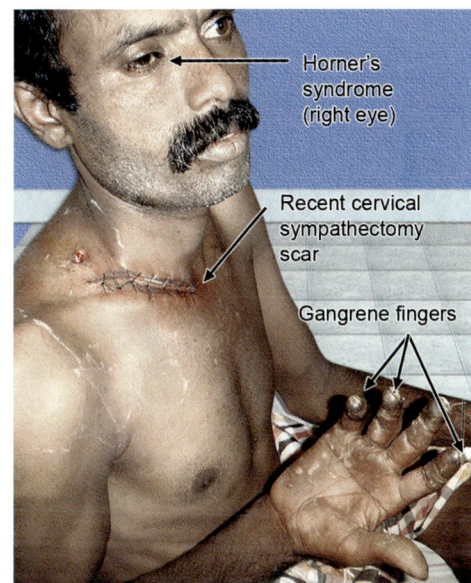

Fig. 6-10 Cervical sympathectomy through neck approach done for gangrene fingers. *One can observe the Horner's syndrome developed due to cervical sympathectomy.*

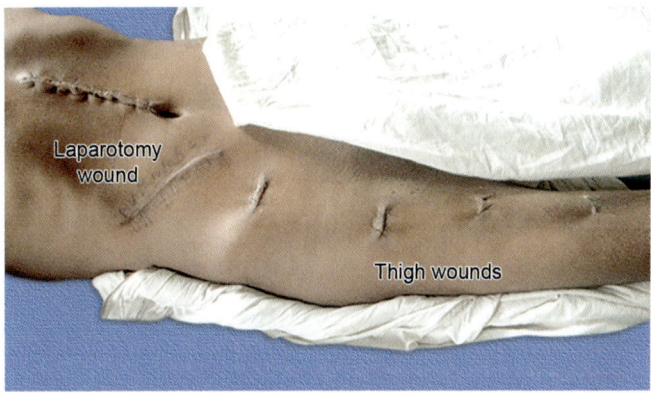

Fig. 6-11 *Patient has undergone omentoplasty recently.* Note the sutured wounds of laparotomy and thigh. Laparotomy is done to harvest the omentum. Mobilized omentum is brought down along the subcutaneous plane towards leg.

valvular disease. Atrial fibrillation in mitral stenosis may precipitate thrombosis in left atrium and subsequent embolism. Common sites of subsequent embolism in this situation are left middle cerebral artery, superficial femoral artery but can occur anywhere in the body like upper limbs, bowel (mesenteric), etc.

Past history suggestive of autoimmune disease, cold sensitivity, Raynaud's disease should be asked for.

Personal History

History of smoking—beedi or cigarettes; duration of smoking; number of cigarettes per day; whether smoking is discontinued and since when. History of chewing *pan* or using any other products (like snuff) with duration is important as both these causes tobacco abuse which predispose TAO.

> **Smoking index (SI)** is number of years of smoking × number of cigarettes/bidis smoked per day.
> **Pack year index (PYI)** is number of years of smoking × number of packets of cigarettes smoked per day.

Family History

Any family history suggestive of atherosclerosis or vascular diseases or diabetes mellitus should be asked.

GENERAL EXAMINATION

Pulse-rate, rhythm, character, condition of vessel wall is noted; blood pressure of both arms and if possible of both lower limbs is checked; attitude of limbs is noted. Other detailed general examination is very essential. Anemia; pedal edema; jaundice; clubbing; lymphadenopathy; rise in temperature; attitude of the patient; nutritional assessment by skin texture, subcutaneous fat, weight, body mass index; any other relevant findings should be mentioned.

LOCAL EXAMINATION

- *While doing local examination, both limbs should be kept side by side for comparison; limbs should be exposed entirely from toes to groin in lower limb and from fingertips to shoulder, scapular region and neck in upper limb.*
- Lower limb is examined in order from below upwards for lesion, from toes to ankle, from ankle to knee, from knee to groin, then abdomen. Similarly upper limb is examined from fingers to wrist, wrist to elbow, elbow to shoulder, neck.

Inspection

Inspection of Both Limbs

- It is done keeping both the limbs side-by-side as comparison is needed during clinical examination.
- *Entire length* of the limb is inspected. Systematic examination initially of the lesion and then of the limb above the lesion is done.

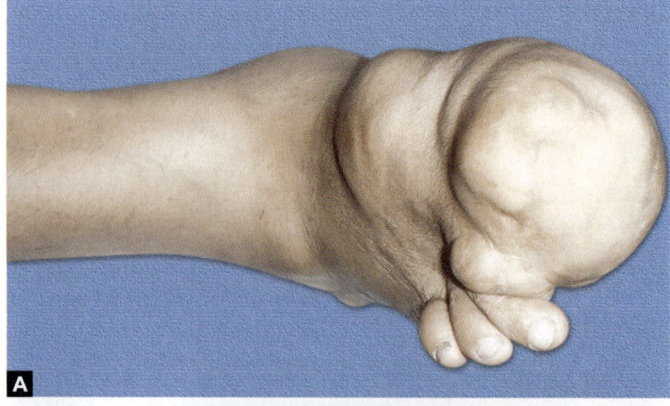

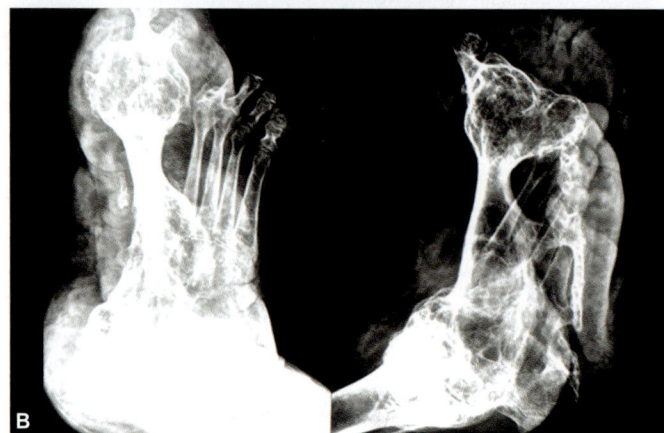

Figs. 6-12A and B Arteriovenous malformations of the foot mainly great toe. X-ray of same patient shows new bone formation due to hypervascularity. *Localized gigantism is typical.*

- Limb is looked for *signs of ischemia.*
- Limb length and girth may be increased in congenital arteriovenous malformations (congenital AVF) **(Figs. 6-12A and B)**. (Measurement of limbs should be done in such patient during palpation).

Change in Color of Limb

- It is very important sign of ischemia. Pallor should be observed by keeping both limbs adjacent **(Fig. 6-13)**. Marked, sudden severe pallor suggests acute arterial obstruction like embolism or severe vasospasm as in Raynaud's phenomenon.
- Presence of cyanosis/purple color/congestion suggest impending gangrene; whereas blackish discoloration suggests established gangrene.
- In gas gangrene, the skin and the wound will be brick red/green/brown. Skin is pale and dry in chronic ischemia.
- Color proximal to gangrene area/ischemic area (usually ischemic area is paler) should be noted.
- One should remember that crusts, black colored traditional applicants or ointments will cause black discoloration and may mimic gangrene.

Change in Texture of Skin and Appendages

- Features of ischemia such as thin shiny skin; loss of subcutaneous fat; hair loss and its extent; nail changes like

Chapter 6: Examination and Clinical Approach in Arterial Diseases

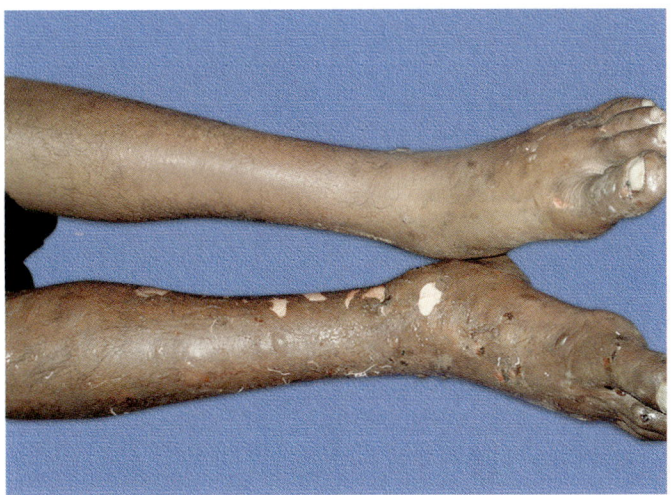

Fig. 6-13 Right leg embolic gangrene. *Note the extent and discoloration.*

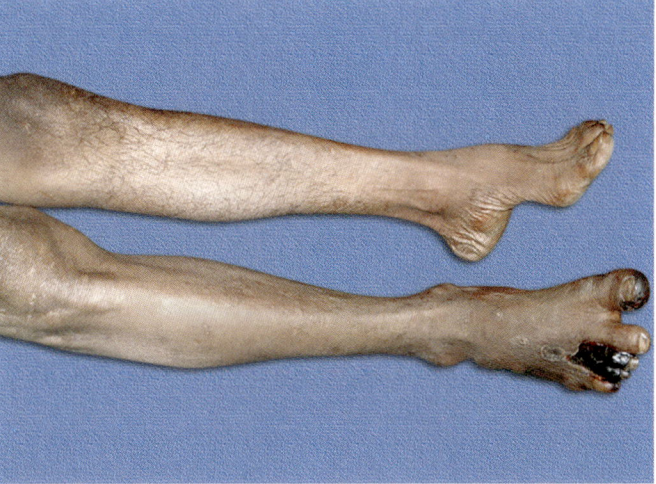

Fig. 6-15 Ischemic changes in the right leg. 3rd and 4th toes are gangrenous with line of demarcation. Great and little toes are partly gangrenous. There are ischemic features in the right foot and *leg like hair loss/skin changes/wasting.*

brittle nail/transverse ridges in the nail any loss of normal lustre should be noted.
- Superficial small ulcerations, ulcers on pressure areas should be noted.
- Skin is dry, shriveled and limb appears mummified in dry gangrene; but edematous, turgid in wet gangrene with multiple blebs and ulcers (in embolic gangrene).
- Plantar aspect of the foot should be inspected for any infective focus/abscess/callosities/skin changes; superficial ulcers in heel/malleoli/toes. Hair loss is due to diminished hair growth as a result of ischemia at hair root **(Figs. 6-14 to 6-16).**

Change in Shape of the Limb (Muscle Wasting)

- ***Muscle wasting*** in the foot/leg/thigh should be observed and should be compared with the other limb. (It is measured using a tape from a fixed bony point at the same levels in both limbs and compared).
- Marked wasting is seen in dry gangrene whereas limb is swollen and edematous in wet gangrene.

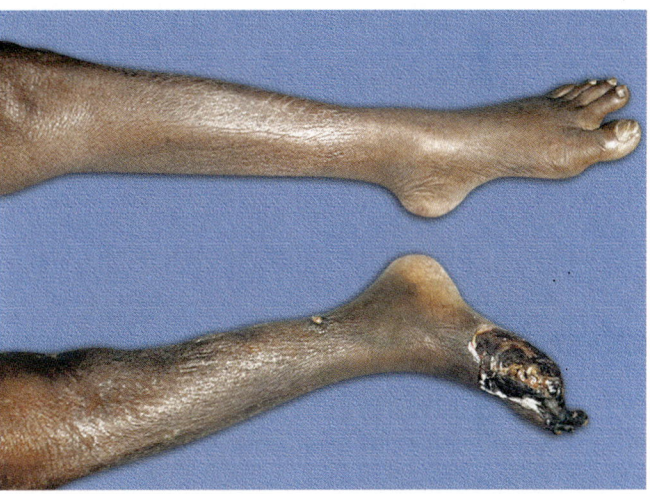

Fig. 6-16 *Gangrene* of distal right foot (forefoot) with *pregangrene* of proximal foot and distal leg; *early ischemic changes on the left leg.*

- Local gigantism/hypertrophy of the limb is seen in congenital AVF.

Gangrene

Gangrene is death with putrefaction of macroscopic part of the tissue *in situ.* **Putrefaction is decomposition of the organic matter by bacteria.** Gangrene may be established in toe/toes/foot/leg, its extent, discharge from area, type of gangrene—*dry or wet* is noted.
- **Line of demarcation** is the line between viable and nonviable tissue. It is defined by a *band of hyperemia and of hyperesthesia.* Line of demarcation is *well-defined* in dry gangrene (separation by *aseptic* ulceration). It is *ill-defined and unclear* in wet gangrene (separation by *septic* ulceration). Line of demarcation—its type; level; depth; involving skin muscle or bone/proximal extent should be checked.

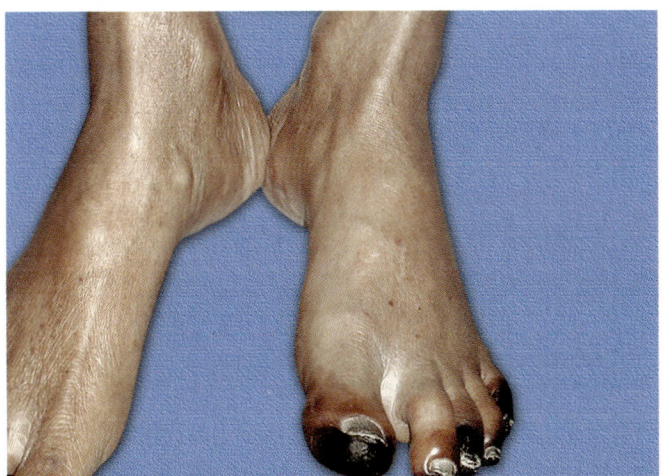

Fig. 6-14 Gangrene of all toes at their distal phalanges. *All ischemic features are obvious.*

- *Color of gangrenous area is noted*—black/purple/greenish black/reddish black [in gas gangrene (H_2S)]. *Odor* of discharge from gangrenous area is noted.
- Patchy ulcers *proximal to gangrenous area*—***skip lesions***, which are usually black and patchy should be looked for.
- ***Pregangrene*** shows color changes (red but cyanosed), edema and hyperesthesia, with or without ulceration (with history of rest pain) **(Figs. 6-17 to 6-20)**.

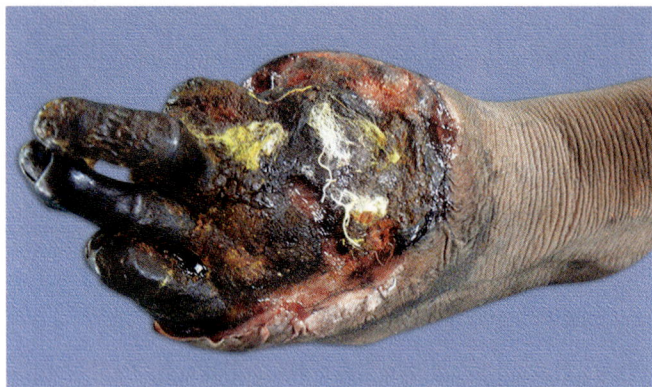

Fig. 6-17 *Dry gangrene* foot.

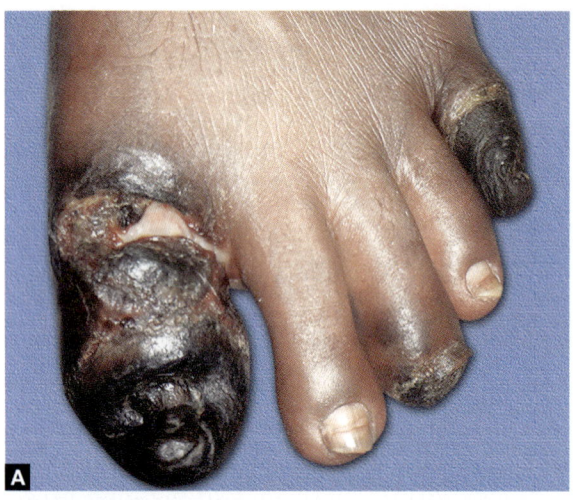

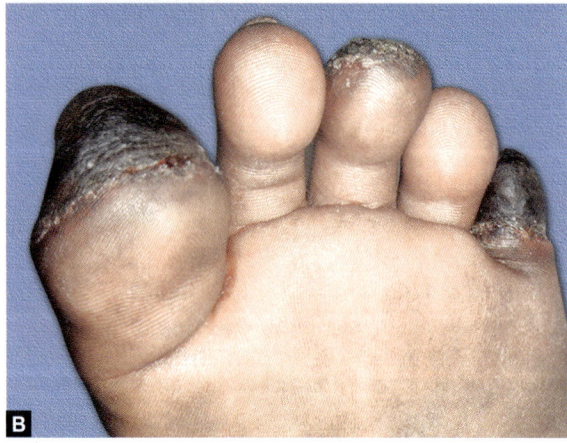

Figs. 6-18A and B Dry gangrene showing *line of demarcation*.

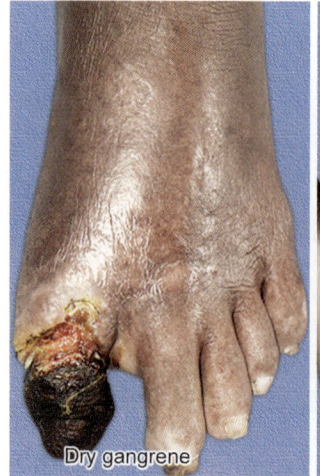 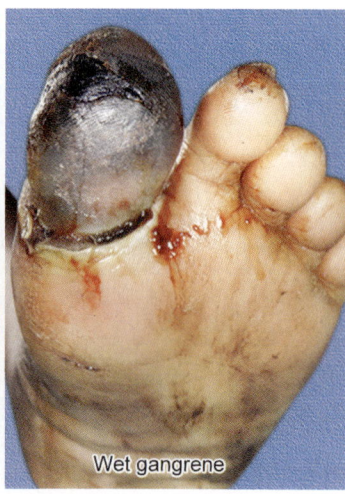

Fig. 6-19 *Dry* gangrene and *wet* gangrene of great toes in two different patients.

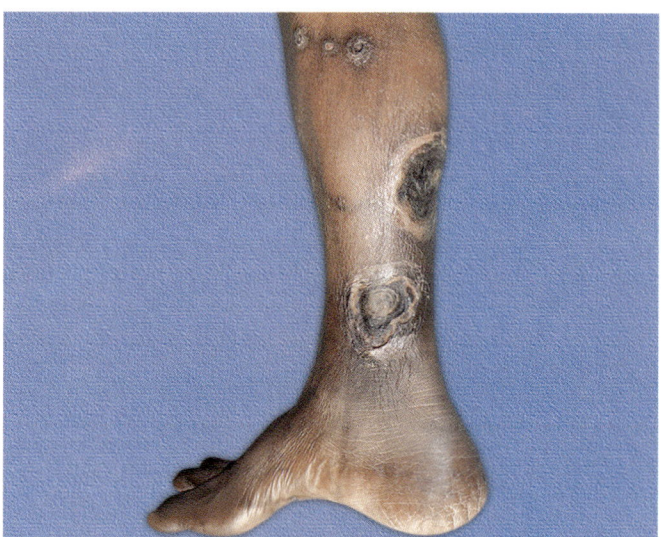

Fig. 6-20 Typical *skip lesions* in an ischemic limb.

Ulceration

Ulceration in the limb with its extent; discharge; size; shape; floor; surrounding area is noted **(Fig. 6-21)**. ***Swelling, sinus,*** when present is to be described. Patchy ulcers proximal to gangrenous area—***skip lesions*** which are usually black patchy lesions should be looked for.

Features of pregangrene:
- Rest pain
- Elevation pallor
- Dependent rubor/congestion
- Hyperesthesia
- Cold and tender ischemic tissue
- Thickening and scaling of the skin
- Wasting of the pulps of the toes or fingers **(Fig. 6-22)**
- Guttering of veins
- Poor capillary refilling

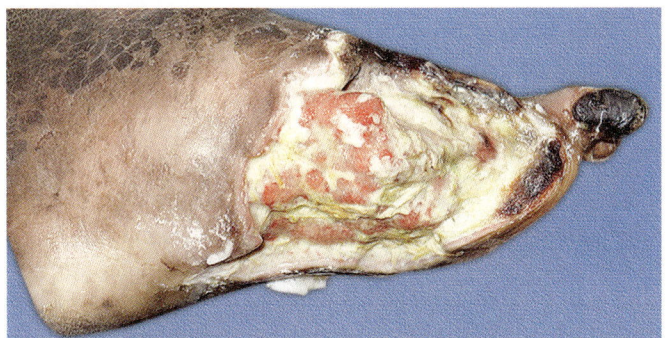

Fig. 6-21 Ischemia with *ulceration* of foot.

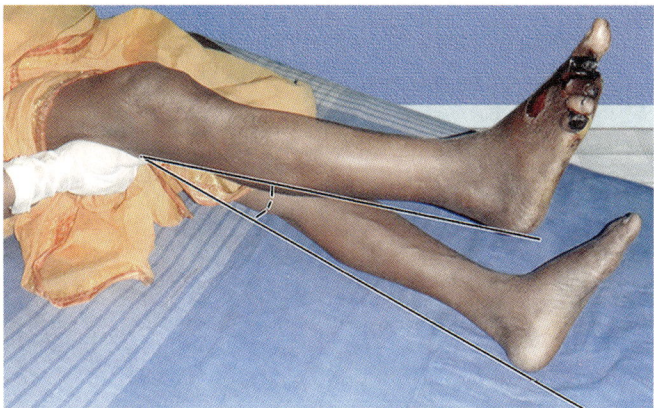

Fig. 6-23 Buerger's angle of *vascular insufficiency*.

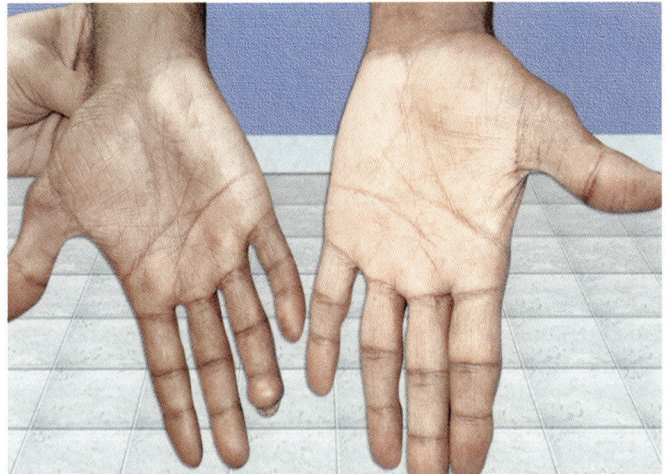

Fig. 6-22 *Wasting of muscles* of right hand because of ischemia. Color differences in both hands should be noted.

Edema

Edema in the foot/feet/legs suggests inflammation/congestion. Edema in the proximal area is common and is due to inflammation and thrombophlebitis.

Buerger's Postural Test

Patient in supine position is asked to raise his legs one after another with knee kept straight. Normal limb remains pink even after 90° elevation without any pallor. Diseased limb shows marked pallor after elevation (over foot) with **empty-guttered veins**. The angle at which pallor develops (between limb and ground) is called as **Buerger's vascular angle of insufficiency** (**Fig. 6-23**). In severe ischemia, this angle will be *less than* 30°. If foot does not become pale or when in doubt after limb elevation (supported by clinician) repeated flexion and extension of ankle and toes is done until (fatigue point is reached) it becomes pale (***cadaveric pallor***) with *empty-guttered veins* on the dorsum of foot and cyanotic congestion appears after lowering the foot in three minutes. Test is useful only in fair skinned people. It should be done in proper day light. Test is useful in patient's who present with claudication; not very much significant in whom there is rest pain and gangrene.

Limb Elevation and Dependency

On elevation, pallor and blanching occurs (**elevation pallor/cadaveric or marble white pallor**) with emptying and guttering of veins; on dependence, reddish purple congestion may occur (**dependent rubor**), i.e. after observing elevation pallor, patient is asked to lower the foot to dependency to observe the appearance of rubor which is a sign of ischemia and is due to release of local metabolites by ischemia causing vasodilatation.

Status of the Superficial Veins

Superficial venous status is to be noted, normally veins are filled but it appears pale/discolored/guttered in ischemic limb. **Guttering of vein** is observed in ischemic limb while raising the leg to 15° due to **complete collapse** of the veins, whereas in normal individual, veins are only **partially collapsed** while raising the leg.

Capillary Filling Time

Earlier elevated limbs are made to hang down off the bed. Limb will remain normal and pink in elevated as well as in dependent position because, of rapid capillary filling time in normal (nonischemic) limb. In ischemia, limb initially becomes pale on elevation and gradually very slowly becomes pink and then purple-red in more than 20 seconds. Purple pink color is due to deoxygenated blood. Prolonged capillary filling time signifies severe ischemia.

Venous Refilling Time

Elevated limb when laid horizontal on the bed, venous refilling occurs normally within 5 seconds. It is delayed in ischemic limb (>20 seconds). Delayed venous refilling causes collapse of veins called as *guttering of veins*. In ischemic limb, even elevation of 10° causes guttering of veins whereas in normal limb guttering develops only at 90° or above elevation.

Limb Deformity

Type of deformity, severity, gait, and attitude is noted. Often patient is seen sitting with holding the foot with his both hands to relieve the pain. By holding the limb, touch or pressure sensation is transmitted to the patient's brain through spinothalamic tract which temporarily blocks the pain transmission.

Note: Examination of supraclavicular fossa—for any abnormal fullness is observed. Cervical rib and subclavian aneurysm may show fullness in this area.

Palpation

Palpation should be done meticulously by wearing gloves.

Temperature

Temperature of the skin is an important factor in ischemic limb. Temperature is checked using **dorsal surface of the phalanges** (middle phalanx is better) as dorsal skin of fingers is thin, lax and contain more temperature receptors. Ischemic part is felt cold; up to what extent the limb is cold and where exactly limb/part becomes warmer proximally should be assessed. Level of temperature change from distal colder to proximal warmer area is important for eventual assessment of level of amputation, if needed. Temperature should be compared with opposite limb; if both lower limbs are diseased, then it should be compared with upper limbs. One has to carefully observe and remember that an uncovered limb will be cooler than covered limb (with blankets or clothes). Limb will be warmer in congenital arteriovenous malformation due to increased vascularity. Limb may also feel warmer due to local infection and cellulitis.

Tenderness

Site; extent; severity should be assessed. Tenderness **along the line of limb vessels** should be checked by palpation. Tenderness is due to inflammation and nerve irritation. Gangrenous area is cold, nontender, and devoid of sensation. Limbs at line of demarcation and above, may be hypersensitive, paresthetic and tender due to inflammation and irritation of nerve endings.

Sensation

There will be **hyperesthesia** in the ischemic area due to nerve irritation and nerve ischemia. Gangrene area is insensitive.

Edema

Pitting edema is checked which may be due to superficial thrombophlebitis or other inflammatory condition.

Gangrenous Area

Gangrenous area should be palpated for extent; whether it is dry and shriveled or whether it is wet and edematous **(Figs. 24A and B)**. Presence or absence of *crepitus* in gangrenous area (gas gangrene which is khaki colored, foul smelling) should be checked. Crepitus is due to presence of gas (H_2S) in the muscles in gas gangrene. Temperature, tenderness and sensation is checked in the gangrenous area. Gangrenous area is cold, nontender and insensitive.

Limb above the Gangrenous Area

Limb above the area is again checked for pitting edema, temperature changes, tenderness, sensation (hyperesthesia/paresthesia). Level where cold part of the limb becomes warm proximally should be found out carefully. Proximal ischemic part may be tender.

Capillary Refilling

Tip of the nail or pulp of the finger or toe is pressed onto the nail bed to blanch it and pressure is released (in 2 seconds) to make it pink again. Time taken for blanched area to turn pink is *capillary refilling time*. It is prolonged (>2 seconds) in ischemic limb. It gives the indirect evidence about the rate of blood flow and pressure within the capillaries **(Figs. 6-25A and B)**.

Harvey's Venous Refilling Test

Two index fingers (or index or middle fingers of one hand) are placed over the vein and pressure is applied over it. Proximal finger is moved for about 5–7 cm proximally without releasing the pressure. Vein between the fingers gets emptied completely and becomes flat. Distal finger (away from the heart) is now released to see the flow of the blood and its refilling is observed, whether good or poor. It is poor in ischemic limb. Venous refilling is rapid in arteriovenous fistula **(Figs. 6-26A to D)**.

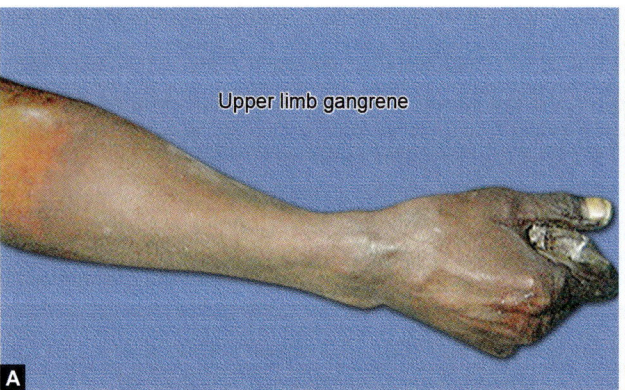
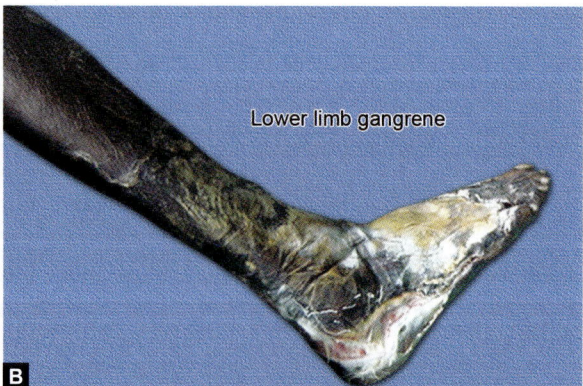

Figs. 6-24A and B Gangrene of upper and lower limbs in two different patients. Upper limb gangrene is *wet type due to embolus*; lower limb gangrene is *dry type due to atherosclerosis*.

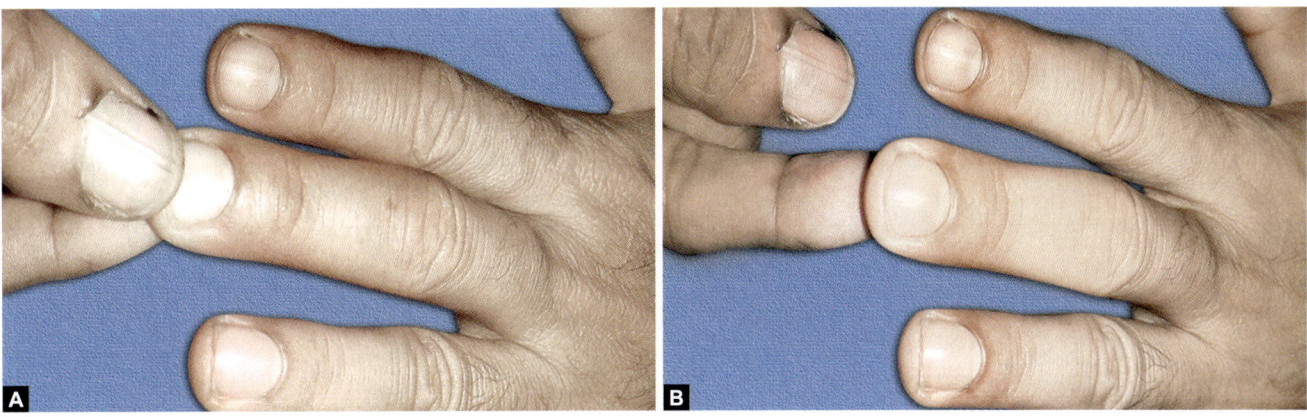

Figs. 6-25A and B *Capillary refilling test.*

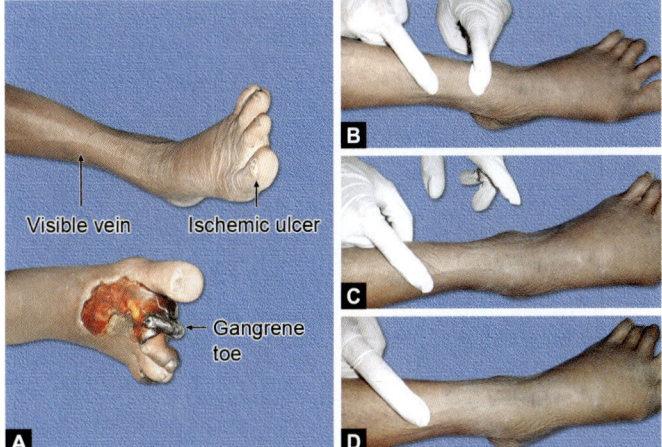

Figs. 6-26A to D *Harvey's venous refilling test.*

Palpation of Blood Vessels

Palpation of peripheral pulses is the ***most important clinical examination*** in vascular diseases. It gives the idea about the level of occlusion and severity. Rate, rhythm, tension, volume, condition of the vessel wall (thickening) and tenderness over the vessel should be checked. All pulses should be compared to opposite sides and *documented in a table as right and left*. Whether it is present or absent or feebler should be mentioned. When a specific pulse is absent, false feeling of pulsation is felt which may be actually surgeon's own pulsation at his finger level. In such situation, surgeon should palpate his own radial or superficial artery pulsation to counteract this false feeling. Artery may be *tender* in embolic vasospasm, acute thrombosis, inflammation (may occur in TAO during recent thrombosis) and vasculitis. ***Expansile pulsation*** in an artery suggests aneurysm. Usually in a vascular case, pulses are examined from below upwards, i.e. from lower limb to upper limb. ***Thrill over an artery*** should be palpated. It suggests turbulent flow through a narrowed vessel. ***Thrill*** may usually be felt at femoral, subclavian or carotid artery (later these areas should be auscultated for bruit for similar reason). Carotid and subclavian thrill may be due to aortic valvular disease. Cimino fistula, surgically created AVF for hemodialysis is the commonest cause for thrill in peripheral vessels of forearm.

Sign of disappearing pulse: Pulse is felt initially (for example, dorsalis pedis artery). Patient is asked to do muscular exercise by walk or pushups for several minutes; pulse is examined again. In normal individual, pulse will become bounding with increased rate but in an ischemic limb, pulse may disappear or will never become bounding. Again after 2–3 minutes of rest, pulse is palpated; pulse will reappear. It is a sign of ***unmasking the pulse*** in an ischemic limb.

- ***Dorsalis pedis artery*** is felt just lateral to the extensor hallucis longus tendon at the proximal end of first webspace, against the navicular and middle cuneiform bones. It is absent in 10% cases. In edematous foot, it may not be felt. Great toe is dorsiflexed by the patient to make better feeling of the extensor hallucis longus tendon **(Fig. 6-27)**. One should remember that it should be felt over the proximal part of the dorsum of the foot where artery dips into the space between the bases of the 1st and 2nd metatarsals. Often dorsalis pedis artery pulsation may be feeble or absent and clinician may get confused with his own pulsation; in such situation using other hand clinician should palpate the radial artery pulsation of the patient simultaneously to avoid confusion **(Figs. 6-28 and 6-29)**.
- ***Anterior tibial artery*** is felt anteriorly above and in the midway between the two malleoli (intermalleolar/ankle joint line) against the lower end of tibia just above the ankle joint lateral to tibialis anterior/extensor hallucis longus tendon. Patient is asked to dorsiflex the foot to identify these tendons. The artery is felt on the surface of the lower end of tibia above the ankle joint line above the extensor retinaculum wherein artery passes deep to retinaculum to become dorsalis pedis artery **(Figs. 6-30A to C)**.
- ***Posterior tibial artery*** is felt against the calcaneum just behind the medial malleolus midway between it and medial border of the Achilles tendon. Foot should be dorsiflexed and inverted **(Fig. 6-31)**.
- ***Peroneal artery*** is felt 1 cm medial to lateral malleolus. In 5% of individuals, it replaces the anterior tibial artery.
- ***Popliteal artery*** is difficult to feel. It is palpated better (***most reliable method***) in ***prone position*** with knee flexed

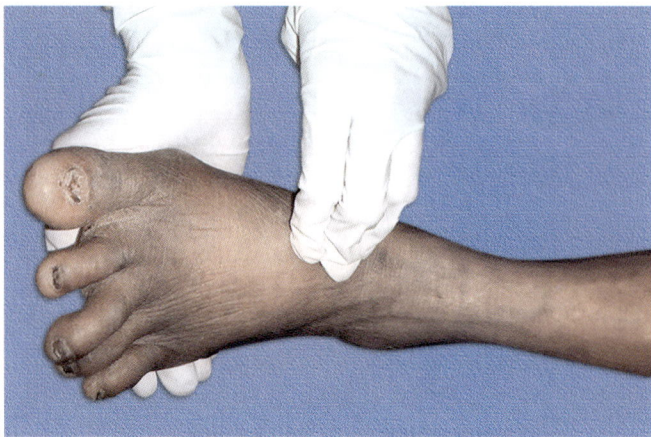

Fig. 6-27 Palpation of *dorsalis pedis artery* pulsation.

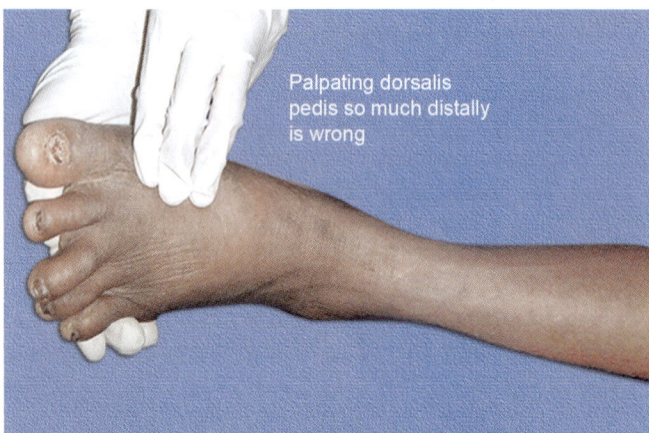

Fig. 6-28 *Wrong way of palpating the dorsalis pedis artery;* it is not possible to palpate close to the 1st webspace as artery enters deep much proximally.

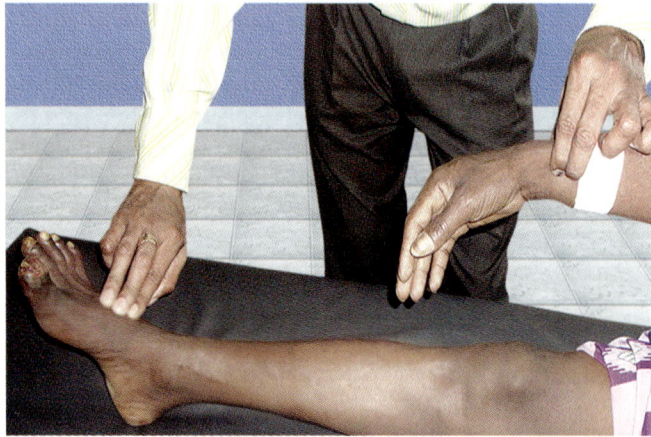

Fig. 6-29 Often dorsalis pedis artery pulsation may be feeble or absent and *clinician may get confused with his own pulsation;* in such situation using other hand clinician should palpate the radial artery pulsation of the patient simultaneously to avoid confusion.

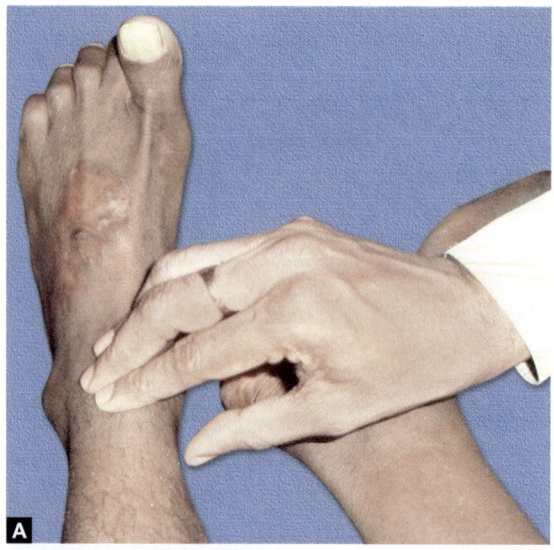
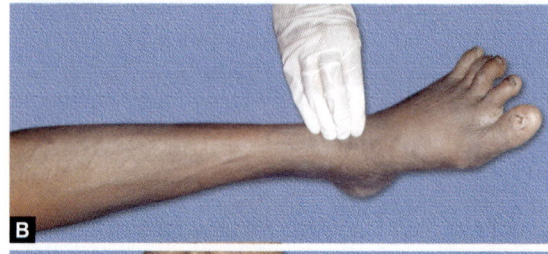
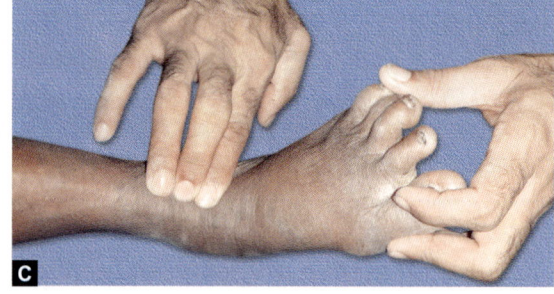

Figs. 6-30A to C Palpation of *anterior tibial artery*.

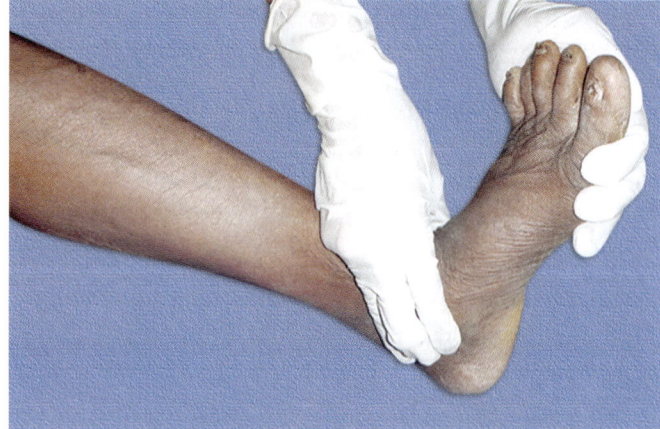

Fig. 6-31 Palpation of the *posterior tibial artery*.

at about 45° to relax popliteal fascia. It is felt in the lower part of the popliteal fossa over the flat posterior surface of upper end of tibia. Artery is not felt in upper end of the fossa, as there is no bony area in intercondylar region (of lower end of femur). It can also be felt in supine position with knee flexed at 90° (***most convenient method***) to relax the popliteal fascia so that pulsation can be felt over the lower part of the popliteal fossa against posterior surface

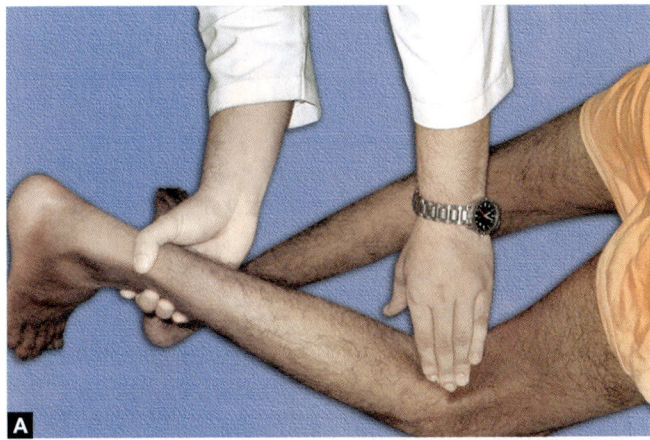

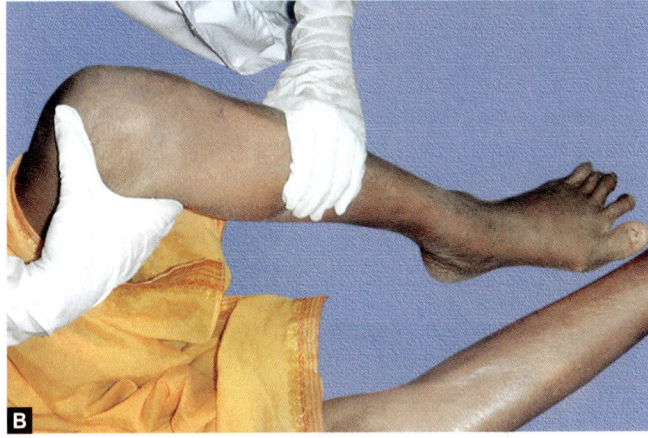

Figs. 6-32A and B Palpation of popliteal artery *both in supine* and *prone positions. Prone position is always better.*

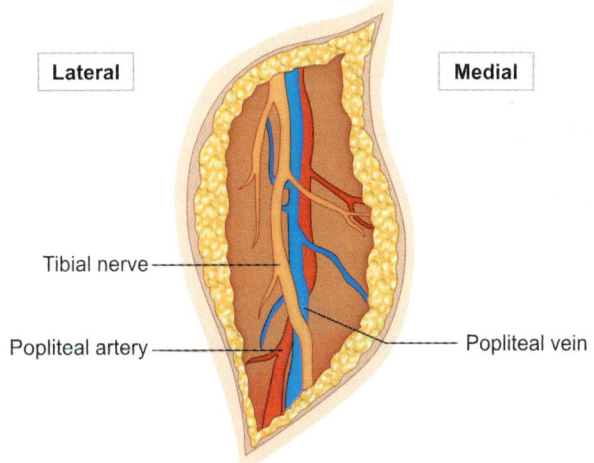

Fig. 6-33 Anatomical location of the *popliteal artery*.

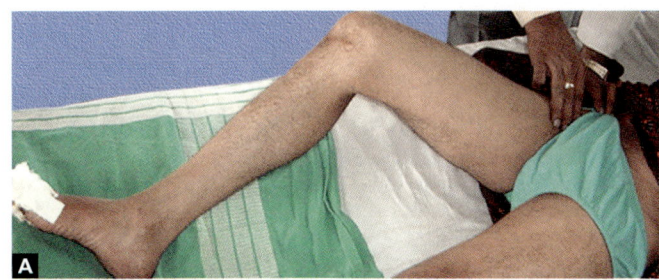

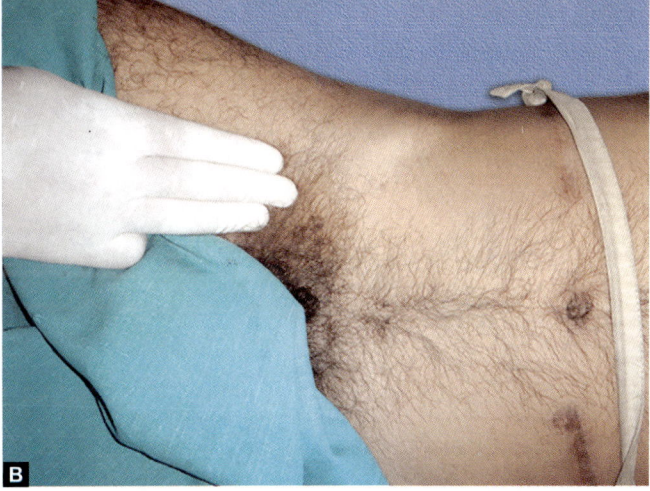

Figs. 6-34A and B Palpation of *femoral artery*.

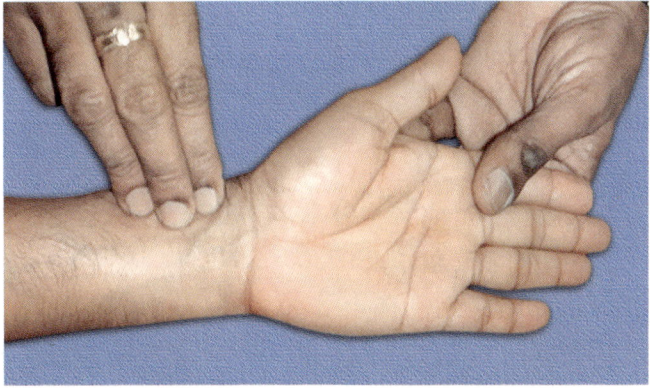

Fig. 6-35 Palpation of *radial artery*.

of upper part of the tibial condyles **(Figs. 6.32A and B)**. Surgeon stands in front of the patient with patient's heel resting on the table to relax popliteal fascia and muscles around; thumb is placed over the tibial tuberosity; fingertips are insinuated in the lower part of the popliteal fossa from side towards midline to feel the popliteal pulse. Third method occasionally may be used; initially with leg straight at knee, fingertips are placed on midline over popliteal fossa with one hand round; knee joint is hyperextended against clinician's hand and touch to feel the popliteal pulse. Clinician should be well aware of the anatomical location of the popliteal artery in the popliteal fossa **(Fig. 6-33)**.

- **Femoral artery** in the groin is felt just below the inguinal ligament, midway between anterior superior iliac spine and pubic symphysis (mid-inguinal point). Often hip has to be *flexed* for about 10–15° with abduction and external rotation to feel it properly. It is felt against the neck of the femur. In posterior dislocation of the head of the femur, femoral artery pulse is not felt—*Narath's sign* **(Figs. 6-34A and B)**.
- **Radial artery** is felt just above the wrist on the lateral aspect against lower end of the front of radius, lateral to the tendon of flexor carpi radialis **(Fig. 6-35)**.
- **Ulnar artery** is felt just above the wrist on the medial aspect against lower end of the front of ulna **(Fig. 6-36)**.

- **Brachial artery** is felt in front of the elbow just medial and behind the biceps brachii tendon against humerus **(Fig. 6-37)**.
- **Axillary artery** is felt on lateral aspect of the axilla against upper end of the shaft and neck of the humerus with raised arm **(Fig. 6-38)**.
- **Subclavian artery** is felt against first rib just above the middle of the clavicle in supraclavicular fossa while patient is lifting the shoulder to relax deep fascia **(Fig. 6-39)**.
- **Common carotid artery** is felt medial to sternomastoid muscle at the level of thyroid cartilage against carotid tubercle (*Chassaignac anterior tubercle*) of transverse process of 6th cervical vertebra (in carotid triangle) **(Fig. 6-39)**.
- **Facial artery** is felt against body of mandible at the insertion of masseter in lower face **(Fig. 6-40)**.
- **Superficial temporal artery** is felt just in front of the tragus of the ear against the zygomatic bone **(Fig. 6-41)**.

All pulsations of both right and left side should be written in a tabular form:

Pulse	Right	Left
Dorsalis pedis	Should be mentioned as present/absent/feeble	Should be mentioned as present/absent/feeble
Posterior tibial		
Anterior tibial		
Popliteal		
Femoral		
Radial		
Ulnar		
Brachial		
Axillary		
Subclavian		
Carotid		
Superficial temporal		

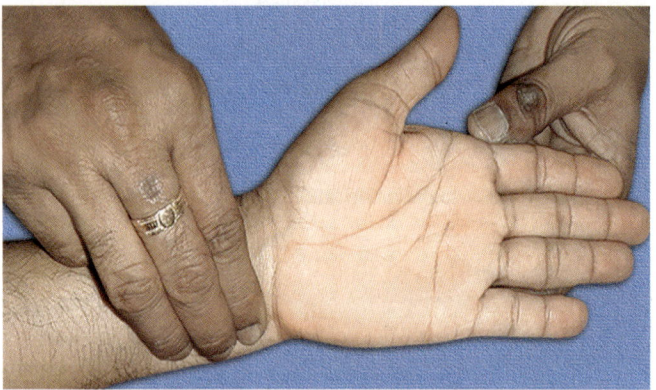

Fig. 6-36 Palpation of *ulnar artery*.

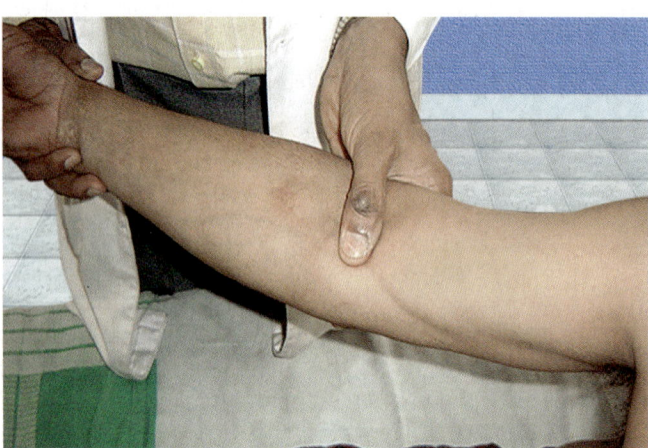

Fig. 6-37 Palpation of *brachial artery*.

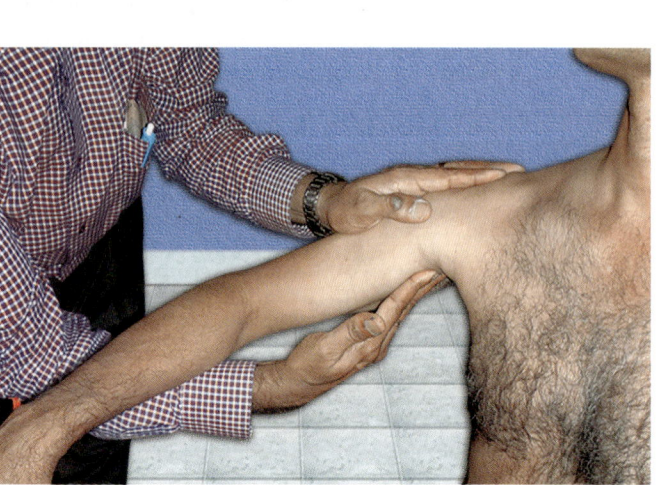

Fig. 6-38 Palpation of *axillary artery*.

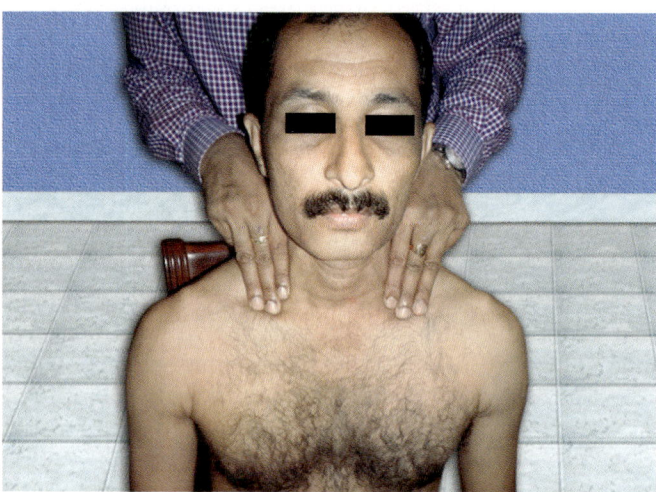

Fig. 6-39 Palpation of *subclavian artery*.

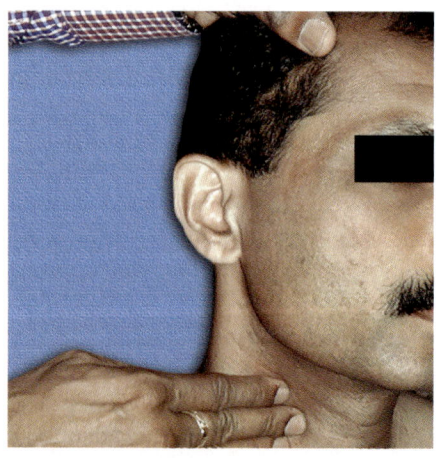

Fig. 6-40 Palpation of *common carotid artery*.

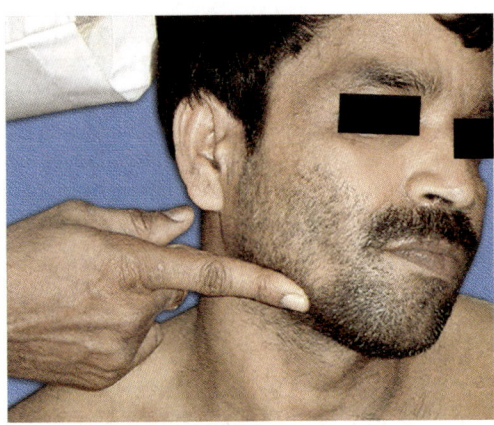

Fig. 6-41 Palpation of *facial artery*.

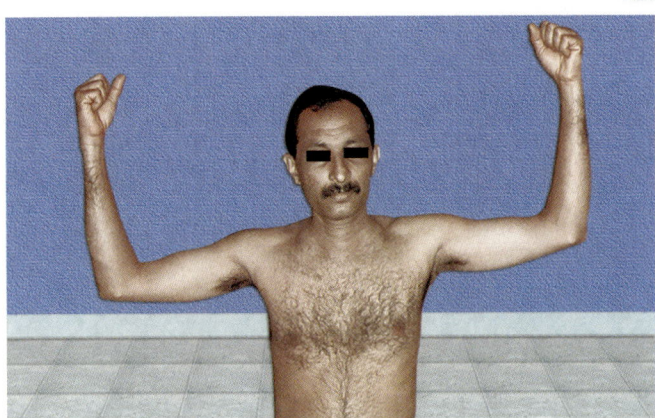

Fig. 6-43 Elevated arm stress test (*EAST*).

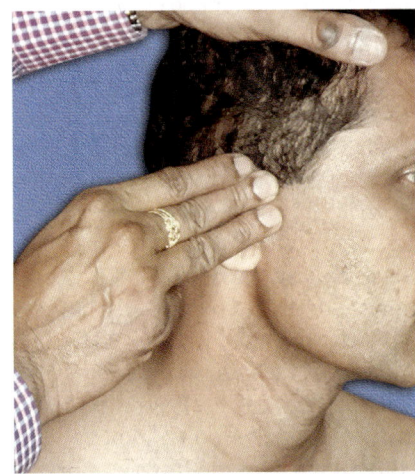

Fig. 6-42 Palpation of *superficial temporal artery*.

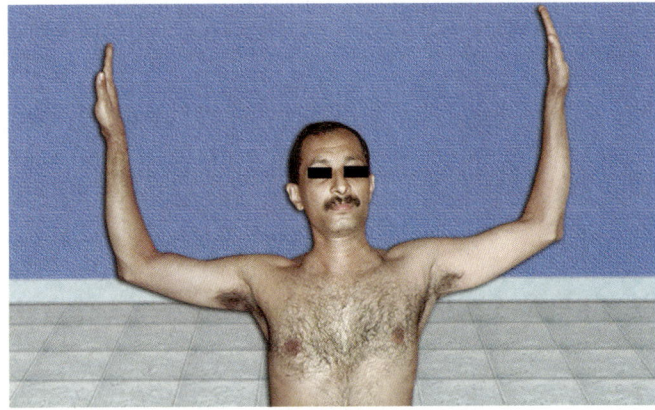

Fig. 6-44 *Roos test.* Shoulder is elevated to 90° with arms externally rotated and kept for 5 minutes; patient with thoracic outlet syndrome develops extreme fatigue on the side.

Special Tests for Upper Limb Ischemia

1. *Elevated arm stress test (EAST)*
   Both shoulders (arms) are abducted to 90° with arms fully externally rotated and the elbows braced backwards. Patient will open and close (clinch and unclench) the hands rapidly for 3–5 minutes. Normal individual can do this without any discomfort and pain. Patient with thoracic outlet syndrome develops pain in neck, back and shoulders; fatigue, paresthesia of forearm with tingling and numbness of fingers which is gradually progressing. Patient will not be able to continue the test for 5 minutes. This test can also differentiate thoracic outlet syndrome from cervical disc prolapse disease **(Fig. 6-43)**.

2. *Roos test*
   Patient is asked to elevate and abduct the shoulders to 90° along with external rotation of arms and keep it for 3–5 minutes. Patient feels fatigue on the diseased side **(Fig. 6.44)**.

3. *Costoclavicular compression maneuver (Falconer test)*
   While palpating the radial pulse of the patient in standing position, he is asked to move his shoulder backwards and downwards (exaggerated military position) which may cause absence/feeble radial pulse and a bruit may be heard while auscultating the supraclavicular region—military attitude test **(Fig. 6-45)**. This is due to compression of subclavian artery between clavicle and first rib. Similarly *Halstead maneuver* is done by 45° abduction and extension of arm with downward pushing of the shoulder with neck turned opposite side to make the pulse feebly palpable.

4. *Hyperabduction maneuver (Wright test)*
   While palpating the radial pulse, arm on the diseased side is passively hyperabducted by the clinician causing feeble or absence of radial pulse **(Fig. 6-46)**. This is due to compression of artery by pectoralis minor tendon (*pectoralis minor syndrome*). An axillary bruit may be heard on auscultation adjacent to anterior axillary fold (in front or behind).

5. *Adson's test*
   After asking the patient to sit on a chair/stool, the radial pulse on the affected side of the patient is palpated; clinician will stand by the side of the patient; patient is asked to take deep breath and turn his extended neck/head towards the same side and to take deep breath so as to compress the thoracoaxillary channel. Adson's test is said to be positive when pulse becomes feeble or absent as in thoracic outlet syndrome/scalenus anticus syndrome. While taking deep breath, thoracic cage moves upwards

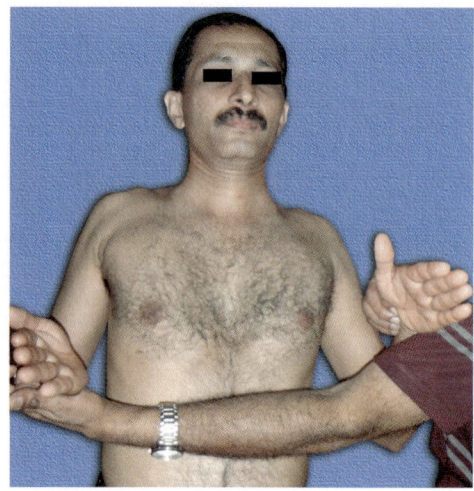

Fig. 6-45 Costoclavicular compression maneuver (*Falconer test*).

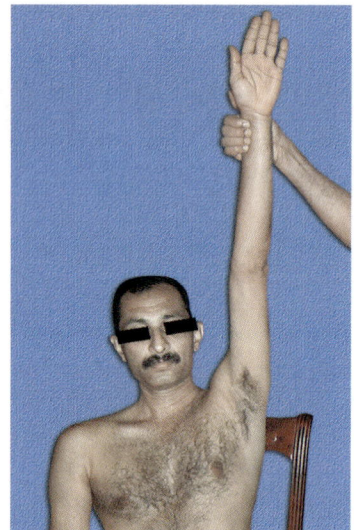

Fig. 6-46 Hyperabduction maneuver (*Wright test*).

and narrows the space aggravating the compression of subclavian artery by scalenus anterior muscle. Contraction of scalenus anterior further aggravates the feature (by turning neck towards same side). Test can be modified by turning the head towards opposite side (to stretch the scalenus anterior muscle)—***modified Adson's test***. Test should be done on opposite side also for comparison **(Figs. 6-47A to C)**.

6. *Allen's test*

   It is used in hand to find out the patency of radial and ulnar arteries. Both radial and ulnar arteries of the patient are felt and pressed firmly at the wrist **(Figs. 6-48A to E)**. Patient clinches his hand firmly (often repeated clinching) and holds it tightly. After one minute, clinch is released to open the palm of the hand which looks pale. Pressure on radial artery in the wrist is released to see area of distribution of the radial artery. Normally it becomes flushed with pink color. If there is block in radial artery, the area will remain white. Test is repeated again. This time pressure on the ulnar artery is released to check the patency of it. Area will be pale and blanched after releasing in case of ulnar artery block. Otherwise it becomes pink after releasing in normal individual.

7. *Cold and warm water test*

   It is commonly done to confirm Raynaud's phenomena. Patient is asked to dip hands in ice cold water to trigger and precipitate the vasospasm; hand will become white due to severe vasospasm. Patient is now made to dip his hand in warm water; it leads into sudden capillary dilatation making hand blue colored—***Raynaud's phenomenon***.

8. *Examination of supraclavicular fossa*

   Mass, if any is palpated for warmth, tenderness, mobility, consistency, pulsatility, etc. Vascular swellings are warm, tender, pulsatile whereas cervical rib is felt as bony hard swelling.

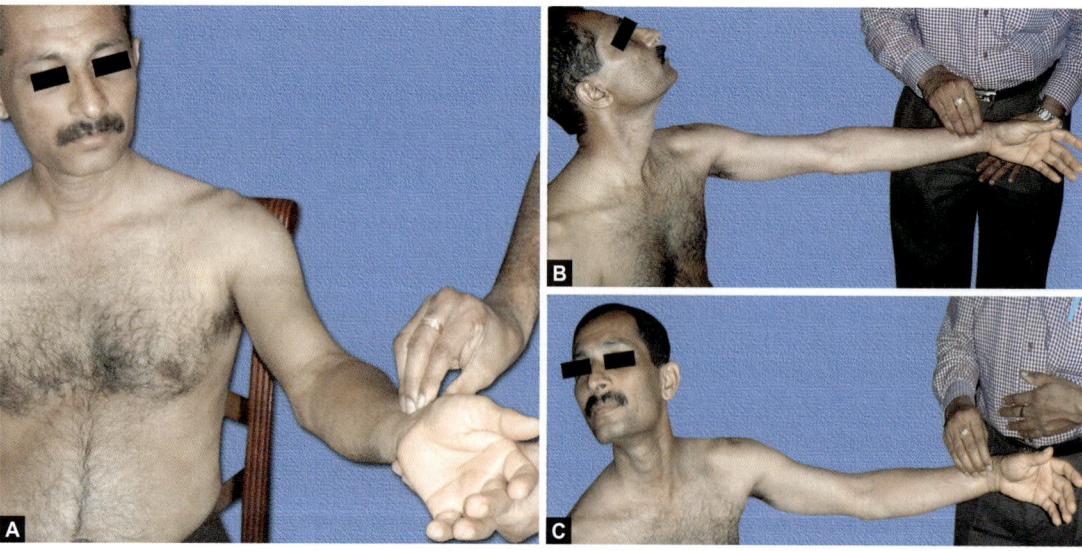

Figs. 6-47A to C *Adson's test*—palpating radial pulse by deep inspiration and turning the neck towards same side with extension, pulse either disappears or becomes feeble (A and B). In modification, patient turns his neck towards opposite side with extension and deep inspiration (C).

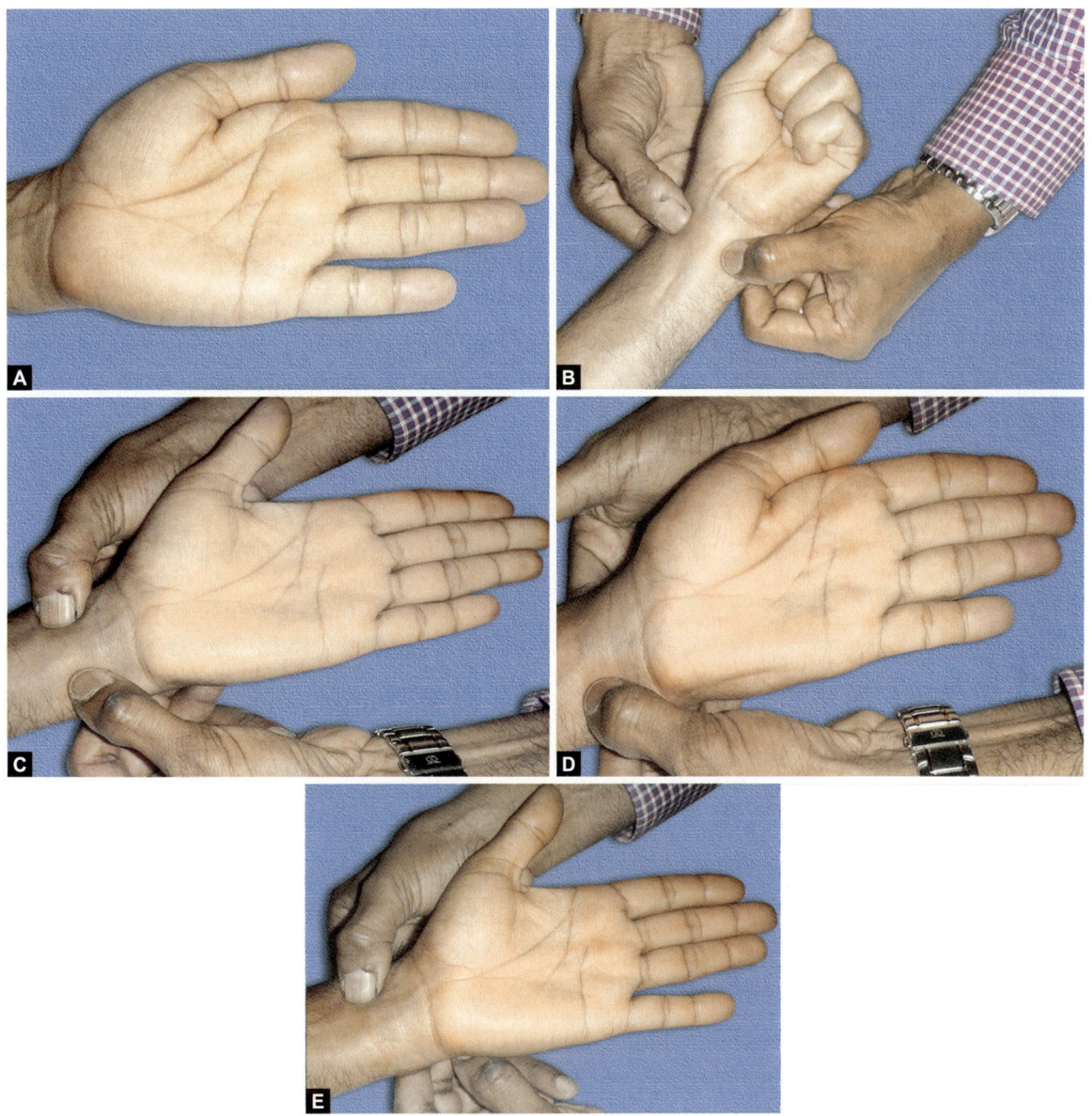

Figs. 6-48A to E *Allen's test.*

Special Tests for Lower Limb Ischemia

1. ***Crossed leg test*** *(Fuchsig's test)*
   Patient is asked to sit with the affected leg crossed above the other so that the popliteal fossa of the affected leg lies against the knee of the other leg. Test is done after diverting the patient's attention. Oscillatory movements of foot can be observed synchronous with the popliteal artery pulsation. If the popliteal artery is blocked, oscillatory movements will be absent. Oscillatory movements are more prominent in popliteal artery aneurysm **(Figs. 6-49A and B).**

2. ***Disappearing pulse syndrome***
   The limb is exercised after feeling the pulse. Pulse will disappear once patient develops claudication in ischemic limb. It is because of vasodilatation and increased vascular space that occurs due to exercise wherein arterial tension cannot be kept adequately and so results in disappearance of pulse (***unmasking the arterial obstruction***). By resting again for few minutes, pulse will reappear. Whereas in normal individual, pulse will be increased and bounding after exercise.

3. ***Buerger's postural test*** *(Leo Buerger—Urologist)*
   Patient lying down on his back is asked to raise the leg forward for two minutes. In normal individual, limb (plantar aspect of foot) remains pink even after raising to 90° angles. Ischemic limb, when elevated shows marked pallor and empty veins. The angle in which pallor develops is called as *Buerger's angle of vascular insufficiency. Less than 30° angles indicate severe ischemia. Ischemic height* of the heel in relation to the sternal angle where pallor develops in heel signifies the severity of the disease. This height in centimeter is equal to the arterial pressure in the foot in mm Hg. After that, patient is asked to keep the legs below the bed to fill the vessels. Time taken for the leg

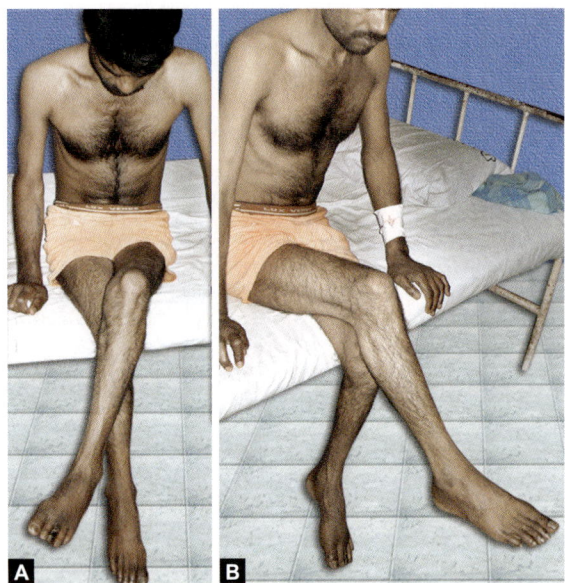

Figs. 6-49A and B Cross leg test— *checking oscillatory movements.*

to become pink is capillary filling time. Filling time more than 30 seconds suggests severe ischemia in the limb. In ischemic limb, after lowering from elevated position, cyanotic hue appears on the dorsum of foot (in 3 minutes of lowering).

4. *Guttering of vein*

 It is usually observed in severely ischemic limb (can be palpated) while raising the leg 15°, due to complete collapse of the veins, whereas, in normal individual, veins are only partially collapsed while raising the leg.

5. *Reactive hyperemia time test (Lewis)*

 The sphygmomanometer cuff is inflated around the thigh up to 250 mm Hg for 5 minutes till significant pallor appears. Release and assess the time of appearing of red flush in skin which signifies the reactive hyperemia time. Normal time is 2 seconds. It is delayed in ischemia. This test is contraindicated in gangrene. This test helps to measure the blood flow. This test is done in patients who are unable to walk. This is done in lying down position in both limbs.

Branham's/Nicoladoni's Sign

In arteriovenous fistula when pressure is applied over the artery proximal to the fistula, there will be reduction in pulse rate, size of the swelling, disappearance of the thrill and bruit, and pulse pressure becomes normal. Distal pulse is felt depending on the location of the arteriovenous fistula either radial in hand or dorsalis pedis/posterior tibial in foot. It should be compared to the opposite side. Tachycardia is common with raised pulse pressure. Artery proximal to the fistula is compressed to cease the shunting of the blood through the fistula; it causes reduction in pulse rate and fall in blood pressure.

Assessment of Wasting of the Limb Muscle

It is important to find out the severity of ischemia. It is done by inspecting the muscle bulk and prominent bony prominences by measurement of the limb girth (circumference is measured using a tape, at the same level in both limbs away from a fixed bony point). *Note:* Measurement of limb length as well as girth should be done in congenital arteriovenous fistula **(Figs. 6-50A and B).**

Muscle Power

It is also checked and graded.
Grade 0: Complete paralysis;
Grade 1: Flicker of contraction, but no movement;
Grade 2: Movement with the elimination of gravity;
Grade 3: Movement against gravity, not against resistance;
Grade 4: Movement against partial resistance;
Grade 5: Normal movement against full resistance where there is local hypertrophy of affected limb **(Fig. 6-51).**

Auscultation

- Auscultation over the artery for **bruit** is done using bell of the stethoscope placed gently over the artery.
- **Bruit** is the sound produced by turbulent blood flow through a stenotic segment of an artery which is transmitted distally along its course. It signifies localized stenosis causing **turbulent** flow **(Figs. 6-52A to C).**
- Continuous buzzing **bruit and machinery murmur** are also heard in arteriovenous malformations/fistulas.
- **Reactive hyperemia test** is done during auscultation also using sphygmomanometer.

Regional Lymph Node Examination

In infection, inguinal or axillary nodes may get enlarged depending on the limb involved.

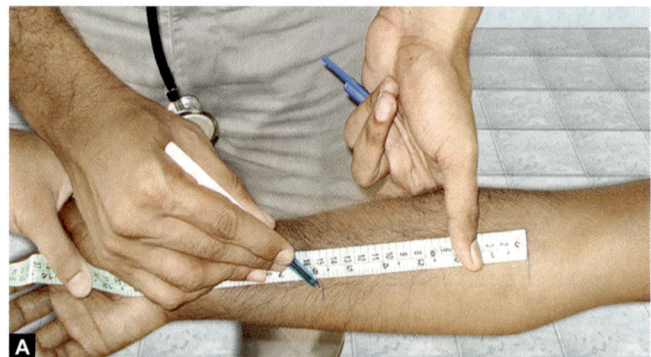
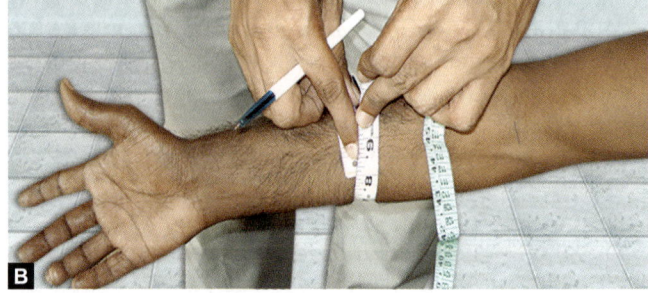

Figs. 6-50A and B *Measurement of girth is important to find out the wasting.* It should be compared to opposite side and measured at a specific distance from a bony prominence.

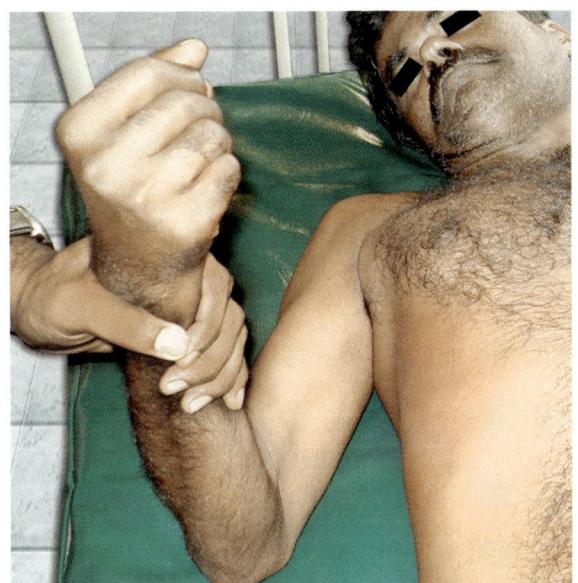

Fig. 6-51 Muscle power *should be checked against resistance* to find out the grade.

myelitis), muscle tone/power at ankle, knee and hip; sensory examination for touch, pain and temperature, reflexes at ankle and knee and plantar should be checked (**Fig. 6-53**).

Abdomen Examination

Abdomen should be examined for the presence of abdominal *aortic aneurysms*. It presents as pulsatile mass above the umbilicus, vertically placed, smooth, soft, nonmobile, not moving with respiration, resonant on percussion. *Expansile pulsation* is confirmed by placing the patient in *knee-elbow or lateral position* (**Fig. 6-54**). *Intensity will be same (unchanged) in expansile pulsation.*

Cardiovascular System

CVS examination is essential part of the arterial system to look for any associated or causative factors. There may be an embolic focus in heart like fibrillation/endocarditis, etc. (**Fig. 6-55**).

Other Relevant Examinations

Other extrinsic abnormality in the course of the artery (cervical rib, bony prominence, any tumor) to be noted. Examination of skeletal system, joints, muscle, veins are essential to rule out arthritis, deep vein thrombosis (DVT) or myositis. Deeper structures like muscle, bone, nerves, joints should be palpated. *Examination of opposite limb should be done thoroughly.*

■ SYSTEMIC EXAMINATION

Neurological Examination

When associated neurological conditions are suspected (like tabes dorsalis, syringomyelia, hemiplegia, transverse

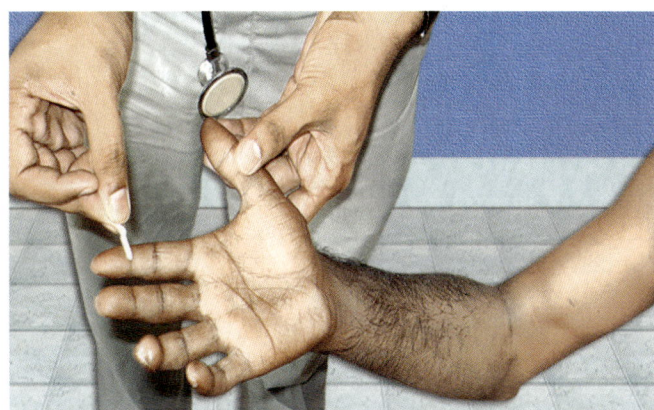

Fig. 6-53 Sensation should be checked for *neurological deficit*—especially in upper limb (cervical rib).

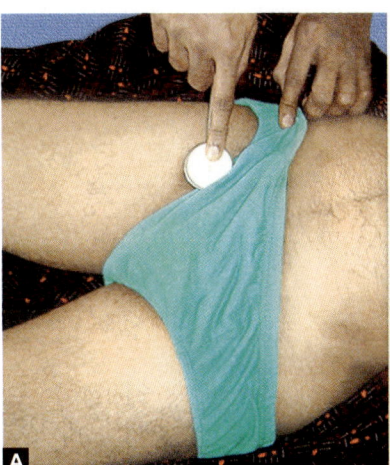
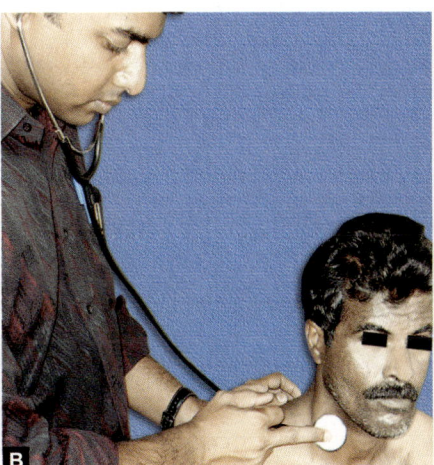
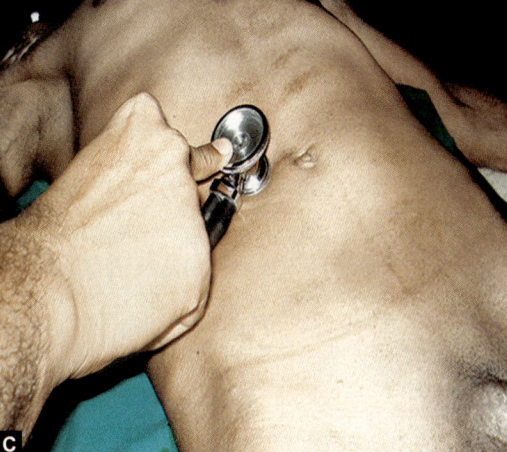

Figs. 6-52A to C Auscultation over the major vessel like femoral/carotid for bruit is important. It *signifies stenosis and turbulence flow of blood*.

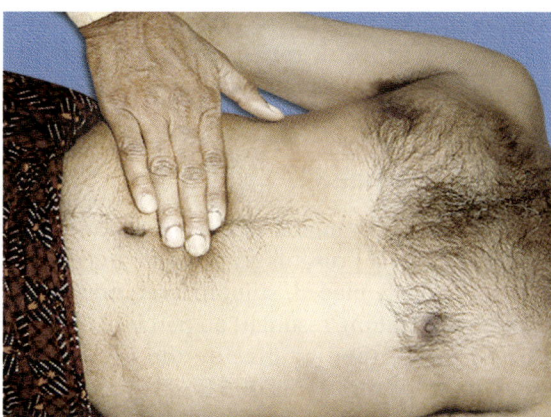

Fig. 6-54 Examination of abdomen for aortic pulsation/aneurysm; old sympathectomy scar are important. Aortic aneurysm is looked for above the umbilicus, in midline. It shows mass with expansile pulsation; vertically placed; above the umbilicus; nonmobile; soft; smooth; resonant; retroperitoneal (*does not change in intensity—in knee-elbow position*).

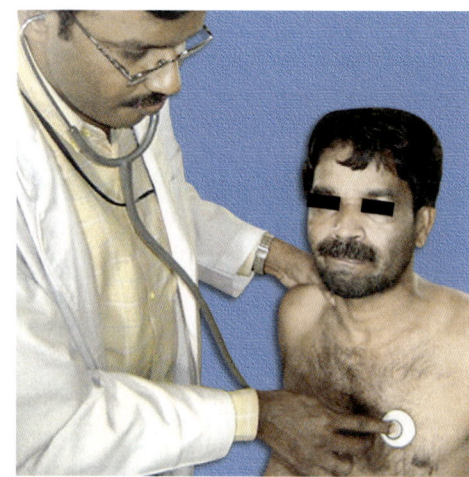

Fig. 6-55 *Cardiovascular system examination is important* to look for mitral stenosis/endocarditis, etc.

Other Systems

Other systems like skeletal and respiratory systems should be examined in detail **(Fig. 6-54)**.

Features of severe ischemia:
- Systolic ankle pressure less than 50 mm Hg
- Systolic toe pressure is less than 30 mm Hg
- Ankle brachial index is less than 0.3
- Buerger's angle of insufficiency less than 30 degrees
- Capillary filling time more than 30 seconds
- Delayed reactive hyperemia time
- Presence of ischemic ulcers, gangrene

Causes of ischemic ulceration:
- **Large artery obliteration**
  - Atherosclerosis
  - Arterial embolism
- **Small artery obliteration**
  - Raynaud's disease
  - TAO
  - Small artery embolism
  - Diabetes mellitus
  - Scleroderma
  - Vasculitis
  - Infective causes
  - Physical agents like pressure, radiation, burns, trauma

Case sheet writing in a patient with peripheral arterial disease

History
Name: Age:
Occupation: Sex: Place/residence:

Chief complaints – Pain; Intermittent claudication; color changes; gangrene.

History of present illness
- Pain – origin, nature, character, duration, time of starting of pain, specific features, severity, aggravating or relieving factors
- Intermittent claudication – distance, location
- Rest pain in detail
- Situation/location of ulcer or gangrene
- Color changes
- Mode of onset and progression
- Discharge – duration, type of discharge, color of discharge, smell
- Fever – type, severity, duration
- History of cold, paresthesia – when started, progress
- History of impotence
- History of chest pain, angina, weakness limb, visual disturbances, postprandial angina, blood in stool, urinary symptoms
- History suggestive of superficial thrombophlebitis

Past history
- Past history of similar complaints
- Past history of trauma
- Tuberculosis, spinal diseases, diabetes, leprosy, malignancies, Raynaud's disease, autoimmune diseases, long-term drug therapy
- Past history of surgery like toe amputation, sympathectomy, vascular surgeries

Family history
- Family tree; history of tuberculosis, diabetes, malignancies; treatment history

Contd...

Contd...

Personal history
- History of smoking – duration
- History of chewing pan or other tobacco products
- History alcohol or other addictions

General examination
Anemia, edema, jaundice, clubbing, lymphadenopathy, pulse, blood pressure, temperature, attitude, nutrition, body weight

Local examination
Inspection
- Both lower limbs should be examined; then both upper limbs
- For signs of ischemia
- Color changes, change in skin texture, edema limb
- Muscle wasting
- Inspection of gangrene – site, extent, type (dry or wet), line of demarcation
- Ulceration, discharge – type, color, odor, foreign body, bone, etc.
- Swelling in the limb
- Surrounding skin – skip lesions
- Buerger's postural test; limb elevation and dependency
- Status of superficial veins; guttering of veins; capillary filling time; venous refilling time
- Limb deformity
- Relevant proximal part inspection – like examination of neck in upper limb ischemia for swelling

Palpation
- Local raise of temperature, tenderness
- Sensation
- Edema
- Gangrenous area – limb above the gangrene
- Capillary refilling; Harvey's venous refilling test
- Palpation of blood vessels – from below upwards – should be in a table
- Special tests for upper limb when indicated – elevated arm stress test (EAST); Roos test; costoclavicular compression maneuver; hyperabduction maneuver; Adson's test; Allen's test; cold and warm test; examination of supraclavicular fossa
- Special tests for lower limb – Crossed leg test (Fuchsig's); disappearing pulse syndrome; Buerger's postural test; guttering of vein; reactive hyperemia time test (Lewis)
- Branham's/Nicoladoni's sign
- Assessment of wasting of limb muscles or lengthening and widening by measurements
- Muscle power assessment
- Palpation of blood vessels for thrill
- Relevant

Auscultation
- Over femorals, renal and carotids for bruit

Examination of regional lymph nodes
Gait and relevant joint movements
Other relevant examination
Systemic examination – abdomen, respiratory, cardiac and central nervous systems

INVESTIGATIONS FOR ARTERIAL DISEASES

- **Blood tests:** Hb%, total count blood sugar, lipid profile, peripheral smear, platelet count, VDRL.
- **Doppler** (*Christian Johann Doppler*—Austrian physicist, 1842) to find out the site of block. Hand held Doppler is used by continuous wave ultrasound signals where transmitted beam and reflected beam will create Doppler shift; this frequency change is converted into an audio signal as a pulsatile sound.
- **Duplex scan:** It is a combination of B mode ultrasound and Doppler study. Difference in transmitted beam of the ultrasound and reflected beam is called as Doppler shift which is assessed and converted into audible signals. It is used to study the site, extent, severity of block, and also about collaterals. Audible sound—with normal flow and sound is important. Turbulence is heard to some extent with stenosed partially blocked artery. Audible sound will be absent if there is complete block. Using Doppler probe, blood pressure at various levels can be assessed. Pulse wave tracing along the artery is also important.
- **Ankle brachial pressure index (ABPI):** Refer Chapter 1.
- **Toe brachial pressure index (TBPI):** Refer Chapter 1.
- **Segmental pressure measurement:** Blood pressures are measured at thighs, calves, arms. *High thigh index <1.0 is suggestive of aortoiliac disease.* Blood pressure cuffs may be placed in the lower limb above the ankle, at midcalf and midthigh. Segmental BP is measured at multiple levels (upper and lower thigh, upper calf and ankle); pressure reductions between levels help to localize the occlusion; normally *pressure increases* as one moves further down the leg (>20 mm Hg gradient abnormal); test is inaccurate in calcified artery walls.
- **Plethysmography:** It measures the blood flow in limbs. Water filled volume recorder, air filled volume recorder or mercury in silastic gauze is used after occluding the venous outflow. It is a noninvasive method. Segmental

plethysmography using occlusion cuffs of 65 mm Hg pressure is placed at thigh, calf and ankle levels and then quantitative measure of pulsation is done.
- **Oscillometry:** For detection of presence/poor/absence of oscillations and identifying the level of block. Sudden drop in oscillations may be due to embolic obstruction. Level of amputation can be decided by this.
- **Angiography** (Enaz Moniz first did carotid angiography in 1927): *Retrograde transfemoral Seldinger angiography*: It is commonly done. It is done only when femorals (at least one of the femorals should be felt) are felt. If femoral pulsation is not felt then angiogram is done either *transbrachially (left brachial artery), or through transaortic direct puncture*. Indications for angiogram are—TAO; atherosclerosis; Raynaud's phenomenon; AV fistulas; hemangiomas; thoracic outlet syndrome (e.g. cervical rib); aneurysms; neoplastic conditions.
- Femoral artery is cannulated; needle is removed; guidewire is passed (under C-arm guidance); cannula is removed; through guidewire Seldinger (Sweden radiologist) arterial polythene catheter (5 French, 1.7 mm) is passed proximally in retrograde direction and water soluble iodine dye (sodium diatrizoate) is injected. A trial of 5 mL is injected initially to observe iodine sensitivity. Later full dose is injected. X-rays are taken to see the block, and its extent in the affected limb. Two types of arteriography are done. Catheter tip is kept in main aorta and 30–50 mL bolus of dye is injected to see main branches and their patterns (entire arterial tree)—is called as *free flush arteriography*. If catheter tip is placed in one of the main specific artery and dye is injected—is called as *selective angiography*. In TAO, *corkscrew* appearance due to dilatation of vasa vasorum is characteristic. *Distal run off through collaterals* (inverted tree/spider leg collaterals); blockage—sites, extent, and severity; *severe vasospasm causing corrugated/rippled artery*—are other specific findings. *Distal run off* is amount of dye filling in the main vessel distal to the obstruction through collaterals. If distal run off is good then ischemia is compensated. If distal run off is poor then ischemia is decompensated. If catheter is passed, still proximally angiogram of opposite side is possible. Seldinger technique can also be used (to study) to do renal angiogram to study renal artery stenosis, renal carcinomas, renal anomalies (vascular). *Complications* of retrograde angiogram are: Bleeding; dissection of vessel wall; formation of hematoma and pseudoaneurysm; atheroembolization into distal vessels (causes *blue toe syndrome*); thrombosis; AV fistula; infection; osmolarity discomfort (osmolarity of contrast agent is eight times of normal plasma); vasodilatation and hypotension; nephrotoxicity; anaphylaxis (4%).
- **Digital subtraction angiography (DSA):** Here artery is delineated in a better way by eliminating other tissues through computer system. AV fistulas, hemangiomas, lesion in circle of Willis, vascular tumors, and other vascular anomalies are well made out. Dye is injected either into an artery or vein. Injecting into a vein is technically easier but requires larger dose of the dye. Injecting into an artery is technically difficult but small dose of dye is sufficient. *Advantages are*—only vascular system is visualized; other systems are eliminated by computer subtraction. Small lesion, its location and details are better observed with greater clarity. *Disadvantages are* cost factor and availability. *Complications* are—anaphylaxis, bleeding, thrombosis.
- **CT angiogram** is very useful in aortic diseases and dissecting aneurysm.
- **Magnetic resonance angiogram (MRA):** MRA with gadolinium enhancement [time of flight (TOF)] is very useful noninvasive method. It is the test of choice for AV malformations.
- **US abdomen:** To see abdominal aneurysm or nature of aorta and other vessels.
- **Plain X-ray of the part:** To see calcifications in atherosclerosis, Monckeberg's arterial calcification; calcification in aneurysm, cervical rib, etc. (Figs. 6-56A and B).
- **Brown's vasomotor index:** Specific nerve of the ischemic limb is anesthetized like posterior tibial nerve or ulnar nerve (local anesthesia or spinal anesthesia is given to anesthetize entire limb). If the ischemic disease is at vasospasm stage (like in TAO), nerve block will relieve the sympathetic vasospasm and skin temperature rises. It is compared to mouth temperature of the patient.

Rise in skin temperature minus rise in mouth temperature divided by rise in mouth temperature is called as *Brown's vasomotor index*. If it is more than 3.5, it is due to vasospasm, and can be relieved by sympathectomy. If less than 3.5, sympathectomy is not beneficial. It can also be done by immersing the both the feet in water at 110°F temperature.
- **Study of blood flow:** Although specific it is less commonly used. Intramuscular injection of Xenon-133 in normal saline or Technetium-99m isotope injection is used to see the *clearance* as an assessment of blood flow in *leg muscles*. If isotope is injected intravenously, using gamma camera, direct visualization of artery is done. Using *electromagnetic flow meter*, rate of blood flow up to 1% also can be detected. But it is technically difficult.
- **Transcutaneous oximetry:** By placing polarographic electrodes over the skin over thigh, leg and foot oxygen tension ($TcPO_2$) can be measured which is reflection of underlying tissue perfusion. Normal $TcPO_2$ in the foot is 50–60 mm Hg. Level less than 40 mm Hg shows inadequate wound healing. Level below 10 mm Hg suggests critical ischemia with complete failure of wound healing.

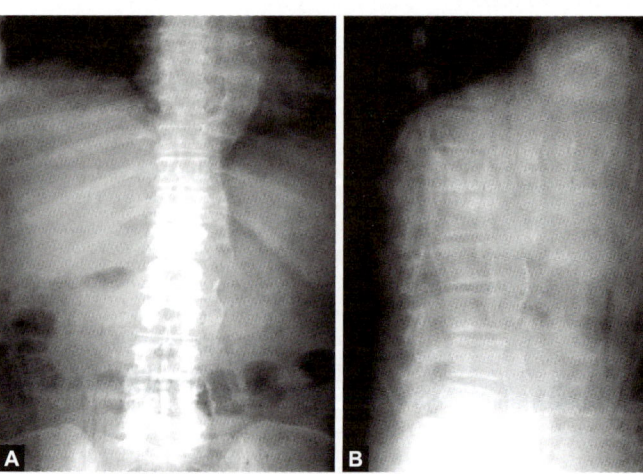

Figs. 6-56A and B X-ray abdomen AP and lateral view showing *calcified aorta*.

- **Treadmill test (TMT)** can be used to measure the claudication distance. TMT is also used for assessing cardiac system. ECG, 2-D echocardiography should also be done.
- **Evaluation of vasculitis:** It is done by doing ESR, C-reactive protein, analyzing the antinuclear antibodies, antibodies against neutrophil granule constituents [Antineutrophil cytoplasmic antibody (ANCA)] either c-ANCA (cytoplasmic) or p-ANCA (perinuclear).
- Intravascular ultrasound (IVUS) and Skin perfusion pressure tests (SAPP test) are other newer specific tests for vascular system.

■ LIMB ISCHEMIA

Functional Limb Ischemia
Here flow of blood is normal when limbs are at rest; but will not be increased during exercise. It presents as claudication. It is defined as *"muscle discomfort in the limb reproducibly produced by exercise and relieved by rest within 10 minutes."*

Critical Limb Ischemia
It is persistently recurring ischemic rest pain for 2 weeks requiring opiate analgesia or ulceration or gangrene of the foot or toes with an ankle systolic pressure <50 mm Hg or toe systolic pressure <30 mm Hg (The TransAtlantic Intersociety Consensus).

Pregangrene
It is the changes in tissue which indicate that blood supply is precarious and it will soon be inadequate to keep the tissues alive and presents with rest pain, color changes, edema, *hyperesthesia* with or without ischemic ulceration. Pallor on elevation, congestion of dependency, guttered veins, tissue tenderness, scaling of skin are the typical features.

Gangrene
It is *macroscopic* death of tissue *in situ* with putrefaction. It can occur in toes, fingers, limbs, localized area of skin and subcutaneous tissues, muscles, organs like appendix, bowel, gallbladder, testis and pancreas. It is black/brown (colored) senseless/painless; pulseless (no perfusion); with loss of temperature; and loss of function.

Classification of gangrene:
Clinical:
1. Dry gangrene
2. Wet/moist gangrene
- *Traumatic:*
  - Mechanical
    - Usually acute except radiation
    - Direct like crushes, splints, plaster
    - Indirect pressure by fracture bone, tourniquet, drug induced (thiopentone, ergot, adrenaline)
  - Chemical corrosives—acid/alkali
  - Thermal—burns, frost bite
  - Electrical
  - Radiation causes chronic type of ischemia/gangrene:
- *Infective:* Usually acute
  - Nonspecific due to boil, carbuncle, cancrum oris, Meleney's postoperative progressive synergistic gangrene
  - Specific—Gas gangrene
- *Occlusive:* Thrombosis, embolism, atherosclerosis, TAO, Raynaud's syndrome, arteritis, aneurysm, compression by cervical rib, tumors, radiation fibrosis
- *Neurogenic:* Tabes dorsalis, syringomyelia, leprosy, hemiplegia
- *Others:* Diabetes mellitus, polycythemia rubra vera, systemic lupus erythematosus (SLE), polyarteritis nodosa, scleroderma

Dry gangrene: It is dry, desiccated, mummified tissue caused by gradual slowing of bloodstream. There is a line of demarcation between dead and viable tissue and is localized. It is noninfected gangrene.

Wet gangrene: It is due to both arterial and venous block or sudden arterial blockade with superadded putrefaction and infection. It spreads proximally and there is no or unclear line of demarcation. It spreads faster. It is infected gangrene. It is soft and boggy greenish, bluish, or purplish color with blister having offensive smell.

Features of ischemia:
- Marked pallor, purple blue cyanosed appearance
- Thinning of skin
- Diminished hair
- Loss of subcutaneous fat
- Brittle nails, with transverse ridges
- Ulceration in digits
- Wasting of muscles
- Tenderness and temperature (cold)

Note: Pressure at arterial end of capillary is 32 mm Hg; pressure at venular end of capillary is 12 mm Hg.

Necrosis: It is *microscopic* cell death.
Sequestrum: It is dead bone *in situ*.
Slough: It is dead soft tissue.
Eschar: It is dried thick dead tissue/slough; seen in burns.
Atheroma *(Greek-gruel):* It is raised, focal, intimal fibrofatty plaque containing a core of lipid with fibrous cap.
Embolus *(Greek-peg):* It is an abnormal, intravascular solid/liquid/gaseous material which is undissolved, transported from its site of origin to distant site/sites.
Arteriosclerosis is thickening of arterial wall with loss of elasticity of arterial wall.

■ DISEASES OF THE ARTERIES

Classification of arterial diseases

Congenital: Berry aneurysm; arteriovenous malformations—*Robertson giant limb*
Traumatic: Mechanical, chemical, thermal, electrical, radiation
Infective: Nonspecific (mycotic), specific
Occlusive:
- *In the lumen:* Thrombosis, embolism
- *In the wall:*
  - Degenerative: Atherosclerosis, Monckberg sclerosis
  - Vasospastic: Raynaud's disease, TAO, acrocyanosis, drug induced like ergots/lead/arsenic
  - Inflammatory: Syphilis, idiopathic arteritis
  - Dilatation: Aneurysm, livedo reticularis
  - Altered vasomotor status: Erythromelalgia
- *Outside the wall:*
  - Congenital: Cervical rib
  - Traumatic: Radiation fibrosis, malunited fracture
  - Inflammatory mass compressing
  - Neoplastic: Tumor pressing over artery
  - Others: Ainhum

Atherosclerosis

Risk factors for atherosclerosis: *Firm causes:* Hypercholesterolemia, hypertriglyceridemia and hyperlipidemia;

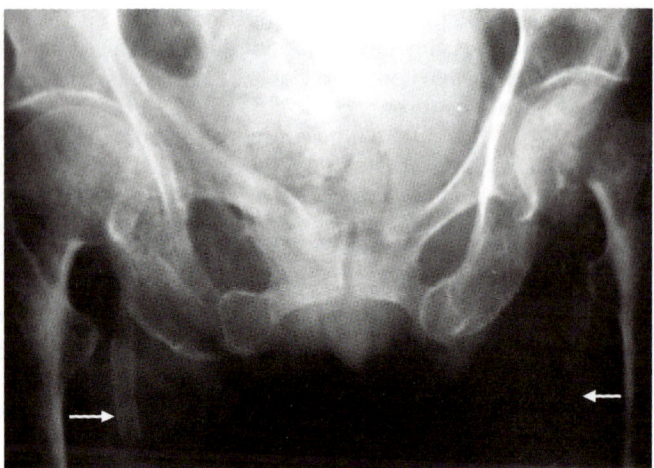

Fig. 6-57 Plain X-ray showing *calcified femoral arteries* due to atherosclerosis.

cigarette smoking; hypertension; diabetes mellitus. *Relative causes:* Elderly; male; sedentary life; family history; hyperhomocystinemia. Atherosclerosis can cause ischemia at various levels—foot, leg, thigh, entire limb and can be bilateral disease; upper limb ischemia—depends on the vessel involved and extent of block it has caused (Fig. 6-57).

Thromboangiitis Obliterans (TAO/Buerger's Disease, Leo Buerger—Urologist)

It is a disease exclusively seen in *males* of young age group (not common in females due to genetic reason). It is seen only in smokers and tobacco users. Usually starts in lower limb, may start on one side and later on the other. Upper limb involvement occurs usually after lower limb is diseased. It is a panvasculitis.

Pathogenesis: Smoke contains *carbon monoxide and nicotinic acid* → causes initially vasospasm and hyperplasia of intima → thrombosis and so obliteration of vessels occur. Commonly medium sized vessels are involved. *Panarteritis* is common. Usually involvement is segmental. Eventually artery, vein and nerve are together involved. Nerve involvement causes rest pain. Patient presents with features of ischemia in the limb. Once blockage occurs, plenty of collaterals open up depending on the site of blockage, either around knee joint or around buttock. Once collaterals open up, through these collaterals, blood supply is maintained to the ischemic area. It is called as *compensatory peripheral vascular disease*. If patient continues to smoke, disease progresses into the collaterals, blocking them eventually, leading to severe ischemia and is called as *decompensatory peripheral vascular disease*. It is presently called as *critical limb ischemia*. It causes rest pain, ulceration, gangrene. It is common in lower socioeconomic group. It is probably an autoimmune disease with often familial susceptibility. Claudication is *common in foot and calf*. Later ischemia, rest pain, ulcers, gangrene develop. Claudication is less common in thigh and buttock. Retrograde Seldinger angiogram shows blockage—sites, extent, severity is noted; *corkscrew* appearance of the vessel due to dilatation of vasa vasorum; inverted tree/spider leg collaterals; *severe vasospasm causing corrugated/rippled artery; distal run off* is amount of dye filling in the main vessel distal to the obstruction through collaterals. If distal run off is good then ischemia is compensated. If distal run off is poor then ischemia is decompensated.

Raynaud's Phenomenon

It was first described by Maurice Raynaud in 1862. It is an episodic recurrent vasospasm, i.e. arteriolar spasm. It leads to sequence of clinical features called as Raynaud's syndrome. It is common in digits. It is spasmodic contraction of digital arterioles precipitated on exposure to cold or stress causing initial pallor, later cyanosis with pain and paresthesia; eventually hyperemic response causing marked rubor.

Raynaud's syndrome: It is sequence of clinical features due to *arteriolar spasm*.
1. *Local syncope:* It is due to vasospasm, causing white, cold palm and digits along with tingling and numbness.
2. *Local asphyxia:* It is due to accumulation of deoxygenated blood as the result of vasospasm causing bluish discoloration of palm and digits with burning sensation (it is due to accumulated metabolites).
3. *Local recovery:* It is due to relief of spasm in the arteriole, leading to return of blood to the circulation causing flushing and pain in digits and palm (Pain is due to increased tissue tension).
4. *Local gangrene:* If spasm persists for more than ischemic time (more than one hour in upper limb), then digits go for ulceration and gangrene. Does not occur regularly but is an occasional event in the cycle.

> **Causes for Raynaud's phenomenon**
> 1. *Raynaud's disease:* It is seen in females, usually bilateral. It occurs in upper limb with normal peripheral pulses. It is due to arteriolar spasm in upper limb (hand) due to abnormal sensitivity to cold. Patient develops blanching, cyanosis and later flushing as Raynaud's syndrome. Occasionally if spasm persists, gangrene may develop. Symptoms can be precipitated and observed by placing hands in cold water.
> 2. *Working with vibrating tools:* Like pneumatic road drills, chain saws, wood cutting, and fishermen traveling in machine boats—seen in males.
> 3. *Collagen vascular diseases:* Like Scleroderma, rheumatoid diseases causing vasculitis (all autoimmune diseases).
> 4. *Other causes:* Cervical rib, Buerger's disease, Scalene syndrome. It is often associated with CREST syndrome (Calcinosis cutis, Raynaud's phenomenon, Esophageal defects, Sclerodactyly, Telangiectasia).

■ ACUTE ARTERIAL OCCLUSION

Causes: (1) Trauma; (2) Embolism.

Traumatic Acute Arterial Occlusion

- Causes: (1) Thrombus due to trauma; (2) Subintimal hematoma; (3) Acute compartment syndrome; (4) During femoral or brachial arterial catheterization, either for diagnostic or therapeutic procedures.
- *Pathophysiology:* Brain tolerates ischemia only for 4 minutes; heart for 20 minutes; limbs for 6 hours in profound acute ischemia. Skin and bone are relatively resistant to ischemia compared to nerves. Nervous system is most sensitive for ischemia. When peripheral nerve is affected by ischemia, it causes pain, paresthesia and paralysis. Muscles play a major role in limb ischemia as muscles account for the 75% of limb weight.

- *Features:* History of trauma; *pain, swelling at the site, pallor, pulselessness, cold limb (pallor).*
- *Acute compartment syndrome*: There is sudden increase in compartment pressure more than capillary perfusion pressure (30 mm Hg) causing impairment of tissue perfusion. It is common in anterior compartment of leg and in front of forearm. Here because of the closed compartment, pressure increases following fracture, hematoma which compresses over the vessel. It leads to blockade of vessel causing acute ischemia of the limb presenting with severe pain, pallor, pulselessness. Measurement of *intracompartmental pressure* by placing a needle cannula directly into the compartment and using pressure transducer is ideal way to confirm the condition as Doppler still may show strong signal of pulse.

Embolism

- It is due to a solid material which is floating and traveling in the bloodstream, eventually blocking the vessel on its pathway.

> **Features of embolism:**
> - Earlier history of claudication is absent but history suggestive of disease for source of emboli will be present
> - Sudden, dramatic, rapid development of pain with numbness
> - Limb becomes rapidly cold and mottled with blebs
> - Loss of sensation and movements
> - Absence of distal pulses but forcible, expansile, prominent proximal pulse. For example: Prominent femoral artery pulsation with embolic block at popliteal level
> - Toxic features

- **Arterial emboli:** *Cardiac source (80%)*—due to mural thrombus following mitral stenosis and atrial fibrillation (50%); myocardial infarction (25%); others (5%). *Noncardiac (10%)*—aneurysms (5%); others (4%); paradoxical (1%). *Idiopathic* is 10%. Cervical rib causing poststenotic dilatation of subclavian artery can cause emboli. *Venous emboli* are due to DVT causing pulmonary embolism. *Fat and air embolism are other types.*
- Complete sudden embolic block causes cool, waxy-white pallor whereas a partial occlusion causes pallor on elevation and rubor on dependency. *Commonest site of arterial emboli—common femoral artery (40%)*; aortic bifurcation, cerebral vessel, iliac vessels account for 15% each; upper limb and popliteal vessels are 10% each; visceral/mesenteric is 5%.
- **Saddle embolus:** It is an embolus blocking at *bifurcation of aorta.* Causes: Mural thrombus after myocardial infarction and mitral stenosis with atrial fibrillation; aortic aneurysm. The embolus which blocks at aortic bifurcation is usually large.
- **Fat embolism:** It is commonly seen after *fracture femur, tibia, or multiple fractures* and occasionally following electroconvulsive therapy, usually occurs in 24–72 hours. It is due to aggregation of chylomicrons, derived from bone marrow, causing fat embolism. *It is often a fatal condition.* Features: Cerebral: Drowsy, restless, disoriented, constricted pupils, pyrexia, and coma. *Pulmonary:* Cyanosis, tachypnea, right heart failure, froth in mouth and nostrils, fat droplets in sputum, eventually respiratory failure. *Cutaneous:* Petechial hemorrhages in the skin. *Retinal artery emboli is the earliest sign to appear, causing striae hemorrhages, fluffy exudates confirmed on fundoscopic examination. Kidney*: Blockage of renal arterioles results in fat droplets in urine.
- **Air embolism:** *Causes:* Through venous access like IV cannula; during artificial pneumothorax; during surgeries of neck and axilla; traumatic opening of major veins sucking air inside causing embolism; during Fallopian tube insufflation; during illegal abortion. Amount of air required to cause air embolism is *50 mL.* When the air enters the right atrium, it gets churned up forming foam which enters the right ventricle and blocks the pulmonary artery.

Aneurysms

- It is dilatation of localized segment of arterial system. It is due to weakening of the wall of artery. *True* aneurysm contains all three layers of artery. *False* aneurysm contains single layer of fibrous tissue as wall of the sac and it usually occurs after trauma.
- Types: *(a) Fusiform*—uniform dilatation of entire circumference of arterial wall; *(b) saccular*—dilatation of part of circumference of the arterial wall; *(c) dissecting*—through a tear in the intima, blood dissects between inner and outer part of tunica media of the artery.
- Causes: *Acquired*: (1) *Degenerative:* Atherosclerosis (*commonest cause*); mucoid degeneration of intima and media (in South African young Negroes). (2) *Traumatic:* Direct; indirect like in post stenotic dilatation by cervical rib; traumatic AV aneurysmal sac; aneurysm due to irradiation (due to dryness and destruction of vasa vasorum causing weakening of the wall). (3) *Infective:* Syphilis; mycotic; tuberculosis (in lung); arteritis; polyarteritis nodosa; acute sepsis. (4) *Collagen diseases* like Marfan's syndrome, Ehlers-Danlos syndrome. *Congenital*: Berry aneurysm; cirsoid aneurysm; congenital AV fistula.
- *Sites:* Aorta; femoral; popliteal; subclavian; cerebral, mesenteric, renal, splenic arteries. *Commonest is true, fusiform, atherosclerotic, aortic aneurysms. Berry's aneurysms are* multiple aneurysms occurring in circle of Willis.
- *Clinical features of aneurysm:* (1) *Asymptomatic.* (2) *Symptoms: Swelling* which is pulsatile; *pain* may be dull aching/severe acute type due to sudden stretching of artery/bursting type when it ruptures or forms a hematoma; referred pain due to pressing over adjacent nerves may be seen; *features of ischemia* of the distal limb; painful, *cyanotic distal edema* due to venous compression. (3) *On palpation:* Swelling at the site is *pulsatile (expansile)*, smooth, soft, warm, compressible, with thrill on palpation and bruit on auscultation. Swelling reduces in size when pressed proximally; moves sideward but not along the line of artery. There is often altered sensation due to compression of nerves; erosion into bones, joints, trachea or esophagus; aneurysm with thrombosis can throw an embolus causing gangrene of toes, digits, often extending proximally also.
- *Differential diagnosis*: (1) Pyogenic abscess: Abscess has to be always confirmed by aspiration; especially in axilla, popliteal region, and groin. (2) Vascular tumors. (3) Pulsating tumors: Sarcomas, pulsating secondaries.

(4) Pseudocyst of pancreas mimics aortic aneurysm. (5) AV fistula.
- **Abdominal aneurysms:** *Abdominal aortic aneurysm is the commonest aortic aneurysm. It has got 2% incidence. Causes:* Atherosclerosis: 95%. Others: Syphilis, dissecting, traumatic, collagen diseases. *Classification I:* (1) Infrarenal—commonest 95%. (2) Suprarenal 5%. Classification II: (1) *Asymptomatic:* Found incidentally either on clinical examination or on angiography or on ultrasound. Repair is required if diameter is more than 5.5 cm on ultrasound. (2) *Symptomatic without rupture*: Present as *back pain, abdominal pain, mass abdomen* which is smooth, soft, nonmobile, not moving with respiration, vertically placed above the umbilical level, pulsatile both in supine as well as in knee-elbow position with same intensity, resonant on percussion. GIT, urinary, venous symptoms can also occur. Hypertension, diabetes, cardiac problems should be looked for and dealt with. If aneurysm is *more than 5.5 cm then surgery is the choice.* (3) *Symptomatic ruptured aortic aneurysm:* Risk of rupture is 1%, if diameter is within 5.5 cm in size. Risk increases to 20% once the diameter ≥7 cm. It may be *anterior rupture* (20%) into the free peritoneal cavity causing severe shock and very early *death*; or *posterior rupture* (80%) with formation of *retroperitoneal hematoma* of large size causing severe back pain, hypotension, and shock, absence of femoral pulses and with palpable mass in the abdomen. Emergency management is needed.
- Effects of aneurysm: Thrombosis and emboli formation; peripheral ischemia; rupture; erosion into adjacent structures like bone, bowel, pressure on organs like esophagus (causing dysphagia); sexual dysfunction; aortoduodenal fistula; aortovenacaval fistula; spinal cord ischemia; infection.
- **Peripheral aneurysms:** Popliteal aneurysm is the commonest (70%) peripheral aneurysm. It is 65% bilateral. Twenty-five percent cases are associated with abdominal aortic aneurysm. Seventy-five percent causes complications in 5 years. Presentations are—swelling in popliteal region which is smooth, soft, pulsatile, well-localized, warm, and compressible, often with thrill and bruit. *It may mimic a pyogenic abscess.* Thrombosis and emboli from popliteal aneurysm can cause distal gangrene which may spread proximally and may lead to amputation. Rupture may cause torrential hemorrhage.
- **Dissecting aneurysm:** It is the dissection of media of the aorta after splitting through intima creating a channel in the *media of* the vessel wall. *Causes:* Hypertension (It is associated in 80% of dissecting aneurysms); cystic medial necrosis; Marfan's syndrome and collagen diseases; trauma; weakening of the elastic layers of the media due to shear forces. It is always seen in thoracic aorta, common in ascending aorta (70%).

Classification (*DeBakey's*): *Type I:* Dissection begins in ascending aorta and extends into descending thoracic aorta (70%). *Type II:* Dissection origins and extends only up to the origin of the major vessels. It is safer type with fewer complications. *Type III:* Dissection begins in the descending thoracic aorta beyond the origin of the left subclavian artery. Dissecting aneurysm can be acute, chronic, healed dissecting aneurysm which communicates distally again to aorta as *double barreled aorta*.

- **Mycotic aneurysm:** It is a *misnomer*. It is not due to fungus but due to *bacterial* (commonly *Staphylococcus, Streptococcus*) infection. Origin of bacteria may be from any site of infection in the body. Common etiology is bacterial *endocarditis* but could be any infective site. Common vessels involved are aorta, visceral, head and neck and intracranial. Commonly it is saccular, multilobed, with a narrow neck. Patient presents with fever, toxemia and tender pulsatile mass if it is in the periphery.

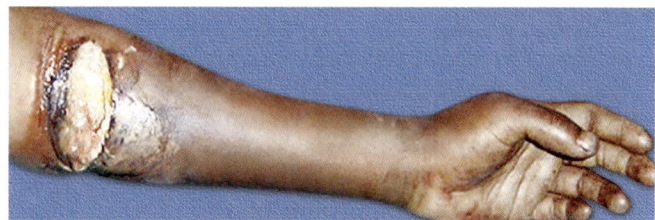

Fig. 6-58 *Gas gangrene.*

Other Conditions

Condition and Pathology	Features
Acrocyanosis (Crurum Puellarum Frigidum): Due to chronic persistent arteriolar constriction with slow rate of blood flow in young females often with endocrine dysfunction.	Persistent, painless, cyanosis seen in fingers, and often in legs aggravated on exposure to cold; paresthesia and chilblains.
Erythromelalgia/Erythralgia: It is severe, episodic burning pain and redness in the feet. Sensation of heat is so severe that patient keeps the feet in cold water to reduce it.	Flushing in the feet; prominent veins; warmness in the skin; severe hyperesthesia is typical; even touching can be painful.
Subclavian Steal Syndrome: Following obstruction of the first part of subclavian artery, vertebral artery provides collateral circulation to the arm by reversing its blood flow.	This causes *cerebral ischemia with syncopal attacks, visual disturbances, and diminished blood pressure in the affected limb.* Symptoms will be aggravated by arm exercise.
Takayasu's Pulseless Arteritis: It is progressive, initially symptomless panarteritis involving aortic arch and branches of aorta of unknown etiology, probably immunological. It is common in young females (85%); common in Japan; commonly involves subclavian artery; involves all layers of arteries of upper limb and neck; often bilateral.	Fever, myalgia, arthralgia, upper limb claudication; absence of pulses in upper limb/limbs; neck; hypertension; fainting on turning the neck or change in position; atrophy of face; thrill/bruit along major arteries of upper limb and neck are the features. Optic nerve atrophy without papilledema; weakness and paresthesia of upper limb; cerebral softening, convulsions, hemiplegia, myocardial infarction, embolism can occur.

Contd...

Contd...

Infective Gangrene: It is development of gangrene commonly due to bacterial infection causing infective thrombosis of local end arteries leading into gangrene of that particular area.	Cancrum oris; gas gangrene; carbuncle; Fournier's gangrene are the examples. It can involve both upper and lower limbs.
Diabetic Foot and Diabetic Gangrene: Callosities; ulceration; abscess and cellulitis of foot; osteomyelitis of different bones of foot—metatarsalls, cuneiforms, calcaneum; diabetic gangrene; arthritis of joints.	Pain in the foot; ulceration; absence of sensation; absence of pulsations in the foot (dorsalis pedis and posterior tibial); loss of joint movements; abscesses; change in temperature and color when gangrene sets in.
Cancrum oris (Noma): *Discussed in oral cavity*	
Gas Gangrene: Infective gangrene caused by clostridial organisms (*Clostridium welchii, C. oedematiens, C. septicum, C. histiolyticum*) mainly affecting skeletal muscles. It can be fulminant, massive, single muscle or of subcutaneous tissue **(Fig. 6-58)**.	*Incubation period*: 1-2 days; Toxemia, fever, tachycardia, pallor; wound under tension with foul smelling discharge; *Khaki brown* colored skin due to hemolysis; Exposed muscle typically brick red/ green/ black colored; Crepitus felt; liver dysfunction, renal failure.
Frostbite: Due to exposure to cold wind or high altitude (below freezing point) there will be arteriolar spasm leading to protein denaturation and cell destruction.	Part is edematous with blistering, deep ulcer and gangrene, painless and waxy; common in old age during cold spells.
Chilblains (Perniosis): Exposure to intense cold causes cutaneous arteriolar constriction.	Only superficial ulcers.
Ainhum: A fissure at the interphalangeal joint of the toe develops which forms fibrous/constriction band that encircle the digit causing necrosis and dry gangrene of toe which eventually leads to autoamputation of the toe **(Fig. 6-59)**.	Common in males but do occur in females; common in Blacks and Negroes; often bilateral; common in 5th toe.
Morvan's Disease: *Painless whitlow* seen in fingers in patients with syringomyelia. May be associated with type I Arnold Chiari malformation. Olivier d'Anger described syringomyelia in 1824 wherein there is formation of cavity in spinal cord along with fourth ventricle with thinning of neural tissue component.	Neuropathic ulceration/gangrene in fingers. There are sensory disturbances in upper limb, weakness of hands and loss of pain and temperature sensation in hands, progressive kyphoscoliosis.
Upper Limb Ischemia: Rare entity when compared to lower limb ischemia. *Causes*: Thoracic outlet syndrome; Raynaud's phenomenon; embolism due to causes like arterial fibrillation; trauma; TAO; atherosclerosis, Takayasu's arteritis; scleroderma.	Upper limb claudication; ischemic rest pain; ischemic features with ulcers and gangrene in fingers; Adson's test +ive; hyperaddduction test +ive; Roos test+ ive; Allen's test is useful. *Investigations*: Arterial Doppler, subclavian angiogram, investigations to confirm vasculitis; blood sugar; lipid profile.

Arteriovenous fistula (AVF)	*Congenital AVF*	*Traumatic AVF*

Abnormal communication between artery and vein
Types:
• Congenital
• Acquired
  1. Traumatic
  2. Therapeutic (*Cimino fistula*) **(Fig. 6-60)**
	Sites:
	Limbs either part [fingers or toes] or whole; lungs; circle of Willis in brain; bowel, liver
	Features:
	• Lengthening of limb
	• Limb girth is increased [*Robertson's giant limb*]
	• Warm; with continuous thrill; and machinery murmur all over the lesion
	• Dilated arterialized varicose veins; bone erosion
	• Because of hyperdynamic circulation–increased cardiac output and congestive cardiac failure
	Complications:
	Hemorrhage; thrombosis; cardiac failure
		Changes at the level of fistula—
		A dilatation with a fibrous sac between artery and vein—*aneurysmal sac*—warm, pulsatile, smooth, soft, compressible swelling which reduces in size, with reduce in thrill and bruit when pressure applied to the artery proximal to fistula (*Nicoladoni's sign or Branham's sign*)
		Changes below the level of fistula—distal part becomes ischemic due to diversion of blood flow; arterialization of high pressure veins and valvular incompetence results in varicose veins
		Changes proximal to fistula—
		Cardiac failure due to hyperdynamic circulation

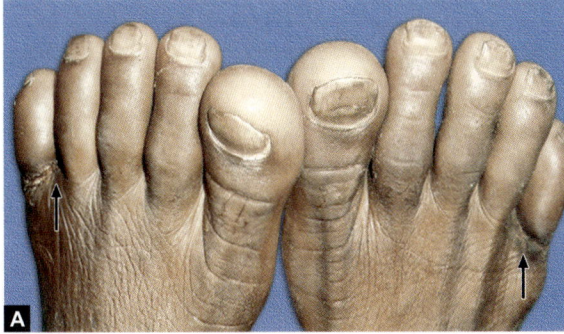 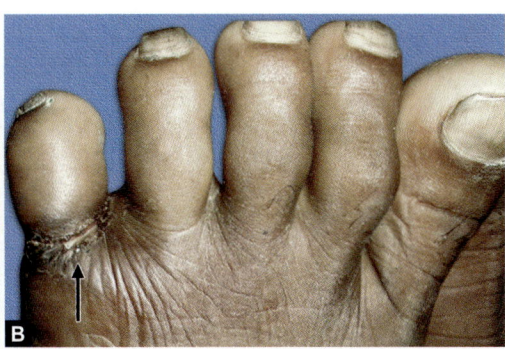

Figs. 6-59A and B Typical Ainhum. Note: It is bilateral. Note *the constriction ring in the little toe*. It may go for autoamputation. It needs Z-plasty. It is common in Blacks and Negroes.

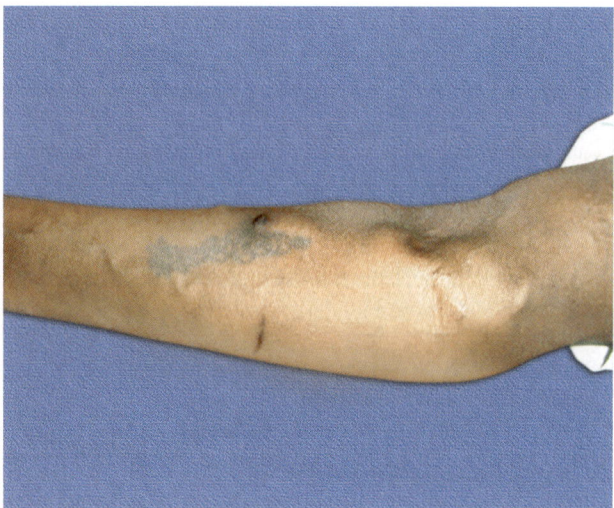

Fig. 6-60 AV fistula done for hemodialysis *(Cimino fistula)*.

CASE DISCUSSION

A 55-year-old male smoker presents with vague pain in the epigastric region with persistent back pain. He also has got claudication in the both thighs and legs. He is diabetic and hypertensive on medications. There is no relevant family history. There are no syncope attacks.

What all possibilities you will think of?
It is probable a case of atherosclerosis involving aorta and its branches. Epigastric pain could be due to aortic aneurysm in relation to his back pain or due to chronic mesenteric ischemia. It is better to ask the history of recurrent colicky abdominal pain, bloody stool.

How will you examine this patient?
Both limbs should be examined in detail for features of ischemia. Peripheral pulses should be examined from below upwards on both sides. Muscle wasting should be assessed. Abdomen is examined for aortic aneurysm which is pulsatile, vertically placed in the midline; smooth, soft, non-mobile, resonant, pulsation will not alter with change of position or knee elbow position; located above the umbilical level. Upper limb and neck pulsations should be checked. Palpable thrill at femoral and carotid area should be looked for. Auscultation for bruit at femoral, renal, subclavian and carotid area should be checked.

How you will evaluate?
Hematocrit, blood sugar, renal parameters (important in relation to aortic aneurysm), lipid profile are basic but essential tests. Ultrasound abdomen, duplex scan (arterial Doppler), CT abdomen with CT angiogram are other essential investigations needed. Aneurysm size, extent, status of renal arteries, presence of thrombus in the aneurysm, status of iliofemoral segments, distal run off, collateral status should be checked.

CHAPTER 7

Examination and Clinical Approach in Venous Diseases

Competency: SU27.5; SU27.6; AN19.3; AN20.5; AN20.9.

Venous disease is a morbid disease. Deep venous thrombosis (DVT), varicose veins, venous ulcers are the most commonly seen venous diseases even though congenital anomalies and rare syndromes are also often seen in clinical practice. Venous anatomy of the limbs is more complex with variations compared to arterial anatomy. Venous physiology is also more complex (Figs. 7-1 to 7-3).

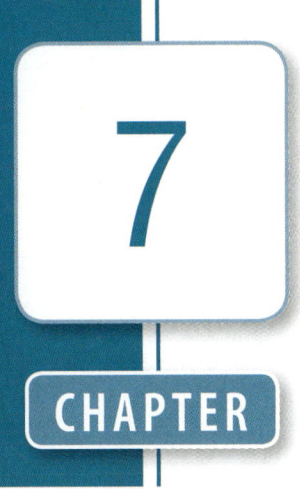

Fig. 7-1 Deep venous thrombosis with *venous gangrene*.

- Varicose vein is **dilated, tortuous and elongated** superficial vein with reversal of blood flow due to incompetence of valves as a result of continuous dilatation under pressure in a course of time. It **is inelastic, pouched and friable with permanent loss of valvular efficiency**. It is seen only in human beings due to erect posture. It is not seen in animals.
- Incidence of varicose veins is 5–20% in general population.
- It is common in females due to progesterone hormone, which relaxes venous wall; it is common in those who stand for long time—conductors, nurses, doctors, athletes (due to muscle contraction); common after superficial thrombophlebitis which causes venous valve destruction; secondary causes like pregnancy, abdominal tumors, ovarian cyst, fibroid, retroperitoneal tumors, retroperitoneal fibrosis, ascites, loaded colon can cause varicose veins. Arteriovenous fistula, congenital or acquired can cause varicose veins.

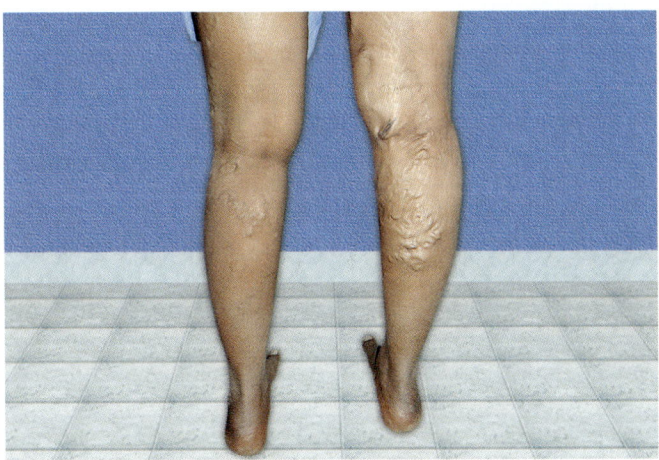

Fig. 7-2 *Varicose* veins in both lower limbs.

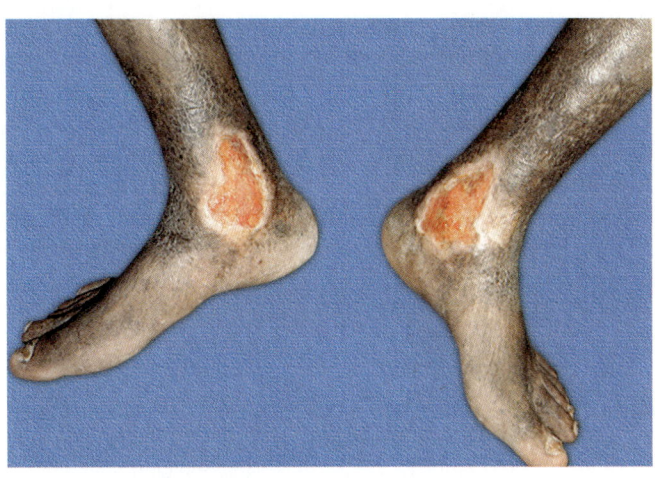

Fig. 7-3 *Venous ulcers* in both legs.

- Other than lower limb, varicose vein can also occur as esophageal varices (submucosa of lower 1/3rd of esophagus), gastric fundal varices, hemorrhoids (submucosa of anal canal), varicocele (pampiniform plexus of veins) or vulval/ovarian varices.
- Varicose vein/venous diseases are more complex condition with more morbidity.

Types of varicose veins
- Long saphenous vein varicosity.
- Short saphenous vein varicosity.
- Varicose veins due to perforator incompetence.
- Thread veins (dermal flares): Are small varices in the skin usually around ankle which look like dilated, red or purple network of veins of < 1 mm in size.
- Reticular varices: Are slightly larger than thread veins located in subcutaneous region 1–3 mm in size.
- Combinations of any of above.
- **It can be**—Primary varicose veins; Secondary varicose veins; Reticular veins (Venulectasia); Telangiectasias (Spider veins, Hyphen webs, Thread veins).
- *Corona phlebectatica* are blue telangiectasias on the medial aspect of the *foot below the malleolus* around ankle level.
- More than five such lesions are the best independent predictor of the skin changes.

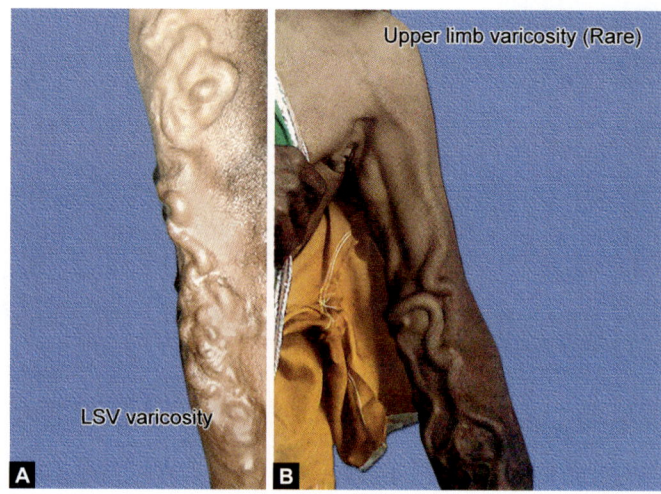

Figs. 7-4A and B (A) Varicose vein leg of great/long saphenous vein. It is *tortuous, elongated, dilated* vein. (B) Upper limb venous varicosity is a rare entity.

History of working in computer for long time is important as it may cause thrombosis of the deep veins *(e-thrombosis)*.

Chief Complaints

- Pain in the leg/thigh/foot of significant duration present on one or both side.
- Feeling of tiredness and aching sensation in lower limb especially during night.
- Swelling/*dilated veins* in the leg of significant duration.
- Swelling around ankle during evening.
- Itching of skin/pigmentation/ulceration in the leg with duration **(Figs. 7-4 and 7-5)**.

History of Present Illness

Pain

- History of pain in the leg/foot/or thigh with duration should be noted. Origin of pain and its severity, nature

■ HISTORY

Name:

Address: It is not commonly seen in Africa. Deep vein thrombosis is more common in cold countries.

Age: Varicose veins are often seen in adults and middle aged individuals but can occur in young individuals due to congenital vascular abnormality.

Sex: Varicose vein is more common in females (10:1).

Occupation: Varicose veins are more common in people who stand for long hours like bus conductors, nurses, doctors, surgeons, manual labourers, watchmen, athletes, traffic policemen, etc. Occupation also may exacerbate the condition.

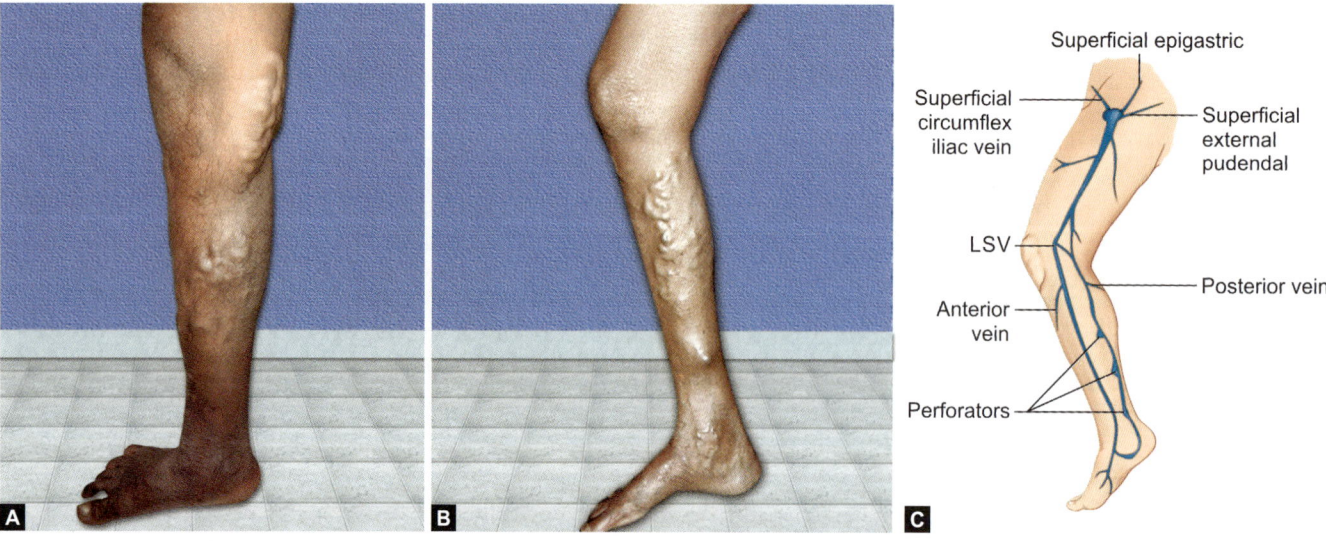

Figs. 7-5A to C Long saphenous vein varicosity. *Note the prominent veins and blow outs.* Note the diagrammatic representation of varicose veins.

of onset whether acute or insidious should be asked. Character of pain—*dull aching or cramping* should be asked. Whether pain gets aggravated by walking/standing should be noted. Dull aching pain along the line of the vein is typical and usually gets aggravated in the evening and relieved by lying down. Pain in calf of short duration, may be due to co-existing deep vein thrombosis *(DVT)*. Pain also can be due to ulcer/periostitis/infection.

- Often severity of the symptoms is not related to the severity of varicose veins. Small varicose veins may be more symptomatic than large one. In bilateral varicose veins, only one limb may be symptomatic and other limb may not.
- Bursting severe pain while walking may be due to deep vein thrombosis.
- Crampy pain during night *(night cramps)* is very common in these patients.
- Feeling of heaviness is common.
- History of difficulty in walking and standing should be asked.

Pigmentation

It is due to stasis and release of chemicals and usually occurs around ankle region. It is associated with itching and often ulceration. Its duration, exaggeration or relieving factors should be asked for.

Ulcer (Figs. 7-6A and B)

History of mode of onset, duration, site of onset should be asked. *Ulcer* on the medial aspect of the ankle is due to long saphenous vein varicosity; on the lateral aspect is due to short saphenous vein varicosity. **History of discharge from ulcer**—its type, smell, quantity signifies the severity of the infection. History of itching and bleeding in the ulcer bed are also (important) to be noted. **Painful ulcers** in leg are seen in arteriovenous fistula (AVF).

Other History:
- **History of fever** suggestive of thrombophlebitis.
- **History of trauma**—Often minor trauma precipitates ulcer formation in patients with varicose vein.
- **History of bleeding from the vein/ulcer** is an important presentation.
- **History of lump in the abdomen**: Pelvic mass (uterus/ovary/rectum) pregnancy may compress IVC/iliac veins and cause bilateral varicose veins. If compression is one side iliac veins, then varicose vein is unilateral.
- **History of similar complaints on the other leg**: Varicose veins are often bilateral.

Swelling

Swelling around the ankle is often noticed which may be due to venous congestion around the area. Its duration; whether regressed any time with or without any medication; or progressive; relation to work/standing/lying down should be noted. History suggestive of difficulty/altered gait due to pain/swelling/deformity should be noted. Area where complications of venous diseases occur—handbreadth around the ankle is called as **gaiter's area** (gaiter means cloth or leather used to cover the ankle).

Past History

Past history of pelvic surgery, fracture femur or pelvis, major abdominal surgeries, laparoscopic surgeries, bed-ridden status due to any cause should be asked in detail. All these are precipitating factors for deep vein thrombosis (DVT). Past history suggestive of pulmonary embolism (sudden chest pain, breathlessness, hemoptysis, hypotension, fever); history of organic heart disease; earlier therapy with heparin or oral anticoagulants should be noted. History suggestive of earlier deep vein thrombosis like pain, calf swelling and fever should be noted. History of typhoid fever should be asked where DVT is common.

Treatment History

History of previous surgery for varicose vein, drug intake like warfarin for DVT, injection therapy—sclerotherapy, wearing stockings/crepe bandages should be noted.

> **History**
> Pain, soreness, aching, burning, throbbing, heavy legs; muscle fatigue, pruritus, muscle cramps, "restless legs"; history of venous insufficiency; presence or absence of predisposing factors; history of oedema.
>
> History of any prior evaluation or treatment; history suggestive of superficial or deep vein thrombosis; history of any other vascular disease; family history of vascular disease.

Personal History

In females, history of varicose veins in pregnancy, and post-delivery period, use of oral contraceptive (may cause deep vein thrombosis) should be noted. History of smoking/alcohol/working pattern should be noted. History of obesity to be noted.

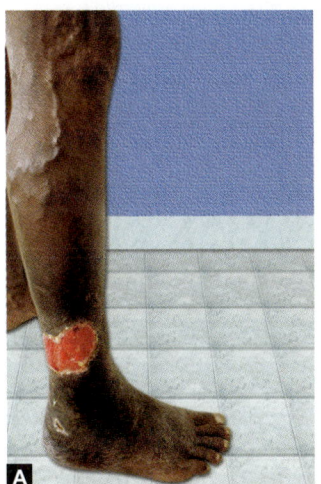
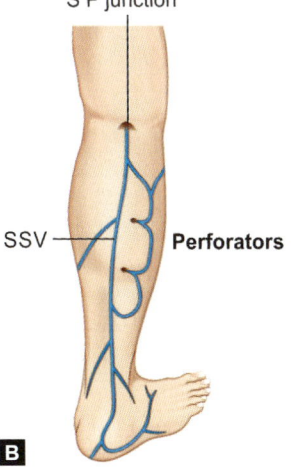

Figs. 7-6A and B Photograph and diagrammatic representation of short saphenous vein. Venous ulcer over the lateral malleolus with short saphenous vein varicosity. *Area around ankle (handbreadth) where complications of venous diseases occur is called as Gaiter's area* **(refer also Fig. 3-24).**

Family History

Varicose veins may be familial, which are bilateral and severe, observed in young individuals. Valves are absent/defective in these patients.

GENERAL EXAMINATION

Pulse—Rate/rhythm/character/condition of vessel wall should be noted; blood pressure is measured. Other detailed general examination is done for anemia/edema/jaundice/clubbing/lymphadenopathy. Raise in temperature/attitude of the patient/nutritional assessment by skin texture, subcutaneous fat, weight, body mass index/any other relevant findings should be mentioned.

LOCAL EXAMINATION

Examination of lower limbs—*symptomatic limb should be examined first.*

Inspection

Examination of limbs in standing position is the first method in varicose veins **(Figs. 7-7A and B)**. Limbs are scrutinized from umbilicus to toes. Both in front (long saphenous vein) and back of the legs should be inspected otherwise short saphenous vein varicosities may be overlooked **(Figs. 7-8 and 7-9)**. Possible perforating veins should also be observed **(Fig. 7-10)**. Dermal flare (< 1 mm), reticular subcutaneous varices (1–3 mm), varicozed tributaries, skin changes should be observed **(Figs. 7-11 and 7-12)**. Lower abdomen and pubes should also be inspected.

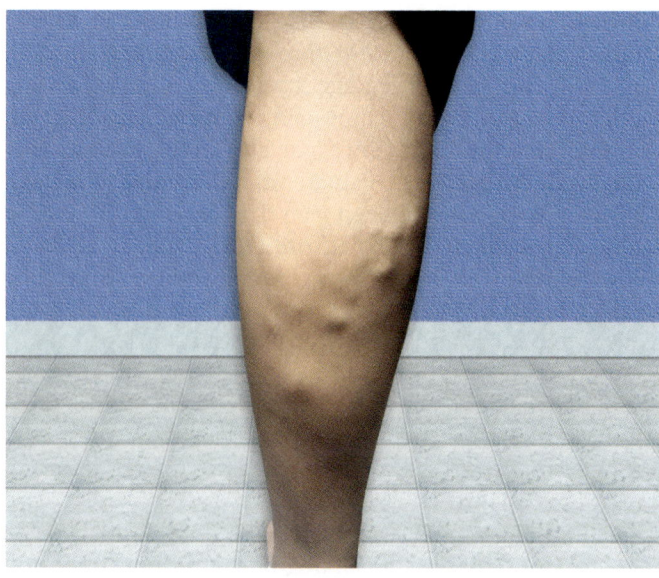

Fig. 7-8 Typical perforators in the calf—'*Blowouts*'.

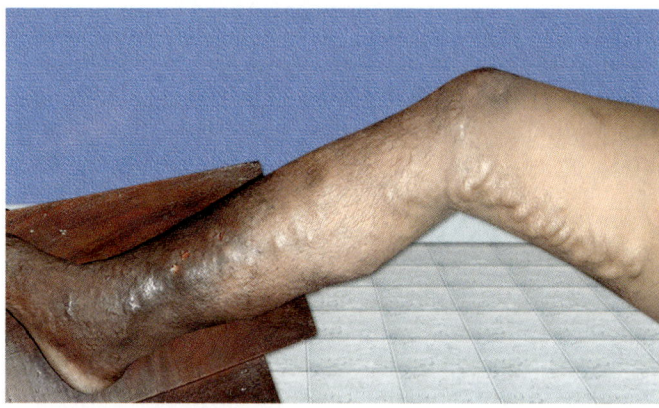

Fig. 7-9 Long saphenous vein incompetence with varicose vein with *skin changes and tiny ulcers (C-7).*

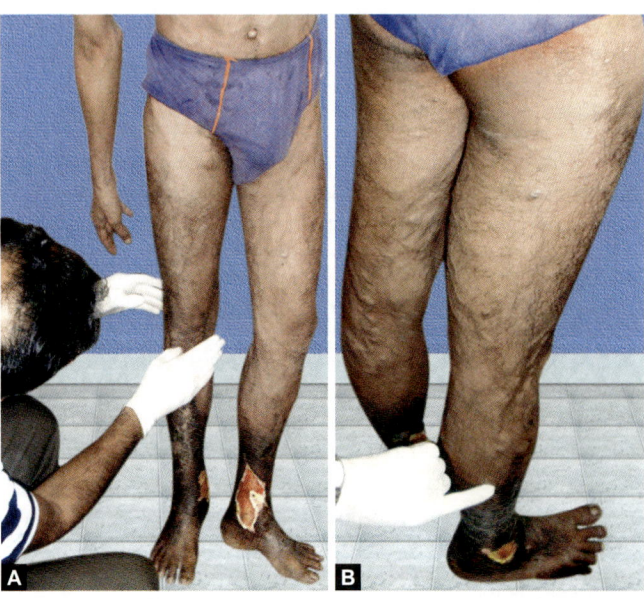

Figs. 7-7A and B *Inspection of varicose veins should be done in standing position.* Great saphenous veins on both sides should be inspected along medial aspect in standing position. *Short/small saphenous vein should be inspected from behind.*

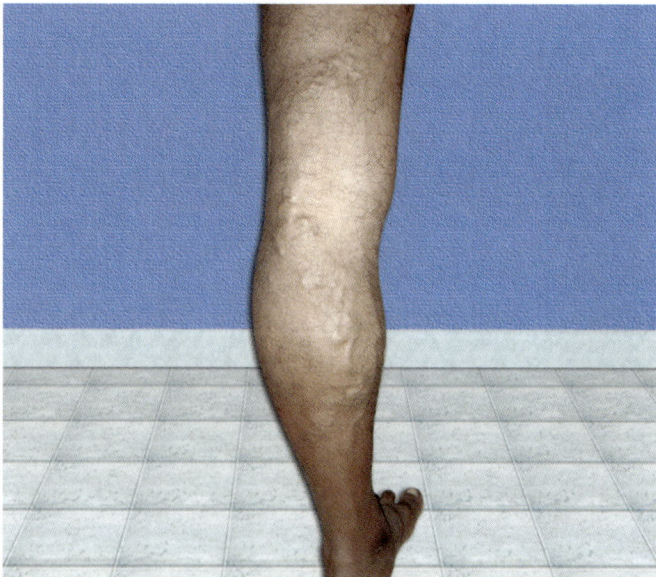

Fig. 7-10 A tributary vein which is varicose running from posterior medial part of the calf above; it could be *posterior arch vein* or a variant tributary which is not uncommon.

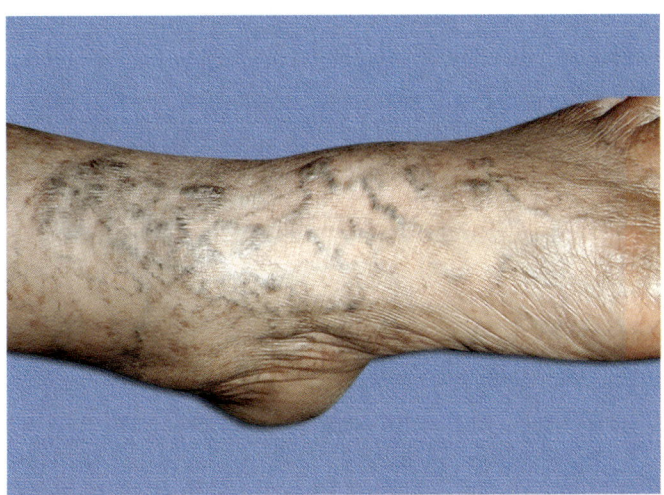

Fig. 7-11 *Typical ankle flare*. Thread veins are dermal and are <1 mm in size (0.5 mm). Reticular veins are subcutaneous and are between 1–3 mm in size.

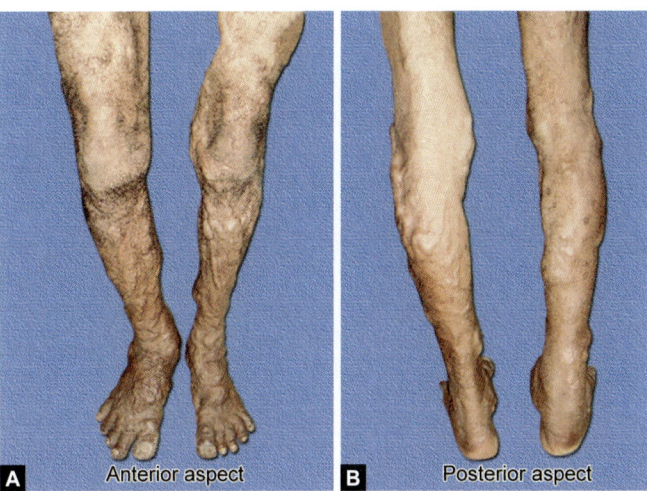

Figs. 7-13A and B Bilateral varicose veins involving *both great and small saphenous veins*.

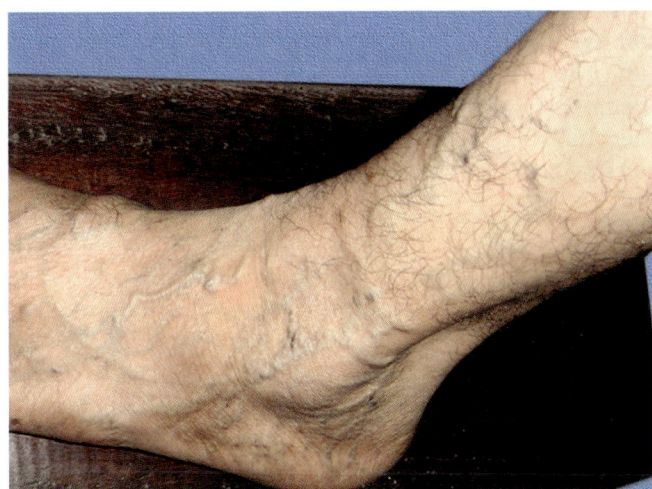

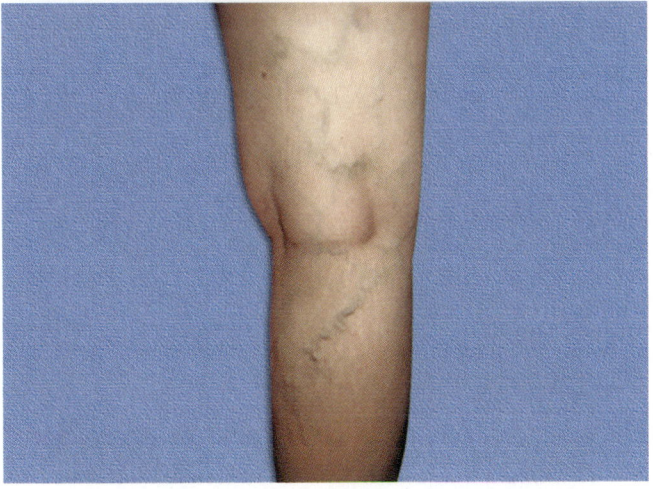

Fig. 7-12 *Dilated reticular* veins causing varicosity.

Limb

Limb is looked for dilated long saphenous vein on the medial side and for short saphenous vein on posterior and lateral side. Other communicating veins are also looked for. Beginning of the varicosity in the foot, later its extent above also should be examined. Great saphenous vein tortuosity often extends into the thigh whereas short saphenous vein varicosity ends at popliteal region. Always limb is looked for skin changes, pigmentation, edema, ankle flare, and ulcer. Ulcer should be examined in the similar way as explained in Chapter 3. Extent, size, shape, floor, margin, edge, discharge in an ulcer and surrounding area, deformity should be noted. Cough impulse at saphenous opening (**Morrisey's**) may be significant, (checked in lying-down position). Effects and complications of venous diseases occur at ankle and handbreadth above it which is called as **Gaiter's area** [Gaiter (French) is leather/cloth covering used to cover lower leg/ankle (in military personnel or horse riders)]. Chronic inflammation, thickening, pigmentation, induration around a ankle and lower leg with contracted skin and subcutaneous tissue but with prominent calf muscle gives the typical look like **inverted beer bottle (sign) or champagne bottle (sign)**; it is more common in postphlebitic limb. It causes tissue hypoxia, recurrent ulceration leading into a poor morbid status (**Figs. 7-13 to 7-16**).

Swelling

In superficial varicose veins it may be a localized swelling in leg/segmental tortuous vein in leg. Diffuse swelling in leg may be due to edema/DVT.

Skin Changes

Color changes: It may be linear redness/reddish blue color in superficial thrombophlebitis; massive edema with pallor and tenderness in—**Phlegmasia alba dolens** (due to DVT of femoral vein with lymphangitis and palpable pulse); limb is swollen and blue in **Phlegmasia cerulea dolens**—it is limb with cyanotic mottled skin with massive tight edema due to occlusion of major veins (iliofemoral vein) and collaterals

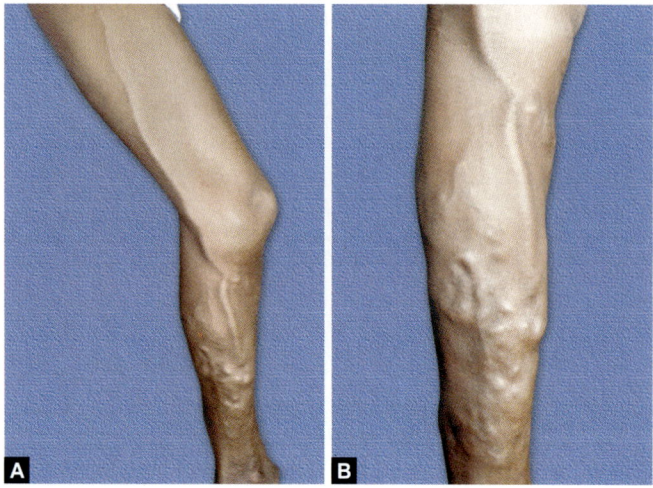

Figs. 7-14A and B Long saphenous vein varicosity. Note the prominent of veins and blow outs.

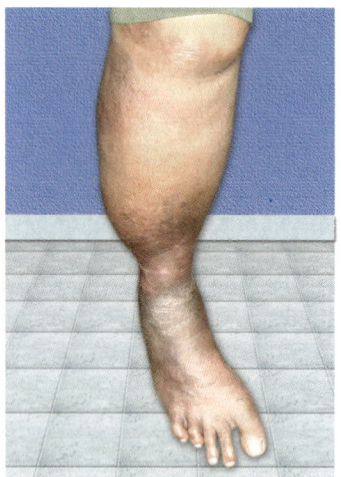 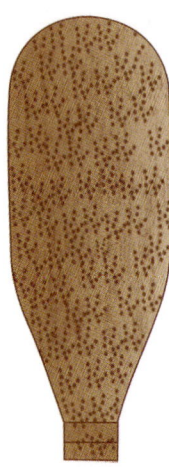

Fig. 7-15 *Champagne bottle sign/inverted beer bottle sign* is seen in *lipodermatosclerosis* due to prominent calf with narrow ankle contracted skin and subcutaneous tissue. Sign is often observed in DVT also.

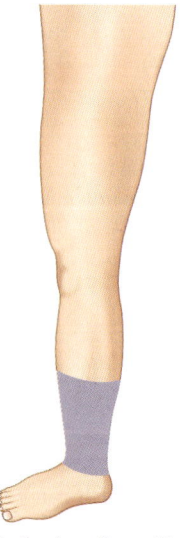

Fig. 7-16 *Gaiter's zone* is the handbreadth area around ankle where problems/complications/ulceration of venous disease occur.

with absence ankle pulses, may cause venous gangrene. In **port wine discoloration of skin** with varicose vein one has to suspect AVF.

Texture of the skin: Skin may be stretched shiny, edematous (in DVT); may also present with eczema; ulcers and scar around the ankle, mostly over the medial aspect over the lower part of leg. Loss of hair and increased nail brittleness may be feature of impending venous gangrene or chronic varicosity.

Venous flare: Finely dilated visible veins just beneath the surface of skin due to incompetence of perforators.

Venous stars: Red nodular lesions over the feet, leg, back and chest; present in persons with vena caval obstruction and pregnancy. Digital pressure squeezes the blood from the lesions but on sudden release fills from the center.

Cough Impulse

Morrissey's cough impulse—Here patient is asked to cough and impulse on coughing is observed at the saphenous opening—***saphena varix***. It is done in lying down position after emptying the vein with limb elevated to 30° (**Figs. 7-17A and B**).

Ulcer

If present should be described with tenderness, induration, warmness, mobility, fixity to the underlying bone, etc. Any palpable indurations of the skin and subcutaneous tissue around ankle which is suggestive of ***lipodermatosclerosis***, that develops at late stage of disease should be looked for.

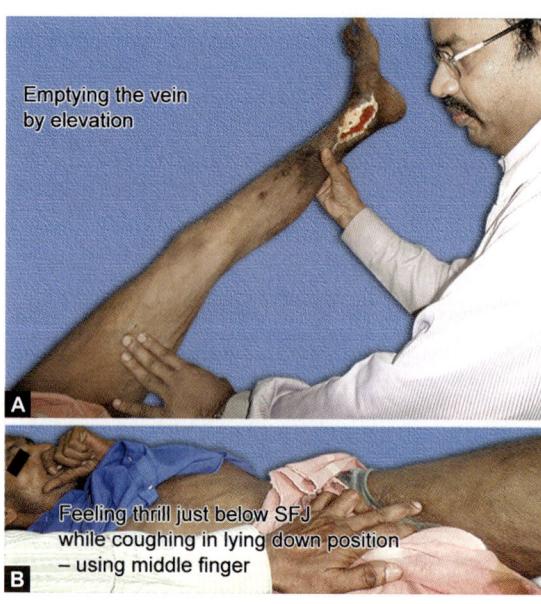

Figs. 7-17A and B *Morrissey's cough impulse*. After emptying the vein, a fluid thrill will be felt on the pulp of middle finger kept on the saphenous vein just below the saphenofemoral junction in case of SFJ incompetence while coughing.

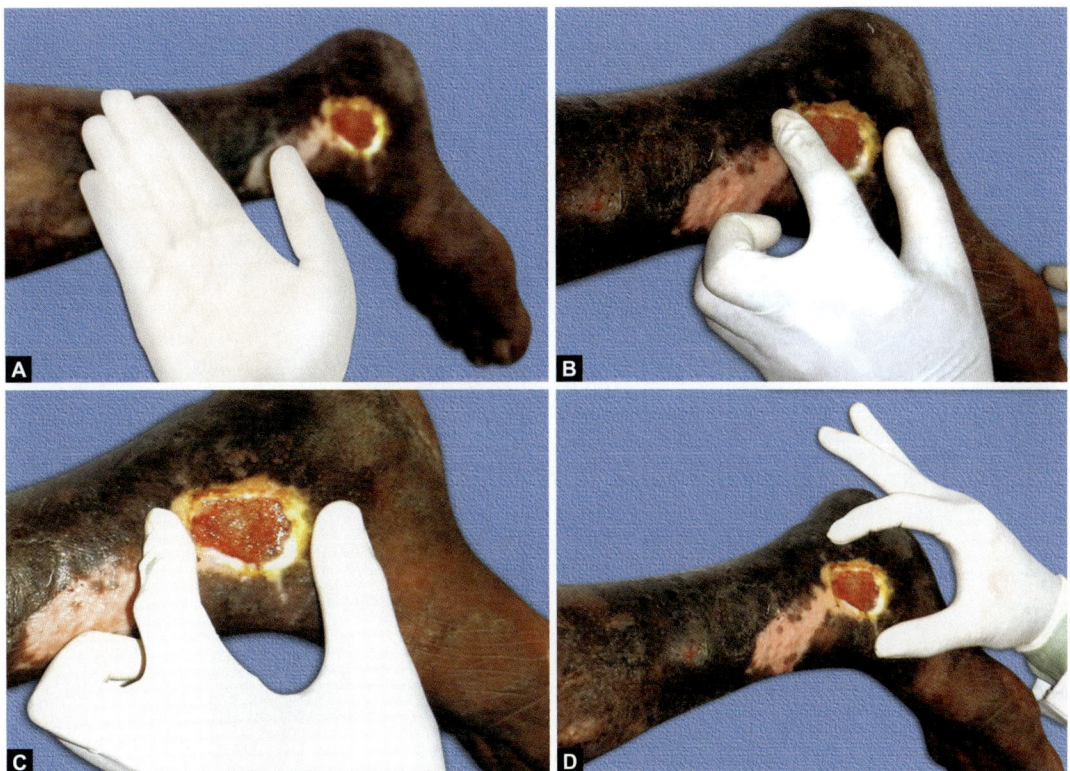

Figs. 7-18A to D Venous ulcer should be examined for *warmness of surrounding area, tenderness, induration, mobility/fixity*.

Palpation

The limb is palpated for **(Figs. 7-18A to D).**:
- Temperature: Warm in venous stasis, thrombophlebitis and AVF.
- Tenderness: Tenderness in calf muscles is seen in DVT; tenderness over the veins is seen in thrombophlebitis.
- Thickness of skin is noted when lipodermatosclerosis sets in.
- Edema: If pitting on pressure is seen over the medial malleolus, it is venous edema if not then it is lymphatic edema.
- Ulcer in detail **(Refer Chapter 3)**

Specific Tests for Varicose Veins

Brodie-Trendelenburg Test (Brodie 1846; Friedrich Trendelenburg 1924)

Vein is emptied by elevating the limb and milking the vein proximally in lying down position; a tourniquet is tied just below the saphenofemoral junction (or saphenofemoral junction can be occluded using a thumb). Saphenous opening is located 3.5 cm below and lateral to the pubic tubercle. Pubic tubercle is palpated along the adductor longus tendon which is identified by adducting the thigh against resistance. Patient is asked to stand quickly. When tourniquet or thumb is released, rapid filling from above signifies saphenofemoral incompetence. ***This is Trendelenburg test I***.

In Trendelenburg test II, vein is emptied again in lying down position and tourniquet is applied at saphenofemoral junction. After standing without releasing the tourniquet, the limb is observed. Filling of vein rapidly from below upwards can be observed within 30-60 seconds. It signifies perforator incompetence **(Figs. 7-19 to 7-21)**.

Tourniquet Test for Short Saphenous Vein

Tourniquet is applied at saphenopopliteal junction after emptying the short saphenous vein by elevation. Saphenopopliteal junction is not in constant position and so it is better applied at the level of lower boundary of popliteal fossa. The tourniquet is released in standing position to look for the rapid filling from above which suggests saphenopopliteal incompetence **(Figs. 7-22A to C)**. Long saphenous vein should be occluded together at SFJ to have accuracy.

Three/Multiple Tourniquet Test (Oschner's Mahoner's Test)

To find out the site of incompetent perforators, three tourniquets are tied after emptying the vein—(1) Just below saphenofemoral junction; (2) Above knee level; (3) Another below knee level; (4) Additional tourniquets may be applied at below-knee and above ankle level. Patient is asked to stand; filling of veins and site of filling is looked for. Then tourniquets are released from below upwards to look again for incompetent perforators. Individual perforators may be tested by repeating the procedure. On standing if veins become prominent between upper most and second tourniquets, it means adductor canal perforator incompetence. Prominent veins between middle and lower signifies below knee perforator incompetence; and prominent veins below lower tourniquet, signifies incompetence of lower leg perforators **(Figs. 7-23A to F)**.

188 Section 1: Examination in General Surgery

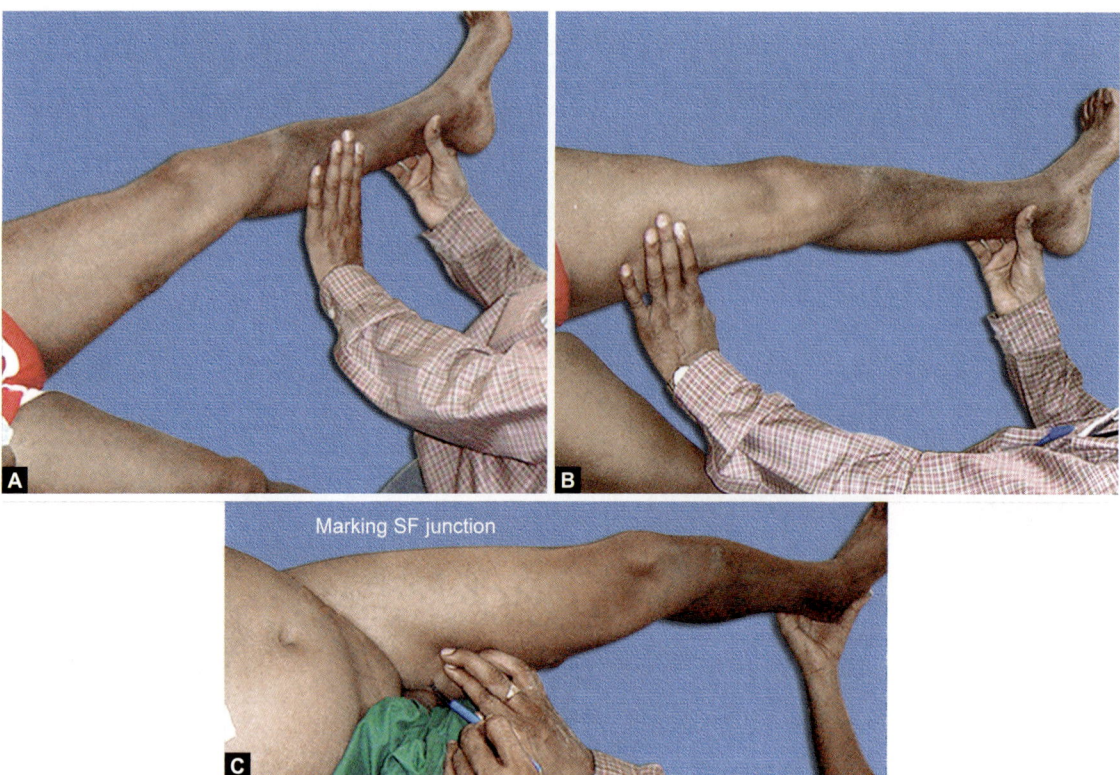

Figs. 7-19A to C *Emptying of the superficial varicose vein is important in all tourniquet tests for varicose veins. It is done in lying down position with elevating and milking the vein. Emptying is not done in modified Perthe's test. Note the marking of the saphenofemoral junction before applying the tourniquet, which is important.*

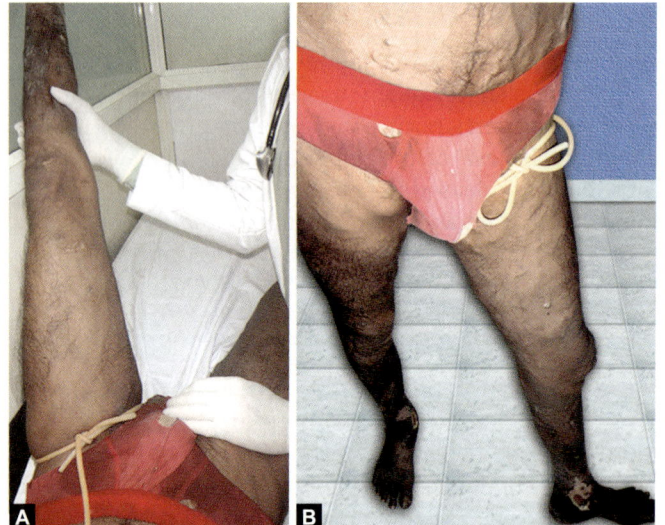

Figs. 7-20A and B *Note the site of applying the tourniquet at saphenofemoral junction. It is 3.5 cm below and lateral to pubic tubercle. Pubic tubercle is identified—by palpating the inguinal ligament from lateral to medial end and first bony point reached is marked as pubic tubercle; it can also be identified by feeling the attachment of the adductor longus tendon to the pubic bone and pubic tubercle is lateral to the attachment. Alternatively palpation begins from pubic symphysis extending laterally to reach pubic tubercle as most lateral one.*

Pratt's Test

It is done to locate the site of perforator. Esmarch bandage is applied to the leg from below upwards with a tourniquet tied at saphenofemoral junction. With tourniquet in situ, bandage is released later to see the perforators as *'blow outs'*.

Fegan Test (George Fegan, Dublin)

Line of the varicose vein is marked; patient is made to lie down and examining limb is raised; heel is made to rest on the upper chest of the examiner. Marked line of the varicose vein is carefully palpated for the gaps in the deep fascia which are felt as circular opening with sharp edges (crescentic). These gaps/openings are the sites of perforator veins. Blow outs may be visible in these points often in standing position **(Figs. 7-24A to D)**.

Schwartz Test

It is a **percussion test**. In standing position, when lower part of the vein in leg is tapped, impulse is felt at the saphenous junction or at the upper end of the visible part of the vein. It signifies continuous column of blood and all valves between two fingers are incompetent. Positive test is usually found in gross venous varicosity **(Fig. 7-25)**.

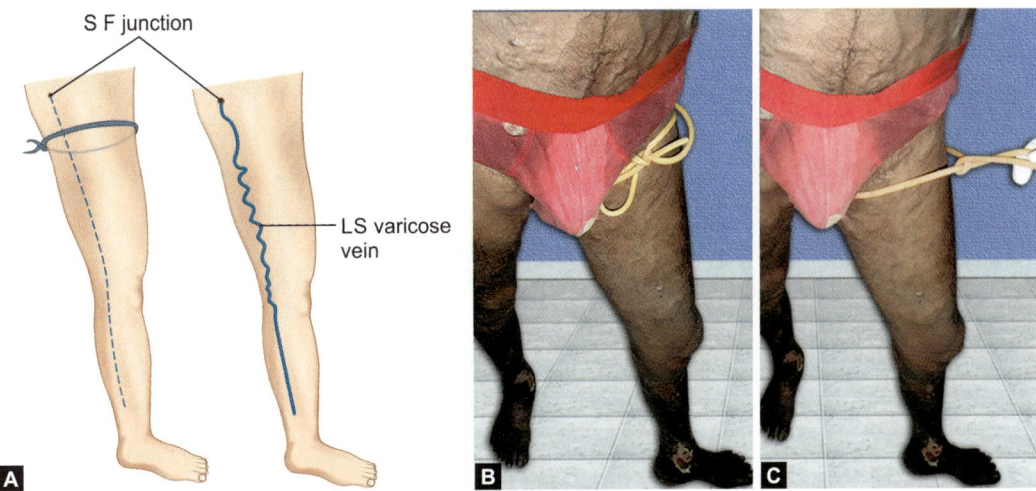

Figs. 7-21A to C *Tourniquet test.* Tourniquet is applied after emptying the vein by elevating the leg and milking. Patient is asked to stand, tourniquet is released immediately and saphenous vein is observed. Rapid filling of vein from above signifies LSV varicosity with saphenofemoral incompetence—Trendelenburg test I. In test II—tourniquet applied after emptying is retained and limb is observed in standing for rapid filling of the vein from below upwards in 1 minute. It means perforators are incompetent.

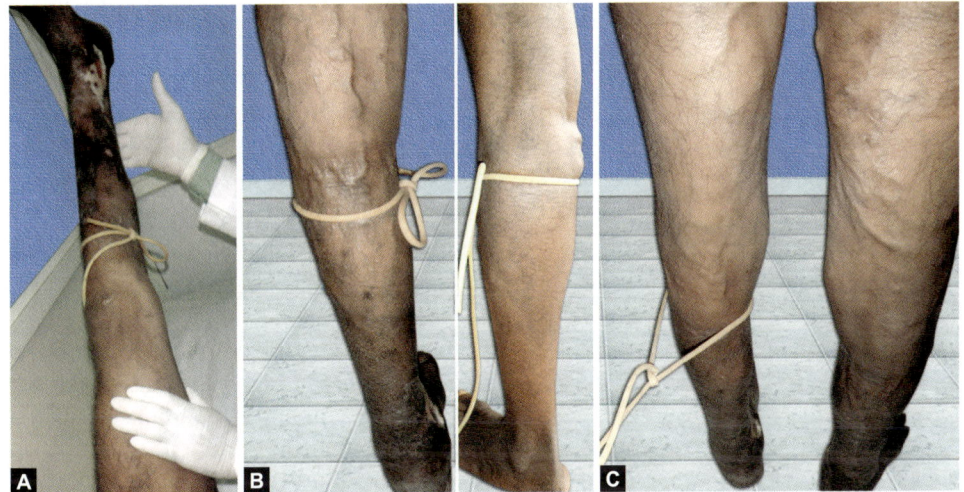

Figs. 7-22A to C *Small/short saphenous vein varicosity can be present* along with other types like of GSV or perforators. Occasionally, it can be isolated small saphenous vein varicosity. Saphenopopliteal junction is variable; but since usual site is in the lower part of the popliteal fossa, tourniquet is applied at the lower line of popliteal fossa after emptying the vein by elevation. On standing and releasing the tourniquet, rapid filling of small saphenous vein is obvious from above downwards signifying saphenopopliteal incompetence.

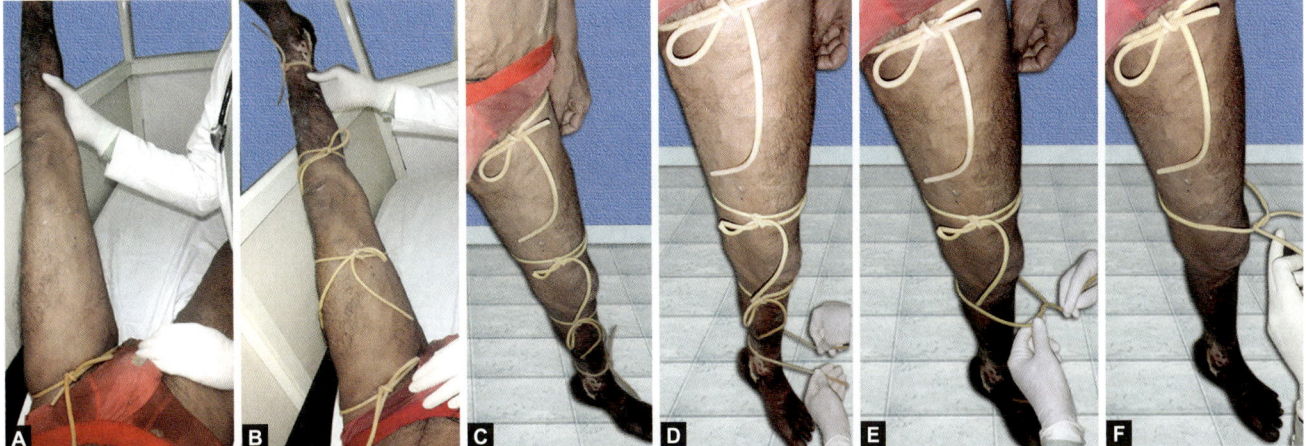

Figs. 7-23A to F *Multiple tourniquet test;* after emptying the vein by elevation patient is made to stand; gaps in between tourniquets are observed for any blow outs. Tourniquets are released from below upwards in standing position to visualize any perforators.

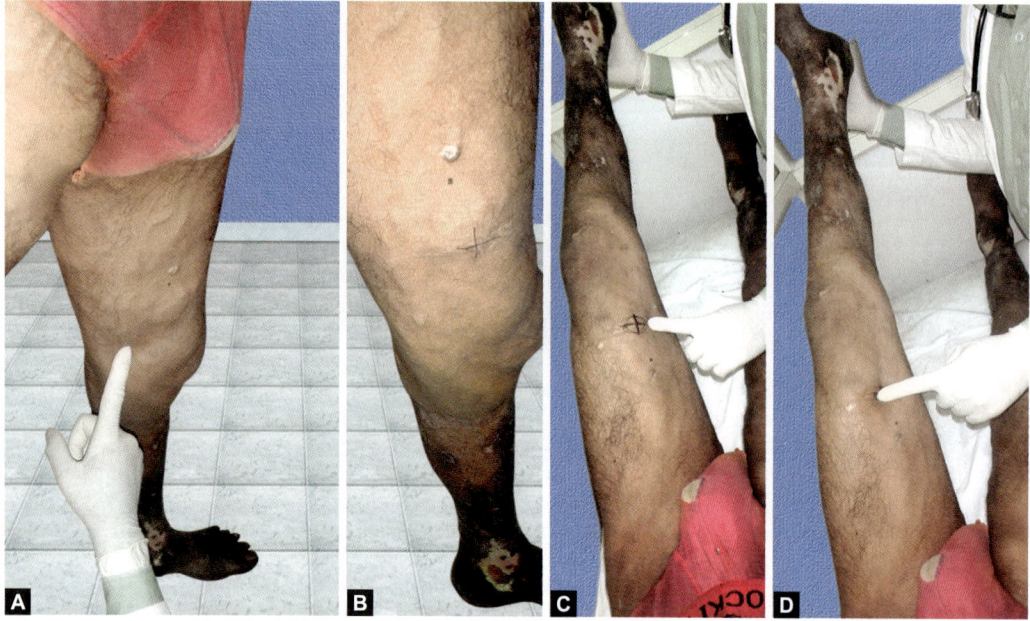

Figs. 7-24A to D *Fegan's test* to find out the site of perforator. It is done both in standing and lying down position. It is done prior to surgery to have a clear idea about the site of the perforator.

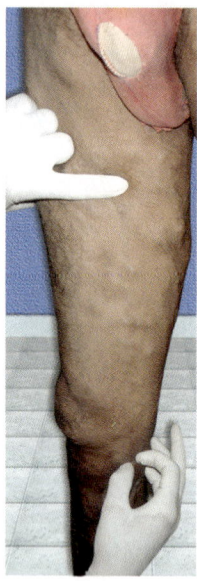

Fig. 7-25 *Schwartz test* is done to confirm the presence of continuous column of blood.

Ian-Aird Test

On standing, proximal segment of long saphenous vein is emptied with two fingers. Pressure from proximal finger is released to see the rapid filling from above which confirms saphenofemoral incompetence **(Figs. 7-26A and B)**.

Morrissey's Cough Impulse (Cough Impulse Test)

After emptying the vein ***in lying down position***, patient is asked to cough forcibly. Impulse, if felt at the fingers kept just below the saphenous opening/at saphenofemoral junction indicates incompetence of the valve at saphenofemoral junction. A fluid thrill is imparted at this point under the palpating fingers. It is observed that cough impulse test is the more reliable clinical test of saphenofemoral incompetence and long saphenous vein varicosity.

Cruveilhier's Sign of Saphena Varix

When patient coughs or blows his nose ***in standing position***, palpating finger over the saphenous opening feels a tremor

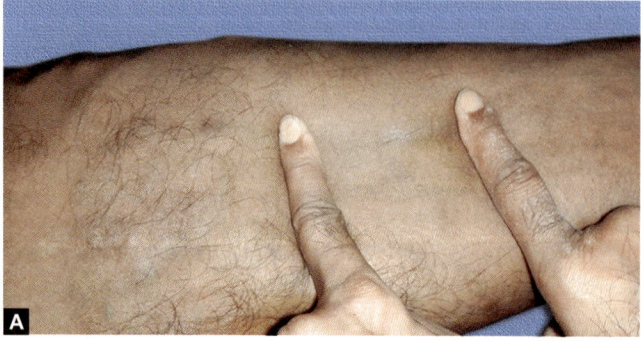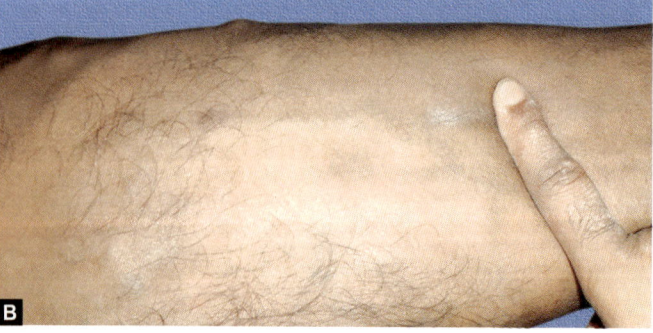

Figs. 7-26A and B *Ian-Aird test.* It is done in standing position; after emptying the vein between two fingers when proximal (upper) finger is released, rapid filling (reversal flow) of blood from above towards lower finger is observed.

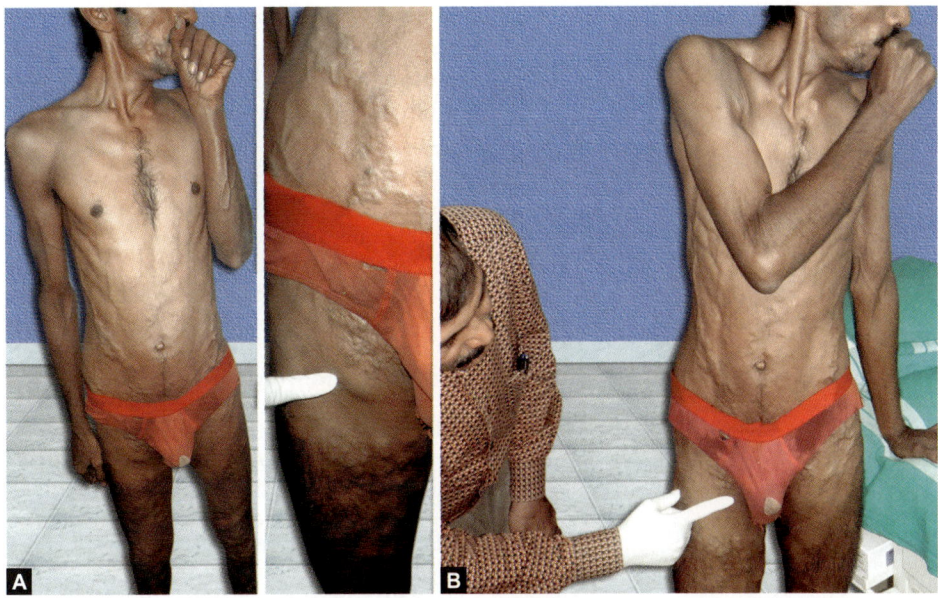

Figs. 7-27A and B *Cruveilhier's sign.* It is done in standing; while patient coughs palpating finger feels a tremor like a fluid jetting back into a pouch.

as if a jet of water entering and filling the pouch **(Figs. 7-27A and B)**.

Chevrier Percussion/Tap Sign

In standing position, left hand fingers are placed by the clinician just below the saphenous opening; main bunch of the varicosities is tapped using right middle finger once by the clinician; an impulse will be felt on the left fingers placed just below the saphenous opening. It is almost similar to Schwartz test.

Note: Saphena varix often mimics femoral hernia as both gives impulse on coughing and disappears on lying down. But saphena varix is softer compared to femoral hernia; it shows positive Morrissey's, Cruveilhier's and Chevrier tap signs; it shows a thin blue discoloration of the overlying skin **(Figs. 7-28A and B)**.

Raju Test

Venous pressure is measured in hand and foot in supine position by inserting a cannula to the dorsal vein of foot/ hand and connecting it to a saline manometer using three way stopcock; normally foot pressure is equal or only around 5 mm Hg more than hand pressure. In venous obstruction, pressure difference is more than 10 mm Hg.

Tests for Deep Vein Thrombosis

a. Perthes Test

The affected lower limb is wrapped with elastic bandage and the patient is asked to walk around and exercise. Development of severe crampy pain in the calf signifies DVT. Test is often subjective.

b. Modified Perthe's Test

Tourniquet is tied just below the saphenofemoral junction ***without emptying the vein***. Patient is asked to do a ***brisk walk*** which precipitates *bursting pain* in the calf and also makes superficial veins more prominent. It signifies DVT **(Fig. 7-29)**.

c. Homan's Test

Passive dorsiflexion of the foot elicits pain/tenderness in the calf (it exerts slight traction on the posterior tibial vein which if involved by thrombosis causes pain in calf) which suggests DVT **(Fig. 7-30)**.

d. Mose's Sign

With the knee flexed around 90°, calf muscle is grasped near tendo-Achilles and squeezing is done gently from below upwards along the muscle bulk to elicit tenderness which confirms DVT mainly in soleus muscle. Relaxed main calf muscle is then squeezed forward and sideward to elicit pain/tenderness which is indicative of posterior tibial vein thrombosis. Test should be done very gently to avoid clot dislodgement and pulmonary embolism **(Figs. 7-31A and B)**.

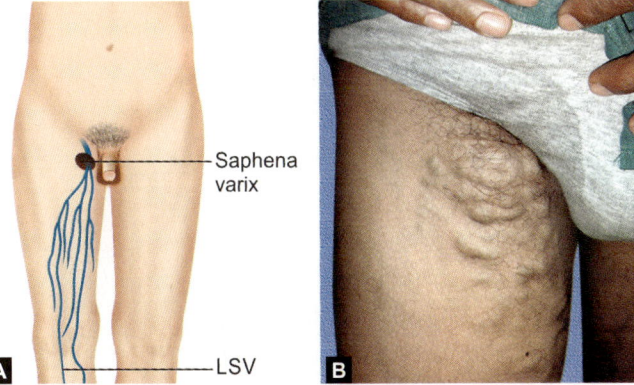

Figs. 7-28A and B *Saphena varix in the groin* – near the saphenous opening.

e. Other Signs

On deep palpation of the calf, thickening and tenderness is felt in the calf—*Neuhof's sign*. After applying tourniquet at saphenofemoral junction, patient is made to walk and without removing the tourniquet, limb is elevated—persistent prominent superficial veins will be observed in DVT—*Linton's test*. Swollen leg mainly at calf with tenderness, warmness and induration with mild fever, pain while moving the calf are also often other features.

Note:
- DVT is contraindicated for any surgical intervention of superficial varicose veins. It is also contraindicated for sclerosant therapy.
- Point also to be remembered is that in case of acute DVT, Homan's/ Mose's tests should not be done as it will precipitate the dislodgement of the clot and embolism.

Bone Thickening

Bone thickening in the shin (tibia and ankle bones) is important which signifies periostitis. It is checked by running the thumb along the shin and malleoli (**Figs. 7-32A and B**).

Measurement and Markings

Measurement of limb length and girth is done especially in arteriovenous malformation with varicose veins where the length and girth is increased and also to find out deformities. Always varicose veins and perforators **should be marked**

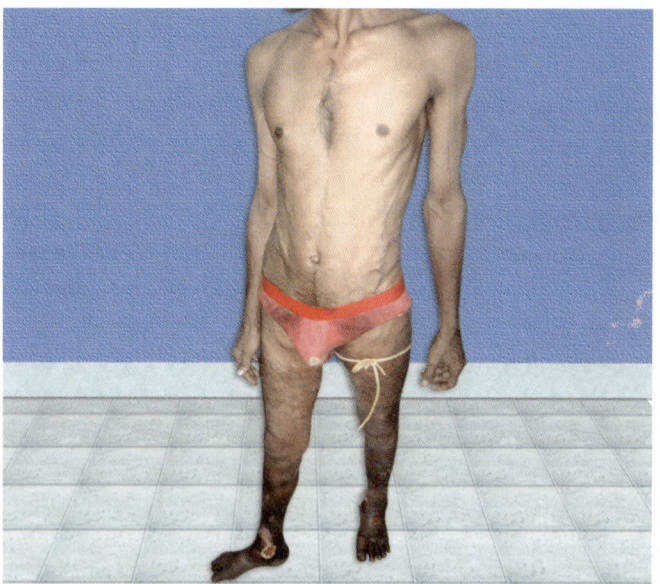

Fig. 7-29 *Modified Perthes' test*. Without emptying the vein, after applying tourniquet, patient is asked to have brisk walk for 3 minutes. In patient with DVT patient develops bursting pain with prominent superficial veins.

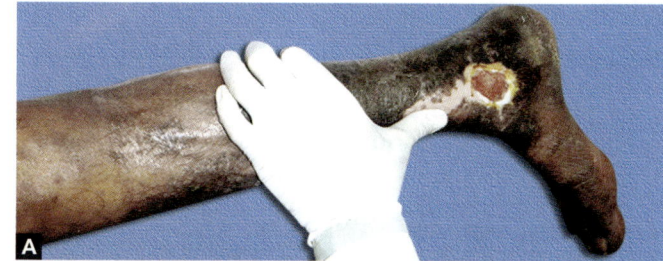

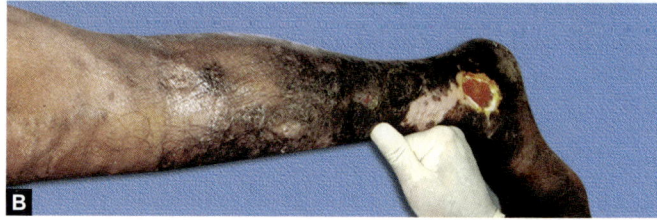

Figs. 7-32A and B *Bone thickening* is checked over tibia, malleoli and often ankle bones using thumb. It suggests periostitis.

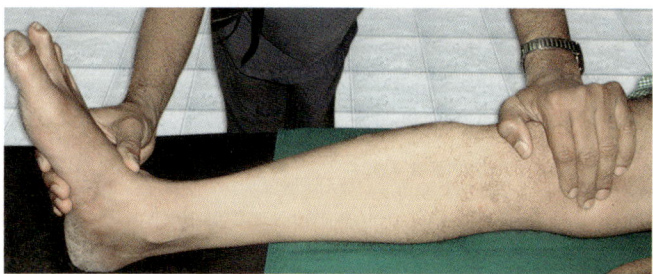

Fig. 7-30 *Homan's test* is done to find out acute DVT. In Homan's, foot is dorsiflexed to elicit pain/ tenderness in the calf.

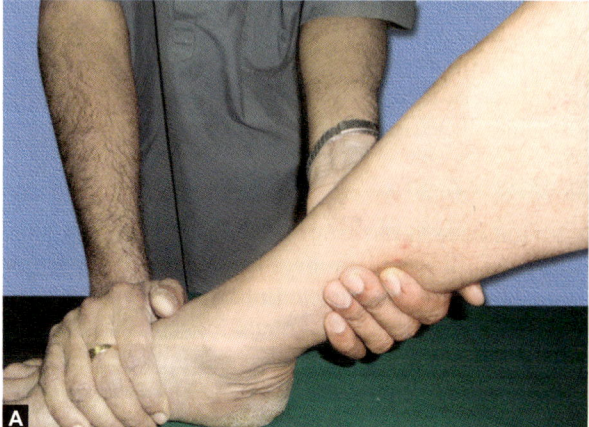
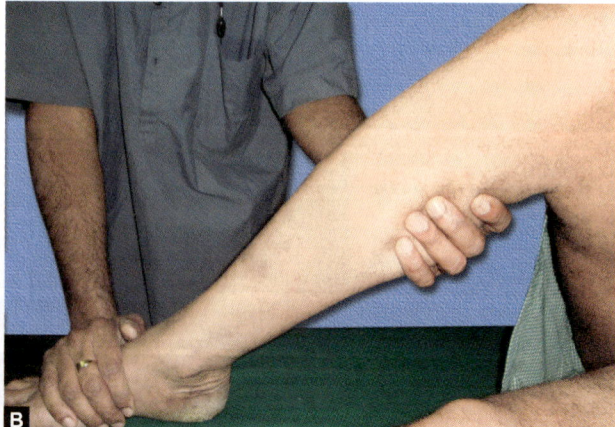

Figs. 7-31A and B Squeezing the relaxed calf muscles sideward to elicit pain/tenderness is *Mose's sign*. Foot is rested on the ground; tendoachilles is squeezed gently initially; then squeezing is done upwards over the soleus gently to elicit tenderness.

with a marking ink especially prior to surgery after taking consent. Marking is ideally done in standing under duplex scan—Doppler guidance.

> **Symptoms in varicose veins:**
> - Dilated tortuous vein—asymptomatic but cosmetic
> - Dragging pain
> - Heaviness/tiredness in the legs
> - Night time cramps—usually late night—typical
> - Edema/itching/thickening/eczema feet and leg
> - Discoloration/ulceration in the feet/painful walk
> - Bleeding blow outs
> - Symptoms are not proportional to the size of varicose veins.
>
> **Signs:**
> - All different positive tests
> - Blowouts—localized dilated vein segment suggests incompetent perforator—Fegan's test
> - Superficial thrombophlebitis
> - Ankle flare
> - Dermal flare (thread veins) < 1 mm—it is within the skin
> - Reticular veins (1–3 mm) in the subcutaneous tissue
> - *Saphena varix*—A large varicosity in the groin (of GSV; often of anterolateral thigh vein)
> - Talipes equinovarus
> - *Champagne bottle sign* (inverted beer bottle look)—contraction of ankle skin and subcutaneous tissue with prominent edematous calf.

Auscultation

Auscultation of the vein for bruit/venous hum over the saphenofemoral junction is done; machinery murmur is heard in arteriovenous fistula (AVF) **(Fig. 7-33)**.

Examination of Peripheral Pulses

Peripheral pulses should be examined as venous and arterial diseases may coexist; will worsen the situation each other; (dorsalis pedis/anterior tibial/posterior tibial/popliteal/femoral) **(Fig. 7-34)**.

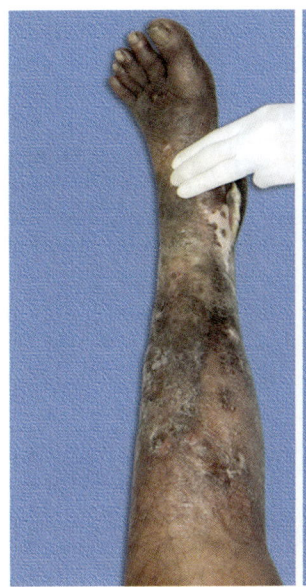
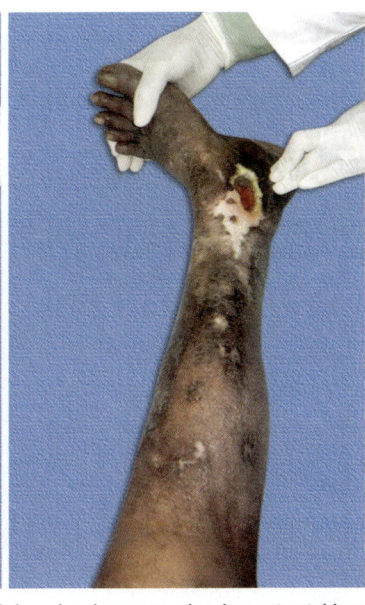

Fig. 7-34 Examination of *peripheral pulses are also important*. Here note the examinations of dorsalis pedis and posterior tibial artery pulsations.

Examination of Regional Lymph Nodes

Vertical group of inguinal nodes and external iliac nodes (above and medial aspect of the inguinal ligament) are palpated. It suggests the infection and its severity **(Figs. 7-35A and B)**.

Joint Examination

Ankle joint movements (plantar and dorsiflexion) are checked for any restriction. Inversion and eversion are elicited in subtalar joint. Restricted joint movements can occur due to chronic inflammatory fibrosis of soft tissues around the joint (fibrous ankylosis) **(Figs. 7-36A and B)**.

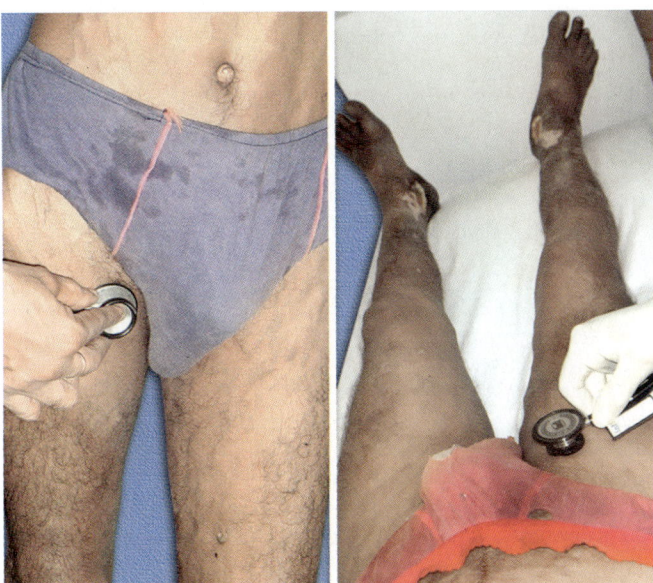

Fig. 7-33 Auscultation over the groin for *venous hum/bruit* (of AVF) is done when needed *'Bell of the stethoscope'* is better.

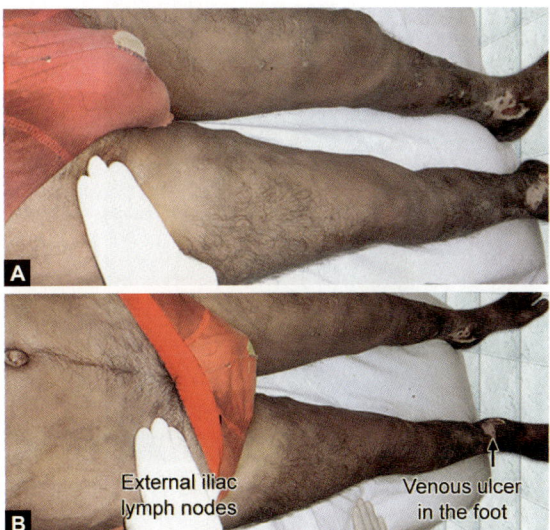

Figs. 7-35A and B Lymph nodes in the region/groin (*vertical inguinal nodes*) should be examined in case of presence of complications like ulcer. *External iliac nodes* (above and medial aspect of the inguinal ligament) are also should be palpated whenever required.

Examination of the Opposite Limb

Opposite limb should be examined both in standing and lying down position; in front and from behind (should not be forgotten).

Examination of the Abdomen

Abdomen should be examined for any mass (gravid uterus, uterine mass, carcinoma cervix, ovarian mass) which might be compressing the inferior vena cava (IVC) or iliac veins causing varicose veins. Digital examination of the rectum is needed **(Figs. 7-37 and 7-38)**.

Examination of Other Systems

Other systems like cardiac and respiratory systems also should be examined. In arteriovenous malformations or fistula patient may develop cardiac failure due to hyperdynamic circulation. DVT may cause pulmonary embolism so respiratory system should also be examined **(Fig. 7.39)**.

> **Complications of varicose veins:**
> - Hemorrhage: Venous hemorrhage can occur from the ruptured varicose veins or sloughed varicose veins, often torrential, but can be controlled very well by elevation and pressure bandage

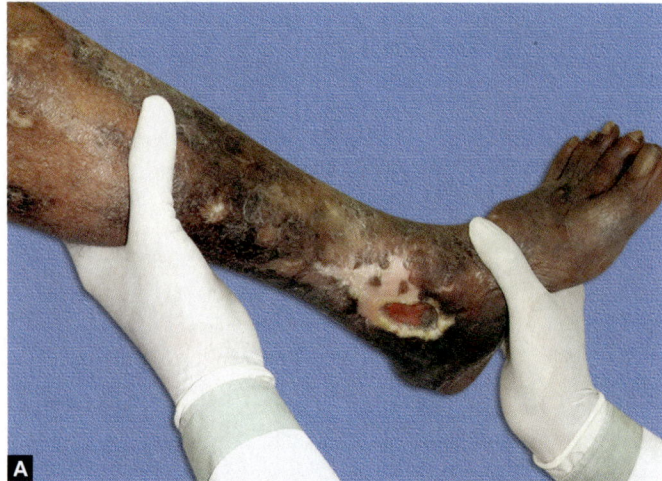
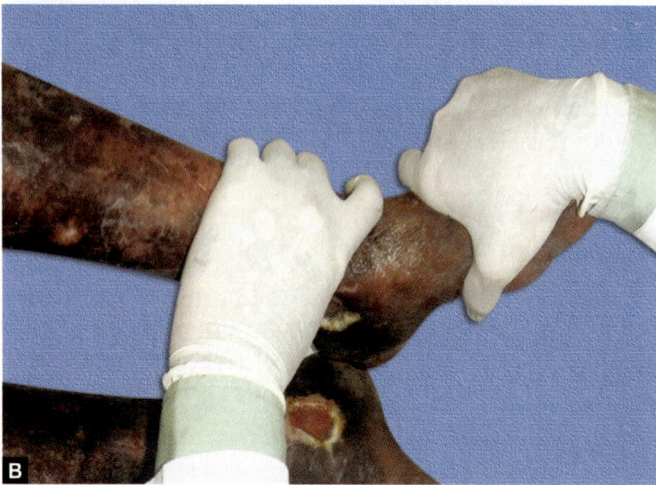

Figs. 7-36A and B *Ankle (dorsiflexion and plantarflexion) and subtalar (inversion and eversion) joint movements* should be checked. Often movements of these joints are restricted in venous ulcer due to fibrous ankylosis of the joints.

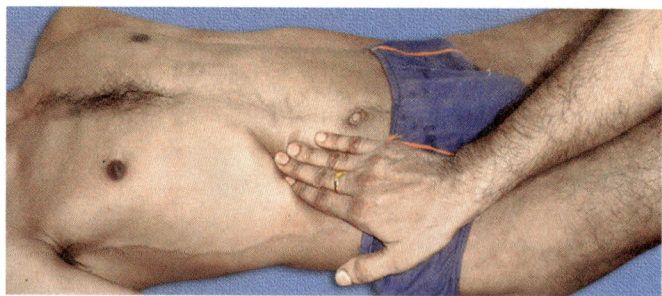

Fig. 7-37 Abdomen should be palpated for mass and ascites. *Mass may compress the major veins causing lower limb varicose veins.*

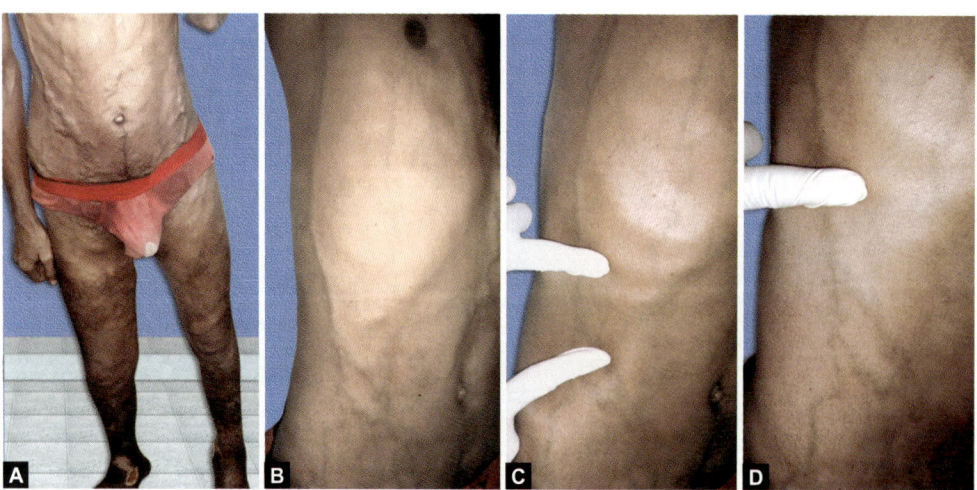

Figs. 7-38A to D Bilateral lower limb varicosity with features of IVC obstruction. *Veins on lateral and front aspect of abdomen and chest veins become prominent with flow from below upwards.* (Normal flow is away from umbilicus. Below the umbilicus flow is downwards; above it is upwards). Venous flow direction should be confirmed using two fingers keeping apart.

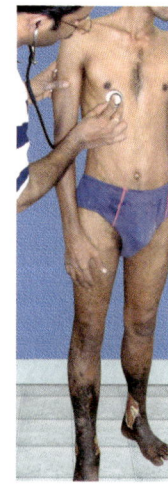

Fig. 7-39 Chest (cardiac and respiratory systems) should be examined. *It is relevant in AV fistula/IVC obstruction.*

- Eczema and dermatitis
- Periostitis causing thickening of periosteum
- Venous ulcer
- Marjolin's ulcer – due to *unstable scar of long duration*—very well differentiated squamous cell carcinoma
- Calcification
- Lipodermatosclerosis
- Ankylosis of the ankle joint
- Talipes equino varus
- Deep venous thrombosis—rare

Complications of venous ulcers:
- Hemorrhage
- Marjolin's ulcer
- Infection
- Talipes equino varus
- Periostitis is common over the tibia/calcaneum/other foot bones

- Disability
- Calcification
- DVT

CEAP classification is used currently for varicose veins especially while planning the therapy.
C (Clinical) – Grade 0 = no visible or palpable signs; Grade 1 = Telangiectases, reticular veins, malleolar flare; Grade 2 = Varicose veins; Grade 3 = Edema without skin changes; Grade 4 = Skin changes due to venous disease like pigmentation (4a)/lipodermatosclerosis or atrophia blanche (4b); Grade 5= Skin changes with healed ulceration; Grade 6 = Active ulceration.
E (Etiological) – Ec = Congenital; Ep = Primary; Es = Secondary; En = No venous etiology.
A (Anatomical) – As = Superficial; Ad = Deep; Ap = Perforator; An = no venous location identified.
P (Pathophysiological) – Pr = Reflux; Po = Obstructive; Pr,o = Both; Pn = No pathophysiology identified.

Case sheet writing in a patient with Varicose Veins

History
Name: **Age:**
Occupation: **Sex:**   **Place/residence:**

Chief complaints
- **Pain in the leg – duration**
- **Dilated veins in the leg – duration**
- **Pigmentation and ulcer – duration**

History of present illness
- Pain – origin, nature, character, duration, time of starting of pain, specific features, severity, aggravating or relieving factors
- Pigmentation - Situation / location
- Ulcer - Mode of onset and progression; Discharge from ulcer – duration, type of discharge, color of discharge, smell
- Bleeding from the dilated veins
- Fever – type, severity, duration
- History swelling underneath – when started, progress

Past history
- Past history of varicose vein surgery, pelvic surgery, embolism, DVT
- Past history of trauma
- Tuberculosis, spinal diseases, diabetes, leprosy, malignancies
- Past history of surgery like laparotomy and details; treatment history

Family history
- Family tree; history of tuberculosis, diabetes, malignancies, varicose veins, DVT; number of pregnancies, oral contraceptives, treatment history in the family members for varicose veins or related to it

Personal history
- History of alcohol, smoking, obesity, working pattern

General examination
Anemia, edema, jaundice, clubbing, lymphadenopathy, pulse, blood pressure, temperature, attitude, nutrition, body weight.

Local examination
Inspection – Examination of both limbs in standing is a must. Expose both limbs adequately.
- *Dilated veins* – medially in the leg; laterally and all around. Its extent below and above. Inspection for saphena varix in saphenous opening
- Skin changes, pigmentation
- Ulcer, size, shape, surrounding area, discharge in detail
- Surrounding skin, venous flare, skin changes
- Swelling – edema; Champagne bottle sign
- Morrissey's cough impulse in lying down position; inspection on Valsalva maneuver mainly at SFJ

Palpation
- Local raise of temperature, tenderness
- Palpation of ulcer in detail
- Thickening – skin, bone thickening for periostitis

Contd...

Contd...

Special tests
- Brodie – Trendelenburg test I and II; tourniquet test for saphenous vein
- Multiple tourniquet test (Oschner Mahoner's); Pratt's test (using Esmarch's bandage)
- Fegan's test; Schwartz test; Ian – Arid test; Morrissey's cough impulse test in lying down position; Cruveilhier's sign of saphena varix in standing position
- Tests for DVT (deep venous thrombosis) – Perthe's test (using crepe bandage); modified Perthe's test; Homan's test; Mose's sign; Neuhof's sign; Linton's test

Percussion – Schwartz test
Auscultation over veins – for bruit/venous hum
Examination of peripheral pulses
Movements of ankle and subtalar joints
Measurements of limb girth and length
Gait
Examination of regional lymph nodes

Systemic examination – abdomen, respiratory, cardiac and central nervous systems

Investigations – ***Venous Doppler with B mode Duplex scan,*** X-ray of the part; ultrasound abdomen; blood tests

■ INVESTIGATIONS FOR VARICOSE VEINS

Laboratory Studies

No currently available lab tests are useful in the diagnosis or treatment of varicose veins. It is mainly to assess presence/absence of DVT, which is absolutely essential prior to intervention.

Specific Tests

Venous Doppler: With the patient standing; the Doppler probe is placed at saphenofemoral junction and later wherever required. Basically by hearing the changes in sound, venous flow, venous patency, and venous reflux can be very well identified. A uniphasic signal means flow is in one direction. A *biphasic signal* means flow in both forward and reverse direction suggesting incompetence. Reversal can often be better appreciated by releasing a tourniquet applied earlier at saphenofemoral junction (Fig. 7-40).

Special tests for varicose veins (not commonly used now)
- **Venography/Phlebography:** Ascending venography was a very common investigation done earlier to Doppler period. A tourniquet is tied above the malleoli and the vein of dorsal venous arch of foot is cannulated. Water soluble dye injected, flows into the deep veins (because the applied tourniquet prevents its flow into superficial veins). X-rays are taken below and above knee level. Any block in deep veins, its extent, perforator status can be made out by this. Note: In the presence of Duplex scan, ascending venography is not a necessary investigation. Descending venogram is done when ascending venogram is not possible and also to visualize incompetent veins. Here contrast material is injected into the femoral vein through a cannula in standing position. X-ray pictures are taken to visualize deep veins and incompetent veins.
- **Plethysmography:** It is a noninvasive method which measures volume changes in the leg.
- *Photoplethysmography:* Using probe transmission of light through the skin, venous filling of the surface venules, which reflects the superficial venous pressure, is measured. Initially patient performs dorsiflexion at ankle for 10 times to empty the venules and pressure tracing falls on photoplethysmography. Patient takes rest and refilling occurs. In normal people, it occurs through arterial inflow in 20–30 seconds. In venous incompetence filling also occurs by venous reflux and so refilling time is faster than normal.

Disadvantage: Site of reflux cannot be localized by this method.
- *Air plethysmography:* Patient is initially in supine position with veins emptied by elevation of leg.
- Air filled plastic pressure bladder is placed on calf to detect volume changes. Minimum volume is recorded. Patient turned to upright position and venous volume is assessed. Maximum venous volume divided by time required to achieve maximum venous volume gives the venous filling index (VFI). VFI is a measure of reflux. Ejection fraction is volume change measured prior and after single tip-toe maneuver which is a measure of calf pump action. Residual venous fraction is an index of overall venous function which is venous volume in the leg after 10 toe-tip maneuvers divided by venous volume prior to maneuver. A patient with increased VFI and diminished ejection fraction will benefit from surgery.
- **Ambulatory Venous Pressure (AVP):** It is an invasive method. Needle inserted into dorsal vein of foot is connected to transducer to get its pressure which is equivalent to pressure in the deep veins of the calf. Ten tip-toe maneuvers are done by the patient. With initial rise in pressure, pressure decreases and eventually stabilizes with a balance. Pressure now is called as ambulatory venous pressure (AVP). After stopping exercise, veins are allowed to refill with return of pressure to baseline. Time required for pressure to return to 90% of baseline is called as venous refilling time (VRT). Raise in AVP signifies venous hypertension. Patients with AVP more than 80 mm Hg has 80% chances of venous ulcer formation.
- **Varicography:** Here non-ionic, iso-osmolar, non-thrombogenic contrast agent is injected directly into the variceal vein to get a detailed anatomical mapping of the varicose veins. It is used in recurrent varicose veins or with anatomical variations.
- **Arm-foot Venous Pressure:** Foot pressure is not more than 4 mm Hg above the arm pressure. Foot venous pressure will be as high as 10-15 mm Hg above of hand venous pressure—Raju test.
- **D-dimer Test:** Patients with varicose veins may have spuriously positive D-dimer test result because of chronic low level thrombosis within varices.
- **Reflux Assessment:** Muscle pump ejection fraction assessment may be useful to demonstrate reflux.
- **Radioactive Fibrinogen Test:** Sodium iodide 100 mg orally is given to the patient 24 hours before the test to block the thyroid activity. I125 labelled fibrinogen 100 μ curies is injected intravenously. First radioactivity of heart is measured by placing the scintillation counter over the precordium. Reading obtained by this is adjusted as 100%. After that legs are elevated using

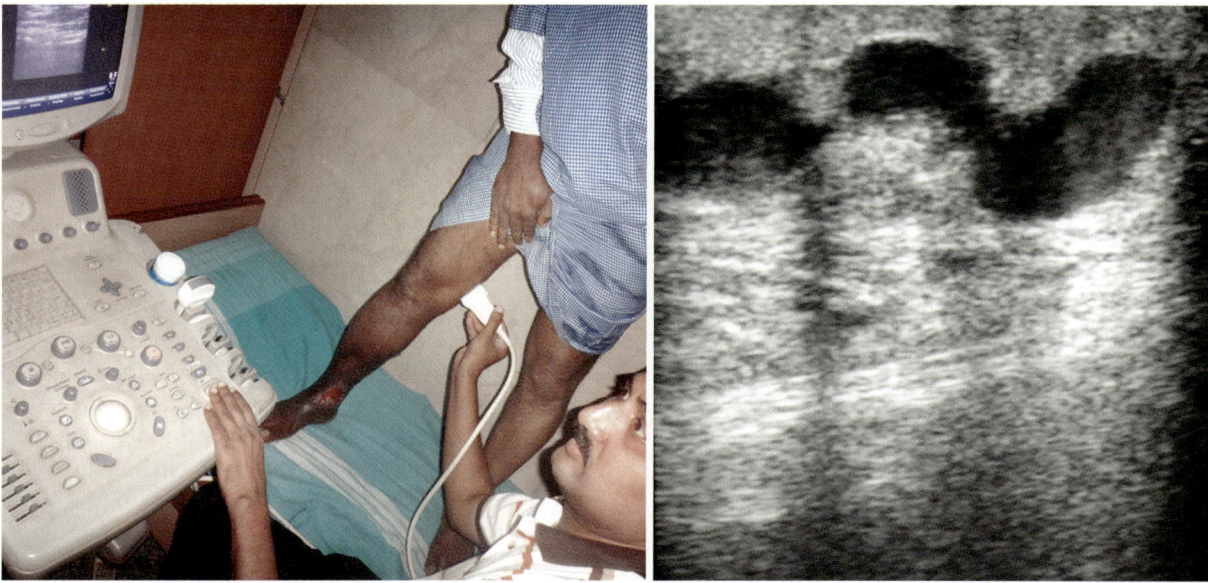

Fig. 7-40 Doppler duplex scan is being done for varicose veins. *Scan should be done in standing position.* Saphenofemoral junction is often called as saphenous eye sonologically. DVT, reflux, compressibility, and venous blood flow should be looked for.

adjustable stands and to prevent venous pooling, scintillation counter is placed over the calf. Counting in the leg is done from below upwards at 5 cm intervals. Procedure is done in preoperative period; on 1st, 3rd and 6th postoperative days. A 20% or more rises in percentage value suggests deep vein thrombosis in leg. I125 labeled fibrinogen is used (earlier I131 labeled fibrinogen was used) because it has got shorter radioaction and its detectability is possible with much lighter and mobile apparatus.

Ultrasound abdomen: U/S abdomen, peripheral smear, platelet count, and other relevant investigations are done depending on the cause of the varicose veins.

Investigating the venous ulcer: If venous ulcer is present, then the discharge is collected for culture and sensitivity, biopsy from ulcer edge is taken to rule out Marjolin's ulcer, plain X-ray of the part is taken to look for periostitis (Figs. 7-41A and B).

Routine Investigations

Hematocrit, blood urea, serum creatinine, blood sugar; Chest X-ray, ECG. It is mainly done to prepare the patient for surgery-for anesthesia purpose.

■ SURGICAL ANATOMY OF LOWER LIMB VEINS (FIG. 7.42)

Superficial venous system—It is located in the saphenous compartment which is between subcutaneous plane and deeper aponeurotic plane. GSV and SSV are in this plane.

Great (Long) saphenous vein (GSV) derived from word "*saphena*" (Arabic) means easily seen: Being the longest vein in the body it runs from the medial end of the dorsal venous arch up along the anteromedial aspect of the leg and thigh until it empties into the femoral vein. There is one valve at this junction—is called as ostial/terminal valve and reflux through it is called as *ostial reflux*. There is one more valve proximal to the main junctional tributary veins and is called as

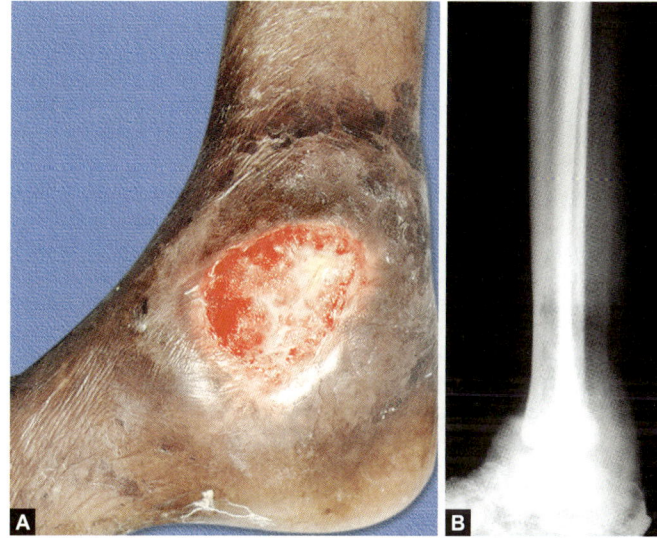

Figs. 7-41A and B Venous ulcer *showing periostitis* features in the X-ray taken.

preterminal valve. More than 50% reflux occurs at preterminal valve (*preterminal reflux*).

Small (Short) saphenous vein (SSV): It runs from the lateral end of the dorsal venous arch up along the posterolateral aspect of the calf until it passes through the popliteal fossa behind the knee and empties into the popliteal vein just above the knee.

Tributaries are located in the subcutaneous plane which joins the saphenous system. Superficial circumflex vein (often joins AAGSV), superficial external pudendal vein, superficial inferior epigastric vein, anterior vein of the leg, posterior arch vein of the leg (joins GSV), posterolateral venous chains of leg—are different tributaries. Long intersaphenous communicating vein often exists between cranial extension of SSV to join GSV and can be varicose and pathological and is called as *communicating vein of Giacomini-Cruveilhier*.

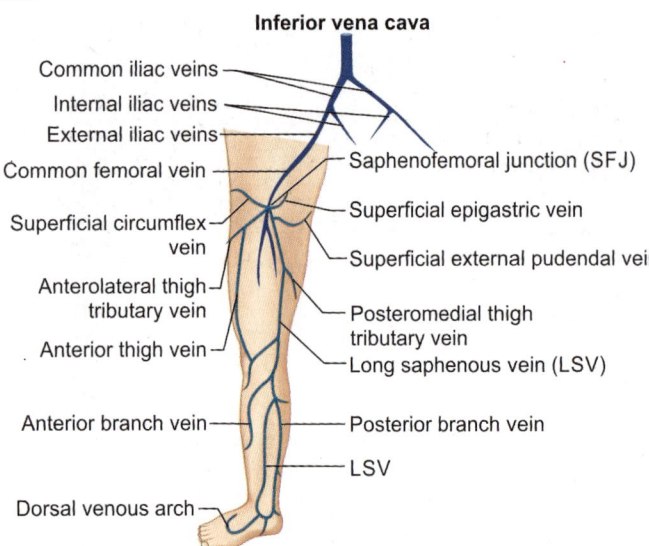

Fig. 7-42 Diagrams showing *venous anatomy* of the lower limb. Also note the functioning of the valve in the vein.

Anterior accessory great saphenous vein (AAGSV, Anterolateral vein of thigh) is communicating vein into the GSV anteriorly and laterally. AAGSV communicates into GSV usually just proximal to preterminal valve (60%); often at confluence (39%); rarely onto femoral vein (1%). In many patients with varicose veins it is this vein which is diseased than GSV. It often receives superficial circumflex vein before joining the GSV.

Different Types of Perforators: Para Achillean (Bassi); Ankle perforators: (May or Kuster); Lower leg perforators between deep veins and posterior arch vein (Cockett): I (posteroinferior to medial malleolus), II (10 cm above the medial malleolus), III (15 cm above medial malleolus); Gastrocnemius perforators between GSV and deep veins—upper proximal paratibial (Boyd)—below knee; Lower and medial paratibial (Sherman); '24' cm perforator between deep veins and GSV; Mid-thigh perforator between deep vein and GSV (Dodd); Hach perforator in the posterior thigh; Hunter's adductor canal perforator in the thigh **(Fig. 7-43)**.

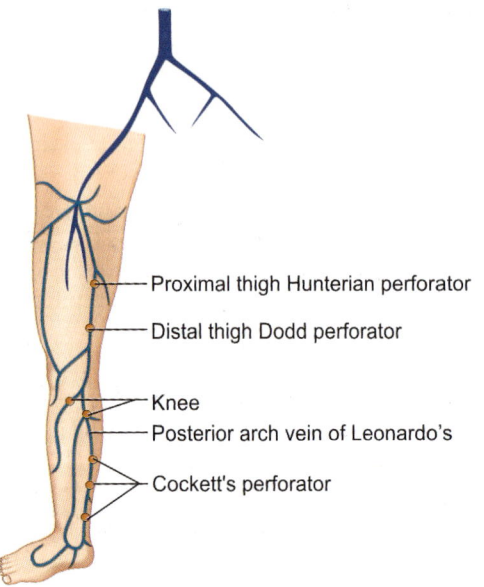

Fig. 7-43 Diagram showing *different perforators*.

Note: IVC does not have any valves. Common, external and internal iliac veins have usually one valve each. Superficial and deep femoral have 3-4 valves; popliteal have 2; posterior tibial 15-19; anterior tibial 8-11; peroneal 8-10. Great and small saphenous veins have 8-10 valves (usually distal to entry of tributary); perforator veins have 1-2 valves deep to deep fascia; communicating vein will have only one valve or valveless. GSV has got 15-20 valves; SSV has got 5-15 valves.

Varicose Veins

It is ***dilated, tortuous and elongated*** superficial vein with reversal of blood flow due to incompetence of valves. It is seen only in human beings due to erect posture. It is not seen in animals. A varicose vein is one which has **permanently** lost its valvular efficiency. As a result of continuous dilatation under pressure in course of time, varicose vein becomes elongated, tortuous, pouched, thickened, inelastic and friable structure. Incidence of varicose veins is 5% in general population.

It is more common in females (10:1). It is much more common in females with a family history. Often it is familial. ***Familial varicose veins*** begin in younger age group and are seen bilaterally, involve all veins including deep veins. Presents with visible dilated veins in the leg with pain, distress, ***nocturnal cramps***, feeling of heaviness, muscle fatigue, throbbing heavy legs, (restless legs), soreness, burning, pruritus. Often there is pedal edema, pigmentation, dermatitis, ulceration, tenderness, restricted ankle joint movement, bleeding, and positive cough impulse at the saphenofemoral junction. Thickening of tibia occurs due to periostitis. It may present with DVT, especially in pregnancy. Local gigantism may be the presentation in varicose veins due to congenital AV malformation.

Note: Extent of valvular incompetence is not related to the presence and severity of the symptoms.

Varicosities are more common in lower limb. Because of erect posture long column of blood has to be supported, which can lead to weakness and incompetence of valves leading to varicosities.

Types:
1. ***Primary varicosities are due to:*** Congenital incompetence or absence of valves; weakness of valves; weakness or wasting of muscles; stretching of deep fascia. It is precipitated by prolonged standing and recurrent thrombophlebitis.
2. ***Secondary varicosities are due to:*** Recurrent thrombophlebitis; occupational—standing for long hours; obstruction to venous return like abdominal tumor, retroperitoneal fibrosis, pelvic mass; ascites; lymphadenopathy; pregnancy (due to progesterone hormone); acquired AV fistula (due to surgery/trauma). It may be due to previous deep venous thrombosis.

Congenital: Congenital A-V malformations; Klippel-Trenaunay syndrome; Avalvulia.

Lipodermatosclerosis and development of different problems in varicose veins: Fibrin deposition, scarring and tissue hypoxia due to chronic venous hypertension around ankle joint is called as ***lipodermatosclerosis***. It is irreversible

Chapter 7: Examination and Clinical Approach in Venous Diseases

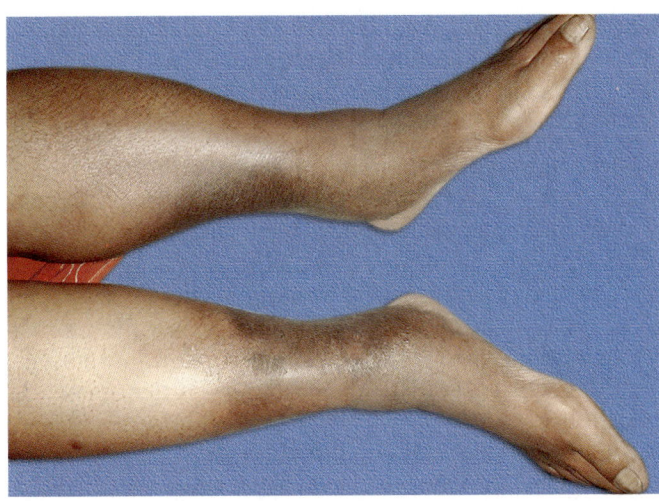

Fig. 7-44 *Lipodermatosclerosis* – a complication of varicose vein with narrow ankle and prominent calf.

change in the soft tissue which eventually leads into ulceration **(Fig. 7-44)**.

Venous Ulcer

It is the complication of varicose veins or deep vein thrombosis **(Figs. 7-45A and B)**. Varicose veins or DVT which are recanalized, eventually causes chronic venous hypertension around ankle → causes hemosiderin deposition in the subcutaneous plane from lyzed RBC's, Eczema → dermatitis and lipodermatosclerosis → fibrosis →anoxia → **ulceration. Area where venous ulcer commonly develops, is around and above the medial malleoli** because of presence of large number of perforators which transmit pressure changes directly into superficial system. This area is called as *Gaiter's zone*. It can be seen on both malleoli. Ulcer is often large, nonhealing, tender, recurrent with secondary infection. Vertical group of inguinal lymph nodes are usually enlarged and tender. Often it leads to scarring, ankylosis, *Marjolin's ulcer* formation. Sloughing from the ulcer bed may give way causing venous hemorrhage. **Periostitis is common** which also prevents ulcer from healing. Due to regular walking on toes to get relief from pain, causes contraction and extra articular fibrosis of Achilles tendon–*talipes equino varus*.

Deep Vein Thrombosis (DVT)

All deep veins in the lower limb have valves except sural veins (veins in soleus muscle). At rest as the blood flow through the sural veins is sluggish it is the commonest site for thrombosis. Pelvic veins are other common site for DVT. Thrombosis of the deep venous system, can be **acute** or **recurrent**. It can be **occlusive** or **non-occlusive**. It can be **free** thrombus or **fixed** thrombus. It can **be propagative** which propagates proximally and has higher chance of formation of embolism or **nonpropagative**. Factors—**Virchow's triad (1856):** Stasis; Hypercoagulability; Vein wall injury. Thrombus may start in a venous tributary which may eventually extend into the main vein causing DVT.

Causes: Following **childbirth;** trauma; muscular violence; **prolonged immobility**; debilitating illness, obesity, bed rest, pregnancy, puerperium, oral contraceptives, and estrogens.

Polycythemia vera, thrombocytosis; deficiencies of antithrombin III, protein C, protein S; factor V of Leiden, antiphospholipid syndrome, thrombophilia, recent myocardial infarction, heart failure, nephrotic syndrome, e-*thrombosis* (in people who sit on computer for long time) are other causes.

Postoperative thrombosis: Common after the age of 40 years. Incidence following surgeries is 30%. In 30% of cases both legs are affected. Usually it is seen after prostate surgery, hip surgery, major abdominal surgeries, gynecological surgeries, cancer surgeries. Bedridden for **more than 3 days** in the postoperative period increases the risk of DVT.

Spontaneous thrombosis is common in visceral neoplasm like carcinoma pancreas or carcinoma stomach. It is often migrating type.

Axillary vein thrombosis: Upper limb DVT (5% of total DVT) can occur spontaneously, following compression by cervical rib, by various causes of thoracic inlet syndrome, or arm being in the hyperabduction state for prolonged period (e.g painting the ceiling, athletes, swimmers), after axillary lymph node block dissection, after radiotherapy to axilla, occasionally as a complication of venous cannulation. Idiopathic upper limb DVT may be due to some occult malignancy in the body. Even though upper limb DVT is less common chances of pulmonary embolism is more—33% of upper limb DVT can lead into pulmonary embolism.

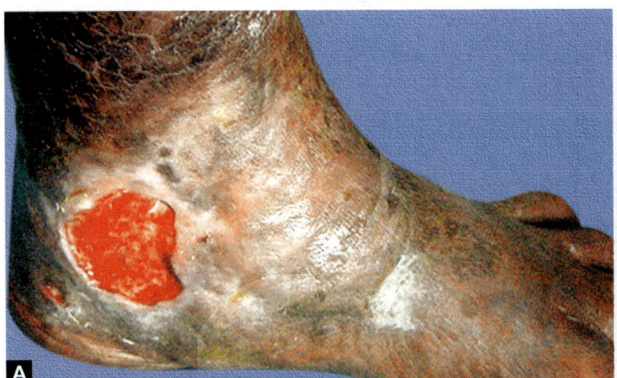 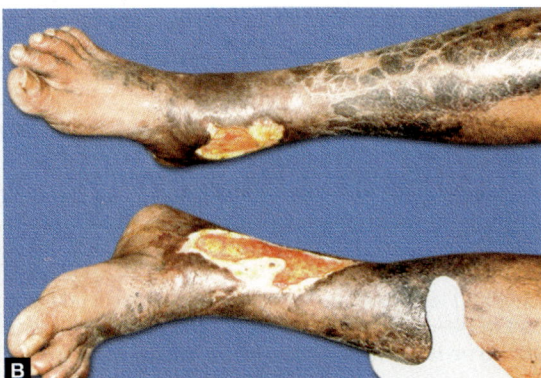

Figs. 7-45A and B *Typical site of venous ulcer*. Often venous ulcer can be bilateral.

> Sites: (1) Pelvic veins—Common. (2) Leg veins—Common in femoral and popliteal veins (Common on left side). (3) Upper limb veins—Not uncommon (Axillary vein thrombosis).
>
> **Phlegmasia alba dolens:** It is DVT of **femoral vein** (deep femoral vein commonly) causing painful congestion and edema of leg, with lymphangitis, which further increases the edema and worsens the situation (**White leg**). **Phlegmasia cerulea dolens:** It is extensive DVT of **iliac and pelvic veins** causing **blue leg** with either venous gangrene or areas of infarction.

Clinical features: Fever is the earliest and common symptom. Pain and swelling in the calf and thigh, commonly associated with fever. Pain is often so severe that the patient finds difficult to flex or move the leg. Leg is tense, tender, warm, pale or bluish with stretched and shiny skin.

Positive Homan's sign: Passive forceful dorsiflexion of the foot with extended knee will cause tenderness in the calf. Positive Homan's sign is confirmative sign of DVT; but absence of Homan's sign is not a reliable indicator of absence of DVT.

Mose's sign: Gentle squeezing of lower part of the calf from side-to-side is painful. Gentleness is very important otherwise it may dislodge a thrombus to form an embolus.

Neuhof's sign: Thickening and deep tenderness is elicited while palpating deep in calf muscles.

Linton's test: After applying proximal tourniquet: with elevation after walk; superficial veins are still prominent. Most often, DVT is *asymptomatic (60%)* and presents suddenly with **features of pulmonary embolism** like **chest pain, breathlessness and hemoptysis.**

Complications and sequelae of DVT: pulmonary embolism (15%), secondary varicose vein, venous ulcer, venous gangrene, partial recanalisation causing chronic venous insufficiency (CVI), recurrent DVT.

Superficial Thrombophlebitis

It is thrombosis with inflammation of superficial veins **(Figs. 7-46A and B)**. It can be acute—due to IV cannulation, trauma, minor injury/infection, hypercoagulability; spontaneous—due to polycythemia, polyarteritis nodosa, TAO; migratory thrombophlebitis (***Trousseau's sign***—1876—Trousseau himself had migratory thrombophlebitis due to advanced carcinoma) is due to underlying gastrointestinal malignancy commonly carcinoma pancreas. ***Mondor's disease*** is superficial thrombophlebitis of subcutaneous veins of breast and chest wall. Clinical features are pain, occasionally fever, redness, tenderness, and cord-like thickening of veins. ***Complications are***—DVT, venous valve destruction and incompetence, infection like cellulitis, embolism.

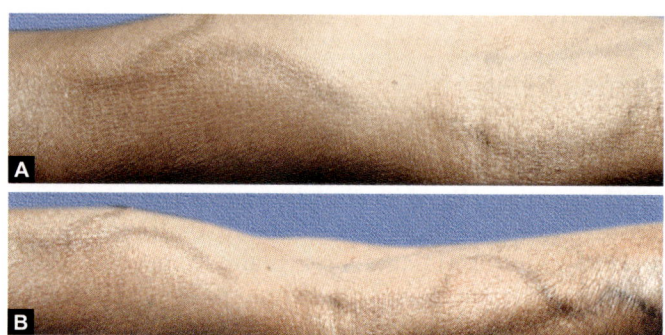

Figs. 7-46A and B Superficial *thrombophlebitis* forearm and arm.

CASE DISCUSSION

A 40-year-old female presents with dilated veins in the both leg since 4 years and ulcers with around both ankles since 4 months. Ulcers are over the medial malleoli of both legs of around 5 × 4 cm in size with discharge. Dilated veins are over the medial side of the both legs suggestive of long saphenous vein. Trendelenburg test both parts showed saphenofemoral and perforator incompetence.

What is your clinical diagnosis? What further clinical examinations you will do?
Clinical diagnosis is varicose ulcers on both ankles due to saphenofemoral and perforators incompetence. Multiple tourniquet tests should be done to identify the location of the perforators. Fegan's test is done to mark out the perforators. Other tests done are Morrissey's cough impulse test, Schwartz test, modified Perthe's test. Ulcer should be examined in detail. Abdomen and cardiovascular system examinations should be done. Deep vein thrombosis (DVT) should be ruled out. Peripheral pulses (dorsalis pedis, posterior tibial, popliteal) should be checked to rule out associated peripheral vascular disease.

What essential investigations are required in such patients?
Venous Doppler with duplex scan of both lower limbs is essential to rule out DVT, to find out the incompetence and perforator status. Ultrasound abdomen should be done. Venous hemodynamic mapping is done prior to intervention. Discharge study, X-ray part is also done.

CLINICAL PEARLS

- Varicose vein is a *more morbid disease*; intervention should be done with caution as recurrence and complications are higher.
- Patient should be examined in *standing position*.
- Trendelenburg test, multiple tourniquet test, Fegan's test and modified Perthes' tests are important clinical tests.
- *Venous Doppler with duplex* scan should be done in all patients also in **standing position**.
- DVT *should be ruled out* in all patients.

CHAPTER 8

Examination and Clinical Approach to Lymphatic System

Competency: SU27.7; SU27.8; AN10.6; AN10.7; AN20.4; AN23.7; AN35.5; PA.19.1; PA19.2; PA19.4; PA19.5.

There are about 600–800 lymph nodes in the body. Lymph nodes are distributed as—around 200–300 in the neck; 100 in the thorax; 50 in axilla; 250 in the abdomen and pelvis; 50 in the groin area.

Lymphatic watershed area: There are 6 lymphatic watershed areas in the body—three on each side. First above the clavicle drains into the neck nodes; second from clavicle to umbilical line which drains into axillary lymph nodes; third from umbilical line below which drains into inguinal/groin nodes.

Microanatomy of lymph nodes: Lymph node contains cortex, paracortex and medulla. Cortex contains follicles with B lymphocytes, macrophages. Germinal center of the cortex is surrounded by small B lymphocytes. Paracortex contains T lymphocytes.

Function of the lymph nodes and lymphatics: It filters the intravascular proteins and recirculates them back to circulation. It also maintains humoral and cell-mediated immunity.

Extranodal lymphatic structures in the body are: *Waldeyer's ring (Inner* = adenoids, tubal tonsils, palatine tonsils, lingual tonsil; *Outer*); *thymus; spleen; Peyer's patches* in the intestine; appendix.

Different diseases involve the lymph nodes and lymphatics. They are—lymphadenitis, tuberculosis, other infections (like HIV, infectious mononucleosis), lymphoma, metastatic to nodes, lymphedema which may be filarial or congenital or malignant or after nodal surgery or after radiotherapy (Figs. 8-1 to 8-6).

Fig. 8-1 Elephantiasis due to *filariasis*.

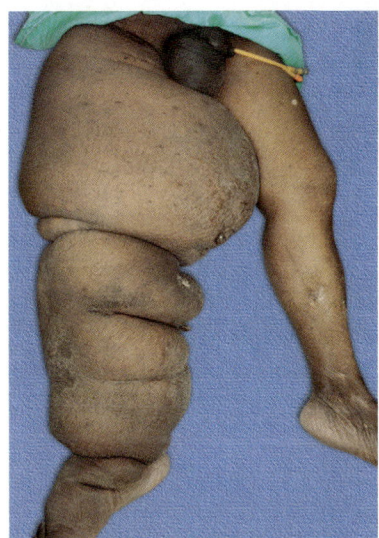

Fig. 8-2 *Advanced lymphedema* foot with vesicles and ulceration.

HISTORY

History taking includes:

Name:

Address: Filarial lymphedema is more common in tropical countries. In India it is common in coastal areas. Odisha is the most affected state in India.

Age: Tuberculous lymphadenitis occurs in young age group. It is common in neck nodes. Hodgkin's lymphoma occurs both in young and elderly with bimodal age occurrence. Malignant secondaries in lymph nodes is common in old age. Nonspecific adenitis, HIV infected lymphadenopathy can

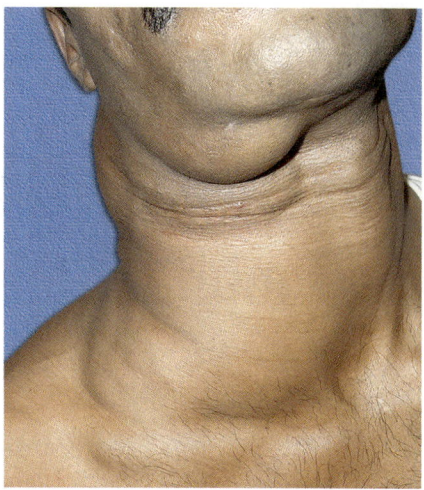

Fig. 8-3 Lymphoma neck. It shows *India rubber consistency*.

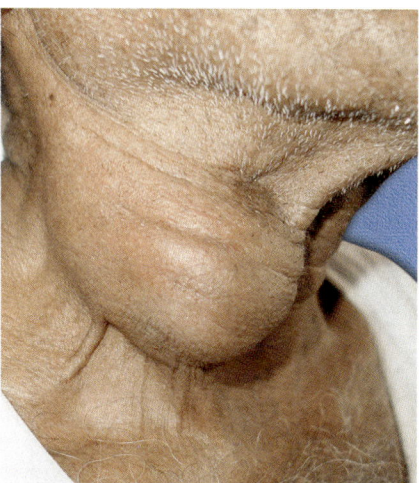

Fig. 8-4 Lymph node *secondaries (metastases) in the neck*. Note the fixity.

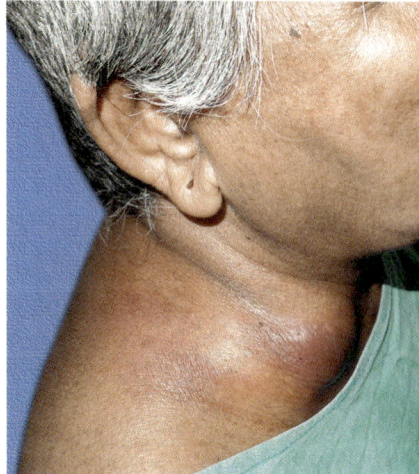

Fig. 8-5 *Cold abscess* in the neck due to caseating type of tuberculous lymphadenitis.

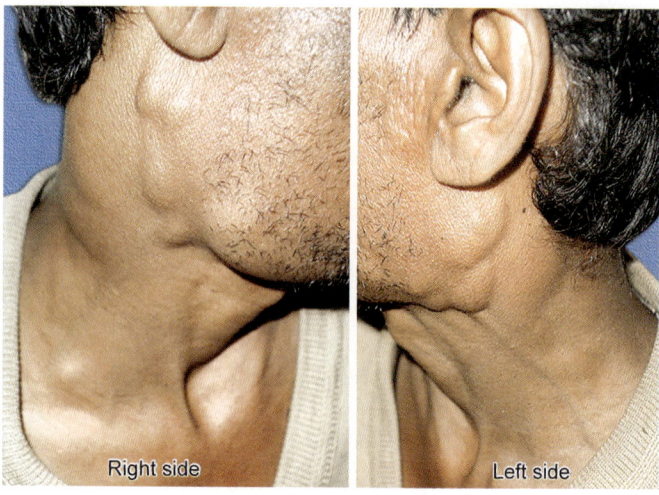

Fig. 8-6 Bilateral neck lymph nodes. It could be *tuberculosis or lymphoma*.

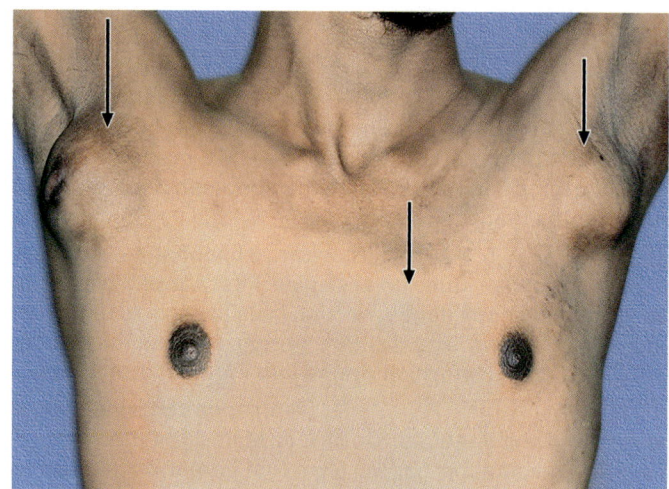

Fig. 8-7 Bilateral axillary lymph nodes—lymphoma. *Entire lymphatic system has to be examined thoroughly.*

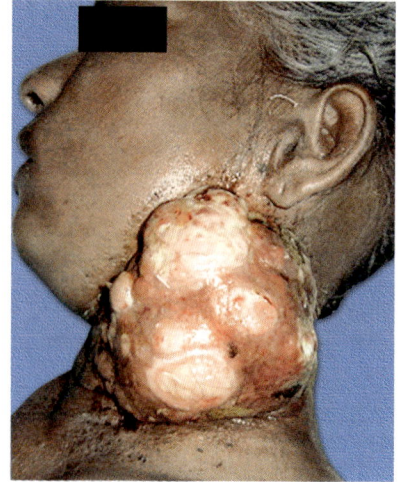

Fig. 8-8 *Fungating secondaries* in the neck.

occur in any age group. Filarial lymphadenitis is common in any age group especially in certain parts of India and other developing countries. It commonly affects inguinal lymph nodes. Primary lymphedema occurs in younger age group; secondary lymphedema occurs in middle aged and elderly (**Figs. 8-7 to 8-11**).

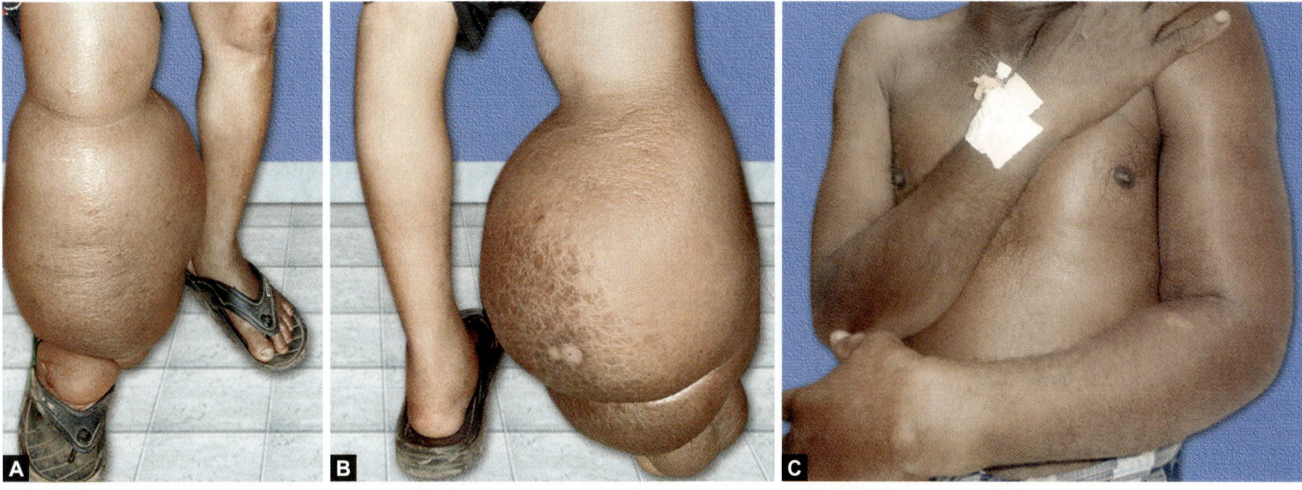

Figs. 8-9A to C Filarial lymphedema—*elephantiasis* left leg. Also *upper limb lymphedema* left side.

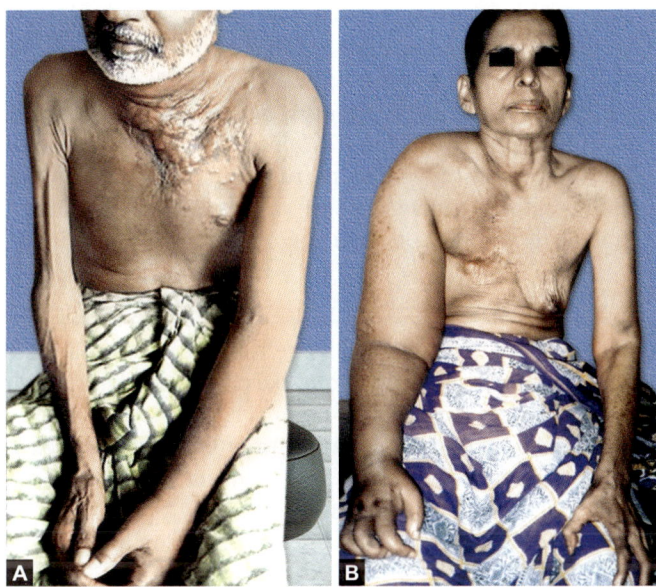

Figs. 8-10A and B Lymphedema left sided in a male patient due to studded *advanced cancer in left axillary nodes* and chest wall. In photo B, female patient having lymphedema right upper limb following *mastectomy with axillary clearance*.

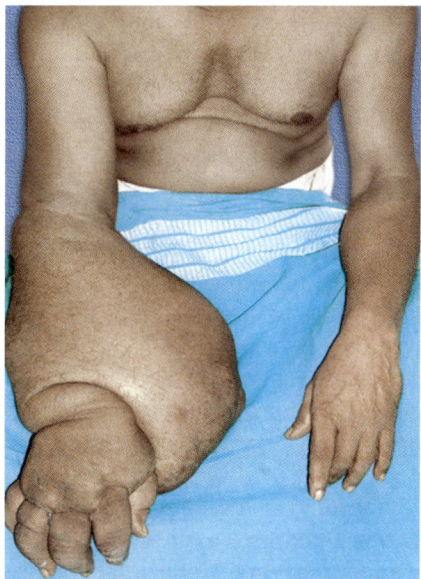

Fig. 8-11 *Right upper limb lymphedema* in a male who underwent reduction surgery for the same.

Sex: Lymphedema, primary or secondary is more common in females.

Occupation:

CHIEF COMPLAINTS

- History of swelling and duration.
- History of pain and duration.
- History of fever.

History of Present Illness

Swelling

Swelling is the commonest presentation in lymphadenopathy.
- **Which group has enlarged** first is to be noted.
- Traumatic origin and inflammatory origin involves only one group whereas generalized lymphadenopathy can occur in leukemia and lymphoma.
- Tuberculosis and Hodgkin's lymphoma is common in cervical lymph nodes.
- Filarial lymphadenitis is common in superficial inguinal lymph nodes. Its progress, presence of pain, whether reduced in size has to be noted.
- Enlarged lymph node if reduces in size after some time means it is of inflammatory origin; there is no spontaneous reduction in size in neoplastic conditions.
- *Number* of swellings is also important. Lymphoma may show multiple groups of nodal enlargement. *Site* of the origin of first swelling is important. If it is in the upper neck, then probably it may be either due to tuberculosis or secondaries with primary in the oral cavity/pharynx/larynx. If it is in the lower neck then it may be secondaries from malignancy in esophagus/bronchus, etc.
- *Duration*—acute lymphadenitis is of short *duration* with pain and fever (with features of acute inflammation—redness, warm, pain, and loss of function at the site).

Malignancy in the lymph node either primary lymphoma or secondaries (metastases) are also of short duration (in few weeks). But initially it is painless. It is rapidly progressive and later may become painful. Lymph nodes of tuberculosis, syphilis, brucellosis and sarcoidosis are of long duration and are often painless. In syphilis lymph node enlargement occurs in secondary type. Syphilis, brucellosis, sarcoidosis are rare now. Tuberculous lymphadenitis is still common condition in developing countries like India. Tuberculous lymphadenitis is much more common in HIV infected or immunosuppressed patients.

Pain

- Acute lymphadenitis is painful.
- Tuberculosis is painless. If there is secondary infection pain can occur. Malignant lymphoma and secondaries in lymph node are initially painless but can be painful once there is fixity, necrosis, infiltration into deeper planes and nerves or fungation or secondary infection.
- Enlarged syphilitic lymph nodes are painless.

Fever

- Continuous high grade fever occurs in acute lymphadenitis with suppuration.
- Evening rise of temperature is seen in tuberculous disease. But many patients with tuberculous lymphadenitis may not show any fever (fever is necessarily not always seen in tuberculous lymphadenitis).
- In Hodgkin's lymphoma intermittent fever *(Pel-Ebstein fever)* may be present which also decides prognosis and staging.
  Pel-Ebstein fever is also seen in brucellosis. Fever is not common in secondaries but can occur due to sepsis, tumor necrosis, and fungation.

History Relevant in Relation to Drainage Area

When lymph nodes of particular region are enlarged, history suggestive of any disease in that particular drainage area should be asked for. Examples—in enlargement of axillary nodes, symptoms pertaining to pathology in upper limb, chest wall, abdomen above the umbilicus area, breast should be asked.

Other Relevant History

- *History of cough, hemoptysis, chest pain* in tuberculosis (tuberculous lymphadenitis may often be associated with pulmonary tuberculosis); *hoarseness of voice* due to pressure on recurrent laryngeal nerve either by lymph nodes in tracheoesophageal groove or by mediastinal nodes on left side compressing the left recurrent laryngeal nerve; *dysphagia* due to compression over esophagus; *swelling of face and neck* due to compression of superior vena cava by superior mediastinal lymph nodes; *stridor or dyspnea* by pressure on the trachea or bronchus. If nodes are secondaries, hoarseness/dyspnea/dysphagia may be features of primary tumor in larynx/bronchus/pharynx or esophagus. Often tuberculous cervical lymphadenitis may be associated with laryngeal tuberculosis causing hoarseness of voice.
- Upper limb edema may be present due to compression in axillary node enlargement. Inguinal lymph node enlargement may cause **lower limb lymphedema or venous edema** due to compression or lymphatic block or infiltration by malignant lymph node. Retroperitoneal nodal enlargement can cause compression/encasement of IVC/iliac vessels causing **edema of lower limbs**.
- *History of bleeding gums* is common in leukemia, lymphomas, and blood dyscrasias.
- *History of trauma* is often important in acute lymphadenitis.
- *History of loss of appetite* and reduced weight is important in lymphomas, advanced secondaries, AIDS, etc. Tuberculous lymphadenitis when associated with pulmonary or abdominal or miliary tuberculosis, patient will have loss of appetite and weight.
- *History of night sweats, rigors, pruritus, and bone pain* are important symptoms in lymphoma. Bone pain may be observed in the sternum, ribs, vertebra could be due to metastases. *Jaundice* may suggest liver secondaries; *hemoptysis* and *chest pain* may suggest lung secondaries.

Past History

- Past history of any disease like tuberculosis, treatment received, earlier investigations like chest X-ray, fine needle aspiration cytology (FNAC), biopsy.
- Earlier treatment for malignancy with radiotherapy or chemotherapy should be asked for. History of BCG vaccination may be relevant.
- History of diabetes mellitus and hypertension is also asked for.

> **In lymph node enlargement following history is important:**
> - Fever, weight loss
> - First node involved, later other nodal regions involved like of axilla, groin in case of neck nodes
> - Pruritus, pain, pain in relation to alcohol, bone pain, anemia, icterus
> - Family members suffering similarly
> - Cough, hemoptysis, chest pain, dyspnea, abdomen mass and fullness
> - History related to skin lesions—scaly elevated red patches are seen in mycosis fungoides

Personal History

History of smoking—its duration, number of cigarettes; alcohol intake—duration, quantity; chewing pan—duration, placing quid in the cheek; snuff abuse; dietary habits; history of sexual contact in case of HIV infection, syphilis, etc.

Family History

History suggestive of any disease or treatment taken for any specific condition by the family members is important.

Tuberculosis can occur among many family members. Lymphoma can run in families.

GENERAL EXAMINATION

Detailed general examination is very essential. Anemia/edema/jaundice/clubbing/lymphadenopathy should be noted. Radial pulse/blood pressure/raise in temperature must be recorded. Attitude of the patient/nutritional assessment by skin texture, subcutaneous fat, weight, body mass index/any other relevant findings should be mentioned. Cachexia signifies advanced malignancy or tuberculosis. Increased pulse rate and fever suggests swelling with inflammatory pathology.

LOCAL EXAMINATION

Inspection

Swelling

Detailed inspection for swelling as is discussed in *swelling* chapter should be done. **Number**—multiple lymph nodal enlargement occurs in lymphoma, tuberculosis, lymphatic leukemia, sarcoidosis, brucellosis, etc; **Size**—it is important in staging metastatic nodal status (N stage); **Shape**—globular, hemispherical, oval; **extent** from a bony part, **Surface**—smooth in lymphoma and tuberculosis, irregular in secondaries; **Margin**—well-defined or ill-defined; **Pulsation**—as transmitted pulsation due to compression over adjacent major arteries like aorta/femoral/abdominal aorta; **Peristalsis**—may be visible in mesenteric lymphadenitis causing subacute obstruction; **Impulse on coughing**—may be present in swellings in relation to cavities like thorax; **Dilated veins over the swelling**—may be visible due to compression over the major veins in the neck or SVC in the mediastinum; *edema* over the swelling or distal to it like in the limbs may be seen; **venous engorgement** of face can be seen in neck swelling **(Fig. 8-12)**. Tuberculosis and Hodgkin's lymphoma usually involve the neck lymph nodes; filariasis and lymphogranuloma venereum (LGV L1, 2, 3) usually involve groin lymph nodes. Epitrochlear and suboccipital nodes are involved in secondary syphilis. Epitrochlear nodes can also get involved in non-Hodgkin's lymphoma (NHL) **(Figs. 8-13 to 8-15)**.

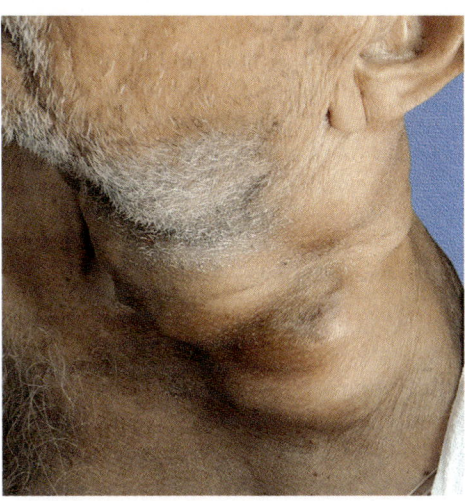

Fig. 8-13 *Lymphoma of neck lymph nodes*; note the number and surface.

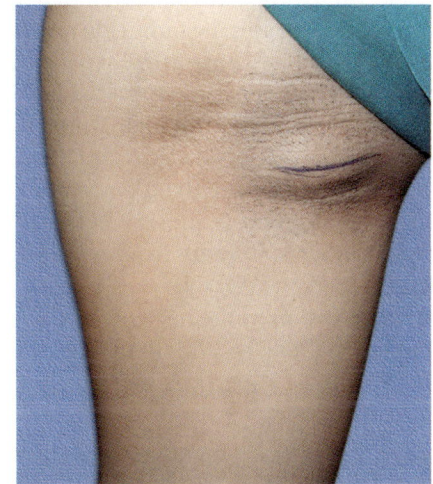

Fig. 8-14 *Typical location* of inguinal lymph nodes.

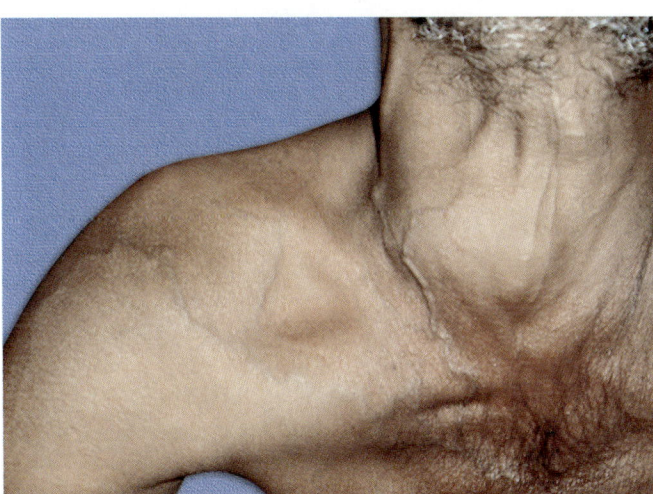

Fig. 8-12 Dilated veins in the neck left side with enlarged lymph nodes. It could be lymphoma/secondaries with mediastinal node enlargement compressing SVC.

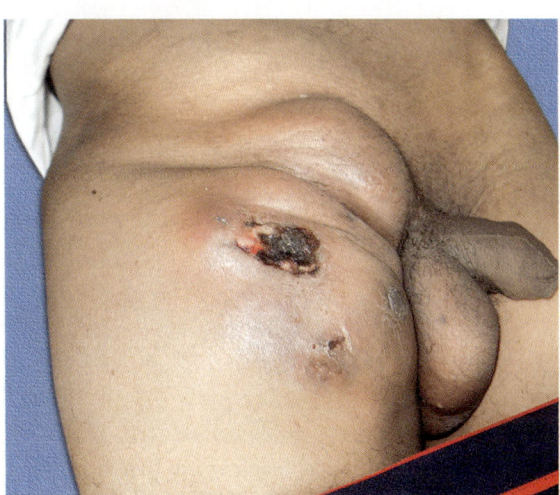

Fig. 8-15 *Extensive inguinal lymph node enlargement* with iliac nodes with fixation to skin and deeper structures.

Skin Over the Swelling

Skin over the swelling is red, inflamed, edematous in acute lymphadenitis. It may be tense, shiny with often dilated veins in rapidly growing lymphosarcoma. **Skin ulceration; skin adherence to swelling** underneath when skin gets infiltrated gives the typical '*Peau d'orange*' appearance; ***fungation***— all common in secondaries in lymph nodes. **Scar, sinus, ulcer** may suggest tuberculosis, malignancy or LGV. **Scar of previous surgery** over the swelling may be present; its length, color, site should be mentioned; scar might have been due to old surgery for drainage or biopsy or excision of similar swelling or different swelling.

Features Suggestive of Pressure Effects

- Diffuse swelling of face and neck with dilated veins in this region suggests compression over major veins in neck or **superior vena cava (SVC)** obstruction in mediastinum.
- Axillary lymph nodes when enlarged may cause upper limb venous edema.
- Neck nodes causing compression over subclavian vein also cause similar effect.
- Compression on **hypoglossal nerve (Fig. 8-16)** (causes deviation of tongue towards the same side with hemiparesis of tongue **muscles of same side**)/**spinal accessory nerve** (causes defective shrugging of shoulder against resistance with wasting of trapezius muscle)/**cervical sympathetic** chain (causes **Horner's syndrome**— enophthalmos due to decreased aqueous humor and pressure, miosis, anhydrosis, ptosis and loss of ciliospinal reflex) can be evident in large fixed neck nodes due to secondaries.
- **Tracheal compression** by the neck nodes causes **stridor**.
- Lower limb edema may be evident in iliac or caval nodal enlargement.

Palpation

> Normal lymph nodes are usually not palpable.

Swelling

- *Local rise of temperature:* It is seen in acute lymphadenitis, and often in vascular tumors like lymphoma. Lymph node secondaries may show local rise in temperature when infection develops in it. Increase in vascularity also may add for the cause **(Fig. 8-17)**. Tuberculous lymph nodes are usually *not warm and not tender* unless there is secondary infection.
- **Tenderness** over the swelling is present in acute lymphadenitis, advanced/late stage secondaries. Enlarged nodes due to tuberculosis, syphilis and sarcoidosis are usually nontender.
- **Number, size, shape** and extent should be assessed by palpation. Symmetrical and consecutive group of lymph node involvement is seen in Hodgkin's lymphoma. Asymmetrical involvement of lymph nodes is common in NHL. It is better to measure the swelling in two dimensions.
- Margin is assessed, whether it is well-defined or ill-defined. Often some part of the margin may be clear and in such occasion the part of margin which is not clear should be mentioned. In the neck if lower margin is not clear then it is considered that it may be extending into the superior mediastinum.
- **Surface** should be felt whether it is smooth or nodular. It may be smooth in lymphoma, nodular in secondaries, typically matted in tuberculous lymphadenitis (due to periadenitis in caseating tuberculous lymphadenitis). Lymph nodes may be adherent to each other in lymphoma and secondaries. Discrete lymph nodes are often observed in lymphoma and hyperplastic tuberculous lymphadenitis. Discrete lymph

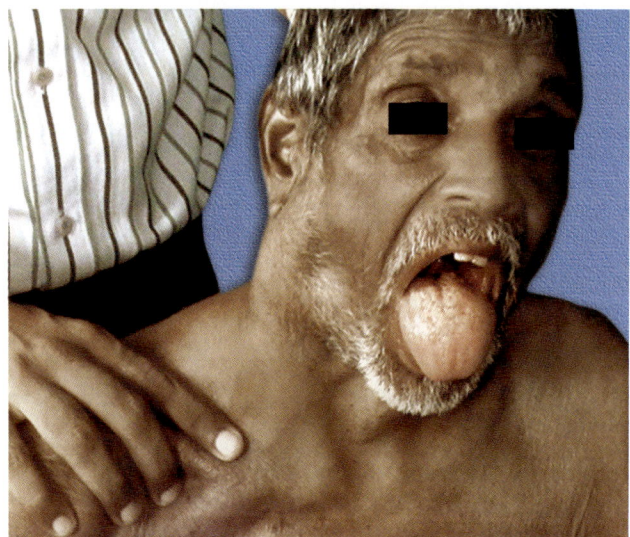

Fig. 8-16 Related neurological involvement (nerve infiltration by malignant tumor) causing altered sensory and motor functions. Example—*hypoglossal nerve involvement by neck secondaries* can cause deviation of tongue towards same side.

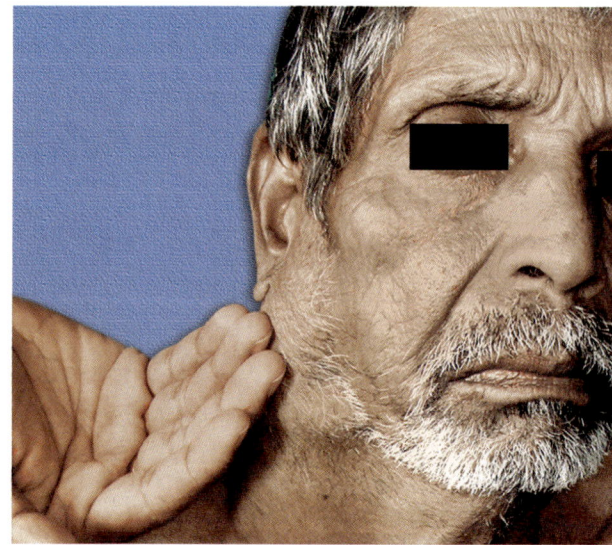

Fig. 8-17 *Warmness* should be looked for in lymph node enlargement.

nodes are also observed in lymphatic leukemia, sarcoidosis, brucellosis, HIV infection and syphilis.
- **Consistency** is very important finding to decide the pathology of the lymph node. It may be **soft and fluctuant** in cold abscess, suppurated lymph node or where there is tumor necrosis usually over summit (here remaining part of the swelling may be hard). In Hodgkin's lymphoma it has typical **India rubber consistency** with firm and elastic nature. In non-Hodgkin's lymphoma it may be **soft/firm/hard or variable in consistency**. **Shotty discrete** lymph nodes are observed in syphilis.
- **Mobility** of swelling should be checked in two perpendicular directions. Once it is checked muscle in relation to it should be contracted and mobility should be checked to find out the fixity.
- **Fixity** of swelling can occur to overlying skin; adjacent muscle either superficial or deep; deep fascia; bone in the deeper plane; vessels and nerves. Swelling is non-mobile when nodes are fixed to bone in deeper plane. Swelling when adherent to the muscle show mobility, but mobility reduces when the muscle is contracted. Skin fixity is checked by moving the skin over the swelling or by pinching the skin **(Figs. 8-18 and 8-19)**.
- **Fluctuation test** is important when it is soft or tensely cystic. Fluctuation is observed in cold abscess (tuberculosis), when there is suppuration in lymph node with abscess formation, and when there is tumor necrosis. It is done with fingers after fixing the swelling or by Paget's method of eliciting the fluctuation.
- **Plane of the swelling** should be assessed. Whether it lies superficial/deep to deep fascia; deep to muscle should be assessed. It is done by stretching the deep fascia or by contracting the muscle underneath against resistance **(Fig. 8-20)**.
- **Involvement of neurovascular bundle** should be assessed. Carotid and superficial temporal artery pulsation in neck nodal mass **(Figs. 8-21 and 8-22)**; femoral artery or distal arteries of the lower limb in groin nodes; radial artery pulsation in axillary nodes should be checked. Infiltration to adjacent nerve should be assessed by checking sensory and motor function. Carcinomatous involvement of upper deep cervical nodes may cause hypoglossal nerve palsy which can be demonstrated by asking the patient to protrude the tongue out—deviation of tongue occurs to *the same side* of the lesion.
- **Transillumination test** is negative in most of the lymph nodal enlargement. Only cystic hygroma in infants and acquired lymph cyst in any age group are brilliantly transilluminant.

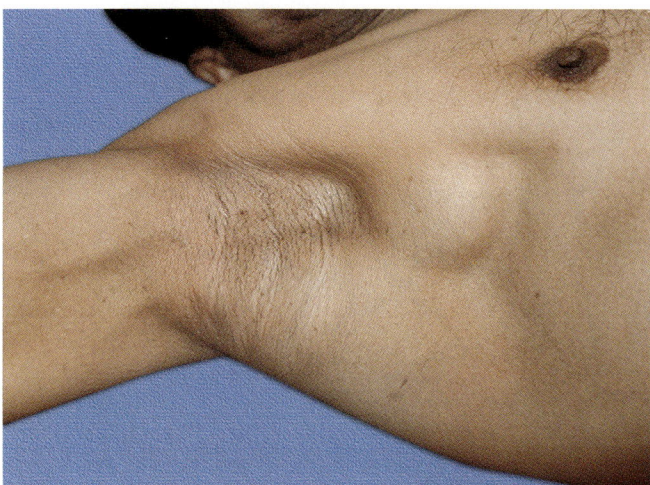

Fig. 8-19 Axillary node—central group. *Note the location, shape and size.*

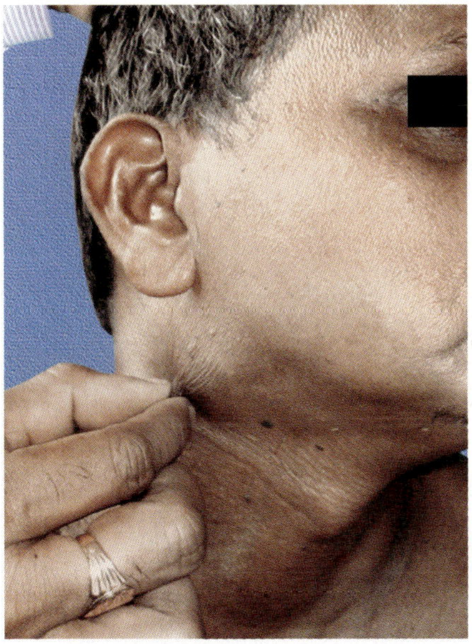

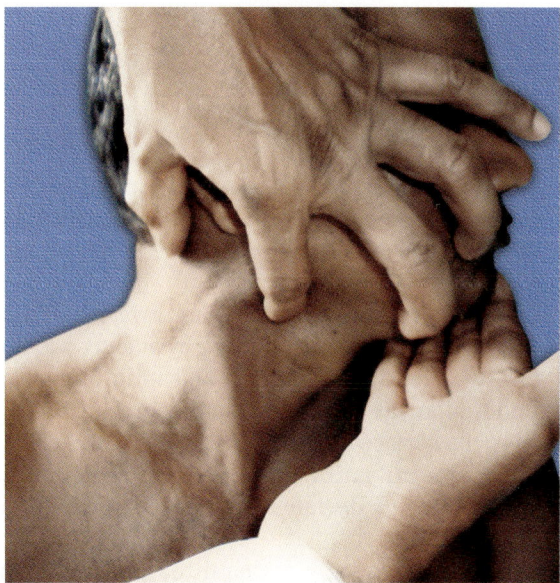

Fig. 8-18 Skin over the swelling is adherent to node underneath or not should be checked by *pinching the skin.*

Fig. 8-20 First mobility of the node/swelling is checked in relaxed position. *Muscle underneath is then contracted against resistance* to check the change in mobility. If node is adherent to muscle, mobility will be restricted.

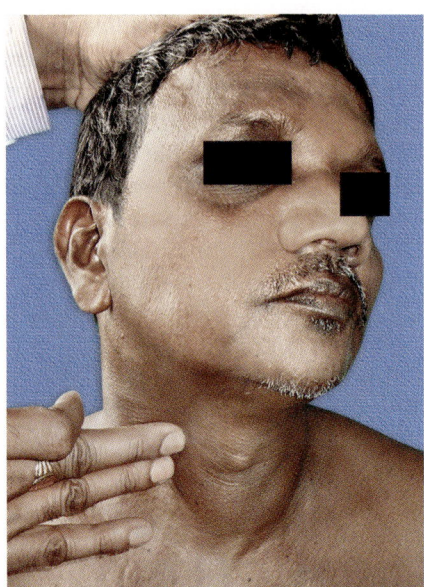

Fig. 8-21 *Palpation of carotid pulse.* Neurovascular bundle should be examined in nodal enlargement.

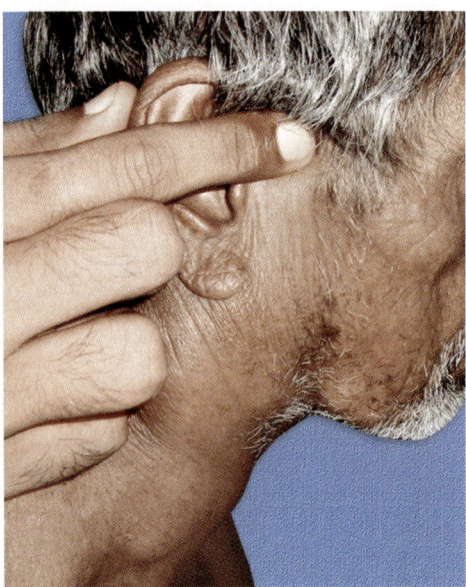

Fig. 8-22 *Pulse distal to the node should be examined* for compression at the nodal level. Palpation of superficial temporal artery is done in neck node enlargement.

- **Transmitted pulsation** may be evident in large node sitting on the major artery. It is confirmed by placing two fingers on the swelling. In transmitted pulsation fingers move perpendicular (as raised without separating apart and away) to the surface but not apart.
- In expansile pulsation (due to arterial disease like aneurysm) fingers deviate apart (raised and separated) properly.
- Para-aortic nodes show transmitted pulsation due to close proximity to the aorta. The pulsation is checked in supine position and later confirmed in lateral and knee elbow position. In transmitted pulsation (nodal mass), pulsation reduces or disappears by changing position whereas expansile carotid (arterial) pulsation will remain same as before.

Examination of Drainage Area

Drainage area of lymph nodes should be examined. It suggests the origin of the disease in the lymph node (secondaries from carcinoma or melanoma/tuberculosis/lymphadenitis) from a primary focus in the drainage area and for pressure signs (lymphedema).

Lymph Nodes in the Groin (Inguinal Nodes)

Patient exposed from mid thigh to nipple line is made to lie supine with hip slightly flexed to relax muscle and fascia. They are palpated in supine position in relation to inguinal ligament in relaxed position **(Fig. 8-23)**.
- Inguinal lymph nodes are divided into superficial and deep group.
- **Deep group** contains 2–3 lymph nodes and superior most is called as **Cloquet's node**, lies deep to fascia lata along the femoral vein. Deep node of **Cloquet lymph node** drains deep tissues of lower limb, glans penis, scrotum, vulva and clitoris. It is the uppermost deep lymph node of the inguinal region; it is located on the Cooper's ligament; it drains above to external iliac nodes.
- **Superficial lymph nodes** are divided into vertical and horizontal groups, lie beneath and parallel to inguinal ligament. Vertical group lie along the upper end of long saphenous vein drains the lower limb, scrotum and penis.
- Horizontal chains are divided into medial and lateral. Horizontal chain of inguinal lymph nodes drain (from umbilicus to toes) lower limb, *perineum, penis, scrotum, vulva, anus, buttock, lower anal canal, lower urethra, vagina, skin over lower abdomen below the umbilicus.*
- In carcinoma penis, inguinal nodes are divided into five zones (*zones of Rouviere*) by a vertical and horizontal line centering at saphenous opening. Zone 1-superolateral; zone

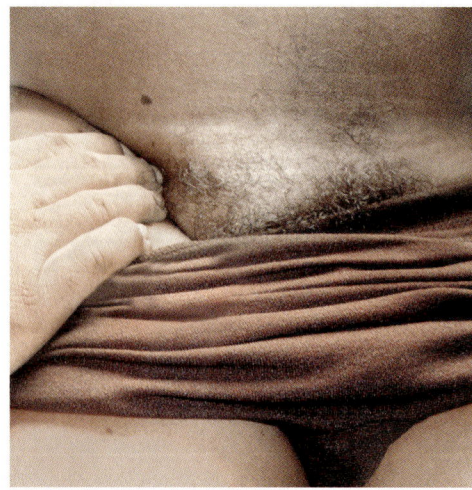

Fig. 8-23 *Inguinal lymph node* palpation.

2-superomedial; zone 3-inferomedial; zone 4-inferolateral; zone 5 is central. Superomedial zone 2 contains sentinel *saphenoepigastric node of Cabanas*.

Axillary Lymph Nodes

They drain entire upper limb, trunks, breast, and chest wall from the clavicle to umbilicus. Axillary lymph nodes are divided into three levels in relation to pectoralis minor muscle. ***Berg's levels***—Level I: below the pectoralis minor; Level II: behind the pectoralis minor; Level III: above the pectoralis minor.

Examination of axillary lymph nodes

Patient will be seated on a stool, examiner will sit/ stand in front of the patient. Patient is uncovered from neck to limb. Right axilla is palpated using left hand and vice versa. Both axillae should be examined always **(Fig. 8-24)**. Conditions which cause axillary lymph node enlargement are carcinoma breast, tuberculosis, lymphoma, lymphadenitis, any inflammatory or neoplastic pathology in upper limb, trunk, above umbilicus. While palpating number, size, surface, discrete or adherent, tenderness, consistency, mobility, fixity should be assessed. For staging in carcinoma breast (N staging), fixity/mobility of nodes, whether discrete or not are important features to be assessed. Which groups are enlarged is not important for staging. Palpable nodes are commonly significant in carcinoma breast; but nonpalpable situation does not confirm the absence of metastases. 50% of clinically impalpable axillary nodes show histologically positive features after axillary dissection in carcinoma breast **(Fig. 8-25)**.

Palpation of axillary lymph nodes

There are five groups—central, apical, anterior, posterior and lateral.

Anterior group (pectoral group) is situated behind the anterior axillary fold. The patient's arm is raised from her/his side and extended fingers of the right hand (for left axillary node) is passed into the axilla and insinuated beneath the pectoralis major. Pulp of the fingers is directed forwards and arm of the patient is lowered to rest in relaxed position over the forearm of the examiner's right hand. Pectoral nodes are palpated between thumb in front and fingers behind the muscle **(Figs. 8-26A and B)**.

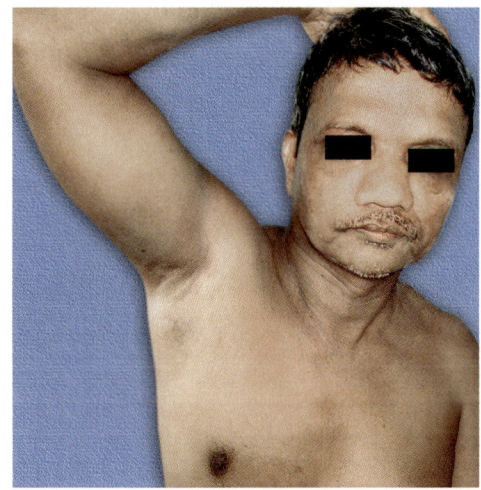

Fig. 8-24 Axilla should be inspected with *arm raised above in sitting position*.

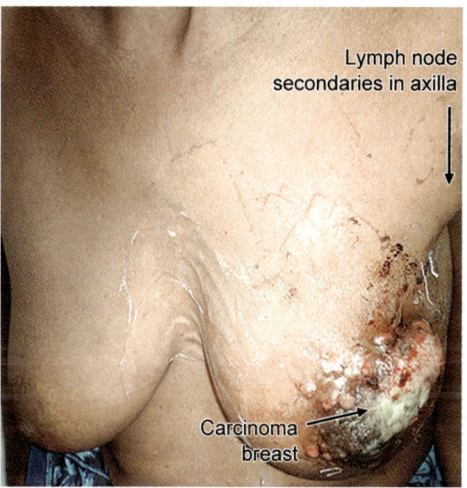

Fig. 8-25 *Carcinoma left breast* with axillary lymph node secondaries (*metastatic deposits*).

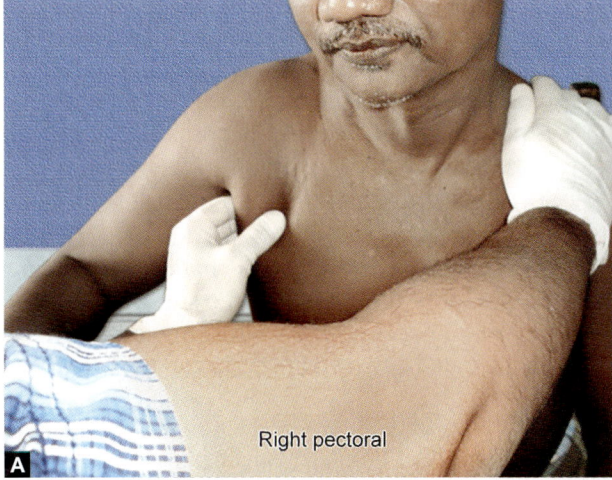

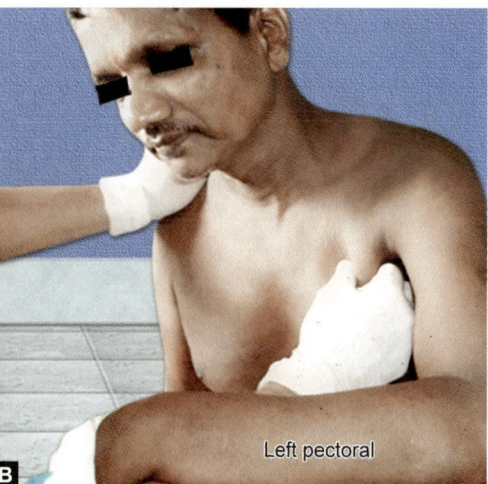

Figs. 8-26A and B Examination of pectoral nodes.

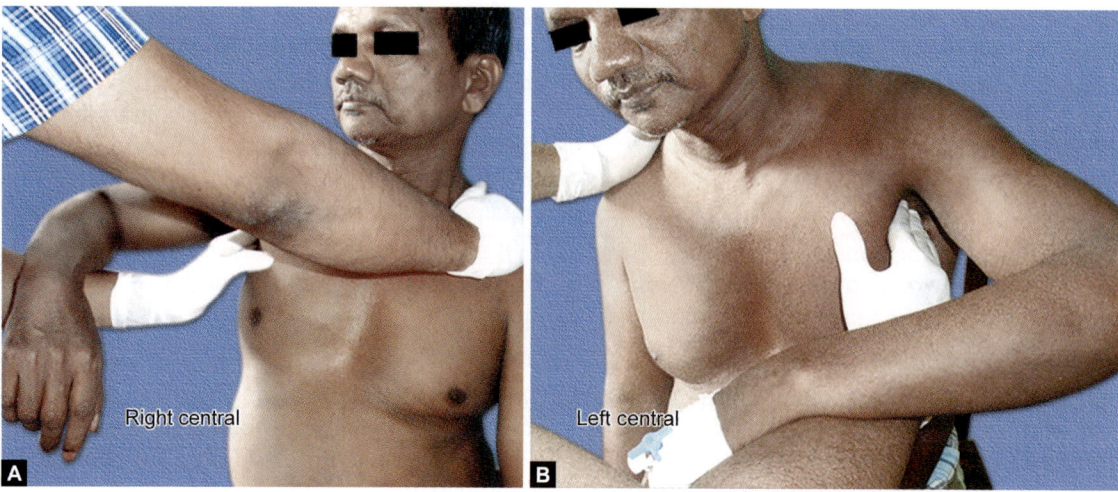

Figs. 8-27A and B Examination of *central group* of lymph nodes.

Central group is over the lateral thoracic wall. The patient's arm is raised from side and extended fingers of the right hand of the examiner are invaginated and passed high up to the apex of left axilla of the patient **(Figs. 8-27A and B)**. Palm and fingers are directed towards the lateral thoracic wall. Patient's arm is relaxed down and forearm rests and relaxed on the examiner's forearm. Non-examining hand (left hand) of the examiner is placed on the right shoulder of the patient to steady and control the examination. Hand and fingers in the axilla are still pushed high up; hand is cupped with fingers sliding and moving over the lateral thoracic wall to feel the slipping of the lymph nodes between fingers.

Lateral/brachial axillary nodes are situated over the axillary vein. The examiner uses right hand for right side of the patient and vice versa. After slightly abducting the patient's arm, the hand and fingers are placed high in axilla, palm and fingers are directed laterally over the humerus beneath the insertion of the pectoralis major over third part of axillary vessels. Opposite hand of the examiner depresses the patient's shoulder for better assess **(Fig. 8-28)**.

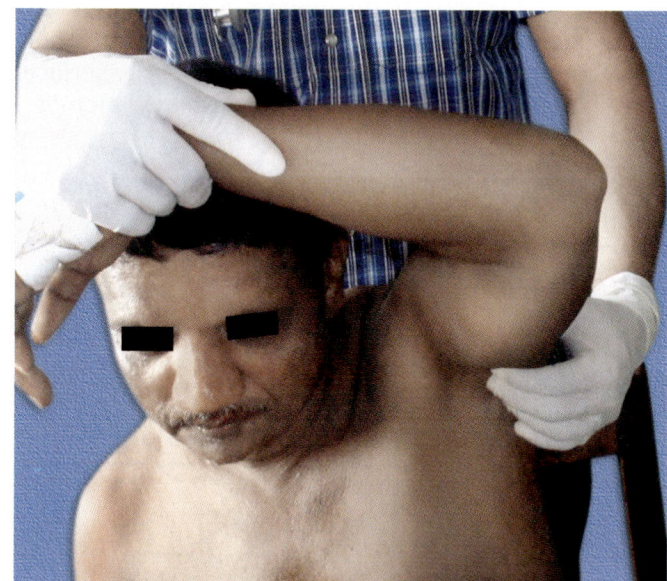

Fig. 8-29 Examination of *subscapular group* of lymph nodes.

Subscapular lymph nodes are located in the posterior axillary fold in relation to latissimus dorsi muscle. It is examined from behind. Examiner stands behind the patient. Respective examiner's hand is used for palpation of respective side of the subscapular group of lymph node. With pulp of fingers directed backwards placed over the anteroinferior aspect of the posterior axillary fold using other hand patient's arm is partially lifted. Nodes are palpated between thumb and fingers **(Fig. 8-29)**.

Apical group of lymph nodes are palpated using examiner's opposite hand. Finger tips are pushed very high up in the axilla and finger tips of another hand of the examiner is placed on the same shoulder over the supraclavicular fossa of the patient to depress downwards. Any enlarged lymph nodes are palpated between finger tips of two hands.

Cervical Lymph Nodes

Cervical lymph nodes drain from lymphatics of head, neck, face, oral cavity, nasal cavity, paranasal sinuses, pharynx,

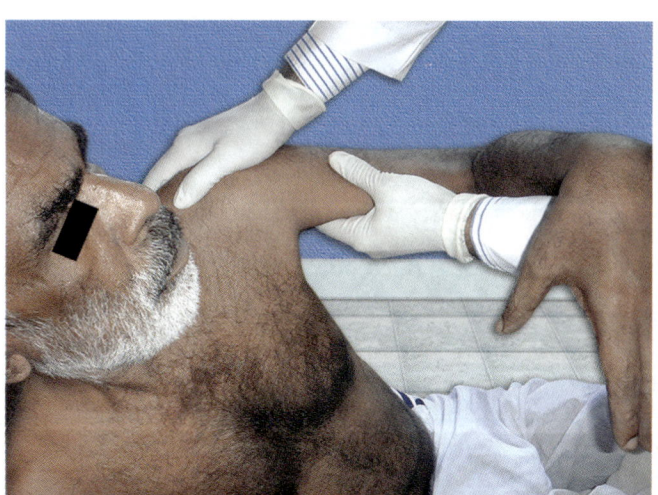

Fig. 8-28 Examination of the *lateral/brachial group* of axillary nodes. Posterior and lateral groups of axillary nodes are palpated by the corresponding hand of the examiner.

larynx and thyroid. Left supraclavicular nodes receive from left upper limb, left side chest wall, left breast, abdomen and both testes. Cervical lymph nodes can be superficial (submental, preauricular, postauricular, external jugular, occipital) or deep (submandibular, upper anterior cervical, upper posterior cervical, lower anterior cervical, lower posterior cervical, supraclavicular along the accessory nerve). Nodes are placed in different levels (Sloan-Kettering)—level I to level VI. Level VII is mediastinal node. Level I—submental and submandibular nodes; level II is upper deep cervical; level III is middle deep cervical; level IV is lower deep cervical; level V is posterior triangle nodes; level VI is central nodes (paratracheal and laryngeal). Level I and level II are further divided into a and b. Ia is submental; Ib is submandibular. Level Va above the spinal accessory level; level Vb is below it **(Figs. 8-30 to 8-32)**.

Cervical lymph nodes are palpated both from front and behind (better and ideal) the patient preferably examiner standing behind the patient. With the patient seated comfortably on a stool with head tilted to the side to be examined so as to relax platysma and neck fascia, examiner uses right hand to right side. Initially palpation is done with flat of finger to find out the presence of node later with tips of finger details of the node is noted. Opposite side of neck should also be examined. ***One side should be examined first; then opposite side (from behind).***

Waldeyer's ring (Waldeyer's-Pirogov ring)

Waldeyer's (German anatomist Heinrich Wilhelm Gottfried von Waldeyer-Hartz) lymphatic ring is a collection of lymphatic tissue in the neck as outermost and innermost circles.

- ***Outer Waldeyer's ring***—occipital; postauricular; preauricular; parotid; facial [superficial (upper, middle, lower) and deep]; submandibular, submental, superficial cervical and anterior cervical.
- ***Inner Waldeyer's ring***—it is the lymphatic ring present around the pharynx—adenoids (nasopharyngeal tonsils), tubal tonsils (overlying the Eustachian tube and its orifice), palatine (faucial) tonsils and lingual tonsils (one on each side of the posterior third of the tongue) **(Fig. 8-33)**.

In generalized lymphadenopathy, all nodal groups on both sides should be examined. ***Epitrochlear (Sigmund gland/node)*** popliteal nodes should be examined. These nodes may get enlarged in NHL. Epitrochlear node may also be enlarged in syphilis, glandular fever. ***Epitrochlear nodes*** are examined in sitting position with elbow partially flexed; in the region 2–4 cm above the medial epicondyle in the groove between biceps and brachialis in the subcutaneous plane medial to the basilic vein **(Figs. 8-34A and B)**. ***Popliteal***

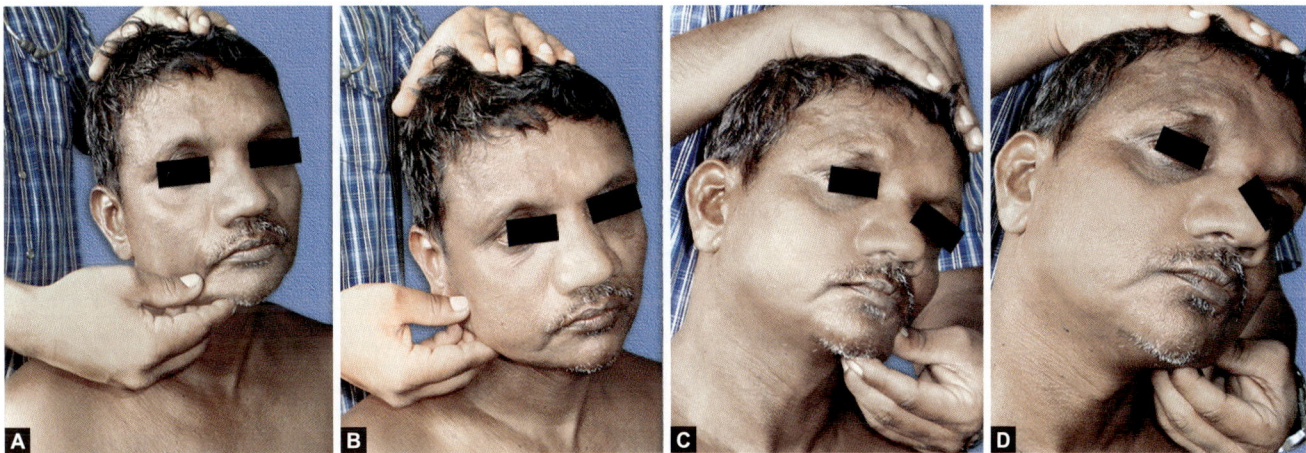

Figs. 8-30A to D Palpation of *submental and submandibular* lymph nodes on both sides.

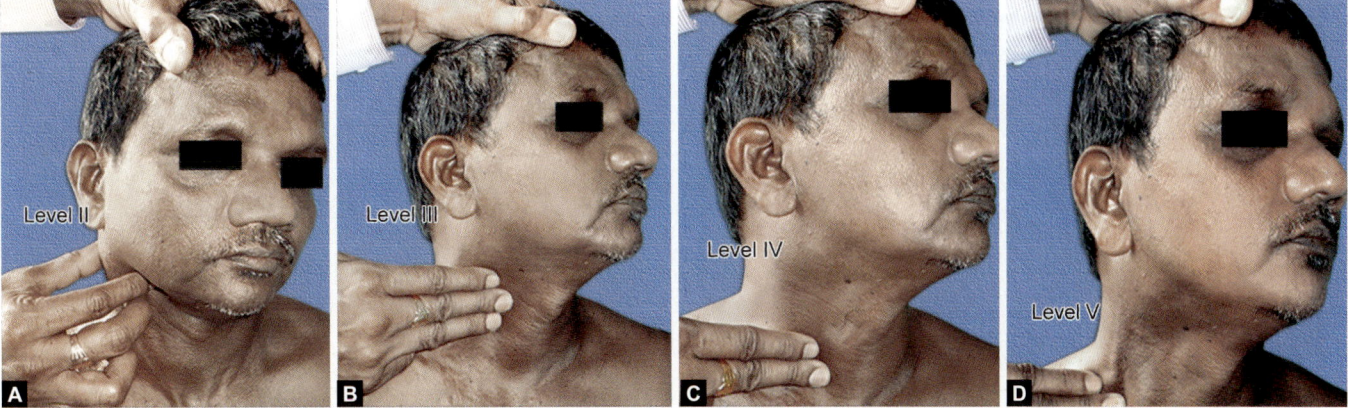

Figs. 8-31A to D Examination of level II, III, IV, V *nodes* in the neck.

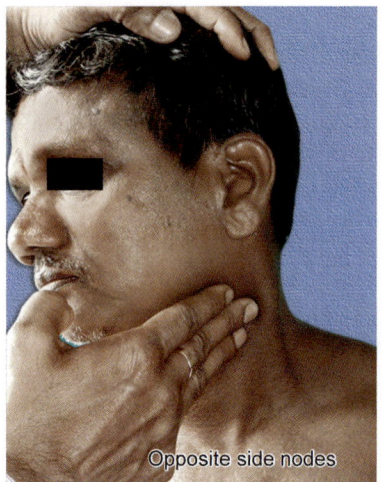

Fig. 8-32 *Opposite side neck* also should be always examined for any enlargement of lymph nodes.

nodes are palpated ideally in prone position with knee flexed to relax the popliteal fascia. It is felt in the lower part of the popliteal fossa over the upper part of flat tibial surface. Lungs should be examined for pleural effusion. Para-aortic nodes, iliac nodes, liver and spleen enlargement should be looked for **(Figs. 8-35A and B)**. Examination of spine is also mandatory.

Percussion

- Sternal tenderness should be checked by direct method. It is elicited in lymphoma and leukemias. Change in percussion note over the sternum (direct or indirect method) suggests superior mediastinal lymph node mass or other superior mediastinal tumors like retrosternal goiter, thymoma, and aneurysm.
- Percussion over the abdomen to look for free fluid is essential.
- Percussion in respiratory system is done to find out pleural effusion **(Figs. 8-36A and B)**.

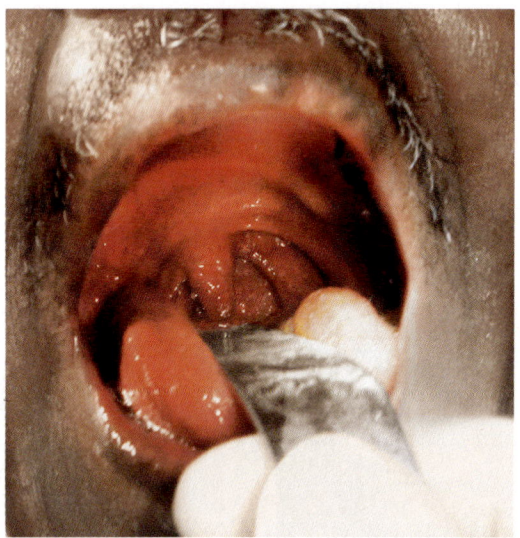

Fig. 8-33 *Inner Waldeyer's ring* should be examined in lymphadenopathy. It is significant in tuberculosis and NHL.

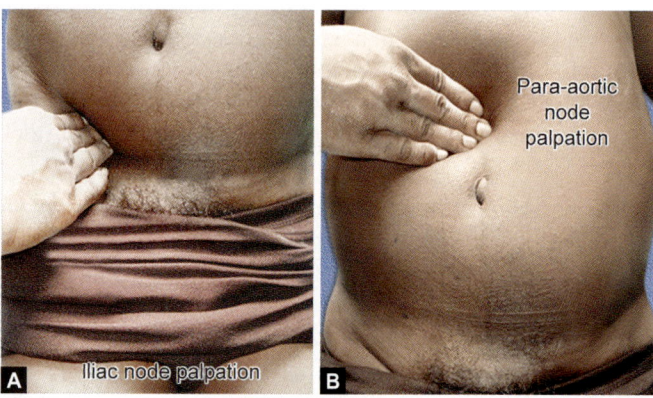

Figs. 8-35A and B Iliac and para-aortic nodes should be examined in *generalized lymphadenopathy*. Iliac nodes are palpated above and medial to inguinal ligament. It is enlarged in lymphoma, secondaries, etc. Para-aortic nodes are palpated in epigastrium above the umbilicus. It is resonant, non-mobile mass, vertically placed. It is felt on deep palpation.

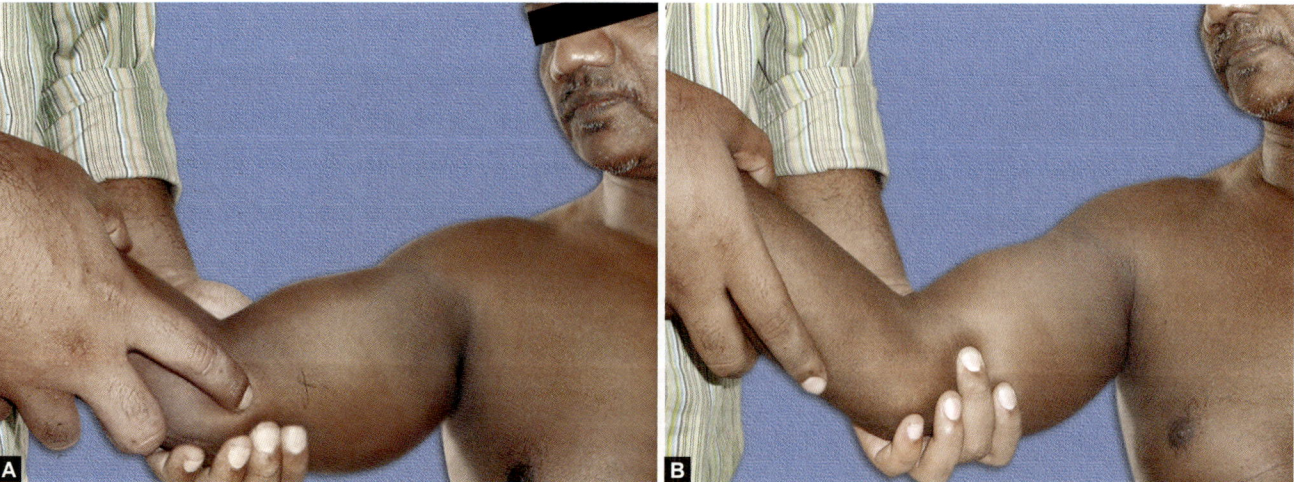

Figs. 8-34A and B *Epitrochlear lymph node* palpation—2 cm above the medial epicondyle.

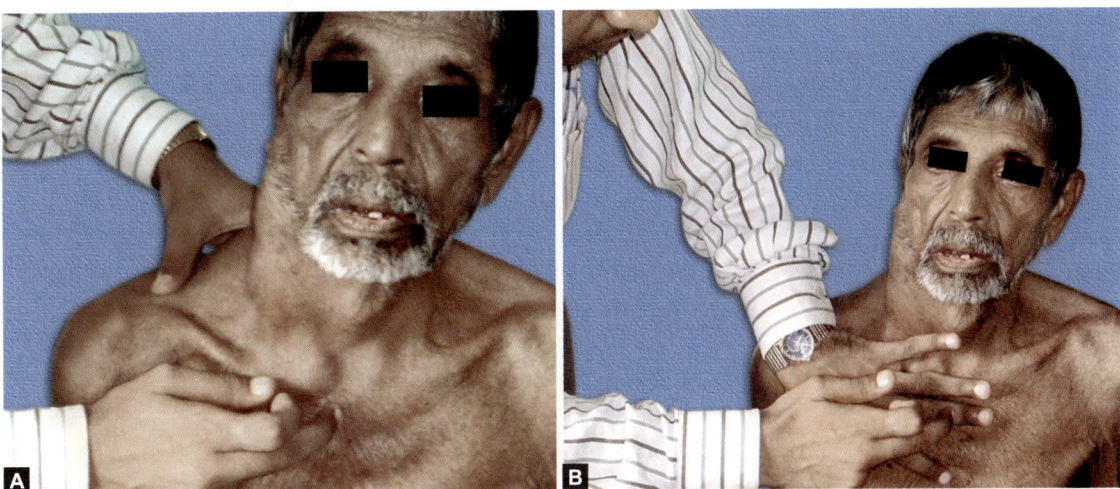

Figs. 8-36A and B *Sternum should be percussed for tenderness and note.* Sternal tenderness is significant in lymphoma and leukemia. Normal note on percussion over the sternum is resonant. It becomes dull if there is mass lesion like lymph nodes in the superior mediastinum. Percussion is done by direct method to check tenderness. To find out the note either direct or indirect method may be used.

Auscultation

Auscultation over the mass is done to find out any bruit due to compression.

Systemic Examination

- *Respiratory system examination* is done to look for pleural effusion, or any altered breath sounds; *abdominal examination* is done to look for palpable liver, palpable spleen, para-aortic nodes, iliac nodes, ascites, etc. **(Figs. 8-37A to E)**.
- *Spine* is examined for tenderness, paraspinal spasm, restricted spine movements and neurological deficits. NHL can involve spine causing neurological deficits **(Figs. 8-38A and B)**. There may be altered sensation, altered muscle power in the lower limb with urinary incontinence.

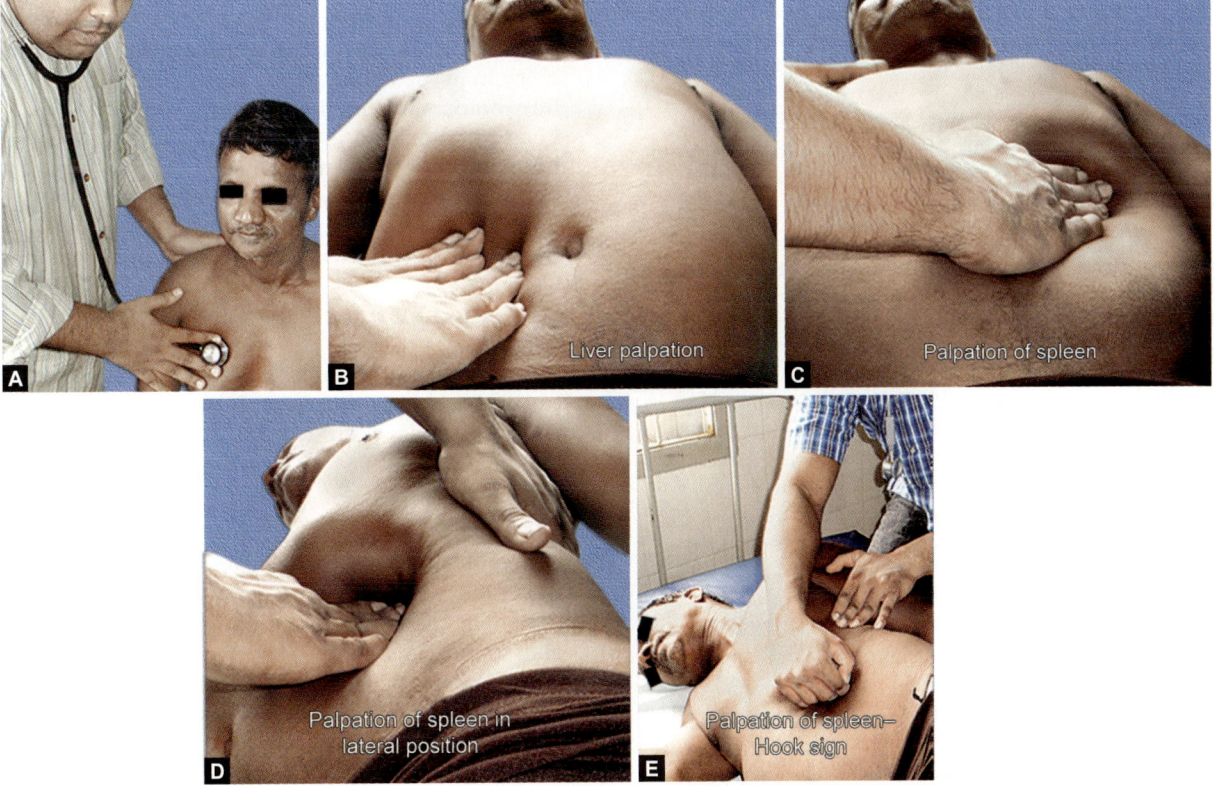

Figs. 8-37A to E Respiratory system is examined for *effusion and altered breath sounds. Abdomen should be examined for liver enlargement, palpable spleen, para-aortic nodes.*

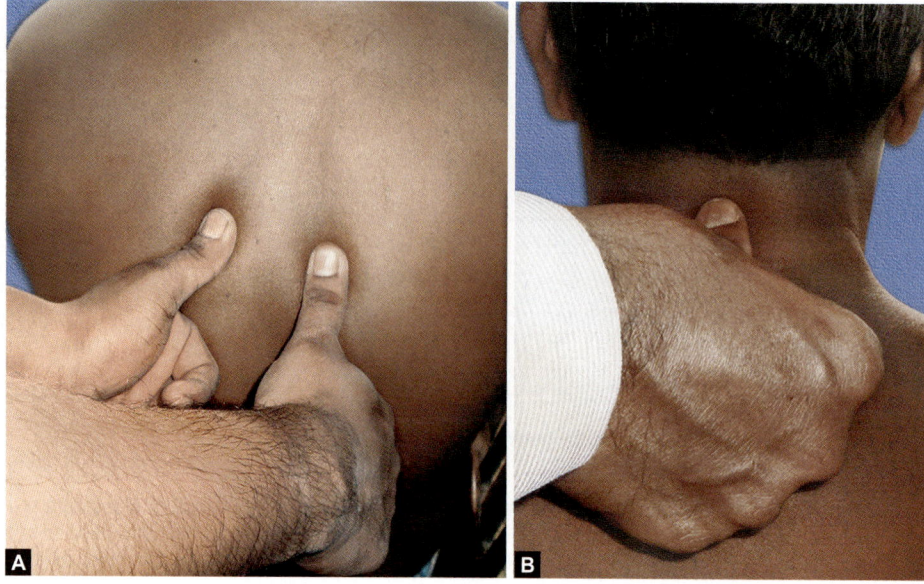

Figs. 8-38A and B Spine should be examined in generalized lymphadenopathy for *tenderness, paraspinal spasm*. It could be lymphoma, chronic lymphatic leukemia, spine tuberculosis.

- It needs urgent radiotherapy/steroid therapy/surgical decompression.

> - **Liver** should be examined in the right hypochondrium, horizontally placed, moves with respiration, cannot insinuate the finger under the right costal margin, upper border cannot be felt, dull on percussion and this dullness continues over liver dullness above.
> - **Spleen** is palpable in left hypochondrium directed towards right iliac fossa, moves with respiration, cannot insinuate the fingers under left hypochondrium, upper border cannot be felt, dull on percussion.
> - **Para aortic lymph node mass** is felt on deep palpation of the abdomen, in the midline, does not move with respiration, nonmobile, all borders may be palpable, transmitted aortic pulsation may be felt over the mass, resonant on percussion.

Three common causes of lymph nodes enlargement

Tuberculous lymphadenitis	Lymphoma	Secondaries in lymph nodes
Matted nodes	Smooth, discrete ovoid node	Nodular nodes
Firm or soft if forms cold abscess	Solid rubbery (India rubber) consistency	Hard (stony)
May form collar stud abscess, sinus	Necrosis, fungation can occur but very rare	Fungation, ulceration occurs eventually
Can be associated with pulmonary or other area tuberculosis	Systemic involvement (extranodal) occurs eventually.	Fixity to deeper structures occurs as stage advances
Dissemination to other systemic areas from lymph nodes can occur in immuno-suppressed people like AIDS	Lymph node fixity is not common.	Further systemic spread occurs depending on the site and type of primary
Jugulodigastric nodes are commonly affected	Posterior triangle nodes are affected commonly (especially in HL)	
Tonsil is the common primary focus in cervical nodal tuberculosis		

INVESTIGATIONS

Blood

- In acute lymphadenitis leukocytosis with neutrophilia is observed. Lymphocytosis is common in tuberculosis, lymphomas, leukemia.
- Peripheral smear may show atypical lymphocytes in lymphatic leukemia. Nocturnal blood smear may show microfilaria in peripheral smear of patient with filariasis.
- Specific blood tests for lymphogranuloma venereum or syphilis or HIV may be carried out. ESR is raised in tuberculosis and malignancies.
- Liver function test is useful in lymphoma to predict the possible involvement of liver. It is also useful during treatment period in case of tuberculosis to assess side effects.
- Hb% is significant in tuberculosis, lymphoma and secondaries.
- Platelet count is needed prior to therapy in case of lymphoma.
- Serological test: Syphilis (VDRL, TPHA, TP immobilization test); LGV (compliment fixation test); infectious mononucleosis (Paul-Bunnel test; tuberculosis (guinea pig inoculation).

FNAC/Aspiration

- It is useful in tuberculosis, malignancy. Caseating material with epithelioid cells is typical feature of tuberculosis. Langhans giant cells, lymphocytes and plasma cells are also found. Secondaries are diagnosed by FNAC.
- FNAC is not much useful in lymphomas as open biopsy is better to assess the type and to do histochemistry.

Lymph Node Biopsy

- It is very useful method of investigation in lymph node enlargement especially in lymphomas. It is also useful in tuberculosis, syphilis.

- *Note:* In metastatic lymph nodal disease, if repeat FNAC is still not conclusive then only open biopsy is done. Routine open biopsy of secondaries in lymph node is avoided as spread can occur to further level of nodes increasing the nodal staging of the disease.
- Lymph node biopsy is done under general anesthesia in the neck as neck is a compact area. But nodes in posterior triangle can be biopsied under local anesthesia with adequate precautions.
- Proper selection of lymph node for biopsy to be taken is essential so that possibility of negative results and need for rebiopsy may be reduced. Large sized/hard lymph node is more likely to be positive than small and soft lymph node.
- Adequate incision, exposure, retraction of deep fascia and soft tissues are needed. Breaking of the capsule is avoided as much as possible. Unnecessary handling of the node during dissection has to be avoided. Lymph node is held with nontoothed dissecting forceps. Ideally entire one lymph node is removed for biopsy. But in adherent node it is often difficult to remove the entire lymph node.
- Imprint films may be taken for cytological study. In tuberculosis cut section of node is yellowish, opaque with caseation in the center.
- Histologically it shows caseating necrosis, epithelioid cells (modified histiocytes), Langhans giant cells, fibrosis, and chronic inflammatory cells. Cut section in lymphoma is fleshy, firm, elastic, grayish with often areas of hemorrhage and necrosis. Histologically (in HL) it shows cellular pleomorphism with features of anaplasia, lymphocytes, lymphoblasts, large multinucleated Reed-Sternberg giant cells with owl eye nuclei. Stroma shows silver stained reticular elements.
- Usually one intact lymph node is removed; if two nodes are removed one is sent to pathologist in formalin; other is sent to microbiology in normal saline. Lowenstein Jensen media (LJ media) takes 6 weeks for culture result; selenite media takes only 5 days for culture result.

Other biopsies
Scalene node biopsy, liver biopsy, skin biopsies are done for sarcoidosis, bone marrow biopsy for lymphomas and leukemia.
Bone marrow aspiration and bone marrows biopsy is essential once lymphoma is confirmed to stage the disease and also eventually to see the therapeutic response. It is also important in lymphatic leukemia. It is taken from iliac crest.

Radiological and other Evaluation Methods

Chest X-ray: Chest X-ray is significant to see evidence of pulmonary tuberculosis, pleural effusion, mediastinal lymph nodal mass, calcified tubercular lymph node, primary bronchogenic carcinoma.
Relevant investigations for primary like endoscopies, blind biopsies, CT of the part is also done.
CT Chest: CT chest is more relevant than chest X-ray to detect early lesions either malignancy or inflammatory condition and also mediastinal nodes. 30% of lesions in the lungs can be missed in chest X-ray but are well detected by CT chest. CT abdomen is done when needed in individual patient basis.

US Abdomen: US abdomen is done to see liver, spleen and para-aortic, mesenteric, iliac nodes especially in lymphomas. *Dancing filaria* may be evident if US is done directly on the lymph node. US of specific area like axilla/groin/neck is done to assess the size, extent, relations of enlarged lymph nodes and also vascularity, and relation of major vessels in the region.
Lymphangiography: It is done in congenital lymphedema to see aplasia/hypoplasia/hyperplasia; lymphomas (shows reticular pattern) to assess the response for treatment as dye stays for long duration in the lymph node and so node can be assessed by taking repeated X-rays of the area. Patent blue dye or 1 mL isosulphan blue is injected subcutaneously in the web space of the foot. Lymph vessels take up this dye and make it clearly visible. (Using operating microscope, after skin incision, lymphatic vessel is identified and cannulated with 30 G needle. Ultrafluid (ethiodized oil) lipiodol is injected slowly using pressure pump at a rate of 1 mL in 8 minutes. On the whole 7 mL of contrast agent is injected. It takes 24 hours to pass through the lymphatics and reach the lymph nodes—iliac and para-aortic nodes). X-rays are taken to visualize lymphatics and lymph nodes. Lymphomas *show foamy or reticular* pattern. Secondaries show irregular filling defects. (Lymphatic pattern/anomalies can be assessed properly and classify lymphedema as congenital hyperplasia (10%); distal obliteration (80%); proximal obliteration (10%)—*Browse's lymphangiographic classification of lymphedema*). Disadvantages—procedure is invasive, technically difficult, time consuming, dye may not reach the required area, extravasation of dye can cause complications like sepsis, skin necrosis.
In melanoma radiopaque phosphorus is added to the dye during lymphangiography which will destroy malignant cells in lymph nodes and is called as *endolymphatic therapy*.
Isotope Lymphoscintigraphy: It has got 90% sensitivity; 100% specificity. It is useful to differentiate lymphedema from other causes of limb swelling. It is simple, safe, reproducible and there is low exposure to radioactivity (5 mCi).
Radio-labeled human albumin or Technetium 99m labeled sulphur colloid is injected into the web space. It migrates in skin and subcutaneous lymphatics and is monitored using whole body gamma camera. It gives clear images of lymphatics, and nodes in the inguinal, iliac, para-aortic region. Later it gives image of thoracic duct also. Amount of radiotracer is assessed in the inguinal nodes in 30 and 60 minutes. Normal uptake is 0.6 to 1.6%. An uptake less than 0.3% in 30 minutes is diagnostic of lymphedema. In edema due to venous diseases, uptake is rapid and shows more than 2% in 30 minutes in inguinal nodes. Thoracic duct, liver and other lymphatic organs in the body can be visualized. It is technically easier and faster.
Mediastinal Gallium 67 radioisotope scan can be done to find out whether mediastinal nodes are involved or not.
Laparoscopy/mediastinoscopy/thoracoscopy are useful in difficult cases.
CT/MRI spine to see spine involvement in case of lymphoma.
*Skin test: Mantoux test/*guinea pig inoculation test for tuberculosis; Gordon's biological test for Hodgkin's lymphoma; Frei's intradermal test for lymphogranuloma venereum. (In *Gordon's test* affected lymph node emulsion is injected into the cerebrum of the rabbit which initiates encephalitis in few days in case of Hodgkin's disease. In *Frie's test* pus is collected from an unruptured bubo. It is diluted using saline—1:10; sterilized with 60 degree temperature. 0.1 mL of such solution when injected intradermally will show a reddish papule at the site of injection in case of positive for lymphogranuloma inguinale [LGV- L1, 2, 3]).

DISEASES OF LYMPHATIC SYSTEMS

Generalized Lymphadenopathy

Generalized lymphadenopathy means enlargement of more than one non-contiguous group of lymph nodes for a period of 3 months with each group showing at least one node more than 1.0 cm in size.

Causes for generalized lymphadenopathy are—tuberculosis; lymphoma either Hodgkin's or non-Hodgkin's; lymphatic leukemia; HIV infection; autoimmune diseases as part of collagen disease; secondary syphilis (secondary and primary syphilis; not in tertiary syphilis); infectious mononucleosis; sarcoidosis; brucellosis; toxoplasmosis, etc. Presently tuberculosis, lymphoma, leukemia are common causes. (Other causes can be present but rare). In generalized lymphadenopathy, all groups of lymph nodes should be carefully examined in detail—neck nodes; axilla; groin nodes. Epitrochlear nodes, popliteal nodes should also be examined. Nodes on both sides should be examined. Respiratory system and chest should be examined for change in breath sounds, pleural effusion. Abdomen should be examined for hepatomegaly, splenomegaly and ascites. Looking for sternal tenderness, percussion note on the sternum, and spine examination is must. Fever, itching, weight loss, wasting, jaundice, neurological deficits are important features to be noted (Fig. 8-39).

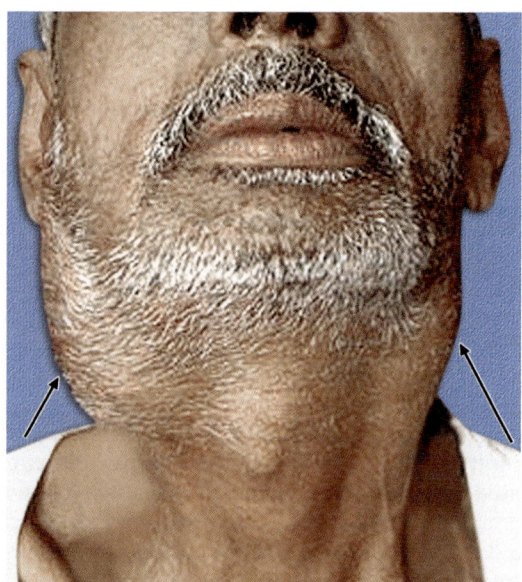

Fig. 8-39 *Generalized lymphadenopathy* in a patient with Non-Hodgkin's lymphoma.

> **Causes of lymph node enlargement**
> a. Inflammatory: **Acute lymphadenitis**; **Chronic lymphadenitis**; **Granulomatous lymphadenitis**: (a) **Bacterial** like tuberculosis, syphilis, tularemia, brucellosis, lymphogranuloma venereum, Cat scratch fever. (b) **Viral** like HIV infection, infectious mononucleosis. (c) **Parasitic** like filarial adenitis, toxoplasmosis. (d) **Fungal** like blastomycosis, histoplasmosis, coccidiodomycosis. (e) **Other causes** like sarcoidosis.
> b. Neoplastic: Lymphomas (HL and NHL); Lymphosarcoma, Burkitt's lymphoma; secondaries in lymph node from most of the carcinomas, sarcomas, malignant melanoma.
> c. Hematological: Chronic lymphatic leukemia.
> d. Immunological: Serum sickness, drug reactions, rheumatoid arthritis, systemic lupus erythematosus, scleroderma, polyarteritis nodosa.

Tuberculous Lymphadenitis

It is common in *neck nodes*. Mediastinal, mesenteric, axillary and inguinal nodes also can get involved. In the neck, nodes are involved commonly through tonsils. *Upper deep* cervical nodes (54%) are commonly involved. Posterior triangle nodes are involved in 22% cases. Often multiple, bilateral nodes may get involved. Axillary nodes are often diseased through retrograde spread from neck nodes of posterior triangle or through blood or from apical lung disease across parietal pleura. Infection also may be following blood spread from primary pulmonary tuberculosis. Occasionally it may be part of miliary tuberculosis also. It is caused by *Mycobacterium tuberculosis*. Infection is more common in HIV, lymphoma, malnourished, immunosuppressed patients. Bacteria evoke inflammation and cell-mediated immunity in the paracortex. Disease passes through *five* stages. Stage 1: Stage of infection and lymphadenitis; lymph nodes are discrete here; Stage 2: Stage of periadenitis and matting; Stage 3: Stage of caseating necrosis and *cold abscess* formation; Stage 4: Stage of *collar stud abscess* formation where caseating material passes through deep fascia into subcutaneous tissue and gets adherent to the skin; Stage 5: Stage of sinus formation. Fibrosis and calcification can occur in this node. Types: Type 1: *Caseating tuberculous lymphadenitis* which is 80% common. It causes caseation, matting due to periadenitis, cold abscess and sinus formation. Here body resistance is less and drug may not reach in effective concentration into the area of caseation and so resistance and residual disease is common to develop. Type 2: *Hyperplastic tuberculous lymphadenitis* is 20% common. It is firm, nontender, discrete node without central caseation. Cold abscess and sinus will not occur. Host resistance is good and so shows good and rapid response to drugs. Gross features of caseating tuberculous lymphadenitis are firm, matted, node with yellowish central caseation on cut section. Histologically it contains *epithelioid cells* (are modified histiocytes—diagnostic feature), Langhans giant cells, macrophages and lymphocytes. Clinically, presents as firm swelling, which is not warm, nontender, matted, usually mobile, can be adherent to adjacent muscles. Cold abscess is soft, nontender, smooth, fluctuant, non-transilluminating, well localized, often nonmobile swelling with free non-adherent skin over the surface. Skin will be adherent at collar stud abscess stage. Tonsils and lungs should be examined for primary focus. Secondaries, lymphoma, chronic lymphadenitis, lymph cyst, HIV, branchial cyst are *differential diagnosis*.

Lymphomas

They are progressive neoplastic condition of lymphoproliferative system arising from stem cells. They are 3rd most common malignancy in children comprising 15% of pediatric cancers. It is often genetically predisposed. It is commonly associated with Sjogren's syndrome,

Wiskott-Aldrich syndrome, ataxia telangiectasia, Epstein-Barr virus infection, celiac sprue, *H. pylori* infection (MALT lymphoma), ionizing radiation.

Types: Hodgkin's lymphoma (HL); Non-Hodgkin's lymphoma (NHL). WHO modified REAL (Revised European American Lymphoma) classification of lymphoma—Type 1. B-cell neoplasms—*subtype I*—of precursor B cell—acute lymphoblastic leukemia (ALL), lymphoblastic leukemia (LBL); *subtype II*—of peripheral B cell—all B cell related NHL. Type 2. T cell putative NK cell neoplasms—*subtype I*—of precursor T cell—ALL, LBL T cell related; *subtype II*—of peripheral T cell and NK cell includes all T cell related NHL. Type 3. Hodgkin's lymphoma—*subtype I*—predominant HL-nodular lymphocyte type; *subtype II*—classical HL-nodular sclerosis, lymphocyte rich, mixed cellularity, lymphocyte depletion.

Hodgkin's lymphoma (HL—Thomas Hodgkin): It is the *commonest* type of lymphoma having fleshy, pinkish gray, rubbery/elastic lymph nodes on gross; with malignant lymphocytes, reticulum cells, histiocytes, giant cells with two large mirror image nuclei [*Reed-Sternberg giant cells* (RS cells are also observed occasionally in other conditions like glandular fever)] on microscopy. Predominant and classical HL are the *types*. *Rye's classification* includes lymphocytic predominance; mixed cellularity; nodular sclerosis (commonest); lymphocytic depletion. *Features:* It is common in males; common in young and elderly (bimodal); presents as painless enlargement of lymph nodes which are smooth, discrete, firm (*India rubber consistency*), non-tender. Neck is the commonest location (80%); commonly seen in lower deep cervical and posterior triangle nodes. Axillary, mediastinal, inguinal, abdominal—are the other groups which may be involved. Consecutive and symmetrical involvement; *splenomegaly* (45%) is common. Hepatomegaly, jaundice, *constitutional symptoms* (stage B – weight loss, fever, night sweats), pruritus, anemia, bone pain are other features. Mediastinal involvement may cause SVC obstruction. Bone involvement may present with sternal tenderness, vertebral pain. Anemia, pancytopenia is common. *Ann Arbor clinical staging* (Ann Arbor is a place): *Stage I*: Confined to one group of lymph nodes; *Stage II*: More than one group of lymph nodes on one side of the diaphragm; *Stage III*: Nodes on both sides of the diaphragm; *Stage IV*: Extranodal involvement like liver, bone marrow. 'S' is added to stage if spleen is involved; 'B' is added for presence and 'A' for absence of constitutional symptoms. 'E' is added for extranodal spread. Stage III (1) is nodes above the renal vein and stage III (2) is below.

Non-Hodgkin's lymphoma (NHL): It occurs in middle-aged and elderly. It is more aggressive than HL. Lymph node involvement is asymmetrical and non-contiguous. General condition is poor. Inner Waldeyer, epitrochlear and peripheral nodes are commonly involved. Hepatomegaly is common. Spleen is not commonly involved. Vertebral involvement and paraplegia can develop which warrants radiotherapy for spine. Cachexia, secondary infection and immunosuppression are more common. *Rappaport and working classifications* are used. It can be nodular or diffuse. It can be B cell or T cell type. It can be precursor cell type or peripheral cell type. It can be small, large, cleaved, uncleaved, etc. It can be low grade, intermediate grade or high grade. Carcinoma or sarcomas can mimic NHL often.

Burkitt's lymphoma (malignant lymphoma of Africa): It is common in South Africa and New Guinea; common in children; *Epstein-Barr virus* may be the cause; often associated with infectious mononucleosis; common in malaria endemic area. It is common in jaw either upper or lower; neck nodes are commonly involved; multifocal, rapidly growing, painless lesion. Other group of lymph nodes also can be affected. Often bilateral renal involvement (75%) is common. Ovaries are commonly affected in females. Histology shows primitive lymphoid cells with large clear histiocytes *(starry sky pattern)*. It can be *endemic African type*—common in jaw; *non-endemic sporadic type*—common in abdomen; *aggressive type*—seen in HIV patients.

Cutaneous T-Cell lymphoma: Cutaneous T cell lymphoma comprises *mycosis fungoides, Sezzary syndrome*, reticulum cell sarcoma of skin and other skin lymphocytic dysplasias. Mycosis fungoides is commonest among them. Cutaneous T cell lymphoma can be indolent (commonly mycosis fungoides); aggressive (Sezzary syndrome); provisional (granulomatous/panniculitis like T cell lymphoma). Initial macular/patch/plaque phase slowly changes into tumor phase with painful, pruritic erythroderma often with visceral spread. Alopecia mucinosa and follicular mucinosis are common in mycosis fungoides. Lymph nodes may get involved.

Secondaries in Lymph Nodes

Metastatic disease in regional lymph nodes occurs by lymphatic spread usually be permeation up to first nodal level and later by embolization. Commonly affects old age group. Head and neck cancers account for 80% of neck nodes secondaries. In axilla, carcinoma breast is the common cause; others are skin malignancies in upper limb, chest wall, etc. Carcinoma in lower limb, perineum, penis, scrotum, genitalia spreads to groin lymph nodes. These lymph nodes are *stony hard* (Fig. 8-40), with nodular surface, initially non-tender but soon become tender by tumor necrosis, nerve infiltration, and fungation. In neglected cases fungation, foul smelling mass is seen (Fig. 8.41). They are initially

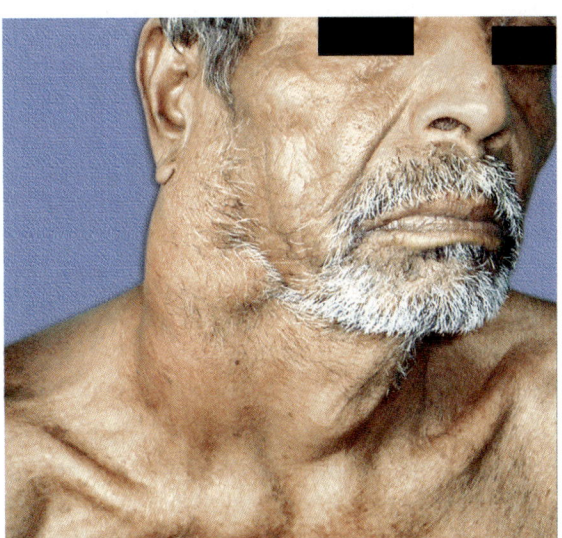

Fig. 8-40 Secondaries in cervical node. It is fixed advanced disease. It is *stony hard in consistency*.

Section 1: Examination in General Surgery

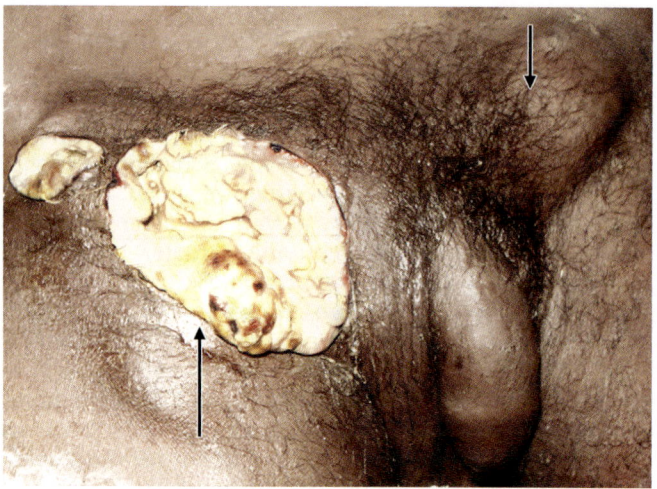

Fig. 8-41 Fungating secondaries in inguinal lymph nodes on the right side. *It is an advanced disease.*

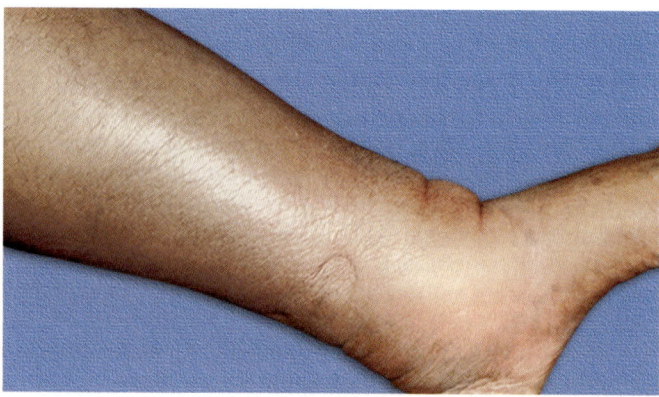

Fig. 8-42 Early lymphedema left side. It is *pitting in nature*.

mobile, but eventually become fixed and nonmobile as it gets adherent to muscle, bone and even to skin. *Infiltration to regional major vessels* causes absence of pulsation (example—carotid in neck), *nerve infiltration* causes neurological deficits (infiltration of hypoglossal nerve causes its palsy leading to deviation of tongue towards same side and wasting of tongue muscle of that side/spinal accessory nerve infiltration causes poor shrugging of the shoulder); *venous obstruction* causes edema of distal part (groin secondaries can cause venous edema of lower limb). Few sarcomas (rhabdomyosarcoma, synovial sarcoma) can cause secondaries in lymph nodes in later stage. Secondaries from malignant melanoma are usually pigmented but not stony hard due to rapid growth.

Others Conditions

Condition	Features
Lymphoedema: Accumulation of protein rich interstitial fluid/lymph in extracellular and extravascular compartment, commonly in subcutaneous tissue. **Kinmonth Classification: Primary; Secondary.**	1. *Primary lymphoedema:* (1) Lymphoedema congenita; Present at birth; < 2 years. Familial type—*Nonne-Milroy's disease;* (2) Lymphoedema praecox; Present in puberty; 2-35 years; Familial type-*Letssier- Meige's syndrome;* (3) Lymphoedema tarda; Present in adult after 35 years. 2. *Secondary lymphoedema*—More common; Factors—trauma, inguinal/axillary block dissection, filarial lymphoedema, tuberculosis, syphilis, fungal infection, advanced fixed nodal malignancy in axilla, groin; radiotherapy; DVT, chronic venous insufficiency. *Wuchereria bancrofti* is the cause of filarial lymphoedema **(Fig. 8-42)**.
Acute Lymphangitis: It is the *bacterial infection of the lymphatic system* from a focus in the draining area. Common in upper and lower limb with primary focus may be small in digits or fingers or nail bed or inter digital space or plantar aspect or foot. *Staphylococci* and *streptococci* are the causative organisms.	Fever, with raised, thin, painful tender visible streaks of lymphatic vessels, blanching on pressure is typical; tender palpable lymph nodes in axilla and groin. **Complications:** Cellulitis; toxemia; septicemia.
Lymphadenitis: **Acute:** Commonly bacterial origin from a focus in the drainage area; neck is the common site; other sites are – axilla, inguinal area. **Chronic:** It is chronic inflammation may be from a chronic focus; often may become acute. **Reactive:** Occurs as a reaction may be viral, autoimmune or other causes. It is hyperplastic response in germinal center to existing disease in the drainage area may be malignancy recurrent infections.	*Acute:* Fever, painful, tender, soft enlarged lymph node(s). Often it gets suppurated forming an abscess depends on the bacteria and its virulence. *Chronic:* Firm or hard, nontender lymph node enlargement often long standing; should be differentiated from tuberculous lymphadenitis or lymphoma or secondaries. *Reactive:* Discrete, nontender, firm, mobile palpable lymph nodes in drainage area.
Filarial Lymphadenitis: Common in filarial endemic areas; common in males; common in inguinal nodes. Firm, tender, enlarged lymph nodes, periodic fever, thickening of spermatic cord (*funiculitis*), thickened epididymis (*epididymitis*), thickened scrotum, filarial limb.	*Tender, recurrent node enlargement with fever is typical. Lymphangitis in the drainage area (limbs) is common.* *Night blood sample*—may show microfilaria. *US of lymph nodes*—typical dancing microfilaria; biopsy may reveal adult worm. *Eosinophilia* is common.

Contd...

Contd...

Infectious mononucleosis (Glandular fever): Acute self-limiting disease caused by *Epstein-Barr* virus; common in young adults.	Fever, sore throat, rashes, tender, elastic lymphadenopathy (initially neck lymph nodes later axillary, inguinal, mediastinal nodes); splenomegaly; abnormal lymphocytes (atypical mononuclear cells) in the peripheral smear; subclinical hepatitis. *Paul-Bunnel test* is positive during early phase and disappears in 2 months— diagnostic for recurrent and new infections.
Cat scratch fever: A type of *psittacosis* caused by *Chlamydia psittaci* after cat scratch or droplet infection. It causes inflammatory reaction at the site, fever, malaise, anorexia, regional lymph node enlargement after 2 weeks which suppurates and burst to release sterile pus.	Mimics chronic/tuberculous lymphadenitis. *Skin test* using human lymph node pus is diagnostic. *LCL bodies* are seen in pus, tissue smears, spleen, lungs and brain. *Complications*: Flu like syndrome, fatal pneumonia, meningoencephalitis, endocarditis, pericarditis.
Sarcoidosis: It is granulomatous condition of unknown aetiology; Noncaseating granuloma with epithelioid cells; positive *Kveim-Siltzbach test (80%)*; H*igh levels of serum angiotensin converting enzyme (SAGE).*	Initially painless, discrete involvement of submental, submandibular, preauricular, occipital, supratrochlear nodes; bilateral hilar lymphadenopathy; involvement of lungs, liver, spleen, lacrimal gland, parotid gland, CNS. CT chest; mediastinoscopy; nodal biopsy; slit-lamp examination of eye-- necessary investigations.
Chronic lymphatic leukemia: It is a hematological disorder with generalized lymphadenopathy, splenomegaly, bleeding tendencies (bleeding gums), fever, anemia, decreased weight.	Peripheral smear (lymphocytosis) and bone marrow aspiration and biopsy is diagnostic.

CASE DISCUSSION

A 20-year-old male presents with multiple swellings in the neck of one month duration. Swelling is painless. There is no fever, no jaundice, no itching. Appetite is normal. No history of back pain, respiratory symptoms or abdominal fullness. Pallor is present on general examination. On local examination of the neck, multiple, rubbery, firm, discrete, mobile swellings are present on both sides of the neck of varying sizes. Swellings are confirmed as level II, III and level V nodes which are deep to sternocleidomastoid muscle.

What other examination will you do?
Oral cavity should be examined for tonsillar enlargement (inner Waldeyer's ring). Other groups of lymph nodes should be examined namely axillary, epitrochlear, inguinal, iliac and popliteal nodes on both sides and para-aortic nodes. Respiratory system is examined for pleural effusion, altered breath sounds; abdomen is examined for hepatosplenomegaly; sternal tenderness should be checked; spine is examined for tenderness, paraspinal spasm, altered movements.

What is the likely diagnosis? What are all differential diagnoses?
It is most probably Hodgkin's lymphoma (HL). Other possibilities have to be thought are non-Hodgkin's lymphoma, tuberculosis, HIV infection, nonspecific lymphadenitis (less likely as it is not tender). As HL is common in the neck, and multiple lymph nodes are palpable which are discrete and rubbery HL is more likely. In tuberculosis, lymph nodes are matted but in hyperplastic type discrete nodes are observed. Once lymphoma is considered all other groups of nodes should be examined. In NHL, involvement of asymmetrical nodes, epitrochlear, popliteal nodes and Waldeyer ring is common. In HL, symmetrical node involvement and splenomegaly is common.

How you will evaluate?
Hematocrit, *peripheral smear* is done. FNAC is done for initial screening only but confirms tuberculosis and secondaries. *Open lymph node biopsy* is a must in lymphoma. Liver function tests, chest CT scan, ultrasound or CT abdomen (as per need but CT is better), MRI spine, *bone marrow biopsy* are investigations needed in lymphoma.

9. Examination and Clinical Approach to Peripheral Nervous System

Competency: AN10.6; AN12.8; AN12.11; AN12.12; AN12.13; AN18.3; AN29.2.

■ HISTORY

Name:

Address:

Age: Deformity of brachial plexus is seen in newborn and infants.

Sex:

Occupation: Occupational hazard like working in lead and arsenic-related industries can cause neurological problems.

Complaints and History of Present Illness

Swelling

Mode of onset (spontaneous/traumatic); duration and progress is asked.

History of Trauma

Trauma is the most common way by which a nerve is gets inured. Nature of trauma will give an idea of site, nature of injury. Incised/penetrating/deep wounds can cause nerve injury. Sometimes fracture/dislocation can cause adjacent nerve injury. Fracture of shaft of humerus can injure radial nerve; supracondylar fracture of humerus can cause median/ulnar or radial nerve palsy; fracture of medial epicondyle of humerus can cause ulnar nerve injury; axillary nerve may be injured in subcoracoid shoulder dislocation or fracture neck of humerus; sciatic nerve (commonly common peroneal part) is injured in posterior dislocation of hip or supracondylar or subtrochanteric fractures of the femur. Fracture neck of femur may injure lateral popliteal nerve.

Traction injury can cause avulsion, neuropraxia or other types of nerve injuries causing typical lesions often, seen in injuries to brachial plexus. Forcible increase in angle between neck and shoulder can cause injury to upper trunk of brachial plexus. During difficult labor, fetal head is pulled out with traction against shoulder causing typical upper trunk brachial plexus injury. Upper trunk lesion is called as **Erb-Duchenne palsy**. Injury to lower trunk of brachial plexus can occur when the arm is forcibly hyperabducted causing typical **Klumpke's palsy**.

Pain

May be dull aching or intense or burning type as in **causalgia**. It may develop immediately or much later after trauma. Pain is worst during night in **carpal tunnel syndrome**.

Specific Complaints

Impairment of muscle function may be partial (paresis) or complete (paralysis) due to involvement of nerve by inflammation or neoplasm, e.g. parotid neoplasms causing facial nerve palsy; ***impairment of sensation***—may present with tingling sensation, numbness or paresthesia.

Entrapment neuropathy can cause typical nerve lesions due to compression. *Tardy ulnar palsy* occurs due to trapping of ulnar nerve at medial epicondyle in the callus formed after fracture of medial epicondyle and supracondylar fracture presenting with pain, tingling, numbness, and muscle weakness.

Ulcer—history of trophic ulcers over foot due to neuropathy may be seen.

Deformity—in the form of claw hand, foot drop, wrist drop may be present.

Skin changes—complains of dryness in complete lesion or increased perspiration in incomplete lesion.

Treatment History

History of taking injections into the arm or thigh may cause irritation of adjacent nerve causing nerve injury. In the arm, axillary nerve may be affected causing paralysis of deltoid. In the thigh sciatic nerve may get injured by injections. History of INH (isoniazid) therapy for tuberculosis should be taken.

History of trauma in the past for which tight bandages or plaster cast was applied, crutches were used. History of diabetes mellitus and leprosy, its course of treatment should be asked.

Note: *Leprosy (Hansen's disease)* is still common cause of peripheral nerve deficits in developing country including India.

Personal History

Alcohol intake and tobacco consumption are also important in nerve lesions. Earlier history of diphtheria was significant as it may cause diphtheritic paralysis.

EXAMINATION

General Examination

Look for anemia, evidence of malnutrition (B_1 deficiency can cause peripheral neuropathy), cachexia in malignancy. Syphilitic and lepromatic stigmata, old scars should be noted.

Skin changes—dry, wrinkled, lusterless in old lesion whereas in recent injury the skin appear pink, due to vasodilatation. Skin is red, glossy, perspiring in incomplete lesion due to irritation (*causalgia*).

Nails—are observed for curvature, ridging, change in color, luster.

Gums are specifically seen for blue line indicating lead poisoning.

Gait—may be high stepping in foot drop.

> **Causalgia**
> - It is severe burning pain in the distribution of a peripheral nerve due to *incomplete injury* to the peripheral nerve.
> - *Sites:* Common in upper limb, seen in brachial plexus or median nerve injuries. In the lower limb it can be seen in sciatic nerve or tibial nerve distribution.
> - Clinically, there will be hyperesthesia and severe, *disabling burning pain* along the distribution of the nerve.

LOCAL EXAMINATION

Inspection

Attitude and Deformity

Erb's palsy/Obstetrician's paralysis: 'Policeman receiving the tip' or 'Porter's tip hand' attitude occurs in injury to upper trunk of brachial plexus **(Figs. 9-1A and B)**. It occurs due to traction injury; often in obstructed labor or during anesthesia. *Here junction of C5 and C6 is affected* (Erb's point). Nerve to subclavius, suprascapular nerve, and nerve to serratus anterior, dorsal scapular nerve to rhomboideus emerge close to this point. Muscles paralysed are—biceps, deltoid, brachialis, brachioradialis; partly supraspinatus, infraspinatus and supinator. Here arms hang by the side of the body adducted and medially rotated; forearm extended and pronated. There is loss of abduction and lateral rotation of the shoulder; loss of flexion and supination of forearm; absence of biceps and supinator jerks; loss of sensation over the skin over lower part of the deltoid.

Klumpke's paralysis: Here injury is to lower trunk of brachial plexus. It is due to undue abduction of the arm after fall from a height while clutching something with hands. *Here C8 and T1 nerve roots are involved.* Muscles paralysed are intrinsic muscles of hand, ulnar flexors of wrist and fingers. It causes **claw hand**; cutaneous anesthesia and analgesia along *the medial border of the forearm and hand*; Horner's syndrome causing ptosis, miosis, anhydrosis, enophthalmos and loss of ciliospinal reflux which is due to injury to sympathetic innervations of head and neck that leave spinal cord through T_1; vasomotor changes in the anesthetized skin like warmness, dryness, absence of sweating and; trophic changes.

Claw hand—there will be hyperextension of all fingers including thumb at MP joint and flexion of IP joint.

Wrist drop is seen in radial nerve palsy where there is paralysis of extensor muscles **(Fig. 9-2)**; **winging of scapula** with prominent vertebral border and inferior angle of

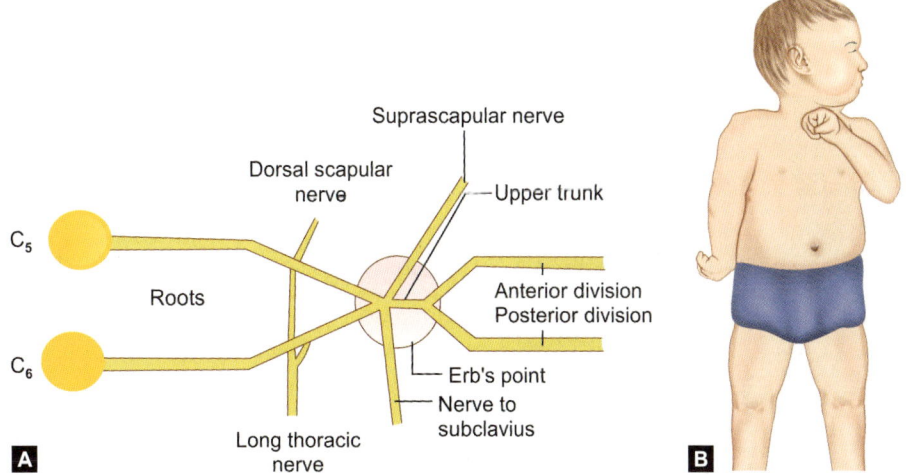

Figs. 9-1A and B Erb's point and Erb's palsy. Note the typical *'policeman receiving tip'* sign.

scapula is seen in paralysis of serratus anterior due to injury to long thoracic nerve of Bell; *'ape thumb'* deformity is due to paralysis of opponens pollicis in median nerve palsy; *'pointing index'* is due to paralysis of lateral half of the flexor digitorum profundus supplied by median nerve. Paralysis of dorsiflexors and evertors due to lateral popliteal nerve injury causes *foot drop*.

Wasting of Muscles

Atrophy of particular muscles supplied by the nerve will be obvious. It is compared to opposite side in unilateral lesion (**Fig. 9-3**). Wasting is often observed in interossei, thenar and hypothenar muscles, forearm, arm muscles, calf and thigh muscles. Muscle girth should be measured at specific point and compared to opposite side.

Inspection of the Skin over the Affected Area

Skin is inspected for dryness, glossiness, loss of skin folds and subcutaneous fat—features of paralysis. Vasomotor changes, cyanosis, excess sweat, brittle nails are observed in partial injury of the nerve. Wound if present should be inspected for its depth, site and other features. Similarly, scar of old wound should be inspected. Nerve related to this wound or scar may be damaged.

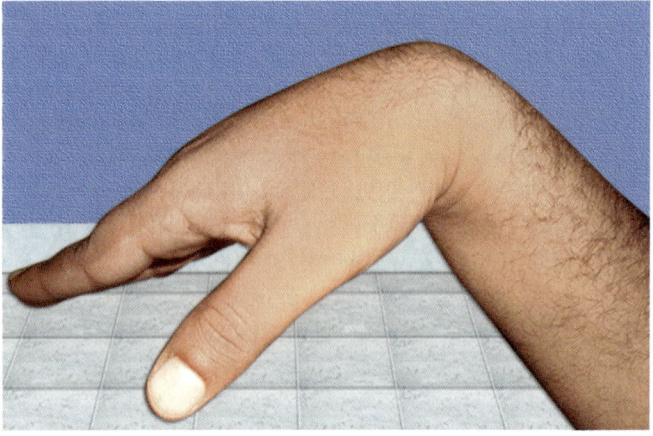

Fig. 9-2 *Wrist drop*—due to radial nerve palsy.

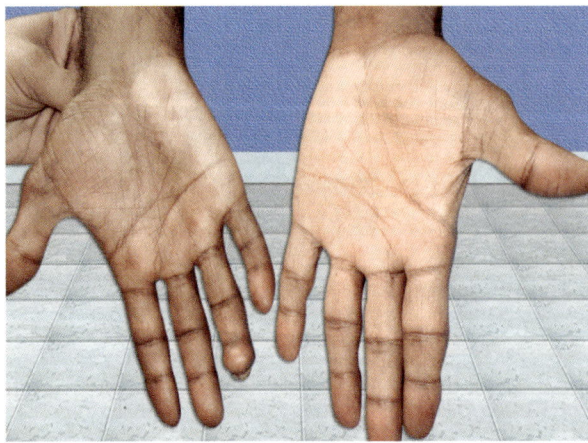

Fig. 9-3 *Wasting in the right* hand especially over thenar eminence.

Palpation

- ***Temperature:*** Paralyzed limb is colder than normal.
- ***Sensation:*** Light touch, pressure, localization, two point discrimination, pain, temperature, sense of position, size, recognition of shape and form of the object, vibration sense—all should be checked in nerve injury/diseases. Sensations are checked ***from impaired area towards*** normal area. ***Light touch*** is epicritic sensation used to locate accurate area of loss of sensation. It is done using cotton wisp. ***Gross touch*** is protopathic sensation which is checked by fingertip. Sensation *of **two point discrimination*** is checked using a compass points. Normally points of 2 mm separation can be made out which is impaired in a nerve injury. It is transmitted through posterior column of spinal cord. ***Superficial pain*** sensation from the skin is elicited using sharp pin. ***Deep muscular or bone pain*** is elicited by gentle pressure or squeezing. ***Temperature*** is checked using warm and cold water in test tubes. Inability to recognize the size, shape and form of the object is called as ***astereognosis***. ***Position sense*** is joint's spatial orientation. It is usually checked in great toe or other toes; thumb or other fingers. Position sense is checked with patient eyes closed and the joint movements are elicited passively by holding its outer aspect (laterally); and the patient is asked what position the joint is held. Position sense is often lost with astereognosis in posterior column lesions. Only astereognosis with normal position sense and light touch is seen in parietal lobe injury. ***Vibration sense*** is checked using tuning fork of 128 Hz placing over the bony surface (bony protuberance). Vibration sense is lost in tabes dorsalis, peripheral neuritis, and posterior column disorders (**Fig. 9-4**).
- ***Anesthesia over the area*** of sensory supply of that particular nerve is typical. In axillary nerve injury paralysis of deltoid muscle will be present along with loss of sensation over the lower part of the deltoid. Often muscle

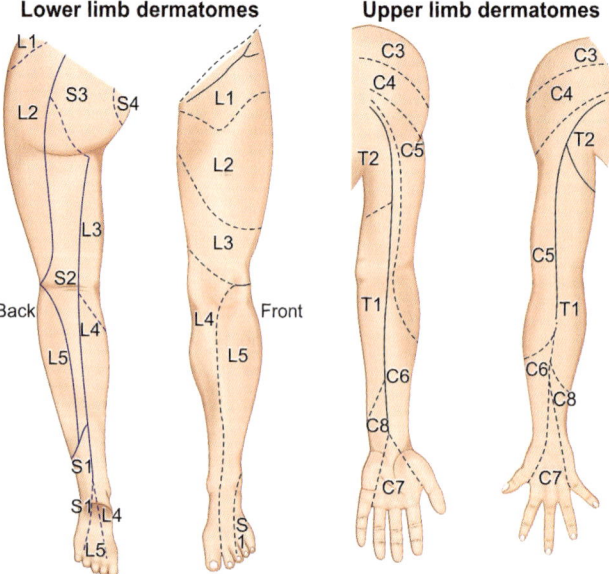

Fig. 9-4 Upper limb and lower limb *dermatomes*.

paralysis or power cannot be assessed due to traumatic fracture of the particular site like shoulder dislocation or fracture neck of humerus in axillary nerve injury. Shifting of hyperesthesia along the distribution of the peripheral nerve is the sign of nerve regeneration.

- **Loss of touch, pain and temperature** is seen in purely sensory nerve section. In motor nerve lesion, joint sensation and vibration is affected. In mixed nerve lesions all sensations are affected.
- **Tenderness:** Wound or scar should be palpated for tenderness. Scar tenderness may signify nerve entrapment or adhesion.
- **Palpation of affected muscles:** Paralysed muscle is soft, and flabby. It shows reduced muscle bulk and texture. They are tender in incomplete lesion, nontender in complete lesion.

Movements (Figs. 9-5A to D)

- **Muscle power:** Muscles which are exclusively supplied by a particular nerve should be checked for altered power. Muscle power of that particular muscle is checked by the movement against resistance across the joint it acts.
- **Medical Research Council graded the muscle power:** 0—complete paralysis; 1—flicker of contraction; 2—contraction of muscle with gravity eliminated; 3—contractions against gravity alone; 4—contraction against gravity and some resistance alone; 5—contraction against powerful resistance.
- **Trapezius** is checked by shrugging the shoulder against resistance. There will be wasting of trapezius with flat shoulder. It suggests spinal accessory nerve palsy. It is observed in advanced fixed neck lymph node secondaries; after radical neck dissection; trauma.
- **In hypoglossal nerve palsy**, patient is asked to protrude the tongue. There will be wasting of tongue on the side of the lesion; tongue will deviate towards the same side of the injury. Hypoglossal nerve palsy occurs in advanced secondaries in neck (upper nodes); after submandibular salivary gland excision (1%); surgery to submandibular salivary gland malignancy.
- **Serratus anterior muscle** is checked by pushing the outstretched hand against wall. Its paralysis causes prominent vertebral border and inferior angle of the scapula will stand out of the chest wall. It is called as '**winging of scapula**'. It is due to injury to long thoracic nerve of Bell. It is derived from the C_5, C_6, C_7 nerve roots of brachial plexus. It may be injured in brachial plexus injury or chest wall/breast surgeries.
- **Deltoid muscle** is checked with elbow flexed at right angle and abducting the arm (through shoulder joint) against resistance. Muscle contraction should be checked by palpation with the other hand.
- **Brachioradialis** muscle is checked by asking the patient to flex the elbow against resistance keeping forearm in midprone position. It originates from upper 2/3rd of lateral supracondylar ridge of the humerus above the origin of the extensor carpi radialis longus and inserted on to the lateral side of the radius just above the styloid process. It is *flexor* of forearm in **midprone** position; supinator of fully pronated forearm. It is supplied by radial nerve $C_{5,6,7}$. It is paralysed in radial nerve injury but its action is intact in posterior interosseus nerve injury **(Fig. 9-6)**.
- **Extensor muscles of wrist:** Extensors of the wrist are supplied by posterior interosseous nerve except extensor carpi radialis longus (supplied by radial nerve). Injury to posterior interosseous nerve will cause wrist drop with inability to extend the wrist. Wrist is extended against resistance to check the power of these muscles

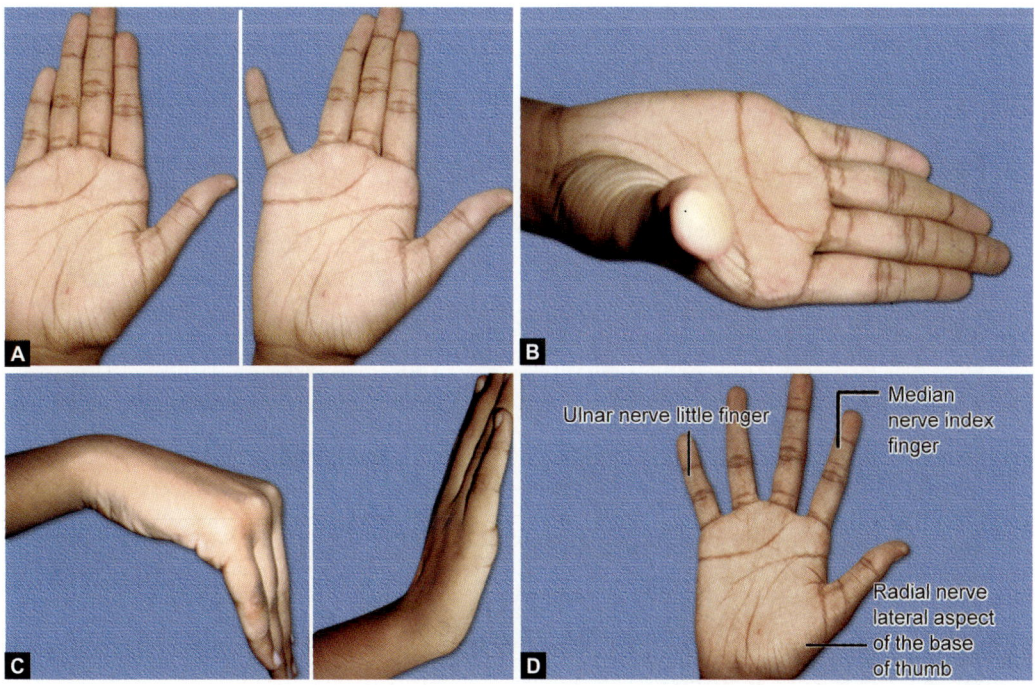

Figs. 9-5A to D *Quick tests for motor and sensory nerves* in the hand—ulnar, median and radial nerves. A, B, C—Motor, D—Sensory.

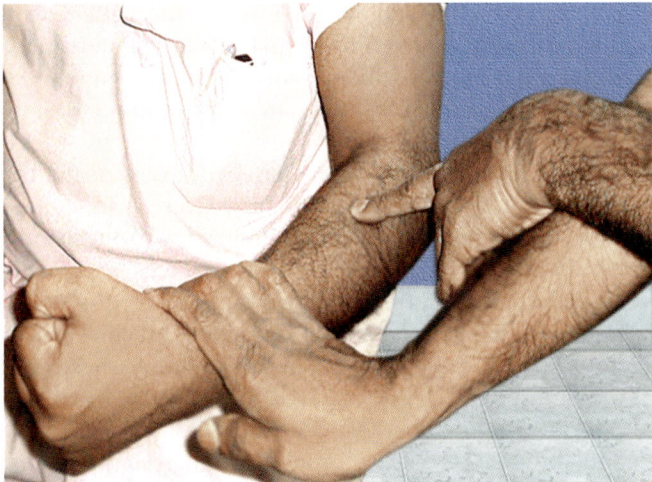

Fig. 9-6 Checking the brachioradialis muscle power *in mid-prone position*. It is paralysed in radial nerve injury. It is intact in posterior interosseous nerve injury.

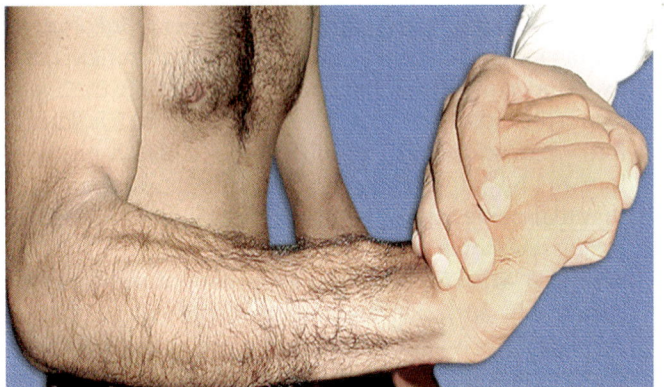

Fig. 9-7 Extension of the wrist should be checked *against resistance*.

(Fig. 9-7). Patient can extend the fingers using interossei. Brachioradialis is intact in posterior interosseous nerve lesion but it will be paralysed in above elbow injury of radial nerve. Extensor carpi radialis longus, extensor carpi radialis brevis, extensor digiti minimi, extensor carpi ulnaris, extensor digitorum and anconeus are common extensors of the wrist. Extensor digitorum from its common extensor origin in the dorsum of hand divides into four slips of tendons one for each of medial four fingers. It extends into the dorsum of proximal phalanx as dorsal digital expansion. Intermediate slip attaches to middle phalanx dorsally. Two side ward tendon slips later join again to attach to dorsum of base of distal phalanx. Interossei and lumbricals pass through the tunnel to enter the dorsal expansion as wing tendons. Extensor digitorum is extensor of metacarpophalangeal joint and interphalangeal joints. Interossei and lumbrical are also flexors of the interphalangeal joints.

- *Flexor pollicis longus:* It originates from upper 3/4th of anterior surface of shaft of radius and anterior surface of interosseous membrane; gets inserted into the palmar surface of the distal phalanx of the thumb; supplied by anterior interosseous nerve; flexor of the distal phalanx of thumb. Its power is checked by asking the patient to steady the proximal phalanx, and to bend the terminal phalanx of thumb against resistance **(Figs. 9-8A and B)**.
- *Flexor digitorum superficialis (sublimus):* Its humeroulnar head originates from medial epicondyle of humerus and tubercle on the medial border of the coronoid process and ulnar collateral ligament; radial head from anterior border of radius; it ends as four tendons one each to medial four fingers; opposite the proximal phalanx each splits into two and gets attached to medial and lateral part of the base of middle phalanx. It is the main flexor of the proximal interphalangeal joint. It is supplied by median nerve.
- *Flexor digitorum profundus (FDP):* It originates from upper 3/4th of anterior and medial surface of ulnar shaft, olecranon and coronoid process of ulna and anterior surface of the interosseous membrane; it ends as 4 tendons one for each medial 4 fingers; each after passing through the split sublimes attaches to base of the distal phalanx in front. It is the chief flexor of the distal phalanx. It is a composite hybrid muscle wherein medial two tendons

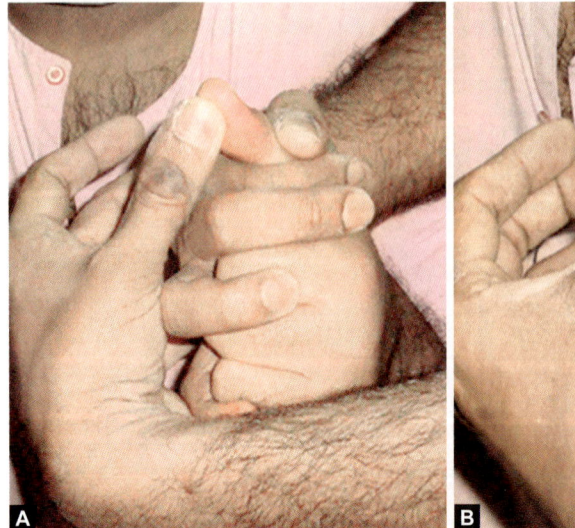 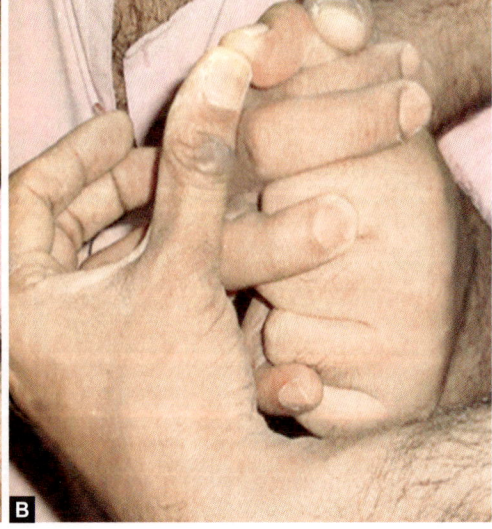

Figs. 9-8A and B *Test for flexor pollicis longus*. Flexion of distal phalanx of thumb against resistance is checked.

are supplied by ulnar nerve and lateral two tendons are supplied by anterior interosseous nerve. Both sublimes and FDP has got synovial folds called as *vincula longa and vincula brevia*.

- **Ochsner's clasping test:** If the patient is asked to clasp the hands, index finger of the affected side fails to flex and remains as ***pointing index***. It suggests median nerve injury **(Figs. 9-9A and B)**.
- **Abductor pollicis brevis:** It originates from the tubercle of the scaphoid, crest of trapezium, flexor retinaculum; gets inserted to lateral side of base of proximal phalanx of thumb. Its nerve supply is median nerve (C_8, T_1). It abducts the thumb at metacarpophalangeal joint and carpometacarpal joints with associated medial rotation. Its power is tested by moving the thumb upwards at right angle to the palm of the hand with palm laid flat on the table. Patient is asked to keep his hand flat supine on the table. A pen tip is kept near thumb in front at higher level; patient is asked to abduct his thumb to touch the pen held. In normal functioning muscle patient can touch the pen otherwise he cannot. It is called as ***'pen test'*** **(Figs. 9-10 and 9-11)**.
- **Opponens pollicis:** It originates from crest of trapezium and flexor retinaculum; gets inserted to lateral half of the palmar surface of the first metacarpal bone; supplied by median nerve (C_8, T_1). It causes opposition of thumb with combination of flexion and medial rotation. It is checked by swinging the thumb across the palm to touch tips of other fingers **(Fig. 9-12)**.
- **Flexor carpi ulnaris:** Its origins is from common flexor origin—humoral head from medial epicondyle; ulnar head from the medial margin of olecranon. It is inserted into the pisiform bone, base of the 5th metacarpal bone, hook of the hamate as pisometacarpal and pisohamate ligaments. It is supplied by ulnar nerve. Its action is flexion of wrist, adduction of wrist. Ulnar nerve passes between two heads

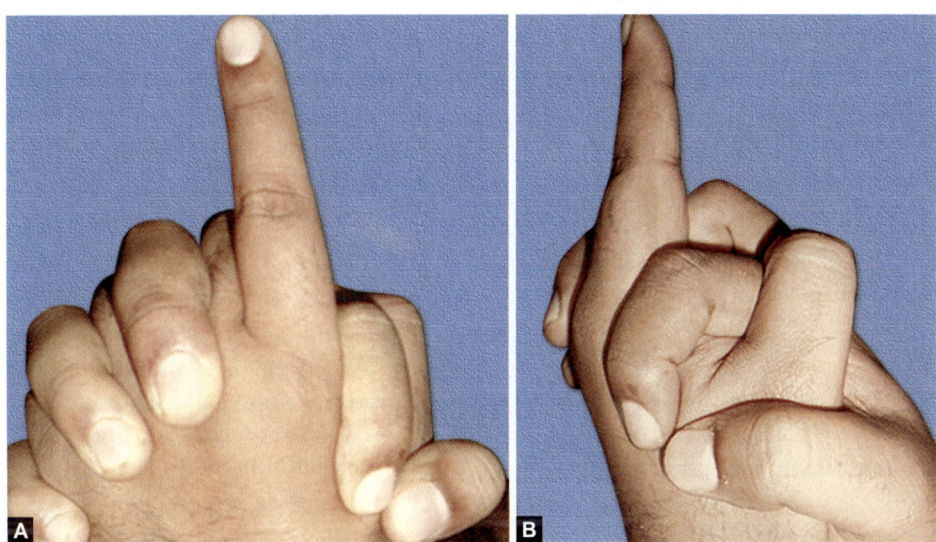

Figs. 9-9A and B *Ochsner's clasping test:* If the patient is asked to clasp the hands, index finger of the affected side fails to flex and remains as pointing index. It suggests median nerve injury.

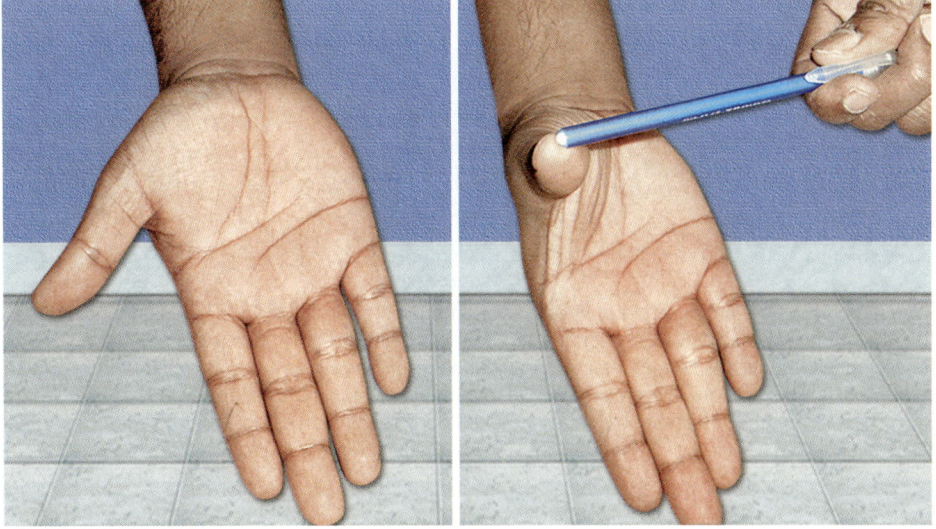

Fig. 9-10 *Pen test* for abductor pollicis brevis—median nerve.

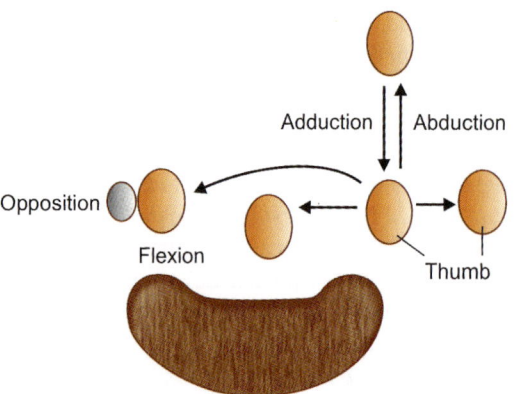

Fig. 9-11 *Abduction and adduction of thumb* occurs in right angle to the plane of flexion and extension of thumb.

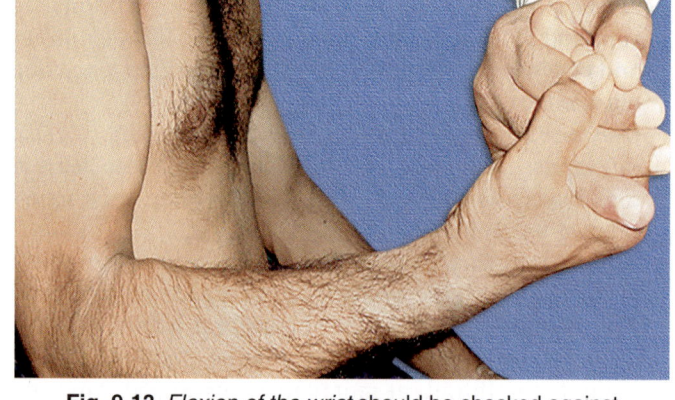

Fig. 9-13 *Flexion of the wrist* should be checked against resistance.

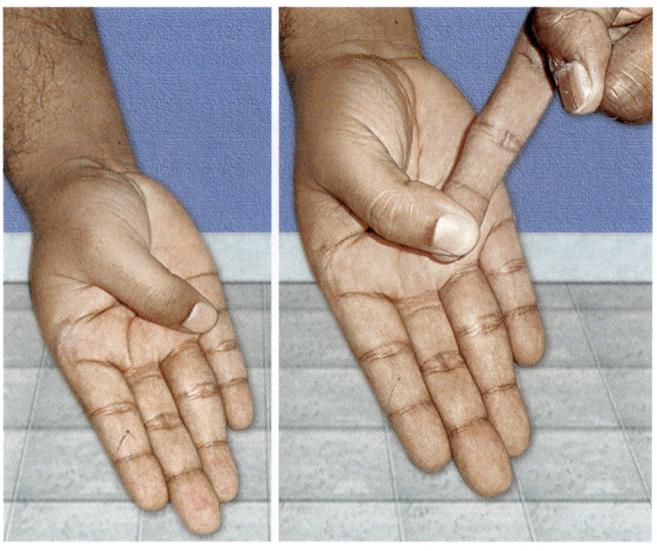

Fig. 9-12 *Checking opponens pollicis* against resistance.

of this muscle. Ulnar vessels and nerve are lateral to its tendon just above the wrist. Pisiform is a sesamoid bone of this muscle. Its power is checked by flexing the wrist against resistance and deviation of hand towards radial side is seen due to defective wrist adduction **(Fig. 9-13)**.

- ***Lumbrical muscles:*** They are four small muscles originating from tendons of the flexor digitorum profundus numbering of which is done from lateral to medial—1, 2, 3 and 4. Their origins are shown in **Figure 9-14**. They are inserted into the 2nd, 3rd, 4th and 5th dorsal digital expansions of the proximal phalanges on their lateral sides. 1st and 2nd lumbricals are supplied by median nerve (C_8, T_1); 3rd and 4th lumbricals are supplied by deep branch of ulnar nerve (C_8, T_1). Along with interossei they extend to proximal and distal interphalangeal joints; and also flex the metacarpophalangeal joints.
- ***Palmar interossei:*** They are 4 small muscles between metacarpals numbered as 1st, 2nd, 3rd and 4th from lateral

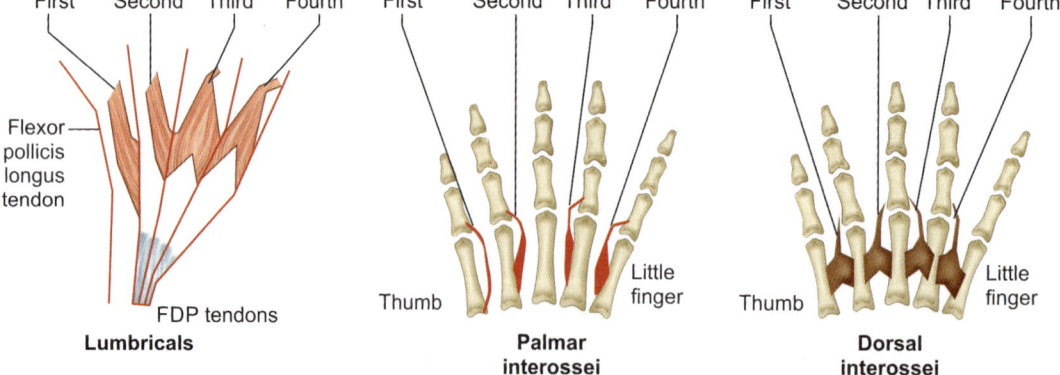

Fig. 9-14 *Figure showing attachments of lumbricals and interossei*. Lumbricals after origin from FDP tendons get inserted to lateral aspects of extensor hoods of medial four fingers. 1st and 2nd palmar interossei are attached to medial aspect of the proximal phalanx of thumb and index; 3rd and 4th are inserted into the lateral side of the ring and little fingers; no palmar interossei is attached to middle finger. 1st and 2nd dorsal interossei are inserted to lateral aspects of base and dorsal expansion of proximal phalanges of index and middle fingers. 3rd and 4th interossei are inserted to medial aspect of proximal phalanges of middle and ring fingers. Middle finger has got on either sides insertions of 2nd and 3rd dorsal interossei.

to medial. 1st muscle originates from *medial side* of the base of 1st metacarpal bone and gets inserted to medial side of the proximal phalanx of thumb. 2nd muscle originates from *medial side* of shaft of 2nd metacarpal, gets inserted to medial side of proximal phalanx and dorsal digital expansion of index finger. 3rd muscle has got its origin from *lateral part* of the shaft of the 4th metacarpal inserting into the base of proximal phalanx and dorsal digital expansion of the ring (4th) finger. 4th muscle begins from *lateral part* of the shaft of 5th metacarpal gets inserted into proximal phalanx and dorsal expansion of little (5th) finger. There is no palmar interosseous to middle finger. It is supplied by deep branch of the ulnar nerve (C_8, T_1). *Actions:* All palmar interossei adduct the finger *(PAD)* with middle finger as the center line. They also flex the metacarpophalangeal joint and extend the interphalangeal joints along with lumbricals **(Figs. 9-15 and 9-16)**.

Dorsal interossei: They are 4 small muscles between metacarpals numbered from lateral to medial. 1st originates from shafts of 1st and 2nd metacarpals; 2nd from shafts of 2nd and 3rd bones; 3rd from shafts of 3rd and 4th bones; 4th from shafts of 4th and 5th bones. First is inserted to lateral aspect of dorsal digital expansion and base of proximal phalanx of index finger; second to lateral aspect of middle finger; third to medial aspect of middle finger; fourth to medial aspect of ring finger. Dorsal interossei is not inserted to thumb and little fingers. Middle finger has got two dorsal interossei insertions on either side. Dorsal interossei are supplied by deep branch of ulnar nerve (C_8, T_1). **Actions:** They are abductors *(DAB)* of the fingers with middle finger as center line of action. Thumb and little finger has got their own abductors and so they do not need dorsal interossei. Abduction of fingers occurs in the plane of the palm whereas abduction of thumb occurs in a plane right angle to the plane of the palm **(Fig. 9-14)**.

Adductor pollicis: Oblique head has origin from capitate bone and bases of 2nd and 3rd metacarpal bones; transverse head from palmar part of 3rd metacarpal bone. It is inserted into medial side of the base of the thumb. It is supplied by deep branch of ulnar nerve (C_8, T_1). It adducts the thumb from abducted or flexed position assisted by first palmar interossei **(Fig. 9-17)**. It helps in forceful gripping. Patient is given a book to hold between extended thumb and fingers. If ulnar nerve is normal, he can hold the book with extended thumb using adductor pollicis and first palmar interossei. If there is ulnar paralysis, grip on book is assisted by flexing the terminal

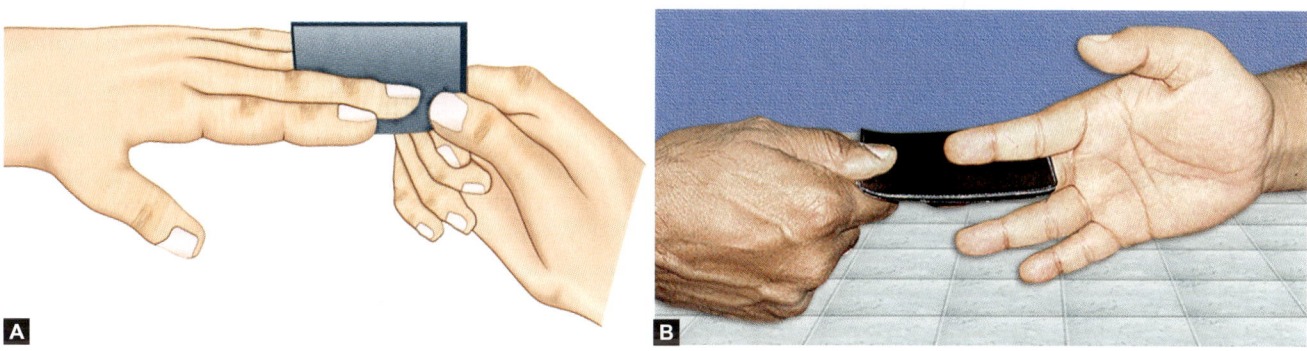

Figs. 9-15A and B Card test: A card is placed between the two fingers of the patient to grasp. In weak palmar interossei, patient cannot grasp (palmar interossei are adductors of the fingers—PAD).

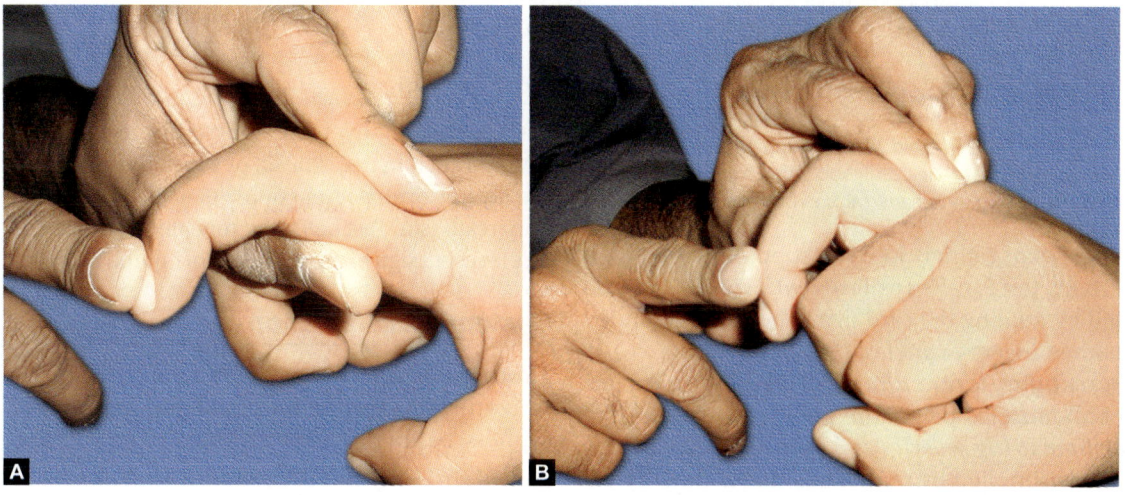

Figs. 9-16A and B *Extension of interphalangeal* joint should be checked against resistance by fixing.

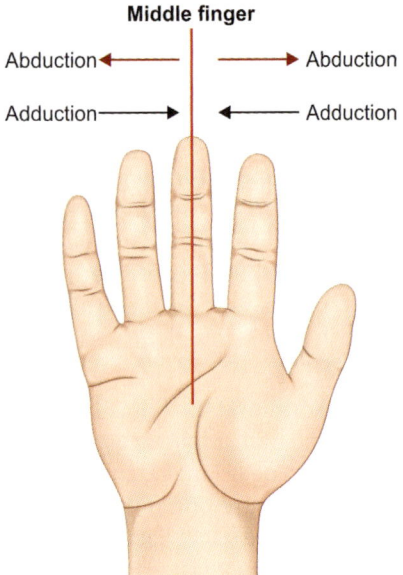

Fig. 9-17 Plane of finger movements is along the middle finger. *Palmar interossei are adductors of the fingers (PAD); dorsal interossei are abductors of the fingers (DAB).*

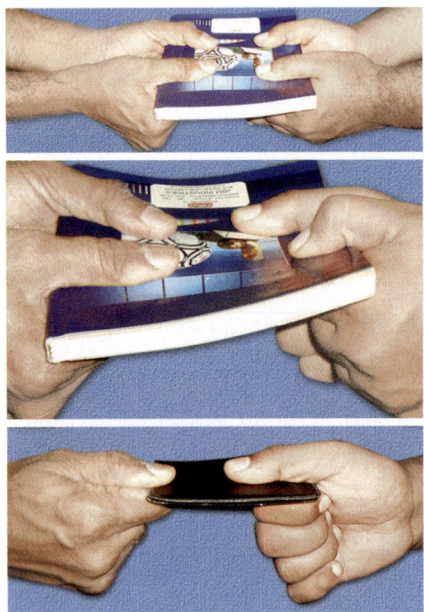

Fig. 9-18 *Froment's test and card test for ulnar nerve—adductor pollicis.* Thumb has to be flexed in paralysed adductor pollicis by over action of flexor pollicis longus to have grip on book or card.

phalanx using flexor pollicis longus (supplied by median nerve). This book test is called as **Froment's sign**. It can also be confirmed by holding the card firmly between extended thumb and other fingers—*card test* (**Fig. 9-18**).

Sciatic nerve injury is rare. When it develops it is complete paralysis of all muscles below the knee and some of the muscles, the **hamstring muscles** and sensory loss below the leg except those supplied by saphenous nerve. Incomplete lesion commonly involves common peroneal nerve (lateral popliteal nerve). There is paralysis of extensor and peroneal muscles of the leg below the knee and short extensors of toe causing **talipes equino varus** and inability to dorsiflex and evert the foot with undue lifting of the foot to clear **'dropped foot'** high from the ground—**'foot drop'** with (**'high stepping gate'**). Patient cannot dorsiflex foot/toes. Tibial nerve supplies the plantar flexors of the ankle joint and intrinsic muscles of sole of foot. Patient will not be able to plantar flex the ankle joint and toes and invert the foot against resistance causing **'talipes calcaneo valgus'**. Ankle jerk is absent. Patient finds difficult in removing the shoes from the affected foot and is unable to stand on tip toe. Sensory loss will invariably lead to trophic ulcer.

Reflexes like biceps, supinator, triceps, knee, plantar, ankle should be checked for changes. Reflexes are *stretch reflexes* and are indicators of the integrity of the spinal segments. Tendon is stretched using a rubber hammer. Often patient is asked to clench the teeth or interlock fingers so that site to be tested is relaxed properly. Biceps—$C_{5,6}$; Triceps—$C_{6,7}$; Finger jerk—C_8; Supinator—C_8; Knee jerk—$L_{2,3,4}$; Ankle jerk—$S_{1,2}$; Plantar reflex—L_5, S_1, S_2; Abdominal reflexes—T_8, T_9, T_{10} and $T_{10,11}$; Cremasteric reflex—L_1 segment. In plantar reflex, lateral aspect of the sole of the foot when scraped causes a withdrawal reflex and flexion of the great toe. Great toe extension (upward) occurs in upper motor neuron lesion. Abdominal reflexes are elicited by stroking upper and lower abdomen which causes contraction of rectus abdominis muscle. In cremasteric reflex inner side of the thigh is stroked to contract cremaster muscle.

Movements of the related joint should be checked. Both active and passive movements should be checked. In paralysed muscle passive movements are increased more than active movements (Normally passive and active movements are near equal; passive movement is elicited by the examiner; active movement is done by the patient himself).

Palpation of area of deformity and confirming it is also necessary. Palpation of injured area; scar; peripheral pulses; regional lymph nodes should be done. Nerve thickening, sensation over a skin patch may need to check in case of leprosy.

Percussion

Gentle tapping over the course of the peripheral nerve is done to elicit hyperesthesia or sensation of 'pins and needles' ideally performed after couple of weeks and noted the level of hyperesthesia. Test has to be repeated regularly. Distal shift of this level is a sign of regeneration of injured nerve—**Tinel's sign**.

Systemic Examination

Examination of respiratory system; examination in relation to features of alcoholism, diabetic neuropathy, neuritis, syphilis, beriberi, lead poison, arsenic poison are essential.

Examination of spinal cord and central nervous system is essential.

RELEVANT INVESTIGATIONS

Blood tests for diabetes; peripheral smear; hemoglobin. Urine analysis. Nasal scraping, skin biopsy, nerve biopsy for leprosy. Usually *sural nerve biopsy* is done. It is done under local anesthesia by making incision over the lateral aspect of the leg or adjacent to lateral malleolus. Nerve abscess and AFB staining will confirm the Hansen's disease.

Radiological

X-ray chest—for evidence of tuberculosis/Pancoast tumor.

X-ray neck/cervical spine—for cervical rib/fracture dislocation.

X-ray of lumbosacral region—for prolapsed intervertebral disc.

Nerve conduction study: It is demonstration of nerve potentials. It is used to find out nerve regeneration. It is useful to differentiate from cervical spondylosis, carpal tunnel syndrome or cervical rib syndrome with neurological manifestations.

Electrical stimulation: It is to assess reaction of degeneration. It begins in 4th day of nerve injury and establishes in 2 weeks. It is seen in denervated muscle. Normally cathodal/kathodal closure contraction (KCC) is stronger than anodal closure contraction (ACC). In muscle denervation, there is no response to Faradic stimulation but weak galvanic response on reverse—Anodal closure contraction has become stronger than Kathodal closure contraction.

Other relevant investigations related to cause—MRI, serum tests, etc.

PERIPHERAL NERVE INJURIES

Injuries may be: (1) open type—due to accident or operative trauma (incised/lacerated/crushed injury), (2) closed type—acute injury from compression or stretching in fracture dislocation; chronic type as in undue stress, strain, deformity. Cut end of the nerve forms proximally *neuroma* and distally *glioma*.

Neuromas may be—True neuroma or False neuroma; End neuroma or Side neuroma.

The types of injury are classified as:

Seddon's Classification

Neuropraxia: It is temporary physiological paralysis of nerve conduction. Here recovery is complete in few hours to weeks with no residual effects.

Axonotmesis (Incomplete division): It is division of nerve fibers or axons with intact nerve sheath. It is an incomplete nerve injury. Wallerian degeneration occurs distally. Patient can present with sensory loss, paralysis of muscles or causalgia.

Neurotmesis: Here complete division of nerve fibers with sheath occurs, usually following penetrating wound. Degeneration occurs proximally up to the first node of Ranvier (retrograde degeneration) as well as distal to the injury. Recovery cannot be spontaneous and is incomplete even after nerve suturing. There is complete loss of motor and sensory functions with loss of reflexes.

Sunderland's Classification

I. Conduction block—temporary neuronal block.
II. Axonotmesis but endoneurium is preserved.
III. Axonotmesis with disruption of endoneurium but perineurium is preserved.
IV. Here there is disruption of endo and perineurium but epineurium is intact.
V. Neurotmesis with disruption of endo, peri and epineurium.

Clinical Features: Loss of sensory, motor, autonomous and reflex functions; secondary changes in the skin and joints.

Prognostic factors in healing of the nerve injury: Higher the lesion worse the prognosis; more the gap between the cut ends worse the prognosis; associated injuries alter the prognosis; children do better with nerve injury; type of the injury also decides the prognosis.

Tinel's sign: It is the clinical sign (prognostic indicator) used to assess the level of regeneration. It is elicited 3 weeks after the nerve injury (Regeneration begins after the completion of nerve degeneration). It is done by tapping over the course of the nerve *from distal to proximal* to elicit a sensation of *'pins and needles' or hyperesthesia*. If sensation is felt at the site as well as distally along the distribution of the nerve that means *good recovery* can be expected. If sensation is felt only at the site of tapping, then result is *equivocal*. If no sensation is felt it means *no recovery*.

> **Causes of Peripheral Nerve Lesions**
> - Nerve injury/disease may be single nerve disease (mononeuropathy) or multiple nerve diseases (Polyneuropathy).
> - Traumatic: Either closed or open injury.
> - Inflammatory: Leprosy, herpes zoster, diphtheria.
> - Compression neuropathies.
> - Lead and arsenic poisoning.
> - Alcoholism.
> - Metabolic: Diabetes mellitus, B1 deficiency (Beriberi), Porphyria.
> - Neurofibroma and other neural tumors.
> - Idiopathic.

BRACHIAL PLEXUS INJURY

It can be—Supraclavicular injury—65%; Infraclavicular injury—25%; Combined—10%.

It can be:
- *Pre-ganglionic injury* like avulsion injury; more dangerous; extends into the spinal cord.
- *Post-ganglionic injury*—usually less severe; better recovery.

Type of nerve lesion	Etiology	Features
Median nerve injury: **Median nerve** arises from lateral (C$_{5,6,7}$) and medial cord C$_8$ and T$_1$ **(Fig. 9-19)** • In the forearm it supplies pronator teres, flexor carpi radialis, palmaris longus, and flexor digitorum superficialis • Anterior interosseous branch of the nerve supplies lateral half of flexor digitorum profundus, flexor pollicis longus, pronator quadratus • In the wrist, abductor pollicis brevis, opponens pollicis, flexor pollicis, lateral two lumbricals • Sensory supply to lateral three and half fingers **(Fig. 9-20)**	Affected in supracondylar fracture of the elbow; fracture-dislocation of elbow; direct cut injury; leprosy; carpal tunnel syndrome; as a part of brachial plexus injury	**High median nerve palsy**— • Paralysis of flexors of thumb, index, middle finger, flexor of wrist on the radial aspect (hand deviates to ulnar side when flexed against resistance) and pronator muscle; • Wasting of thenar eminence; • Loss of sensation in lateral three and half fingers **Ochsner's clasping test**: Hand shows flexed little, middle and ring finger but *pointing index* finger because of inactivity of flexor digitorum superficialis and lateral part of flexor digitorum profundus **Ape/Simian thumb deformity**: • Due to overaction of adductor pollicis thumb comes in same plane of the metacarpals. • *Pen test:* Pen held in front of hand and cannot be touched by thumb as abduction not possible due to paralysis of abductor pollicis brevis • **Low median nerve palsy**—as flexor digitorum profundus is not paralysed pointing index not seen
Carpal tunnel syndrome **Compression neuropathy of median nerve** in the carpus deep to flexor retinaculum **Carpal tunnel**—formed by carpal bones behind, flexor retinaculum in front contains median nerve and long flexor tendons of fingers and thumb	• Lunate dislocation, malunited Colle's fracture; radio carpal arthritis; flexor tendon tenosynovitis; myxedema; acromegaly; pregnancy. • Common in females; often bilateral	• Tingling, numbness, paresthesia and burning sensation in lateral three and half fingers, aggravated in night. • Ape thumb deformity, wasting of thenar muscle, weakness of opponens pollicis and abductor pollicis brevis • Light touch and two point discrimination is affected in palm and lateral 3 and 1/2 fingers
Ulnar nerve injury **Ulnar nerve** arises from medial cord of brachial plexus (C$_8$ and T$_1$) Supplies flexor carpi ulnaris, medial half of flexor digitorum profundus, all muscles of hypothenar eminence, adductor pollicis of thenar eminence, 3rd and 4th lumbricals, all interossei of the hand, sensory supply to medial part of hand and medial one and half finger	Affected in supracondylar fracture; injury to medial epicondyle; tardy ulnar palsy; leprosy; cubitus valgus deformity **Types:** a. *Low ulnar palsy*: Lesion in the wrist; deformity is more b. *High ulnar palsy*: Deformity is less as FDP is also paralysed **Ulnar paradox:** In ulnar palsy higher the lesion lesser the deformity (FDP is also paralysed), lower the lesion more the deformity (as FDP is intact, more flexion, aggravates claw hand)	• **Claw hand deformity** (marked in low lesion); • Weakness of all muscles supplied by ulnar nerve. • **Card test:** Card placed between two finger cannot be grasped firmly due to weakness of interossei muscles (palmar interossei-PAD). • Abduction of fingers is also affected. • **Froment's test/sign**: A book placed to grasp between fingers and thumb; normally the thumb will be straight by the action of adductor pollicis. But in ulnar palsy as it is paralysed grasp is achieved by flexor pollicis longus and there will be flexed thumb
Claw hand • It is the hyperextension of metacarpophalangeal joint with flexion of interphalangeal joint • Flexion of MCP joint and extension of IP joint is brought about be lumbricals and interossei (extensor hood) which are affected by ulnar nerve palsy, so develops claw hand **(Fig. 9-21)**	• Leprosy; trauma; entrapment neuropathy; tardy ulnar palsy; Klumpke's palsy. • It is a deformity due to loss of motor function–intrinsic muscle power loss (*intrinsic minus deformity*) **Note:** *Intrinsic muscle plus deformity* is due to muscle fibrosis and contracture	• Loss of sensation along the ulnar nerve distribution. • Inability to grasp card between fingers • While holding book between fingers and thumb gets flexed- **Froment's sign** **Types:** • *Ulnar claw hand*: Only medial 2 and ½ fingers involved. • *Median claw hand*: Lateral two fingers involved. • *Combined*: All four fingers involved
Radial nerve lesions Radial nerve derived from posterior cord of brachial plexus [C$_{5,6,7,8}$, T]	**In the axilla**—neuropraxia due to fracture of upper end of humerus; bony or soft tissue growth.	**Wrist drop (Fig. 9-22)** • Inability extend wrist; • Inability to extend MCP joint (extension of IP joint normal);

Contd...

Contd...

Type of nerve lesion	Etiology	Features
In the arm it supplies triceps, anconeus, brachioradialis, extensor carpi radialis longus, part of brachialis; posterior and lower lateral cutaneous nerve of arm, posterior cutaneous nerve of forearm. *Superficial branch* in the forearm ends up forming 5 digital nerves giving sensory supply to lateral side of the thumb, related part of thenar eminence, radial three and half finger on dorsal aspects; *deep branch (posterior interosseous nerve)* supplies supinator, extensor carpi radialis brevis; short branches to- extensor digitorum, extensor digiti minimi, extensor carpi ulnaris, long branches—to abductor pollicis longus and extensor pollicis brevis; extensor pollicis longus and extensor indicis	**In the radial groove**—pressure or compression on the arm from the edge of table/chair or by fall **Saturday night palsy**—due to alcohol over consumption compresses his arm over a chair. **Tourniquet palsy**—prolonged application of tourniquet. Fracture of shaft of humerus Rarely intramuscular injection. **In the elbow**—due to dislocation or fracture neck of radius	• Inability to extend forearm; • Inability to extend thumb; • Difficult to flex elbow in mid-prone position against resistance due to weakness in brachioradialis; • Loss of sensation in arm, forearm, hand, lateral three and half fingers **(Fig. 9-23)**. **Posterior interosseous nerve injury** will not affect sensation as it is purely motor and brachioradialis muscle is not affected as it is supplied by radial- so flexion of elbow in mid-prone position against resistance is possible
Common peroneal nerve lesion Common peroneal nerve supplies extensor and peroneal group of muscles and sensory supply to skin over the front and lateral aspect of leg and dorsum of foot **(Fig. 9-24)**	Fracture neck of fibula; leprosy; lead poisoning; iatrogenic	**Foot drop with high stepping gait;** • Talipes equino-varus deformity; • Loss of sensation in the lateral side of the leg and dorsum of foot
Foot drop Inability to dorsiflex and evert the foot as a result of paralysis of extensor and peroneal group of muscles due to injury to common peroneal nerve **(Fig. 9-25)**	Fracture neck of fibula; leprosy; lead poisoning; iatrogenic	High stepping gait; Loss of sensation over lateral and dorsum of foot
Medial popliteal nerve Supplies soleus, gastrocnemius, popliteus, tibialis posterior, flexor digitorum longus, flexor hallucis longus	Rarely injured by trauma or any disease	Inability to plantar flex; claw toes; loss of sensation in the sole of foot
Axillary nerve injury Axillary nerve supplies deltoid, teres minor and sensory supply over upper lateral aspect of arm	Fracture neck of humerus; dislocation of humeral head; intramuscular injection into deltoid	Loss of abduction of shoulder; loss of sensation over lateral part of the arm
Long thoracic nerve injury Long thoracic nerve supplies serratus anterior **(Fig. 9-26)**	Infiltration from malignancy; injury during surgery to breast, chest wall, axilla	When with outstretched arm pushed against a wall, inferior angle of scapula becomes more prominent—**winging of scapula**

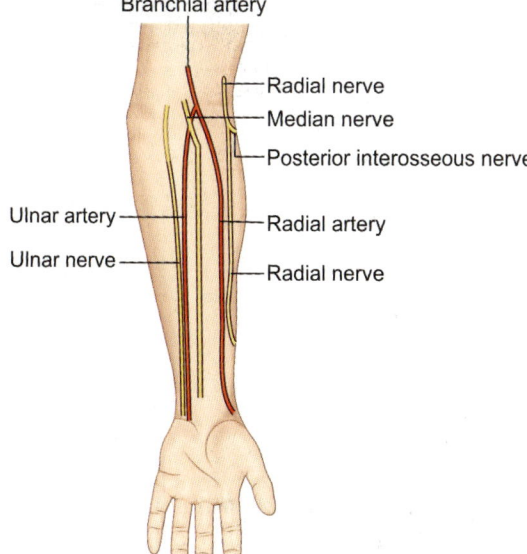

Fig. 9-19 Nerves of forearm—*ulnar, median, radial and their branches.*

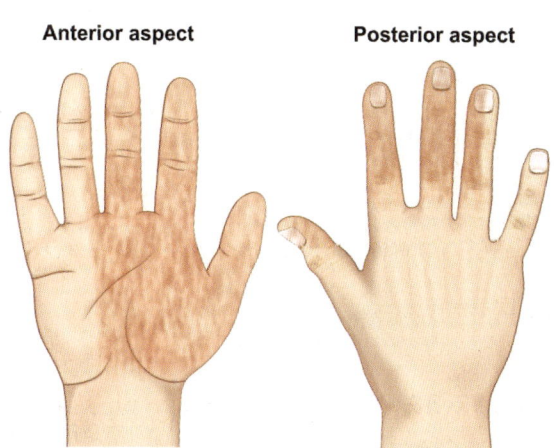

Fig. 9-20 *Sensory loss* in median nerve injury.

Section 1: Examination in General Surgery

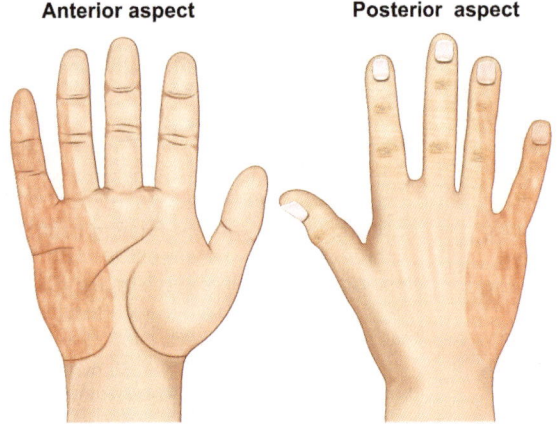

Area of sensory loss in ulnar nerve injury

Fig. 9-21 *Sensory loss* in ulnar nerve injury.

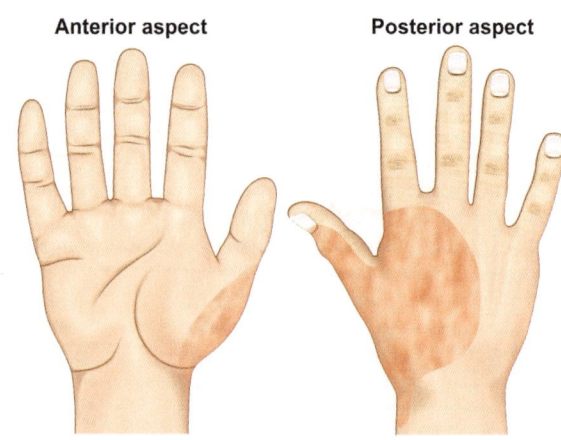

Area of sensory loss in radial nerve injury

Fig. 9-23 *Sensory loss* in radial nerve injury.

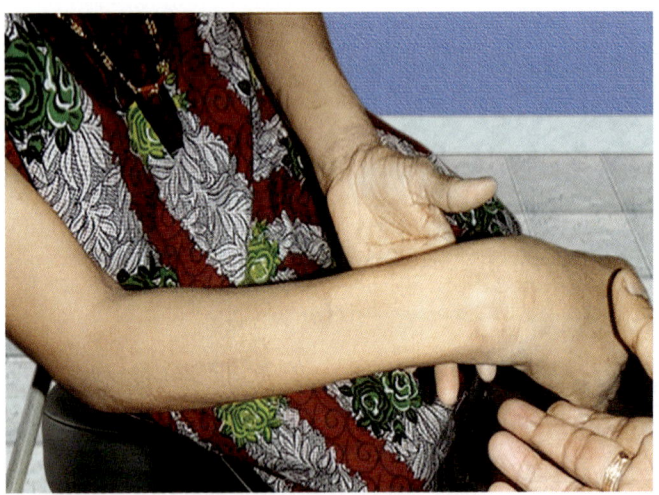

Fig. 9-22 Traumatic radial nerve injury *causing wrist drop*.

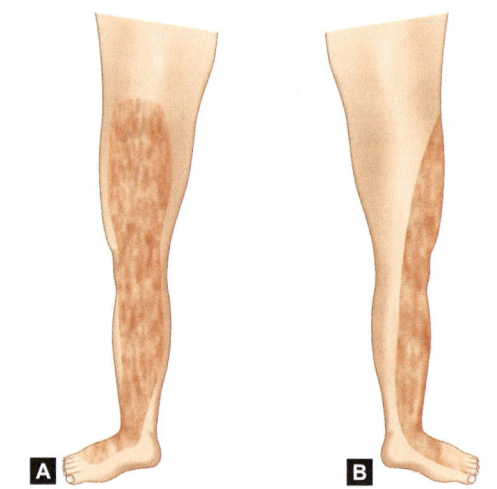

Figs. 9-24A and B *Sensory loss* seen in lateral popliteal nerve/common peroneal nerve palsy.

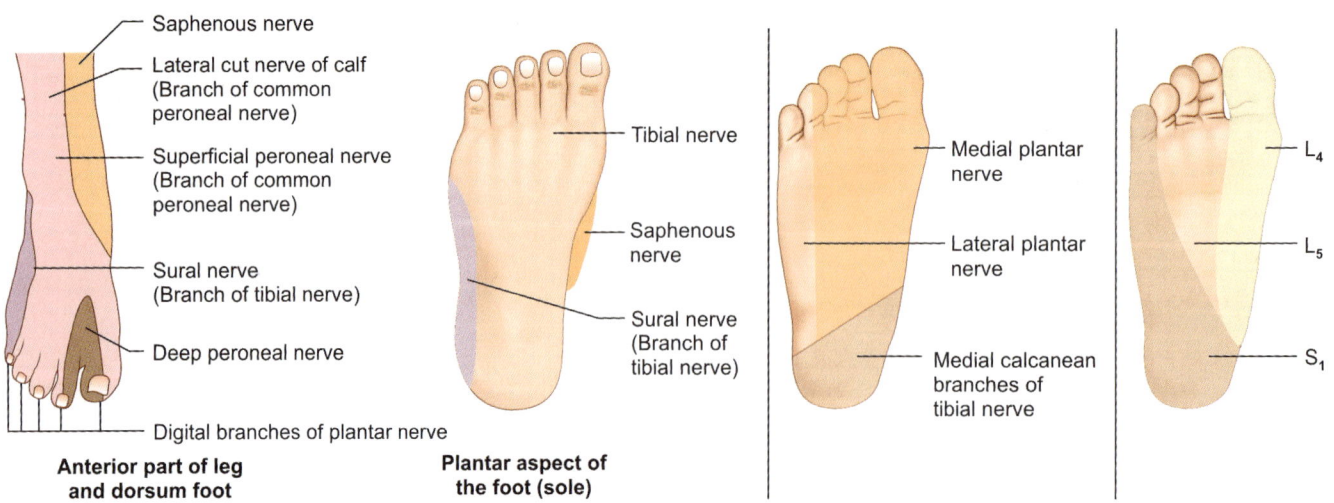

Fig. 9-25 *Sensory nerve supply of foot*, sole with sole dermatomes.

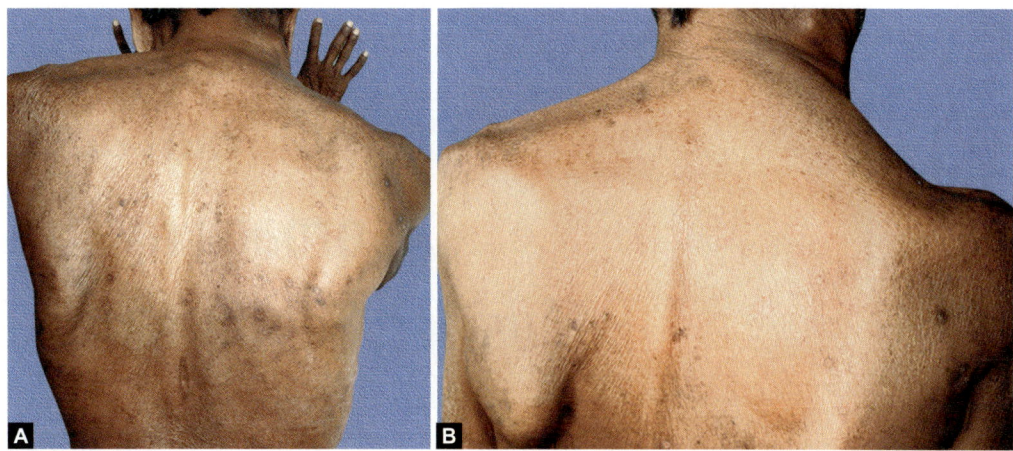

Figs. 9-26A and B *Winging of scapula* is injury to long thoracic nerve of Bell—paralyzing the serratus anterior muscle.

Different Joints with their Innervation and Various Muscle Actions

Joint	Action	Roots	Muscles and Nerves
Shoulder	Flexion	$C_{5,6}$	Nerve to pectoralis major, circumflex nerve to deltoid
	Extension	$C_{5,6}$	Thoracodorsal nerve—latissimus dorsi
	Abduction	$C_{5,6}$	Deltoid muscle—axillary nerve
	Adduction		Pectoralis major, latissimus dorsi, biceps
Elbow	Flexion	$C_{5,6}$	Brachialis, biceps, brachioradialis—musculocutaneous nerve
	Extension	$C_{6,7,8}$	Triceps, anconeus—radial nerve
Wrist	Flexion	$C_{6,7,8}$	Flexor carpi radialis, flexor carpi ulnaris—median and ulnar nerves
	Extension	$C_{6,7,8}$	Extensor carpi radialis longus, extensor carpi radialis brevis, extensor carpi ulnaris—radial nerve
	Abduction		Flexor carpi radialis, extensor carpi radialis longus and brevis, abductor pollicis longus and extensor pollicis brevis
	Adduction		Flexor carpi ulnaris, extensor carpi ulnaris
Hip	Flexion	$L_{2,3,4}$	Psoas major, iliacus—lumbar and femoral nerves
	Extension	$L_5, S_{1,2}$	Gluteus maximus and hamstrings—inferior gluteal nerve
	Abduction	$L_{4,5}, S_1$	Gluteus medius and minimus—superior gluteal nerve
	Adduction	$L_{2,3,4}$	Adductor longus, brevis, magnus—obturator nerve
	Medial rotation		Tensor fascia lata, anterior fibers of gluteus medius and minimus
	Lateral rotation		Two obturators, two gemelli, quadratus femoris
Knee	Flexion	$L_{4,5}, S_{1,2}$	Biceps femoris, semitendinosus, semimembranosus—sciatic nerve
	Extension	$L_{2,3,4}$	Quadriceps femoris—femoral nerve
Ankle	Dorsiflexion	$L_{4,5}, S_1$	Tibialis anterior—deep peroneal nerve (anterior tibial nerve)
	Plantar flexion	$L_5, S_{1,2}$	Gastrocnemius and soleus—posterior tibial nerve (tibial nerve)
Foot	Inversion (is more than eversion)	$L_{4,5}$	Tibialis anterior and tibialis posterior
	Eversion	L_5, S_1	Peroneus longus and peroneus brevis—superficial peroneal nerve

CASE DISCUSSION

A 40-year-old female presents with progressive numbness and pain in her both hands; but right side pain is more; thumb is mainly affected; she drops objects suddenly from her right hand due to numbness. History of trauma or family history is not present. She is not diabetic.

What are the differential diagnoses?
It could be carpal tunnel syndrome or cervical spondylosis or thoracic outlet syndrome. Intracranial lesions (infarcts) are less likely but should be ruled out.

What other relevant history you will ask?
Carpal tunnel syndrome (CTS) is due to median nerve compression at carpal tunnel. Exaggeration of symptoms at night time is common. CTS is more common in diabetes, myxedema, hyperthyroidism, pregnancy, malunited Colles' fracture, arthritis of the wrist. Direct digital pressure on the median nerve point at carpal tunnel will produce symptom in 30 seconds. Thenar wasting, decreased vibration sense loss, loss of abductor muscle resistance of thumb, positive Phalen's test are typical. 50% of patients CTS is bilateral.

What investigations are done in CTS?
Electromyography (EMG) is very useful; nerve conduction studies, X-ray wrist and cervical spine; MRI wrist—are other useful methods of evaluation. In doubtful cases, CT head and CT thoracic outlet may be needed.

Examination and Clinical Approach in Diseases of Muscles, Tendons and Fasciae

Competency: AN12.10; AN12.11; AN12.14; SU17.7.

Sound clinical knowledge of muscle and tendon diseases is essential. It also needs a good anatomical knowledge of the muscle, its origin, insertion, actions and nerve supply.

HISTORY

Pain: Pain is the main feature in degenerative diseases of the tendons, muscles, ligaments or fasciae. Pain in epicondyles in ***tennis elbow*** (lateral) or ***Golfer's elbow*** (medial) is common. Pain of the tendon is felt in tendonitis like patellar or Achilles' tendons. In tenosynovitis, pain is felt along the tendon in de Quervain's tenosynovitis. Rest pain along the distribution of the median nerve is common in carpal tunnel syndrome.

Deformity: It is the symptom as well as the inspectory finding. Patient always observe the deformity and tells the history.

GENERAL EXAMINATION

Pallor and other associated relevant features should be looked for along with nutrition, neurological examination, etc. Specific deformities are seen often in conditions like leprosy.

LOCAL EXAMINATION (LOOK/FEEL/MEASURE/MOVE)

Inspection

Deformity is the commonest and specific for certain conditions. In ***Dupuytren's contracture*** there is flexion of ring and little fingers. ***Volkmann's ischemic contracture*** causes extension of wrist and metacarpophalangeal joints with flexion of interphalangeal joints. When the wrist is fully flexed, fingers can be extended—***Volkmann's sign***.

Swelling is seen in torn muscle. Tenosynovitis causes swelling of the tendon.

Skin over the area or swelling for scar/color/edema/sinuses/asymmetry, abnormal wrinkles, etc. should be asked for.

Wasting of the muscles should be inspected. Shape, wasting, hypertrophy, irregularity, displacement of the muscle should be looked for. Muscle should be inspected ***at rest as well as with contraction.*** It should be compared to other muscles and opposite side muscles.

Length of the limb, discrepancies on inspection should be observed and noted.

Palpation

Look for rise in skin temperature/presence of pitting when edema is there.

Tenderness is elicited at the sites of the degenerative pathology whether it is epicondylitis or tendinitis.

Palpation of the swelling for all its features like any other swelling (*see* **Chapter 4: Examination and Clinical Approach of a Swelling/Lump**) should be carried out.

Measure the real and apparent lengths of the limb and compare to opposite side.

Muscle should be palpated at rest as well as with contraction. When muscle is at rest intramuscular swelling moves in right angle to the length of the muscle; when muscle is contracted intramuscular lump becomes immobile. Ruptured muscle when felt will be tender often with a swelling. There will be a depression when relaxed; but a firm swelling over the edge of the ruptured muscle with a sharp depression at the site of tear is typical while contraction is typical. Hematoma may be felt in a ruptured muscle **(Fig. 10-1)**.

Movements of the joints: Active movement is the one which patient does and shows to the examiner; whose range, abnormal mobility or restrictions should be observed. Passive movement is the one which examiner elicits using his hands.

Neurological Examination

Neurological examination should be done like in carpal tunnel syndrome for median nerve palsy. Motor power and reflexes should be checked.

Peripheral pulses should be examined for blood supply.

Relevant Systemic Examination

Relevant systemic examination is a must. CNS, spine, respiratory system or other systems should be examined in detail.

Diseases of Muscles, Tendons and Fasciae

Carpal Tunnel syndrome: It is the classical example of stenosing tenosynovitis (Refer for detail Chapter 9).

Dupuytren's contracture: It is localized thickening of palmar aponeurosis with fibrous *nodule* formation causing flexion of ring and then little fingers. Terminal phalanx is not affected as palmar aponeurosis does not extend into terminal phalanx. It begins at and mainly involves medial aspect of the palmar aponeurosis. Eventually all fingers may get involved; joints also may be involved causing arthritis and stiff joints. Skin gets adherent to thickened palmar aponeurosis. It is often familial and bilateral (45%). It is common in males (10 times). Pain is not common; but stiffness is usual. Taut fibrous strands are seen and felt especially along the line of ring and little fingers. By flexing the wrist flexion deformity *will not get reduced. Garrod's pads* of fat develop over the knuckles of proximal interphalangeal joints. Dupuytren's contracture is often associated with—plantar fasciitis (5%–*Ledderhose* disease); mediastinal and retroperitoneal fibrosis; *Peyronie's* disease of penis (3%); nodules in the face and ear; *Pellegrini Steida's* disease (Myositis ossificans with calcification of commonly superior part of medial collateral ligament of knee joint). *Galezia triad* is Dupuytren's contracture; retroperitoneal fibrosis; Peyronie's diseases of penis. Dupuytren's contracture may be due to repeated minor trauma, cirrhosis, alcoholism, epileptics on phenytoin therapy, diabetes mellitus and other metabolic conditions. It can be often familial—autosomal dominant. Condition causes restriction of hand function and arthritis of joints.

Volkmann's Ischemic contracture: It is development of muscular infarction initially acute later chronic causing subsequent contracture. There is shortening of the long flexors of the forearm due to ischemic fibrosis of the muscle (aseptic muscle necrosis and fibrosis). *Causes:* Supracondylar fracture (commonest) injuring brachial artery which bleeds or undergoes spasm causing raised pressure in the compartment which again further compromises the blood supply of the muscle; a tight plaster which compresses the artery blocking the blood flow; arterial embolism. Burns, closed forearm crush injury, intravenous chemotherapy are other causes. *Features in acute phase:* Condition is common in young individual; history of trauma is evident; pain in the forearm and fingers (under the plaster is typical); loss of finger movements (mainly finger extension); cold skin; paresthesia (due to ischemia of median and anterior interosseous nerves) severe burning pain or pins and needles sensation due to ischemic neuritis; absence of radial pulse; pallor; edema of the forearm (puffiness). *Chronic phase:* Once acute phase subsides gradually, pain disappears but deformity persists with inability to extend fingers. By flexing the wrist fingers can be extended—*Volkmann's sign*. There is claw hand deformity. Fingers are in acutely flexed position. Forceful passive finger extension is uncomfortable and often painful. Metacarpophalangeal joint is extended (Fig. 10-2).

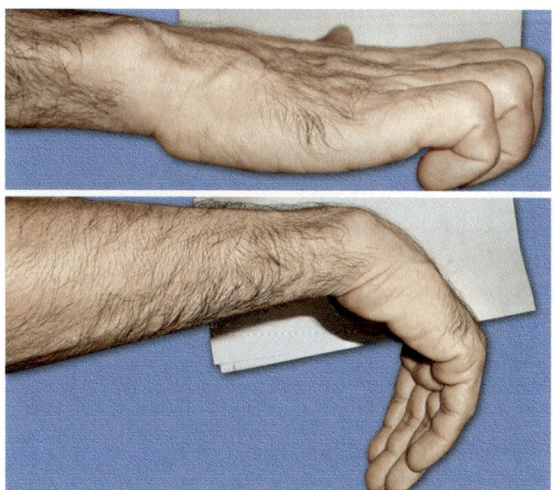

Fig. 10-2 *Volkmann's sign* in Volkmann's ischemic contracture. When wrist is flexed fully fingers can be extended at interphalangeal joints. It is not possible in Dupuytren's contracture.

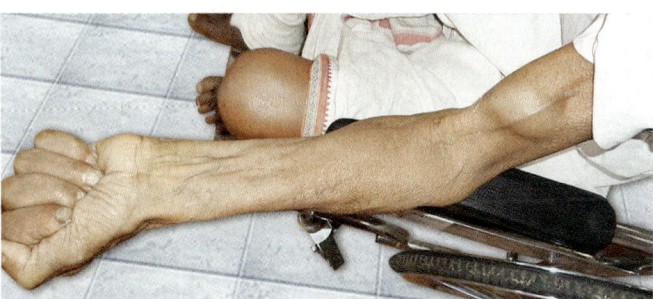

Fig. 10-1 Old ruptured biceps brachii muscle.

Types and etiological factors	Clinical features
Stenosing Tenosynovitis/Tenovaginitis 1. *Trigger finger:* Unknown; Commonly seen in middle/ring finger; common in middle aged women. Thickened nodule in the long flexor tendon sheath adjacent to head of metacarpal or constricting band in the synovial sheath. 2. *Trigger thumb/snapping thumb:* Rare, seen in neonates and infants. 3. *de Quervain's stenosing tenosynovitis:* Common tendon of extensor pollicis longus and extensor pollicis brevis involved.	Extension of affected finger is difficult; finger gets '*locked*' in flexed position; can be extended with a "sudden click" like a trigger of a pistol using excessive effort often with other hand. Finger appearance and sensation normal. Thumb is similarly affected. Orange pip-like swelling felt over head of the first metacarpal bone. Bulge seen or felt in radial styloid process or anatomical snuff box. Abduction and extension of thumb is difficult, adduction of thumb is painful.
Congenital contracture of little finger: Bilateral, seen in childhood with contracture of soft tissues.	Palmar aponeurosis is normal; ring finger not involved; hyperextension of proximal phalanx, flexion of middle and distal phalanges; straightening of finger not possible.
Burns contracture of finger: Burn injury.	Permanent contracture of fingers and wrist.
Mallet finger/Base ball finger: Rupture of extensor tendon of distal phalanx or avulsion fracture of the base of distal phalanx as a result of injury by a hard ball or object onto the tip of finger.	Fixed flexion deformity (20 degrees) of terminal/distal phalanx. Distal IP joint can be flexed to 90 degrees and when extended it comes up to 20 degrees beyond which cannot be extended and straightened.
Rupture of extensor pollicis longus: Due to attrition of extensor pollicis longus tendon causing sudden rupture with a snap while working. Common in females, seen in Rheumatoid arthritis; as a complication of Colle's fracture.	Thumb remains in adducted position with inability to extend the terminal phalanx.
Heberdon's nodes: Nonspecific cause; in females commonly associated with osteoarthrosis; in males may be traumatic in origin by sports like baseball/cricket.	Immobile bony swelling close to distal interphalangeal joint both in palmar and dorsal aspect; with a small adventitious bursa between the swelling and the skin may be seen. All fingers except thumb is involved. Index finger most affected. Radial deviation of distal phalanx with osteoarthritis of distal IP joint.
Rupture of muscle fibres: Unusual sudden contraction of normal muscle or normal contraction of degenerated muscle. Common in young athletes, or in old people. Adjacent joints/arterial/nervous system to be examined. Usually spontaneous in elderly due to degenerative disease. a. *Rupture of long head of biceps brachii:* Seen in elderly due to degenerative disease as spontaneous. b. *Rupture of supraspinatus tendon:* Spontaneous I elderly as degenerative disease. c. *Rupture of Achilles' tendon:* In athletes, football players where violent undue contraction of calf muscle occurs.	Biceps brachii, quadriceps femoris –commonly affected. Can complete/partial. Initially pain, bruising, swelling, later muscle weakness with limp In partial tear, depression in the muscle at the site of tear is felt when in relaxed state; when contracted a firm swelling is seen/felt at the edge of depression with no independent mobility. Movement of muscle is absent in complete tear Sudden pain in upper arm or swelling (due to bunching of muscle) when elbow is flexed. Sudden pain; absence of initiation of abduction (initiation done by body leaning to the affected side), later part of the abduction is normal. Swelling is seen/felt in the posterior part of lower leg with plantar flexion of the ankle.
Intramuscular haematoma: Direct injury with tear in muscle along with injury to intramuscular blood vessels. Common in patients on anticoagulants and with blood dyscrasias. *Gastrocnemius is the commonest muscle affected.*	Pain at rest, aggravated with movement. Firm/hard, well localised, tender swelling is felt in the muscle when relaxed, which is longitudinally ovoid, and parallel to muscle fibres. The swelling becomes soft once liquefaction occurs. The swelling becomes indistinct when the muscle contracts.
Muscle hernia: Common in lumbar region and calf. Swelling is obvious in muscle having thick fibrous covering as in anterior compartment of leg, lateral abdominal and back muscles. Size of hernia depends on the amount of contraction in the muscle.	Bulging out of muscle during contraction through a defect in its fibrous covering; bulge disappears when muscle is relaxed but a distinct defect can be palpable in the fascia. These are *two essential features* to diagnose muscle hernia.
Intra- and intermuscular lipoma: Lipoma within the muscle or in between the muscle.	Smooth, soft –firm swelling with lobulation is felt in the muscle when relaxed, becomes indistinct, immobile and hard when contracted. Occasionally some unpalpable swelling becomes suddenly painful, palpable during exercise due to bursting out through muscle fibres. Usually single, common in back of trunk, slow growing to attain a large size.
Myositis ossificans: Calcification and eventual ossification of injured muscle; associated with fracture of adjacent bone. Fracture strips the periosteum causing haematoma which is invaded by the osteoblasts causing calcification and post traumatic ossification. It is a misnomer; as it is not myositis Example: (1) Lower part of brachialis after supracondylar fracture (2) Quadriceps femoris after fracture femur.	Inability to use the muscle, stiff adjacent joint with features of old fracture, painful forced movements. Ossified part attains the involved muscle shape, fixed to the underlying bone, continuous with the callus underneath.

Contd...

Contd...

Types and etiological factors	Clinical features
Tennis elbow: *Lateral epicondylitis* of the humerus involving common extensor origin which is due to repetitive stress disorder caused by overloading of the wrist extensor origin against resistance.	Pain and localized tenderness at lateral epicondyle of humerus at the attachment of common extensor tendon of forearm, aggravated when wrist is extended against resistance.
Golfer's elbow: *Medial epicondylitis* due to repetitive stress disorder of common flexor origin over medial epicondyle; opposite of tennis elbow.	Pain and tenderness over medial epicondyle adjacent to origin of common flexor tendon of forearm, aggravated by flexing the wrist against resistance.
Plantar fasciitis: Tear or bony spur at the attachment of plantar fascia to calcaneum.	Unbearable pain in the heel while walking.
Supraspinatus tendinitis: Compression of degenerated and calcified supraspinatus tendon between the head of humerus and acromion during abduction of the shoulder; common in middle aged/elderly males.	Pain in the shoulder during middle third of abduction and external rotation of the shoulder. First 60° abduction is painless followed by next 60° of painful abduction beyond [>120°] which once again becomes painless—**painful arc syndrome.** Development of stiffness of shoulder—**frozen shoulder.** Pain gradually subsides while stiffness increases; later stiffness persists but pain subsides in 3 months; in further 3 months stiffness also slowly subsides. Spontaneous rupture of the degenerated supraspinatus tendon can occur. Calcification in the tendon can be confirmed by X-ray.
Rheumatoid arthritis of hand: Hands are commonly involved in rheumatoid arthritis. Hypertrophy of the *synovial* membrane of the joints is the initial feature. Overlying skin becomes shiny and atrophic. Wasting of muscles with swollen, spindle shaped/fusiform joints and later development of deformities occurs. Metacarpophalangeal joint is first to get affected; later proximal interphalangeal joint **(Figs. 10-3 and 10-4)**.	Deformities are—deviation of finger towards ulnar side at metacarpophalangeal joint (*varus deformity of 45°–60°*)—*ulnar drift*; fixed flexion deformity of wrist with ulnar deviation; fibrotic contraction of interossei and lumbricals causing hyperextension of the proximal interphalangeal joint and flexion of distal interphalangeal. Joint—*swan neck deformity*; flexion of proximal interphalangeal joint and hyperextension of distal interphalangeal joint due to attrition of middle slip of the extensor tendon—'*boutonniere' deformity*; rupture of extensor tendons at wrist level causing dropped finger.

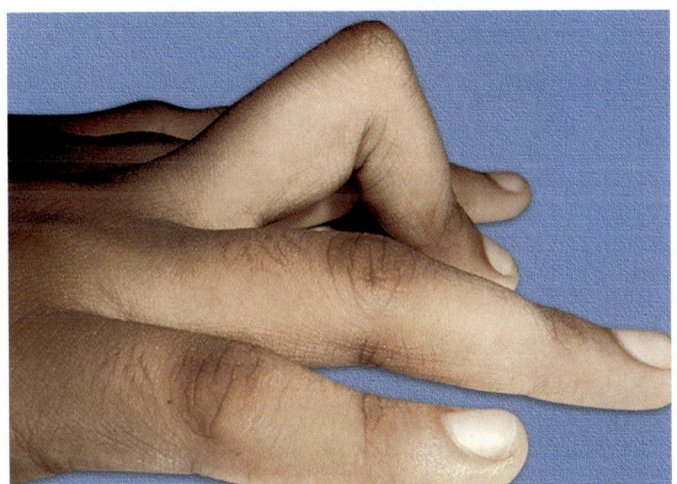

Fig. 10-3 *Button hole*/Boutonniere deformity. There is flexion of proximal interphalangeal joint and hyperextension of distal interphalangeal joint.

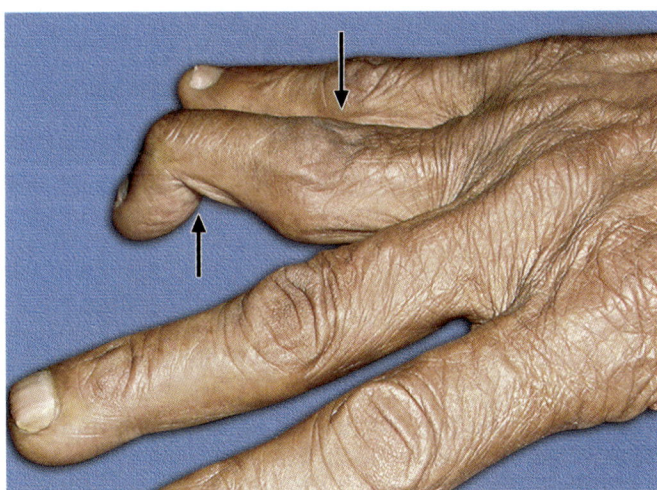

Fig. 10-4 *Swan neck deformity.* It is hyperextension of proximal interphalangeal joint and flexion of distal interphalangeal joint.

11 CHAPTER

Clinical Approach and Examination of Oral Cavity

Competency: SU20.1; SU20.2.

Oral cavity is a wide area which includes lips, vestibule, gums, teeth, cheeks, tongue, palate, and floor of the mouth. Vestibule is a smaller outer portion bounded externally by lips and cheeks; internally by teeth and gums. Parotid duct opens into the cheek opposite the crown of upper 2nd molar tooth. Numerous mucus glands that are situated in the submucosa of lips and cheeks open into the vestibule.

■ HISTORY

History taking begins with:

Name:

Age: Cleft lip and palate are seen in newborns. Tongue tie is often seen in infants. Mucus cysts can occur at any age group. *Oral cancers* occur usually in middle age and later age groups.

Sex: Carcinoma oral cavity is more common in males.

Occupation: Agriculturists who are constantly exposed to sunlight are prone to develop carcinoma lip—*countryman's lip*.

Address: *Australian Caucasians commonly develop lip cancers. It is less common in Negroes.*

History of Present Illness

History of swelling: Mucus cyst of lip or cheek presents as painless swelling of long duration. Duration, progress, presence of pain should be asked for. Carcinoma often can present as swelling of short duration. Lip cancer is slowly progressive and so may be of long duration whereas carcinoma of cheek and tongue is rapidly progressive and is of short duration. Minor salivary gland tumor in palate and lip presents as a swelling **(Figs. 11-1 to 11-4)**.

History of ulcer: Ulcer in the oral cavity is common. It can be aphthous ulcer/syphilitic ulcer/traumatic ulcer/tuberculous ulcer/malignant ulcer. Aphthous ulcer is painful. Malignant

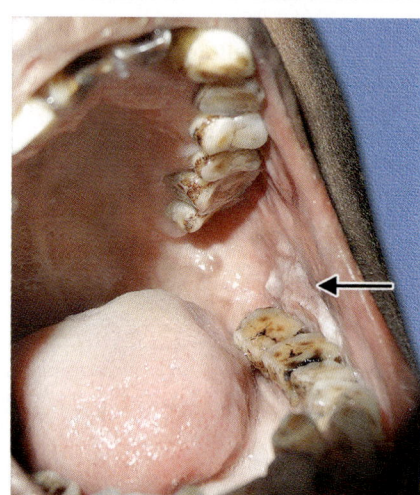

Fig. 11-1 Carcinoma cheek (buccal mucosa). *It is the commonest site of oral cancers in Indian subcontinent.*

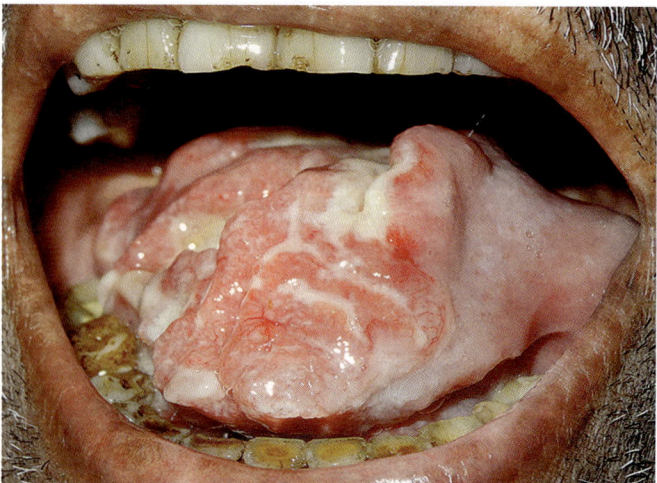

Fig. 11-2 Carcinoma tongue involving extensively; there is *ankyloglossia* (inability to protrude the tongue out), ulceration; lesion crosses the midline. Such lesion spreads to bilateral cervical lymph nodes.

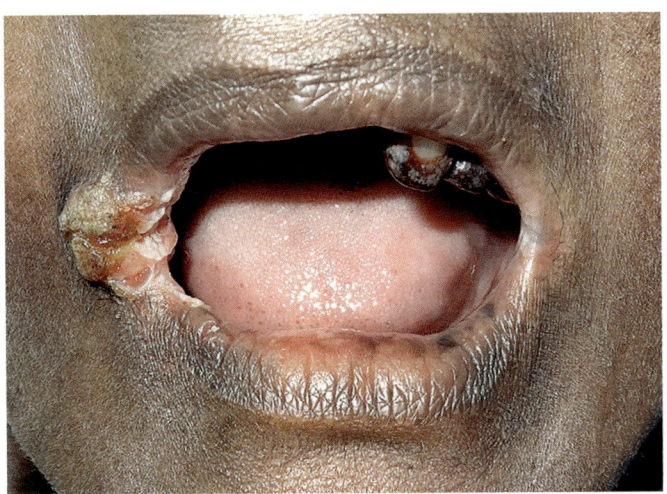

Fig. 11-3 Carcinoma involving the angle (right) of the mouth; it could be *verrucous carcinoma*; it also extends into buccal mucosa.

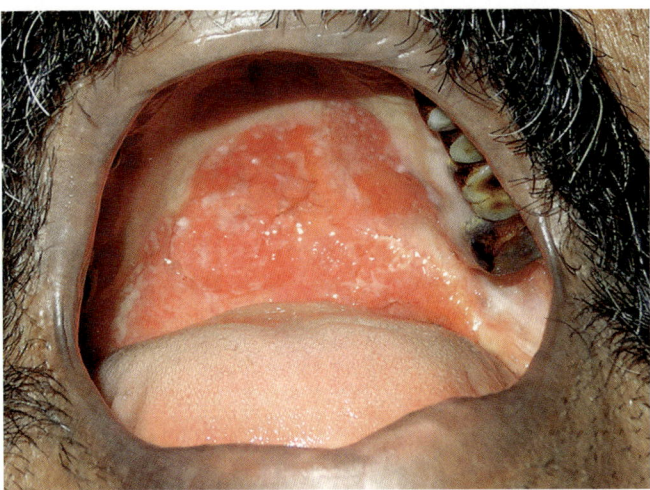

Fig. 11-4 *Carcinoma palate*; note the extensive local involvement and crossing the midline.

ulcer is painless to begin with, but becomes painful once it infiltrates or gets infected. Origin of ulcer, duration, progress should be asked for.

History of pain: Site of pain, radiation, referred pain, severity of pain, pain over the adjacent mandible, whether pain restricts mouth opening or swallowing should be asked for. Pain may radiate or gets referred to ear through lingual nerve or inferior alveolar nerve (through auriculotemporal branch of mandibular nerve). Dental ulcer on the margin of the tongue is painful. Aphthous ulcer is painful. Tuberculous ulcer may not have any pain. Retention cyst, leukoplakia, early oral cancers are painless. In late cases of carcinoma, pain develops due to deeper infiltration (to nerves) and sepsis.

Excessive salivation (sialorrhea) is common in oral cancers, especially in carcinoma tongue.

Inability to protrude the tongue out is common in carcinoma tongue involving floor of the mouth or infiltrating the genioglossus muscle; also seen in tongue tie.

Deviation of tip of tongue when protruded out is also asked for.

Difficulty in speech is common in carcinoma tongue. It is also often seen in painful aphthous ulcers.

Voice change or dysphagia may be the feature of carcinoma posterior third of tongue.

Dentition, recent history of loosening of teeth, falling of teeth is important as it may be due to underlying carcinoma.

Bleeding, halitosis (foul-smelling breath), **altered taste sensation,** cough, hemoptysis are other history to be asked. History of fever suggests infection, bronchopneumonia (due to aspiration, especially in carcinoma tongue).

History of symptoms suggestive of local invasion (difficulty in opening the mouth, mandibular pain, loss of sensation in the chin or gums); cervical lymph nodal spread (swelling in the neck, duration, pain, ulceration) are asked for.

Past History

Past history of oral ulcers, recurrent stomatitis, treatment received in the form of surgery, radiotherapy, chemotherapy has to be noted. History suggestive of leukoplakia also should be asked.

Personal History

Smoking, alcohol intake, spicy food, pan chewing (betel nut, supari, khaini, etc.) are important causes for carcinoma. It is also important to note how long patient keeps the pan in the cheek which will increase the irritation. **Reverse smoking** is often related to carcinoma hard palate.

> **Etiology for oral cancers:**
> *Tobacco chewing* (betel nut, betel leaf, tobacco, smoked lime); smoking; alcohol. *Six 'S'* are—spices, spirit, smoking, sepsis, sharp tooth, syphilis. Risk is 8 times more in tobacco chewer; with quid it is 10 times; keeping quid in the buccal mucosa/gingivolabial sulcus overnight raises the risk to 30 times
> *Human papilloma virus (HPV)*—seen in 70–90% of oral carcinomas. Epstein-Barr virus may also play a role
> *Deficiency* of vitamin A, iron deficiency anemia, poor dental hygiene are other factors

■ GENERAL EXAMINATION

Detailed general examination is very essential. Anemia/edema/jaundice/clubbing/lymphadenopathy/radial pulse/blood pressure/raise in temperature/attitude of the patient/nutritional assessment by skin texture, subcutaneous fat, weight, body mass index/any other relevant findings should be mentioned. *Cachexia* signifies advanced malignancy. *Halitosis* may be found. Temperature may be raised.

■ LOCAL EXAMINATION

Inspection

Inspection of the oral cavity should be done using proper and adequate light. *A spatula* should be used eventually to inspect

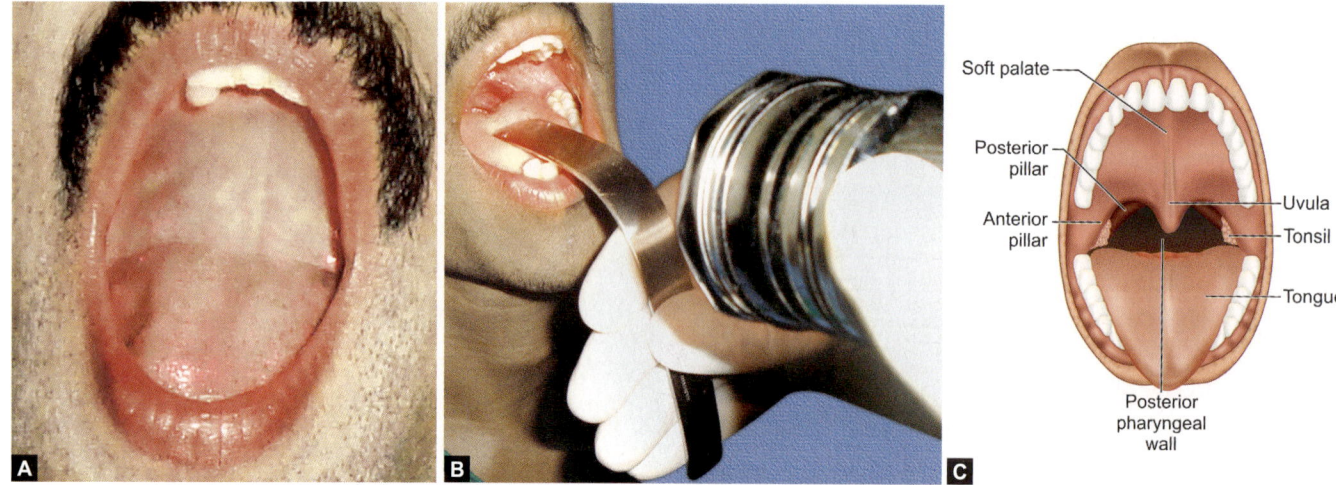

Figs. 11-5A to C *Proper inspection of the oral cavity is essential part of the examination.* Often spatula/tongue depressor and a good light source should be used to inspect the oral cavity.

posterior aspect of the oral cavity. Inspection is done in order—lips, cheeks, teeth, gums, tongue, floor of the mouth, palate, tonsils, posterior aspect **(Figs. 11-5A to C)**.

Inspection of the Lip

Lips are two fleshy folds lined by skin outside and mucous membrane inside. Upper lip is bounded by nose and nasolabial groove. Lower lip is bounded by cheek and labiomental groove. Orbicularis oris forms the muscular bulk of the lip which encircles the lip and is supplied by facial nerve. **Frenulum** in the midline in upper and lower lips joins lip to the gums. **Vermilion border** is red border of the lip where skin part merges gradually into the mucous membrane part. It contains wet line inside and a dry line outside. Small rounded nodule at the center of the lowest part of the upper lip is called as **tubercle**. A depression running from tubercle to nostrils is called as **philtrum**. The corner where upper and lower lips meet at right and left angles are called as **commissures** of lip. 5 mm elevation of mucous membrane posterior to commissure is called as **commissural papule**. Upper lip drains into upper deep cervical nodes. Center of lower lip drains into **submental nodes** then to upper deep cervical nodes. Lateral part of lower lip drains into submandibular lymph nodes then *to middle cervical nodes*. Lymph from angles of mouth drains into both nodes of upper and lower lips. Lips are red or reddish brown in young. It is often brownish in smokers.

Cleft lip and **cleft palate** are obvious **(Fig. 11-6)**. Its type, side, extent should be noted down. Cleft lip may be complete (when it extends into the nostril) or incomplete (when not extending into the nostril). It may be unilateral/bilateral. When there is bilateral cleft lip with palate there is protuberant premaxilla.

Macrocheilia is enlarged lip which is common in upper lip may be due to lymphangioma or hemangioma (soft, bluish with compressibility and emptying is typical) **(Figs. 11-7 and 11-8)**.

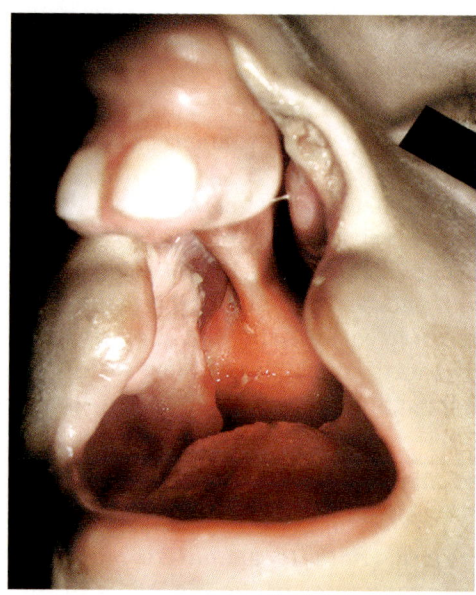

Fig. 11-6 *Cleft lip and palate* in a child.

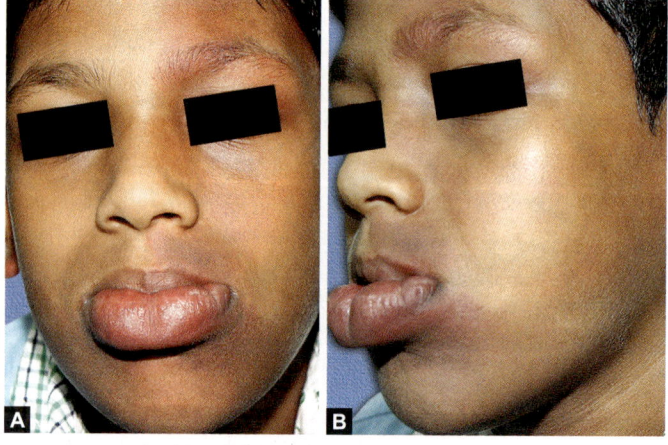

Fig. 11-7 Hemangioma lower lip. *It is compressible swelling.*

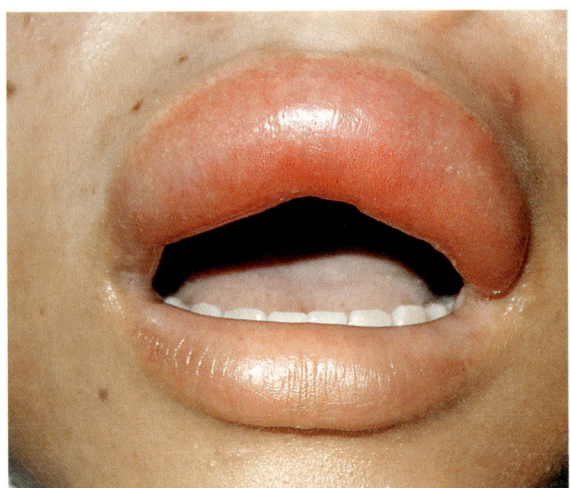

Fig. 11-8 Inflammatory edema of upper lip. It subsides usually on its own.

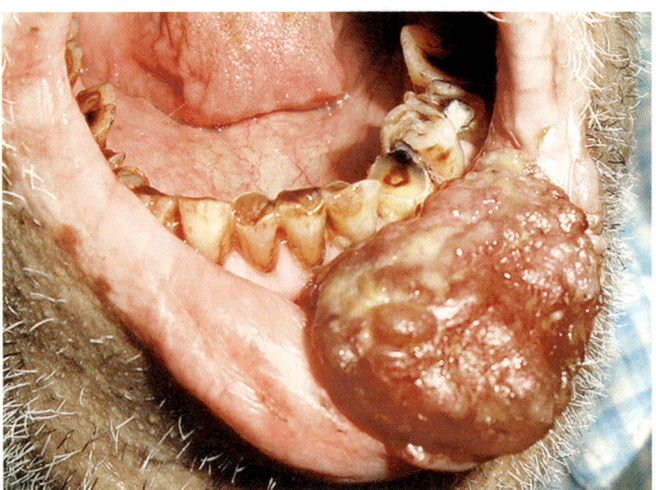

Fig. 11-10 Carcinoma lip—*proliferative lesion*.

Pigmentation—Blackish pigmentation can occur in lip or cheek in Addison's disease. *Bluish* pigment spots are seen in lower lip, cheek or palate in Peutz-Jegher's-syndrome along with multiple polyps in the small bowel, occasionally in colon inherited as autosomal dominant familial disease. Other causes of pigmentation are metal (Bismuth, lead, mercury): drugs (phenothiazines/antimalarials).

Acute ulcers like **aphthous ulcers** can occur in lip. *Aphthous ulcers* (*aphthous* - Greek—to set on fire; in USA called as '*Canker sore'*) are common in younger age group; self-limiting in 7–14 days; related to stress or nutritional deficiency; folate, vitamin B12 and iron deficiencies; are small, often multiple superficial painful erosive lesions with whitish floor with yellowish and hyperemic margin. In cold weather, lips may get *cracked* mainly in the midline **(Figs. 11-9A and B)**.

Carcinoma lip is common in lower lip. It is slow growing tumor initially may present as a proliferative/nodular or ulcerative lesion with whitish flaques/red areas/necrotic tissues over the surface **(Figs. 11-10 to 11-12)**. This lesion should be inspected in detail for margin (regular/irregular/well-defined/ill-defined); edge (everted/raised); floor; surrounding area; angles of the lip. Often there will be

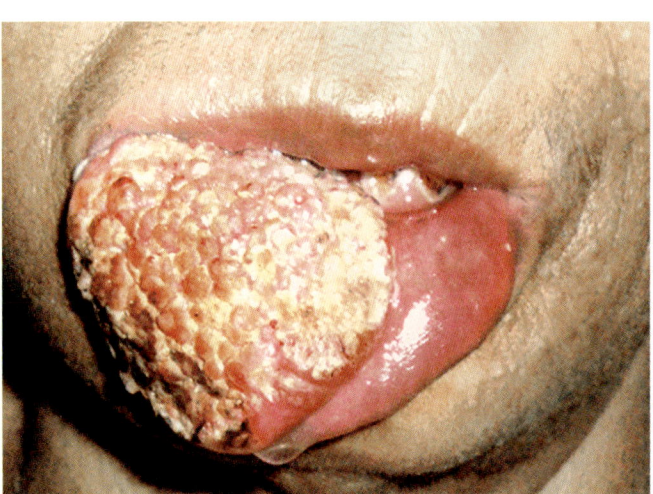

Fig. 11-11 Carcinoma lower lip.

edema surrounding the lesion. Entire lip may get enlarged. *Discharge* on the surface may be serous/serosanguinous/purulent.

Minor salivary gland tumor can occur in upper lip. It usually begins as a swelling in the upper lip; slowly progresses eventually forming an ulcer over the summit of the swelling.

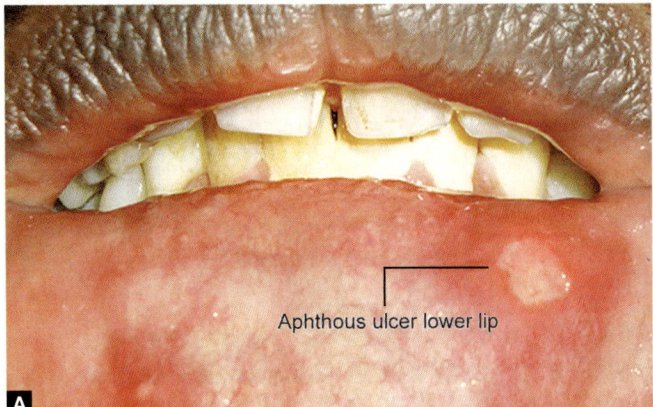

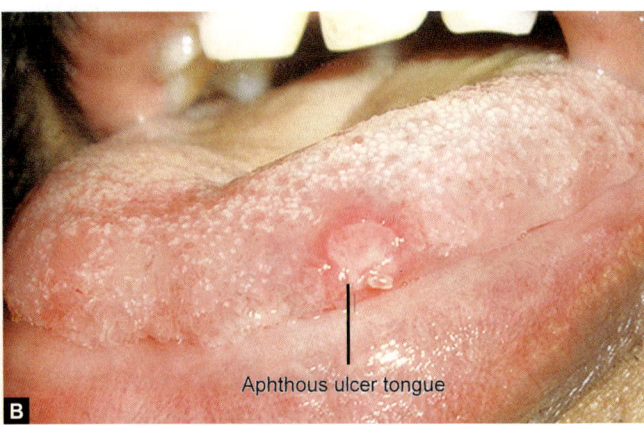

Figs. 11-9A and B *Aphthous ulcer* over the lip and tongue.

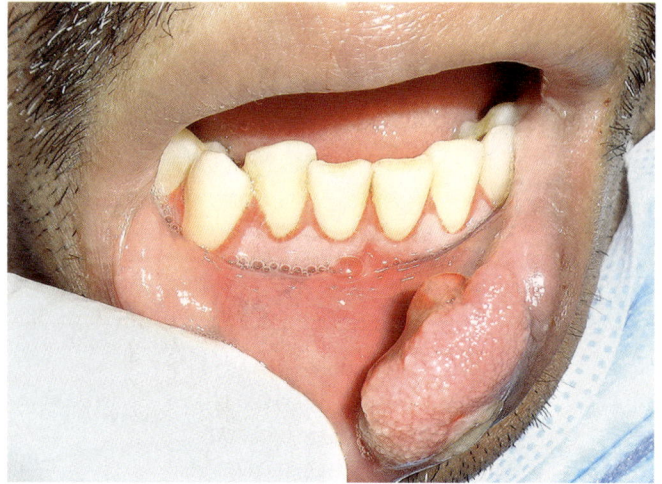

Fig. 11-12 Carcinoma lower lip presenting as swelling.

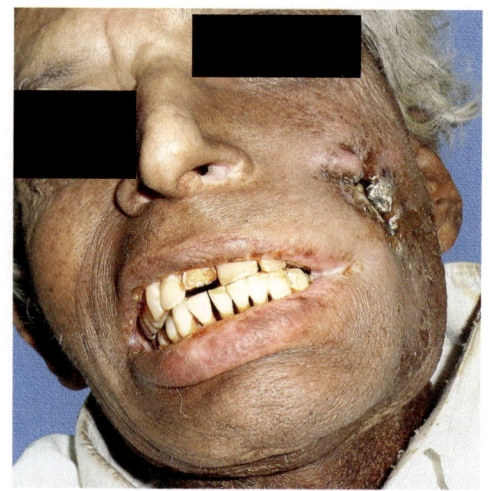

Fig. 11-15 Severe angular cheilitis with carcinoma cheek post-radiotherapy status with trismus.

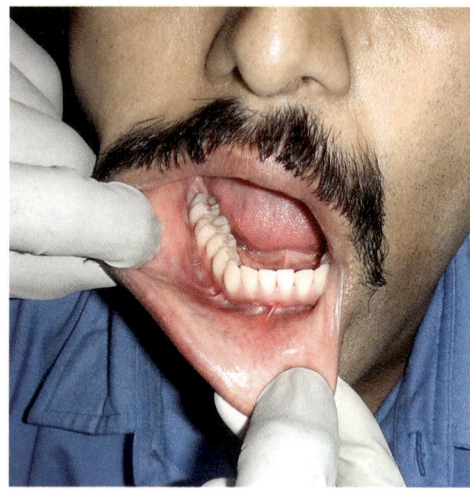

Fig. 11-13 Lip should be examined carefully with *adequate exposure*.

Primary syphilitic chancre in the lip (common in upper lip) is pink painless macule to begin with; becomes papule and later superficial ulcer with thick crust on the floor and often ulcer may be painful. These ulcers eventually heal with a permanent fine superficial scar.

Angular stomatitis (cheilosis), syphilitic ***rhagades*** (secondary syphilis), vitamin deficiency (riboflavin) ulcers, denture induced, cracks due to allergy to dentures/lipsticks can develop in the angles of the mouth (commissures). *Perleche* (French—to lick) is angular stomatitis seen in children as a simple infection which does not extend to mucus surface and heals without scarring. Stomatitis in syphilis extends to mucous membrane and heals with a scar.

Carbuncle of upper lip eventhough now rare; can be dangerous due to development of fatal cavernous sinus thrombosis due to spread of sepsis through dangerous zone. It may cause thrombophlebitis of ophthalmic plexus of veins leading into upper eyelid edema.

Both upper and lower lips should be examined carefully with adequate exposure for cheilitis, necrosis or any other lesions **(Figs. 11-13 to 11-15)**.

Actinic cheilitis, common in lower lip is due to exposure to sun light, present as recurring small blisters with epithelial exfoliation; recurrent lesions are premalignant. ***Keratoacanthoma*** (molluscum sebaceum) can occur in lower lip which is entirely benign but mimics carcinoma.

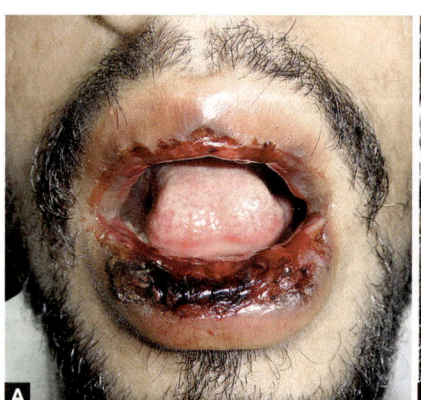 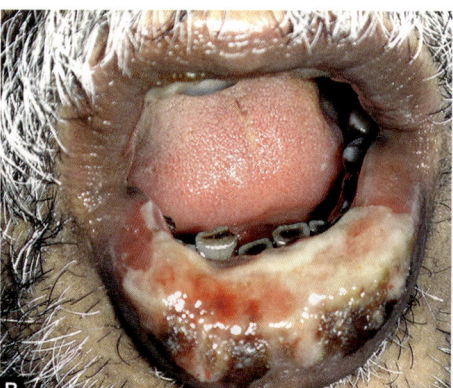 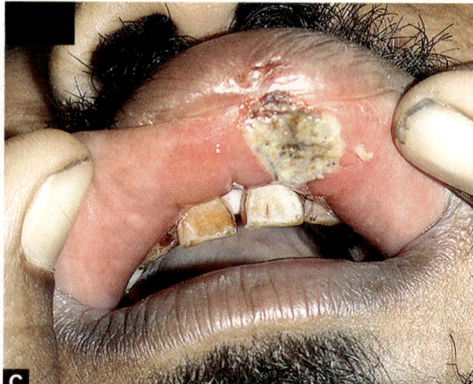

Figs. 11-14A to C *Different inflammatory lip lesions*—(A) Cheilitis, (B) Extensive necrosis and (C) Localized sloughing of the lip.

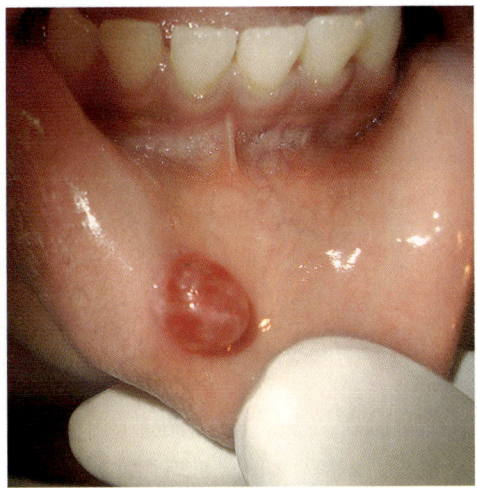

Fig. 11-16 *Mucus cyst* of lower lip.

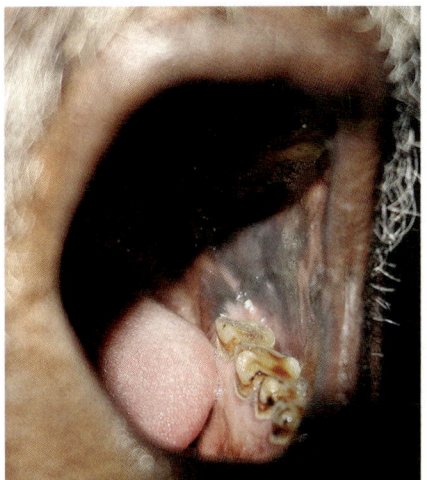

Fig. 11-18 *Pigmentation of cheek.*

Retention mucus cyst is common in lower lip which is blue, well-localized; smooth (fluctuant and transilluminating) (**Fig. 11-16**).

Inspection of the Cheek

It is large fleshy flap one on each side covering the vestibule. It contains skin, superficial fascia with facial muscles, parotid duct, mucus glands, buccinator with buccopharyngeal fascia, submucosa and mucous membrane. Buccal pad of fat lies on the buccinator partly deep and partly in front of masseter.

It is better to use a spatula to inspect the buccal mucosa. One should look for pigmented patches (Addison's diseases), pigmented swelling (hemangiomas), aphthous ulcer (opposite 1st molar tooth is the commonest site), leukoplakia, mucus cyst, papilloma, carcinoma (ulcerative lesion with everted edge).

Cheek is inspected for leukoplakia, mucus cyst, swellings, papilloma, and carcinoma (**Fig. 11-17**). Pigmentation similar to lips can also develop in cheeks. **Leukoplakia** is whitish patch in the mucosa of the oral cavity that cannot be characterized clinically or pathologically to any other disease (**Figs. 11-18 and 11-19**). It is a premalignant disease. It is common in smokers and who chew pan (20%). It has got 4% chances of turning into malignancy.

Erythroplakia, submucosal fibrosis are other conditions to be looked for in cheek.

Often **severe mucositis** can occur in cheek in diabetics and immunosuppressed patients (**Fig. 11-20**).

Carcinoma cheek needs special mention. Cheek is the common site for carcinoma in oral cavity (**Fig. 11-21**). It can be either ulcerative or proliferative lesion. Margin, size, shape, edge, floor of the lesion and surrounding area should be inspected. Once carcinoma infiltrates deep into the pterygoid muscle, ***trismus*** develops.

Mucus cyst often develops on the inner aspect of lower lips and buccal mucus membrane of cheek at the level of bite of teeth.

Trismus is inability to open the mouth adequately. Trismus is decreased inter-incisor distance between upper and lower

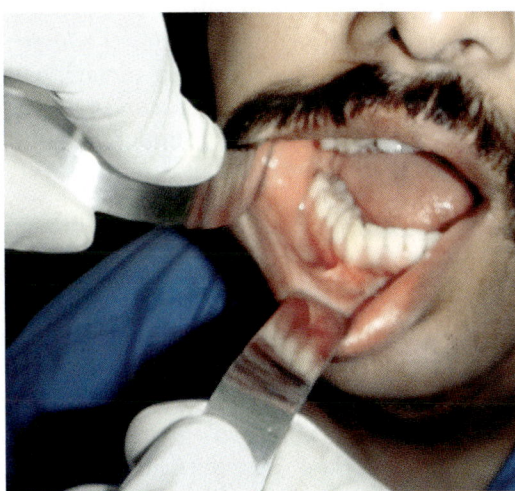

Fig. 11-17 Cheek inspected using *a spatula/depressor*.

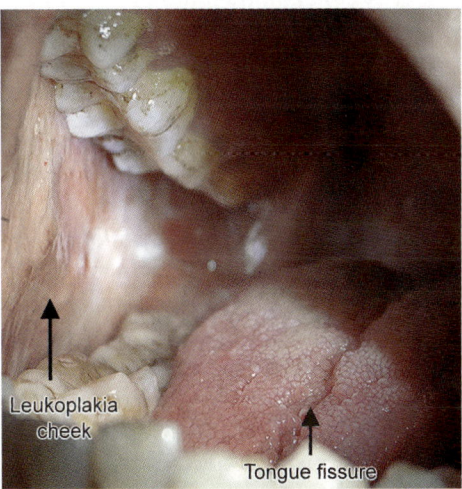

Fig. 11-19 *Leukoplakia right cheek.* Note also fissure in the tongue. Both are premalignant lesions of the tongue.

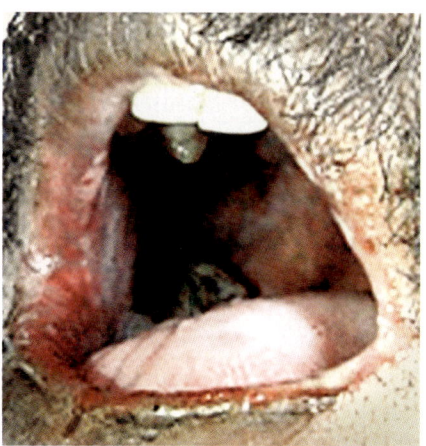

Fig. 11-20 *Severe mucositis* mainly in cheek.

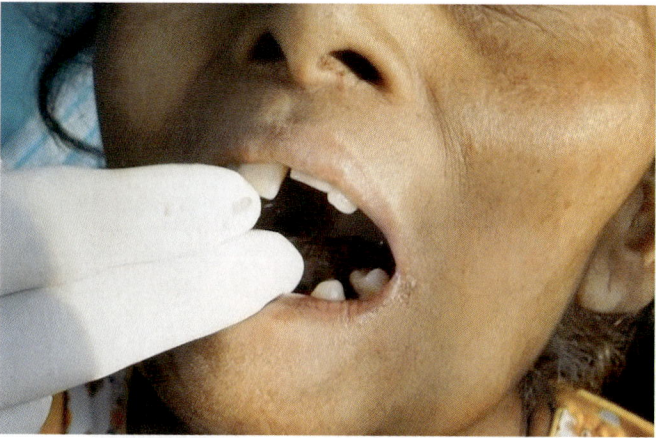

Fig. 11-22 Carcinoma cheek presenting with trismus.

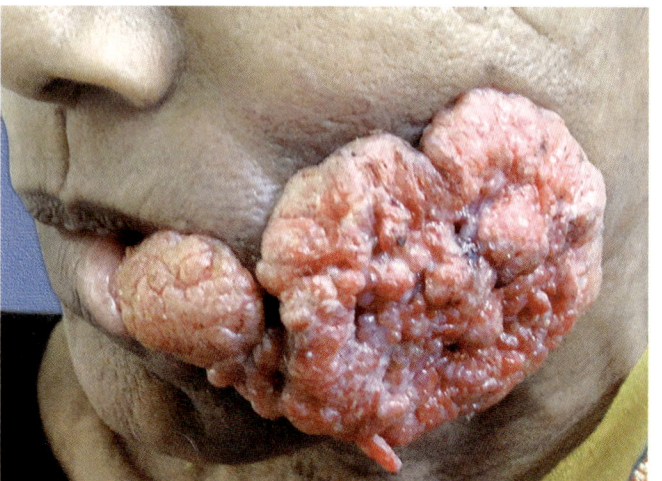

Fig. 11-21 *Carcinoma of lip and cheek.*

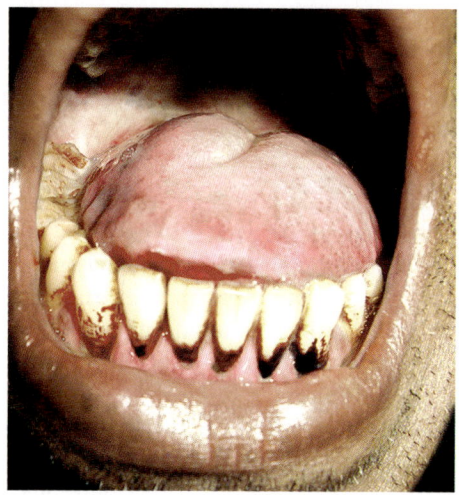

Fig. 11-23 Oral cavity inspection always includes *inspection of dentition properly.*

jaws. **Grading of trismus**: Interincisor distance more than 3.5 cm is—normal. Grade I is between 3.0–3.5 cm. Grade II is between 2.0–3 cm. Grade III is less than 2 cm. **Trismus in carcinoma** is due to involvement of the pterygoids and soft tissues. It is checked by placing fingers (of patient) perpendicularly between opened jaws **(Fig. 11-22).**

Inspection of Teeth and Gums

Artificial dentures are to be removed. Teeth and gums are examined by everting the lips **(Fig. 11-23).** Inspection is further aided by dental mirror and spatula.

Teeth should be counted. Primary dentition is 20 in children. Secondary permanent dentition is 32 in adult. 2 incisors; 1 canine; 2 premolars; 3 molars (2123). Third molar tooth (total four) are last to erupt on each sides at late teenage. One or more tooth may be absent; changed spacing; deformities are common. Teeth may be green in infants with jaundice; tetracycline given in early childhood may stain the teeth. Excess fluorides in drinking water may cause brown or black pits in the teeth. Yellowish brown staining is seen in teeth of chronic heavy smoker. Transverse ridge with curved notching is seen in rickets. *Tartar* (precipitated calcium in saliva) deposition occurs on lingual sides of lower incisors due to constant exposure to calcium-rich saliva from submandibular salivary gland. Tartar may precipitate pyorrhea alveolaris.

Tooth which is prevented from erupting by other teeth is called as *impacted tooth*. Mandibular 3rd molar is commonly impacted tooth (*wisdom tooth*). *Incompletely erupted mandibular 3rd molar commonly suppurates and can be dangerous, and is common cause of trismus. Dead tooth* is less white or bluish gray and insensitive to ice placed over it. *Stigma of congenital syphilis*—Hutchinson's teeth, only secondary dentitions are affected; common in upper central incisor; small notched incisor, which is broader towards gums is typical. *Screwdriver tooth* is also seen in congenital syphilis. *Moon's molar* is dome shaped first molar.

Gingivae *or gums* are mucous membrane covering the alveolar process of the jaws. It is pink in color in healthy person. It is spotted with brown melanin pigment in dark skin people and people from Mediterranean region. It is pigmented in smokers

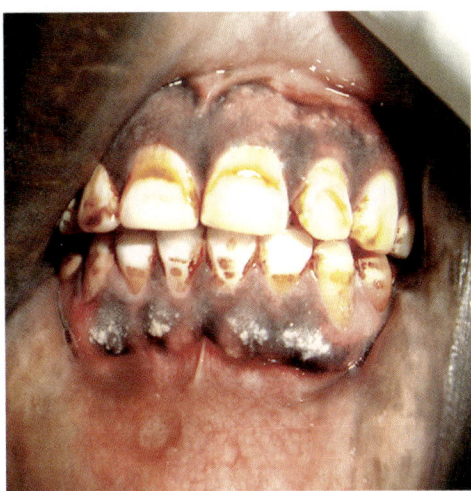

Fig. 11-24 *Gingivitis* with pigmentation and ulcer.

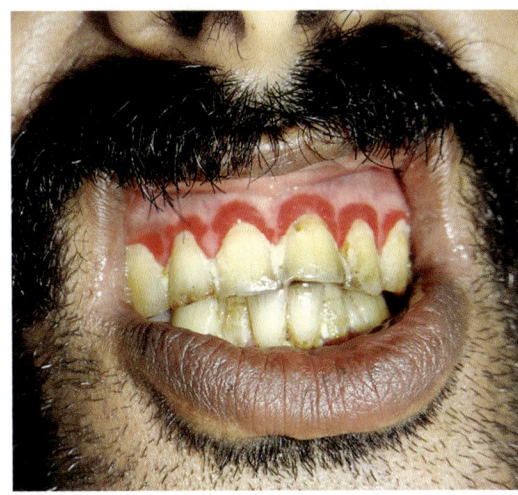

Fig. 11-25 Gums should be inspected properly for *swelling (epulis), color, bleeding.*

and pan chewers. Gingival margin is occlusal border at which gingiva meets teeth. *Free gingiva* is gingival part encircling the tooth forming a gingival sulcus. *Attached gingiva* is mucosa which is firmly bound to the underlying bone. **Alveolar mucosa** is movable vascular mucosa and less attached to bone. Lips should be everted properly to inspect the gums. Proper light is needed. Gums recede as age advances **(Fig. 11-24)**.

Vincent's gingivitis/stomatitis (Trench mouth) is an inflammatory condition with ulcer and *pseudomembrane* in the gums and adjoining mucous membrane. It is due to **Borrelia vincentii** and fusiformis bacteria. In carcrum oris purple red lesion may be evident in gums, commonly over the molar or premolar region, and associated with foul smell. *Cancrum oris (Noma)* is an infective gangrene, rapidly progressing into the bone and soft tissues in cheek with destruction *(Phagaedena)*. It is common in children after measles, gastroenteritis, typhoid, and bronchopneumonia.

Swollen gum is seen in dental abscess. Localized red swelling in the gums is called as *epulis* which can be pedunculated/sessile **(Fig. 11-25)**. *Blue line* in gums is observed in those who work in lead industries. They are better observed using magnifying lens. Similarly bismuth or mercury lines may also be seen.

Swollen, livid, spongy, tender bleeding gums with loose teeth are seen *in scurvy*. *Generalized hyperplastic progressive gingivitis* where the gums are hypertrophied and teeth are buried, is often seen in children on antiepileptic drugs. *Hyperplastic gums* are also seen in children with acute leukemia due to immature granulocytes and secondary infection. Here gums bleed on touch and there may be fever. Localized hyperplasia is seen in ill-fitting dentures **(Figs. 11-26 and 11-27)**.

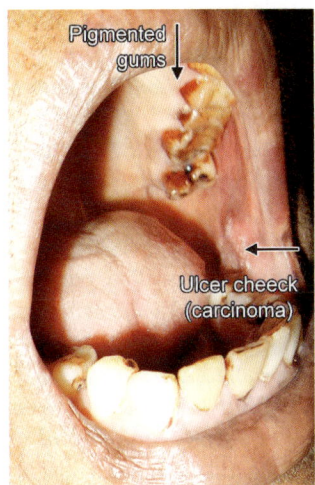

Fig. 11-26 Pigmentation of the gums; teeth and gums should be inspected properly.

Inspection of the Tongue

Tongue is a muscular, glandular, vascular flat organ. Anterior 2/3rd is termed as body; posterior 1/3rd is base/root. Superior surface is **dorsum of the tongue**. It is an essential organ of taste. Tongue is important in speech, mastication and swallowing. *Filiform papillae* are located in anterior 2/3rd of the dorsum of tongue and are numerous, fine, hair-like. *Fungiform papillae*

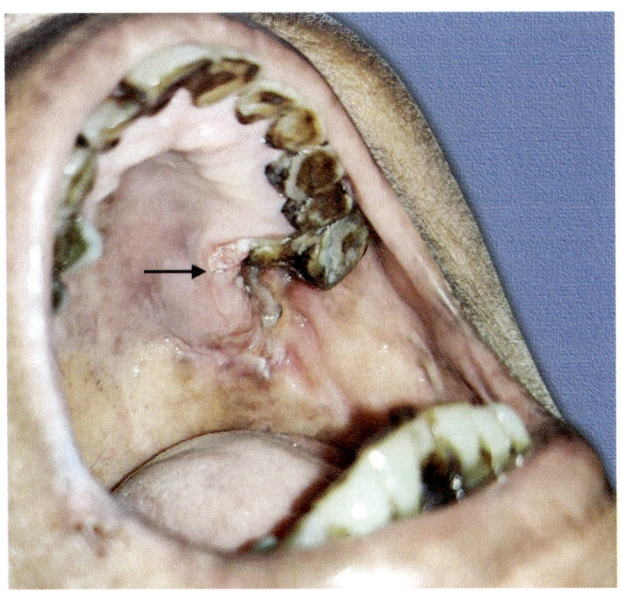

Fig. 11-27 Carcinoma alveolus—typical look. Careful examination of alveolus is essential.

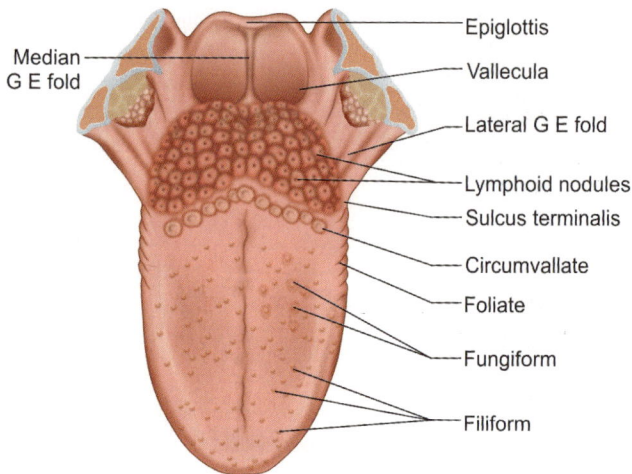

Fig. 11-28 *Anatomy of tongue.*

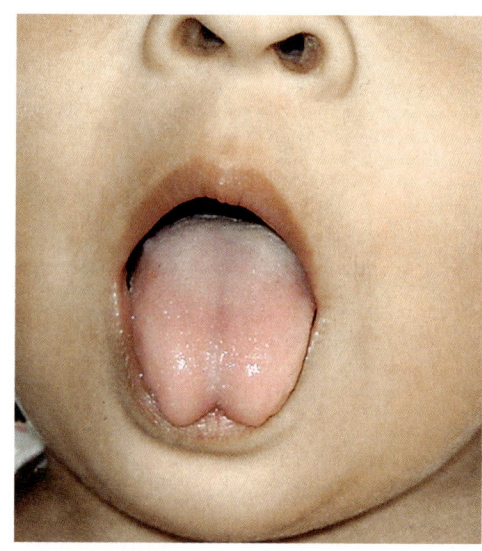

Fig. 11-29 *Tongue tie:* Typical look (*Courtesy:* Dr Sathish, MCh, Plastic Surgeon, Mangaluru, Karnataka).

are mushroom shaped, deep red, larger, sparsely located near the tip of the tongue. Large, red, leaf-like *foliate papillae* are located in posterior third of tongue on lateral aspect which contains taste buds. *Circumvallate papillae* are 8–12 in number mushroom-shaped, arranged in large V-shaped row near posterior third of the dorsum tongue and contains plenty of taste buds. Small circular opening just posterior to this V row in the midline is called as *foramen caecum* which is the remnant of thyroglossal duct **(Fig. 11-28)**. Shallow groove just behind the circumvallate papilla on either sides of the foramen caecum is called as **terminal sulcus**. Numerous mucin glands and lymph follicles in the posterior third of the dorsum of tongue is called as **lingual tonsil**. *Posterior third of the tongue is difficult to inspect;* it needs headlight, and spatula. It is better felt than seen. *Ventral surface* is smooth, has a median fold, *frenulum linguae* and deep lingual veins on either side. *Lingual frenulum* is attached about 10–15 mm below the mandibular central incisor tooth. **Tongue tie** is due to congenital short frenulum which is attached 3–4 mm below the central incisor and is better seen when tip of the tongue is rolled upwards. Here the child may not be able to protrude the tongue out and there may be speech difficulties. Tongue is examined properly often by wrapping it with a damp gauze and pulling it out. Its anterior surface, dorsum, ventral surface, margins should be inspected **(Figs. 11-29 and 11-30)**.

Following features of tongue to be noted on inspection:

a. Size: Macroglossia (*Megaloglossia/pachyglossia*) is a disorder in which the tongue is larger than normal. Macroglossia is usually caused by an increase in the amount (volume) of tissue on the tongue, rather than by a growth, such as a tumor. It is often seen in hemangioma, lymphangioma, muscular macroglossia (in cretins), acromegaly, **Beckwith Wiedemann syndrome** (hypoglycemia, abdominal wall defects, Wilm's tumor, macroglossia, adrenal tumor), **Down's syndrome (Fig. 11-31)**, mucopolysaccharidoses, primary amyloidosis, occasionally plexiform neurofibromatosis. Often it causes functional and cosmetic problems.

b. Color: Pale in anemia, *white* in **chronic superficial glossitis**/leukoplakic patches, **black hairy tongue** (filiform

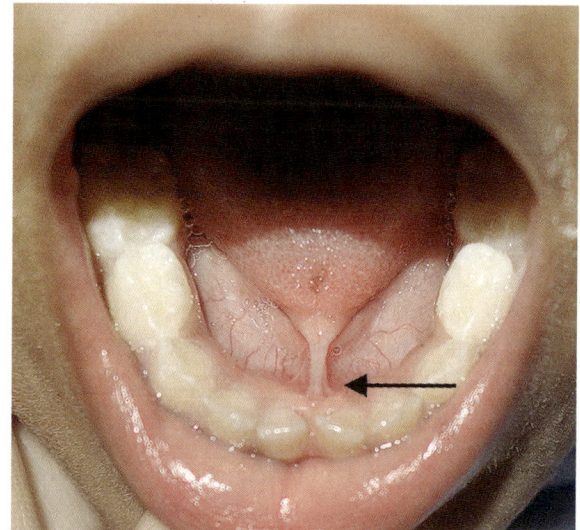

Fig. 11-30 Tongue tie—*typical look on ventral aspect.*

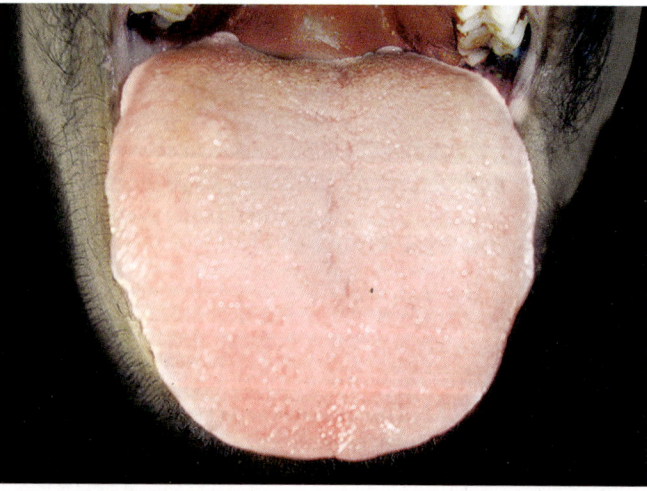

Fig. 11-31 *Macroglossia in a Down's syndrome patient.*

papillary hypertrophy on the back of the dorsum of the tongue with elongated papillae having black particles on the surface with a furry look) in *Aspergillus niger* fungus infection due to mucous membrane hyperkeratosis (now it is commonly seen in HIV infection), *bluish in* venous hemangioma. **Median rhomboid glossitis** is a rhomboid mass in the midline posteriorly in front of the foramen cecum of tongue; probably due to persistent tuberculum impar; extends deep into the tongue muscles; with well-defined margin; without any papillae; with slight induration on it mimicking carcinoma. **Glossitis migrans/ geographical tongue** can be idiopathic in children or secondary to major surgery or peritonitis causing bright red color discoloration of tongue with yellowish white margin. Its location and pattern alters in 2 days. If it is of idiopathic origin and subsides in 7 days; but in secondary type it subsides only when patient recovers from the primary disease.

Leukoplakia in tongue is typical (*leukoplakia* (Greek— white plate). Early lesion is thin, crinkled and pearly. Late lesions are large, creamy white, thick often desquamated with beefy red color. Sir Henry Butlin said 'tongue looks as though it had been covered with white paint that had hardened, dried and cracked'. Early cases are better inspected by pressing a glass slide on the surface.

Lichen planus in tongue are delicate bluish white silver nitrate-like color; often difficult to differentiate from carcinoma; but there are also lesions over the front of wrists and shin.

Excessive furring is seen in stomatitis, tonsillitis, sinusitis, pneumonia; in dehydration, in pyrexia, in tobacco abuse. Tongue may be dry and brown here. **Dry tongue** is seen in dehydration, intestinal obstruction and renal failure. It is due to diminished salivary mucus gland secretions.

Strawberry/raspberry tongue occurs in scarlet fever due to hypertrophy of fungiform papillae; **curdy white** lesions are seen as **mucosal thrush in Candida albicans** (moniliasis) infection **(Fig. 11-32)**; central cyanosis causes **blue tongue**; *bald tongue* may be red and painful which is due to atrophy of papillae and is seen in pernicious and severe iron deficiency

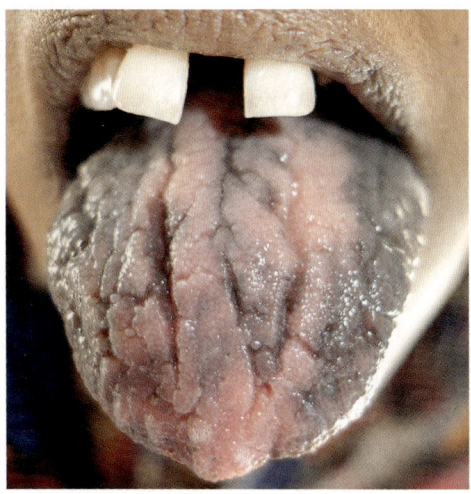

Fig. 11-33 *Fissure tongue* with blackish pigmentation. Congenital fissures of the tongue are transverse; syphilitic fissures are longitudinal; malignant fissure is rare but can occur and is indurated on palpation; it is of recent onset with short duration.

anemia, deficiencies of folic acid and B_{12}—*beefy red tongue* of pellagra, *magenta tongue* of riboflavin deficiency. Painful, red, smooth tongue is seen in **Plummer Vinson (Patterson Kelly)** syndrome when there is also postcricoid web and koilonychia. Consumption of iron causes black tongue; and of black berries and cherries causes purple tongue.

c. Fissure/cracks: Congenital fissure is ***transverse***. It appears at the age of 3 years and persists later for life. Syphilitic fissure is **longitudinal with denuded** intervening epithelium **(Fig. 11-33)**. Carcinoma can present as a fissure **(Figs. 11-34 and 11-35)**.

d. Texture: Whether dry (in dehydration)/moist.

e. Ulcer: Ulcer in tongue when present, its size, location, margin, edge, extension and surrounding area should be inspected. Aphthous/dental ulcers are common on the *lateral margin*. Tuberculous ulcer is common in *tip* of the tongue. Syphilitic gummatous ulcer is common on *dorsum of tongue*. Carcinoma is common in *lateral margin* **(Fig. 11-36)**.

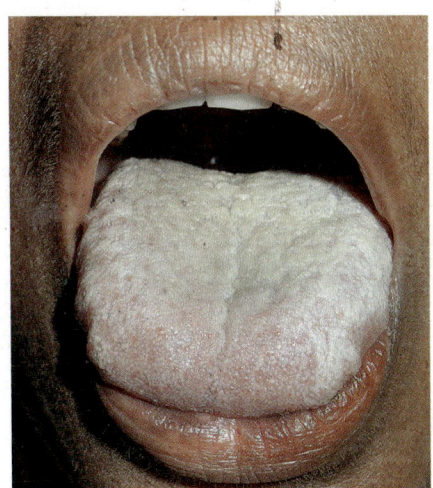

Fig. 11-32 Candida infection of the tongue; *typical curdy white look*; it is common in HIV patients.

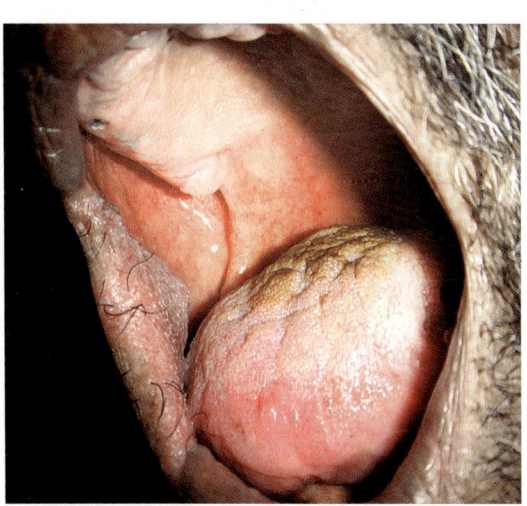

Fig. 11-34 Tongue fissure. It *could be a presentation of carcinoma*.

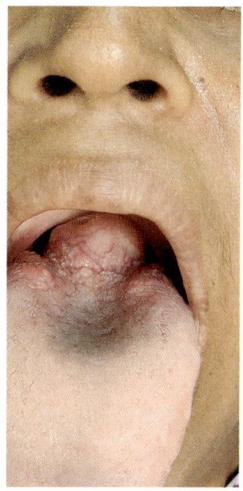

Fig. 11-35 Lingual thyroid—from posterior part of the tongue. (*Courtesy*: Dr Mohan, Consultant Surgeon, District Hospital, Chitradurga, Karnataka)..

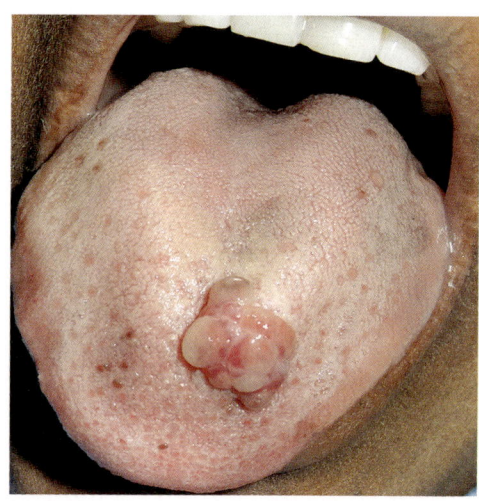

Fig. 11-37 *Papilloma tongue*. It is premalignant condition. It is firm, well-localized swelling which may bleed on touch. It needs excision.

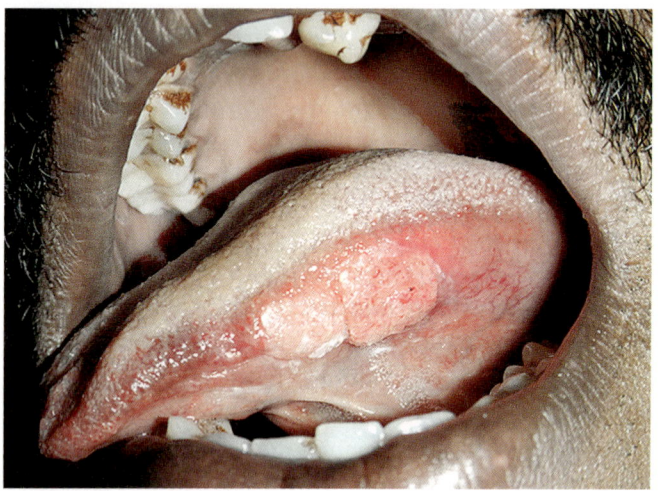

Fig. 11-36 Carcinoma tongue. It is common *on the lateral margin*.

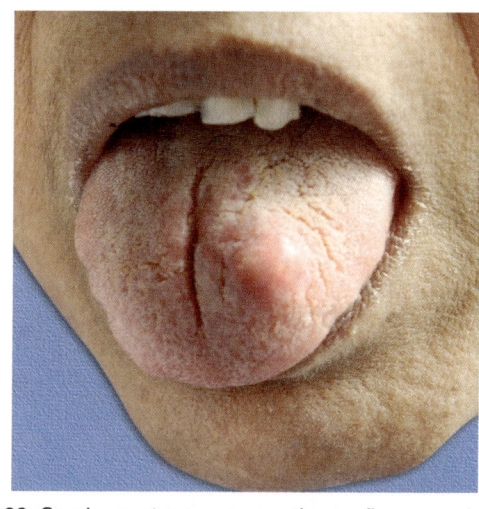

Fig. 11-38 Carcinoma tongue presenting as fissure and swelling; induration will be typical while palpating.

f. Swelling: **Papilloma (Fig. 11-37)**, neurofibroma can occur in the tongue. Size, shape, surface, margin should be mentioned. Lingual thyroid may be the only thyroid existing in the region of foramen *caecum* as a smooth swelling **(Figs. 11-38 and 11-39)**. *Vascular malformations* in the tongue presenting as pigmented, bluish swelling is not common **(Fig. 11-40)**.

g. Movements of the tongue: Inability to protrude the tongue is called as *ankyloglossia* **(Fig. 11-41)**. It is seen in carcinoma tongue infiltrating the floor of the mouth. Tongue may deviate towards same side (with wasting of tongue muscle on the same side) if there is **hypoglossal nerve palsy** due to nodal infiltration or carcinoma tongue infiltrating the nerve **(Fig. 11-42)**. Inability to protrude the tongue out is also seen in tongue-tie. *Tongue tremor* is checked with tongue kept inside the oral cavity (in protruded tongue fasciculation may mimic the tremor).

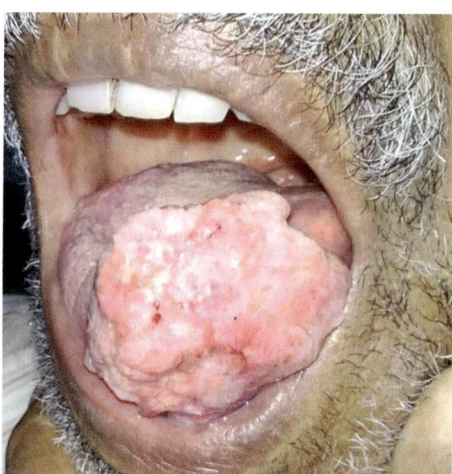

Fig. 11-39 Carcinoma tongue with everted proliferative lesion (swelling) extending into tip of the tongue and crossing the midline.

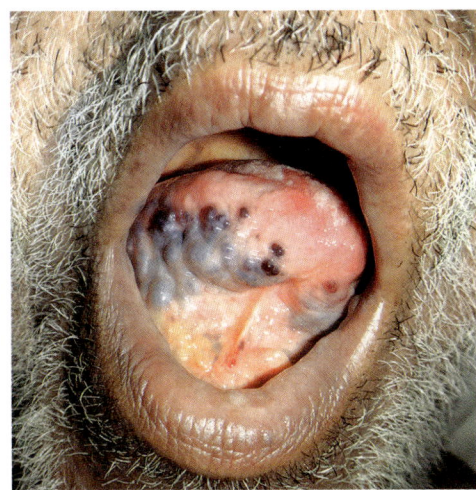

Fig. 11-40 *Vascular malformation* of the tongue on the ventral surface; it is acquired one in this patient.

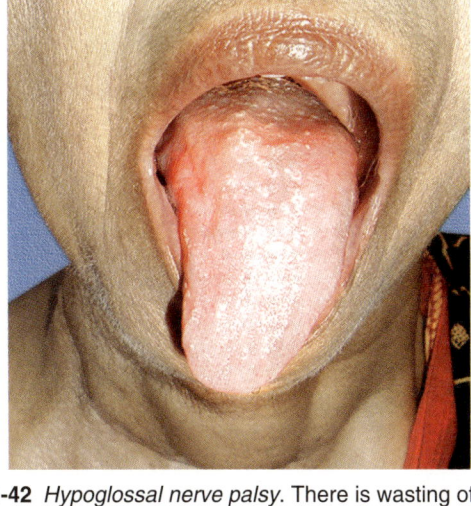

Fig. 11-42 *Hypoglossal nerve palsy.* There is wasting of tongue muscle on same side with tongue deviating towards same side.

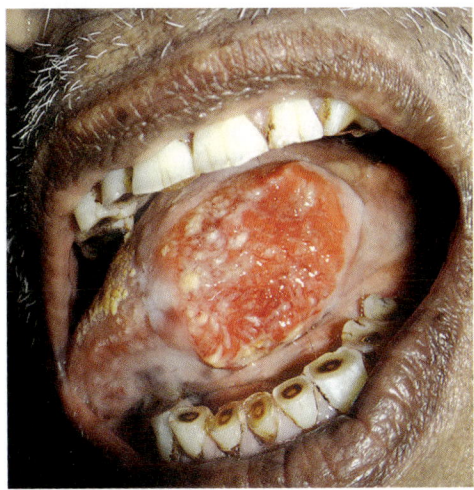

Fig. 11-41 Carcinoma of tongue causing *ankyloglossia* due to involvement of genioglossus muscle.

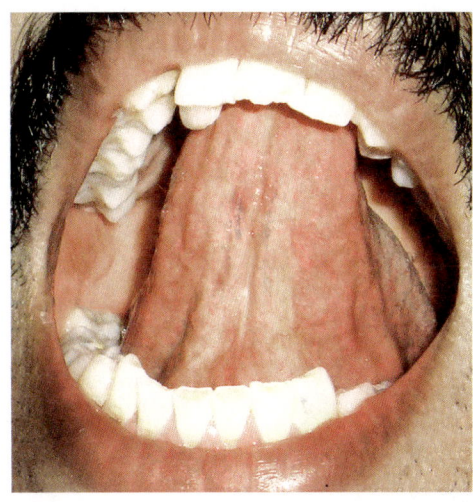

Fig. 11-43 *Inspection of the floor of the mouth.* Tip of the tongue should be kept upwards to touch the palate to inspect the floor of the mouth.

Inspection of the Floor of the Mouth

It is U-shaped area bounded by lower gum and oral tongue. It ends posteriorly at the insertion of anterior tonsillar pillar into the tongue. Sublingual papilla is present on each side of the frenulum; on summit of which is the opening of the duct (Wharton's) of submandibular salivary gland. Laterally and behind this papilla, sublingual fold is present which overlies the sublingual gland. Genioglossus and geniohyoid muscles are deeper to it. On either side mylohyoid muscles forms the muscular part of the floor of the mouth. It arises from mylohyoid ridge of the mandible extending up to the 3rd molar tooth. Submandibular salivary gland rests on the external surface of mylohyoid muscle; only small deeper part extends into the internal surface. Submandibular salivary duct runs about 5 cm between sublingual gland and genioglossus to end in papilla. Lingual and hypoglossal nerves are closely related to gland and duct. Alveolingual sulcus is valley-shaped space between tongue and mandibular alveolar bone. Tip of the tongue should be kept upwards to touch the palate to inspect the floor of the mouth **(Fig. 11-43)**.

Swelling or ulcer in floor of the mouth should be inspected for its extent, size, shape, margin, edge. Extent from the gum margin, whether crossing midline or not are important especially in carcinomatous ulcer. Unilateral bluish localized swelling may be ranula. **Ranula** extending into the submandibular region across mylohyoid is called as *plunging ranula*. **Sublingual dermoid** is in the floor of the mouth *midline* often extends into submental region externally **(Figs. 11-44A and B)**.

Inspection of the Palate

Roof of the mouth is formed by hard palate and soft palate. **Hard palate** is firm anterior part of the roof of the mouth ending opposite 3rd molars anterior to fovea palatine. **Soft palate** is mobile posterior part of the roof of the mouth. Junction between hard and soft palate is called as *vibrating line*. Small

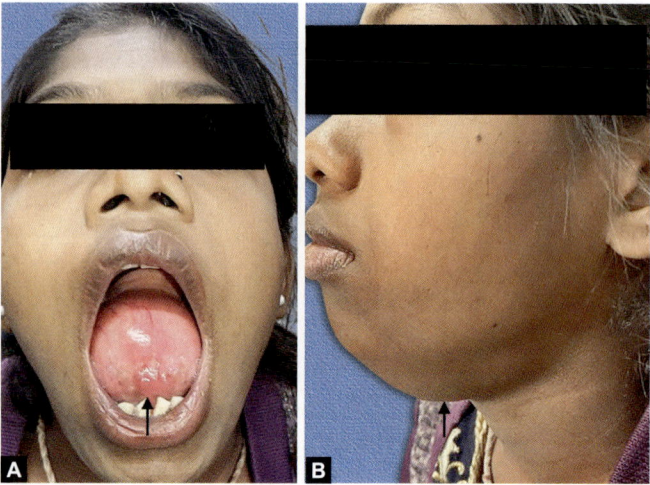

Figs. 11-44A and B Sublingual dermoid presents usually as midline swelling in the floor of the mouth often it may be visible in front of the neck—midline in submental triangle (*Courtesy*: Dr Achaleshwar Dayal, Professor, Department of Surgery, Itarsi, Madhya Pradesh).

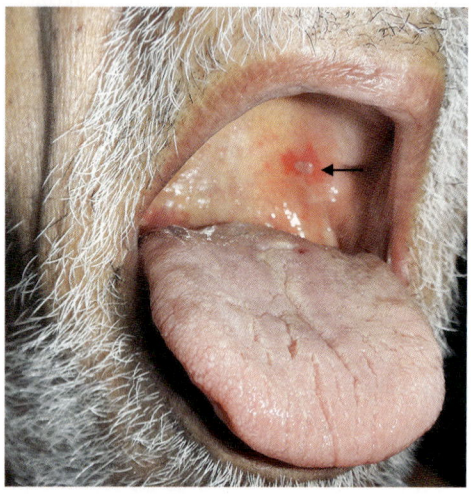

Fig. 11-45 Palate should be examined properly; it could be SCC or minor salivary gland tumor.

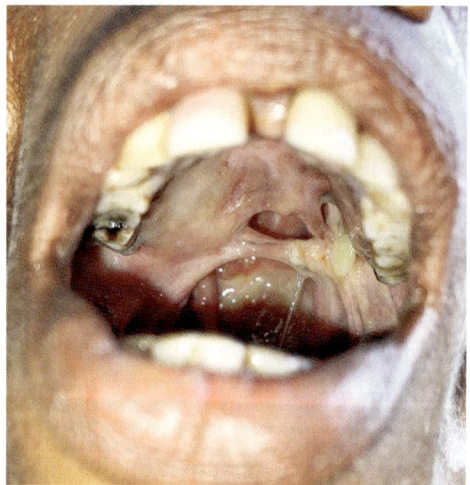

Fig. 11-46 Perforated palate due to syphilitic gumma. (*Courtesy*: Dr Rajat Chowdhary, MS).

rounded elevation of tissue on the midline behind the central incisors is called as **nasopalatine papilla** which is over incisive foramen through which nasopalatine nerve traverses to supply anterior hard palate. Slightly elevated central line is called as **palatine raphe**. Here mucosa is firmly adherent to underneath periosteum without any fat and so it is harder area of hard palate. Sides of hard palate contain fat and minor salivary glands (there are around 350 minor salivary glands in posterior hard palate). Series of elevations in hard palate are called as **palatine rugae** useful for food positioning and aiding tongue to produce specific sounds. Hard palate is partition between nasal and oral cavity. Anterior 2/3rd formed by palatine process of maxillae; posterior 1/3rd by horizontal plates of palatine bones. Anterolateral margins continue with alveolar arches and gums. Posterior margin attaches to soft palate (**Figs. 11-45 to 11-47**).

Soft palate is redder than hard palate due to its vascularity. There is no bone in soft palate behind vibrating line. Soft palate vibrates or moves. It is mobile muscular fold. It has got anterior and posterior surfaces, superior and inferior margins. Uvula is small fleshy part projecting from center of the posterior margin of the soft palate. Pair of pits on either side of the center of the soft palate just behind the vibrating line is called as *fovea palatini* to which palatine mucus glands opens. Side of the uvula has got anterior and posterior folds. Anterior palatoglossal arch contains palatoglossus muscle which ends as anterior pillar of fauces (in front of tonsils). Posterior palatopharyngeal arch contains palatopharyngeus muscle which ends as posterior pillar of fauces (behind tonsils). Soft palate contains mucus glands and taste buds. Soft palate contains following muscles—tensor veli palati, levator veli palati, musculus uvulae, palatoglossus and palatopharyngeus. All muscles except tensor palati are supplied by pharyngeal plexus through cranial part of accessory nerve; tensor palati is supplied by the mandibular nerve. General sensory nerves are derived from middle and posterior palatine nerves which are branches of maxillary nerve and from glossopharyngeal nerve. Gustatory special sensations are carried through lesser

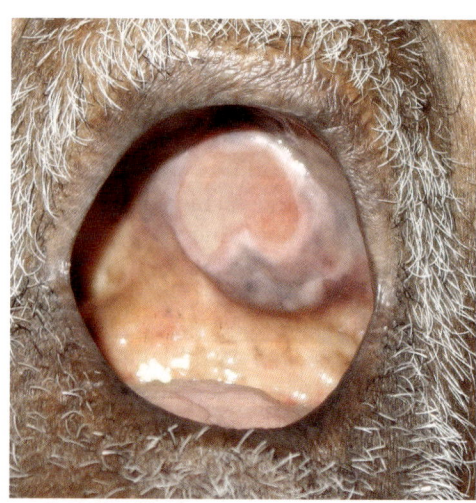

Fig. 11-47 *Carcinoma palate.*

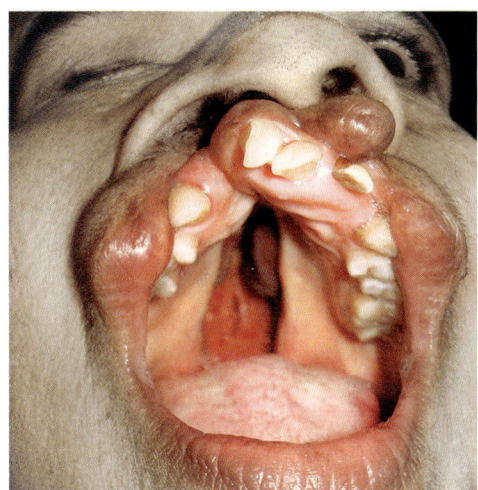

Fig. 11-48 *Cleft lip and palate* in an adult.

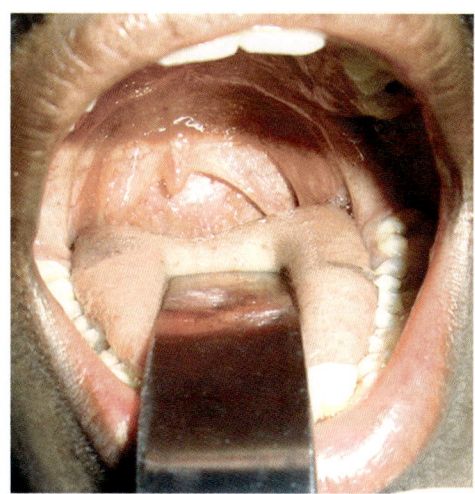

Fig. 11-50 Inspection of fauces is done *using tongue depressor*.

palatine nerve → greater petrosal nerve → geniculate ganglion of facial nerve → nucleus of solitary tract. Secretomotor fibers are derived from superior salivatory nucleus through greater palatine nerve and lesser palatine nerves. **Paralysis of the soft palate** *(vagus nerve lesions) causes nasal regurgitation of liquids, nasal twang in voice, flattening of palatal arch.*

Cleft palate is a congenital defect of uvula, soft palate or hard palate along with nasal septal defect or with cleft lip which should be looked for carefully **(Fig. 11-48)**. *Swelling* in the palate may be minor salivary gland tumor. Detailed inspection of such swelling should be done. *Ulcer* palate could be due to carcinoma/syphilis/tuberculous origin. Gummatous ulcer is painless with punched out edge and often with perforation. Carcinomatous ulcer is with everted edge whereas tuberculous is with undermined edge. It is also important to check *uvular movements* and sensations.

Inspection of Tonsils and Fauces

Inspection of tonsils and fauces should be done to look for ulcers/tubercles/growth/leukoplakia, etc. **(Figs. 11-49 and 11-50)**.

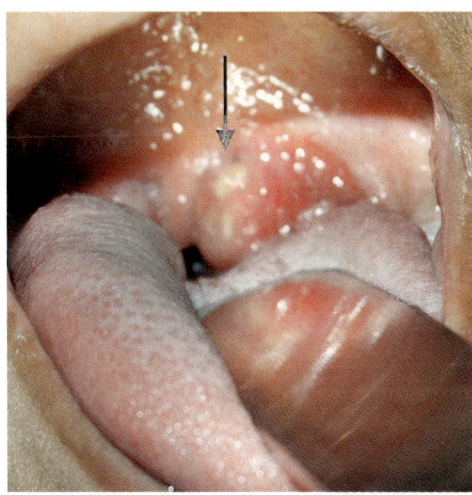

Fig. 11-49 *Carcinoma left tonsil on inspection.*

Note: Examination of the angle of the mouth with oral cavity should be done properly.

Palpation

Palpation of Lip

Both upper and lower lips should be examined. Usually carcinoma lip is nontender initially. Later it becomes stony hard in consistency. Indurated edge is typical. Extent of lesion should be assessed carefully; whether it crosses the midline, whether extends into cheek, angles of mouth are important in deciding the surgical intervention **(Figs. 11-51A and B)**. Lesion is held with fingers of one hand and with other hand, lip is held to check the mobility. Carcinoma is always fixed. Benign lesions like mucus cyst are mobile. Mucus cyst will be fluctuant and transilluminant. Hunterian chancre is rubbery hard in consistency.

Palpation of Cheek

Cheek should be palpated for any ulcer and swelling. Ulcer due to carcinoma will show induration of edge, base and surrounding area. Its extent should be checked. Posterior extent is important. If it extends beyond retromolar trigone, it means it is advanced. Involvement of soft tissues, mandible, and skin over cheek should be checked. **Retromolar trigone** is the anterior surface of the ascending ramus of the mandible. It is triangular in shape with the base being superior and apex lying inferior behind the third molar tooth. How much gap is present between growth and alveolar margin should be checked. Other part of the oral cavity should also be palpated.

Mandible is palpated using two fingers. Index finger of one hand is placed inside the mouth to feel over the lingual surface of the mandible. Finger of other hand is placed over outer surface of the mandible. Fingers are run along the surface of the mandible to feel for tenderness, irregularity, thickening or any fracture site (features of mandibular involvement by carcinoma)—**bidigital palpation of the mandible**. Mandible is involved by direct extension or through subperiosteal lymphatic plexus which are communicating with oral lymphatics **(Figs. 11-52 to 11-55)**.

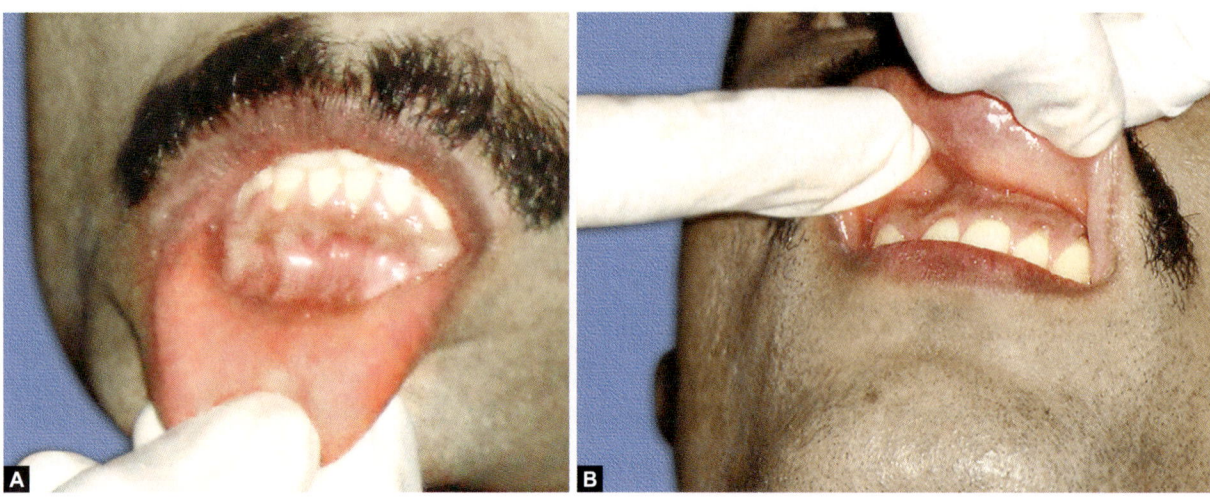

Figs. 11-51A and B *Examination of lip*—methods.

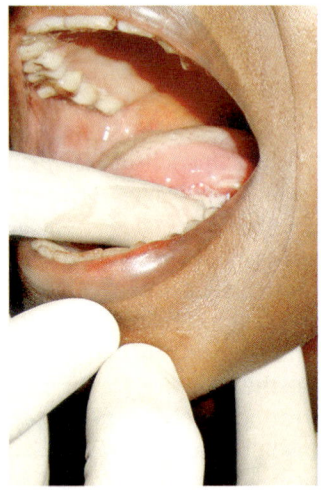

Fig. 11-52 Bidigital palpation of the mandible for tenderness, *thickening, irregularity and fracture site* should be done in all oral carcinoma—to assess the involvement.

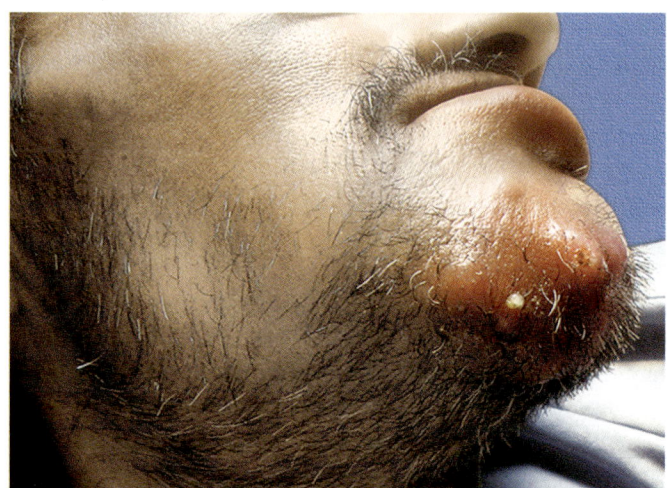

Fig. 11-53 Oral carcinoma *infiltrating through the mandible* extending externally.

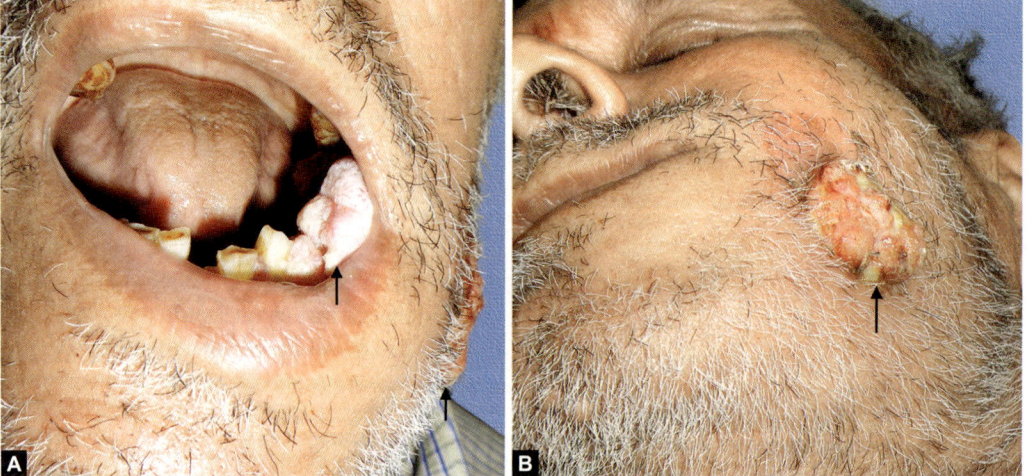

Figs. 11-54A and B Carcinoma buccal mucosa extending across soft tissues to skin presenting outside as proliferative cauliflower like lesion/swelling.

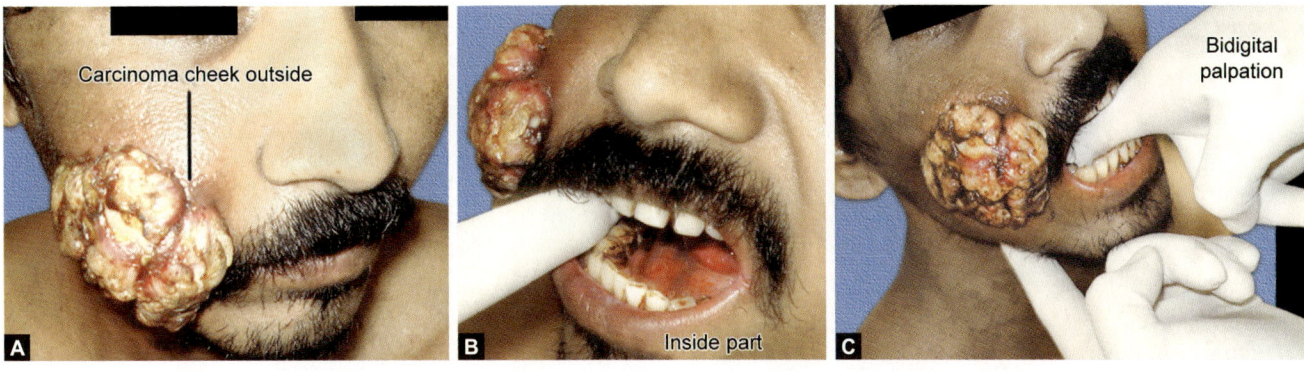

Figs. 11-55A to C Carcinoma of cheek involving skin and soft tissues—*locally advanced malignancy.*

Palpation of Gums and Teeth

Gums are examined by everting the lip fully. Posterior part of the gums is examined using spatula; head mirror is better for proper examination.

Bleeding from the gums on palpation is an important finding. It may be due to growth, leukemia, uremia, scurvy, epulis. When any lesion is present either swelling or ulcer its size, shape, extent, tenderness, induration, mobility should be checked.

Palpate the teeth to look for any loose tooth. Also palpation is done with a probe to find out erosion of enamel. In dental caries, involving the pulp a characteristic pain can be elicited using hot/cold water. Gums are palpated for tenderness. Gums are edematous and tender in pyorrhea alveolaris, Vincent's stomatitis, alveolar abscess where on pressure, pus may exude out (**Figs. 11-56 and 11-57**).

Palpation of Tongue

Tongue should be ***kept within the oral cavity*** while palpating as the protruded tongue feels harder due to contraction of muscles mimicking induration. Palpation for any sharp tooth is done in benign traumatic ulcer. Gummatous ulcer often may be indurated. Tuberculous ulcer is not indurated. It is painful, tender, often multiple. Palpation of tongue ulcers is very important to know the extent of induration/invation. Bleeding on palpation, extent of induration, whether lesion is crossing the midline, tongue movements, floor of the mouth in relation to the lesion should be checked. Entire length of lateral margins should be palpated carefully. Often cheek is retracted using a spatula to palpate the tongue. Recess between lateral base of the tongue and anterior pillar of the fauces is examined (**Figs. 11-58 to 11-64**).

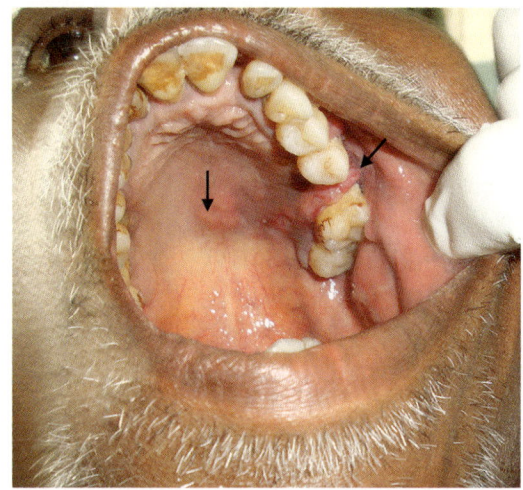

Fig. 11-57 Carcinoma alveolus (left sided) extending into the palate. Carcinoma alveolus is common in India due to tobacco (pan) usage; it is aggressive; bone should be clinically palpated for involvement and local spread; neck nodes should be examined.

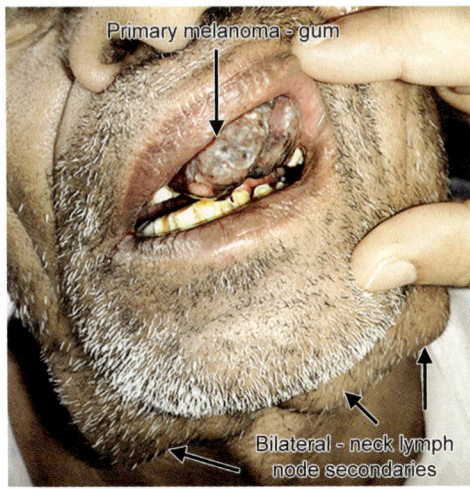

Fig. 11-56 *Pigmented lesion in upper gums*—melanoma gum with bilateral neck secondaries.

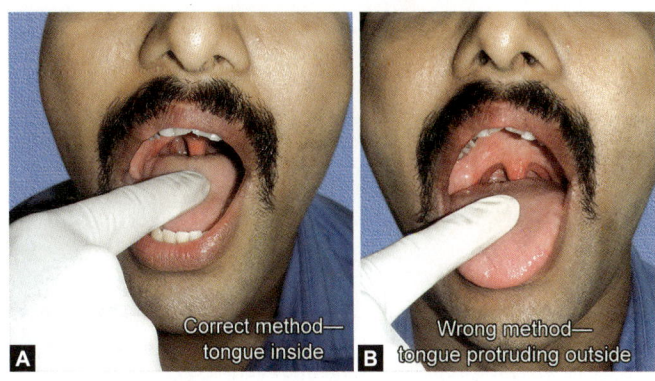

Figs. 11-58A and B *Tongue should be palpated with tongue laid within the oral cavity.* Otherwise induration is difficult to assess. Protruded tongue will be firm normally while palpation.

254 Section 1: Examination in General Surgery

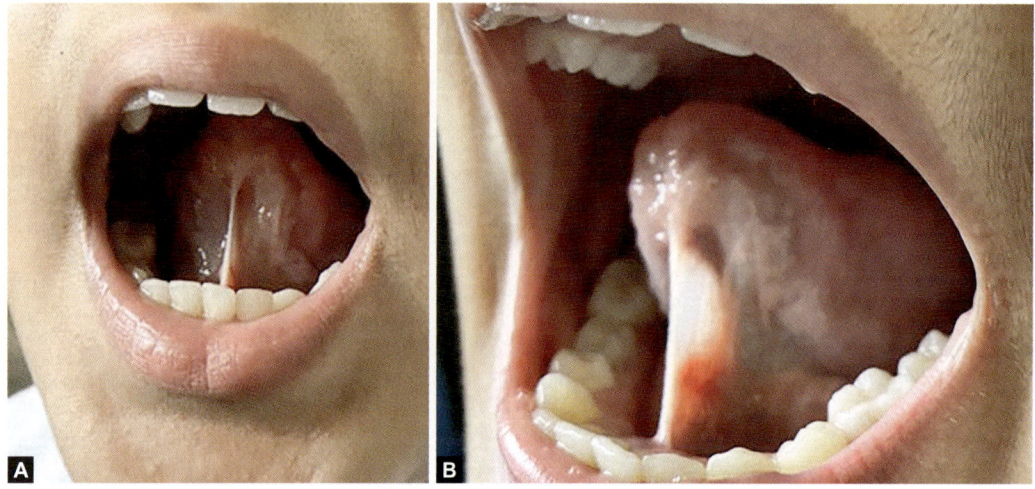

Figs. 11-59A and B Typical tongue tie. (*Courtesy*: Professor Shankar, Consultant Neurologist, Mangaluru, Karnataka).

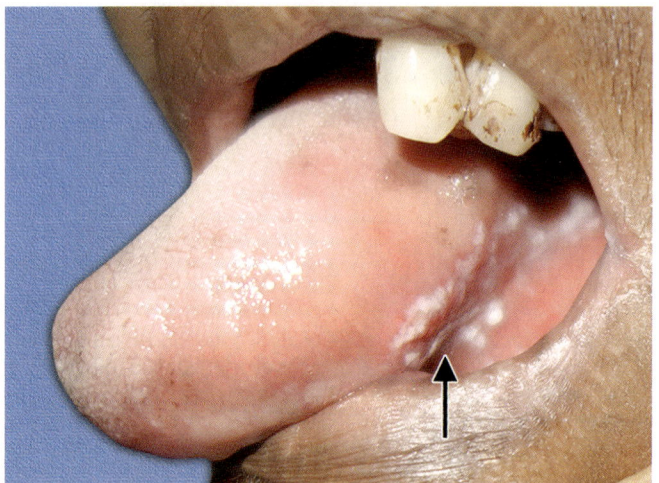

Fig. 11-60 *Leukoplakia* tongue.

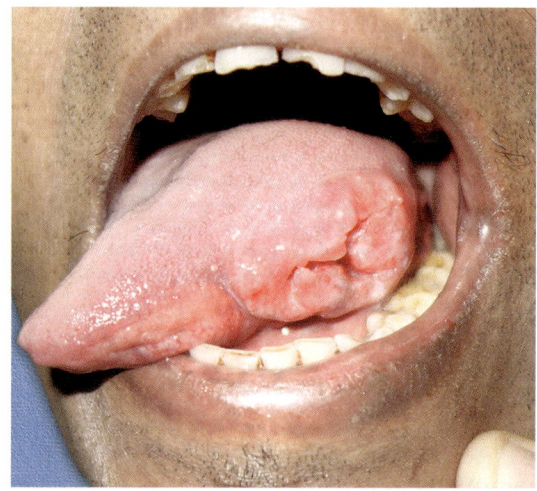

Fig. 11-62 *Carcinoma tongue*—ulcerative lesion in the lateral margin.

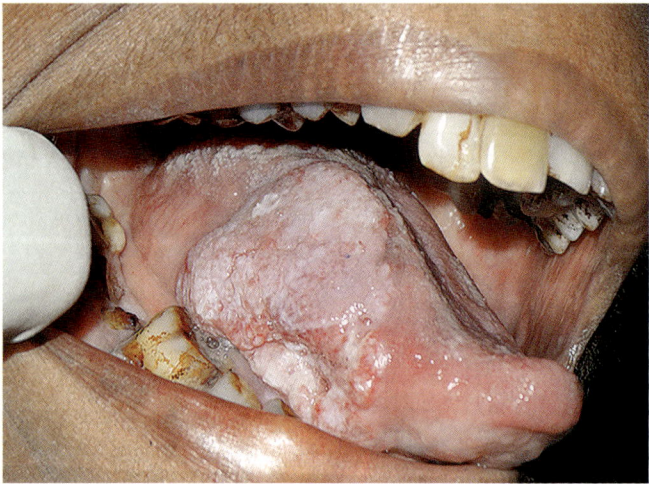

Fig. 11-61 Carcinoma tongue occurring on the lateral margin; *it is the commonest site (50% of cases).*

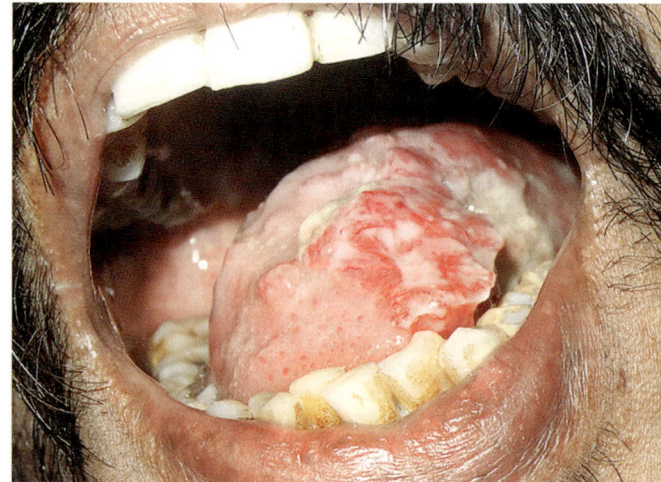

Fig. 11-63 Carcinoma tongue involving extensively and causing *ankyloglossia*; lesion extends towards the alveolus and floor of the mouth.

Chapter 11: Clinical Approach and Examination of Oral Cavity

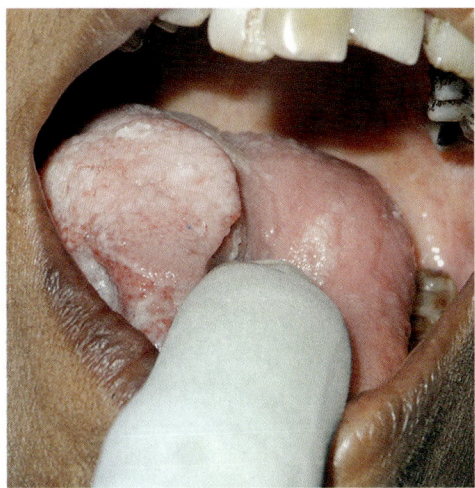

Fig. 11-64 Palpation of tongue in carcinoma for *induration, edge*. Tongue should be palpated with tongue inside.

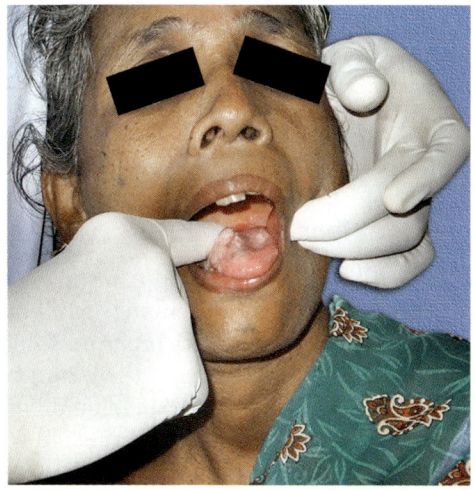

Fig. 11-65 *Palpation of posterior third of the tongue.*

Palpation of posterior third of the tongue is often difficult. Often no growth is visible in this site or only part of the growth is visible. When hyperactive gag reflex is present, local anesthetic spray can be used prior to examination. Patient is asked to open the mouth widely. All left hand fingers of examiner are kept straight and stiff and are pressed firmly over the patient's cheek so that they intervene between upper and lower teeth. Palpation is done using examiner's right index finger over posterior part of the tongue. Left hand fingers prevent biting of the right examining finger by the patient. By reflex patient may bite only his pushed cheek **(Figs. 11-65 and 11-66)**.

Examination of the tongue:
- Tongue should be inspected *both* with tongue inside and protruded outside. Tip, margins, dorsum, ventral aspect should be inspected; holding the tip of tongue using gauze and pulling the tongue gently outwards and sideward facilitates better inspection of the margins
- Posterior third of the tongue is difficult to inspect and needs spatula and good illumination; it is better felt actually
- Tongue is palpated *with tongue inside*

- Tongue should be examined on its *undersurface* without fail; patient is asked to put tip of the tongue on the palate to visualize its undersurface; both inspection and palpation should be done
- *Examine*—size (macroglossia); restricted mobility (ankyloglossia due to genioglossus involvement); altered movements (deviation towards *same side* in hypoglossal nerve palsy); inability to tilt tongue tip upwards (tongue tie); lateral borders; posterior third of the tongue
- *Examine for*—leukoplakia, fissure, lichen planus (looks like delicate, bluish white lesions as if mucosa with silver nitrate coat; but always examine associated lesions in wrist and shin), ulcer, induration, hemangioma, black hairy tongue, lingual thyroid
- *Ulcer in the tongue* may be aphthous, dental (elongated, painful, tender ulcer on the margin or undersurface; in chronic type edge of the ulcer is heaped), carcinomatous (everted edge), gummatous ulcer (rare; in midline anterior 2/3rd punched out, painless with wash leather slough), nonspecific ulcer, tuberculous ulcer (almost always in the tip or sides of the anterior 2/3rd of the tongue; can be multiple; severe pain interferes with mastication and speech; ulcer is shallow, undermined with pale granulation tissues in the floor)
- *Palpation of the posterior third* needs special method by placing the left hand fingers between jaws outside and right hand index finger is used to palpate the tongue; it prevents biting of the

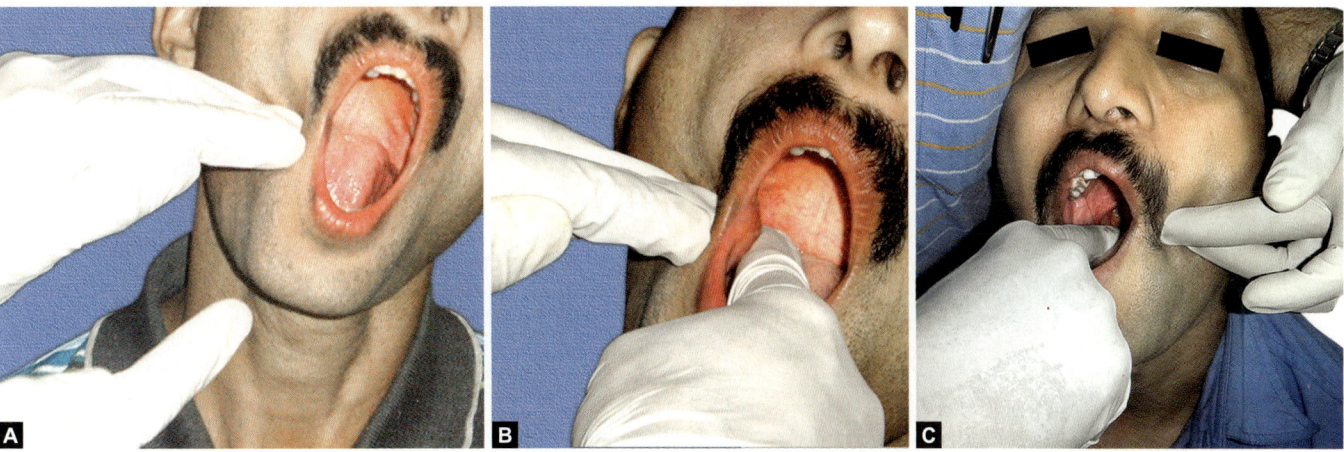

Figs. 11-66A to C *Examination of posterior part of the tongue* needs special method (See text).

examining finger; examiner stands on the side of or behind the patient; local anesthetic (xylocaine) spray may be useful
- *Mirror examination* may be needed to assess posterior 1/3rd (base) of the tongue. (*Note:* Mirror examination is also used to visualize pharynx and larynx)

Palpation of the Floor of the Mouth

It is palpated by asking the patient to put the tip of the tongue on the roof of the mouth with head bending slightly backwards. **Ranula** is an extravasation cyst arising from sublingual or mucus glands. It is smooth, soft, fluctuant and brilliantly transilluminant. When it extends into submandibular region across posterior margin of mylohyoid muscle with cross fluctuation, it is called as **plunging ranula. Sublingual dermoid** is usually midline swelling in the floor of the mouth with extension outside into submental region. It is smooth, soft, fluctuant but not transilluminant. Carcinoma floor of the mouth is stony hard with indurated edge and base. Mandibular thickening may be felt. It is often fixed (**Figs. 11-67 and 11-68**).

Palpation of Palate

Palate is examined with mouth fully opened with proper light source illumination. Head should be tilted backwards. Patient is asked to say 'Ah' while checking for the soft palate movements. Such normal movement of the soft palate allows the proper visualization of the palatine tonsils. Movement in one half of the soft palate will be lost in vagus nerve lesion or infiltrating nasopharyngeal carcinoma. Entire soft palate paralysis is seen in bulbar poliomyelitis. Palpation is done using index finger with patient's mouth open. Normal palate shows 4–6 transverse ridges in the hard palate called as palatal rugae which is more prominent in newborn (helps in sucking); it flattens in aged. Cleft palate is common in newborn.

Any ulcer/swelling when present are examined in usual systematic way. Leukoplakia or erythroplakia may be evident. Carcinoma of maxillary antrum pushes the palate downwards. Alveolar abscess in the upper jaw may be felt

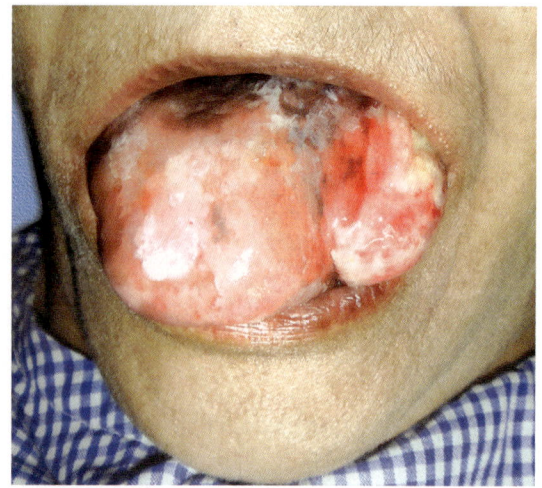

Fig. 11-68 *Carcinoma floor of the mouth* extending into tongue margin and gums.

as tender fluctuant swelling near the alveolar margin. Minor salivary gland tumor is common in palate. Palatal squamous cell carcinoma can also occur. Carcinoma is ulcerative or ulceroproliferative lesion (**Fig. 11-69**) whereas minor salivary

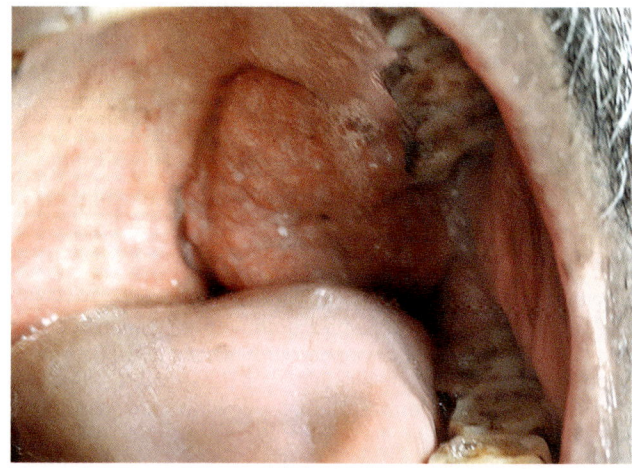

Fig. 11-69 *Carcinoma palate.*

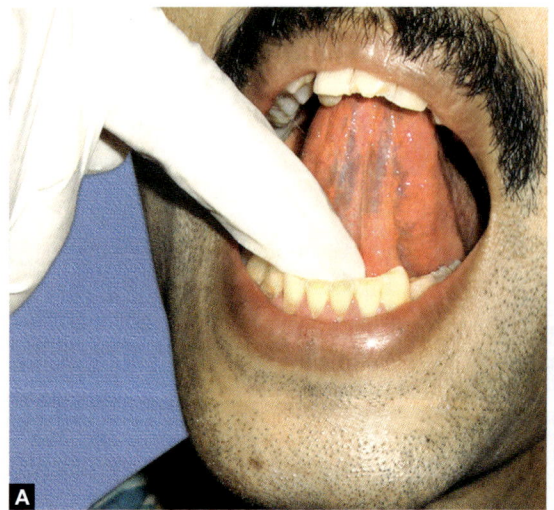 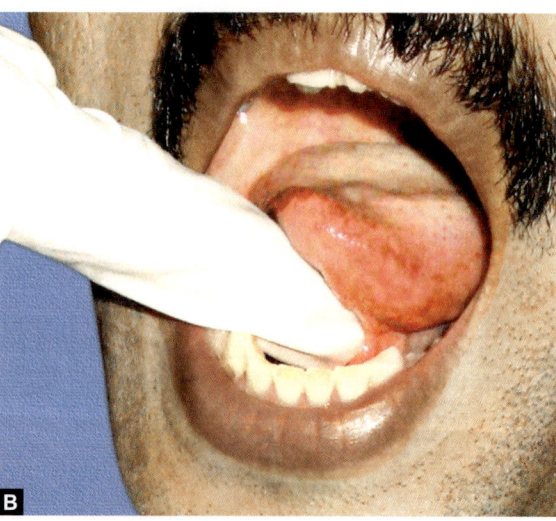

Figs. 11-67A and B Palpation of the *floor of the mouth*.

tumor of palate is swelling with ulceration over its summit due to necrosis. Minor salivary gland tumor may be adenoid cystic or mixed (pleomorphic) type but more commonly malignant compared to major salivary gland tumors. Any lesions in the palate should be palpated for tenderness, margin, edge, surface, consistency, induration, mobility. Initially lesion may be mobile, but soon gets adherent to the palatal bone to make it immobile as mucosa is adherent to periosteum (mucoperiosteum). Nasal cavities and maxilla should be examined always. Palatal lesions may be on one side or in the midline; it is important to observe whether lesion is crossing the midline or not. Syphilitic gumma (tertiary syphilis) is usually in the midline, initially present as painless, soft, nontender swelling which later forms a gummatous ulcer which is deep seated punched out, nontender which later may perforate the palate forming a rounded perforation (hole); but this condition is rare now. Palatal perforation can also occur after radiotherapy for carcinoma. Advanced malignancy also cause palatal perforation. Both malignant minor salivary tumor and carcinoma can invade deeper plane to involve base of skull also. Initially these lesions are painless and nontender but become severely painful and tender once it invades deeper structures; invasion of cranial nerves can occur causing severe pain along the distribution of the nerves. Palatal mucus cyst can occur as smooth, well-localized, transilluminant swelling but is rare.

Palpation of Tonsils and Fauces

It should be done in posterior growths of cheek and tongue and in tuberculosis. Surface ulcerations, induration should be looked for. Peritonsillar abscess, carcinoma tonsil, carcinolymphoma (lymphoepithelioma)/lymphosarcoma of tonsil should be kept in mind.

Method of examination of tonsils: Tongue is depressed using a spatula (tongue depressor) and using another spatula anterior pillar of the tonsil is gently pressed to visualize the tonsillar bed (palatine/faucial) for any pathology. Adequate illumination using a light source is essential. Patient is asked to tell '*Ah*' to make tonsils better visible by making soft palate to move upwards and backwards **(Figs. 11-70 to 11-74)**.

Points to Remember:
- History of tobacco abuse, smoking, alcohol intake
- History of loosening tooth of recent onset
- History of tooth extraction and absence of healing of the socket; difficulty in placing dentures
- History of pain, swelling, ulceration
- History of ear pain due to lingual nerve irritation radiating along the auriculotemporal nerve; sensation of cotton wool pad in the ear
- History of difficulty in swallowing, opening the mouth and protruding the tongue
- History of bone pain (mandible and maxilla)
- History of halitosis—foul-smelling breath which is due to release of tryptophan from necrotic tumor cells
- History of profuse salivation due to irritation of taste fibers
- Oral cavity should be inspected properly using a tongue depressor with adequate light source **(Figs. 11-75A to J)**
- Trismus, ankyloglossia should be assessed

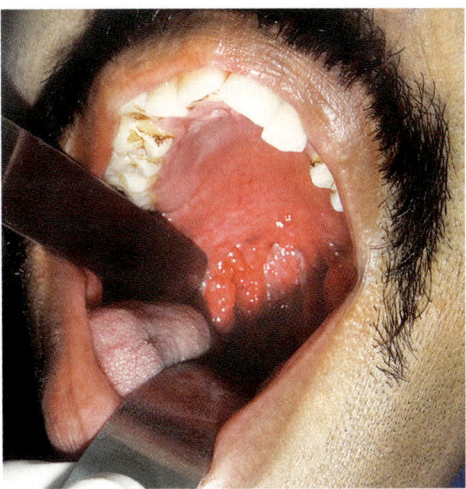

Fig. 11-70 *Tonsil is examined using spatula, ideally two—one over the tongue and another on the anterior pillar of the tonsil. Patient should tell 'Ah' to move soft palate above and behind and make tonsils visible properly.*

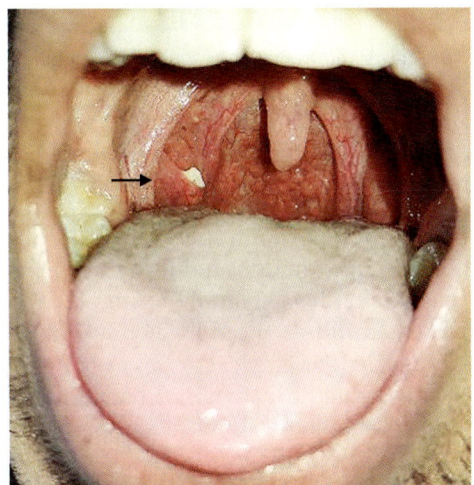

Fig. 11-71 Tonsillar keratosis—right sided.

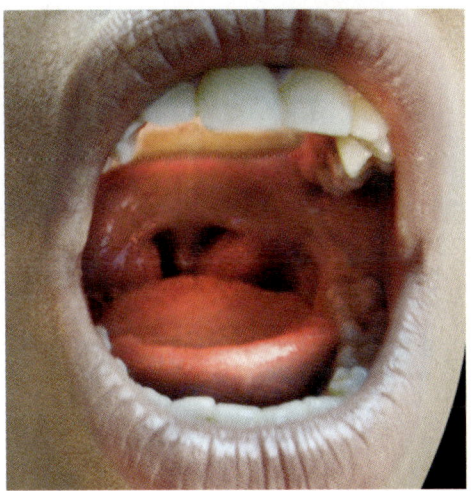

Fig. 11-72 *Bilateral enlargement of the tonsils*; it is chronic tonsillitis which needs tonsillectomy.

- Tenderness, ulcer edge, base surrounding area, induration crossing the midline or not should be checked for
- Posterior 1/3rd tongue, tonsils, fauces should be examined carefully
- Mandible should be palpated for tenderness, thickening, irregularity, fracture site by bidigital examination
- Cervical lymph nodes should be examined methodically
- Respiratory system should be examined for bronchopneumonia and occasionally for metastases

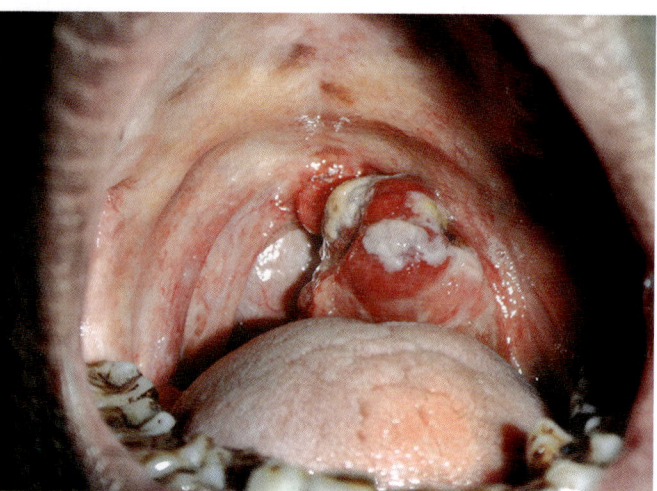

Fig. 11-74 Large *lymphoepithelioma* of the tonsil— left sided.

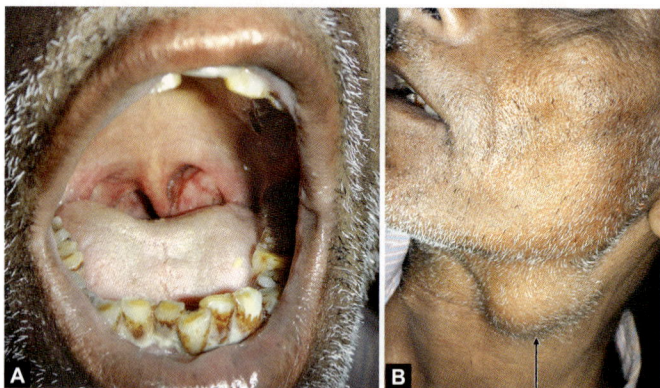

Figs. 11-73A and B *Growth in the tonsils* with left jugulodigastric (level II) lymph node enlargement.

EXAMINATION OF CERVICAL LYMPH NODES

Cervical lymph nodes should be examined. Submental, submandibular, upper, middle and lower deep cervical and posterior triangle nodes should be examined. Size, shape, mobility, fixity, number should be checked. Both sides should be examined for cervical nodes as lymphatics cross communicate especially in carcinoma tongue and floor of the mouth. All levels should be examined properly **(Figs. 11-76 and 11-77).**

SYSTEMIC EXAMINATION

Eventhough metastatic (blood spread) disease is rare in oral carcinomas, respiratory system examination is important as aspiration pneumonia is common in oral carcinoma, especially in carcinoma tongue. Melanoma, lymphoma, rarely aggressive carcinoma can spread to bone, liver through blood. Abdominal and musculoskeletal system examination should be completed **(Fig. 11-78).**

INVESTIGATIONS

Biopsy of ulcer: *Wedge biopsy* is done. Usually two biopsies are taken. If it is on the anterior aspect it can be done under local anesthesia. Posterior lesions are biopsied under general anesthesia. Suction apparatus should be used during biopsy. Biopsy area may be apposed using catgut sutures to prevent bleeding. Malignant *squamous cells with epithelial pearls (Keratin pearls)* are the histological features of carcinoma. Broder's histological

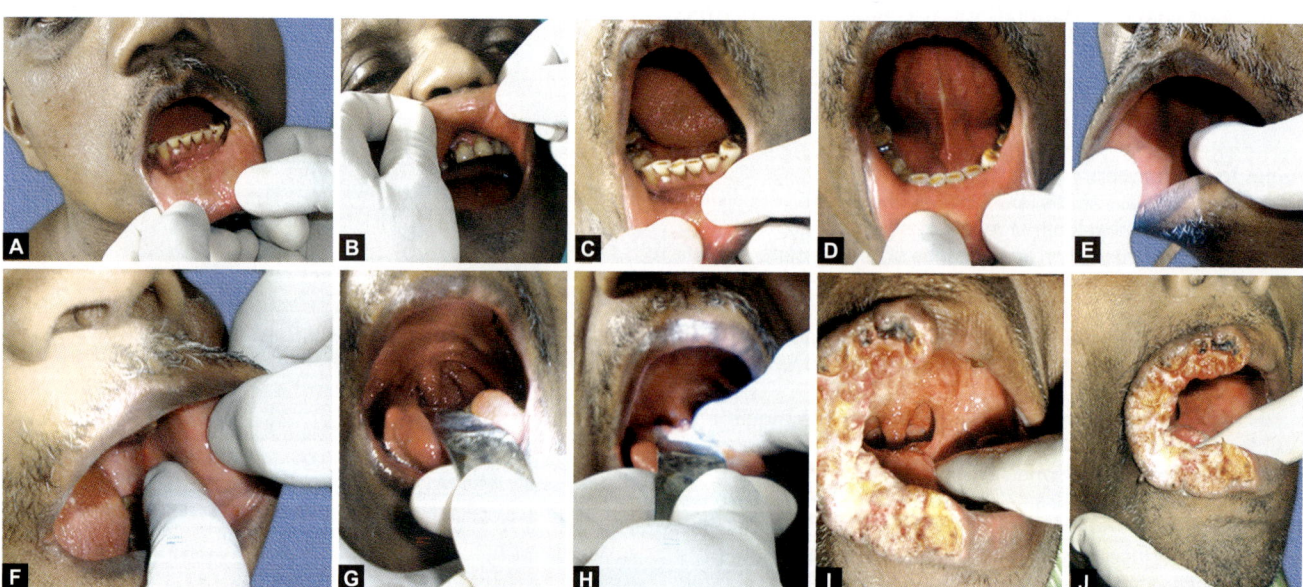

Figs. 11-75A to J Examination of oral cavity should be methodical—*lips, gums, cheeks, tongue, floor of the mouth, palate, posterior aspect of the oral cavity.*

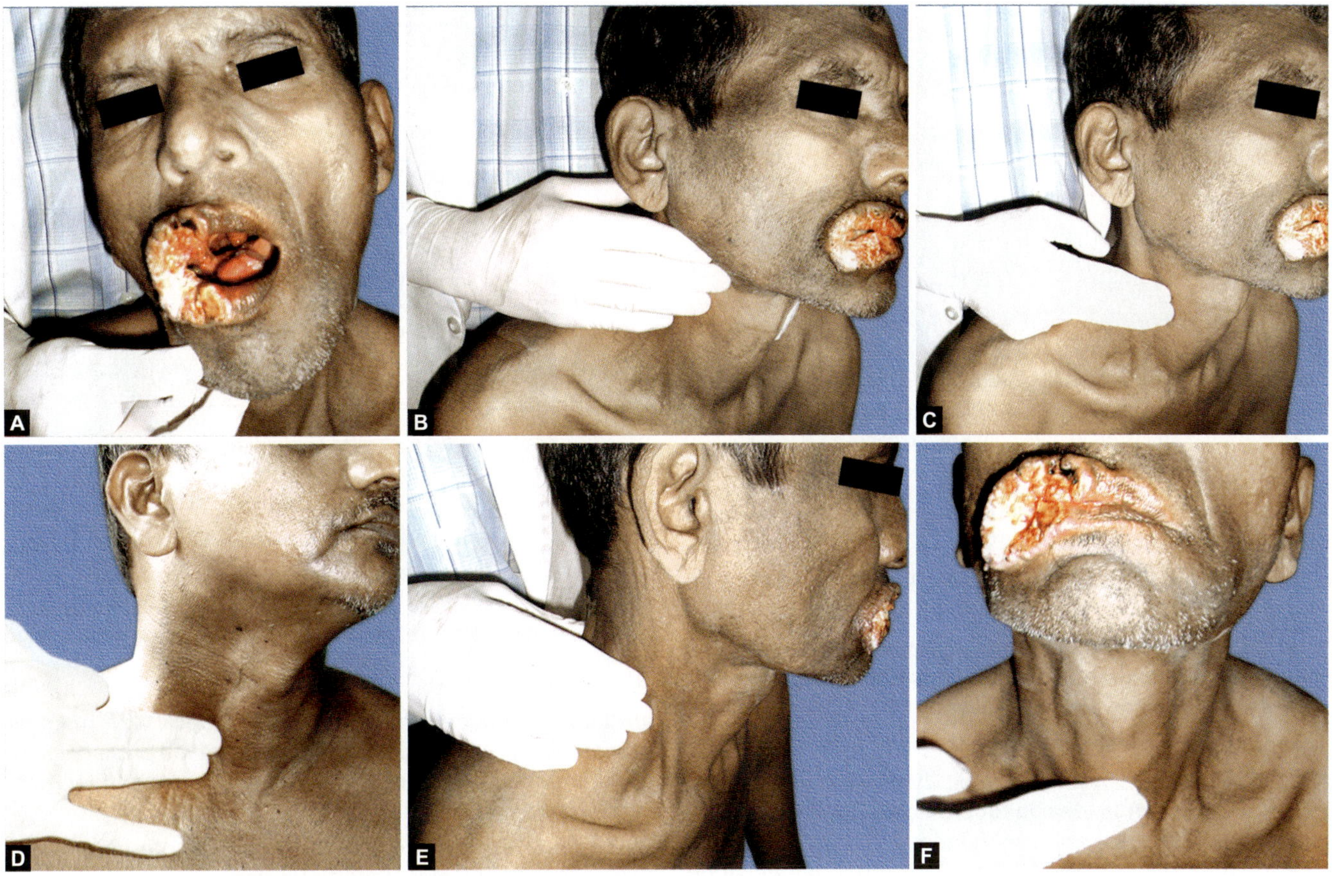

Figs. 11-76A to F Examination of *different levels of neck nodes*—Level I; II; III; IV; V; VI.

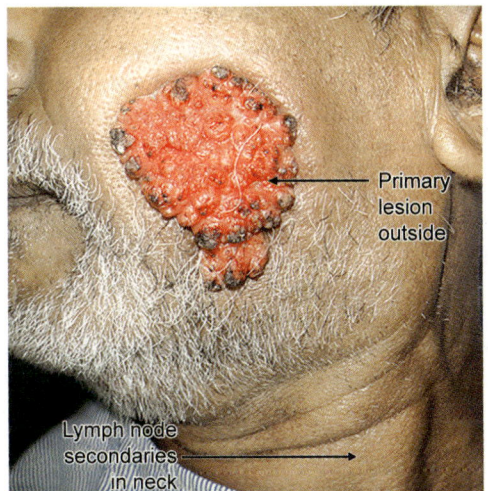

Fig. 11.77 *Carcinoma cheek* extending from inside mucosa to outside skin with *cervical lymph node spread*.

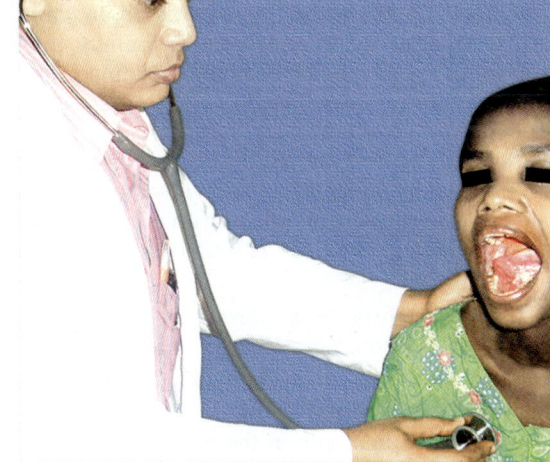

Fig. 11-78 Respiratory system should be examined for the possible development of *bronchopneumonia* in oral carcinoma, especially of tongue.

grading: (1) Well differentiated: >75% epithelial pearls; (2) Moderately differentiated: 50–75% epithelial pearls; (3) Poorly differentiated: 25–50% epithelial pearls; (4) Very poorly differentiated: <25% epithelial pearls. 1% toluidine blue staining with Lugol's iodine counterstaining is used to identify the appropriate area for tissue biopsy.

Orthopantomogram (OPG): OPG is a must in all oral carcinomas to see mandibular involvement. Cortical thinning, and bone destruction are looked for. It is plain X-ray mandible showing entire mandible in a single plane. It is a rotational tomogram showing dentition, inner and outer plates of mandible and joints. It is done in jaw tumors, osteomyelitis

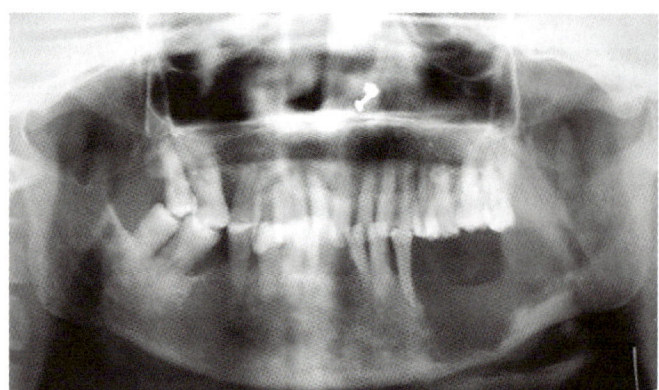

Fig. 11-79 *Orthopantomogram* is a must to see mandibular invasion in carcinoma oral cavity.

of mandible, fracture mandible and to see spread from carcinoma oral cavity (Fig. 11-79).

Dental occlusion X-rays or intraoral X-rays often may be needed.

Chest X-ray is done to look for bronchopneumonia which is more common in carcinomas in the posterior part of the oral cavity and tongue and also whenever there are ankyloglossia.

Ultrasound neck to identify the neck lymph nodes.

FNAC of the cervical nodes is done. US or CT-guided FNAC is more sensitive. It is ideal in tuberculosis (Langhans giant cells, epithelioid cells) and secondaries in lymph node. It is done in lymphoma as an initial tool but open lymph node biopsy is ideal for confirmation, grading, histochemistry and types.

CT scan is very useful in identifying cervical and retropharyngeal lymph nodes; bone invasion; in identifying posterior lesions; useful in patients with trismus, mandible spread, when marginal mandibulectomy is planned, pterygoid involvement, base of skull extension. *CECT* (contrast enhanced computerized tomography) scan has got *highest specificity* in evaluating the oral cancers. However, *MRI* is better in identifying the soft tissue involvement. A positron emission tomography (PET) scan can identify the biological function of the tumor. PET–CT is better tool than only PET scan.

MRI is useful mainly to assess soft tissue spread, retropharyngeal spread. Surgical clearance can be planned using MRI.

Cone beam CT scan (CBCT): It is cone-shaped millimeter by millimeter cross sections of the mandible, maxilla, soft tissues, nasal cavities, sinuses, dentition, etc. It gives better visualization of the tissues than OPG; but not as good as CECT or MRI in relation to resolution. It is mainly used for benign lesions currently.

Indirect laryngoscopy, posterior rhinoscopy, direct laryngoscopy are commonly used simple evaluation methods in posterior tumors (Refer Chapter 15).

Triple endoscopy/Panendoscopy: Direct laryngoscopy, bronchoscopy and esophagoscopy is useful in oral carcinoma as in 10–15% of patients, synchronous carcinomas

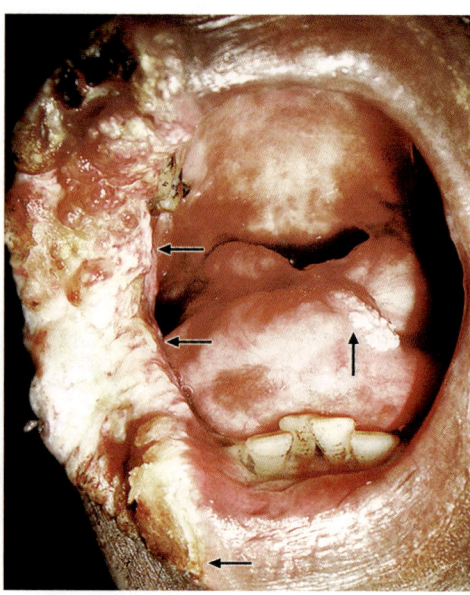

Fig. 11-80 Carcinoma of lip, cheek and tongue. Patient was earlier (3 years early) operated for carcinoma cheek. Now metachronous growths appeared in lip, cheek and tongue.

are known to occur. In secondaries in neck with unknown primary to identify the possible location of the primary lesion, triple endoscopy is useful. It is often also done in laryngeal carcinoma.

Blood tests like hemogram, ESR; *serology* to identify HIV, VDRL for syphilis may need to be done. *Study of discharge* is also useful.

General Features of Oral Carcinoma

Oropharyngeal cancer is the most common cancer (Fig. 11-80)—40% in Indian subcontinent. In Western countries, it accounts for 4% only. *Risk factors*—tobacco and related products; alcohol; areca nut; human papilloma virus; Epstein-Barr virus; Paterson-Kelly syndrome; nutritional deficiency. Patient may develop a second primary (15%) in the oropharynx in different site at the same time or within 6 months of the existing primary (*synchronous*—4% prevalence; 20% of second primaries) or after 6 months of first primary (*metachronous*—80% of second primaries). Metachronous second primary is more common than synchronous second primary and it usually occurs in 2 years. In India cheek is the commonest site, then followed by tongue, floor of the mouth, palate and lips. In western countries, tongue, floor of the mouth, lip and cheek is the order of occurrence of oral carcinoma. *Problems with oral carcinoma*: Upper airway obstruction, especially posterior growths; bronchopneumonia; feeding difficulties; malnutrition; infection; torrential bleeding due to erosion of vessels like lingual; fixity of secondaries; fungation; disability and psychological discomfort.

Carcinoma Cheek

Squamous cell carcinoma is the most common carcinoma of the cheek. Occasionally it can be adenocarcinoma arising from the minor salivary glands or mucus glands. It may be also rarely melanoma.

Precipitating factors: All 'S'—Smoking, Spirit, Syphilis, Sepsis, Sharp tooth, Spices. It is common in Chutta smokers (Tobacco enrapped in a tobacco leaf). Chutta carcinoma is common in Andhra Pradesh and Orissa. Pipe smoking (buccal carcinoma); snuff use (floor of the mouth); different mouthwashes may be other etiologies.

Premalignant conditions: Leukoplakia, erythroplakia, submucosal fibrosis, hyperplastic candidiasis. *Betel nut chewing* (Pan, with pan quid kept in cheek pouch for a long time) is an important causative factor of carcinoma cheek. Types: Ulcerative; proliferative (exophytic); verrucous.

Verrucous carcinoma: It occurs as a superficial proliferative exophytic lesion with minimal deep invasion. Lesion has got white, dry, velvety or warty, keratinized surface. It is of low grade, very well-differentiated squamous cell carcinoma, which is locally malignant without any lymphatic spread. It is a curable malignancy. It is common in females. It may be related to human papillomavirus. It is often multicentric. Invasive carcinoma also may develop in other sites.

Biological behavior of carcinoma cheek: Carcinoma cheek is common in posterior half of cheek than anterior. It spreads into the deeper plane to involve buccinator, pterygoids; into the retromolar trigone, base of the skull, pharynx. It spreads outwards to involve the skin causing fungation, ulceration, orocutaneous fistula formation. Mandible is commonly involved either by direct extension or through subperiosteal lymphatic plexus which communicates freely with oral lymphatics. Lymph nodes commonly involved are submental, submandibular, deep cervical and often lateral pharyngeal groups. Nodal spread is observed in 50% of cases. Infection of the tumor area and soft tissues around is common, causing fever, foul-smelling ulcer, halitosis. Respiratory infection is common in these patients. Once tumor extends into the retromolar region, soft palate, pharynx, dysphagia will occur.

Clinical features: Ulcer in the cheek which gradually increases in size in a patient with history of chewing pan, and smoking. *Pain* occurs when it involves the skin, bone or if secondarily infected. Referred pain into the ear signifies involvement of lingual nerve. *Involvement of retromolar trigone* indicates that it is an advanced disease, as the lymphatics here communicate freely with the pharyngeal lymphatics. *Everted edge, induration* are the typical features of the ulcer. Mandible is examined bidigitally for thickening, tenderness, and sites of fracture. *Trismus and dysphagia* signifies involvement of pterygoids, or posterior extension. Occasionally, it may extend into the *upper alveolus and to the maxilla* causing swelling, pain and tenderness. Submandibular lymph nodes and upper deep cervical lymph nodes are involved which are hard, nodular, and initially mobile but later gets fixed to each other and then to deeper structures. Once lymph nodes get fixed it may infiltrate into hypoglossal nerve (tongue will deviate towards the same side), spinal accessory nerve (defective shrugging of shoulder) and cervical sympathetic chain *(Horner's syndrome)*. Compression over external carotid artery causes absence of superficial temporal artery pulsation. Eventually it causes fungation and bleeding from major vessels—*carotid blow out*.

Features of advanced carcinoma cheek: Involvement of retromolar trigone; extension into the base of skull and pharynx; fixed neck lymph nodes; extension to the opposite side.

Carcinoma Lip

It is common in men; common in old age; common in *lower lip (90%);* upper lip 5–10%; less common in Negroes; common in white Caucasians. It is commonly due to exposure to sunlight (ultraviolet rays); common in pipe smoker. It is slowly progressive tumor; it spreads to submental nodes and later to other neck nodes on both sides; usually it is a *well-differentiated squamous cell carcinoma*.

Causes: UV rays, smoking, cheilitis, solar keratosis, papilloma, leukoplakia, tobacco chewing, Khaini chewers (tobacco + lime); agriculturist who are exposed to sunlight—*countryman's lip*, Leukoplakia, actinic chelitis—precancerous lesion.

Carcinoma Tongue

Types: *Gross:* (1) Papillary; (2) Ulcerative or ulceroproliferative; (3) Fissure with induration; (4) Lobulated, indurated mass.

Histologically: Squamous cell carcinoma—commonest. Sites: Lateral margin—commonest—47–50%; posterior third—20%; dorsum—6.5%; ventral surface—9%; tip—10%.

Features: Painless ulcer/swelling in the lateral margin of the tongue which becomes painful later (*Florid, painless, friable, bleeding, everted edge, sloughing yellow gray floor, serosanguinous discharge, induration of edge and base and is extending into surrounding area* are the features). *Pain* in the tongue due to infection or ulceration or due to the involvement of lingual nerve (pain is referred to ear); pain on swallowing, in case of carcinoma of posterior third of tongue; *excessive salivation* (It is due to irritation of nerves of taste buds and ankyloglossia causing difficulty in swallowing saliva); *dysphagia* either due to fixed tongue or due to the involvement of genioglossus or growth in the posterior third of the tongue; v*isible ulcer* in anterior two thirds of tongue with raised everted edge, area of induration is more extensive than visible ulcer area; ulcer may cross the midline or extend into alveolus, floor of the mouth, mandible; bleeds on touch; growth or ulcer in posterior third, is usually *not visible. Ankyloglossia*; inability to articulate; *fetor oris (halitosis)* due to infection and necrosis in the oral cavity; *change in voice* occurs in posterior third tumors. Tumor in posterior third area is more aggressive. Indirect laryngoscopy is often needed to visualize posterior third of the tongue. *Lymph nodes* may be palpable in the neck which are hard, nodular and may get fixed in advanced stages. Features of bronchopneumonia may be present.

Terminal events in advanced cases: Aspiration pneumonia; erosion of major vessels by primary tumor (lingual artery) or by secondaries in neck (carotid artery); cachexia; laryngeal edema; asphyxia; starvation due to inability to swallow.

OTHER MALIGNANT CONDITIONS OF ORAL CAVITY

Type	Features
Carcinoma of floor of the mouth Rare in India; 2nd most common oral malignancy in Western countries	• Aggressive tumor; Invades hyoglossus, mylohyoid, genioglossus and anterior mandible early • Trismus; ankyloglossia; mandibular spread; involvement of bilateral neck nodes—are presentations • Prognosis poor; poor cosmetic result
Carcinoma alveolus Squamous cell carcinoma arising from gums; common in males; common in India; associated with tobacco/pan chewing	Similar to other oral carcinoma with bone involvement by direct spread; lymph node spread also common
Carcinoma of hard palate • Squamous cell carcinoma: common in males; common in reverse smokers due to thermal injury • Hard palate is also a common site for minor salivary gland tumors; commonly malignant; malignant adenoid cystic type is common	• Ulcer with raised, everted edge and induration; fixed; spreads to periosteum, bone, maxilla, sinus, nose. Upper deep cervical lymph nodes involved (25%). • Single, solid, smooth swelling with ulcer over the summit is typical of minor salivary gland tumor. • Edge biopsy; FNAC; CT scan of neck and base of skull are the needed investigation

BENIGN CONDITIONS IN ORAL CAVITY

Ranula *(Rana-frog; look like the belly of frog)* Extravasation cyst, mainly arising from sublingual gland, rarely from mucus gland of *Blandin and Nuhn* in the floor of mouth. Initially retention cyst formed by blockade of sublingual duct, later with increased pressure acini break up to form an extravasation cyst	• Bluish, smooth, soft, fluctuant, nontender, *brilliantly transilluminant* swelling, in the **lateral aspect of floor of mouth** • Extends into the submandibular region through deeper part of posterior margin of mylohyoid—**plunging ranula**—*cross fluctuant* across mylohyoid muscle
Sublingual dermoid They are sequestration dermoid lined by squamous epithelium containing keratin **Types:** • *Median sublingual dermoid—more common.* Derived from germinal epithelium that undergoes ectodermal differentiation at the level of fusion of two mandibular arches. • *Lateral sublingual dermoid*—derived from *first branchial arch*	• Asymptomatic, smooth, soft, cystic, nontender, non-transilluminant (contains cheesy material) midline swelling between two genial muscle above mylohyoid • Cystic swelling in sub mandibular region; in the lateral aspect of floor of mouth
Mucus retention cyst (Fig. 11-81): Due to blockage of duct of small mucous gland in the mucous membrane 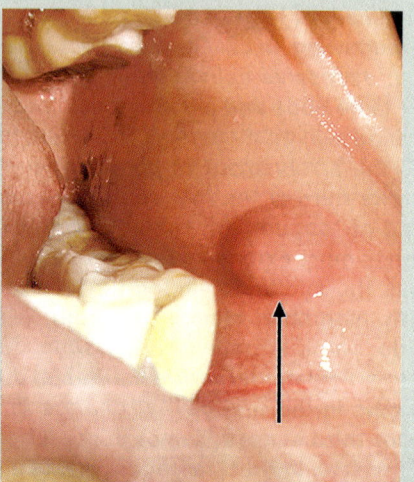 *Fig. 11-81 Mucus retention cyst of the cheek.*	• Common on inner side of lower lip or cheek; seen in any age group. Presents as painless, slowly progressive, soft, smooth, cystic swelling • Pale pink in color with grey glary appearance of visible mucus; becomes white, scarred, obscured colored if overlying mucus is damaged • Not adherent to overlying mucous membrane or underlying muscle. Lymph nodes not enlarged.
Fibroepithelial polyp: Due to repeated trauma to buccal mucosa	Soft, pedunculated, fibrous swelling
Papilloma: Multiple fingers like processes with nodular cauliflower like surface covered with keratinized epithelium; occasionally can turn into carcinoma.	Single/multiple; may occur anywhere in the oral cavity; associated with similar lesion in genitalia, hands and feet
Hemangioma	Bluish, warm, soft compressible well localized swelling; seen in floor of mouth or cheek.
Median rhomboid glossitis: Often mistaken for carcinoma	Rhomboid mass in the midline on the dorsum of tongue in front of foramen cecum.
Geographic tongue: Unknown etiology	Migrating reddish white patches on the dorsum of tongue

PREMALIGNANT CONDITIONS OF ORAL CAVITY

Premalignant conditions of oral cavity are important to identify before it turns into malignancy.

High risk—definite risk of malignant change: Lesions with definitive risk of malignant change. They are—leukoplakia; erythoplakia Chronic hyperplastic candidiasis	Medium risk: Premalignant but not associated with higher incidence of carcinoma. They are—oral submucus fibrosis; syphilitic glossitis; sideropenic dysphagia (sideropenia is iron deficiency without anemia); Plummer–Vinson syndrome	Equivocal risk lesion: Oral lichen planus, congenital dyskeratosis, discoid erythematosus

Type of premalignant lesion	Etiology	Features
Leukoplakia White patch in the oral mucosa that cannot be characterized clinically/pathologically to any other disease. *Types*—homogenous; nodular; speckled (Highly potentially malignant).	**Common causes**: Smoking, spirit, sepsis, superficial glossitis, syphilis, spices, sharp tooth, susceptibility, pan chewing (using areca, tobacco, slaked lime), chronic hypertrophic candidiasis. **Incidence 20%** in smokers and pan chewers, incidence turning to malignancy is **2–4%**	Well localized, white/grayish colored lesion in cheek, palate, tongue, or other areas of oral cavity
Erythroplakia Red velvety appearance of mucosa not characterized to any recognized condition. *Types*—homogenous, speckled, granular	Histologically parakeratosis with severe epithelial dysplasia **17–20 times more potentially malignant than leukoplakia.**	Equal in both sexes; common in lower alveolar mucosa; gingivobuccal sulcus, floor of mouth
Oral submucus fibrosis Progressive fibrosis of the oral cavity	Common in Asians and Indians	• Mucosa of cheek, gingivae, palate and tongue shows mottled/marbled pallor. • Trismus, ankyloglossia.
Chronic superficial glossitis Chronic inflammatory degenerative condition of tongue preceding to carcinoma	**Predisposing factors** Six 's'—syphilis, sharp tooth, smoking, spices, spirit, sepsis	Five phases before becoming carcinoma: 1. Stage of epithelial hypertrophy 2. Stage of leukoplakia 3. Stage of red glazed tongue 4. Stage of cracks and fissure 5. Stage of carcinoma

DIFFERENTIAL DIAGNOSIS OF TONGUE ULCERS

Tongue ulcers	Etiology	Features	Location
Dental ulcers	Jagged tooth or dentures causing mechanical irritation	Elongated, erythematous painful ulcer, with slogh in the floor surrounded by hyperemia	Margin or under surface of tongue
Aphthous ulcer	Autoimmune, deficiencies, anemia, celiac disease, Crohn's disease, stress, HIV infection idiopathic, hormonal, familial	Single/multiple, recurrent, painful ulcers with whitish floor yellow margin, hyperemic zone, common in females	Tip, under surface, anterior part of dorsum of tongue
Types: a. *Minor* b. *Major* c. *Herpetiform*		• <5 mm in size, recurrent, single/multiple, heals spontaneously. • >5 mm in size, lasts longer • Small, painful numerous (20–100) ulcers, eventually coalesce to form large ulcer	
Syphilitic ulcers a. *Primary syphilis* b. *Secondary syphilis*	*Treponema pallidum*—sexually transmitted disease	Painless ulcer (*Hunterian chancre*), rubbery hard, with thick crust covering, leaves a fine superficial scar on healing, shotty discrete lymph nodes in neck. Multiple shallow ulcers often with radiating cracks with fine scar eventually (snail track ulcer). Grayish mucus patches in inner lip, check and anterior pillar of tonsils can occur.	Ventral surface and lateral margin. Middle of the dorsum of tongue
c. *Tertiary syphilis*		*Hutchinson's condyloma* (wart) can occur in tongue. *Gummatous ulcer*—punched out, deep, painless, nontender ulcer (Gumma can occur in tongue, palate, nasal septum and lip also).	Midline, on dorsum of tongue (anterior 2/3rd).

Contd...

Contd...

Tongue ulcers	Etiology	Features	Location
Tuberculous ulcer	Coexist with pulmonary or laryngeal tuberculosis	*Multiple, undermined, painful ulcer*	Margin, tip, dorsum (painful)
Malignant ulcer	*Leukoplakia, erythroplakia, all 'S' factors*	Painless to begin with later painful ulcer with raised rolled out margin, slough in the floor, bleeds on touch, indurated base and enlarged lymph nodes	Lateral margin commonest site
Post-pertussis ulcer	After whooping cough		Frenulum on the ventral surface of tongue
Chronic nonspecific ulcer	Nonspecific etiology	Painless ulcer, indurated mimics carcinoma	Anterior 2/3rd of tongue

STOMATITIS

It is general term used for inflammation of entire lining of the mouth including tongue.

Causes

Local	General
Sharp teeth, poor fitting dentures; smoking; infections like herpes virus, *Candida*, and Vincent's angina; trauma either due to mechanical, chemical, thermal, X-rays	Hematological (anemia, agranulocytosis, purpura, leukemia); vitamin deficiencies (vitamin C), sprue, celiac disease, pellagra, pernicious anemia, tuberculosis, advanced carcinoma drugs (phenobarbitone, phenytoin); poisoning (bismuth, mercury, lead); syphilis

Types	Causes	Features	Site
Infective stomatitis	By opportunistic organisms (streptococci, staphylococci, Vincent's organism or even by true pathogens) when patients defense mechanism is reduced	Foul smelling fluid with redness and pain; common after chemotherapy, radiotherapy	Buccal mucosa, tongue
Catarrhal stomatitis	Associated with acute upper respiratory infection and acute fever	Oral mucosa becomes edematous, red; small ulcers coalesce to form large ulcers	Entire oral mucous membrane involved
Aphthous stomatitis	Unknown	Small painful tender vesicles with hyperemic base which eventually breaks forming small, white, circular deep ulcer	Cheek, lips, floor of the mouth, soft palate
Monilial stomatitis (oral thrush) Associated pharyngeal and esophageal thrush causes dysphagia	Fungal infection—*Candida albicans* Common in children, debilitated individuals, immunosuppressed individuals, (HIV, patients on cancer chemotherapy), antibiotic therapy	Small red patches initially, which turn into curdy white. When patches removed leaves behind multiple painful bleeding ulcer, excessive salivation	Mucosa of cheek and tongue
Ulcerative stomatitis (Vincent's angina)	Anaerobic gram-negative *Borrelia vincentii* and *Fusobacterium fusiformis*	Starts initially as severe gingivitis with swollen, inflamed, painful, peppered gums with small ulcers covered by yellow slough, which later spreads to cheek, tonsils, fauces with gum bleeding, fetor oris, toxicity, ill look, fever, enlarged tender neck nodes	Gums, tonsils, cheek, fauces
Cancrum oris/gangrenous stomatitis (Noma) (Fig. 11-82)	Rare, severe form of Vincent's ulcerative stomatitis, gingivitis with high mortality. Seen in malnourished children, often in patients with measles, kala-azar, typhoid, leukemia	Infective gangrene with Ischemic necrosis and extensive destruction of soft tissues, bone, skin, with toxemia, pyrexia, excessive salivation, fetid odor. **Phagedena**: Destructive ulceration with gangrene; here destruction is with no proliferation in contrast to malignancy	Starts in gum spreads into cheek, bone, soft tissues and skin.
Angular stomatitis (Cheilosis; Perleche) (Fig. 11-83) *Perleche means lick in French*	Constant dribbling of saliva at the corners of the mouth, common in children who constantly rub or lick	Inflamed red brown fissures which heals without scarring	Corners of the mouth

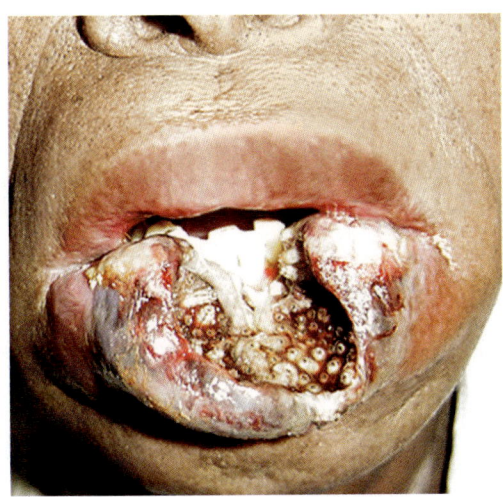

Fig. 11-82 *Cancrum oris* involving gingiva and lower lip extensively with plenty of maggots in it.

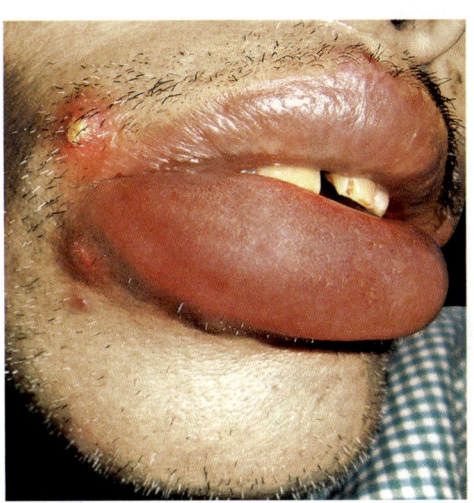

Fig. 11-83 Severe infection of lip (*Cheilitis*), angle of mouth. Patient is also having severe stomatitis.

CASE DISCUSSION

A 50-year-old man who is a tobacco chewer presents with painless progressive ulcerative lesion over his right cheek of 2 months' duration. Lesion started insidiously. Patient used to chew tobacco since childhood. On examination, ulceroproliferative lesion of 3 × 3 cm size is found on the right cheek; its edge is everted, margin is irregular and rounded; indurated edge and base. Few right sided upper deep cervical lymph nodes are palpable which are discrete, nontender, hard, mobile and 2 × 1 cm in sized. Respiratory system is normal.

What is your diagnosis and why?
Probable diagnosis is carcinoma cheek. Reasons are—tobacco chewing, short duration, painless, progressive ulcer which has got everted edge with induration. Significant right sided cervical lymph nodes are palpable.

What is the staging?
It is T2, N1, M0.

How you will evaluate?
Wedge biopsy from the ulcer for tissue diagnosis; FNAC of the palpable lymph nodes. Ultrasound neck may be useful to identify other nodes. Orthopantomogram is done to see the mandible involvement; chest X-ray to identify bronchopneumonia. CT neck and skull base including oral cavity is useful to identify exact local spread and nodal status.

CLINICAL PEARLS

Oral cancer is the one of the commonest cancer in India.

All 'S' with chewing tobacco, loosening tooth, trismus, otalgia, excess salivation, ulcer, ankyloglossia, deviation of tongue, mandibular pain, everted edge, induration, hard nodes in the neck are the essential things to look for with some variations depending on the exact location of the tumor such as cheek, lip, tongue, palate, etc.

Examine oral cavity and neck methodically always.

Wedge biopsy, chest X-ray, OPG mandible, FNAC of lymph node, CT head and neck are essential investigations.

12 Clinical Approach and Examination of Jaw

CHAPTER

Competency: SU19.1; SU19.2; AN30.1; AN30.2; AN33.2; AN33.4; AN33.5.

There are two jaws—upper and lower. Upper jaw is formed by maxilla and lower jaw by mandible.

Mandible is the largest, and strongest bone of the face. It has got horse-shaped body with two rami projecting upwards from its posterior ends. Outer surface of body contains symphysis menti, mental protuberance, mental foramen, oblique line, incisive fossa. Inner surface contains mylohyoid line, submandibular fossa (below), sublingual fossa (above), genial tubercles. Upper alveolar border bears sockets for teeth. Quadrilateral ramus has got medial and lateral surfaces, anterior, posterior, upper and lower borders and coronoid and condyloid processes. Medial surface of ramus contains mandibular foramen above the center of the ramus near the occlusal surface of teeth (transmits inferior alveolar nerve and vessels across mandibular canal to mental foramen on the outer surface); lingula (bony projection of mandibular foramen gives attachment to sphenomandibular ligament); mylohyoid groove (medial pterygoid is inserted below and medial to this groove). Lateral surface of ramus is flat (attachment of the masseter muscle). Upper border of ramus forms curved mandibular notch; lower border containing angle of mandible is the continuation of the base of mandible; posterior border of ramus is thick; anterior is thin. Anterior projection is called as *coronoid process* (temporalis is inserted on its apex and medial surface); posterior projection is called as *condyloid process*. Condyloid process is strong with expanded upward head which articulates with temporal bone to form temporomandibular joint. Anterior part of neck of condyloid process has got pterygoid fovea for the insertion of lateral pterygoid muscle. Oblique line on the outer surface of the body gives origin to buccinator; mylohyoid line on the inner surface of body gives origin to mylohyoid and superior constrictor muscles; upper genial tubercle gives origin to genioglossus and lower to geniohyoid; digastric fossa gives origin to anterior belly of digastric muscle. Investing layer of deep fascia and platysma is attached to lower border (base) of the mandible. Masseteric vessels and nerve passes through mandibular notch; mental foramen transmits mental vessels and nerve; inferior vessels and nerve passes through the mandibular canal; mylohyoid vessels and nerve are related to mylohyoid groove; lingual nerve is related on the medial surface; auriculotemporal nerve is related to medial side of the neck of the mandible. Mandible is the second bone to ossify in the body after clavicle. *Ossification center* (*only one center*) appears in 6th week of intrauterine life, one on each side near mental foramen. Entire *body* ossifies from *membrane* except only one near incisor teeth; ramus *above the mandibular foramen* ossifies from *cartilage*. Site at canine socket is weak and is the *commonest site of fracture* which may involve inferior alveolar nerve causing neuralgic pain and loss of sensation over the distribution of mental nerve (Fig. 12-1).

Maxilla is the 2nd largest bone of the face. Two maxillae form upper jaw. Each maxilla has got body, 4 processes—frontal, zygomatic, alveolar and palatine. Body is pyramidal in shape with base medially at nasal surface; apex laterally at zygomatic process. Body has got 4 surfaces—anterior/facial; posterior/infratemporal; superior/orbital and medial/nasal. Anterior facial surface gives attachments to many muscles of facial expression. Infraorbital foramen transmitting the infraorbital vessels and nerve is above the canine fossa. Posterior surface forms the anterior wall of infratemporal fossa. Maxillary tuberosity gives origin to superficial head of medial pterygoid muscle. Anterior wall of the pterygopalatine fossa is above the tuberosity—grooved by maxillary nerve. Superior surface is orbital surface forming floor of the orbit. It is related to lacrimal crest, inferior orbital fissure, nasolacrimal canal (contains nasolacrimal duct), infraorbital groove, inferior oblique muscle. Medial nasal surface forms the lateral wall of the nose. Posterosuperiorly maxillary sinus opening, and maxillary hiatus is present. Below inferior meatus of nose is present. Behind hiatus, there is greater palatine canal containing greater palatine vessels, anterior, middle and posterior palatine nerves. In the alveolar process canine socket is deepest; molar sockets are widest with each having 3 minor sockets. Palatine process is thick horizontal medial projection forming roof of the mouth and floor of the nasal cavity. Two palatine processes, one on each side forms the anterior 3/4th of the bony palate

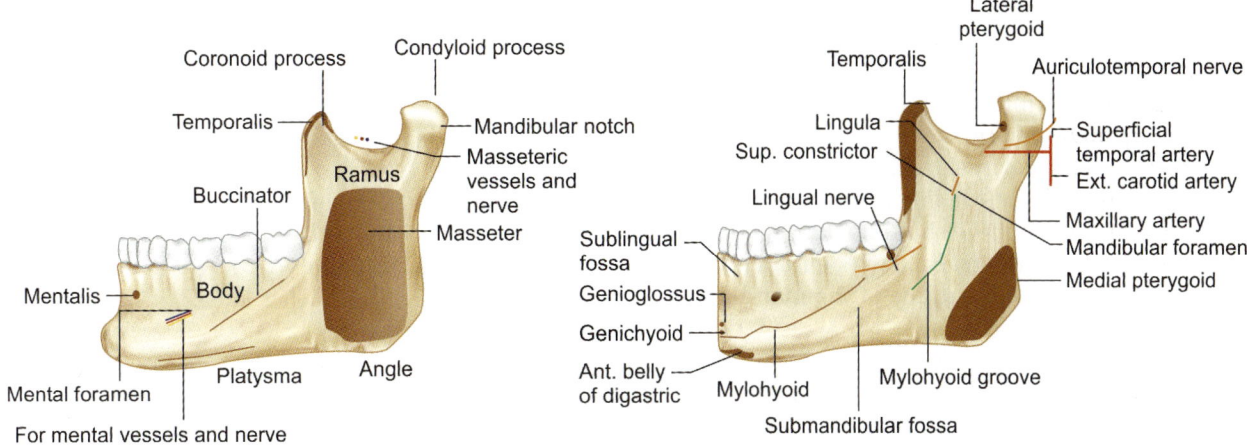

Fig. 12-1 *Anatomy of mandible* showing attachments and relations.

which articulates with the horizontal plate of palatine bone. Greater palatine vessels and anterior palatine nerves are present posteromedially. Maxilla articulates laterally with 1 bone—zygomatic; superiorly with 3 bones—nasal, frontal, ethmoidal; medially with 5 bones—ethmoid, inferior nasal concha, vomer, palatine and opposite maxilla. *Maxillary sinus is the pyramidal shaped cavity inside the body of maxilla with base medially and apex towards zygomatic process. Its roof is floor of the orbit. Its floor is alveolar process of maxilla. It is 3.7 × 3.7 × 2.5 cm in size. Maxillary sinus is first sinus to develop. Maxilla ossifies from membrane from 3 centers. One for maxilla proper is above the canine fossa during 6th week of intrauterine life. Two for premaxilla—one just above the incisive fossa at 6th week; another paraseptal is at 10th week.*

Temporomandibular joint is a condylar synovial joint. Upper temporal articular surface articulates with lower head of the mandible. Joint is covered with fibrocartilage with an intra-articular disc inside dividing the joint into upper and lower parts. Fibrous capsule, lateral temporomandibular ligament, stylomandibular ligament and sphenomandibular ligaments are the supports. Sphenomandibular ligament is related to lateral pterygoid, auriculotemporal nerve, maxillary artery, chorda tympani and pharynx. Laterally joint is related to parotid and temporal branches of facial nerve; medially tympanic plate, internal carotid artery, sphenomandibular ligament and related structures; below maxillary vessels; behind parotid, external auditory meatus, superficial temporal vessels, auriculotemporal nerve.

Movements: Depression (mouth opening) is by lateral pterygoid mainly (gravity muscle) supported by digastric, geniohyoid and mylohyoid; *elevation* is by masseter, temporalis and medial pterygoid (antigravity muscles); *protrusion/*protraction by both lateral and medial pterygoids; *retraction* by posterior fibers of temporalis. *Lateral/side-to-side* movement is by same side lateral pterygoid and opposite side medial pterygoid.

HISTORY

History taking begins with:

Name: **Age:** **Occupation:**
Address:

History of present illness: History of trauma and mode of injury should be asked for. Blood stained saliva after trauma suggests compound fracture especially in mandible as mucoperiosteum is adherent. Pain, swelling in the floor of the mouth (hematoma), difficulty in speech and swallowing, difficulty in moving the jaws are the other history to be asked. History of swelling, its duration, progression of swelling; History of pain, its nature, severity, progression; History of nasal block, nasal discharge, epistaxis; History of visual disturbances (diplopia, eyeball protrusion); History of swelling in the oral cavity; History of headache over the sinuses are other matters to be asked for. Referred pain in the ear can occur though auriculotemporal nerve. Maxillary sinus tumors can present with swelling, nasal problems, visual disturbances, headache. History of ulcer, swelling in the alveolus, palate or gums should be asked. History of epiphora suggests blockage of nasolacrimal duct causing constant overflow of tears. History of bleeding gums, purulent nasal discharge suggests maxillary antral sepsis (empyema); history of caries teeth, persistent severe neuralgic pain are also important. Tumor may invade especially maxillary division of trigeminal nerve causing severe pain. History of swelling in the neck suggests cervical lymph node enlargement suggesting neoplastic or inflammatory pathology. Its duration, progress, presence of pain should be asked.

Past history: Earlier history of similar complaints; treatment of sinus pathology, surgeries done earlier for similar condition; response to treatment should be asked.

Personal history: Alcohol intake, smoking, tobacco chewing history are important points to be noted.

GENERAL EXAMINATION

Anemia, clubbing, pulse, cyanosis, lymphadenopathy, blood pressure should be checked.

LOCAL EXAMINATION

Inspection

Inspection of outer surface of the maxilla, and mandible is done for swelling, ulcer, skin edema; discharging sinus (due to dental infection or osteomyelitis of the bone or due to malignancy or due to previous radiotherapy or due to recurrent tumor), upper and lower lips should be everted to examine jaw properly. Asymmetry in the level of inferior orbital margin is looked for. Any swelling arising from the surface/proptosis (forward pushing of the eyeball) is looked for. Any obvious protrusion from the side of the nose is observed. Nasal cavity should be inspected properly using nasal speculum. Any swelling arising from the walls, deviation of septum, blockage should be observed. Nasal discharge may be evident. Presence of epiphora (overflow of tears) is observed. Inner surface of the mandible and inferior/palatine surface of the maxilla is inspected by opening the mouth widely (using proper light source). Teeth (missing, caries) should be numbered and labeled; ulcers; swelling from inner surface of the bone should be inspected. When swelling is present, its size, shape, extent should be observed. Epulis (swelling arising from gums), odontomes may be evident. Contour of the alveolus; alignment of teeth; trismus should be observed. Ears should be inspected using a speculum **(Figs. 12-2 and 12-3).** Nasopharynx should be examined.

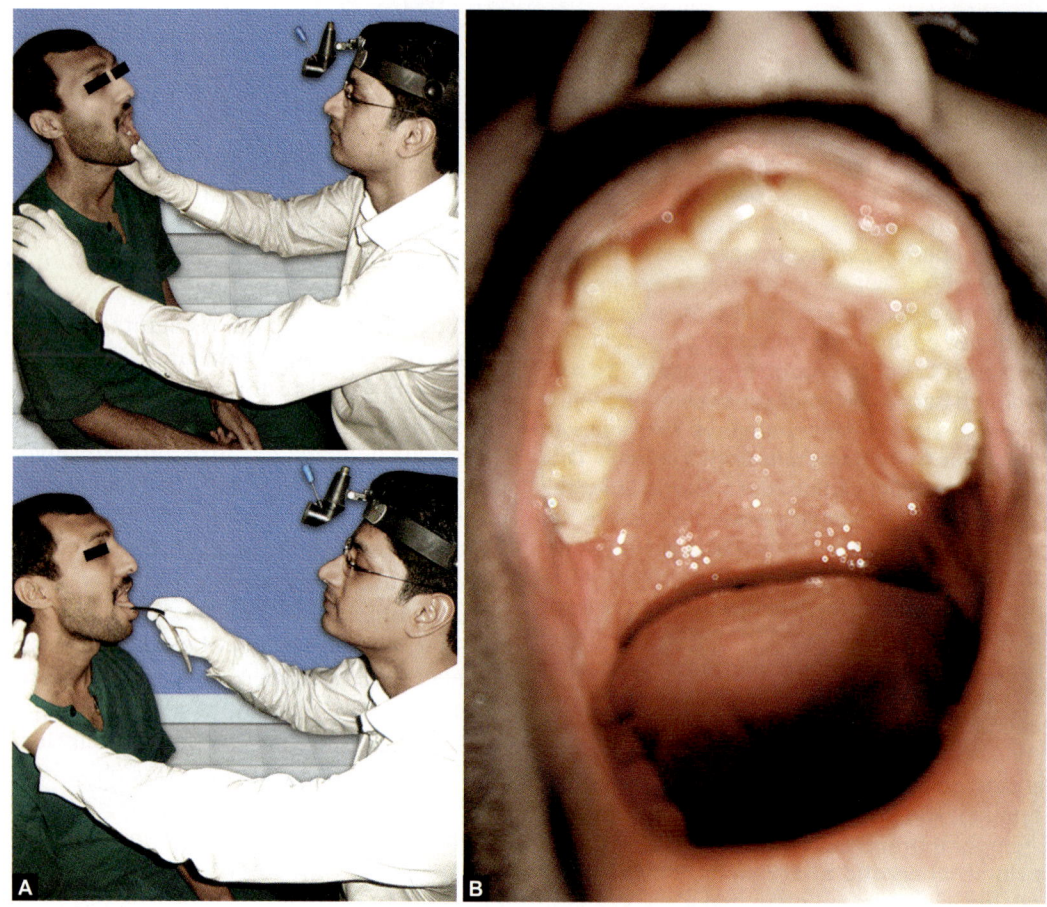

Figs. 12-2A and B *Inspect the oral cavity and palate carefully.* Use a spatula and light source.

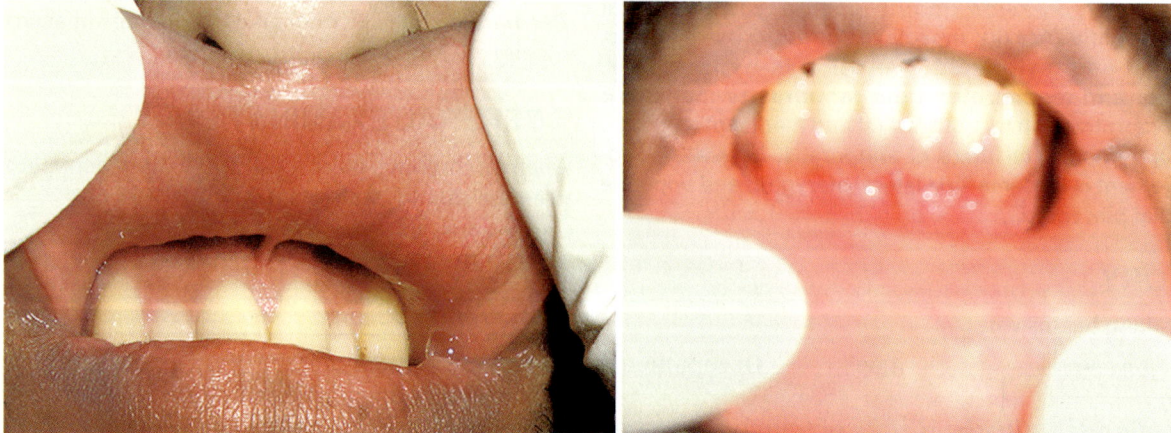

Fig. 12-3 Inspect alveolus by properly *retracting the lips.*

Palpation

Palpation is done initially over the outer surface then inside by wearing a glove. Tenderness over swelling, and fracture site (in mandible there is loss of continuity of lower border and crepitus) should be examined. Surface, consistency, tenderness, mobility, fixity should be ascertained while examining a swelling. Orbital margins of the maxilla should be palpated carefully on both sides for bone erosion, discontinuity, and swelling. Patient is asked to blow through one nostril while closing the other nostril. Free easier blowing means there is no nasal blockage. Only tenderness in the maxillary antrum along with purulent nasal discharge suggests sepsis in the antrum. Area adjacent to loose teeth should be palpated. *Dental cyst* arises from carious tooth; *dentigerous cyst* from unerupted tooth. Entire alveolar margin of both upper and lower jaw should be palpated. Body, angle and lower part of the ramus of the mandible should be palpated from outside and inside. **Bidigital palpation of mandible** is done by placing one finger inside the mouth and fingers of other hand are placed outside to feel tenderness, irregularity, fracture mandible, discrepancies, swelling, and thickening. It should be done on both sides for comparison **(Figs. 12-4 to 12-8).**

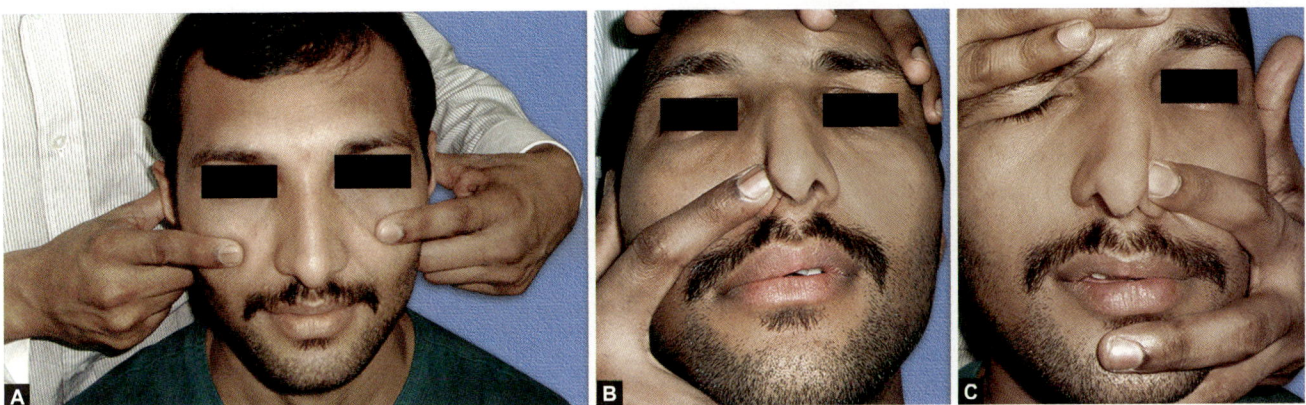

Figs. 12-4A to C *Eliciting the tenderness in maxilla and also checking the nasal blockage.*

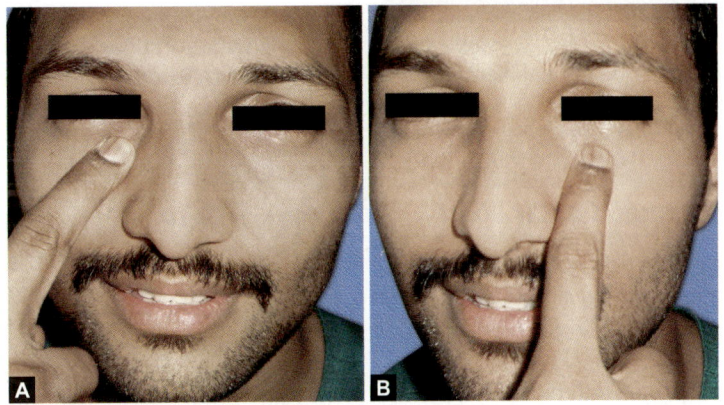

Figs. 12-5A and B Palpating inferior orbital margin for *tenderness or disruption.*

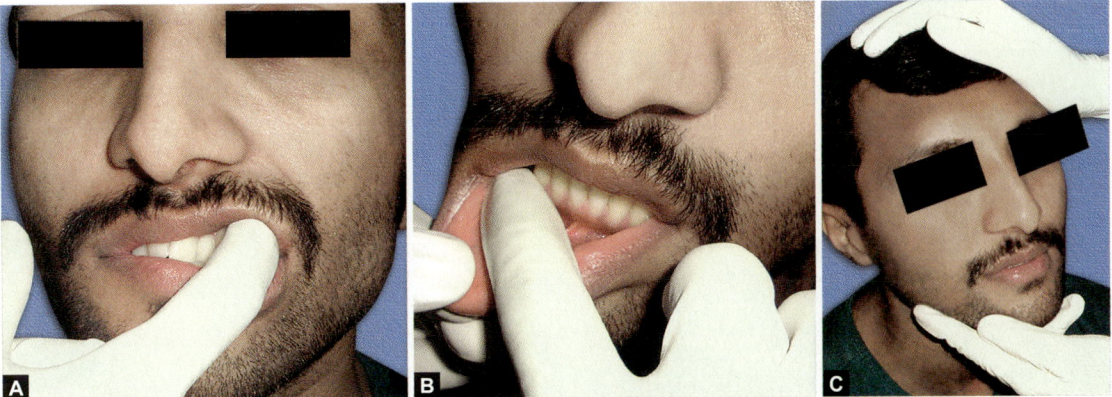

Figs. 12-6A to C *Palpating the alveolar margins of the jaw and lower margin of the mandible.*

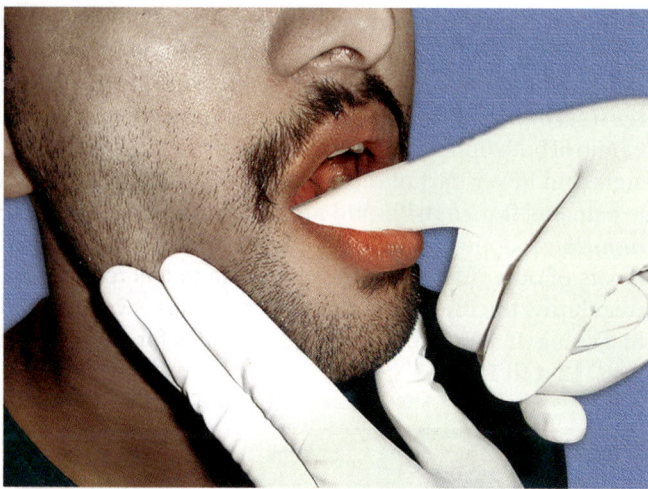

Fig. 12-7 *Bidigital palpation of jaw (mandible) is important.*

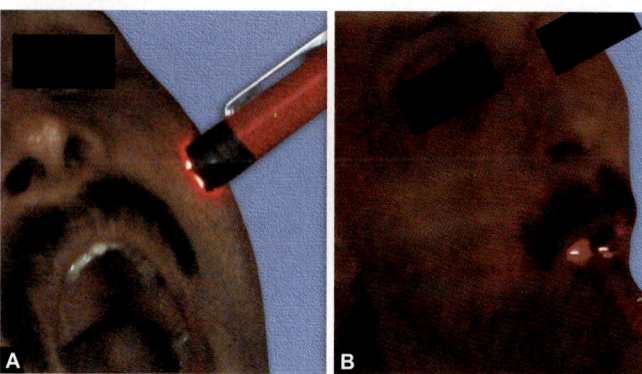

Figs. 12-8A and B *Transillumination of maxilla is done by two methods.* One is by illuminating the torch over the external surface of the maxilla in a darkroom. Another is by placing the tip of illuminating torch into the mouth and mouth is closed in a darkroom to see whether maxilla is transilluminating (normal) or not (pus or tumor).

Movements of the Temporomandibular Joint

Joint can be felt by placing *little finger* in the external auditory canal with pulp facing *forward* and asking the patient to open and close the mouth **(Figs. 12-9A to C)**. Condylar movements cannot be felt in dislocated TM joint. ***Dislocation*** can be unilateral or bilateral. Partially opened jaw with deviation towards opposite side and hollowness behind the dislocated condyle can be felt. In bilateral dislocation mouth is opened and fixed (*prognathous deformity*). In normal opening of the jaw the distance between upper and lower incisor teeth is 2.5 cm. Joint movement is also checked by placing fingers over the joint just below and in front of the tragus. **Crepitus** due to osteoarthritis; ***click*** due to loose bodies can also be felt. **Ankylosis of TM joint** causes restricted mouth opening. Osteoarthritis, fibrosis of soft tissues around (due to chronic ulcer, osteomyelitis mandible, cancrum oris) are the causes. It is often difficult to differentiate it from trismus. **Trismus** is due to muscular spasm (masseter and pterygoids) by inflammation (dental abscess, acute parotitis, partially erupted 3rd molar/wisdom tooth, pharyngeal, peritonsillar abscess); risus sardonicus of tetanus; oral malignancy infiltrating the soft tissues beneath. **Clicking of jaw** also occurs due to displacement of articular cartilage of the TM joint which is common in females. Patient with dislocation of temporomandibular joint presents with open mouth deformity with inability to close. When the mouth is opened widely like in yawning the jaw gets suddenly locked with a snap in the ear; and patient cannot close the mouth later. Later each time opening of mouth causes a click. A small hollow in front of tragus is formed due to dislocation of condyles. Clinical signs are less obvious in unilateral dislocation. The clinician should insert his little finger into the patient's external ear with pulp directed forwards. The condylar movements will not be felt on the side of dislocation when the patient is asked to open and close the mouth.

Sensation over the mental area, infraorbital region and other areas of trigeminal nerve should be checked when needed **(Figs. 12-10A and B)**.

Cervical lymph nodes should be palpated for significant enlargement **(Fig. 12-11)**.

INVESTIGATIONS FOR JAW DISEASE

1. **Orthopantomogram (OPG):** It is a plain X-ray of the mandible which shows the entire mandible and only partly maxilla in a single plane. It is better than X-ray mandible lateral view as it highlights proper dentition, inner and outer plates of mandible (Figs. 12-12A and B). It is a rotational tomogram. *Indications:* Jaw tumors—adamantinoma, dental cyst, dentigerous cyst, osteoclastoma; osteomyelitis of the mandible; fracture mandible; to see infiltration in carcinoma of oral cavity.

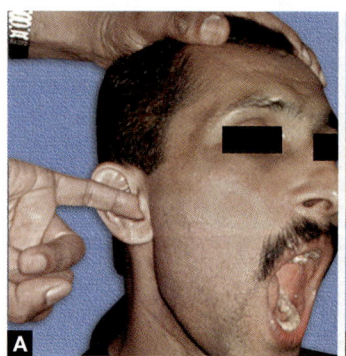
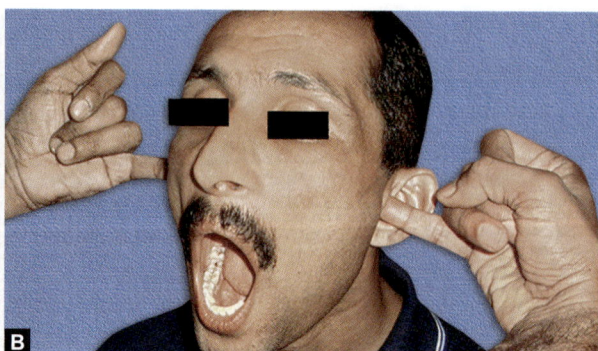
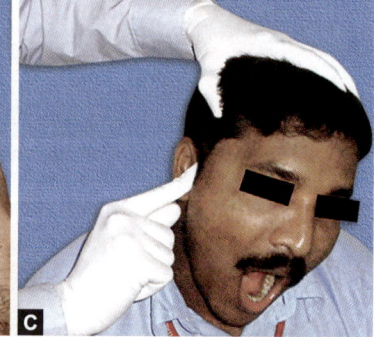

Figs. 12-9A to C *Temporomandibular joint movements* should be checked both by placing little finger inside and from outside the ear.

Chapter 12: Clinical Approach and Examination of Jaw

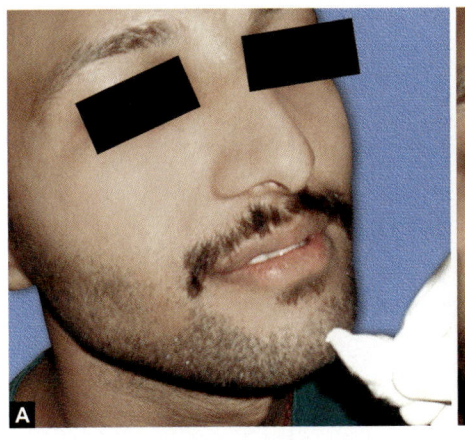
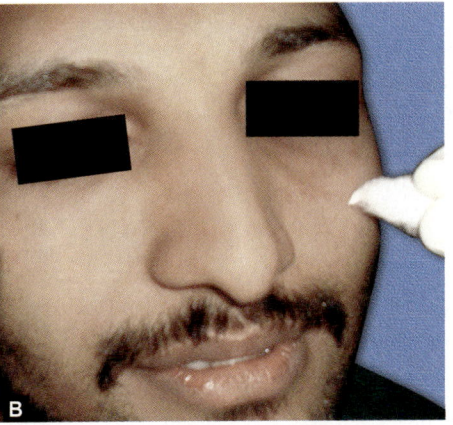

Figs. 12-10A and B *Sensation should be checked* using cotton over the mentum in lower jaw; over the infraorbital region in upper jaw.

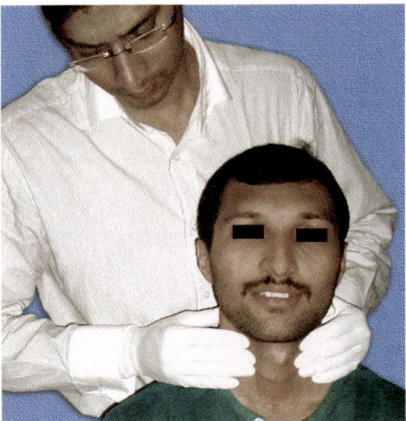

Fig. 12-11 *Cervical lymph nodes* should be palpated in jaw tumors.

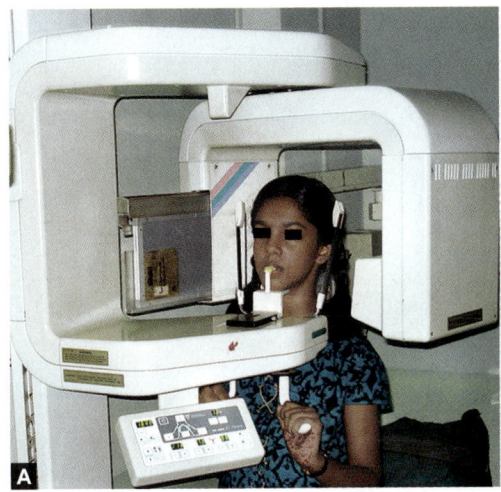
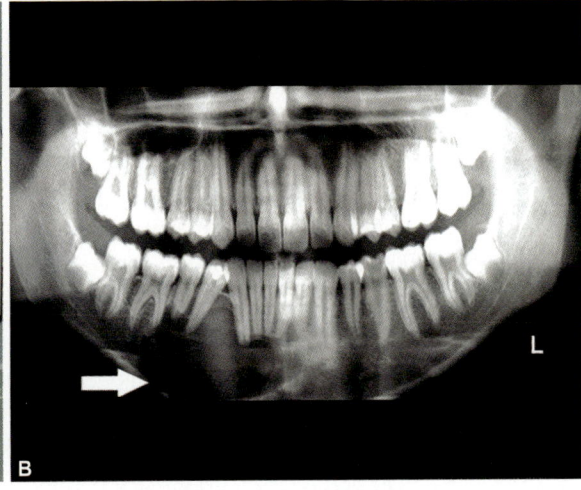

Figs. 12-12A and B *Orthopantomogram* being taken and X-ray OPG look.

2. Water's view for maxilla. It is very useful imaging method for maxilla.
3. CT scan of jaw including neck and base of skull in maxillary diseases, tumors, trauma to assess extent. Sinus endoscopy.
4. Biopsy, discharge study, for sulfur granules in actinomycosis, culture of discharge, FNAC of lymph node.
5. Anterior rhinoscopy for tumors over the medial wall of the maxilla.
6. Posterior rhinoscopy for tumor over the maxillary antrum.

Classification of jaw tumors		
Swelling arising from gums (*Epulis*)	Congenital epulis, fibrous epulis, pregnancy epulis, giant cell epulis, myelomatous epulis, sarcomatous epulis	
Swelling arising from the dental epithelium (*odontomes*)	*Benign:* • Epithelial—Ameloblastoma; calcifying odotogenic tumor; Odontogenic adenomatoid tumor; enameloma; composite odontoma • Mesodermal—Dontogenic fibroma, dentinoma, cementoma, myxoma	*Malignant:* Malignant ameloblastoma, Fibrosarcoma
Cysts arising in relation to dental epithelium	Dental cyst; dentigerous cyst	
Swelling arising from mandible/maxilla	*Benign*—Osteoma; osteoblastoma; fibrous dysplasia	*Malignant*—Osteosarcoma; osteoclastoma; secondaries
Surface tumors		
Maxillary antral tumors		

Upper jaw tumors (Fig. 12-13): Ivory osteoma, osteoclastoma, osteosarcoma, squamous cell carcinoma of maxillary antrum, carcinoma of hard palate are the examples

Lower jaw tumors (Fig. 12-14): Fibrous dysplasia is common in mandible as it develops partly from membrane. Paget's disease of jaw, osteoclastoma, oral malignancy infiltrating the mandible are common types

Section 1: Examination in General Surgery

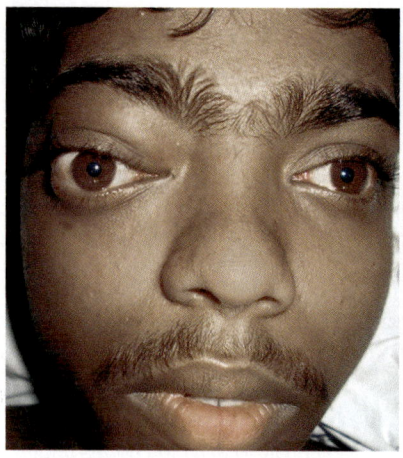
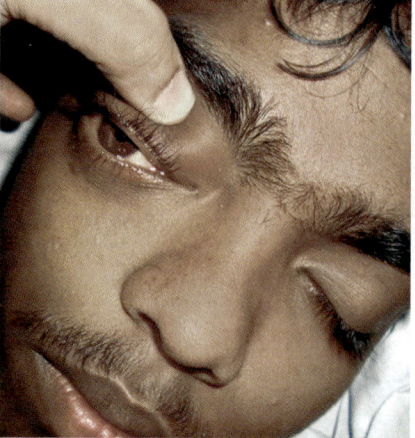

Fig. 12-13 *Upper jaw tumor*—from maxilla causing proptosis.

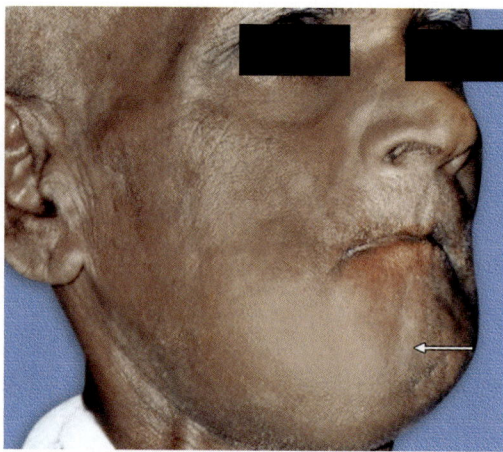

Fig. 12-14 *Lower jaw tumor*—could be adamantinoma mandible.

Maxillary Tumors (Fig. 12-15)

- They are rare. Maxillary sinus is the *commonest site* of malignancy in paranasal sinuses. Ethmoids, and sphenoids are next in order.
- It is common in people working in furniture industries, mustard gas industries, and leather industries. It is common in Bantus in South Africa where snuff with nickel and chromium is commonly used.
- Squamous cell carcinoma is the commonest type—80%. Adenocarcinoma, transitional cell carcinoma, salivary tumors, sarcomas, melanoma and Burkitt's lymphoma also can occur.
- *Behavior and presentation:* Initially may be asymptomatic or may present with *epistaxis or features of chronic sinusitis*. When it spreads to the floor, loosening of the teeth, swelling in the hard palate, necrosis, antro-oral fistula can occur. Extension medially causes nasal block, fungation, nasal discharge, blockage of nasolacrimal duct (epiphora). Extension anteriorly causes pain, anesthesia and swelling in the cheek, ulceration and fungation in the skin of cheek. Spread above into the orbit causes epiphora, diplopia, proptosis. *Posterior spread is most dangerous* as it is not revealed easily. It causes postnasal discharge,

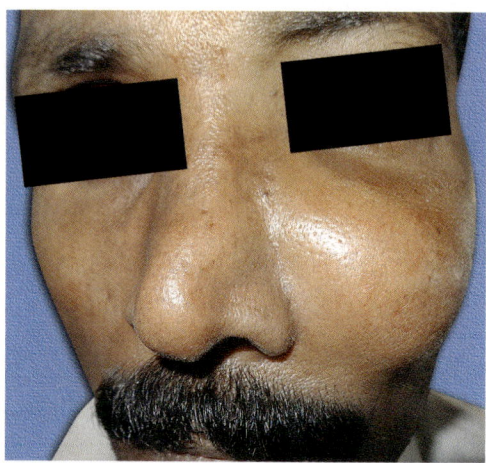

Fig. 12-15 Jaw tumor: *Left maxillary tumor*—presenting as swelling in upper jaw.

which is offensive and purulent, pain, trismus, limitation of movement of temporomandibular joint unrelieved tooth ache. Involvement of upper deep cervical lymph nodes in later stage is common.
- *Differential diagnosis:* Chronic sinusitis.

Epulis

Epulis	Features
a. **Congenital epulis:** Benign condition seen in newborn arising from gum pads; more common in girls	Well localized swelling from the gum, firm, bleeds on touch
b. **Fibrous epulis:** Benign swelling arising from periodontal membrane, commonest type of epulis, can occur in any individual	Painless, well localized, hard/elastic; sessile/rarely pedunculated; slow growing; gray-pink swelling arising from gums that bleeds on touch. Mimics squamous cell carcinoma. Recurrence can occur if root not removed properly. *Investigations:* OPG; biopsy
c. **Pregnancy epulis:** Occurs in pregnant women (3rd month) due to inflammatory gingivitis	Clinically resembles fibrous epulis/pyogenic granuloma that resolves spontaneously after delivery; if not has to be excised
d. **Granulomatous epulis:** Mass of granulation tissue in the gum around carious tooth	Soft, bright red swelling that bleeds on brushing
e. **Myelomatous epulis:** Seen in leukemic patients; other features of leukemia may be there	Investigation: Bone marrow aspiration; peripheral smear, biopsy

Contd...

Contd...

f. **Giant cell epulis:** Osteoclastoma causing ulceration and hemorrhage of gum	Painless expanding swelling in mandibular part
g. **Carcinomatous epulis:** Squamous cell carcinoma of alveolus and gum	Localized hard, indurated swelling, with ulceration
h. **Fibrosarcoma epulis:** Arising from fibrous tissue of gum	Variable consistency, soft, bluish red, progressive swelling that bleeds on touch
Swelling related to dental system and jaw bones	***Features***
Ameloblastoma (Adamantinoma, Eve's disease, multilocular cystic disease of jaw) Common in males in 5th decade. From mandible/maxilla or from the base of the skull in relation to Rathke's pouch. Arises from dental epithelium probably from enamel/dental lamina; can occur from pre-existing dentigerous cyst	Multilocular/can be unilocular. Unilateral; painless, progressive, smooth-hard swelling in the jaw; *inner table intact; outer table expanding*. Histologically basal cell carcinoma. OPG—*'honey comb'* appearance. Locally malignant, neither spread to lymph nodes nor through blood. *Curable with proper surgery.*
Dentigerous cyst (Follicular odontome) Common in *lower jaw in relation to pre-molar or molars* Common in younger age group Arises in relation to dental epithelium from an *unerupted permanent tooth;* Mimics dental cyst, adamantinoma, osteoclastoma	Solitary, unilocular, cystic, painless, smooth, hard swelling containing glairy viscid fluid; *egg shell crackling* as there is expansion of outer table of mandible. Histology: Enamel derived squamous cells. OPG: Well circumscribed translucent area with *soap-bubble/pseudo-trabecular* appearance with unerupted permanent tooth within it.
Dental cyst (Radicular cyst; Periapical cyst Common in adult; Common in *maxilla adjacent to incisor or canine* Develops as infective granuloma under the *root of chronically infected dead erupted tooth;* where there is epithelial proliferation which later gets degenerated to form a cyst filled with mucoid fluid with cholesterol crystals	Smooth, nontender localized swelling, in relation to caries tooth. OPG shows circular radiolucent area with sclerosed margin in relation to tooth
Solitary bone cyst: Occur in premolar or molar region of mandible	Rounded cyst, bulges outwards, contains yellowish fluid with high bilirubin content; bone resorption with bone deposition in the margin
Osteofying fibroma Common in young girls. Occurs exclusively in jaw bones	In upper jaw fills the maxillary antrum, and later present as localized external swelling. Growth is rapid initially, later ceases to grow X-ray- soft tissue shadow with scattered bone deposition
Fibrous dysplasia Common in females. Monostotic (common in long bones)/polyostotic (mandible commonly involved). Self-limiting disease where the medullary/spongy bone is replaced by fibro-osseous tissue **(Figs. 12-16A and B)**. Polyostotic fibrous dysplasia; pigmentation of the skin; precocious puberty in females is—*Albright's syndrome*	Bilateral, presenting as painless swelling in mandible of growing children; expansion of outer cortex with teeth normal. It is crab flesh in color; containing islands of cartilage and cystic spaces. X-ray shows typical are of *'smoke screen translucency'*. Treatment is done only after cessation of skeletal growth
Osteoclastoma (giant cell tumor) of mandible Giant cell tumor arising from epiphysis in young adults. Central part of jaw mandible common, can occur in maxilla also can be; benign/intermediate/malignant. Giant cells are due to fused spindle cells (not due to osteoclasts-misnomer). Giant cell epulis, brown tumor of hyperparathyroidism, dentigerous cyst and adamantinoma are differential diagnosis.	*Expanding swelling towards inner table of the mandible* with cystic spaces; egg shell crackling; discontinuity in inner table. Displaced roots of adjacent teeth, loose tooth common. When malignant can spread to lungs. X-ray, biopsy—investigations
Giant cell reparative granuloma (Jaffe tumor) Common in women. Swelling which occurs due to hemorrhage in the bonemarrow; contains vascular stroma, collagen and connective tissue cells	Painless enlargement of jaw. It is common in women It can be treated by calcitonin (100 units/0.5 mg subcutaneously daily for 12 months) or surgical curettage

Other Conditions of Jaw

Condition	Features
Burkitt's lymphoma Common in Africa; Common in pre-molar and molar area; Multifocal childhood lymphoma; Probably due to *Epstein-Barr virus*	Disease expands outwards involving cheek and soft tissue; lamina dura of teeth lost; neck nodes may enlarge; retroperitoneal mass, hepatomegaly, ovarian tumor, renal, adrenal, pancreatic, nodal involvement occur Spinal nerve involvement, breast, thyroid, bones, intracranial spread, cranial nerve palsies Histology: *Typical starry sky pattern*

Contd...

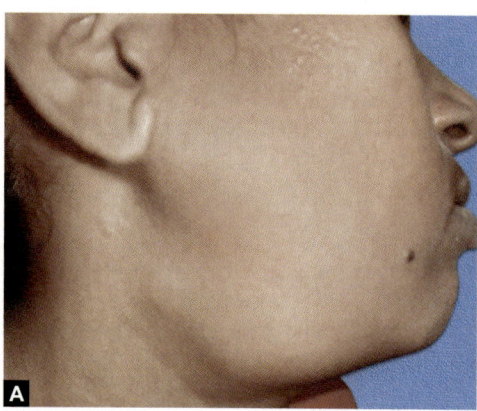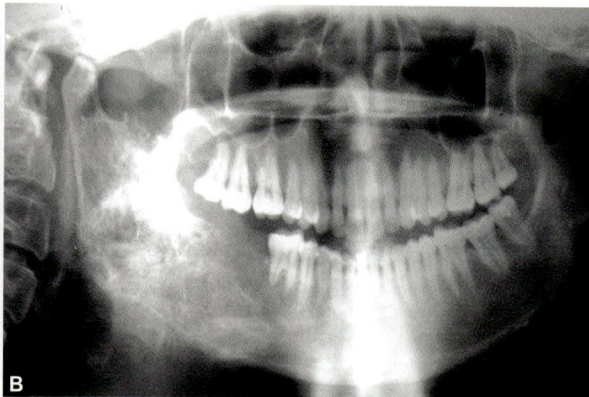

Figs. 12-16A and B *Fibrous dysplasia of mandible* (A) and X-ray picture (B).

Contd...

Alveolar abscess (Dental abscess) Commonest swelling of the jaw arising from the molar teeth of lower jaw; Due to spread of infection from the root of the tooth into the periapical tissues; Periapical abscess formed; initially spread into the cortical part of the soft tissues forming alveolar abscess **Complications:** Septicemia; Ludwig's angina; cavernous sinus thrombosis; chronic osteomyelitis of jaw; Submasseteric abscess; Lower incisor abscess can cause abscess in the chin and later median mental sinus	Diffuse initially later localized swelling with redness and edema of gum Initial pain is dull continuous, later becomes severe excruciating Fever, trismus, often dysphagia, palpable tender lymph nodes Edema, pain in the floor of mouth, swelling may burst outside to form sinus. Alveolar abscess in relation to upper incisor and molar will produce swelling medially not outside **X-ray:** Rarefaction of the root is visible only after 10 days
Osteomyelitis of jaw Can be in maxilla/mandible. **Types** a. **Acute:** Common in children; **Causes:** Alveolar abscess ; recurrent dental infection; trauma; after dental extraction; surgeries of jaw b. **Subacute** (commonest): Common in adults; common in mandible c. **Chronic:** Common in mandible; Chronic dental infection, apical abscess; postradiotherapy osteomyelitis; chemicals like phosphorus, tuberculosis, actinomycosis	Swelling, redness, fullness pus through the nostril if maxilla involved Pain, tenderness, bone irregularity and thickening, numbness over the chin due to compression of inferior dental nerve Pain, irregularity, thickening, discharging sinus, sequestrum in discharge; **X-ray**—osteomyelitis with new bone formation and sequestrum
Actinomycosis Faciocervical commonest; Lower jaw commonly involved; *Actinomycosis israelii* is the infective agent; Infection begins from infected tooth	Indurated gums, multiple discharging sinuses with yellowish sulphur granules in discharge
Cherubism (Cherub—Angelic Being) Autosomal dominant, occurring in first year of life; Commonly bilateral; Commonly seen in angles of mandible and also in maxilla; Giant cell granuloma with fibrous tissue in the jaw; Self-limiting disease	Diffuse enlargement of maxilla, both sides mandible; bulging of cheek pulls the lower eyelid down (babies apprear looking upwards—*winged shaped angelic babies*). Interferes with development and eruption of tooth
Treacher-Collins syndrome: Familial	Mandibulofacial dystosis; hypoplasia of zygomatic bone; and mandible; antimongoloid slant of palpebral fissure; coloboma of lower eyelid; low ear lobule; difficient middle ear
Micrognathism: Undue small mandible **Prognathism:** Mandible is larger than average with protrusion; maxilla is usually hypoplastic	Backward bending of tongue can cause respiratory distress

13

Clinical Approach and Examinations of Pharynx, Larynx, Nasal Cavities and Paranasal Sinuses

CHAPTER

Competency: AN30.1; AN30.2; AN33.2; AN33.4; AN33.5.

■ EXAMINATION OF PHARYNX

Pharynx has *got 3 parts—Nasopharynx; oropharynx; laryngopharynx.*

Nasopharynx is the uppermost part of pharynx situated behind the nose and above the lower border of the soft palate. Anteriorly it communicates with nasal cavities; inferiorly with *oropharynx* through nasopharyngeal isthmus (*Passavant's ridge*). Lateral wall contains opening of the auditory tube; tubal elevation; fossa of Rosenmuller/pharyngeal recess behind the tubal elevation. This is above the upper edge of superior constrictor. Roof continues as posterior wall of nasopharynx. Adjacent to base of occiput, nasopharynx contains lymphoid aggregates called *pharyngeal tonsil* which is small or absent in adults but well-developed in children and *pathologically* can be enlarged as adenoids. *Tubal tonsil* is collection of lymphoid tissue one on each side behind the tubal opening.

Oropharynx is middle part of the pharynx which communicates above to nasopharynx through nasopharyngeal isthmus, in front with the oral cavity through oropharyngeal isthmus (isthmus of fauces), below to laryngopharynx at the level of upper border of epiglottis. *Palatine tonsil* lies in tonsillar fossa in the lateral wall one on each side between palatopharyngeal arches (by palatopharyngeus muscle) behind, palatoglossus arch (palatoglossus muscle) in front. Tonsils are *seen per orally.* Oropharynx is formed behind by superior, middle and posterior constrictors of the pharynx.

Laryngopharynx or hypopharynx is laryngeal part of the pharynx that extends from the upper part of epiglottis above to lower margin of cricoid below. Anterior wall of hypopharynx shows laryngeal inlet, posterior surfaces of cricoid and arytenoids. Posterior wall is formed by constrictors. Middle constrictor overlaps the upper margin of inferior constrictor; superior constrictor overlaps middle constrictor in front (superficially). *Pyriform fossa* is located in the lateral wall of the pharynx as a depression on each side of the laryngeal inlet; bounded medially by aryepiglottic fold, laterally by thyroid cartilage and thyrohyoid membrane. *Carcinoma pyriform fossa* may be silent; or present as difficulty in swallowing saliva as opposed to food, later definitive dysphagia, change in voice, laryngeal fixation (as late feature) or palpable significant cervical lymph nodes. It is beyond reach for digital examination. Laryngeal mirror is essential to visualize and examine it. *Sideropenic dysphagia* and *post-cricoid carcinoma* can also occur.

Examination of Oropharynx

Inspection: It is done under proper illumination either with a torch/head mirror. The head is steadied by the nurse from behind and mouth is widely opened. **Oropharynx is examined** using two spatulas. Tongue is depressed with one spatula and with another cheek is retracted laterally with its tip gently compressing the anterior pillar of the fauces. Tonsillar crypts, size, surface, discharge, surrounding areas should be examined. In adults, tonsils are atrophied and small. But in children, tonsils are often enlarged so much that both sides touch in the midline (*'kissing tonsils'*). Tubercles in the tonsils may be obvious. In peritonsillar abscess, soft palate is grossly inflamed, uvula edematous, swollen and pushed to opposite side. Any ulceration, growth, swelling (retropharyngeal abscess), granulation (pharyngitis), discharge over posterior wall is observed.

Palpation: The anterior pillar of tonsil is pressed with spatula. Type and quantity of discharge is noted. Cheesy white discharge is not of significance, whereas in septic tonsillitis, pus is seen coming out of the crypts.

Ear pain, halitosis, blood stained saliva, hemorrhage, ulceration, fungation, dysphagia, trismus, palpable significant neck lymph nodes are features of carcinoma of tonsils. Lymphosarcoma may develop in the tonsil in young individuals. Painless swelling in throat, thick speech, large pale tonsil are the initial features of lymphosarcoma of tonsil. Extracapsular spread may cause a palpable and often visible swelling behind and below the angle of the mandible as a direct extension of the primary tumor. But sooner cervical lymph nodes get involved in same place as secondaries and become palpable.

Examination of Nasopharynx

Nasopharynx is palpated with patient sitting on a stool. Examiner stands behind the patient with patient extending his neck and head which is supported by examiner's body **(Fig. 13-1)**. After opening the mouth one side index finger pushes the cheek inward from outside (to prevent biting of the examiner's hand). Index finger of the other hand is passed inside, behind the soft palate towards nasopharynx to sweep over the roof (for adenoids) and walls of the nasopharynx (for nasopharyngeal carcinoma). Posterior pharyngeal wall is palpated for retropharyngeal abscess which is felt and only often seen after proper depression of the tongue (can be seen when inspected using a direct laryngoscope). It is felt as an indentable cushion like projection to the finger. Acute retropharyngeal abscess is usually due to retropharyngeal lymph node suppuration and occupies a lateral position. Chronic retropharyngeal abscess is usually due to tuberculosis of cervical spine (C6) and is behind the prevertebral fascia and so situated in midline. However, occasionally tuberculosis of retropharyngeal lymph nodes can occur as a rare entity and in such situation, it will be in lateral position. It also may present as swelling/cold abscess in the neck behind the sternomastoid muscle. Back of the tongue is palpated for growth.

Diseases of Pharynx

Tonsillitis: It is common in children and young adults. *Clinical features*: Sore throat, pain on swallowing. Tonsils are enlarged, congested; studded with multiple yellow spots with pus extruding from the crypts. The faucial pillar, soft palate are red and congested. When both tonsils are enlarged and meet in midline (kissing tonsil), dyspnea, and dysphagia may occur. In septic tonsillitis, pus may be squeezed out of the tonsil with severe constitutional symptoms. Regional lymph nodes are enlarged and tender. In chronic tonsillitis, where there are repeated acute attacks, tonsils are congested; thin creamy pus comes out on pressure. Cervical lymph nodes are enlarged but not tender.

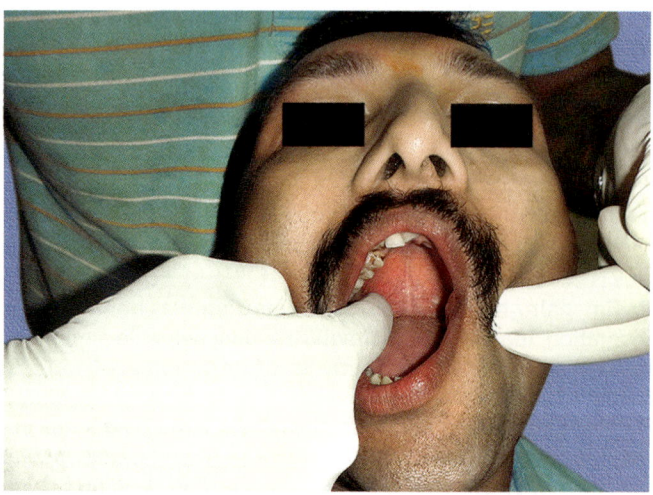

Fig. 13-1 Palpation of nasopharynx *from behind*.

Peritonsillar abscess: Collection of pus between tonsillar capsule and lateral pharyngeal wall following an attack of acute tonsillitis. Here patient is toxic and presents with painful swallowing, fever and trismus. Anterior faucial pillar is red, edematous, swollen along with soft palate which is also edematous, displacing the uvula to opposite side. Regional lymph nodes are enlarged and tender.

Carcinoma tonsil: Rare, seen in old age and unilateral. Presents with severe pain in throat referred to ear due to infiltration of glossopharyngeal nerve, dysphagia, fetor oris, bleeding and enlarged lymph nodes are the features.

Pharyngitis: Severe sore throat with signs of inflammation; pharyngeal mucosa is hyperemic, red, and edematous with enlarged lymph nodes. Patient may be toxic with high fever, associated laryngeal inflammation may be present.

Nasopharyngeal carcinoma: Nasopharynx lies above the level of the soft palate which separates it from oropharynx below. It is also called post-nasal space or epipharynx. Eustachian tube opens on its anterolateral wall. Fossa of Rosenmuller is located above and behind the opening of the Eustachian tube as a small depression. Clinical features: Epistaxis, nasal speech, post-nasal discharge and nasal obstruction; pain in the ear with unilateral deafness due to compression of Eustachian tube with fluid collection in the middle ear; elevation and immobility of soft palate on the same side; pain in the area of distribution of trigeminal nerve due to direct infiltration of the nerve at foramen lacerum; palpable secondaries in upper deep cervical lymph nodes (70%). *Trotter's triad*: Unilateral deafness; immobile elevated soft palate; pain in the distribution of trigeminal nerve. Nasopharyngeal carcinoma is common in China, Taiwan, Hongkong and Mongolia. It is rare in USA. In India, it is common in North East region. It is common in males (2:1). It may be related to Epstein–Barr virus. It is commonly squamous cell carcinoma (85%). Lymphoma, minor salivary tumors and sarcoma are other malignancies that can occur rarely in nasopharynx. Lymphoepithelioma of nasopharynx is called as *Schmincke/Regaud tumor*. Carcinoma can be of proliferative, ulcerative, and infiltrative types. Commonest site is fossa of Rosenmuller in lateral wall of pharynx. It is three times common in males. *HO's triangle* in supraclavicular fossa (bounded by medial and lateral ends of clavicle and point where neck meets the shoulder) is the site where metastatic nodes commonly exist in nasopharyngeal carcinoma. In 50% of cases, nodal involvement is bilateral. Often cervical lymphadenopathy may be the first presentation. Clinical features may be nasal, otogenic, ophthalmoneurogenic (involving most of the cranial nerves with facial pain, squint, diplopia, exophthalmos, and ophthalmoplegia), jugular foramen syndrome (cranial nerves IX, X, XI involvement), nodal spread and distant spread to bones, lungs and liver. Unilateral serous otitis media may be the only presentation.

EXAMINATION OF LARYNX

External Examination

The position of the prominent thyroid cartilage, 'Adam's apple' is noted. It may be shifted to right or left.

Internal Examination

It is done under local anesthetic spray with help of laryngoscope. Good illumination is necessary which is provided by a head lamp or head mirror.

Indirect laryngoscopy (ILS): Examiner sits in front of the patient, who sits upright with head bent slightly forward. Patient opens the mouth widely, any artificial denture, if present, is removed. Local anesthetic spray is used to anesthetize the posterior pharyngeal wall to suppress the gag reflex. The patient is asked to protrude the tongue out which is gently pulled out with a gauze. Meanwhile with one finger, upper lip should be raised. The light is reflected to the pharynx from head mirror. The laryngeal mirror is warmed prior to introducing into the mouth to prevent fogging of the mirror by the breath. It is passed into the posterior aspect of mouth, placed firmly but gently on the soft palate just above the base of the uvula. By tilting the head mirror, the light is directed on various parts of larynx and hypopharynx but the mirror placed on the soft palate should not be moved, as the patient may 'gag' or close the mouth. The reflected light from the head mirror is focused on the laryngeal mirror to visualize the posterior aspect of the mouth as follows in succession—back of the tongue, vallecula, epiglottis, posterior aspect of arytenoids and aryepiglottic fold, vocal cord, pyriform fossa, tracheal rings. Epiglottis is observed as pinkish white margin, overhangs the interior of larynx. Any redness, swelling, ulcer, edema, excess secretion in this region are observed. Aryepiglottic folds and arytenoids should appear smooth, symmetrical and more pink than epiglottis. Smooth glistening, ivory white colored vocal cord should be observed for any congestion, ulceration, papilloma, growth over its edges. Papilloma occurs in children, carcinoma in elderly people over the anterior half of vocal cord **(Figs. 13-2A and B)**.

Movement of the vocal cords: Patient is asked to utter 'E' while the movement of the vocal cord is observed for adduction movement. On quite inspiration, they move outwards to a small extent and on expiration, they move in again but do not reach the midline. Full abduction movement is seen in deep inspiration. Phonation brings the cords together. In bilateral paralysis of cord, they remain immobile in cadaveric position (midway between adduction/abduction). In unilateral paralysis: the affected cord remains immobile in cadaveric position or may sometimes cross the midline.

Direct laryngoscopy: Direct laryngoscopy allows direct visualization of the inlet of the larynx clearly. It is also useful in identifying the movements of the vocal cord **(Fig. 13-3)**.

Neck lymph node examination: Cervical lymph nodes are examined for enlargement as in metastasis:

Systemic examination: Respiratory system is examined for any evidence of tuberculosis/secondaries.

Diseases of Larynx

Edema of glottis: Causes: (1) *Traumatic:* Chemical irritation by corrosives and noxious gases, accidental trauma, irradiation. (2) Spread of infection from surrounding structures like pharynx and larynx. (3) Angioneurotic edema. (4) Renal/cardiac failure. Patient presents with hoarseness of voice and dyspnea.

Vocal nodules: It occurs due to localized hypertrophy of the fibrous element of the edge of the vocal cord. Often bilateral; caused by voice abuse, common in singers, teachers; present with hoarseness of voice or tiredness while speaking.

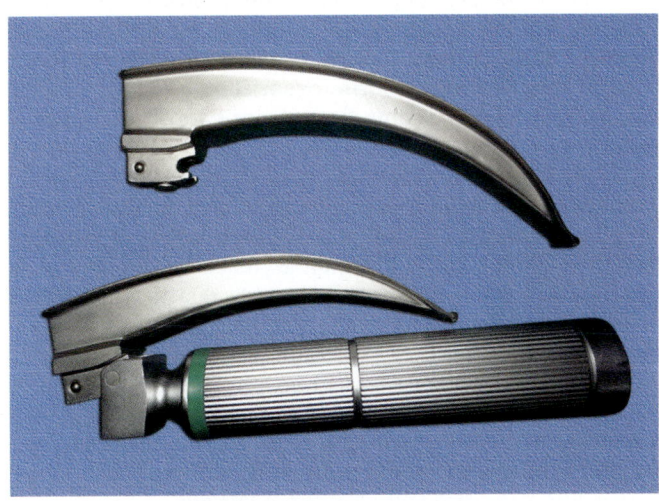

Fig. 13-3 *Direct laryngoscope.*

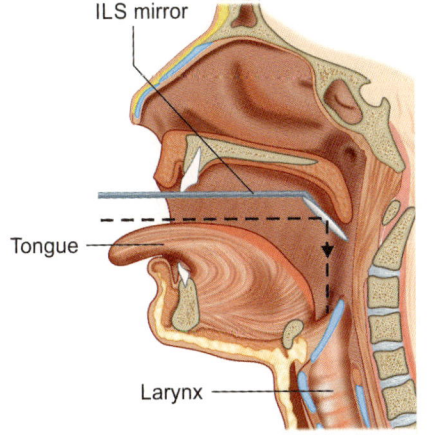
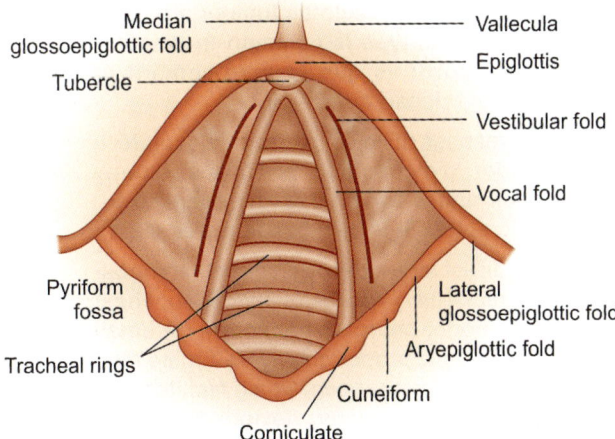

Figs. 13-2A and B (A) *Indirect laryngoscopy* being done; (B) View of the vocal apparatus through the mirror.

Vocal polyp: It is a smooth glistening structure attached to one cord, often pedunculated and may involve entire length of both vocal cords.

Papilloma: More often in children, viral etiology, always multiple, frequently extends into trachea and bronchi. Often presents with hoarseness. Spontaneous regression do can occur before puberty.

Laryngeal Carcinoma

Etiology: Smoking, tobacco, alcohol intake, occupational/industrial exposure to chemicals like mustard gas, asbestos, benzopyrones, petroleum products, previous radiation, genetic Russians develop familial laryngeal cancers, papilloma virus, herpes simplex virus, EB virus, keratosis and malnutrition.

Incidence: Squamous cell carcinoma is commonest (95%); common in males (10:1); common in 5th/6th decade.

Types: Ulcerative; Proliferative.

Anatomical Types: *Supraglottic (25%):* It arises from infrahyoid part of epiglottis, ventricles, and arytenoids. It spreads to neck lymph nodes early (40%) due to rich lymphatics in this area. Throat pain, dysphagia, palpable neck nodes and referred pain are common features. Hoarseness of voice, loss of weight, respiratory obstruction, and halitosis are late features. Carcinoma in epiglottis causes bilateral nodal spread. Local spread occurs to vallecula, base of tongue and pyriform fossa. *Glottic (65%):* It is the commonest type. It begins from upper part or free edge of vocal cords (mid or anterior) often extending 10 mm below. Lymphatic spread is slow (only 4%) as this area has got least lymphatics. Opposite vocal cord can involve as 'kiss cancer'. Vocal cord mobility is unaffected in early cases. Vocal cord fixation signifies spread to thyroarytenoid which is a poor prognostic sign. It presents very early due to hoarseness of voice. Eventual cord fixation causes stridor. Locally it spreads anteriorly to anterior commissure, posteriorly to vocal process and arytenoids, above to ventricle and false vocal cords, below to subglottis. *Subglottic (2%)* is less common involving undersurface of true vocal cords and subglottic space. It spreads to deep cervical and paratracheal nodes (20%). Upward spread is rather late and so hoarseness is not an early symptom in this type. It can spread through cricothyroid membrane or thyroid gland.

Note: In Indian subcontinent, supraglottic tumors are more common than glottic. Glottic type is common in Western countries. Fixation of cords is due to involvement of thyroarytenoid muscle or cricoarytenoid joint.

Clinical Features: Hoarseness of voice; pain and discomfort; cough; dyspnea, stridor, dysphagia in late cases; bloody sputum; palpable neck nodes, which eventually get fixed; absence of laryngeal crepitus. It is common in males (10:1).

Investigations: ILS (Indirect laryngoscopy); direct laryngoscopy and biopsy; CT neck—*very useful investigation;* chest X-ray; FNAC of lymph node; microlaryngoscopy in small lesions to identify and to have proper biopsy; toluidine blue staining to stain early superficial cancers which facilitate the accurate biopsy; Hopkin's endoscopy; flexible, fiberoptic laryngoscopy.

EXAMINATION OF NASAL CAVITIES AND PARANASAL AIR SINUSES

Nasal Cavity

Inspection

The outer surface of the nose is observed for any swelling or ulcer. Any deformity due to deviated nasal septum, or depressed nasal bridge is noted. In rhinophyma, the tip of the nose is enlarged. In lupus vulgaris, there may be ulceration and destruction of the nose. Alae nasi are observed for its movements which collapse on inspiration when there is nasal obstruction. By lifting the tip of the nose, the vestibule, inferior turbinate, anterior part of nasal septum is observed. Any nasal polyp if present is observed.

Anterior rhinoscopy: It is done with the help of **Thudicum's speculum** under bright light. The speculum is held with left hand and inserted into the nasal cavity with the blades closed. It is gently opened to dilate the nostril. The structures that are observed are anterior part of nasal septum, anterior part of inferior and middle turbinates with their corresponding meatus, anterior part of floor of the mouth.

- The mucous membrane is observed for its color (normally pink, pale in anemia, bright red in acute rhinitis); texture (normally moderately wet, but excessive wet in rhinitis and dry in atrophic rhinitis).
- Change in shape of the septum—may be deviated to one side producing 'C/S' shaped deformity; the side to which deviation has occurred, whether it is anterior/posterior; whether obstructing, the cavity markedly is noted.
- Bony/cartilaginous spur may be seen along the upper border.
- Anterior ends of the turbinates (inferior/ middle) are observed for color, membrane covering them (smooth/rough).
- Polyp may be present (often hypertrophied turbinates are mistaken for polyps).
- Ulcer may be present.
- The nasal secretion which is normally clear and mucoid can turn out to be pucopus/pus when there is suppuration in the sinuses.

The middle meatus is observed for any pus suggestive of suppuration in maxillary/frontal/anterior ethmoidal sinuses. Pus between middle turbinate and septum suggests suppuration of the posterior group of ethmoidal sinuses.

Posterior rhinoscopy: Patient is asked to open the mouth. Posterior pharynx is anesthetized by spraying lignocaine. The tongue is depressed with a spatula. Postnasal mirror is inserted after prior warming into the mouth and placed between the uvula and posterior pharyngeal wall. The light is focused over the mirror. The structures that are observed are posterior end of nasal septum is seen as a white pillar, posterior nares, posterior aspect of superior/middle/inferior turbinates, posterior aspect of superior and middle meati, adenoid (over upper posterior wall of nasopharynx), opening of Eustachian tube. Any ulcer, growth, antrochoanal polyp if present is

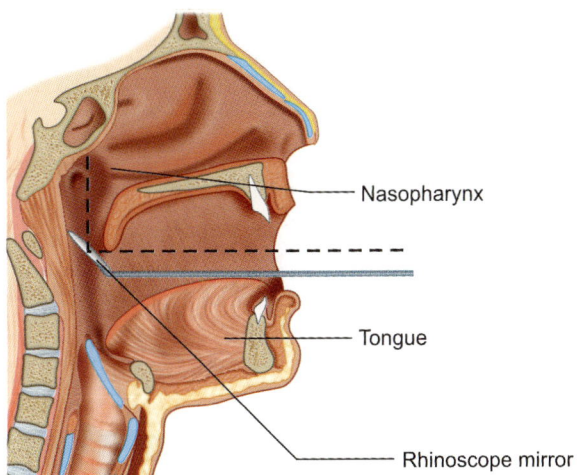

Fig. 13-4 *Posterior rhinoscopy.*

observed. Any pus or secretion in relation to turbinates is observed **(Fig. 13-4).**

Palpation

External surface of nose and sinuses are palpated for tenderness. To elicit tenderness in frontal sinusitis, finger tip is insinuated beneath the roof of the orbit with pressure directed upwards.

Examination of Paranasal Sinuses

Transillumination test for maxillary sinus: It is carried out in a dark room. A torch is inserted into the mouth of the patient and pressed against the middle of the hard palate. Patient is asked to close the mouth. Normally a cherry red glow is seen on either side of the face with crescentic fold of infraorbital margin.

The torch may be placed near the gum-line medial to the last upper molar on each side directed towards the sinus and glow on both sides are compared. Alternatively, the penlight may be placed externally at the inferior portion of each orbit, and the glow may be observed through the palate. It should be obvious that the patient's dentures must be removed. The transillumination results may be reported as opaque, dull, or normal. A unilaterally opaque maxillary sinus is always abnormal. Absence of infraorbital crescent, absence of glow through the lower fornix of conjunctiva, absence of transmission of light through the cheek, all indicate negative transillumination often seen in maxillary sinusitis where there is pus in the sinus with swollen mucous membrane or growth in the maxillary sinus. Fallacies in this test occur due to variation in the bone thickness, asymmetrical development of the sinuses **(Refer Chapter 12: Examination of Jaw).**

Transillumination test for frontal sinus: Torch is placed against the inner corner of the orbit.

Postural test: It helps to find out the definite source of pus when presents in middle meatus. The patient sits upright and the pus is wiped out. Decongestive drug is applied. If pus appears immediately then it comes from frontal sinus, if it comes after some period of time, it is from ethmoidal sinus (anterior/posterior); if the pus comes only when head is bent forward with suspected site above, then it is from maxillary sinus.

Lymph nodes: Submandibular and upper deep cervical nodes should be examined.

Diseases of Nasal Cavity and Paranasal Sinuses

Fracture of nasal bone: Occurs more often, due to blow upon the nose. Two types—depressed fracture and lateral fracture. Hematoma often conceals the fracture. Often careful palpation will reveal it. Nose often looks crooked with history of bleeding from nose after trauma.

Hematoma of nasal septum: Blood is collected under mucoperichondrium, often due to injury but sometimes spontaneous or after trivial trauma in patients with bleeding disorder. Patient often complains of headache. Mouth is held open; nostrils splayed, anterior end of nose widened. Due to stretching, the nasal tip may look pale with blunted sensation over that area due to pressure over anterior ethmoidal nerve. If the hematoma is not evacuated in time, it can lead to necrosis of underlying cartilage. When infected, leads to abscess. Patient presents with fever, throbbing pain and feeling of fullness over the nose, swelling over the nose that has extended onto face.

Septal deviation: It may be traumatic/developmental in origin where the septum is deviated to one or the other side. It may involve upper/lower part of the septum. It may be—cartilaginous/bony. Presents with uni/bilateral nasal obstruction and headache.

Foreign body in nose: Common in children, can be in the form of pebbles, shirt buttons, peas, rubber. Often presents with unilateral obstruction with purulent discharge. In adults, they take the form of rhinoliths, where deposits of calcium over pieces of gauze or other substances are seen. Over considerable period of time, these rhinoliths cause atrophy of mucous membrane.

Rhinosporidiosis: It is caused by *Rhinosporidium seeberi*, a yeast like organism, that gives rise to fleshy nasal polyps having a 'strawberry appearance', over the septum and floor of the nose. Patient complains of nasal obstruction with purulent bloodstained discharge.

Sinusitis: It is an inflammation of the mucous membrane of the sinus; often it is an extension of nasal infection caused by viral followed by secondary bacterial infection. The mucous membrane is thick, polypoidal and edematous in early stage, but in later stage, it becomes similar to granulation tissue. The sinus cavity is filled with pus. Patient presents with temperature, headache, and tenderness over the sinuses.

Maxillary sinusitis: Patient experiences aching over the antrum and over the upper teeth, tenderness in the region of canine fossa.

Frontal sinusitis: Tenderness over the floor of the sinus, tapping over the frontal region may be painful.

Ethmoidal sinusitis: Deep seated headache behind the eyes with tenderness in the region of the inner canthus.

14 CHAPTER

Clinical Approaches and Examination of Salivary Glands

Competency: SU21.1; SU21.2; AN28.10; AN34.1; AN34.2.

Salivary gland diseases are not uncommon. It needs meticulous clinical and surgical approaches to treat many of the salivary gland diseases like sialadenitis, neoplasms otherwise may lead into complications.

Parotid and submandibular salivary glands are commonly involved with different diseases. Acute parotitis like mumps is common in parotid gland. Calculous sialadenitis (formation of stone/stones in submandibular salivary gland with chronic or acute or chronic inflammation) is common in submandibular salivary gland. Neoplasms can occur in both parotid and submandibular salivary glands even though they are much more common in parotid. Tumors are rare in sublingual and minor salivary glands.

■ HISTORY

Name:
Address: Mumps (viral parotitis) can occur as epidemic.
Age:
Sex: Warthin's tumor (adenolymphoma) is commonly seen in males after 40 years of age. Carcinoma parotid is usually equal in both sexes.

History of Presenting Complaints

Swelling: Site and mode of onset, where exactly it started and how it progressed should be asked. Duration, progress, recent increase in size should be asked. Swelling of short duration with pain, trismus could be due to acute parotitis. Pleomorphic adenoma is slow growing tumor of long duration (**Fig. 14-1**). Recent increase in size of swelling is important which suggests malignant transformation probably from a pre-existing pleomorphic adenoma. Adenolymphoma is slow growing tumor from lower pole of the parotid. Often it is bilateral in children due to viral cause (mumps). Bilateral enlargement of parotid along with other salivary glands and

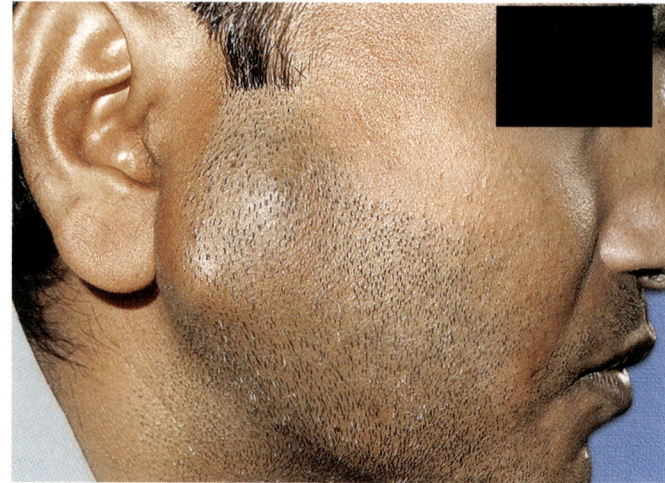

Fig. 14-1 *Typical parotid tumor.* Commonly, it is pleomorphic adenoma.

lacrimal gland is called as **Mikulicz syndrome**. Dry eyes, joint pain along with enlargement of all salivary glands is called as **Sjögren syndrome**. Recurrent painful swelling in the glands during meals is seen in the obstruction of duct by stone (calculi). Sometimes more than one salivary glands (parotid and submandibular both) (**Fig. 14-2**) or both sides are involved; then which gland was involved first should be asked for. Warthin's tumor is often bilateral. Swelling in the submandibular region which increases in size during meals and also becomes painful is probably submandibular salivary gland swelling; it could be due to submandibular sialadenitis, a inflammatory condition. Neoplasm also can occur in submandibular salivary gland (*Enlarged submandibular lymph node is also located in the same site but it is differentiated from submandibular salivary gland as lymph nodes are not bidigitally palpable*) (**Figs. 14-3 and 14-4**).

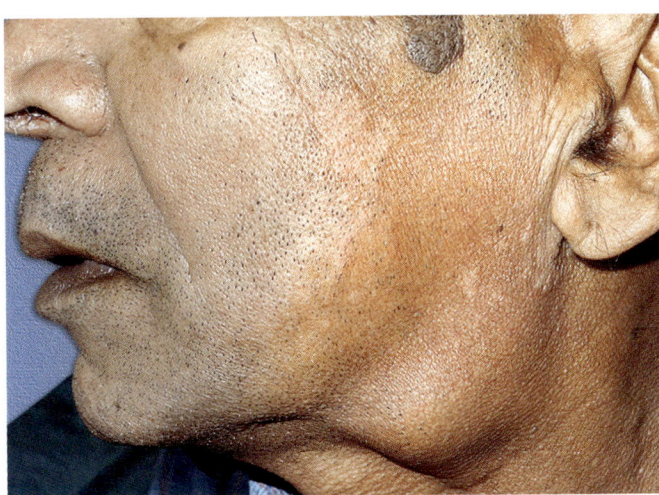

Fig. 14-2 *Submandibular salivary gland tumor.*

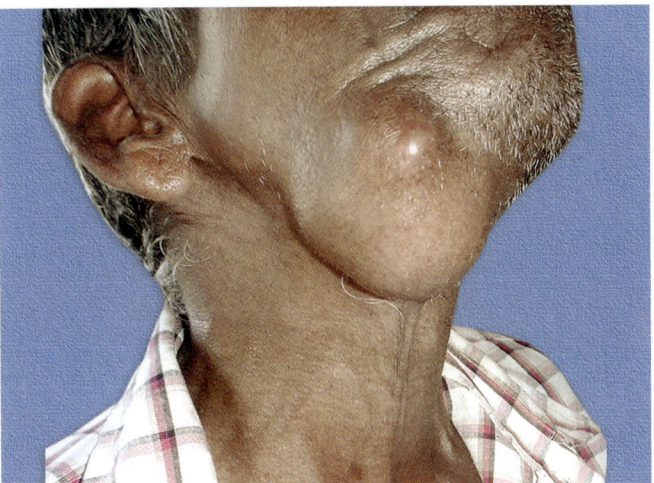

Fig. 14-4 *Submandibular salivary gland tumor.* Here oral cavity should be examined for deep lobe (bidigitally with one finger in the floor of the mouth); Wharton's duct (on either side of the frenulum of tongue); mandibular bone for thickening; hypoglossal nerve and lingual nerve palsy; neck nodes for spread.

Pain: Duration, type, severity, radiation should be asked for. Sudden onset of severe pain is a feature of acute parotitis. Throbbing excruciating pain may be a feature of parotid abscess. Colicky pain during meals is a feature of salivary calculus with sialadenitis ***(Salivary colic)***. Stone is more common in submandibular salivary gland but can also occur in parotid gland. Swelling, which was initially painless and now become painful suggest malignant transformation of the pre-existing tumor.

Fever—It is a feature of acute sialadenitis or abscess. Acute sialadenitis with suppuration is common in parotid. Parotid abscess is usually unilateral. Mumps in children is bilateral. Neoplastic condition, once necrosed can cause fever.

Difficulty in opening mouth (***trismus***): It can occur in acute parotitis, submandibular sialadenitis, and malignancy extending into the soft tissues.

History of excess salivation during meals/more pain during meals/swelling becoming more prominent during meals should be asked. It is a feature of stone in the salivary duct. Excessive secretion of saliva is called as ***ptyalism***; it may be due to stomatitis, reflex irritation of the trigeminal nerve (5th) due to carious teeth, ill-fitting dental plate, foreign body impacted to the gum, ulcerative oral growth or due to drugs like mercury, iodides, bromides, arsenic, etc.

History of discharge from sinus and fistula: Its formation, discharge, etc. should be asked. Discharge from sinus/fistula is usually saliva. Its quantity, duration, color, whether increases while taking food should be clarified. Parotid fistula can occur after parotid surgery like incision and drainage or parotidectomy. Discharge may occur at the opening of the parotid (Stenson's) or submandibular (Wharton's) duct due to sialadenitis; it may be purulent or watery or infected fluid. Here discharge increases during meals **(Figs. 14-5A to C)**.

History of impairment of function like drooling of saliva, inability to close eyes, tears in the eye, asymmetry of face, difficulty in opening of the mouth should be asked which are all features, suggestive of facial nerve palsy which may have started in relation to the swelling (how long after the appearance of the swelling these features are started should be noted).

History suggestive of metastases in case of malignant salivary tumors like of lungs, bone and brain is noted.

Along with the enlargement of the major salivary glands if simultaneous enlargement of lacrimal gland is present, then ***Mikulicz syndrome*** should be suspected. Along with this if there is dry *conjunctiva (sicca)* and multiple joint pains (polyarthritis), then it is called as ***Sjögren's syndrome.***

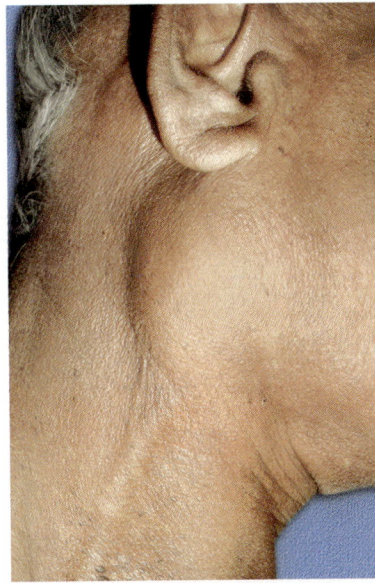

Fig. 14-3 Typical parotid swelling—*pleomorphic adenoma.*

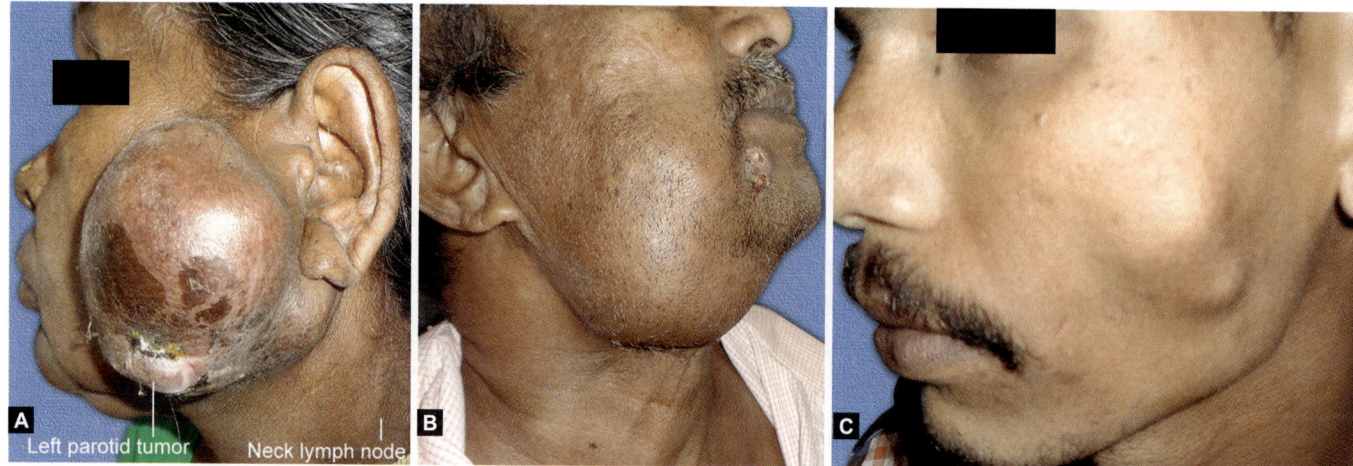

Figs. 14-5A to C (A) Left sided malignant parotid tumour with skin involvement and nodal spread; (B) Right submandibular salivary gland tumor with skin involvement; (C) Left accessory parotid (social parotidis) gland tumor.

Past History

History of surgery for parotid or submandibular swellings should be asked. Recurrent parotid tumors are known to occur in pleomorphic adenoma and malignancies. Detailed history of surgery, evaluation methods, postoperative management should be taken. Past history of radiotherapy in head and neck region; past history of other malignancy in the body should be asked for.

History of recent illness or major surgery may be evident in acute parotitis. History of exposure to HIV (HIV associated sialadenitis) is important.

Personal History

History of alcohol intake, diabetes mellitus, endocrine disorders, bulimia (eating disorder), drug intake (antihistaminics, guanethidine) is relevant in bilateral parotid enlargement.

GENERAL EXAMINATION

It is carried out in usual way. Temperature, pulse rate, hydration of tongue, xerostomia, trismus, blood pressure should be checked. One should remember that suppurative parotitis especially in immunosuppressed individuals can cause septicemia and patient may be in septic shock; along with that dysphagia, breathlessness may also be evident. Such patient may require ICU care and occasionally tracheostomy may be warranted.

LOCAL EXAMINATION

Examination of Parotid Gland

Inspection

Swelling is examined in detail. It may be unilateral/bilateral; single/multiple. Position of the swelling is noted. Parotid swelling lies **below, behind and in front of the ear lobule**. Parotid enlargement shows typical upward **raise in ear lobule**. Normal hollow/depression just below the ear lobule and behind the mandibular ramus is obliterated. By clenching the teeth masseter is contracted and parotid swelling becomes more prominent. Adenolymphoma arises from the lower pole of the gland at the level of lower border of mandible. Size, shape, extent, skin over the swelling should be inspected. The swelling in inflammatory conditions and pleomorphic adenoma takes the shape of the gland. Surface appear nodular/bosselated in pleomorphic adenoma. The edge of the swelling is well defined in tumor but ill-defined in parotitis. *Movement of the swelling on contraction of masseter is observed* **(Figs. 14-6 and 14-7)**.

Skin over the swelling should be inspected. Skin is red and edematous in parotid abscess or inflammatory conditions (sialadenitis). Ulceration or fungation may develop in advanced carcinoma parotid. Scar of earlier surgery may be seen in case of recurrent parotid abscess or recurrent tumor. ***Size of the scar***, features of the scar should be detailed. Scar of the drain placed may also be evident.

Sinus or *salivary fistula* should be inspected for discharge and location. If the fistula lies pre-masseteric then it is from

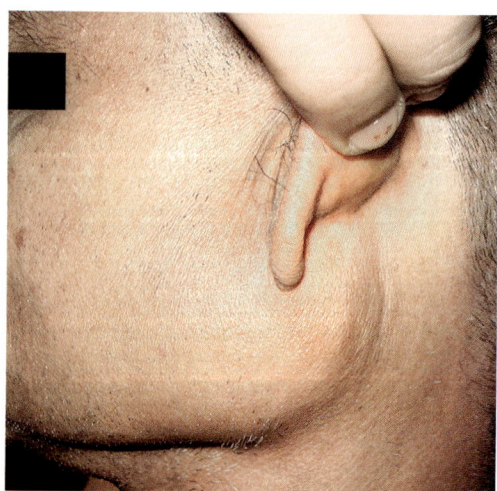

Fig. 14-6 Inspection of parotid should be done carefully *by holding the ear lobule.*

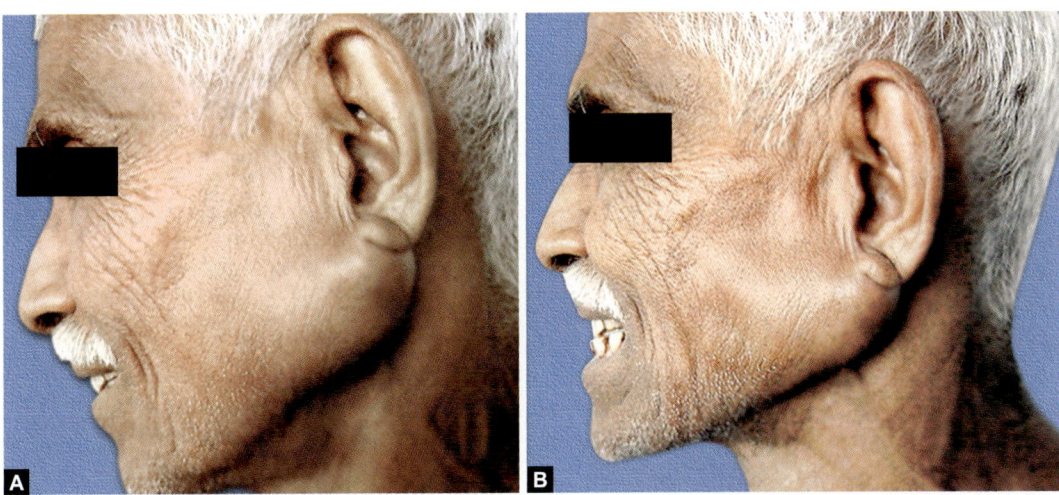

Figs. 14-7A and B Typical parotid swelling with *raised ear lobule*. Swelling is also observed on contraction of the masseter *by clenching the teeth*. Parotid swelling becomes more prominent as it is superficial to masseter muscle.

the duct; if it is masseteric then it is from the gland **(Figs. 14-8 and 14-9)**.

Deep lobe of parotid enlargement is checked by inspecting the oral cavity for any bulge in front of the tonsil and lateral wall of the pharynx and behind the 3rd molar tooth. Tonsil may be pushed medially **(Figs. 14-10A and B)**.

Parotid duct (Stenson's) orifice should be inspected *opposite the crown of the 2nd upper molar tooth*. Duct runs deeper to the

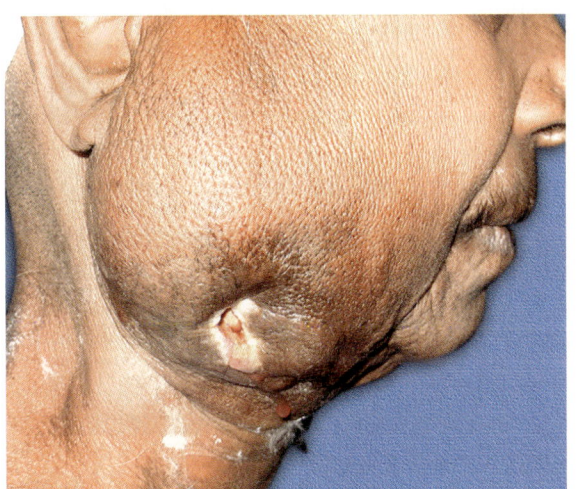

Fig. 14-8 *Parotid fistula.*

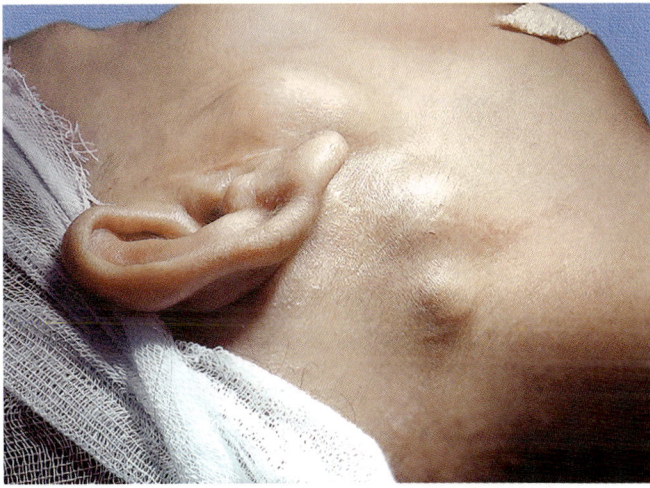

Fig. 14-9 *Recurrent parotid tumor* with visible neck lymph nodes.

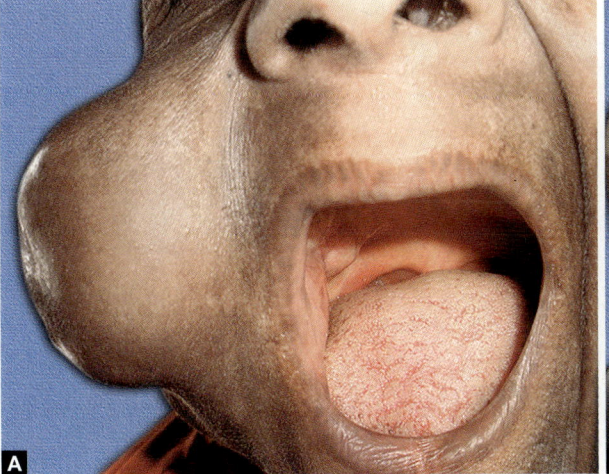

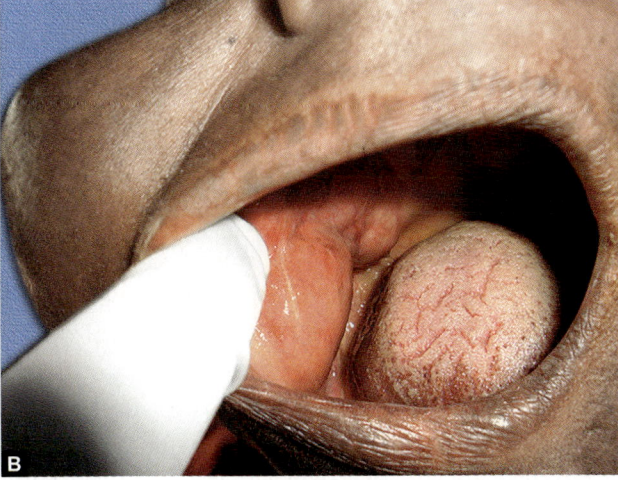

Figs. 14-10A and B *Deep lobe of the parotid* should be inspected from inside.

anterior part of the parotid gland and superficial to masseter muscle; curves inwards and pierces the buccinator muscle to open as parotid duct orifice at the mucous membrane of the mouth opposite to the 2nd upper molar tooth. Duct lies one fingerbreadth below the inferior border of the zygomatic bone. Cheek should be retracted using spatula and with a good light source the duct opening should be inspected properly. In suppurative parotitis, pus may be seen gushing out of the duct orifice after gentle pressure over the parotid gland. Blood in the duct orifice (ampulla of duct) may be due to malignant parotid tumor **(Figs. 14-11A and B)**.

Inspection of the opposite parotid is important. Often Warthin's adenolymphoma of parotid (usually at lower pole) can be bilateral; it is common in males above 40 years of age. Occasionally acinic cell carcinoma of the parotid can be bilateral (2%). Sialectasis, Mikulicz syndrome and Sjögren's syndrome are commonly bilateral. Sialosis, sarcoidosis, HIV-related sialadenitis and benign lymphoepithelial disease and lymphomas are other causes **(Figs. 14-12A and B)**.

Inspection of the neck is also important for cervical lymph node enlargement **(Figs. 14-13A and B)**.

Features of parotid swelling:
- Ear lobule raise
- Swelling in parotid region; deep to parotid fascia; superficial to masseter muscle
- Swelling occupying the groove between posterior part of the mandible and mastoid process
- Obliteration of the hollow below the ear lobule
- Moves upwards up to zygomatic bone—*curtain sign*

Palpation

Swelling should be palpated like any other swelling. *Lower margin should be palpated* to assess its lower extent **(Fig. 14-14)**.

Local rise of temperature and tenderness: There is local rise of temperature in acute parotitis and parotid abscess; tenderness suggests that it could be abscess, necrosis in a tumor or deeper infiltration.

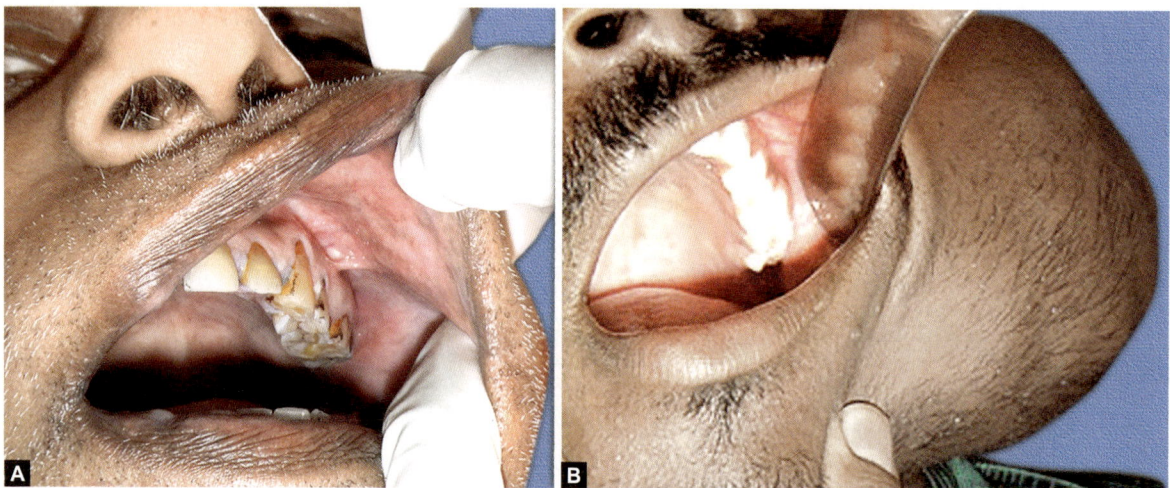

Figs. 14-11A and B *Stenson's parotid duct* should be examined opposite *2nd upper molar tooth*.

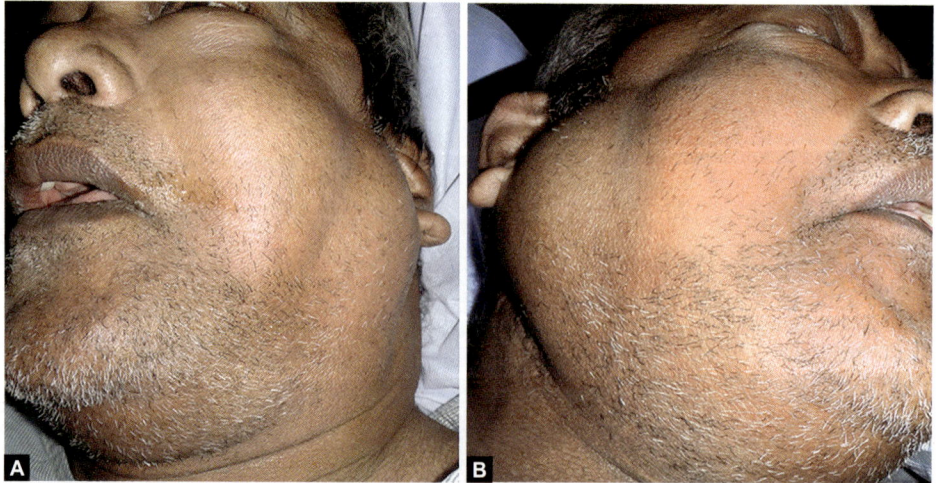

Figs. 14-12A and B *Bilateral parotid swelling* is common in many metabolic conditions such as diabetes, acromegaly, obesity, liver diseases, etc. Bilateral nontender, firm, smooth enlarged gland is typical. It is also seen in Warthin's tumor, Mikulicz syndrome and Sjögren's syndrome.

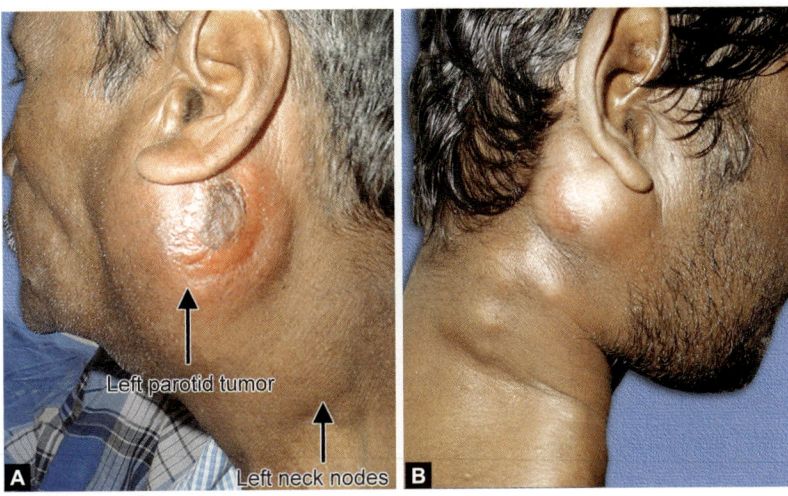

Figs. 14-13A and B Carcinoma parotid with *skin involvement* and cervical *lymph node enlargement*.

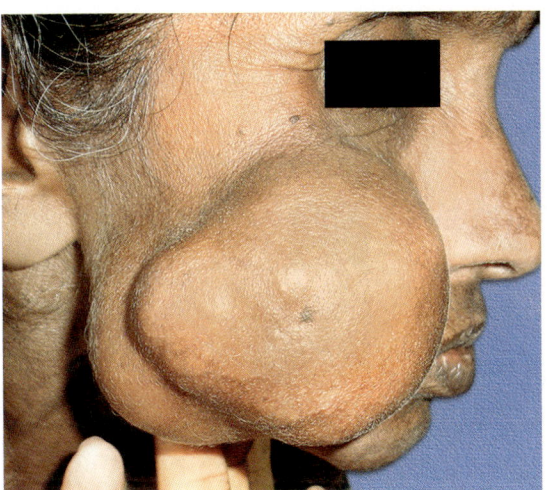

Fig. 14-14 *Lower margin of the enlarged parotid* gland should be assessed.

Surface: Smooth in benign swelling/irregular or nodular in malignant/ill defined in parotitis.

Consistency: It is variable in different conditions—pleomorphic adenoma is firm but can be hard with smooth surface; malignant swellings often have nodular surface and hard consistency; adenolymphoma (Warthin's) is smooth, soft often fluctuant and usually not transilluminant.

Fluctuation: It is seen in parotid abscess and Warthin's tumor.

Mobility: It is checked in both directions—horizontal and vertical. **Curtain sign** often can be elicited (*Curtain sign* is—deep fascia/parotid sheath is attached above to the zygomatic bone. So, swelling arising from parotid gland cannot be moved up beyond zygomatic bone wherein deep fascia acts like a curtain to prevent its further mobility whereas swelling superficial to deep fascia can be moved above, beyond the level of the zygomatic bone).

Skin is free or not is checked—by pinching the skin over the swelling helps to know the infiltration to skin in malignant condition. *Scar, fistula* on the surface should be palpated.

Extension to deeper plane—relation to masseter and mandible: Initially mobility of the swelling is checked in both directions; then patient is asked to clench the teeth so that **masseter gets contracted** and mobility is checked again. If mobility is restricted then swelling is adherent to masseter muscle (**Masseter muscle** with its superficial, middle and deep layers originates from zygomatic arch and inserts to outer surface of the ramus and coronoid process of the mandible; it is supplied by masseteric nerve, a branch of anterior division of the mandibular nerve; muscle elevates the mandible to clinch the teeth). Non-mobile swelling means it is adherent to bone beneath.

Features by which one should suspect the malignancy of parotid are: Fixation, resorption of adjacent bone, pain and anesthesia in the skin and mucosa, muscle paralysis, skin involvement and nodularity, involvement of jaw and masticatory muscle, nerve involvement (facial nerve); mandibular branch of 5th cranial nerve may be involved when tumor tracks along the auriculotemporal nerve to the base of the skull causing severe pain in the distribution area; blood spread to lungs can occur **(Figs. 14-15A and B)**.

Intraoral Examination

Parotid duct is palpated using one finger inside the cheek, near upper 2nd molar tooth and thumb outside the cheek—**bidigital palpation of terminal part of the parotid duct**. Duct can be better felt by rolling the finger after making masseter muscle taut by clenching teeth. Only anterior part of the duct is felt. When mild pressure is applied over the parotid, discharge (watery/purulent in suppuration/blood stained in malignancy) is seen gushing out of the **duct orifice**. Lump or induration may be felt at the duct orifice occasionally. Enlarged **deep lobe of the parotid** can be felt by **bidigital palpation** with index finger of one hand placed inside the mouth in front of the tonsil and behind the 3rd molar tooth and fingers of the other hand placed outside behind the ramus of the mandible **(Figs. 14-16 to 14-18)**. 10% of parotid tumors and 30% of malignant parotid tumors are found in deep lobe.

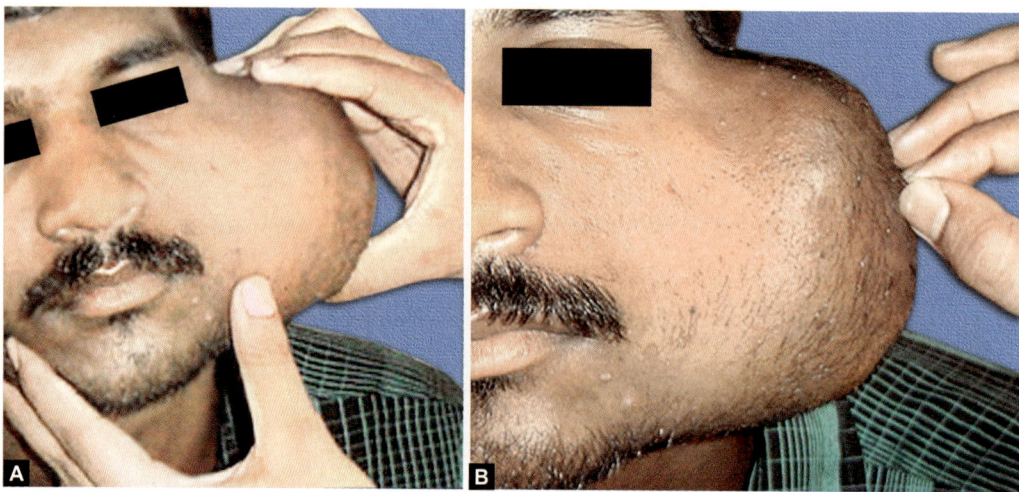

Figs. 14-15A and B *Checking the mobility and skin fixation* of the parotid swelling. Mobility should be checked in two directions. Mobility also should be checked by clenching the teeth to contract the masseter muscle underneath.

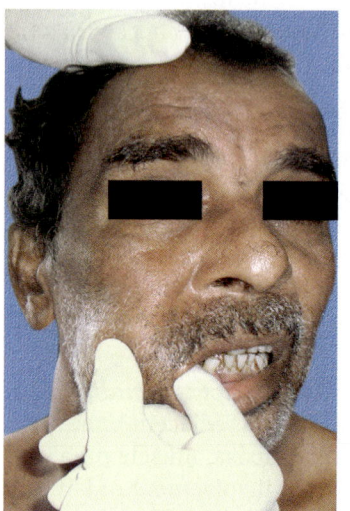

Fig. 14-16 *Parotid duct palpation.*

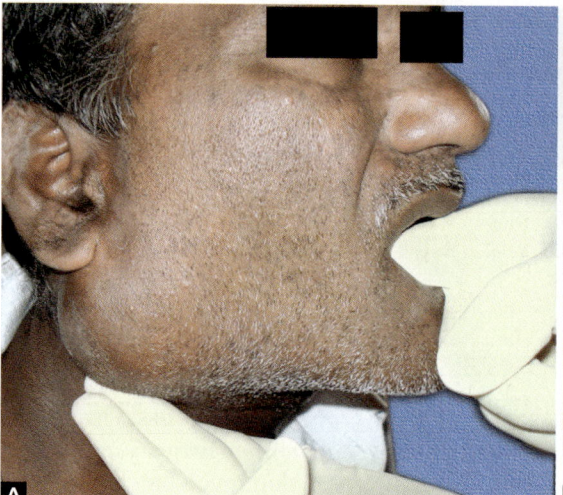

Figs. 14-17A and B Palpation of *deep lobe of the gland.*

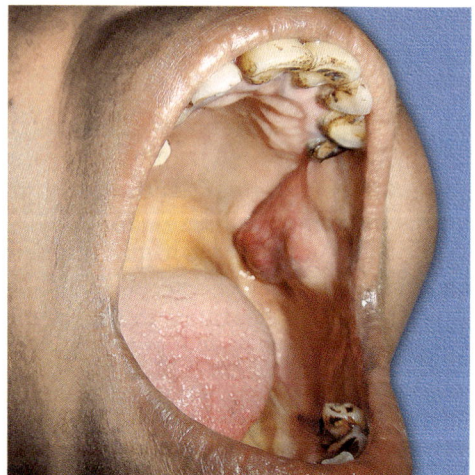

Fig. 14-18 *Enlargement of deep lobe*—in deep lobe parotid tumor it is often obvious.

Examination of Facial Nerve

Functions of facial nerve should be checked. It is involved in malignant growth where nerve is infiltrated. It is involved early in adenoid cystic carcinoma; in carcinoma ex-pleomorphic adenoma. It is involved *only late* in mucoepidermoid carcinoma.

Patient finds *difficulty in closing eyes* (orbicularis oculi); eye contains tear which does not fall; *difficulty in chewing food* (buccinator); difficulty in *talking,* laughing, blowing, and whistling (orbicularis oris).

Facial nerve divides into upper *temporofacial* and *lower cervicofacial* and both divides into branches—temporal, zygomatic (upper); buccal, mandibular, and cervical (lower) called as **pes anserinus** *(goose foot)*. Facial nerve is sandwiched between superficial and deep lobes of parotid gland. **Faciovenous plane of Patey** is the plane where facial nerve is seen superficial to the posterior facial vein (retromandibular vein) in the substance of parotid gland.

Clinical Signs of Facial Nerve Paralysis

Upper Face

Orbicularis oculi: In facial nerve paralysis, tightly closed eyes can be easily opened when tried by examiner **(Fig. 14-19)**.

Frontal belly of occipitofrontalis: Absence of furrowing (normal horizontal wrinkles) in the forehead while looking upwards.

Corrugator supercilii: Absence of corrugation in the forehead while frowning **(Fig. 14-20)**.

Lower Face

Bucccinator: While blowing with closed mouth, tone which is felt in the cheek is weak on the affected side. Paralysed side blow more and on pressing with finger weakness with supple tone of the muscle can be felt **(Fig. 14-21)**.

Buccinator is the muscle of the cheek; upper fibers arise from maxilla opposite molar teeth to reach upper lip; lower fibers from mandible opposite molar teeth to reach lower lip; middle fibers from pterygomandibular raphe first decussate to reach upper and lower lips.

Orbicularis oris: Its weakness causes inability to whistle **(Fig. 14-22)**.

Levator anguli oris: Its weakness causes deviation of angle of mouth towards opposite side while showing teeth **(Fig. 14-23)**.

Platysma: Its weakness causes loss of normal contraction while stretching the neck. It arises from deltopectoral fascia running in front of clavicle to reach in front and base of mandible and behind to lip and lower face skin and continues as risorius **(Fig. 14-24)**.

Other Relevant Examinations

Taste sensation and general sensation (lingual nerve) should be checked. Patient is not allowed to speak but asked to write in a paper. Taste material is instilled on the surface of the diseased

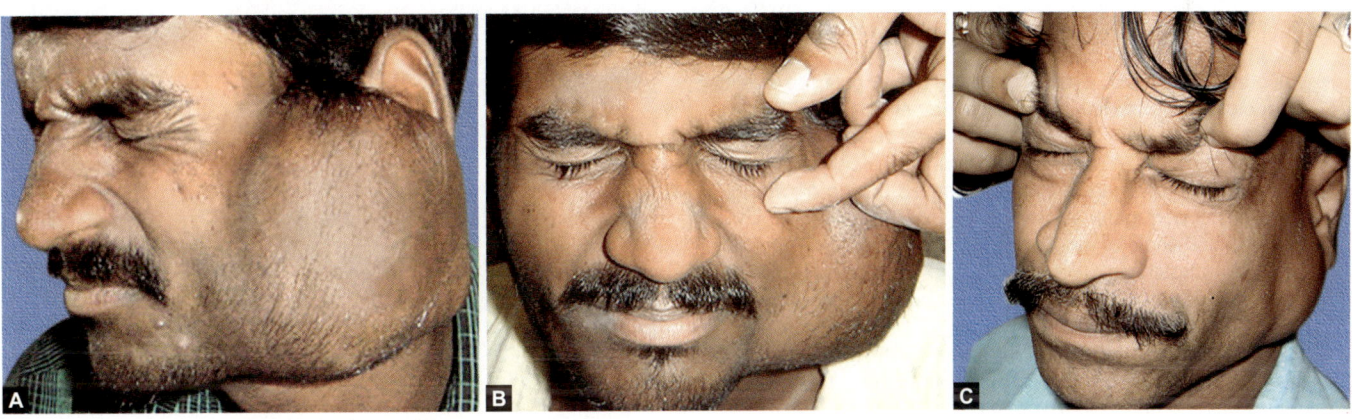

Figs. 14-19A to C Method of checking of failure of closure of eyelids or easily opening of the eyelids after closure—*paralysis of orbicularis oculi.*

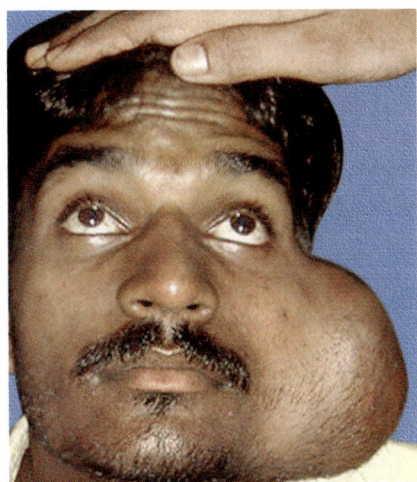

Fig. 14-20 Method of checking of absence of corrugation in the forehead during frowning—*paralysis of corrugator supercilii.*

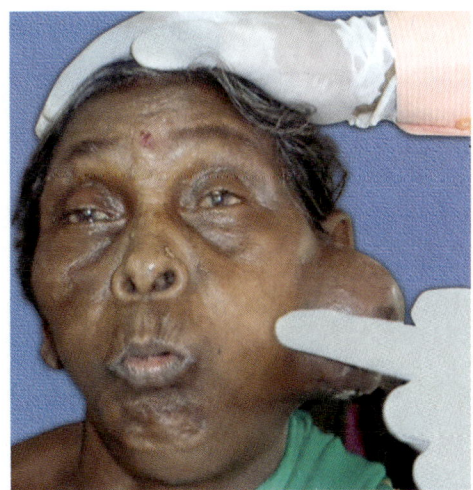

Fig. 14-21 Weakness of the buccinators muscle is checked by pressing the blown cheek using finger.

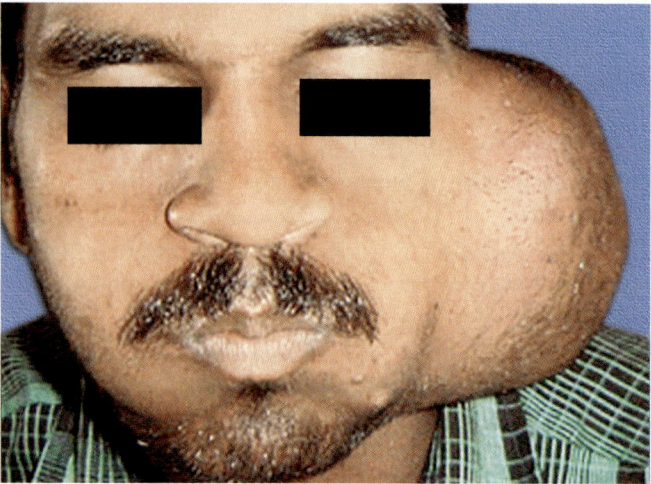

Fig. 14-22 Method of checking of inability to whistle—*paralysis of orbicularis oris.*

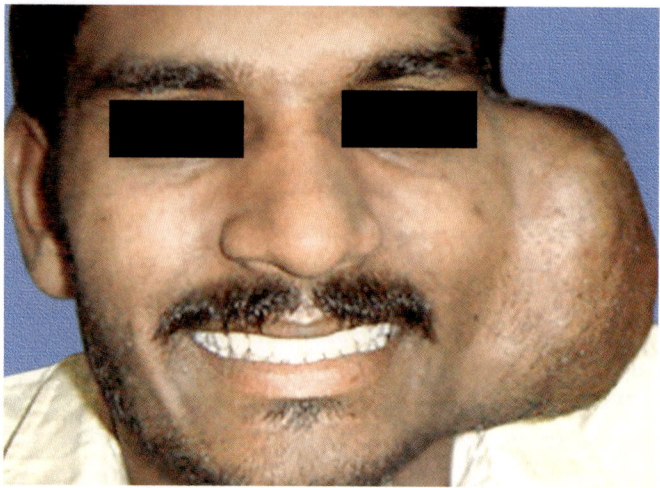

Fig. 14-23 Method of checking of deviation of angle of mouth towards opposite side while showing the teeth—*paralysis of levator anguli oris.*

Features of facial nerve palsy (Figs. 14-25A and B):
- Difficulty in chewing food as food accumulates in vestibule due to buccinator weakness
- Deviation of angle of mouth from the diseased side towards healthy side while talking, laughing, blowing, whistling due to paralysis of orbicularis oris
- Failure of closure of eyelids or easily opening of the eyelids after closure—paralysis of orbicularis oculi
- Absence of furrows while looking upwards (paralyzed side remains immobile)—paralysis of frontal belly of occipitofrontalis
- Absence of corrugation in the forehead during frowning—paralysis of corrugator supercilii
- Deviation of angle of mouth towards opposite side—paralysis of levator anguli oris
- Loss of contraction of platysma in the neck while stretching the neck—paralysis of platysma
- Inability to blow the air by the cheek with paralysed side cheek more bellowing out and on palpation reduced tone of buccinator—paralysis of buccinator
- Inability to whistle—paralysis of orbicularis oris

Note: In supranuclear (upper motor neuron lesion) paralysis upper face escapes due to bilateral cortical representation.
Show the teeth; puff the cheeks; shut the eyes; move the eyebrows upwards

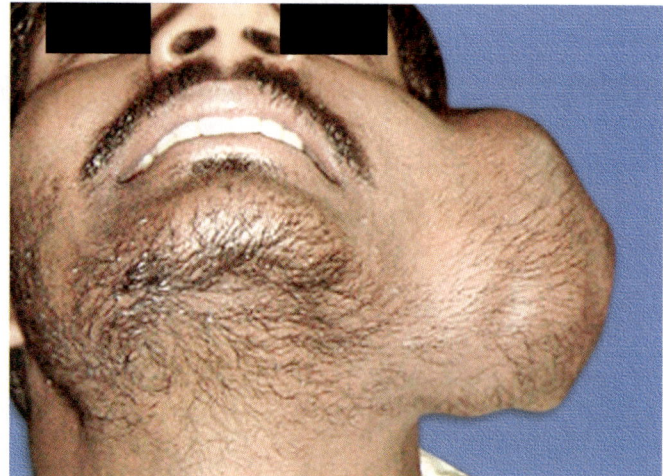

Fig. 14-24 Method of checking of loss of contraction of platysma in the neck while stretching the neck—*paralysis of platysma.*

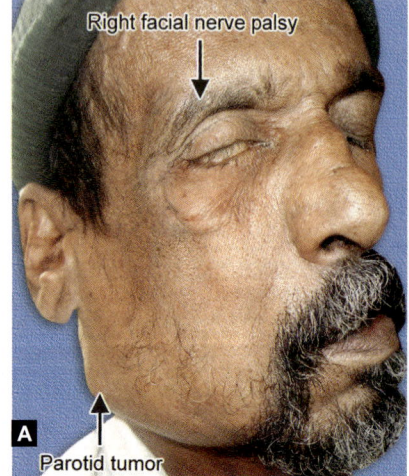
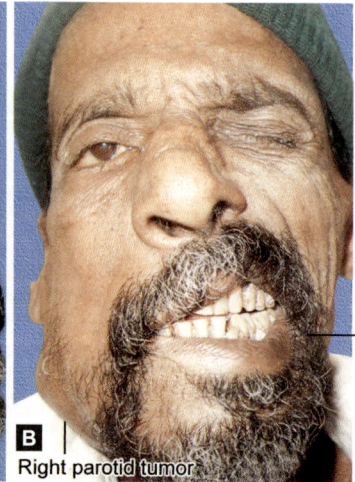

Figs. 14-25A and B *Facial nerve palsy* in a patient with parotid tumor infiltrating the facial nerve.

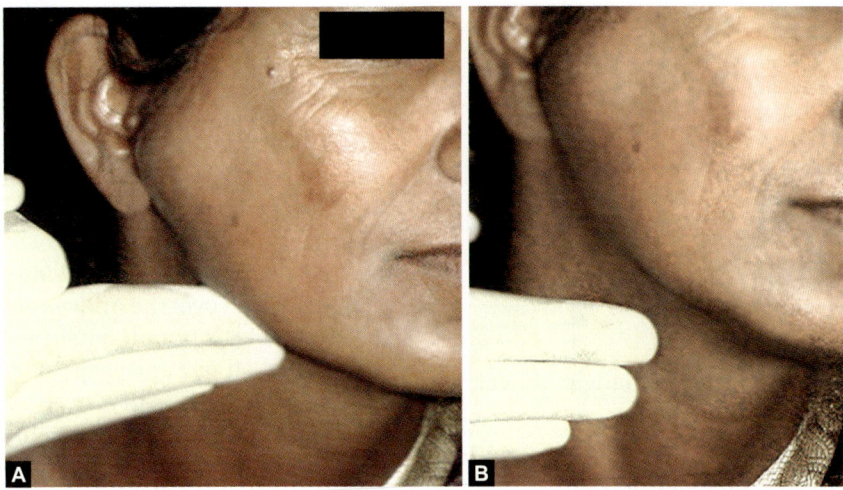

Figs. 14-26A and B *Palpation of neck nodes in a patient with parotid swelling—submandibular and upper deep cervical.*

side first and then normal side. Prior to each instillation patient should wash his mouth with warm water. Usually four substances are used. After 10 seconds patient should identify the substance and write. **Facial nerve serves 3 tastes**—*salt* (rock salt) on the tip of tongue; *sweet* using syrup on the tip of the tongue; *sour* using lemon juice on the lateral aspect of the tongue. *Bitter taste* is mediated by **glossopharyngeal nerve** and is tested using quinine on posterior third of the tongue.

Hypoglossal nerve function is checked by asking the patient to protrude the tongue out and observe the deviation of tongue. **Accessory nerve function** is assessed by asking the patient to shrug the shoulder, done in cases of enlarged upper deep cervical nodes infiltrating the nerve and paralyzing the trapezius.

Palpation of superficial temporal artery pulsation should be done in front of the tragus over the zygomatic bone.

Palpation of cervical nodes for significant enlargement should be done. Upper deep cervical, pre- and post-auricular nodes are enlarged in inflammatory and malignant conditions. Features of Horner's syndrome also looked for in specific patients **(Figs. 14-26A and B)**.

Movements of the jaw—is checked; it is restricted in inflammatory and malignant conditions of the parotid.

Differential Diagnosis for Parotid Enlargement

Parotid tumors: Pleomorphic adenoma is the commonest benign parotid tumor. Mucoepidermoid carcinoma is the commonest malignant parotid tumor **(Figs. 14-27A and B)**.

Idiopathic hypertrophy of masseter muscle: Is a rare entity but presents like a swelling. When teeth are clenched, entire swelling hardens; but when relaxed swelling softens. It often can be bilateral.

Pre-auricular lymph node enlargement: Swelling lies in front of the tragus; normal depression below and in front of the ear lobule is not obliterated; it may be suppuration, adenitis, tuberculosis or lymphoma or secondaries with primary from forehead, eyelid, cheek, scalp or external auditory meatus.

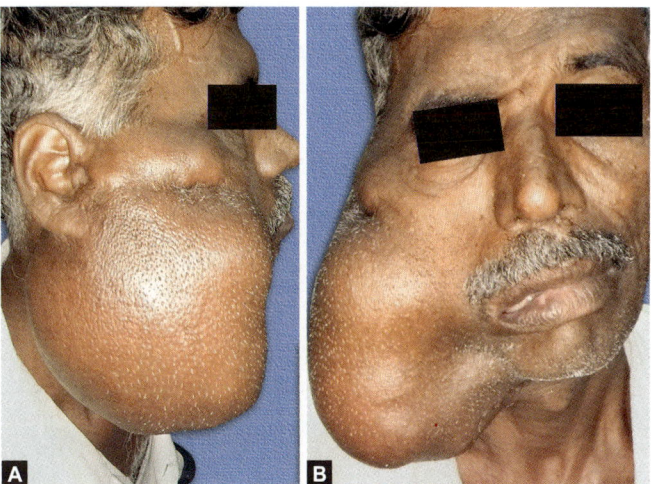

Figs. 14-27A and B *Mucoepidermoid carcinoma* of the parotid – with extensive involvement (*Courtesy:* Professor Prabhu Hubli, VIMS Ballari, Karnataka).

It feels more superficial; as it is outer to parotid capsule. It is freely mobile.

Rarely parotid and paraparotid/subparotid lymph nodes may be enlarged as secondaries from primary from oral mucosa and skin malignancies of head and neck region (but these things are very rare and so students should not consider in usual clinical practice unless it is relevant). Still rarely parotid gland may be enlarged as non-metastatic obstruction of the duct by carcinoma cheek.

> **Palpation of parotid:**
> - *Swelling*—tenderness/temperature/extent/size/surface/consistency/mobility/fixity/plane of the swelling/masseter involvement/facial nerve involvement/skin over the swelling
> - *Parotid duct palpation*—by rolling the finger across the masseter muscle while patient is clinching the teeth to make masseter taut. Terminal part of the duct is palpated bidigitally using index finger inside and thumb outside.
> - *Palpation of oral cavity/*bidigital examination for deep lobe is done with one finger inside the mouth behind the tonsillar fossa and the other outside in parotid region.

- All features of facial nerve palsy—inability to close eye/difficulty in blowing/altered nasolabial groove/clenching of teeth
- Neck nodes should be examined
- Jaw movements should be checked
- Opposite parotid should be examined
- Other salivary glands (submandibular salivary gland) should be examined for the enlargement

Examination of Submandibular Salivary Gland

Inspection

The swelling is seen in submandibular triangle of neck, is examined as any other swelling.

In salivary calculus (submandibular calculus), swelling immediately becomes more prominent when lemon juice or chocolates are given to the patient to drink or eat. Floor of the mouth should be inspected for enlargement of deep lobe of the submandibular salivary gland **(Figs. 14-28A to C)**.

Acute submandibular sialadenitis is (painful) diffuse, attains large size with redness and other features of inflammation; trismus is common; (often dyspnea and dysphagia may develop) **(Fig. 14-29)**.

Inspection of the duct orifice: Opening and course of the submandibular salivary duct *(Wharton's duct,)* should be inspected by asking the patient to open the mouth and raise the tip of the tongue to touch the palate (using a torch/light source). Orifice is situated at the papillae on either side of the frenum linguae. Duct orifice may be inflamed and edematous in severe infection and with slight pressure over the gland pus may be seen discharging from it. Often stone may be visible impacted near the duct orifice. *Lime juice test*: Two small dry swabs are placed over the orifices on each side and stimulant like lemon juice is put on dorsum of tongue; after a minute swabs are taken out and inspected; swab on the side with impacted orifice will be dry; swab over normal orifice will be wet. The salivary flow is blocked in the duct with impacted stone and hence orifice on that side looks dry whereas orifice on normal side looks wet due to normal salivary flow. Wharton's duct (*5 cm in length*) exits from the medial surface of the gland and runs between lateral part of the mylohyoid and hyoglossus muscles and on the genioglossus emptying intraorally in the anterior part of the floor of the mouth lateral to lingual frenum; lingual nerve wraps around the duct from lateral to medial; hypoglossal nerve runs parallel and below the duct **(Fig. 14-30)**.

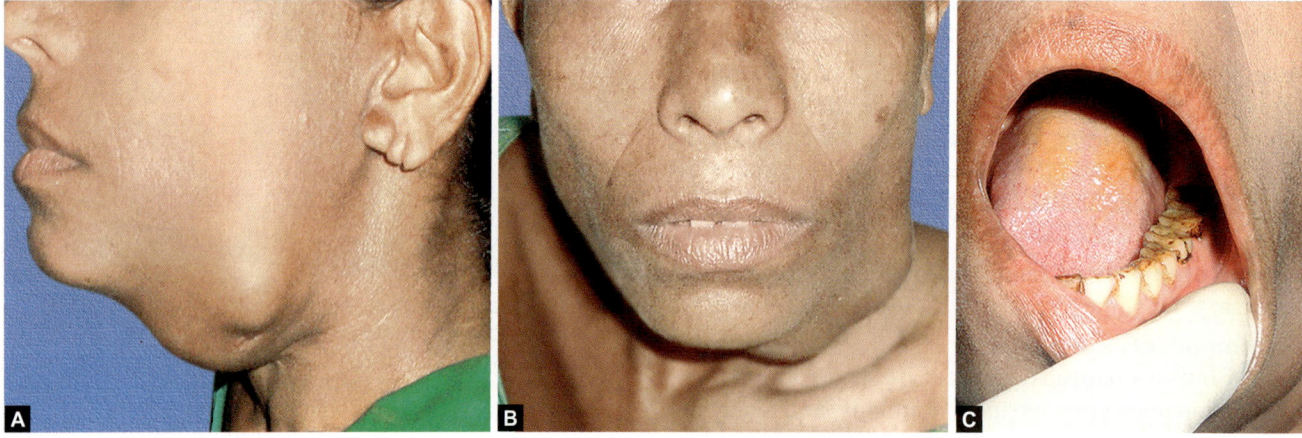

Figs. 14-28A to C *Inspection of submandibular salivary gland swelling.* Oral cavity is also should be inspected.

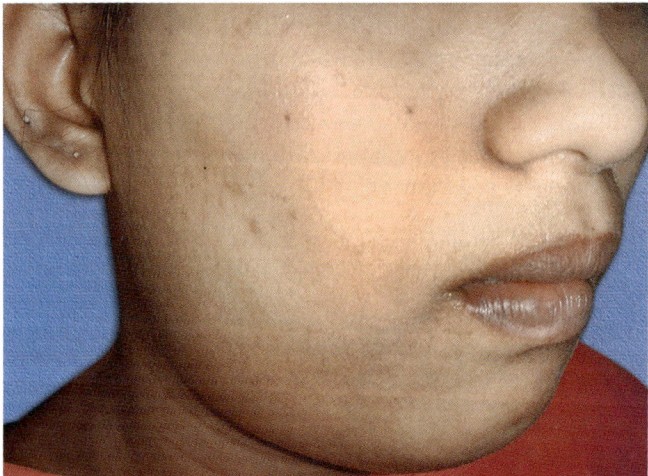

Fig. 14-29 Acute right sided *submandibular sialadenitis* showing diffusely enlarged submandibular salivary gland.

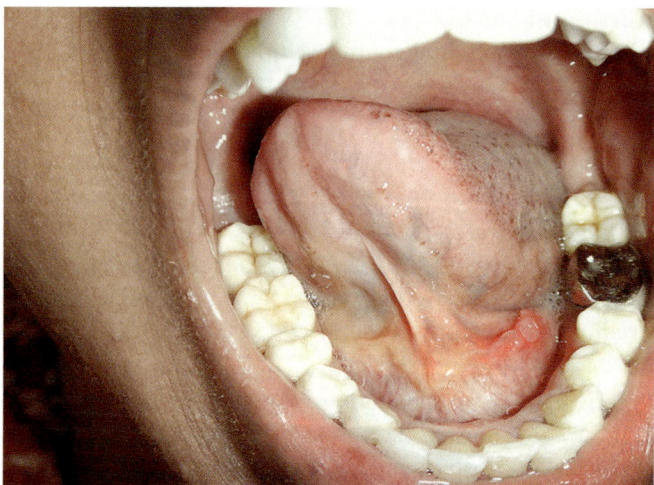

Fig. 14-30 In submandibular salivary gland enlargement *Wharton's duct should be inspected* by raising the tip of the tongue over to palate.

Palpation

First dentures if present should be removed. Best way of palpating the *submandibular salivary gland* is by ***bidigital palpation***. It is because 'C' shaped submandibular salivary gland has got a small deep buccal part above the mylohyoid muscle and a large cervical superficial portion; both are in continuity. Index finger of one hand is placed over the floor of the mouth medial to alveolus and lateral to tongue pushing the finger as deep as possible; fingers of other hand are placed outside under the mandibular margin to push the swelling upwards. By this way the finger inside the oral cavity not only helps to feel the deep lobe of the salivary gland, which is deep to mylohyoid muscle; but also the superficial lobe and often duct can be better assessed by this method. Its medial, posterior extension, relation of the swelling to the lower margin of the body of the mandible should be checked. It confirms that the swelling as submandibular salivary gland. Duct is palpated from behind forwards. Submandibular salivary gland enlargement occurs as a result of chronic sialadenitis or neoplastic conditions. Its surface is usually smooth whereas submandibular lymph node enlargement is usually nodular. ***Submandibular lymph node is not bidigitally palpable*** as it lies outside the mylohyoid muscle, superficial to the gland. Stone in the Wharton's duct also can be palpated by this method. Shape, size, consistency can be assessed by this method **(Figs. 14-31 to 14-36)**.

Differential Diagnosis for Submandibular Salivary Gland Enlargement

Submandibular salivary gland tumor: Pleomorphic adenoma, mucoepidermoid carcinoma and other neoplasms: They are progressive, initially painless, later infiltrates adjacent structures in malignancy. Lymph nodes in the neck may get enlarged eventually.

Enlarged submandibular lymph nodes: Bidigital palpation helps to confirm it. Lymph nodes are not bidigitally palpable.

Enlarged facial lymph node lies adjacent to facial artery at the lower margin of the mandible which can be moved above the level of the margin of the mandible into the face.

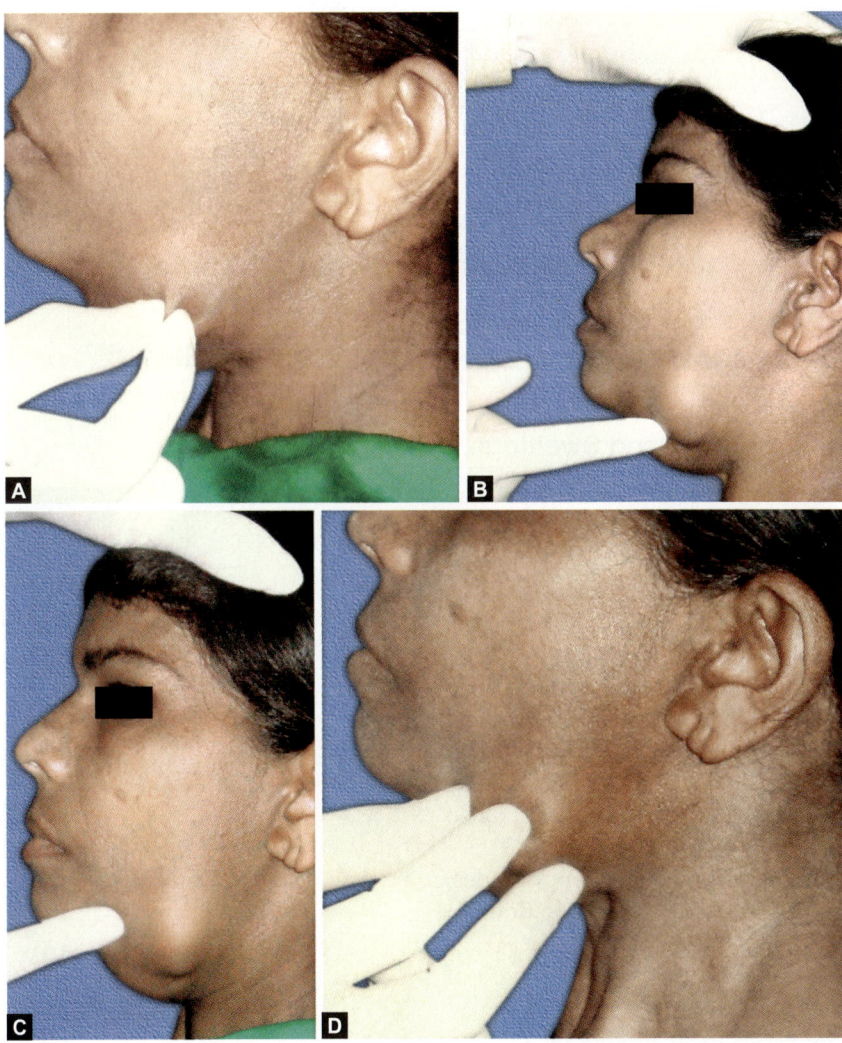

Figs. 14-31A to D Submandibular salivary gland palpation—skin fixity (pinching); extent and margin and mobility. Fluctuation should be elicited in a soft swelling.

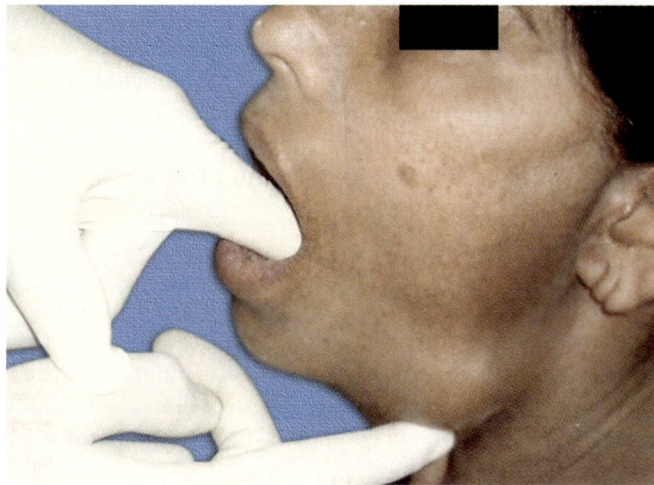

Fig. 14-32 Submandibular salivary gland *bidigital palpation.*

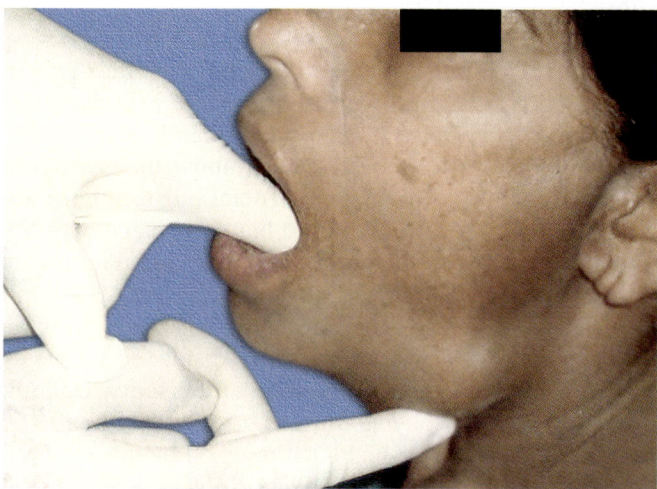

Fig. 14-34 Mandible should be palpated bidigitally for relation of *tumor, thickening, and tenderness.*

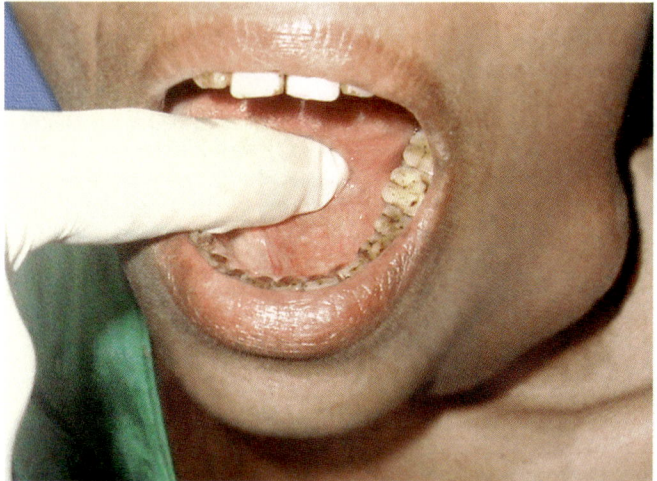

Fig. 14-33 Submandibular salivary duct *should be palpated per orally.*

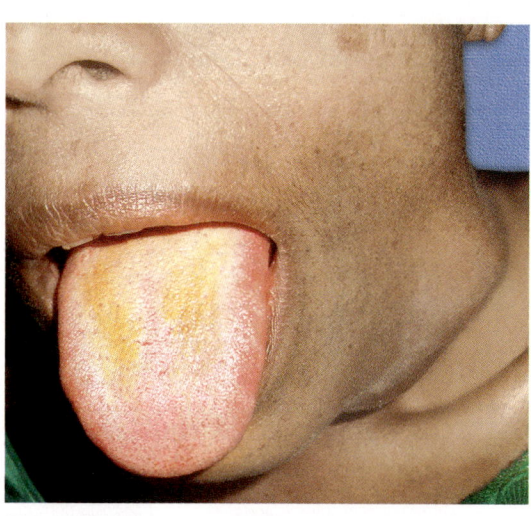

Fig. 14-35 *Hypoglossal nerve should be assessed* in submandibular salivary gland enlargement.

Examination of Minor Salivary Gland Swellings

- Minor salivary glands are around 450 in number; located in lips, palate, floor of the mouth, oropharynx, paranasal sinuses, and larynx.
- Swellings from these glands are usually neoplastic; commonly malignant (90%). History of painless swelling of short duration in the palate or lip which is slowly progressive; often ulcerates over its summit. It is firm or hard, often crosses the midline in the palate, may get adherent to palatal bone or deeper structure making it immobile. It should be examined intraorally in detail like any other swelling or ulcer. Nasal cavities, maxilla also should be examined.
- Oral cavity and neck for enlarged cervical lymph nodes; systemic examination for metastases should be done in detail.
- Adenoid cystic carcinoma is the commonest type of malignant minor salivary gland tumor.
- **Ranula** is mucous cyst arises from sublingual salivary gland or from mucous glands of Blandin and Nuhn.

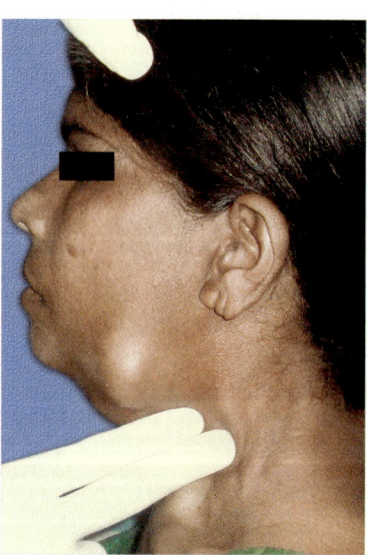

Fig. 14-36 *Cervical nodes should be palpated* in submandibular salivary gland enlargement.

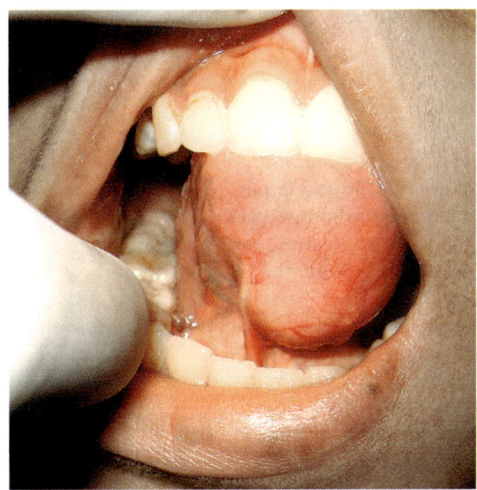

Fig. 14-37 Swelling in *sublingual region*.

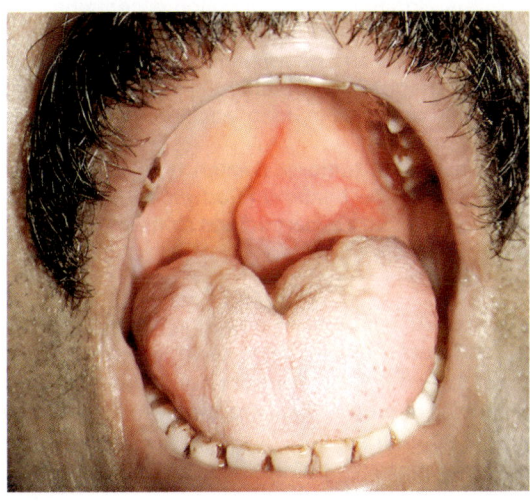

Fig. 14-38 *Minor salivary gland tumor in palate. Palate and lips are the commonest sites.* Minor salivary gland tumors are commonly malignant; adenoid cystic carcinoma is the commonest type. Its surface is smooth; often vascular; sometimes with ulceration on its summit.

Mikulicz disease is also common in sublingual salivary gland **(Figs. 14-37 and 14-38)**.

Note: Students should not get confused with the word *ectopic salivary gland* for minor salivary gland. Ectopic salivary gland is the one which is actually salivary gland in aberrant position, and a migratory gland from one of the major salivary glands.

■ INVESTIGATIONS FOR SALIVARY DISEASES

X-ray of the part: Orthopantomogram (OPG) X-ray or often *intraoral X-ray* is done to look for radiopaque stone in the submandibular region. Usually stones are radiopaque. Ideally X-ray imaging should be done in multiple planes. Extended chin, open mouth posteroanterior view with cheek blown out is used for parotid and its duct. For submandibular salivary gland, extended chin, open-mouthed lateral view with depressed tongue is used (Fig. 14-39).

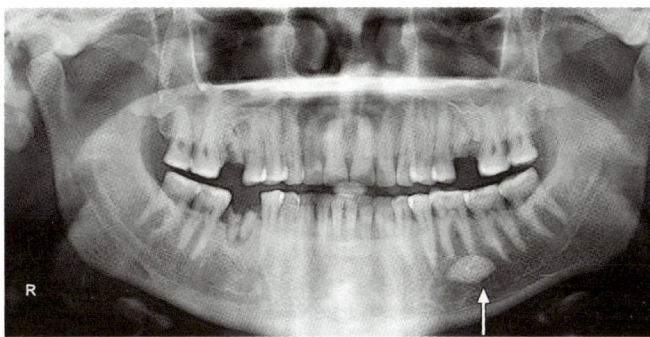

Fig. 14-39 Plain X-ray (orthopantomogram, OPG) showing submandibular salivary gland stone—radiopaque. (*Courtesy:* Dr Jagadish Chandra, MDS, Mangaluru).

CT scan or MRI: Both are very useful; and are taken of the part including neck, base of skull to see extent of the tumor, deep lobe involvement, involvement of bone, relation of tumor to carotid artery and styloid process, adjacent spread and nodal status. CT has got 100% sensitivity; shows entire diseased gland as well as opposite gland. It identifies stones 10 times better than plain X-ray. Tumor invasion, nerve involvement can be identified better with CT. Calcifications can be seen in sialadenitis as well as pleomorphic adenoma; but it is diffuse in sialadenitis. CT is better to identify skull base invasion, to differentiate solid mass from cystic mass. Duct and facial nerve is not clearly made out. MRI may be better for delineating facial nerve and duct (Fig. 14-40).

Role of FNAC: FNAC of the major salivary gland swelling is *ideal*. FNAC of cervical lymph nodes when enlarged is often done.

Note: Incision (open) or core needle/trucut biopsy is *contraindicated* in major salivary gland tumors/diseases due to likely chances of seedling, fistula and facial nerve injury. Incision biopsy is ideal investigation *only for* tumors of minor salivary glands of palate, lip, etc.

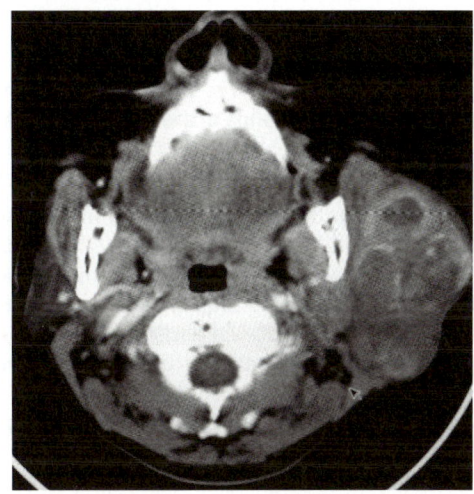

Fig. 14-40 CT scan of pleomorphic adenoma.

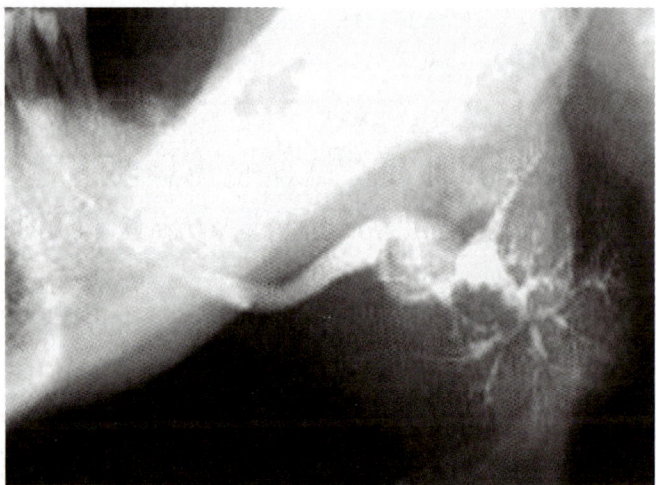

Fig. 14-41 *Sialogram* of submandibular gland.

Ultrasound: Ultrasound using linear, high frequency transducer, which shows high resolution images, are used to identify solid and cystic nature of the swelling during *ultrasound-guided FNAC*.

Radionuclear imaging: 99Tc pertechnetate radioisotope imaging is very useful in detecting Warthin's adenolymphoma of parotid.

Sialography: Sialography is rarely done nowadays. It is done for sialectasis, salivary fistula, Sjögren's syndrome only, congenital conditions, extraglandular masses. It is done for parotid and submandibular salivary gland imaging. Sialography cannot be done for sublingual salivary gland. Preliminary plain X-ray should be taken to identify existing stones. Fine polythene or lacrimal cannula is passed into the orifice. Not more than 1 mL of water soluble iodine dye (if more dye is injected it causes extravasation and chemical sialadenitis) like sodium diatrizoate is injected. X-rays are taken. Digital subtraction Sialography is better in Sjögren's syndrome. Findings: Narrowing, (stricture); grape like cluster appearance (sialectasis); dilatations; communications (Fistulas); mass lesions. Sialography should never be performed in acute inflammation. Sialography is contraindicated in acute suppurative sialadenitis. It is not useful in neoplasm (Fig. 14-41).

Fistulography/Sinusography: It is done by injecting radiopaque dye into sinus/ fistula of the parotid/submandibular salivary gland.

Ultrasound of parotid/submandibular gland/region and neck: It is becoming more useful, simple initial method of evaluation. It can identify tumor, cyst and abscess. US-guided FNAC is ideal. Cervical lymph nodes assessment also can be done. US-guided core needle biopsy is becoming accepted now. *Ultrasound guided core needle biopsy* (USCNB) of parotid or submandibular salivary gland is accepted now especially when surgery is not contemplated. Risk of facial nerve palsy, tumor seedlings is known but very less as per current studies. Linear, high frequency transducer which shows high resolution images are used. *Study of discharge:* Discharge collected from duct orifice is sent for culture and sensitivity and cytology.

SALIVARY NEOPLASMS

Classification
a. Epithelial:
  1. *Adenomas*
     – Pleomorphic adenoma.
     – Monomorphic adenomas.
       - Adenolymphoma (Warthin's tumor).
       - Oxyphil adenomas, oncocytoma.
       - Basal cell adenoma.
  2. *Carcinomas*
     – Mucoepidermoid carcinoma—commonest malignancy.
     – Acinic cell carcinoma—1%.
     – Adenoid cystic carcinoma—very aggressive.
     – Adenocarcinoma.
     – Squamous cell carcinoma—2%.
     – Carcinoma in ex pleomorphic adenoma.
     – Undifferentiated carcinoma.
b. Nonepithelial:
   – Hemangioma—commonly seen in infants, usually in parotids. Spontaneous regression is common.
   – Lymphangioma.
   – Neurofibromas and neurilemmomas.
c. Malignant lymphomas: Common in parotid; NHL type.
d. Secondary tumors from head, neck region; bronchus and skin.
e. Lymphoepithelial tumors: Benign type (5%) is common in females; can be bilateral *(Godwin's tumor)*. Malignant type is rare—occurs in parotid and submandibular salivary glands *(Eskimoma)*.

Incidence: 75–80% salivary neoplasms are in the parotids of which 80% are benign; 80% of these are pleomorphic adenomas. 15% of salivary tumors are in the submandibular salivary gland; of which 60% are benign; 95% of these are pleomorphic adenomas. 10% of salivary neoplasms are in the minor salivary glands—palate, lips, cheeks and sublingual glands. Of these only 10% are benign.

Pleomorphic adenomas (Mixed salivary tumor, 80%): It is the commonest salivary gland tumor. It is more common in parotids. It is of mesenchymal, myoepithelial and duct reserve cell origin. *Grossly* it contains cartilages, cystic spaces, and solid tissues. *Histologically* it shows—epithelial and myoepithelial cells; mucoid material with myxomatous changes; cartilages. Even though it is capsulated, tumor may come out as pseudopods and may extend beyond the main limit of the tumor tissue. When disease occurs in parotid, often it involves superficial lobe or superficial and deep lobe together. But sometimes only deep lobe is involved where it presents as swelling in the lateral wall of the pharynx, soft palate and posterior pillar of the fauces. There may not be any visible swelling in the preauricular region—*Dumb-bell tumor*. This tumor is in relation to styloid process, mandible, stylohyoid, styloglossus, stylopharyngeus muscles. It has got 1:1 male to female ratio; occurs in any age group; usually unilateral. Present as a single painless, smooth, firm lobulated, mobile swelling in front of the parotid with positive curtain sign. It remains free from skin, masseter and facial nerve. The ear lobule is lifted. When deep lobe is involved, swelling is commonly located in the lateral wall of pharynx, posterior pillar and over the soft palate. Facial nerve is not involved.

Long-standing pleomorphic adenoma may turn into carcinoma—(carcinoma in ex-pleomorphic adenoma). Its features are—recent increase in size; pain and nodularity; involvement of skin; involvement of masseter; involvement of facial nerve—*lower facial nerve palsy*; involvement of neck lymph node. Malignant transformation is 3–5%; it may be 10% in long standing (15 years or more) pleomorphic adenomas.

Adenolymphoma (Warthin's tumor, papillary cystadenolymphomatosum): It is a benign tumor that occurs only in parotid (2nd most common), often bilateral (10%) usually in the lower pole/near angle of the mandible; usually from superficial lobe; common in old males (4:1); common in smokers. It is said to be due to trapping of jugular lymph sacs in parotid during developmental period. It is composed of *double layered of columnar epithelium*, with papillary projections into cystic spaces with lymphoid tissues in the stroma. It presents as a slow growing, smooth, soft, cystic, fluctuant swelling, in the lower pole, often bilateral and nontender. Not fixed to skin/masseter. Facial nerve is not involved. It is not seen in Negroes. A *'hot spot'* in 99Technetium pertechnetate scan— *is diagnostic*. Adenolymphoma does not turn into malignancy.

Mucoepidermoid tumor: It is the commonest malignant condition in major salivary glands. It is slowly progressive, often attains a large size and spreads to neck lymph nodes. It contains malignant epidermoid and mucus-secreting cells. It can be *low or high grade*. Facial nerve involvement is rare but can occur *late* in mucoepidermoid carcinoma of parotid. It presents as swelling in the salivary (parotid or submandibular) region, slowly increasing in size, eventually attaining a large size, which is hard, nodular, often with involvement of skin and lymph nodes.

Adenoid cystic carcinoma (10% of salivary tumors): It is common in minor salivary glands. It consists of myoepithelial cells and duct epithelial cells with cribriform or lace-like appearance. It involves facial nerve very early, spreads through the perineural sheath over a long distance more proximally and infiltrates into the perineural tissues and bone marrow. It also invades periosteum and bone medulla early and spreads extensively. It carries poor prognosis.

Acinic cell tumor: It is a rare, slow growing tumor that occurs almost always in parotid and is composed of cells alike serous acini. It is more common in women. It occurs in adult and elderly. It can involve facial nerve or neck lymph nodes. Clinically, it is of variable consistency with soft and cystic areas. It is low grade malignant tumor.

Submandibular Salivary Gland Tumors
- **Benign tumors:** Benign tumors commonly pleomorphic adenomas are smooth, firm or hard, bidigitally palpable, without involving adjacent muscles or hypoglossal nerve or mandible bone. Diagnosis is by FNAC, orthopantomogram and CT scan
- **Malignant tumors:** They are hard, nodular, often get fixed to skin, muscles, hypoglossal nerve, and mandible. Diagnosis is by FNAC of primary tumor and of lymph nodes when involved, CT scan and OPG

Other Salivary Tumors

Minor salivary gland tumors: It is 10% of salivary tumors. It is common in—palate (40%); lip; cheek. 10% are benign—*commonly pleomorphic adenomas*. 90% are malignant—commonly adenoid cystic carcinomas. They present as swelling with ulcer over the summit. If it is malignant, then extension into the palate, maxilla, pterygoids can occur often with involvement of cervical lymph node. *Differential diagnosis*: Squamous cell carcinoma of oral cavity

Parotid lymphoma: Parotid lymphoma can occur from the lymph nodes in the gland or from parotid parenchyma. It can occur in HIV patients; lymphoepithelial diseases and in Sjögren's syndrome. It is common in elderly. Disease may be confined to parotid gland or may involve other nodes in neck, mediastinum. 90% of salivary lymphomas occur in parotid

Note: Lymphoma occasionally can occur in other salivary glands also (10% of all salivary lymphomas)

Other Conditions of Salivary Glands

Condition	Features
Salivary calculus and sialadenitis 80% are in submandibular; 80% are radio-opaque; commonly calcium phosphate and calcium carbonate stones. Calculi in submandibular gland is more common, because the gland secretion is viscous, contains more calcium and also its drainage is nondependent, causing stasis. Secretion from parotid is serous, contains less calcium and so stones are not common	*Features in acute cases:* Pain, swelling, tenderness is seen in submandibular region and floor of the mouth; duct is inflamed and swollen *Features in chronic cases*: Pain is more during mastication due to stimulation. Salivary secretion is more during mastication causing increase in gland size. Firm, tender swelling is palpable *bidigitally*. When stone is in the duct, it is palpable in floor of the mouth as a tender swelling with features of inflammation in the duct. Pus exudes through the duct orifice. In submandibular salivary gland, the stones are multiple, with inflammation of gland *(sialadenitis)* *Differential diagnosis* is salivary neoplasm
Parotitis **Acute** Viral—mumps (commonest cause of parotitis), Coxsackie virus A and B, parainfluenza 1 and 3, Echo and lymphocytic choriomeningitis; Bacterial—*Staphylococcus aureus;* Allergic; HIV infection; Radiotherapy, postoperative period; Specific infections like syphilis; Sjögren's syndrome (bilateral) **Chronic** It can occur due to stone blocking the Stenson's duct presenting as rubbery hard slightly tender recurrent swelling in parotid region which is more during eating, with aching pain. Often it may be bilateral	*Acute*: Continuous, throbbing pain radiating to ear, and side of the head; speaking/eating/any movements of TM joint is painful; fever with chills and rigors; diffuse swelling in front and behind the ear, which is tender smooth firm with brawny induration, redness and warmness; non-mobile becomes prominent by clenching teeth; tender, palpable, upper deep cervical nodes; restricted TM joint mobility; trismus; facial nerve is normal; edematous ductal orifice with discharge

Contd...

Contd...

Condition	Features
Parotid abscess (Suppurative sialadenitis) It is a result of an acute *bacterial sialadenitis* of parotid gland. It is an ascending bacterial parotitis, due to reduced salivary flow, dehydration, starvation, sepsis, after major surgery, radiotherapy for oral malignancies and poor oral hygiene. Organisms are *Staphylococcus aureus, Streptococcus viridans*, and often others like Gram-negative and anaerobic organisms. Parotid fascia is densely thick and tough and so parotid abscess does not show any fluctuation until very late stage	Pyrexia, malaise, pain, trismus; firm swelling is seen in the parotid region which is red, tender, warm, well localized, tender lymph nodes are palpable in neck; Features of bacteremia are present in severe cases. Pus or cloudy turbid saliva may be expressed from the parotid duct opening, which can be sent for culture and sensitivity. Septicemia, severe trismus, dysphagia, rupture into external auditory canal—**complications** **Note:** In suppurative parotitis, patient may develop severe laryngeal or pharyngeal edema and may require steroids, tracheostomy and critical care
Parotid fistula It arises from *parotid gland* or *duct* or *ductules*. It may open inside the mouth as internal fistula; or open outside onto the skin as external fistula. Fistula from the duct has profuse discharge. Fistula from the gland shows only minimal discharge	**Causes:** After superficial parotidectomy; after drainage of parotid abscess; trauma; malignant recurrence of tumor **Features:** Discharging fistula in the parotid region of face; tenderness and induration; trismus
Frey's syndrome (Auriculotemporal syndrome; gustatory sweating) Occurs in 10% of cases, due to injury to auriculotemporal nerve (postsynaptic fibers from otic ganglion become united with sympathetic nerves of superior cervical ganglion) *Starch iodine test:* Involved skin is painted with iodine and dried; dry starch applied over this area turns blue due to more sweat in this area	**Causes:** Surgeries or accidental injuries to parotid Surgeries or accidental injury to temporo-mandibular joint. **Features:** Flushing, sweating, pain, hyperesthesia in the skin over the face innervated by auriculotemporal nerve whenever salivation is stimulated causing great inconvenience to patients
Sjogren's syndrome Autoimmune disease, causing progressive destruction of salivary and lacrimal glands causing keratoconjunctivitis sicca (dry eyes) and xerostomia (dry mouth) **Investigations:** Rheumatoid factor; ANF; Salivary duct antibody; sialography; *Schirmer test*—to detect lack of lacrimal secretion; FNAC of parotid and lacrimal gland; Technetium 99m pertechnetate scan	**Types:** • *Primary:* Common in middle aged women; *with severe dry eyes, dry mouth, enlarged and often tender parotid and lacrimal glands*; superadded infection in mouth (Candida common); Often bilateral parotitis; but no association of connective tissue disorders. Incidence of lymphoma is high • *Secondary:* Common in females (10:1); associated with connective tissue disorders—SLE (30%); rheumatoid arthritis(15%); primary biliary cirrhosis (near 100%)
Mikulicz disease Variant of Sjogren's syndrome; autoimmune disease of salivary and lacrimal gland with infiltration of glands with round cells; glandular tissues are replaced by lymphocytes	**Triad:** 1. Symmetrical enlargement of all salivary glands (parotid, submandibular, sublingual, accessory parotid) 2. Narrowing of palpebral fissure due to enlargement of lacrimal gland 3. Parchment like dryness of mouth; but patient is not thirsty
Sialosis It is enlargement of the salivary gland due to fatty infiltration as a result of various metabolic causes like diabetes, acromegaly, obesity, liver disease	Bilateral diffuse enlargement of parotids, which is smooth, firm, nontender
Sialectasis It is an *aseptic dilatation of salivary ductules* causing *grape-like* (cluster-like) dilatations. It is a disease of unknown etiology with destruction of parenchyma of gland accompanied by stenosis and cyst formation in the ducts	It is common in parotids; often bilateral; presents as a smooth, soft, fluctuant, non-transilluminant swelling, which increases in size during mastication; tender initially; lasts for many days with a long symptom free period of the disease. Sialogram is diagnostic (*grape cluster* look)

Anatomy of Parotid Gland (Para-around, Otis-ear)

Parts of the Parotid Gland: Superficial part (80%): Lies over the posterior part of the ramus of mandible. Deep part lies behind the mandible and medial pterygoid muscle. Parotid gland is pyramidal shaped with upper pole just below the zygomatic bone and wedged between external auditory meatus and the mandibular joint. Anterior border is over the masseter; lower pole is below and behind the angle of the mandible and indented by sternomastoid. Parotid is covered by dense parotid fascia, which is derived from investing layer of deep fascia. *Accessory parotid* is prolongation of the gland along the parotid duct. Accessory parotid is also called as social parotidis; it is located above the parotid duct. Parotid (*Stensen's*) duct is 2–3 mm in diameter, emerges from the anterior border of the gland runs horizontally across masseter and passes through the buccinator muscle and opens into the oral mucosa opposite upper second molar tooth. *Facial nerve* emerges from the stylomastoid foramen lying between external auditory meatus and mastoid process. It passes around the neck of the condyle of mandible and becomes superficial, later dividing into *temporofacial and cervicofacial branches*, which in turn, divides into many branches. Some of these may be interconnected as *pes anserinus (goose foot)*. Branches are—temporal (auricularis anterior and superior part of frontalis), zygomatic (frontalis and orbicularis oculi), upper buccal and lower buccal (buccinator, orbicularis oris, elevators of the lip), mandibular (lower lip muscles) and cervical (platysma).

Blood supply is from external carotid artery; venous drainage is to external jugular vein. Nerve supply is from autonomic nervous system; parasympathetic is secretomotor from auriculotemporal nerve; sympathetic is vasomotor from plexus around external carotid artery. *Faciovenous plane of Patey* of retromandibular vein is of surgical importance as facial nerve branches lie superficial to it. *25% of saliva* is from parotids.

Great auricular nerve (cutaneous sensory around angle and lower part of the ear lobule) and auriculotemporal nerve which is from mandibular division of trigeminal nerve (secretomotor to parotid gland) are other nerves present in relation to parotid gland.

Secretomotor Fibers: Secretomotor preganglionic fibers from *inferior salivary nucleus* → glossopharyngeal nerve → tympanic branch → tympanic plexus → lesser superficial petrosal nerve → otic ganglion → post-ganglionic fibers → auriculotemporal nerve, branch of mandibular division of trigeminal nerve → parotid gland.

Submandibular Salivary Gland

Parts: *Superficial part* lies in submandibular triangle, superficial to mylohyoid and hyoglossus muscles, between the two bellies of digastric muscles. *Deep part* is in the floor of the mouth and deep to the mylohyoid. Submandibular (*Wharton's*) duct (5 cm), comes from the deep part of the gland, enters the floor of the mouth, on a papilla beside the frenum of the tongue. Lingual nerve and submandibular ganglion are attached to upper pole of the gland. Facial artery emerges from under surface of the stylohyoid muscle, enters the gland from posterior and deep surface reaching its lateral surface crossing the lower border of mandible to enter the face. Venous drainage is to anterior facial vein. *70% of total saliva* is from submandibular salivary gland.

Secretomotor fibers of submandibular salivary gland: Preganglionic fibers from *superior salivary nucleus* → facial nerve → chorda tympani nerve → lingual nerve → submandibular ganglion → post-ganglionic fibers → submandibular and sublingual salivary glands.

Minor Salivary Glands

There are around 450 minor salivary glands which are distributed in lips, cheeks, palate and floor of the mouth. Glands also may be present in oropharynx, larynx, trachea and paranasal sinuses. They contribute to 10% of total salivary volume. Sublingual salivary glands are minor salivary glands one on each side; located in the anterior aspect of the floor of the mouth in relation to mucosa, mylohyoid muscle, body of the mandible near mental symphysis. Gland drains directly into mucosa or through a duct which drains into submandibular duct. This duct is called as *Bartholin duct*. Mikulicz disease is common in sublingual salivary gland. Minor salivary glands are *not present* in gingivae and anterior portion of the hard palate.

Ectopic Salivary Gland

Ectopic salivary gland also called as aberrant salivary gland/migrant salivary gland is nothing but ectopic lobe of the juxtaposed salivary gland. It is commonly seen in relation to submandibular salivary gland. Commonest ectopic salivary tissue is *Stafne bone cyst*. It is invagination of the juxtaposed submandibular salivary gland into the mandible bone on its lingual aspect. X-ray shows radiolucent area due to the cyst below the angle of the mandible, lower to inferior dental vessels and nerve. Jaws, eyelids, middle ear, paranasal sinus, nose, rarely skin of face and neck are other sites wherein ectopic salivary tissue can be demonstrated.

CASE DISCUSSION

A 40-year-old male comes with history of progressive, painless swelling in front of the right ear for 2 years. There is no excessive salivation, no fever. No history of any other swelling in the neck and opposite side of the face. On examination, swelling in front of the right ear in the face of 5 × 4 cm with raised ear lobule and obliteration of the hollow below and behind the mandible. Swelling is non-tender without any local rise of temperature. Surface is nodular with hard consistency. Skin is free; it is mobile in both directions with positive curtain's sign in upward movement. It is not attached to the masseter. Features of facial nerve palsy are not found. Neck nodes are not palpable clinically. Opposite side of the face and neck are normal. Oral cavity looks normal. There is no deviation of the uvula and tonsillar pillars towards opposite side. Parotid duct on palpation looks normal. Systemic examinations are normal.

What is the probable diagnosis and why?
It is right sided pleomorphic adenoma. Swelling is situated in front of the right ear; raised ear lobule; obliteration of the groove behind the ear. It is slowly progressive swelling hence benign.

Which lobe is probably involved?
Right superficial lobe is involved; deep lobe is not involved as there is no deviation and bidigitally not palpable.

What are the features of malignant transformation in benign parotid tumor?
Rapid increase in size, skin, masseter muscle and facial nerve involvement and cervical lymph gland enlargement—are the features.

How to investigate?
FNAC, CT neck and parotid region, MRI to check in selected patients.

What is the treatment?
Superficial parotidectomy is the surgical treatment.

What are the complications?
Facial nerve injury, bleeding, Frey's syndrome, flap necrosis, salivary discharge are complications.

15

Clinical Approaches and Examination of Neck

CHAPTER

Competency: AN35.5; AN35.9; AN43.5; PA19.1; PA19.2.

Neck is a complex anatomical area comprised of many compartments, triangles, tubes (trachea, esophagus), vessels and lymph nodes. Thorough anatomical knowledge of the area is essential for safe clinical and surgical practice. Student should read the specific anatomical book for the same.

■ HISTORY

History taking begins with:

Name: **Address:**   **Sex:**

Age: *Cystic hygroma, branchial cyst* and *fistula* are congenital in origin. Sternomastoid tumor, a misnomer seen in infants and children, due to organized hematoma in sternomastoid muscle leading to fibrosis of its muscle fibers following a birth trauma. *Cystic hygroma* is seen in infants (newborn). *Branchial fistula* is present since birth and is often bilateral also. *Branchial cyst* is seen in adolescents or in early adult age group. *Tuberculous lymphadenitis* occurs in young adults, *carcinoma/secondaries* in lymph nodes usually occur in elderly. *Hodgkin's lymphoma* is seen in children/adolescents or elderly like bimodal presentation. Benign swellings like lipoma, osteoma, aneurysms occur in middle aged.

Occupation: *Laryngocele* is common in trumpet blowers, glass blowers.

History of Present Illness

Swelling: Swelling is the commonest presentation in the neck. *Lymph nodal mass is the commonest* type of swelling in the neck. It could be due to lymphadenitis (nonspecific bacterial infection and inflammation); tuberculosis; malignancy; AIDS, viral causes. Other swellings which can occur in the neck are cystic swellings, carotid body tumor, cervical rib, carotid aneurysm, etc. History **(like in Chapter 4: Examination and Clinical Approach of a Swelling/Lump)** should be asked in detail. History associated with swelling like mode of onset, progress, duration, recent increase in size, number, etc. should be asked. Acute inflammatory swellings are of very short duration with signs of acute inflammation. Swelling of short duration is commonly malignant. Malignancy may be lymph node secondaries or lymphoma. It takes few months for tuberculous cold abscess to evolve in a tuberculous lymphadenitis. Presence of similar swelling elsewhere in the body like in axilla, abdomen, and groin suggests that it could be lymphoma.

Note: Thyroid swelling is the 2nd commonest swelling in the neck.

Pain: Time of onset of pain, whether it was present at the beginning, whether initially painless later became painful (sepsis, infiltration, tumor necrosis) should be asked for. Acute conditions are painful to start. Malignancy is initially painless. *Ludwig's angina* is inflammatory edema of submandibular region and floor of the mouth due to streptococcal infection causing diffuse swelling with pain, fever, trismus, brawny edema and often may cause laryngeal edema. *Submandibular abscess* due to infection and suppuration of the lymph gland is also not uncommon **(Fig. 15-1)**.

Fever: Fever suggests acute inflammatory condition; mild fever with occasional evening rise of temperature is seen in tuberculous lymphadenitis. But one should remember that fever is not necessarily a feature in all patients with many tuberculous lymphadenitis.

Sinus/fistula: Often associated with discharge. The duration, mode of onset, history of surgery in the past, type of discharge should be asked.

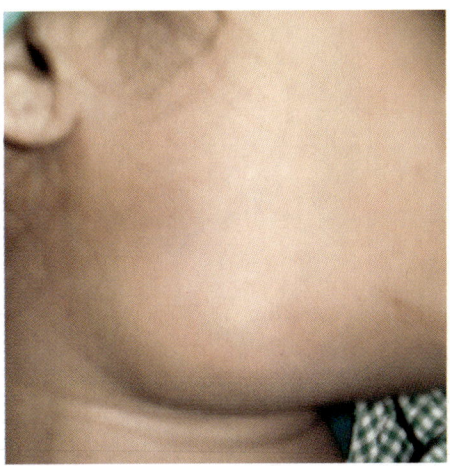

Fig. 15-1 Abscess in the right submandibular region. *It is inflamed, red, diffuse swelling.*

Relevant histories like cough, hemoptysis (tuberculosis, lymphoma and carcinoma), voice change, dyspnea, dysphagia, abdominal discomfort are important.

Hoarseness—carcinoma larynx, thyroid
Dysphagia—carcinoma posterior 1/3rd of the tongue, pharynx, esophagus
Hemoptysis, cough, dyspnea—carcinoma lung
Ear pain, deafness—nasopharyngeal carcinoma

Past History

Past history of treatment for tuberculosis, their details, treatment for malignancy (surgery, chemotherapy, radiotherapy) are important. History of diabetes mellitus and syphilis is important.

Personal History

History of smoking, alcohol consumption, dietary habits, decreased appetite and loss of weight (in advanced carcinoma and lymphoma and in tuberculosis) should be asked.

GENERAL EXAMINATION

Anemia, clubbing, jaundice, cachexia are checked. Pulse, and blood pressure are recorded; nutrition, and built are assessed. Lymph nodes on other sites are examined to rule out generalized lymphadenopathy.

LOCAL EXAMINATION

Inspection

Neck should be exposed up to the nipples for proper examination. Entire neck including all triangles should be examined. The commonest cause of neck swelling is lymph node enlargement. ***Both sides of the neck should be inspected carefully*** (Figs. 15-2 to 15-4).

Swelling

Swelling is the commonest presentation in the neck. Its number, site, size, shape, extent, surface, dilated veins, skin changes like redness, edema, ulceration or fungation should be inspected.

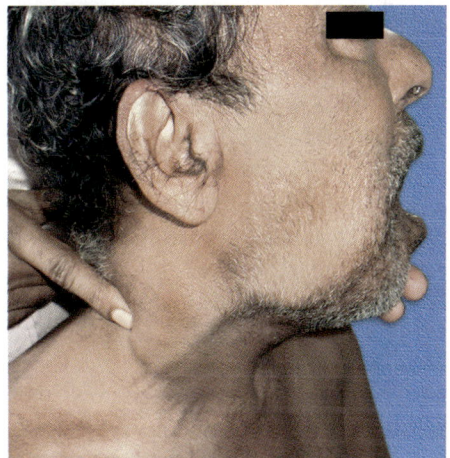

Fig. 15-2 *Proper inspection* of the neck is essential.

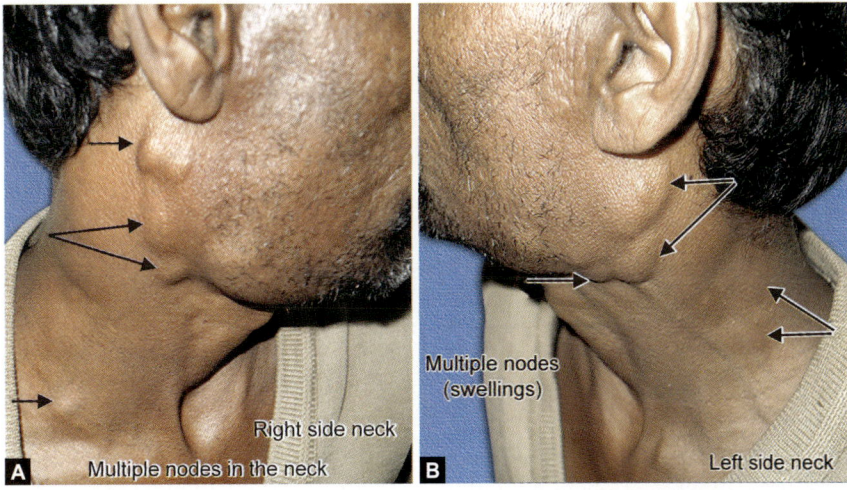

Figs. 15-3A and B *Neck should be examined both sides carefully under inspection.* Bilateral neck nodes are common. Lymph node enlargement is the *commonest swelling* in the neck.

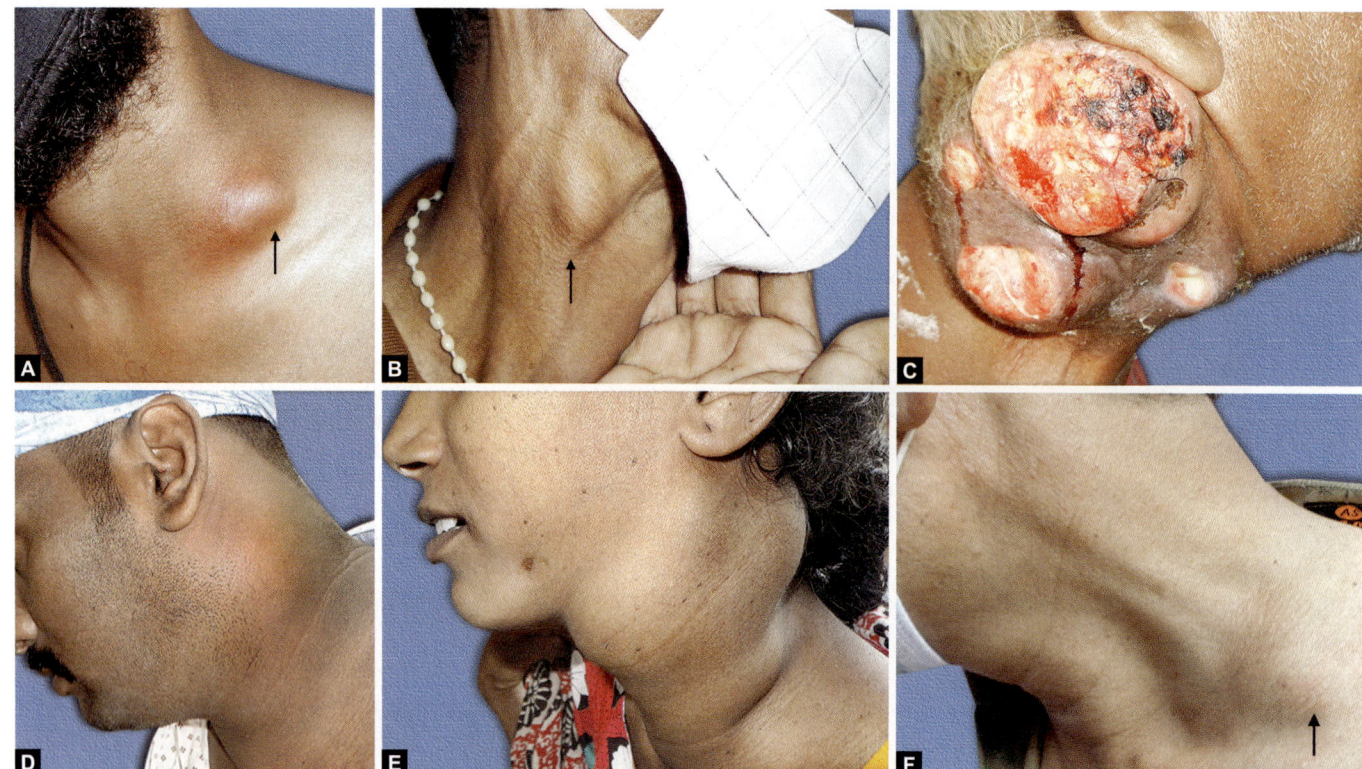

Figs. 15-4A to F Different neck swellings: (A) Cold abscess; (B) Swelling (lymph node) in relation to sternocleidomastoid muscle; (C) Fungating secondaries in neck; (D) Lymphoma neck in a male patient; (E) Hodgkiin's lymphoma in female patient; (F) Cervical rib in posterior triangle.

Site: Branchial cyst is located at the junction of upper 1/3rd and middle 1/3rd of the sternomastoid muscle with posterior ½ of the swelling lying underneath the sternomastoid muscle **(Fig. 15-5)**. Cystic hygroma occurs in supraclavicular fossa. *Dermoid cyst* can occur below the chin, in *space of Burns* in the midline at the line of embryonic fusion. *Cervical rib, cystic hygroma, subclavian artery aneurysm* occur in posterior triangle of the neck. *Carotid artery aneurysm* is usually seen in carotid triangle or along the line of carotid artery. *Carotid body tumor* is seen in carotid triangle. Lymph nodes can get enlarged in any area in neck. *Plunging ranula* can occur in upper neck (submandibular triangle).

Size: It is mentioned in centimeters usually vertical X horizontal or longitudinal X transverse dimensions. It should be confirmed later by measurement also.

Extent of the swelling: It is more relevant than the size (even though size signifies the staging, severity of the disease in malignancy). Extent should be assessed in anteroposterior and superoinferior directions which should be confirmed later by palpation. Extent is mentioned with reference to bony points like of mandible, clavicle or mastoid and also in relation to sternocleidomastoid muscle.

Number: Often neck swellings are single but lymph node swellings are multiple. Most of the neck swellings are unilateral, but lymph node swelling can be unilateral/bilateral (as in secondaries of midline primary). Tuberculous lymphadenitis can show multiple nodal enlargements, lymphoma can show enlargement of bilateral nodes **(Figs. 15-6A and B)**.

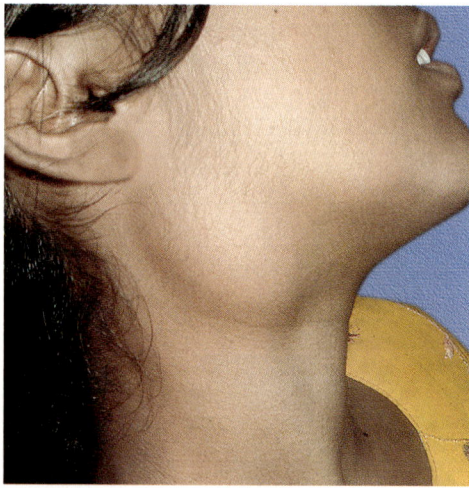

Fig. 15-5 Branchial cyst. It is *located at the junction of the upper 1/3rd and middle 1/3rd of the sternocleidomastoid muscle* level.

Surface: Nodular in secondaries and tuberculosis, smooth in lymphoma. Cold abscess and branchial cyst shows smooth surface on inspection.

Edge: Well defined in benign swelling but can be well or ill defined in malignant condition.

Mobility (on inspection): Swelling should be differentiated from thyroid swelling by checking *movement with deglutition*. Thyroid swelling, thyroglossal cyst, subhyoid bursa all move with deglutition as these swellings are directly/indirectly adherent to pretracheal fascia. Usually lymph node mass will

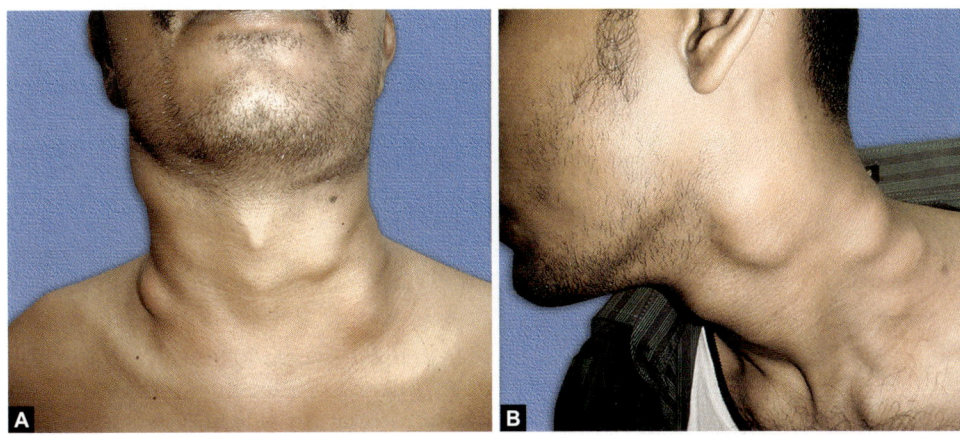

Figs. 15-6A and B Often swellings in the neck can be *multiple and bilateral*; it is commonly observed when lymph nodes in the neck are enlarged. It could be due to tuberculosis or Hodgkin's lymphoma.

not move with deglutition. Tuberculous/malignant lymph nodes that are adherent to larynx and pretracheal fascia may move with deglutition. Pretracheal or prelaryngeal lymph nodes move with deglutition.

Skin over the swelling: Dilated veins are seen in malignancy like sarcoma and vascular swellings, redness (inflammation), edema (inflammation or malignancy), discharging sinus/fistula, ulcer, scar are looked for. Undermined tuberculous ulcer/sinus/adherence to skin are known to occur in tuberculous lymphadenitis. Syphilitic gummatous ulcer may be seen in sternomastoid muscle (now rare). Sinus, ulceration, fungation may be feature of advanced fixed secondaries in the lymph node. Skin puckering is often seen in secondaries involving the platysma. Fungation can occur on the surface of the malignancy. ***Surrounding skin*** should be inspected. Multiple nodules may be seen in the surrounding skin in secondaries (metastases) **(Figs. 15-7 to 15-10)**.

Visible veins in the neck—is important; one should find out whether it is unilateral or bilateral. Increased vascularity (dilated veins), compression on the vein (dilated prominent veins) (internal jugular vein) can cause visible veins in the neck. Lymph node mass, neoplasm or aneurysm can cause unilateral visible veins. Raised CVP (central venous pressure), overhydration cause bilateral visible veins. Retrosternal goiter, thoracic outlet syndrome by compression of superior vena cava (SVC) cause **dilated visible veins** on both sides of the neck.

Visible pulsation—seen in carotid body tumor and aneurysm-pulsatile swellings; it could be transmitted like in carotid body tumor or expansile like in carotid aneurysm.

Expansile impulse on coughing and reducibility— Laryngocele shows expansile impulse or becomes prominent while blowing/coughing **(Fig. 15-11)**.

Parts proximal and distal to swelling—face, neck and chest are observed for any pressure effects of the swelling. **Dilated/engorged veins** in head, neck and chest wall suggest mediastinal compression by tumor/nodes (secondaries) or malignant tumor overlying the carotid sheath.

Muscle wasting: Wasting of trapezius **(Fig. 15-12)**, sternomastoid, and other neck muscles should be noted; *torticollis* (chin turns towards opposite side, neck towards same side due to spasm/contraction/fibrosis of sternomastoid muscle)—in sternomastoid tumor. **In torticollis**, face often is

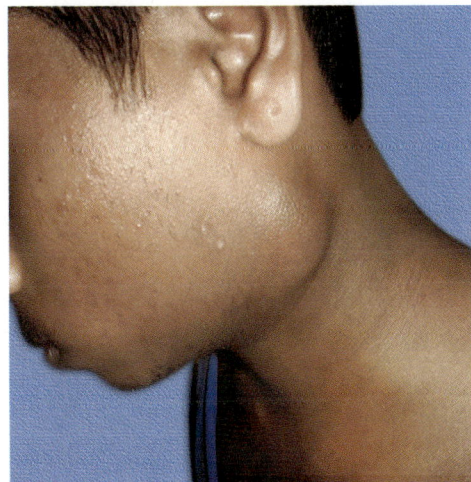

Fig. 15-7 Pyogenic abscess neck due to *suppurative lymphadenitis*; note the swelling with redness and features of acute inflammation.

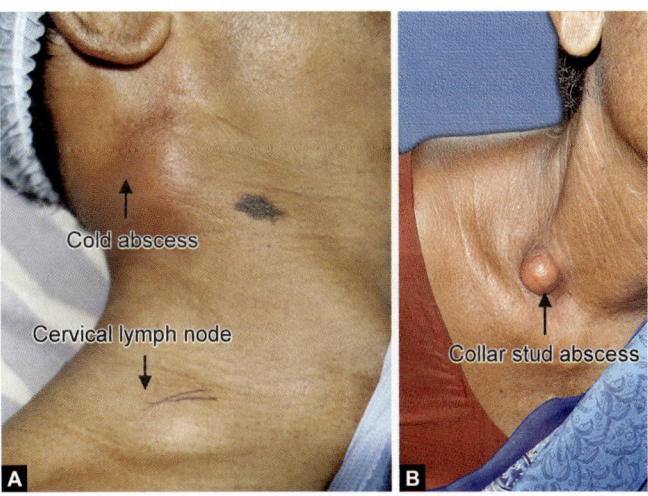

Figs. 15-8A and B (A) *Cold abscess* in the neck due to tuberculous lymphadenitis; (B) *Collar stud abscess* which is adherent to the skin.

less developed on the affected side. When patient attempts to straighten the neck, *sternal head* of sternomastoid stands out taut and firm with inability to straighten the head. Asymmetry of skull can be detected by examining the head and neck from behind. *All swellings should be inspected carefully with its relation to sternomastoid muscle.*

Fistula/Sinus

Discharging sinus or fistula should be inspected for its location, number, type of discharge and any swelling underneath; often it may be bilateral like in branchial fistula.

Branchial fistula is located at junction of middle 1/3rd and lower 1/3rd of the sternomastoid muscle along the anterior margin **(Fig. 15-13)**; ***thyroglossal fistula*** in the midline lower 1/3rd; tuberculous sinus can occur anywhere in the neck depending on the location of the underlying tuberculous lymphadenitis; chronic pyogenic osteomyelitis of the mandible can cause discharging sinus over the lower margin of the mandible; ***actinomycosis*** of the mandible

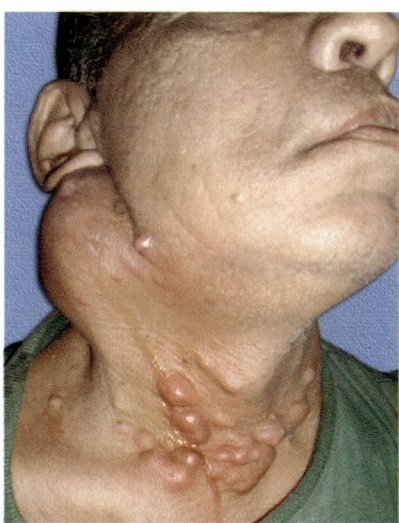

Fig. 15-9 Large secondaries in the neck with *multiple nodules in the surrounding skin.*

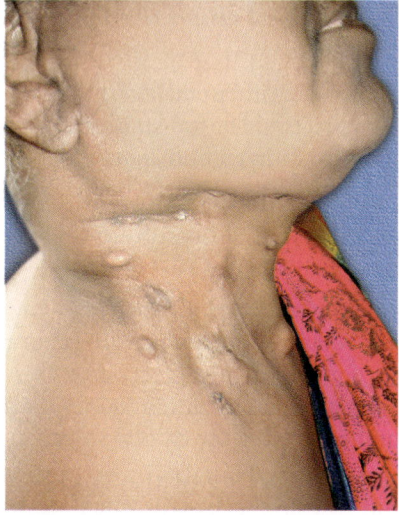

Fig. 15-10 *Skin nodules, scar of previous surgery, sinuses in the skin.* This patient has earlier undergone surgery (radical dissection) for lymph node secondaries. Now it is recurrence.

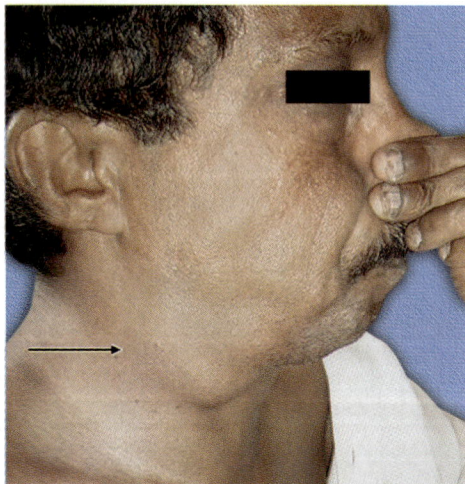

Fig. 15-11 *Laryngocele* shows expansile impulse on coughing. X-ray when taken will show radiolucent area in the region.

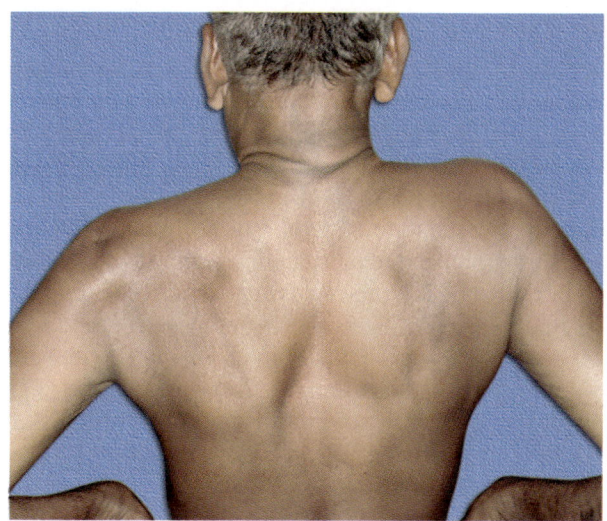

Fig. 15-12 *Wasting of the trapezius muscle* is obvious due to spinal accessory nerve involvement.

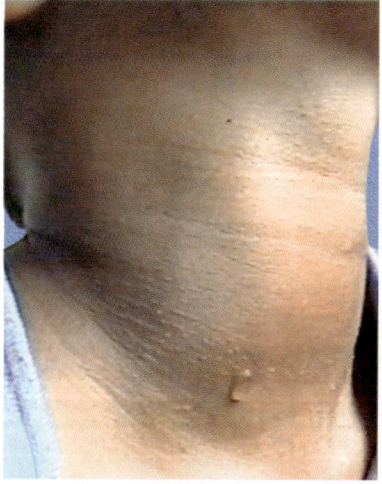

Fig. 15-13 Branchial fistula *secreting gel like fluid*. It is located at the junction of the lower 1/3rd and middle third of the sternocleidomastoid muscle. It is usually present since birth as a congenital entity.

causes multiple sinuses with discharge containing sulphur granules. After **therapeutic radiotherapy** to oral cavity region osteoradionecrosis is possible distressing complication. It causes caries teeth, osteomyelitis of the mandible presenting with severe pain, tenderness, diffuse swelling with a single sinus located at the base of the mandible; occasionally sinus may be multiple.

Palpation

Palpation of neck is done with patient sitting on a stool and examiner standing behind the patient. Initially, palpation is done from side with examiner also sitting comfortably; then it is continued from behind (*as palpation from behind is better*). Thumb is placed on the occiput with neck passively flexed to relax muscles and deep fascia. Neck is more flexed towards the side of the examination **(Fig. 15-14)**.

> First *always ascertain the relation of the swelling to sternomastoid by palpation*. With examiner standing behind the patient, patient is asked to push his chin against examiner's hand firmly to make the sternomastoid muscle tense; with the other hand examiner should palpate the sternomastoid muscle from below upward along its anterior border and ascertain the swelling in relation to the muscle. Commonest cause of neck swelling is cervical lymph node enlargement. Cervical lymph nodes are also examined *from behind*. Patient should flex the neck to relax the muscle and fascia to make the swelling easy for palpation. Usual order of palpation of lymph nodes are Level I, II, III, IV, V and VI. Submandibular group of nodes are felt with neck flexed towards same side. In posterior triangle both supraclavicular and suboccipital nodes are palpated. Often supraclavicular lymph nodes are palpated from front. *Virchow's node* is the left supraclavicular lymph node which is the harbinger of abdominal malignancy.

During palpation of the swelling one should look for temperature, tenderness, location, size, shape, surface, consistency, plane of the swelling, margin, reducibility, impulse on coughing, and mobility.

Temperature—raised in inflammatory swelling (abscess), highly vascular swelling like sarcoma, and AV malformations.

Tenderness—is seen in acute lymphadenitis and acute abscess.

Surface and edge (margin)—cystic and benign swellings have smooth surface and well defined edges (cystic hygroma, branchial cyst, dermoid cyst, laryngocele); tuberculous lymph nodes have matted surface, lymphoma have smooth surface, lymph node secondaries have irregular surface and irregular well-defined or ill-defined edges.

Consistency—soft in all cystic swellings (cystic hygroma, branchial cyst, laryngocele, lymph cyst, dermoid cyst, cold abscess), firm **India rubber like consistency** is seen in lymphoma, firm to hard in carotid body tumor, **stony hard nodular** swelling in secondaries in lymph nodes. Consistency may be uniform or variable.

Plane of the swelling: It is checked by placing the hand below the chin opposite to the side of the swelling and then the patient is asked to turn the chin to opposite side against resistance of the examiner's hand thereby contracting the sternomastoid **(Fig. 15-15)**. Alternatively examiner's hand (can be fisted hand) can be placed under the chin (**chin test**) of the patient who is asked to push/nod the chin downwards against resistance offered by the examiner's hand (here sternomastoid on both sides contract and become prominent) and swelling is palpated to check whether it is deep to sternomastoid or not. The plane is checked on both sides simultaneously. If the swelling is in deeper plane, when muscle is made taut it reduces in size with restricted mobility. If the swelling is in superficial plane, it becomes more prominent remains mobile over the muscle after muscle contraction. Swelling is freely mobile but mobility will be restricted while contracting the muscle if swelling is arising from the muscle or fixed to muscle.

Fixity to skin: Pinching the skin/gliding the skin over the swelling should be done to assess the fixity to skin. Skin is often fixed to swelling in lymph node secondaries, tuberculosis forming collar stud abscess and acute lymphadenitis **(Figs. 15-16 and 15-17)**.

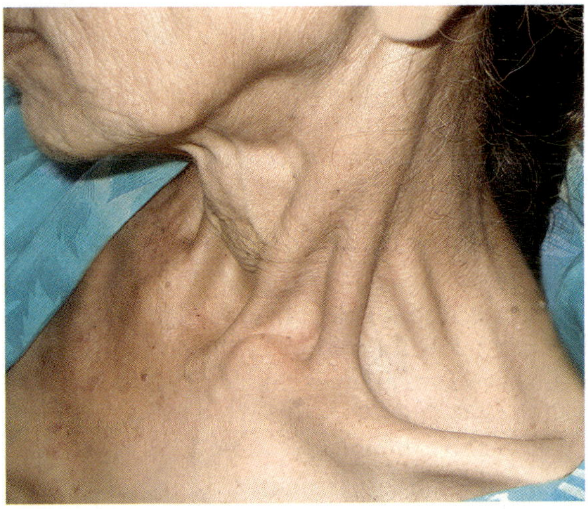

Fig. 15-14 One should always *ascertain the relation of the swelling to sternocleidomastoid muscle.*

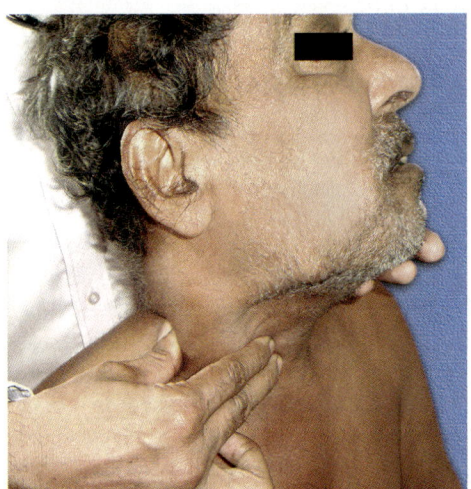

Fig. 15-15 *Method of checking the relation of sternomastoid muscle to swelling by palpating from behind and by contracting the muscle against resistance.*

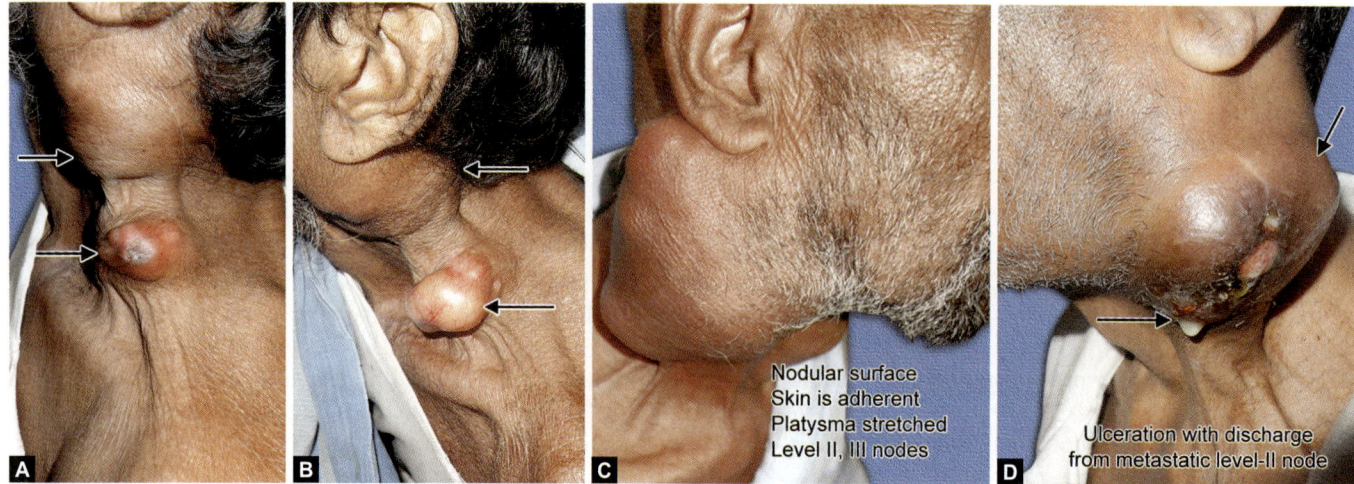

Figs. 15-16A to D Different secondaries in cervical lymph node (metastatic). *Nodularity, skin involvement, fixity, adherent to sternocleidomastoid muscle, ulceration, discharge*—are observed.

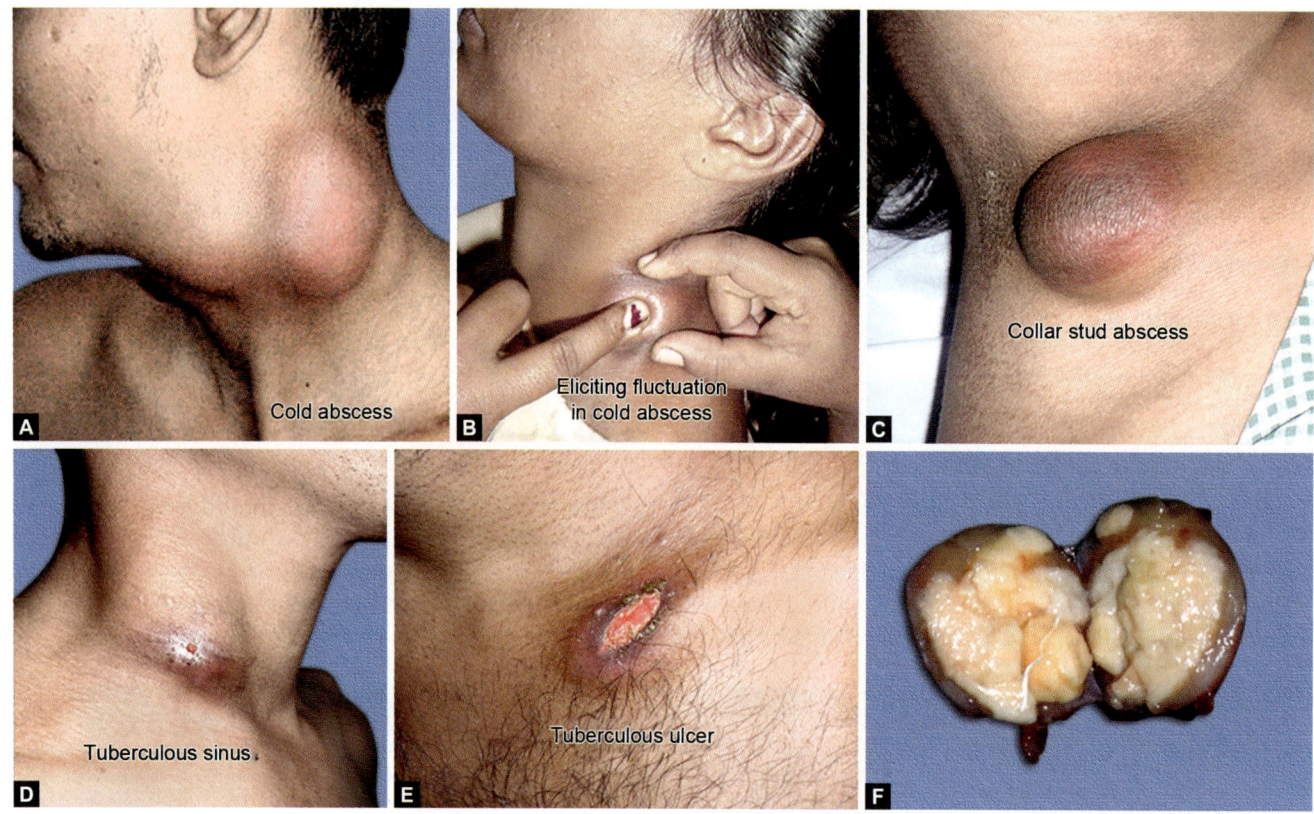

Figs. 15-17A to F *Cold abscess, eliciting fluctuation (Paget's); collar stud abscess; tuberculous sinus; tuberculous ulcer*—due to cervical tuberculous lymphadenitis (different stages). Note the cut section of tuberculous lymph node showing caseation.

Mobility: It should be checked in both directions. Carotid body tumor and carotid aneurysm move *only* horizontally not in the line of the artery. **Swelling will be completely immobile** if it is fixed posteriorly to paravertebral region as seen in advanced secondaries in neck **(Figs. 15-18A to E)**. Bony swelling is immobile; example—cervical rib in supraclavicular region.

Fluctuation—checked in two directions. Both patient and clinician should be sitting comfortably in stools. Small swellings need Paget's test to be done to check for fluctuation. Cold abscess, cystic hygroma, lymph cyst, branchial cyst, dermoid cyst, subhyoid bursa, thyroglossal cyst are *fluctuant*.

Transillumination: Cystic hygroma and lymph cyst are **brilliantly transilluminant** as they contain clear fluid. Branchial cyst is often transilluminant. Cold abscess is not transilluminant. Transillumination is checked in a dark room using pen torch and *transilluminoscope* **(Figs. 15-19 and 15-20)**.

Pulsation—expansile/transmitted; carotid aneurysm shows **expansile** pulsation; *carotid body tumor* shows **transmitted** pulsation. A rare tumor (neurofibroma) can occur from vagus nerve on the posterior aspect of the carotid sheath which

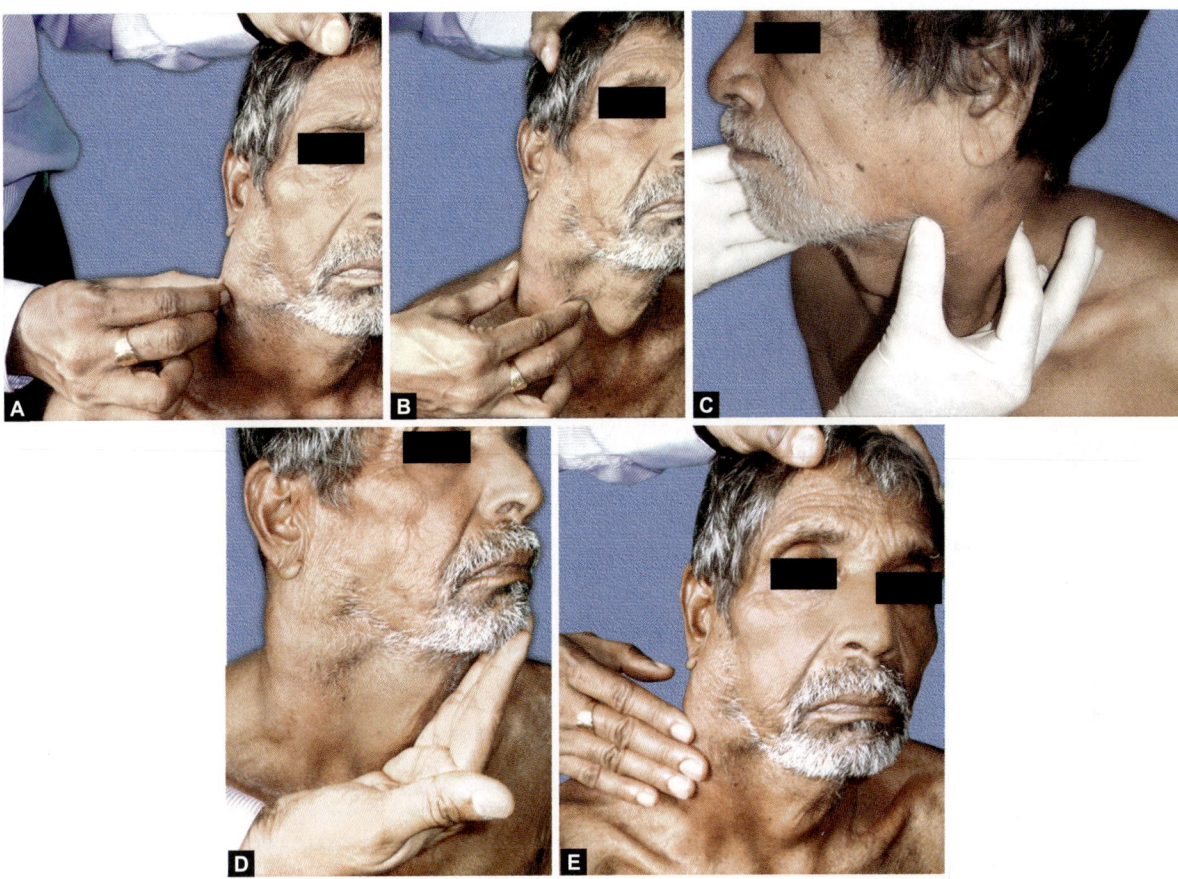

Figs. 15-18A to E *Skin pinching (for fixity); mobility; contraction* of sternomastoid against resistance towards opposite side to find out the plane of the swelling; palpation from all directions of the swelling are essential.

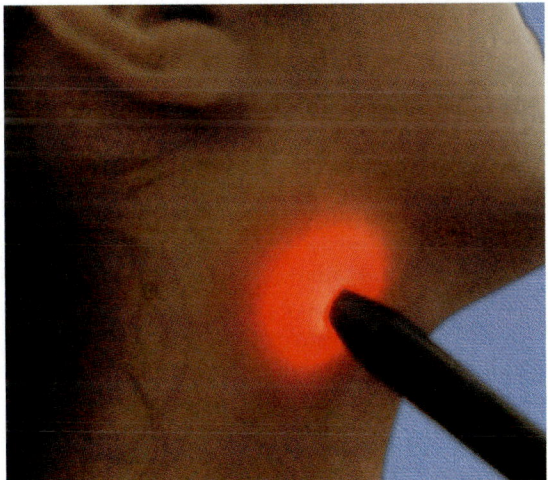

Fig. 15-19 Transilluminant swelling in the neck; it could be acquired lymph cyst. Branchial cyst often may be transilluminant.

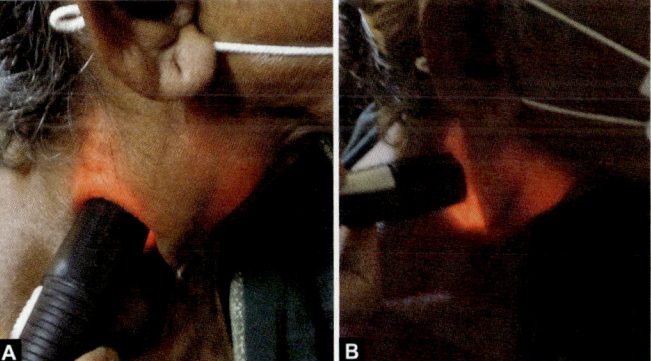

Figs. 15-20A and B Transilluminant swelling in the neck in adult probably lymph cyst. Transillumination should be checked ideally in dark room.

causes cough sensation while palpation; and this swelling is only horizontally mobile, firm, with typical transmitted pulsation. Occasionally hypervascular tumors may show expansile pulsation.

Compressibility: Here swelling partially reduces in size on gentle pressure and returns back to its original size after releasing the pressure. Hemangioma, lymphangiomas are compressible.

Expansile impulse on coughing and reducibility—*Laryngocele* may show expansile impulse or becomes prominent while blowing/coughing (expansile impulse is both seen and felt and so should be inspected during inspection).

Crepitation—is felt in surgical emphysema.

Torticollis—It is due to shortening of sternomastoid, should be differentiated from ocular torticollis. Head is clasped by examiner's hand and slowly straightened observing the eyes. Straightening of the head makes squint apparent in ocular torticollis **(Fig. 15-21)**.

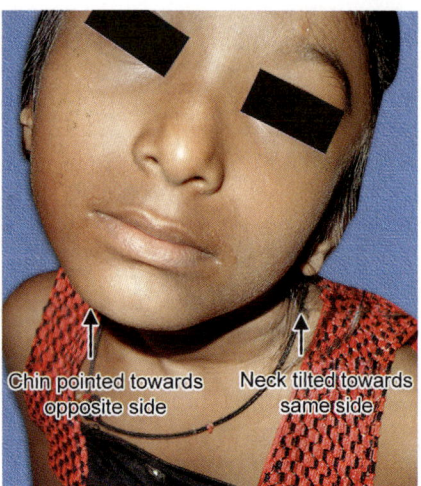

Fig. 15-21 *Torticollis* with head turning towards same side and chin pointing towards opposite side.

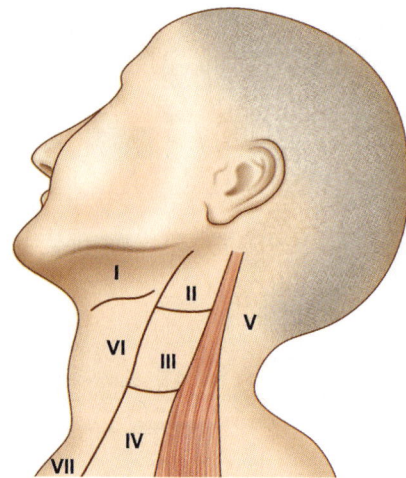

Fig. 15-22 *Levels in cervical lymph nodes.*

Examination of Lymph Nodes of the Neck

This is very important part of the examination of neck as the common cause of swelling in the neck is nodal enlargement. ***Lymph nodes are better examined from behind. One side is examined first then later on the other side***. Initial palpation can be done from the side of the patient. It is better to use four fingers of the hand while palpating the lymph nodes of the neck **(Figs. 15-22 to 15-30)**.

ANATOMY OF LYMPHATICS OF HEAD AND NECK

Nodes are arranged in levels (Sloan Kettering Memorial Hospital, USA)—Level I to level VI.
1. Level I—submental and submandibular nodes; Ia is submental; Ib is submandibular.
2. Level II is upper deep cervical (extends from base of skull to hyoid bone). Level IIa is below the spinal accessory nerve (in sternomastoid muscle) and IIb above the nerve.
3. Level III is middle deep cervical (extends from hyoid bone to omohyoid muscle).
4. Level IV is lower deep cervical (extends from omohyoid muscle to clavicle).
5. Level V is posterior triangle nodes. Level Va is above the spinal accessory level (in posterior triangle) and level Vb is below it.
6. Level VI is central nodes (paratracheal and laryngeal).
7. Level VII is mediastinal node.

Note: Retropharyngeal nodes, facial nodes, post-auricular nodes are not included in these levels.

Waldeyer rings
- *Inner Waldeyer's ring* which includes adenoid, tubal tonsils, faucial tonsils, lingual tonsils also should be examined.
- *Outer Waldeyer's ring* (outer circular chain of nodes) includes occipital, post-auricular, preauricular, parotid, facial, submandibular, submental, superficial cervical and anterior cervical.

Healy's classification of lymph nodes in neck
- SH—superior horizontal chain; IH—inferior horizontal chain; PV—posterior vertical chain; IV—intermediate chain; AV—anterior vertical chain.

Drainage areas
- *Submandibular lymph nodes drain:* The side of the nose, cheek, angle of the mouth, entire upper lip, outer part of the lower lip, the gums, side of the tongue.

- *Submental lymph nodes drain:* From the central part of the lower lip, floor of the mouth and apex of the tongue.
- *Superficial cervical nodes:* They lie on outer surface of the sternomastoid around the external jugular vein. They drain the parotid region and lower part of the ear.
- *Deep cervical lymph nodes:* Upper deep cervical lymph nodes—*jugulodigastric nodes*; lower deep cervical lymph nodes—*jugulo-omohyoid nodes*; middle deep nodes. They drain from that half of head and neck and finally form a *jugular lymph trunk* from lower deep cervical to join thoracic duct on the left side and junction of right subclavian and right jugular vein on right side.

Other Relevant Examinations to Look for

Spinal accessory nerve: Shrugging of shoulder is difficult
Hypoglossal nerve: Tongue deviates to same side with wasting
Sympathetic chain: Horner's syndrome with miosis, anhidrosis, upper eyelid droop (pseudoptosis), enophthalmos and loss of spinociliary reflex.

Nerve involvement: Patient is asked to protrude the tongue to look for hypoglossal nerve palsy (tongue deviates towards affected side); defective shrugging of shoulder with wasting of trapezius is seen in spinal accessory nerve involvement; features of Horner's syndrome in cervical sympathetic chain involvement **(Fig. 15-31). Also refer Chapter 29, Page 523.**

Vessel involvement—palpation of carotid artery pulsation, superficial temporal artery pulsation (over zygomatic bone) should be done **(Figs. 15-32 and 15.33)**.

Neighboring organ involvement: Tracheal palpation; *laryngeal crepitus* (normally it is present, but absent in advanced laryngeal carcinoma—***Bocca's sign***) should be checked. Laryngeal crepitus is present in normal individual; it is elicited by holding the larynx with thumb and fingers and transversely moving the larynx **(Fig. 15-34)**. Crepitus in larynx is derived from the cricoarytenoid joint of the larynx.
Examination of the trachea: Trachea should be examined using three fingers for deviation. ***Oliver's sign*** is tracheal tug

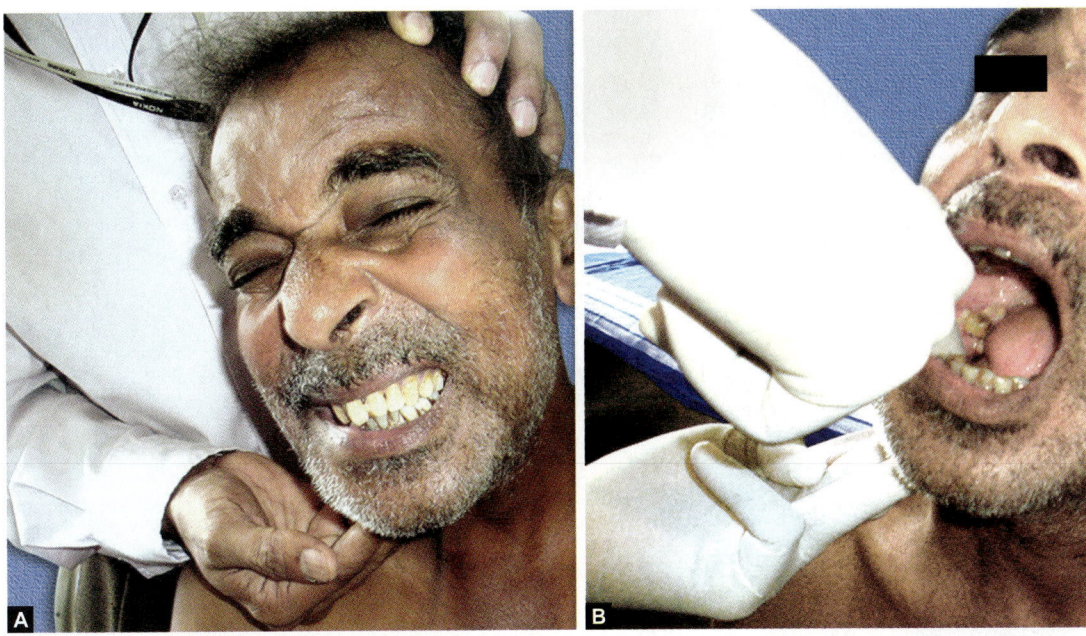

Figs. 15-23A and B *Submandibular lymph nodes are examined from behind with flexion of the neck. Bidigital palpation is* done to confirm it as lymph nodes not as submandibular salivary gland. Lymph nodes are not bidigitally palpable; submandibular salivary gland is bidigitally palpable.

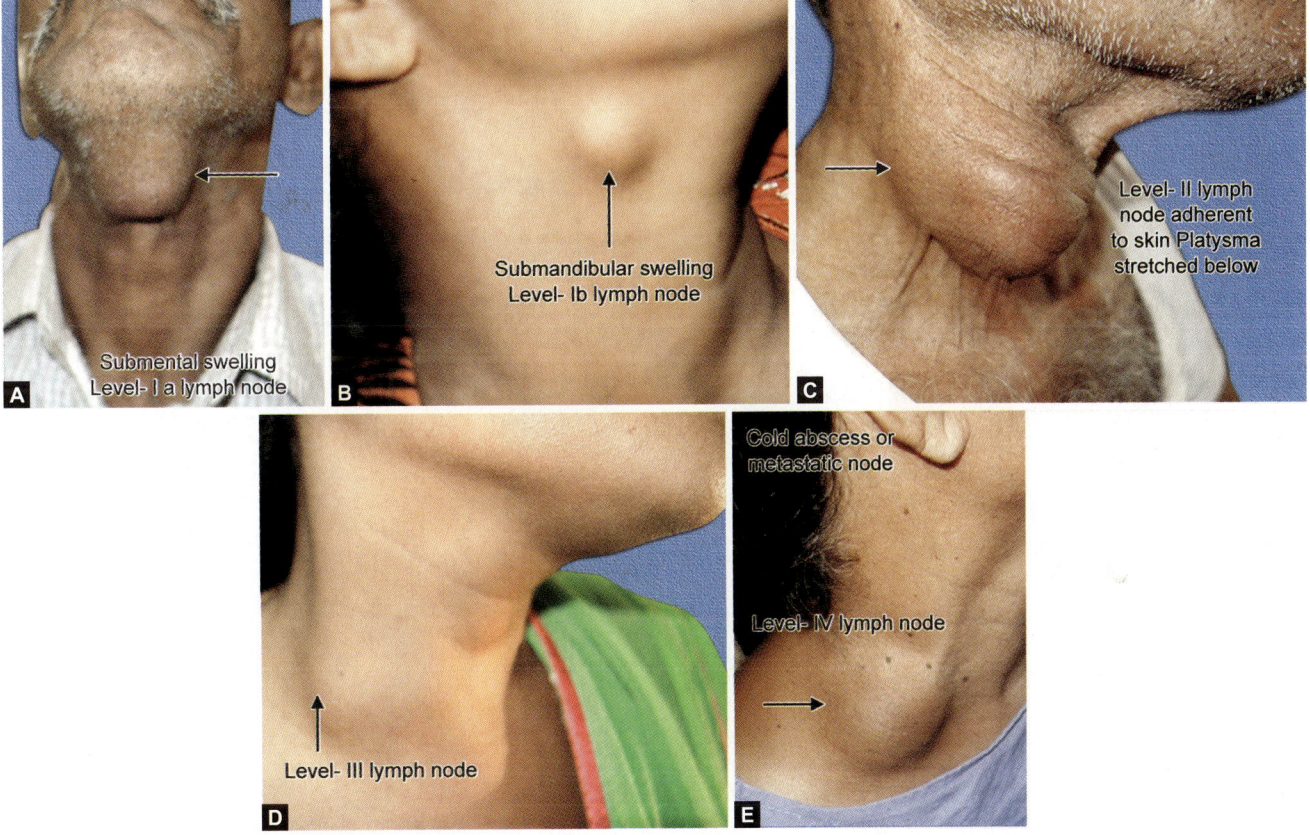

Figs. 15-24A to E *Neck nodes at different levels.* (A) Level I a—submental node (it could be cystic swelling in the midline or lipoma); (B) Level II b—submandibular node; (C) Level II—upper deep (jugulodigastric) lymph node; (D) Level III—middle deep cervical lymph node; Level IV—lower deep cervical node.

felt due to compression over the bronchus by aortic aneurysm **(Fig. 15-35)**.

Oral cavity should be examined in all neck swellings especially when swelling is thought to be lymph node. Tonsils may show tubercles in case of tubercular lymphadenitis. Retropharyngeal abscess in tuberculosis is chronic and is in midline **(Fig. 15-36)**.

Drainage area of the specific lymph nodes which are palpable should be examined. *Cervical lymph nodes*

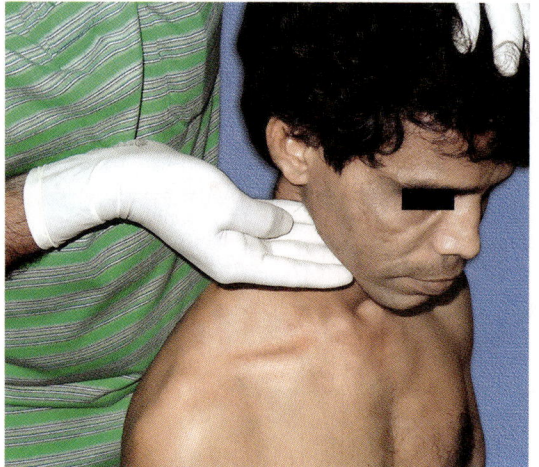

Fig. 15-25 Palpation of *level 1* lymph nodes.

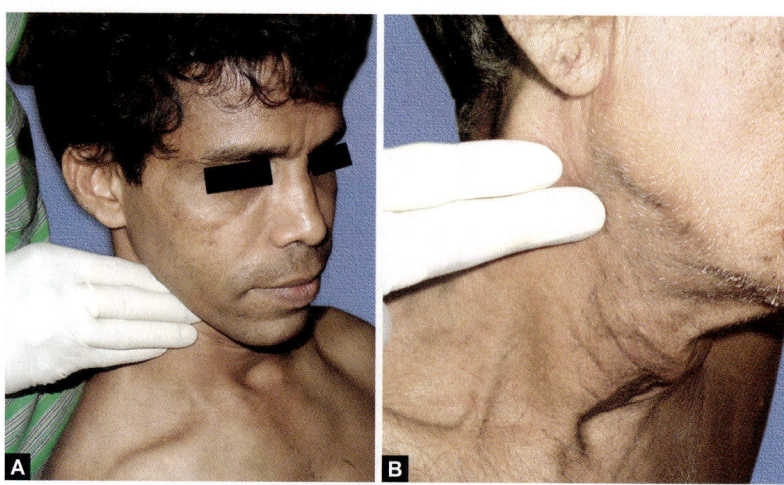

Figs. 15-26A and B Palpation of *level 2* lymph nodes.

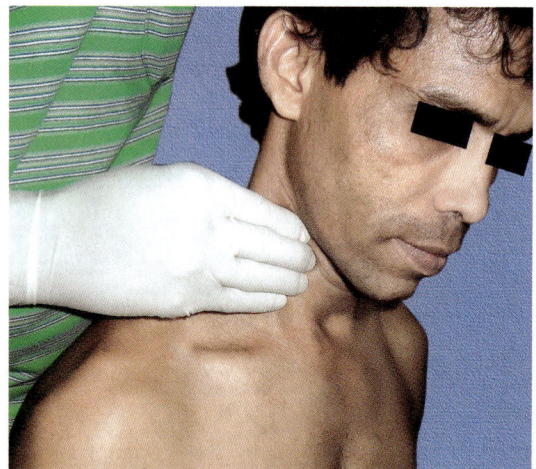

Fig. 15-27 Palpation of *level 3* lymph nodes.

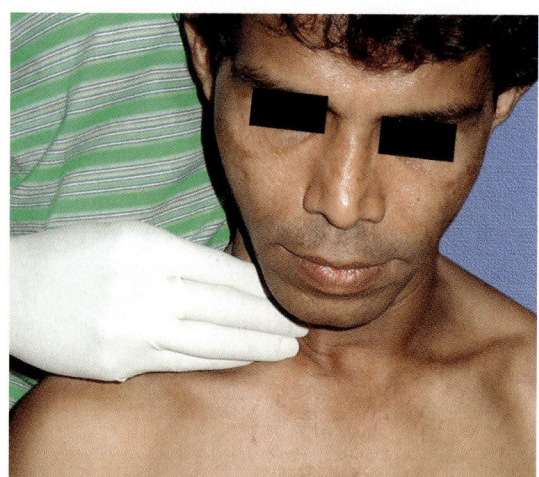

Fig. 15-28 Palpation of *level 4* lymph nodes.

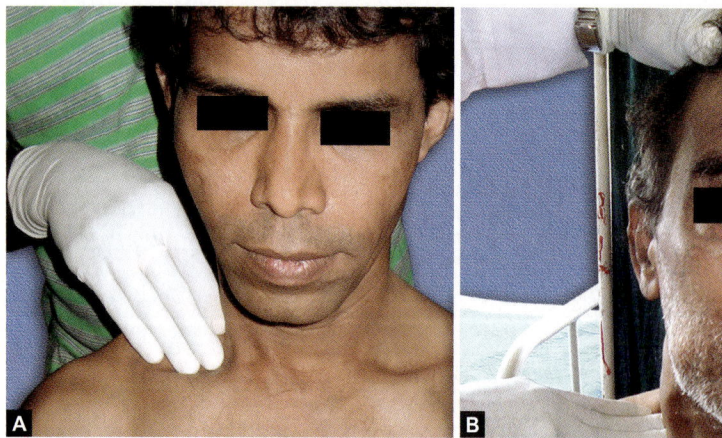

Figs. 15-29A and B Palpation of level 5 lymph nodes. It is palpated both from behind and front.

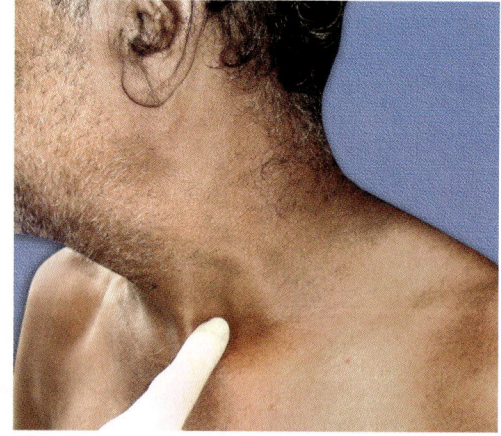

Fig. 15-30 Palpation of *Virchow's lymph node* in the neck in supraclavicular region.

drain from lymphatics of head, neck, face, oral cavity, nasal cavity, paranasal sinuses, pharynx, larynx and thyroid. Left supraclavicular nodes receive from left upper limb, left side chest wall, left breast, abdomen and both testes.

In females (rarely in male) carcinoma breast may be the cause of neck node enlargement, so breast should be examined in suspected cases.

Other lymph nodes in the body should be examined—axillary, para-aortic, iliac, inguinal, epitrochlear (above the

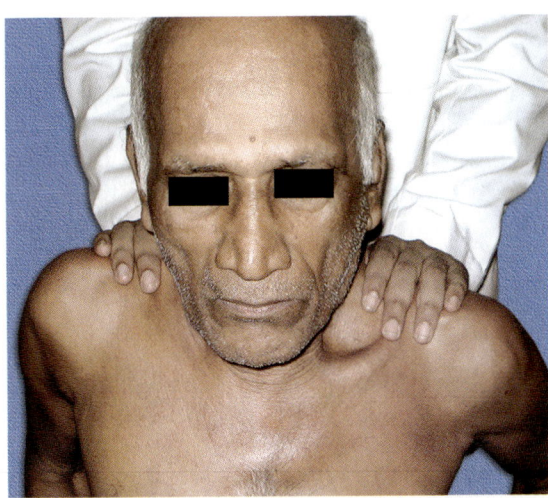

Fig. 15-31 *Shrugging of shoulder against resistance* to check trapezius paralysis due to infiltration of spinal accessory nerve.

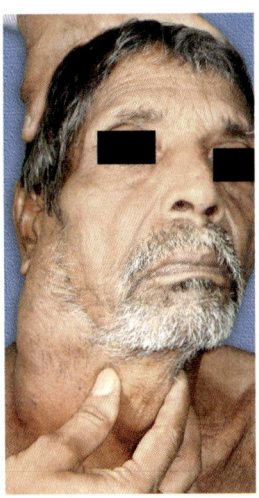

Fig. 15-34 *Laryngeal crepitus* is present normally. It will be absent in advanced carcinoma larynx.

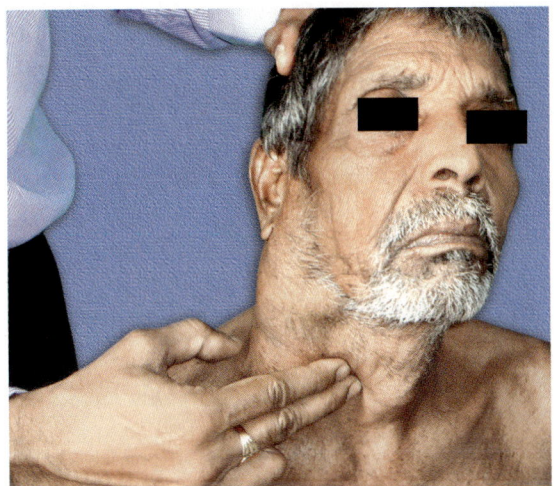

Fig. 15-32 *Carotid pulsation* should be checked to confirm whether it is infiltrated/encased by tumor/presence of thrill (suggests stenosis) and also should be auscultated for bruit.

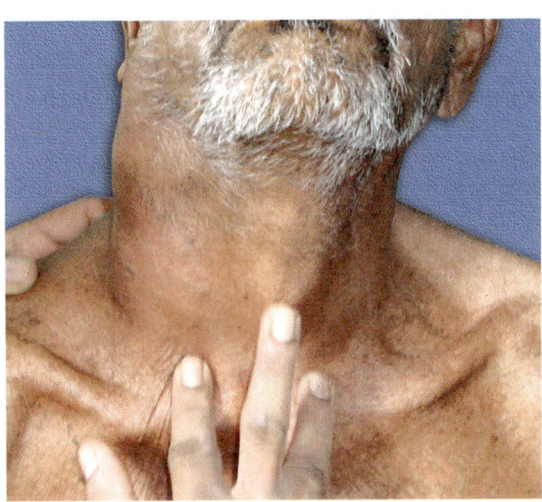

Fig. 15-35 Trachea should be examined *for deviation*.

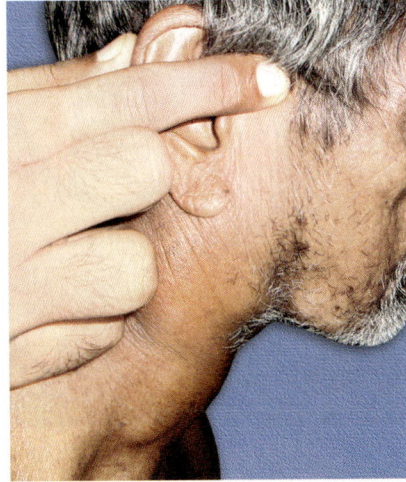

Fig. 15-33 *Superficial temporal artery* pulsation should be checked in front of tragus over zygoma.

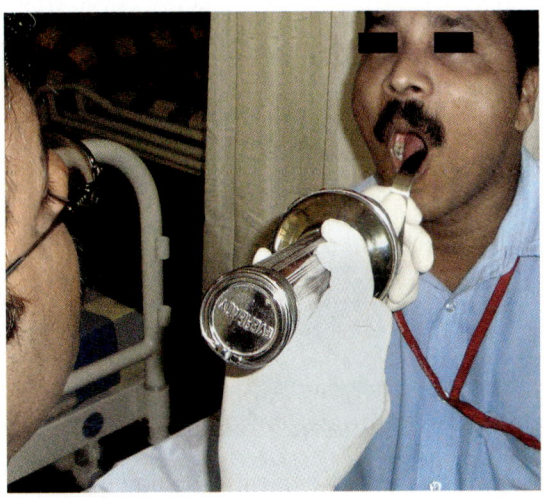

Fig. 15-36 *Oral cavity should be examined* in all neck swelling patients thoroughly.

medial epicondyle and on the medial aspect of the arm), and popliteal lymph nodes. Lymphoma may cause generalized lymphadenopathy **(Figs. 15-37A and B)**. Preauricular, buccal/parotid lymph nodes should be examined.

Percussion

In laryngocele tympanic note may be heard on percussion. Percussion over the sternum is important to elicit tenderness in lymphoma (bone marrow involvement—Stage IV) and also in mediastinal nodal mass, when present will elicit dullness **(Fig. 15-38)**.

Auscultation

Auscultation is done to hear *bruit over carotid* in carotid artery aneurysm; over supraclavicular region in subclavian artery aneurysm.

Examination of the Larynx, Pharynx, Nasal Cavities, Paranasal Sinuses and Ear

Laryngeal mirror is essential to visualize and examine it.
Nasopharynx is palpated with patient sitting on a stool. Examiner stands behind the patient with patient extending his neck and head which is supported by examiner's body. After opening the mouth one side index finger pushes the cheek inward from outside (to prevent biting of the examiner's hand). Index finger of the other hand is passed inside towards nasopharynx to sweep over the roof and walls of the nasopharynx **(Fig. 15-39)**.

Retropharyngeal abscess is always felt and only often seen after proper depression of the tongue (can be seen when inspected using a direct laryngoscope). It is felt as an indentable cushion like projection to the finger. Acute retropharyngeal abscess is usually due to suppuration of retropharyngeal lymph node and occupies a lateral

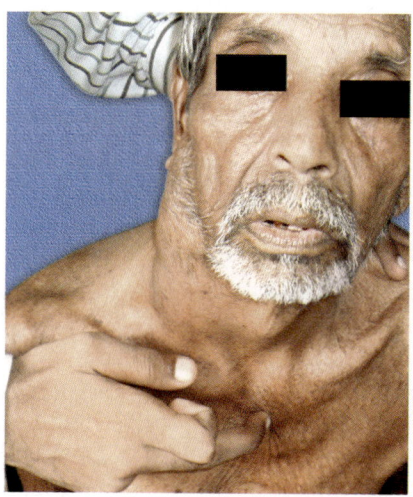

Fig. 15-38 *Percussion over sternum for tenderness* (in lymphoma and lymphatic leukemia) *and dullness* for mediastinal mass.

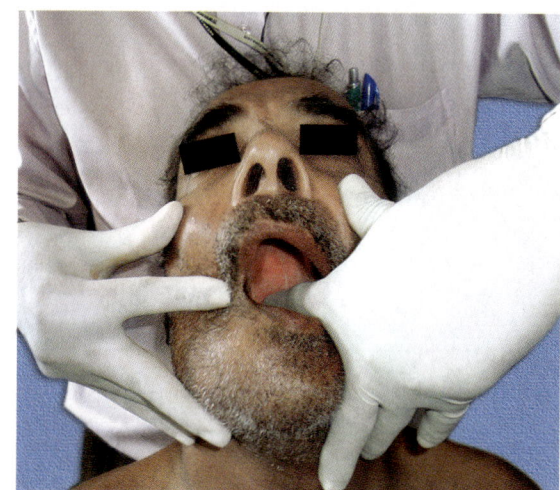

Fig. 15-39 Palpation of nasopharynx *from behind*.

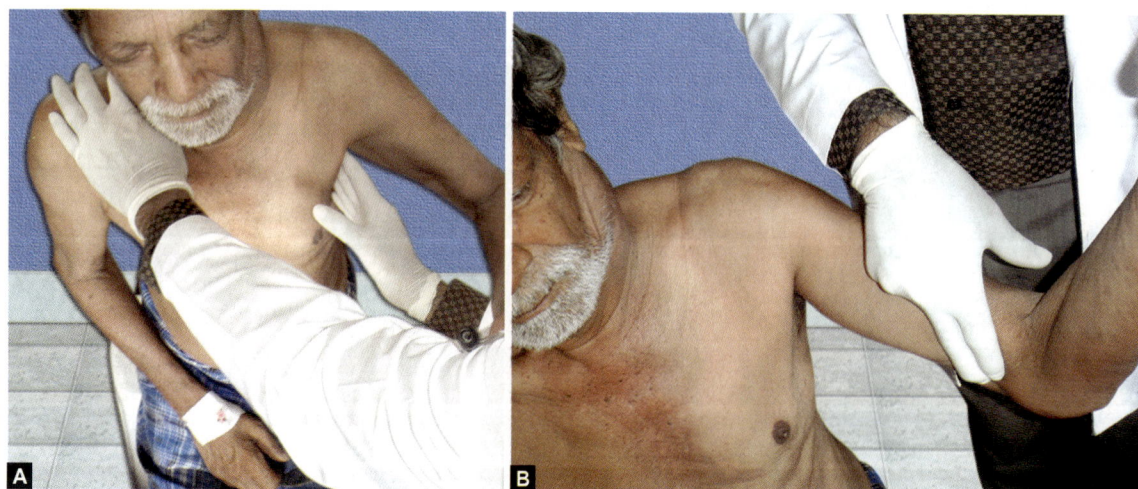

Figs. 15-37A and B Other lymph node regions like *axilla, groin, abdomen* should be examined for significant palpable lymph nodes.

position. Chronic retropharyngeal abscess is usually due to tuberculosis of cervical spine (C6) and is situated behind the prevertebral fascia in midline. However, occasionally tuberculosis of retropharyngeal lymph nodes can occur as a rare entity and in such situation, it will be in lateral position. It also may present as swelling/cold abscess in the neck behind the sternomastoid muscle.

Nasal cavities should be examined using a nasal speculum. Frontal, ethmoidal and maxillary air sinuses should be examined for fullness, swelling, tenderness. Sinusitis is common. Tumors of maxillary and ethmoidal air sinuses should be thought of. Maxillary tumor causes upward displacement of eye; ethmoidal tumor causes lateral displacement of the eye. Neoplasm in frontal air sinuses is practically *rare*. Proper knowledge of surgical anatomy of these areas is essential.

■ SYSTEMIC EXAMINATION

Abdomen should be examined for splenomegaly and hepatomegaly in case of lymphoma; hepatomegaly in case of secondaries **(Figs. 15-40A and B)**.

Respiratory system is examined for pulmonary tuberculosis, bronchogenic carcinoma.

Skeletal system: Spine and long bones should be examined for secondaries and involvement in case of lymphoma. Tenderness, swelling, pathological fracture may be evident.

Neurological deficits and paraplegia with bowel and urinary incontinence may be present in case of spine involvement.

Spine: Cervical spine should be examined (paraspinal spasm, tenderness, deformity, restricted movements) especially in case of tuberculosis of cervical spine. Movements are grossly restricted in acute inflammatory condition and tuberculosis. *Spine should be examined both in standing* and sitting position **(Fig. 15-41)**.

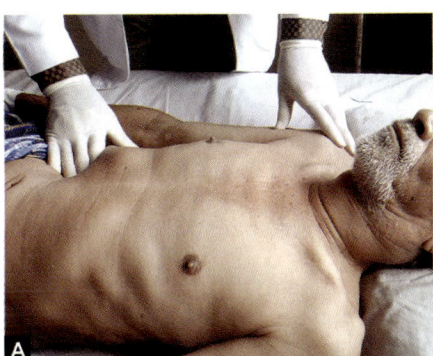
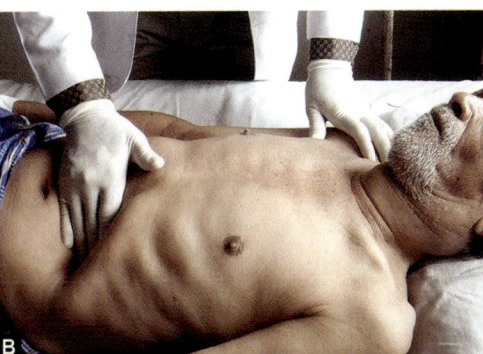

Figs. 15-40A and B Abdomen should be examined for *hepatosplenomegaly* in case of lymphoma.

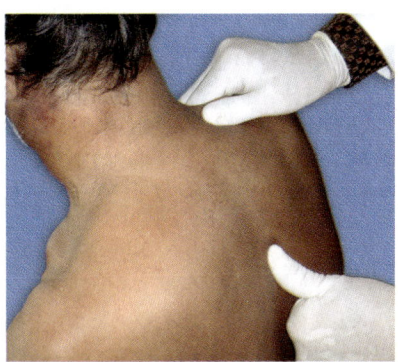

Fig. 15-41 Spine should be examined in neck lymph node enlargement for lymphoma or tuberculosis.

Case sheet writing in a patient with neck swelling
History
Name: Age:
Occupation: Sex: Place/residence:
Chief complaints
History of present illness   • Swelling—duration, mode of onset and progress, site of origin, number, disappearing or reducing in size   • Pain—origin, nature, character, duration, time of starting of pain, specific features, severity, aggravating or relieving factors   • Fever—type, severity, duration   • Other lumps—when started, progress   • Secondary changes like ulceration, fungation   • Loss of function   • Loss of weight   • Pressure symptoms
Past history   • Past history of swelling and treatment for that   • Tuberculosis, spinal diseases, diabetes, leprosy, malignancies   • Past history of treatment and surgery
Family history   • Family tree; history of tuberculosis, diabetes, malignancies; treatment history
General examination   Anemia, edema, jaundice, clubbing, lymphadenopathy, pulse, blood pressure, temperature, attitude, nutrition, body weight

Contd...

Contd...

Case sheet writing in a patient with neck swelling

Local examination

Inspection
- Swelling—location/site (in relation to bony point and sternocleidomastoid muscle), size, shape, extent, color, surface of the swelling, skin over the swelling, number, edge/margin/border of the swelling, movement of the swelling, pulsation, impulse on coughing, sinus, fistula
- Pressure effects—edema, dilated veins, paralysis, deformity, wasting

Palpation
- Local raise of temperature, tenderness
- Size, shape and extent of the swelling, edge of the swelling, surface of the swelling, consistency
- Fluctuation, transillumination test
- Reducibility, expansile impulse on coughing, compressibility, pulsatility, thrill
- Plane of the selling (should be checked in relation to sternocleidomastoid muscle by contracting it), mobility, fixity to skin or deeper structures
- Examination proximal and distal to swelling
- Examination of regional neurological (*spinal accessory, hypoglossal, sympathetic chain*) and vascular systems

Examination of oral cavity (is a must), scalp, ear, nasal cavities, paranasal sinuses

Percussion

Auscultation—bruit over the swelling or carotid or subclavian arteries

Examination of cervical lymph nodes and other regional nodes like axilla, groin, para-aortic, epitrochlear, popliteal

Systemic examination—abdomen, respiratory, cardiac and central nervous systems

INVESTIGATIONS

- Fine needle aspiration cytology (FNAC) of the node. It is useful in secondaries, tuberculosis (epithelioid cells). In branchial cyst cholesterol crystals are seen (Fig. 15-42).
- Lymph node biopsy in suspected case of lymphoma.
- Chest X-ray, X-ray cervical spine in tuberculosis.
- Fistulogram in branchial fistula and other fistulas.
- MR fistulogram.
- CT scan chest and neck for multiple nodal mass.
- Barium swallow or water soluble contrast study (better) in pharyngeal pouch.
- Arterial Doppler in aneurysm, carotid body tumor, subclavian artery aneurysm.
- Carotid or subclavian arteriogram.
- Discharge study for AFB, culture, cytology.
- Wedge biopsy if ulcer is present.
- Laryngoscopy/bronchoscopy/mediastinoscopy/esophagoscopy in relevant causes.

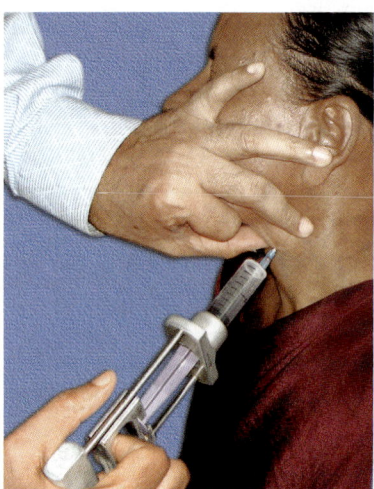

Fig. 15-42 FNAC of neck lymph node is *ideal initial investigation*.

CLASSIFICATION OF NECK SWELLINGS

Neck swellings are grossly classified as midline swellings, lateral swellings and others (*refer table*). Other classifications are—non-neoplastic and neoplastic; Benign and malignant; Inflammatory and non-inflammatory; thyroidal and non-thyroidal; lymph nodal and non-lymph nodal mass/swellings.

Swellings in the neck are also classified as swellings arising *superficial to deep fascia* like–lipoma, sebaceous cyst etc. Swelling arising from structures *deep to deep fascia* which are specific to neck region.

Different Classifications of Neck Swellings

Midline swellings of the neck	Lateral swellings	Others
• Ludwig's angina • Submental lymph node • Sublingual dermoid • Thyroglossal cyst • Subhyoid bursa • Thyroid isthmus swelling • Prelaryngeal and pretracheal lymph nodes • Midline dermoids and lipomas • Suprasternal lymph node	**Submandibular triangle:** • Submandibular salivary gland enlargement • Submandibular lymph node enlargement • Plunging ranula • Jaw tumors extending down **Carotid triangle:** • Carotid aneurysm • Carotid body tumor • Branchial cyst • Branchiogenic carcinoma • Thyroid swelling—lateral lobe • Sternomastoid tumor • Lymph nodal mass	**Acute** • Cellulitis • Lymphadenitis • Ludwig's angina **Chronic** *Cystic:* • Cold abscess • Cystic lesions of thyroid • Branchial cyst • Thyroglossal cyst • Cystic hygroma • Dermoid cyst • Sebaceous cyst

Contd...

Contd...

Midline swellings of the neck	Lateral swellings	Others
	Posterior triangle: • Lymph nodal mass • Cystic hygroma • Pharyngeal pouch • Subclavian aneurysm • Cervical rib • Lateral aberrant thyroid	*Solid:* • Secondaries in neck lymph nodes • Thyroid swelling • Branchiogenic carcinoma • Sternomastoid tumor • Cervical rib • Soft tissue tumor *Pulsatile* • Carotid aneurysm • Carotid body tumor • Subclavian artery aneurysm • Primary toxic goiter

Causes for Neck Swelling
Infectious
- *Bacterial:* Nonspecific—*streptococcal, staphylococcal; Specific*, tuberculous, syphilis, leprosy, plague
- *Viral*—Epstein-Barr, cytomegalovirus, HIV
- *Protozoal*—toxoplasmosis, filarial
- *Fungal*—blastomycosis, histomycosis
- *Chlamydial*—lymphogranuloma venereum (LGV)

Neoplastic
- *Benign*
- *Malignant*—secondaries, lymphoma, lymphatic leukemia

Immunological
- Systemic lupus erythematosus
- Rheumatoid arthritis

Drug induced—allopurinol, phenytoin
Others—sarcoidosis, thyroid swelling

Differential diagnosis for neck lymph node enlargement
- Tuberculous lymphadenitis **(Refer Chapter 8)**
- Secondaries in lymph nodes
- HIV infection
- Lymphomas **(Refer Chapter 8)**
- Chronic lymphatic leukemia
- Nonspecific lymphadenitis
- Infectious mononucleosis
- Sarcoidosis

Note: Lymph node enlargement is the commonest neck swelling (2nd is thyroid enlargement).

COLD ABSCESS (Refer Chapter 8: Examination and Clinical Approach to Lymphatic System)

It is a complication of tubercular disease; commonly observed in neck in relation to caseating tuberculous cervical lymphadenitis. It can occur in relation to spine as cold abscess in the neck (like psoas abscess, paraspinal region or any other area). Cold abscess does not show any signs of acute inflammation.

It is well localized, smooth, soft, fluctuant, nontender, nontransilluminating swelling with free skin in front. It eventually lends into tuberculous sinus. Relevant lymph nodes, oral cavity/tonsils, cervical/thoracic spines, lungs should be examined. Branchial cyst, lymph cyst, suppurated lymph node are the *differential diagnosis*.

SECONDARIES IN NECK LYMPH NODES

Common sites of primary: Oral cavity, tongue, tonsils, salivary glands, pharynx—nasopharynx, larynx, esophagus, lungs, GIT, thyroid. It is commonly from squamous cell carcinoma, but can be from adenocarcinoma, or melanoma. Squamous cell carcinoma is mainly from oral cavity, pharynx. Adenocarcinoma is usually from GIT, commonly involving left supraclavicular lymph nodes.

Features of Secondaries in Neck

- Presents as initially painless swelling with nodular surface, hard, often fixed when it is advanced. Secondaries from *papillary carcinoma of thyroid* can be soft, cystic and contains brownish black fluid. Secondaries can infiltrate into carotids, sternomastoid, posterior vertebral muscles, spinal accessory nerve (shrugging of shoulder is affected), hypoglossal nerve (tongue deviates towards the same side), cervical sympathetic chain (*Horner's syndrome*).
- Secondaries spread into adjacent soft tissues and also to the skin causing fungation and ulceration. Often because of tumor necrosis, softer area develops in the hard node. In advanced cases tumor may infiltrate into the major vessels like carotids, or branches of external carotid artery causing torrential hemorrhage. Dysphagia, dyspnea, hemoptysis, hoarseness of voice, ear pain, and deafness are other features seen depending on the primary site location.

Types of Secondaries in the Neck

1. *Secondaries in the neck with known primary:* Here secondaries are present in the neck and primary has been identified clinically in the oral cavity, pharynx, larynx, thyroid, or other areas. Biopsy from the primary and FNAC from the secondaries has to be taken.
2. *Secondaries in the neck with clinically unidentified primary:* Hard, neck lymph nodes are the secondaries, but primary has not been identified clinically. FNAC of the neck node has to be done and secondaries have to be confirmed. Then search for the primary has to be done

by various investigations. They are nasopharyngoscopy, laryngoscopy, esophagoscopy, bronchoscopy. *Blind biopsies* are taken from the fossa of Rosenmuller, lateral wall of pharynx, pyriform fossa, larynx; FNAC of thyroid and suspected areas are done; CT scan is essential.

3. *Secondaries in the neck with an occult primary (70% in jugulodigastric nodes):* Here secondaries in the neck lymph nodes are confirmed by FNAC, *but primary has not been revealed by any available investigations.* When all the investigations mentioned above do not show any evidence of primary, then only it is called as *occult primary*.

> **Nodal staging in secondaries:**
> N0—nodes not detected
> N1—single node same side <3 cm
> N2a—single node same side 3–6 cm
> N2b—multiple nodes same side <6 cm
> N2c—bilateral/contralateral nodes <6 cm
> N3—node >6 cm

■ THORACIC OUTLET SYNDROME (TOS)

It is syndrome complex due to compression of neurovascular bundle in the thoracic outlet. *Thoracic outlet has got two main spaces—scalene triangle* which is bound by scalenus anterior, scalenus medius and first rib and contains subclavian artery and brachial plexus; *Costoclavicular space* which is bound by clavicle, first rib, costoclavicular ligament and scalenus medius and contains subclavian artery, vein and brachial plexus.

Causes: Cervical rib; long C7 transverse process; anomalous insertion of scalene muscles; scalene muscle hypertrophy; scalene minimus; abnormal bands and ligaments; fracture clavicle or first rib; exostosis; tumors in the region; brachial plexus trauma and diseases.

Differential diagnosis of TOS: Carpal tunnel syndrome, cervical spondylosis, spinal canal tumors, shoulder myositis, angina, Raynaud's disease, spinal stenosis, ulnar nerve compression, epicondylitis.

Features:
- *Neurological:* Paresthesia; pain in shoulder, arm, forearm and fingers; occipital headache as referred pain from tight scalene muscles; weakness in forearm, hand.
- *Vascular:* Claudication, ischemic ulcers and gangrene; poor capillary refilling; absence or feeble pulse.
- *Signs:* Scalene muscle tenderness; pulsatile swelling in supraclavicular region with thrill and bruit (25%); bony mass above clavicle.
- Adson's test, Roos test, elevated arm stress test (EAST), costoclavicular compression maneuver and hyperabduction maneuver are positive (Refer Chapter 6).

Cervical Rib

It is an extension of transverse process of C7 vertebra more than 2.5 cm (normal). It is due to persistent ossification of C7 lateral costal element due to failure of reabsorption of this ossified element. Syndrome caused by it is called as *cervical rib syndrome, thoracic inlet syndrome, thoracic outlet syndrome; scalene syndrome.*

It is 0.5% common, common in females, more on right side; can be *unilateral or bilateral;* can be *asymptomatic or symptomatic.*

Types: (1) *Complete bony:* Cervical rib is radiopaque, anteriorly ends over the first rib or manubrium. (2) *Fibrous:* Cannot be demonstrated radiologically. (3) *Combined:* Partly bony partly fibrous. (4) *Partial bony:* With free end expanding as *bony mass.*

Features:
- Majority of patients are asymptomatic.
- *Neurological features (most common presentation):* It is due to compression of T1 and C8 causing sensory (tingling and numbness in the little finger, medial side of hand and forearm); motor (wasting of thenar and hypothenar eminence with often claw hand and loss of power of the hand).
- Vasomotor with excessive sweating of the hand (Fig. 15-43).
- *Vascular manifestations (more problematic presentation): Pain* is due to ischemia in the muscle; is more during work, exercise and is relieved by rest. *Roos, Adson's, modified Adson's tst, EAST (see above and Chapter 6) are positive.*
- Often *digital gangrene* may be observed. Limb is colder and pallor than the opposite side.
- *Features in the neck:* (a) Hard, fixed, bony mass in the supraclavicular region. (b) *Palpable thrill* above the clavicle in the subclavian artery. (c) *Bruit* on auscultation.

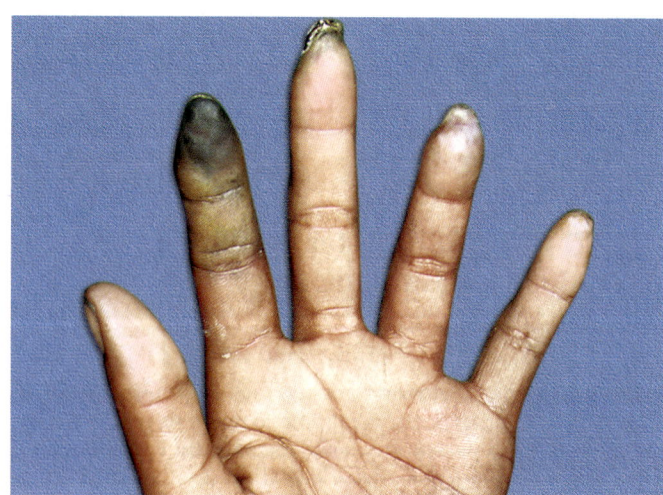

Fig. 15-43 *Cervical rib causing gangrene of digits.*

Conditions	Features
Branchial cyst It is a congenital swelling but present in 2nd or 3rd decade; arises from remnants of second branchial cleft (called as **cervical sinus**) which gets sequestered eventually to form a cyst; contains clear or thick toothpaste like material that contains fat globules and cholesterol crystals; Feels like "*half-filled double hot water bottle*"; histologically lined by squamous epithelium	Swelling in the neck, *beneath the anterior border of upper third of sternocleidomastoid muscle*; smooth, soft/tensely cystic, fluctuant, occasionally transilluminant, not compressible, not reducible. Neck nodes not enlarged
Branchial fistula It is a persistent second branchial cleft that communicates outside with an external opening; commonly *congenital* but could be an *acquired* one due to inadvertent incision/rupture of infected branchial cyst. Track is lined by ciliated columnar epithelium with patches of lymphoid tissues beneath	• *External orifice* is located near the lower third of neck near anterior border of sternomastoid muscle (in congenital type) or in upper 1/3rd of neck (in acquired type); *internal orifice* is located on the anterior aspect of posterior pillar of fauces just behind the tonsils but sometimes fistula may have a blind end • Discharge—mucoid/mucopurulent
Cystic hygroma	*Discussed in Chapter 4: Examination and Clinical Approach of a Swelling/Lump*
Pharyngeal pouch A protrusion of mucosa through *Killian's dehiscence* due to imperfect relaxation of cricopharyngeus muscle causing the increased pressure in the pharynx mainly during swallowing leading to protrusion of mucosa through the Killian's dehiscence (weak area in the posterior pharyngeal wall between cricopharyngeus and thyropharyngeus part of inferior constrictor muscle of pharynx)	• Complains of regurgitation during night or while turning neck, pain, dysphagia, recurrent respiratory infection (pneumonia/lung abscess) • Swelling in the posterior triangle of neck on **left side (commonly)**, smooth, soft, tender. Gurgling noise heard while swallowing is typical • **Complications:** Pouch infection/abscess formation
Laryngocele It is unilateral narrow necked, air containing diverticulum situated in the anterior third of laryngeal ventricle between thyroid cartilage and false cord; can be external/internal/combined; results from herniation of laryngeal mucosa through thyrohyoid membrane, commonly seen in trumpet players, glass blowers, and in patient with chronic cough	Swelling in the neck in relation to larynx adjacent to thyrohyoid membrane; smooth, soft, *resonant* that becomes prominent while blowing. Expansile impulse on coughing is observed. Hoarseness of voice and laryngeal obstruction may eventually develop **Complications**: infection/abscess **Investigations**: X-ray neck; laryngoscopy, CT scan
Sternomastoid tumor It is a misnomer; not a tumor. It is due to birth injury to sternocleidomastoid muscle; hematoma that results from birth injury (breech delivery) undergoes organization to form sternomastoid tumor	• Seen in infants of 3–4 weeks age; swelling occurs in sternocleidomastoid muscle that is smooth, hard, nontender, and adherent to muscle • Infants present with torticollis, with chin pointing to opposite side; head towards same side • In later stage—hemifacial atrophy due to reduced blood supply as a result of compression of external carotid artery; compensatory cervical scoliosis and squint
Torticollis (wry neck) Head is bent to one side with chin pointing towards opposite side **Causes:** • *Congenital*—sternomastoid tumor (due to birth trauma) • *Traumatic*—fracture dislocation of cervical spine • *Inflammatory* pathology of neck nodes • *Spasmodic*—spasm of same side sternomastoid muscle and posterior neck muscle of opposite side • *Burns* contracture • *Rheumatic*—exposure to cold	Mild facial atrophy on the affected side; less arched eyebrow; reduced distance from outer canthus of eye to angle of mouth, flat nose, flat spine
Carotid body tumor (potato tumor/chemodectoma/nonchromaffin paraganglioma) • Arises at the bifurcation of carotid artery from carotid body, cells of which are sensitive to changes in pH and temperature of the blood. Blood supply is from external carotid artery • Locally malignant; 20% regional spread to lymph nodes • Familial, seen in middle age **Shamblin classification**: Type 1—localized, easily resectable (26%) Type 2—adherent, partially surrounding the carotids (46%) Type 3—adherent, encasing the carotids completely (27%) May extend into the cranial cavity along the internal carotid artery—*dumb bell tumor*	• Slow growing tumor, located at the level of hyoid bone deep to the anterior edge of sternomastoid muscle in anterior triangle; vertically placed, smooth, round, firm to hard "*potato*" like swelling • Pulsatile; Moves only side to side but not in vertical direction; thrill may be felt; bruit may be heard • May present with features of transient ischemic attack due to pressure of the tumor over the carotids/feeling of syncope with slowing of heart rate on applying pressure over the swelling—*carotid body syncope* • *Lyre sign*—widening of carotid bifurcation in CT angiogram • Differential diagnosis—carotid aneurysm • *Note: Dumb-bell tumors* are seen in parotid tumor, spinal cord tumor, carotid body tumor
Primary branchiogenic carcinoma Rare, diagnosed by exclusion; arises from remnants of branchial cleft; histological diagnosis	Mimics clinically *secondaries in the neck nodes* but without any primary focus

Contd...

Contd...

Conditions	Features
Ludwig's angina Inflammatory edema of submandibular region and floor of mouth; commonly due to streptococcal infection; common in severely ill and in advanced malignancy	• *Diffuse swelling and brawny edema of the submandibular region*; fever, toxicity, dysphagia, trismus, laryngeal edema causing dyspnea, intraoral edema, putrid halitosis • As the infection is deep to deep facia in closed facial planes it spreads very fast leading to dreaded complications like *jugular vein thrombosis*
Parapharyngeal abscess It is infection of pharyngomaxillary space (base formed by the base of skull, apex by greater cornu of hyoid bone, lateral wall by internal pterygoid, angle of mandible, submandibular salivary gland, medial wall by the superior constrictor muscle); infection arises from the tonsils after tonsillectomy or from submandibular space	• Diffuse swelling in upper neck, trismus, fever, toxicity • **Complications:** Jugular vein thrombosis; erosion of the internal carotid artery causing torrential hemorrhage; septicemia
Retropharyngeal abscess It is due to infection of retropharyngeal lymph nodes located between buccopharyngeal fascia and prevertebral fascia in paramedian position **Acute**: Infection and suppuration of retropharyngeal lymph nodes due to staphylococci and streptococci infection; commonly from tonsils/pharynx; common in infants and children **Chronic**: Features of tuberculosis of cervical spine will be observed	*In acute type*, presentation is as lateral smooth, tender swelling in the pharynx; with dysphagia, dyspnea, cough, toxic features and neck rigidity *In chronic type*, midline swelling in the posterior pharyngeal wall, which is smooth nontender; often abscess may point in the neck in relation to sternomastoid; neurological manifestation in severe disease
Subhyoid bursitis It is inflammation of bursa between posterior surface of hyoid bone and thyrohyoid membrane; inflammation sets due to constant friction	*Horizontally placed swelling* between lower part of hyoid bone and thyrohyoid membrane, smooth, soft, cystic, fluctuant, non-transilluminant that moves upwards with deglutition but not while protruding the tongue out, contains turbid fluid which may get infected to form an abscess *Differential diagnosis*—thyroglossal cyst; pretracheal lymph nodes
Lemeierre's syndrome Enlarged neck lymph nodes, sore throat, peritonsillar abscess by anerobic *Fusobacterium necrophorum*	Bacteria eventually penetrate into the jugular vein causing infective thrombosis in the vein and later septicemia

CASE DISCUSSION

A 20-year-old male comes with the history of mild on and of fever for 2 months. Later he noticed a swelling on the right side of the neck which was painless but progressively increasing in size. Later few more swellings appeared in the same side of the neck. Earlier swelling started becoming well localized and softer. He does not give any history of throat pain, cough or dyspnea. There is no history of loss of appetite and reduced weight. There is no change in voice or difficulty in swallowing. On general examination he had temperature of 99.5°F. He is not anemic. On local examination of the neck, a smooth, swelling of 5 cm sized is seen in right upper part of the neck deep to sternocleidomastoid muscle. It is well localized and smooth. Few more swellings are seen adjacent and below the main large swelling which are of variable size between 2–3 cm. Opposite side of the neck looks normal. Thyroid area is normal. On palpation, large swelling is non-tender without local raise of temperature. It is soft, adherent to sternocleidomastoid muscle which is confirmed by contracting the sternocleidomastoid muscle. Swelling is fluctuant but not transilluminant with restricted mobility. Other adjacent swellings are smooth, firm, discrete, mobile and deep to sternocleidomastoid muscle. Opposite side neck (left) is normal. Thyroid is normal. Oral cavity on examination looks normal; tonsils are normal; oral mucosa is normal; there is no trismus. Axilla, inguinal region, epitrochlear area, abdomen are normal. Liver and spleen are not palpable; ascites (free fluid is not present). Respiratory system is normal. There is no bone tenderness; spine is clinically normal.

What is the probable diagnosis? Why? What are the differential diagnoses?
Probable diagnosis is right sided cervical tuberculous lymphadenitis with cold abscess. Reason is—young age group; mild fiver of 2 months; multiple nodes with soft cystic swelling. Differential diagnoses are—lymphoma, secondaries, nonspecific lymphadenitis, HIV infection. Lymphoma presenting like cold abscess is not common even though it can happen. Secondaries is not common in this age group and it is hard in consistency.

What you will do?
Blood—Hb, Tc DC ESR; peripheral smear; FNAC of the swelling; chest X-ray; USG abdomen; LFT. Epithelioid cells with caseating material with Langhans giant cells are typical in FNAC. Treatment is—antituberculous drug therapy; nondependent drainage of the cold abscess to prevent sinus formation; closure of the wound. Follow up with—regular clinical examination, weight monitoring; monitoring with ESR, Hb, LFT (to observe drug toxicity).

16

Clinical Approach and Examination of Thyroid

Competency: SU22.1; SU22.2; SU22.3; SU22.4; SU22.5; SU22.6.

Thyroid diseases can be congenital or acquired. Congenital thyroid conditions may be like absence of gland causing cretinism or anomalies of thyroglossal tract causing thyroglossal cyst or anomalous location like lingual thyroid. Acquired disorders are inflammatory, neoplastic and metabolic origin. Inflammatory conditions of thyroid like acute/chronic thyroiditis which are rare; of undetermined etiology like Hashimoto's (autoimmune), giant cell thyroiditis, Riedel's thyroiditis, deQuervain's thyroiditis (viral) are not uncommon. Neoplastic conditions can be benign or malignant; malignant can be differentiated (papillary/follicular) or undifferentiated or medullary. Metabolic conditions are physiological, diffuse, colloid, nodular, toxic goiters. *Thomas Wharton in 1656* named the gland as '*thyroid*' which is derived from *Greek word 'thyreoides'* which means '*shield-like*'. The '*goiter* is derived from Latin word '*gutter*', which means throat. Goiter is defined as '*any enlargement of thyroid gland*' (Figs. 16-1 to 16-3).

Fig. 16-1 *Simple goiter*—enlargement of thyroid gland.

HISTORY

Name:

Age: Simple hyperplastic goiter is often seen in girls during puberty. Goiter due to dyshormonogenesis occurs in younger age group. Physiological goiter occurs when there is increased metabolic demand of the hormone like in puberty or pregnancy. Solitary nodule, colloid goiter, papillary carcinoma and primary thyrotoxicosis are seen between 20–40 years. Multinodular goiter, follicular carcinoma, thyroid adenoma, secondary thyrotoxicosis and Hashimoto's thyroiditis are seen in middle aged women. Anaplastic carcinoma is seen in elderly.

Sex: Most of the thyroid diseases like hyperthyroidism (8:1), hypothyroidism, goiters and neoplasms (3:1) are commonly seen in *females*. Hashimoto's thyroiditis is exclusively observed in females.

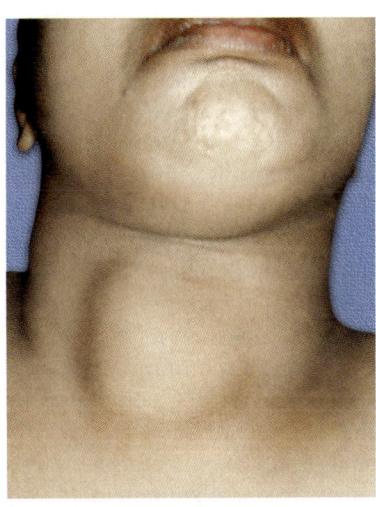

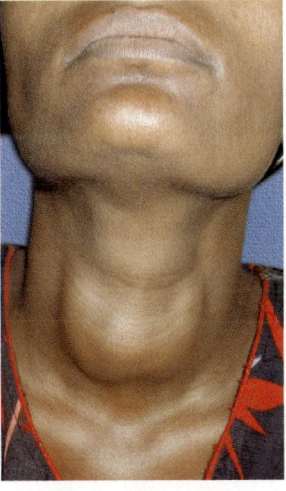

Fig. 16-2 Thyroid swelling (goiter) in a female patient; *note the butterfly shape.*

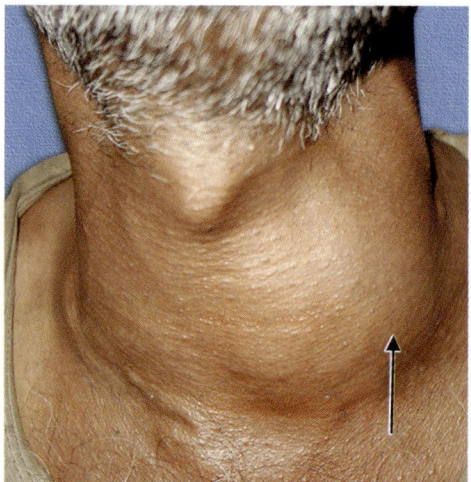

Fig. 16-3 Thyroid nodule in a male patient. *Carcinoma should be suspected in a male patient thyroid enlargement.*

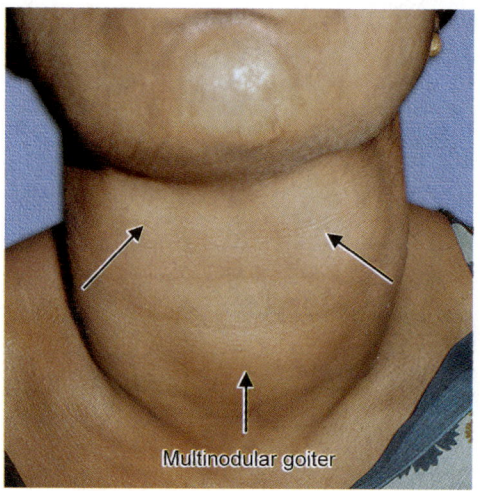

Fig. 16-5 *Multinodular goiter.*

Thyroid swelling is not common in males; but when it occurs in males malignancy (carcinoma) has to be suspected.

Address: Knowing the residential place may be important in certain types of goiters—***endemic goiter***, due to iodine deficiency in water and food which is common in interior areas, mountainous areas like Vindhyas, Himalayas. Goiter is more common in South India than in North India. It is also common in great lakes of North America, banks of river Struma which takes its source from mountains in Bulgaria where the soil is devoid of iodides. Follicular and anaplastic carcinoma may be more common in iodine deficient areas but papillary carcinoma is not related to iodine deficiency. In the United Kingdom, endemic goiter is common in midlands (***Derbyshire neck***). Chalk or limestone producing areas like Southern Ireland and Derbyshire are goitrogenic areas as calcium is goitrogenic. Russia is known for iodine deficiency goiter. Micropapillary carcinoma is more common in France. In India, four million people suffer from goiter; 0.5 million from cretinism; 100 million suffer from iodine deficiency. In India, highest incidence of thyroid carcinoma is in Manipur (Imphal), Mizoram (Aizawl) and Bengaluru **(Fig. 16-4)**. *Himalayan goiter belt* is observed in North East and North West India.

Occupation: Not much related to thyroid diseases. Toxic thyroid may be more seen in people with stressful work **(Figs. 16-5 and 16-6)**.

Chief Complaints

Swelling in front of the neck and its duration; ***pain*** in the swelling and its duration; ***hoarseness of voice*** due to recurrent laryngeal nerve palsy; ***difficulty in swallowing*** or ***breathing***; ***tremor*** in the hands; ***generalized weakness; palpitation; significant loss of weight/weight gain.***

History of Present Illness

Swelling

Its mode of onset, duration, whether sudden or insidious in nature should be asked. Progress of swelling whether gradual (benign) or rapidly progressive (malignancy) or recent rapid increase in an existing swelling (benign turning into malignant) or sudden rapid increase (may be seen in hemorrhage). Hemorrhage or malignant transformation (follicular carcinoma) can occur in a preexisting multinodular

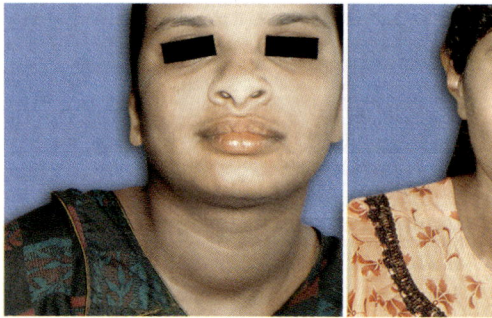

Fig. 16-4 Goiter may occur in many *family members*. Two siblings presented with goiter.

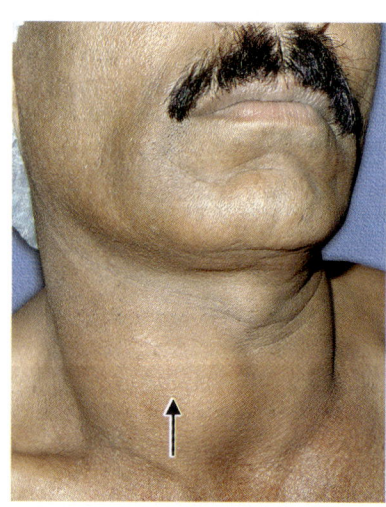

Fig. 16-6 *Solitary nodule in a male.*

goiter. Thyroglossal cyst may be present since childhood. Most of the goiters, solitary nodule, multinodular goiter are slow growing swellings. Anaplastic carcinoma, follicular carcinoma, medullary carcinoma are rapidly growing tumors. Papillary carcinoma which is the commonest thyroid malignancy, even though malignant, is a slow growing tumor often for few years. Swelling may be single/multiple; occupying one lobe, or both lobes or isthmus. In primary thyrotoxicosis, symptoms like irritability, insomnia, loss of weight, tremors appear first (CNS) and later diffuse thyroid swelling (often it is less or insignificant) whereas in secondary thyrotoxicosis thyroid swelling of long duration appears first and later symptoms appear gradually mainly of cardiac manifestations like palpitation, tachycardia.

Note: Any thyroid of any size or any duration or any consistency or in any age group can be malignant unless proved otherwise.

Pain

Its duration, character like dull aching/pricking, site of pain, radiation, factors which alter the pain should be asked for. Usually goiters are painless. Thyroiditis is painful; often with a discomfort in the neck. Thyroiditis may be Hashimoto's, deQuervain's or radiation-induced. Hemorrhage in a existing multinodular goiter, adenoma or cyst can cause pain. Malignancy is initially painless but later becomes painful. Infiltration into surrounding structures (nerves)/necrosis/hemorrhage makes it painful and tender. Anaplastic carcinoma commonly infiltrates into nerves to cause pain.

Fever

Acute thyroiditis causes fever; increase in temperature is observed in toxic goiter.

> **Causes of dyspnea/stridor in thyroid diseases:**
> - Carcinoma thyroid infiltrating recurrent laryngeal nerve/trachea
> - Large, long standing goiter causing tracheomalacia
> - Retrosternal goiter
> - Congestive cardiac failure in thyrotoxicosis

Pressure Symptoms

Dysfunctioning of the neighboring structures occurs due to pressure/infiltration like dysphagia (esophageal compression), dyspnea (tracheal compression), stridor—whistling sound of air as it rushes through the narrowed trachea [due to infiltration into trachea *(stridor at rest)*], hoarseness of voice (recurrent laryngeal nerve compression), prominent neck veins and Horner's syndrome (infiltration of cervical sympathetic chain—ptosis, loss of sweating on same side of face, miosis and enophthalmos). Their duration, onset and progression should be asked. Dyspnea due to intrathoracic retrosternal goiter may be mistaken for asthma. Nocturnal dyspnea, dyspnea precipitated by tilting the neck towards one side are features of retrosternal goiter. Postural cough during sleep may be due to retrosternal goiter. Occasionally hemoptysis unmixed with sputum can occur due to rupture of engorged tracheal vein.

Symptoms/Features of Toxicity

Metabolic: Increased appetite, loss of weight, diarrhea, increased sweating, cold preference, heat intolerance.

Neuromuscular: Irritability, nervousness, sleeplessness (insomnia), hand tremors, proximal muscle weakness in the thigh or arm like fatigue on getting down the steps or lifting weight using arms (myopathy) due to difficulty in isometric contraction and increased muscle metabolism, wasting of muscles.

Cardiovascular: Chest pain aggravated by exercise, palpitation, tachycardia; in late stages features of cardiac decompensation like edema feet, orthopnea, dyspnea.

Genital: Amenorrhea, infertility.

Eye: Visual disturbances with bulging, staring, protruding of the eyes (exophthalmos), inability to close the eyes, double vision, pain in the eye, excessive watering of eyes.

> **Cardinal signs of toxic thyroid:**
> - Palpable thyroid often with thrill and bruit
> - Tremor of hands and tongue
> - Tachycardia
> - Exophthalmos

Skin: Skin is moist with more sweating. **Pretibial myxedema** is a feature of primary thyrotoxicosis. It is a misnomer; it is deposition of myxomatous tissue in the skin over the shin; it is bilateral, symmetrical, shiny, red and dry skin **(Fig. 16-7)**.

In primary thyrotoxicosis, usually symptoms appear first which are more severe than secondary type followed by diffuse thyroid swelling in the neck. Here often swelling in the neck may not be present or may not be obvious. ***In secondary thyrotoxicosis,*** obvious swelling appears first which is nodular followed by symptoms of thyrotoxicosis which are less severe initially as compared to primary thyrotoxicosis, but gradually become more severe. Neurological and eye signs are more severe in primary thyrotoxicosis whereas cardiovascular symptoms (due to cardiac arrhythmias, fibrillation, flutter) are

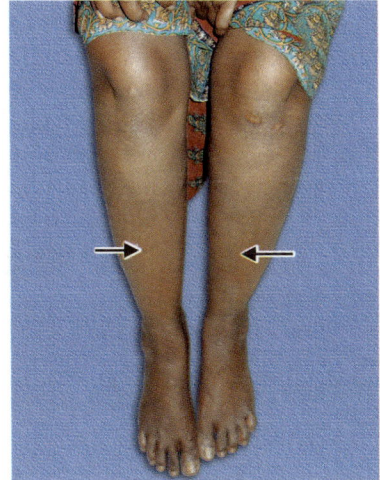

Fig. 16-7 *Pretibial myxedema*; it is a feature of primary thyrotoxicosis—observed in both feet and legs due to myxomatous tissue deposition.

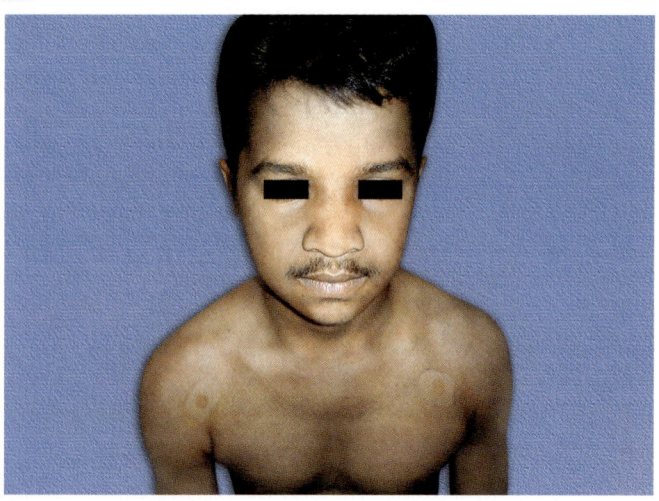

Fig. 16-8 *Myxedema*—hypothyroidism status.

more severe in secondary thyrotoxicosis. **Hyperthyroidism** means toxicity due to hyperfunctioning thyroid (diffuse/nodular) whereas *thyrotoxicosis* is toxicity due to raised thyroid hormone levels either from toxic thyroid or from other sources like ectopic functioning thyroid, struma ovarii, metastatic functioning follicular carcinoma, trophoblastic tumors, thyrotoxicosis factitia.

In thyroglossal fistula, mode of onset, duration, type of discharge should be asked for.

Symptoms/Features of Hypothyroidism/Myxedema (word meaning—mucus swelling) (Fig. 16-8)
It is a clinical state of severe lack of thyroid hormone. It is common in middle aged and elderly females. Previous scar of thyroidectomy may be seen.
- *Metabolic:* Weight gain, poor appetite, constipation, cold intolerance, preference to heat; nonpitting edema; puffy spade like hands which are cold; enlarged tongue.
- *Neuromuscular:* Muscle weakness fatigue, lethargy, less memory, sleepiness, change in voice due to vocal cord edema (deep, hoarse voice) slow speech, slow movement, sluggish ankle jerks with prolonged relaxation period.
- *Cardiovascular:* **Bradycardia** (40–60 beats/minute); low blood pressure.
- *Facial:* Facial swelling, thickening and heaviness of eyelids, dull look, superciliary madarosis (loss of hairs) in lateral half of the eyebrows, loss of hair in scalp; flushed pink orange cheeks (peaches).
- *Skin:* Minimal sweating, thin ragged hairs, elastic nonsweating dry skin; smooth pale yellow creamy skin.
- *Genital:* Menorrhagia, infertility.
- **Myxedema coma** develops eventually with hypothermia, hypotension, hyponatremia, hypoventilation, hypoglycemia, *deadly cold skin* like of a toad; rectal temperature below 24°C. Types of *myxedema*: (1) *Primary* is due to reduced thyroid hormones T3 and T4. (2) *Secondary* is due to reduced levels of TSH at pituitary level due to pituitary tumors or pituitary infarction (*Sheehan's syndrome*). **Myxedema crisis** may develop with acute exacerbation of features.

Past History

History of irradiation should be asked in carcinoma thyroid. Irradiation to head and neck region may have been given for benign lesions like adenoids, tonsillitis, thymus, acne vulgaris or hemangiomas or malignancy in younger age groups like for lymphomas. Chernobyl nuclear disaster in Ukraine in 1986 caused increased incidence of papillary carcinoma of thyroid in that children. *Previous history of having thyroglossal cyst* must be noted which might have been infected causing fistula either due to spontaneous rupture or after surgical drainage of the infected cyst. Previous surgery for thyroid in recurrent thyroid swelling or earlier surgery for thyroglossal cyst in case of thyroglossal fistula should be asked for.

Personal History

History of smoking, alcohol intake or any drugs which may cause alteration in thyroid function should be asked. History of any drug intake like patient may be on thyroxine or on antithyroid drugs or beta-blockers or other drugs like lithium, PAS or sulfonylureas which may alter the thyroid should be noted. Dietary habits should be asked. Vegetables belonging to Brassica family like cabbage, kale and rape are goitrogens. Type of salt consumed may be important; commercial iodized salt or rock salt which is non-commercialized and noniodized. Sea fish, egg and milk are rich in iodine. WHO recommends 150 μg of daily iodine intake in adult and 200 μg in pregnancy and lactation. History of diarrhea in toxic thyroid may be significant; in hypothyroidism, constipation is common.

Family History

Dyshormonogenesis (familial partial enzyme deficiency usually thyroid peroxidase), medullary carcinoma of thyroid can be familial (**MEN syndrome**). Familial tumors can occur in children and adolescents; there is no sex predilection. Endemic goiter and Grave's disease can occur in families. Altered thyroid function may be the cause for infertility.

Menstrual History

History of menarche/menopause; duration of menstruation, history suggestive of menorrhagia, amenorrhea, oligomenorrhea, etc. should be asked for. Hyperthyroidism can cause amenorrhea; hypothyroidism may cause menorrhagia.

Treatment History

History of investigations or treatment undergone, relevant to thyroid disease should be asked for. Patient may be taking L-thyroxine for hypothyroidism (as once a day–small tablet) or may be taking antithyroid drugs like carbimazole or propylthiouracil usually three times a day for hyperthyroidism. History should be detailed whether patient is becoming better after therapy or not (drug response). Often patient may be taking drugs like PAS or sulfonylureas which are goitrogenic. History of intake/usage of drugs for other diseases or investigations should be mentioned (antitussives, contrast X-ray agents like sodium diatrizoate, radiotherapy or surgery.

GENERAL EXAMINATION

Nutrition: Thyrotoxic patient is thin and undernourished in spite of good appetite. Obesity is seen in myxedema. Patient may be cachexic in thyroid carcinoma which is advanced/metastatic.

Facies: The typical 'staring' look of exophthalmos is seen in toxic thyroid patient who appears irritable, agitated, tensed with nervous face. Myxedema face is typical. It is expressionless/lethargic, **mask-like puffy** face. Patient will be dull with low intelligence (*everything is slow*—walking, talking, moving, thinking, and reflex).

Gait: Hasty-rapid gait is seen in hyperthyroid and slow-lethargic gait in hypothyroidism. One has to find out whether **rising from the squatting position** is possible with or without using support of hands; in hyperthyroidism due to proximal myopathy, patient needs support to get up from squatting position. Severe muscular weakness often resembles myasthenia gravis. Inability to get up from chair is called as **Plummer's sign**.

Pulse: Its rate, rhythm, character is noted. Whether it is tachycardia (in thyrotoxicosis), collapsing/Corrigan's/pulsus paradoxus type is noted. Missed beat in ectopic; rapid, irregular pulse in fibrillation has to be looked for. Pulse rate may be slow (bradycardia) in hypothyroidism **(Fig. 16-9)**. *Sleeping pulse rate* is better indicator of severity of thyrotoxicosis and is checked at late night or early morning for three consecutive nights and average is taken. The need of sedating with diazepam or phenobarbitone to check sleeping pulse rate is controversial (better to avoid). Sleeping pulse rate is graded as per Crile's grading.

Blood pressure (systolic) may be high in toxic thyroid.

Crile's grading	Sleeping pulse rate/minute	
I	Up to 90	Mild
II	90–110	Moderate
III	>110	Severe

Note: Those on propranolol, sleeping pulse rate will be irrelevant.

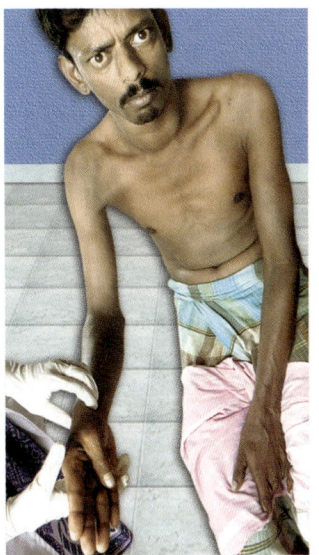

Fig. 16-9 *Palpation of radial pulse* for its count, volume, variations should be done in thyroid diseases.

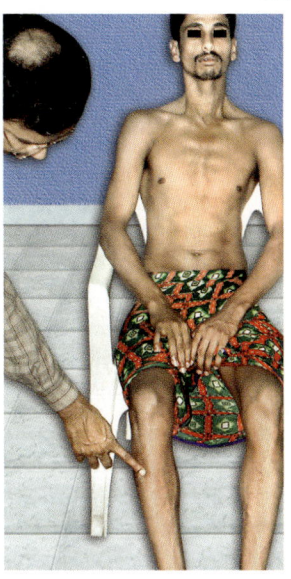

Fig. 16-10 Pretibial myxedema is checked *over the shin and ankle* which is often seen in primary thyrotoxicosis.

Skin: Skin is wet and warm in hyperthyroidism (*moist palm while shaking hands*); dry and cold in hypothyroidism. Anterior aspect of both legs and ankle region should be inspected *for pretibial myxedema*. It is a feature of primary thyrotoxicosis. It is due to deposition of myxomatous tissue **(Fig. 16-10)**.

Hands: In thyrotoxicosis, fine tremors are observed in the outstretched hands with fingers spread forward. Often small object like pen may be kept over the fingers to watch the tremor better. It is due to diffuse irritation of the gray matter. In hypothyroidism, the hands are cold and spade-like, and there is supraclavicular pad of fat **(Figs. 16-11A and B)**.

Tremor:
- Tremor is defined as regular, rhythmic, oscillations of one part of the body from a fixed point in one plane and is due to contraction of antagonistic muscles
- Limbs, neck, tongue, chin and vocal cords may be affected by tremor

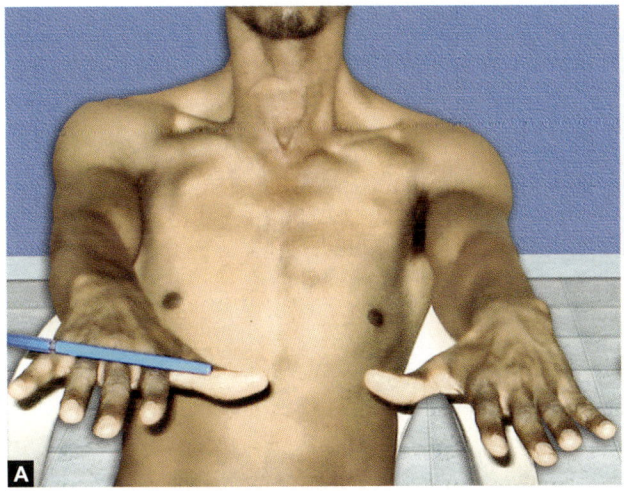
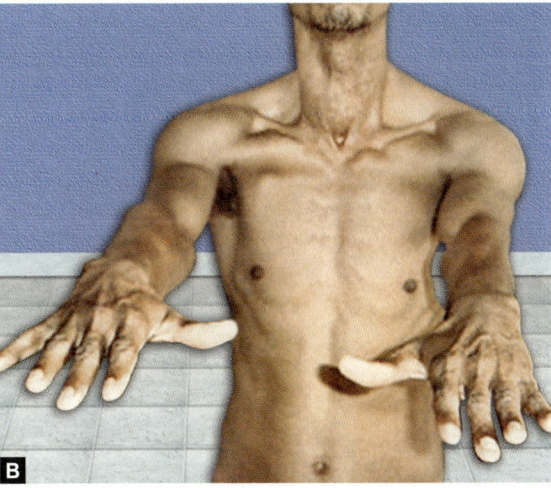

Figs. 16-11A and B *Tremor of the outstretched hands* is a feature of thyrotoxicosis.

- Tremor may be fine or coarse
- Tremor may be resting, postural or intention
- Resting tremor occurs in Parkinson's and Wilson's disease
- Postural can be physiological or essential. It is seen in stress, anxiety, thyrotoxicosis, pheochromocytoma, hypoglycemia, drugs like beta-blockers/theophylline, caffeine, alcohol, amphetamine. Toxic thyroid causes postural fine tremor
- Intention tremor is seen in cerebellar disease, stroke, tumors of brain, multiple sclerosis

Thyroid acropachy is clubbing of fingers and toes in primary thyrotoxicosis; hypertrophic pulmonary osteoarthropathy may also develop.

Mouth: Tongue twitching can be observed by opening the mouth and carefully observing the tongue **(Figs. 16-12A and B)**. Tongue should be kept *within* oral cavity (tip of the tongue should not be beyond the lower lip) to check the tremor as protruded tongue causes fasciculation of intrinsic muscles of tongue which mimic tongue tremor. In hypothyroidism, the tongue is thickened and coarse. *Look for the presence of lingual thyroid* which presents as a swelling on the posterior third of tongue **(Fig. 16-13)**.

Eye: In primary thyrotoxicosis, exophthalmos and all other eye signs are looked for.

1. **Exophthalmos:** In normal individual, both the eyelids partially cover the bulbar sclera. In exophthalmos, *lower bulbar sclera is clearly visible* and lower eyelid lies below and will not cover the bulbar sclera. In severe exophthalmos, sclera will be visible all over, both above and below. Exophthalmos is measured using exophthalmometer. (In **lid retraction,** upper eyelid is above the upper margin of cornea, often with visible upper bulbar sclera due to spasm of involuntary part of levator palpebrae superioris muscle. Here lower eyelid is in normal position. This does not indicate exophthalmos. Lid retraction is only a sign of toxic goiter) **(Figs. 16-14 to 16-16)**.

Severe exophthalmos shows: Eyelid edema, chemosis, conjunctival injection, diplopia, ophthalmoplegia (complete weakness of all extraocular muscles and so no

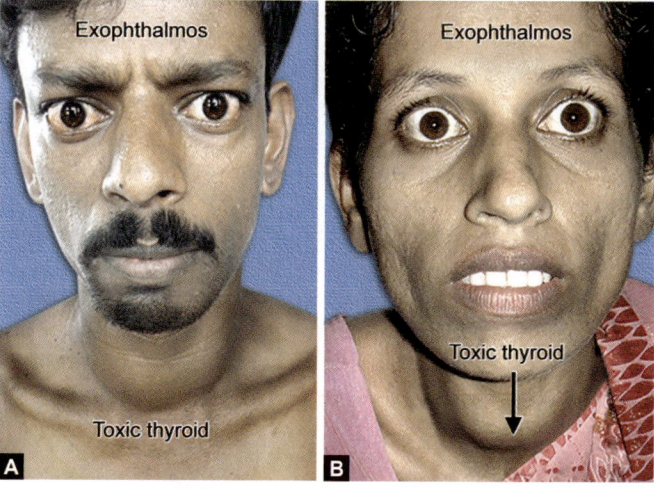

Figs. 16-14A and B Thyrotoxicosis with *exophthalmos.*

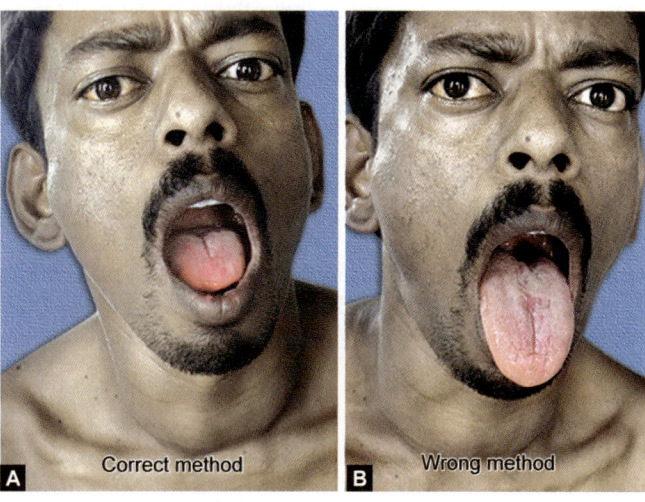

Figs. 16-12A and B *Tongue tremor* should be checked in thyrotoxicosis. (A) Tongue should be inside the mouth, (B) not outside while checking the tremor.

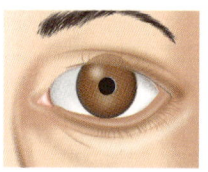

Upper eyelid between upper limbus and pupil

Normal

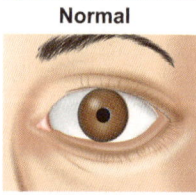

Upper eyelid raised lower eyelid normal

Lid retration

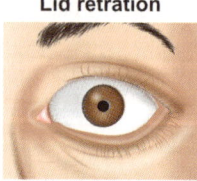

Both upper and lower eyelids away from the center with visible sclera all around mainly below

Exophthalmos

Fig. 16-15 *Looks of eyes in different conditions* including thyrotoxicosis.

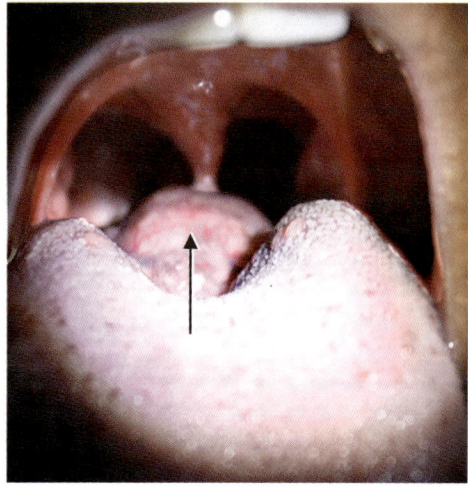

Fig. 16-13 Lingual thyroid.

Chapter 16: Clinical Approach and Examination of Thyroid

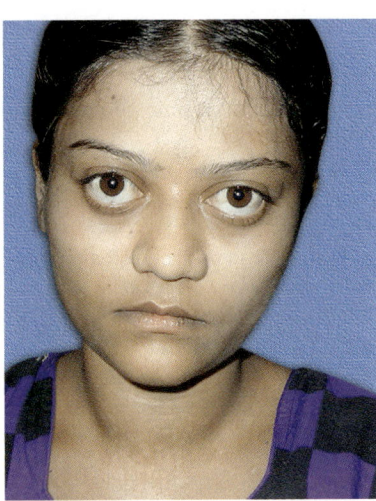

Fig. 16-16 *Lower sclera is visible* in exophthalmos.

movements possible), corneal ulceration; papilledema soon develops; finally it may also cause loss of vision. It is called **malignant exophthalmos** (even though it is neither malignant nor related to any malignancy).

2. **Important Eye Signs**
   Eye signs are common in primary thyrotoxicosis. Lid lag, lid spasm can occur in secondary thyrotoxicosis also.
   i. ***Stellwag's sign:*** It is absence or infrequent blinking, so *staring look*. It is *first sign* to appear. It is due to tonic contraction of striated part of the levator palpebral superioris in toxic thyroid.
   ii. ***Von Graefe's sign/Lid lag sign:*** It is visible white sclera above the corneal margin due to **lid lag** as the upper eyelids cannot keep pace with the eyeball when they look down. Examiner's left hand is placed over the patient's head. Examiner's right index finger placed at the level of patient's eye is slowly brought down and the patient is asked to visually follow the downward moving finger. If the upper sclera is visible then it is positive lid lag sign. Test is repeated few more times for confirmation. Normally upper eyelid follows the finger downwards along with the eyeball but lid lag is observed in primary thyrotoxicosis **(Figs. 16-17A and B)**. It is due to overactivity of involuntary part of the levator palpebrae superioris muscle (Muller's muscle).
   iii. ***Lid retraction:*** Here upper eyelid is higher than normal whereas lower eyelid is in normal position. It is not a sign of exophthalmos. It is due to over activity of involuntary smooth muscle part of the levator palpebrae superioris. It is one of the eye signs of toxic goiter. When it is associated with exophthalmos, sclera adjacent to lower eyelid is also visible. It is a sign of hyperthyroidism.
   iv. ***Naffziger sign:*** Examiner stands behind the patient, and patient's neck is extended and examiner looks from behind along the superior orbital margin of the patient. Eyeball is seen beyond the superciliary ridge in exophthalmos **(Figs. 16-18A and B)**.
   v. ***Dalrymple's sign:*** It is upper eye lid retraction due to spasm of involuntary part of levator palpebrae superioris, so upper sclera is visible.
   vi. ***Joffroy's sign:*** It is absence of wrinkling on forehead when patient looks up (frowns) with the neck flexed as protruded eyeball obviates the necessity for frowning **(Figs. 16-19A and B)**.
   vii. ***Moebius sign:*** It is lack of convergence of eyeball. Defective convergence is due to lymphocytic infiltration of inferior oblique and inferior rectus muscles in case of primary thyrotoxicosis. There will be diplopia. It may be an early sign of eventual ophthalmoplegia. Examiner's left hand is placed over the patient's head. Right index finger from distance is brought towards the root of nose between the eyes and patient is asked to visually follow the approaching finger to look for convergence. If positive, patient will be unable to converge and develops diplopia **(Figs. 16-20A and B)**.
3. ***Chemosis:*** Edema of conjunctiva occurs due to compression of ophthalmic vein and lymphatics by increased orbital pressure often associated with excess watering of eyes.

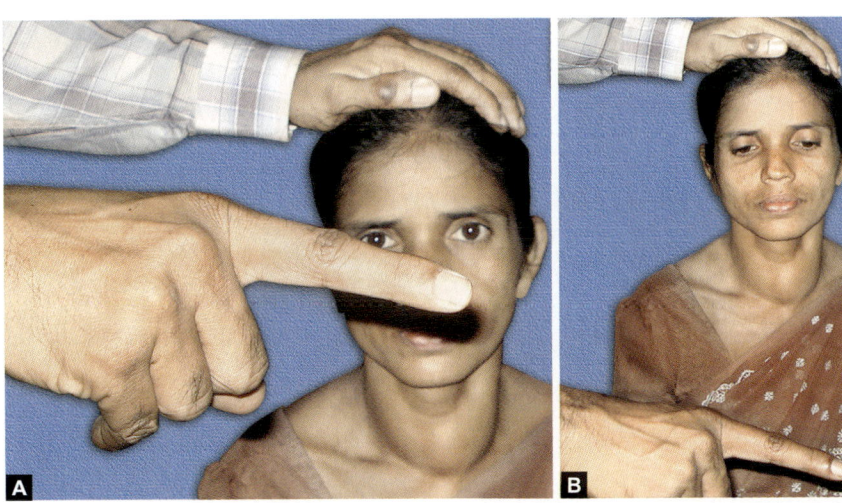

Figs. 16-17A and B *Lid lag* to check in primary thyrotoxicosis.

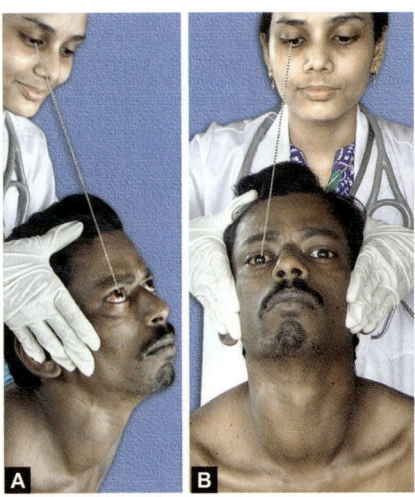

Figs. 16-18A and B *Naffziger's sign.*

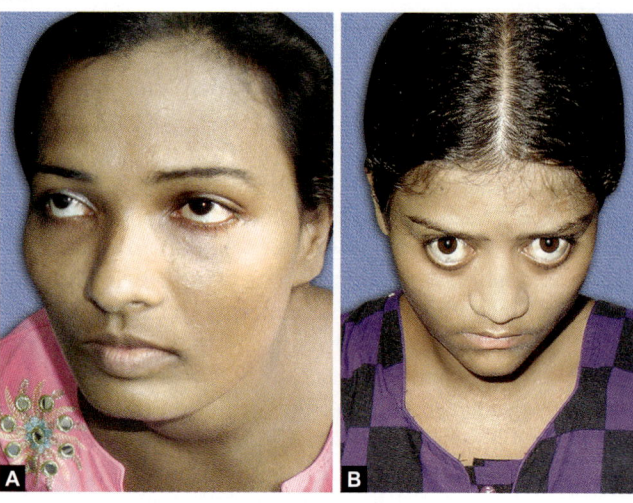

Figs. 16-19A and B *Joffroy's sign.*

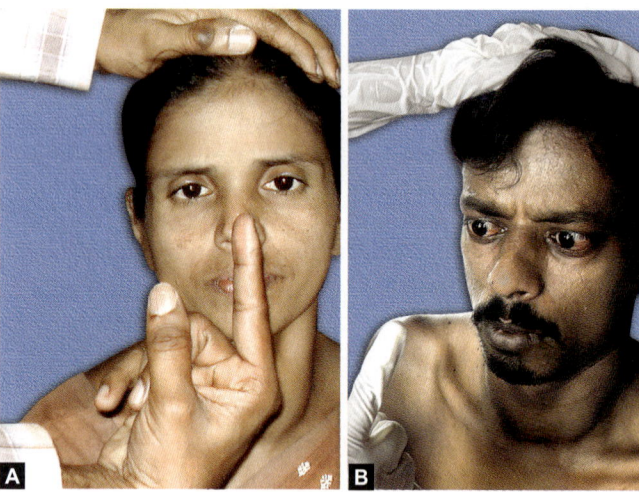

Figs. 16-20A and B *Moebius sign.*

4. **Ophthalmoplegia:** Edema and infiltration of muscle and oculomotor nerve lead to weakness in the movement of the globe by lateral/medial rectus and inferior oblique muscle. All the movements of the eyeball are checked. Patient is specifically not able to look upwards and outwards (**Figs. 16-21A and B**).

Other eye signs: *(Only of academic interest—students do not require to remember these)*

1. *Jellinek's sign:* Increased pigmentation of eyelid margins
2. *Enroth sign:* Edema of eyelids (lower eyelid specifically) and conjunctiva
3. *Rosenbach's sign:* Tremor of closed eyelids
4. *Gifford's sign:* Difficulty in everting upper eyelid in exophthalmos of toxic thyroid. Differentiates from exophthalmos of other causes and from proptosis
5. *Loewi's sign:* Dilatation of pupil with weak adrenaline solution
6. *Knie's sign:* Unequal pupillary dilatation.
7. *Cowen's sign:* Jerky pupillary contraction to consensual light
8. *Kocher's sign:* When clinician places his hands on patient's eyes and lifts it higher, patient's upper lid springs up more quickly than eyebrows
9. *Grove's sign:* Upper lid resistance to downward traction
10. *Rochin's sign:* Reduced amplitude of blinking
11. *Boston's sign:* Uneven jerky movement of the upper eyelid in inferior movement
12. *Mean's sign:* Eye globe lags behind upper eyelid on upward gaze
13. *Griffith's sign:* Lower eyelid lags behind the eye globe on upward gaze
14. *Sainton's sign:* Frontalis contraction after cessation of levator activity
15. *Vigouroux's sign:* Puffiness of lids
16. *Ballet's sign:* Ophthalmoplegia—paralysis of more extraocular muscles
17. *Suker's sign:* Difficulty in maintaining fixation in extreme lateral gaze
18. *Wilder sign:* Jerking of eyes on movement from abduction to adduction
19. *Trousseau's/Payne's sign:* Dislocation of the eye globe
20. *Reisman's sign:* Bruit over eyelid
21. *Snellen/Donder's sign:* Bruit over the eye
22. *Goldzieher's sign:* Deep injection of conjunctiva
23. *Becker's sign:* Abnormal pulsation of the retinal artery on fundoscopy

Note: *In hypothyroidism,* thickening of eyelid, hair loss on outer 2/3 aspect of the eyebrows is noted.

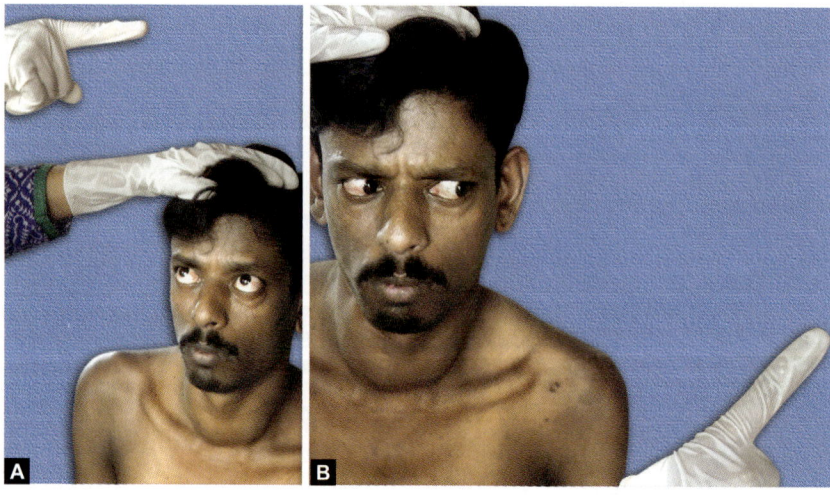

Figs. 16-21A and B *Movements of the eyeball should be checked* in primary thyrotoxicosis with exophthalmos to rule out involving eye ball muscle infiltration by macrophages, inflammatory cells.

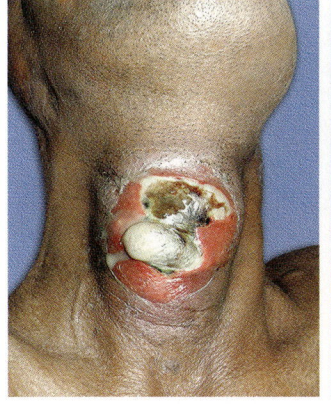 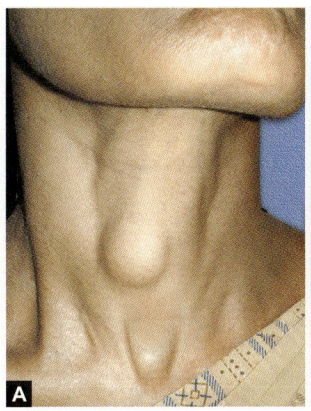 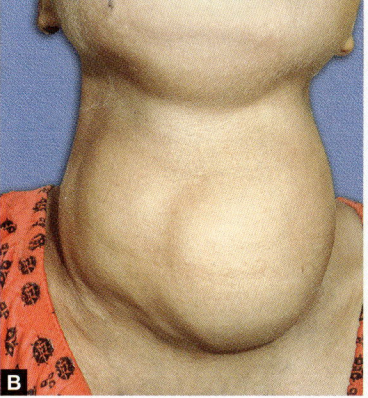 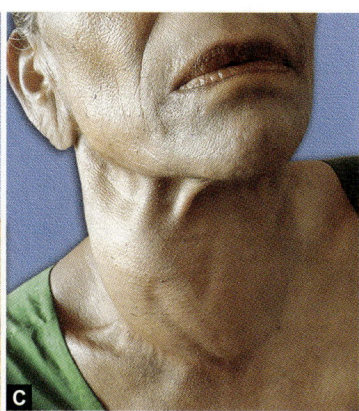

Fig. 16-22 *Acute suppurative thyroiditis* with pus formation and necrosis. It is rare.

Figs. 16-23A to C Different types of goiter—*solitary nodule, multinodular, large goiter (malignancy)*. Inspection of goiter is very important.

■ LOCAL EXAMINATION

Inspection

Thyroid is the only endocrine gland which is properly accessible clinically; only gland that can be involved in all age groups; only gland where malignant tumors are mostly nonfunctioning (**Figs. 16-22 and 16-23**).

Inspectory findings of the swelling should include:
Location: In thyroid region/below in retrosternal goiter; thyroglossal cyst/fistula may be suprahyoid/subhyoid/infrahyoid; lingual thyroid at base of the tongue.

Size: Both vertical and horizontal dimensions of each lobe and isthmus or if it presents as single mass dimensions of the single swelling is noted.

Shape: Butterfly shape if both lobes are involved uniformly as in colloid goiter.

Extent: From posterior border of sternomastoid laterally to midline in single lobe enlargement of gland or from one sternomastoid to opposite side sternomastoid if both lobes are enlarged. Upper extent is usually up to thyroid cartilage. **Lower margin may or may not be clearly visible** during deglutition. Extent of each lobe when enlarged above and below should be mentioned; extent of isthmus should also be examined.

Surface: It is smooth in physiological goiter, primary toxic goiter and Hashimoto's thyroiditis. It is nodular in multinodular goiter. In malignancy, it can be smooth or nodular.

Movement: Upward movement with deglutition is seen in thyroid swelling. Thyroid moves upwards during deglutition due to attachment of the condensed vascular pretracheal fascia *(Berry's ligament)* above, medially and behind to cricoid cartilage and this pretracheal fascia is also attached to larynx/thyrocricoid cartilage → thyroid membrane → hyoid bone with *inferior constrictor muscle which moves upwards during deglutition*; inferior constrictor has got two parts—upper thyropharyngeus and lower cricopharyngeus (**Fig. 16-24**). This movement is restricted in malignant infiltration and inflammation of thyroid. Thyroglossal cyst, subhyoid bursa, prelaryngeal or pretracheal lymph nodes also move with deglutition.

> **Swellings which move upwards with deglutition:**
> - Thyroid swelling
> - Subhyoid bursa
> - Thyroglossal cyst
> - Pretracheal/prelaryngeal lymph nodes
> - Swelling from larynx/trachea

Whether swelling *moves up while protruding the tongue out* should be looked for. The neck of the patient is extended and then asked to protrude the tongue out. Thyroglossal cyst moves upwards with protrusion of tongue. After opening the mouth, with the lower jaw kept still cyst/swelling is held firmly and patient is asked to protrude the tongue outwards. Upward pull of the cyst is felt as a *'tug' like feeling by the palpating* fingers (**Figs. 16-25 and 16-26**).

Skin over the swelling: Skin is stretched and shiny in large goiter. Any scar (of previous surgery) or dilated veins (in toxic goiter, carcinoma thyroid, venous compression, retrosternal

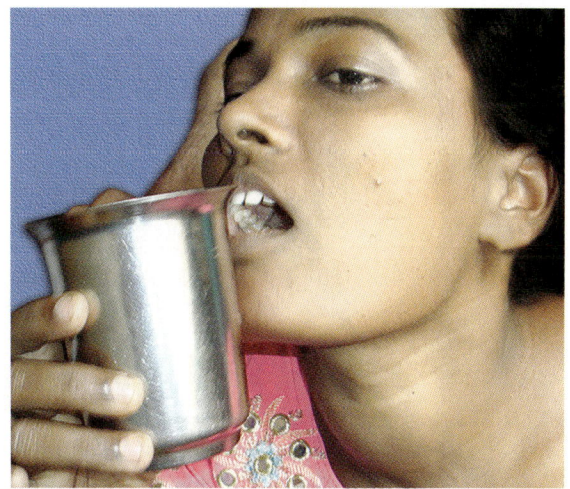

Fig. 16-24 *Thyroid moves upwards with deglutition.* Often it is better to give a glass of water to the patient to drink.

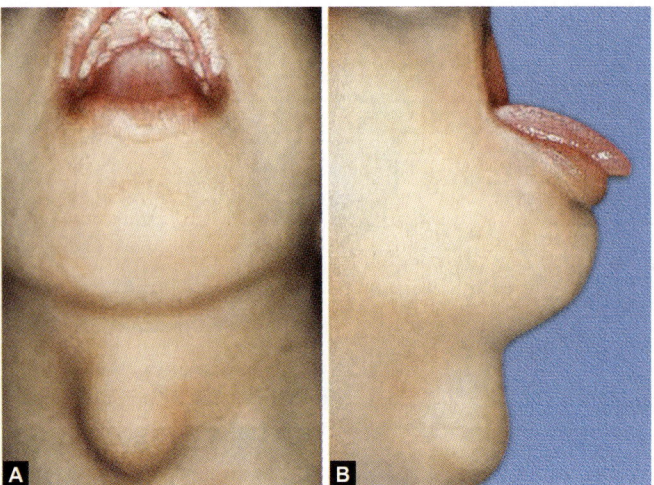

Figs. 16-25A and B *Thyroglossal cyst.*

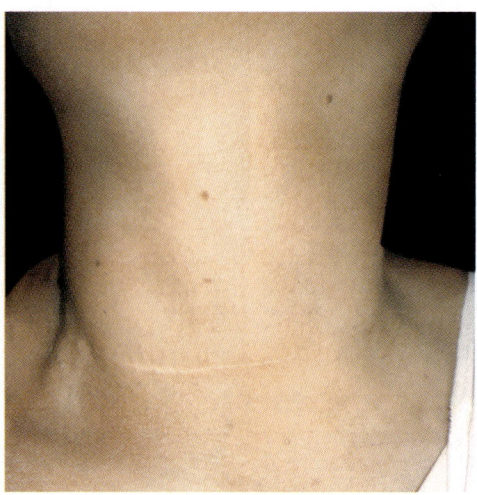

Fig. 16-27 *Scar of previous thyroid surgery* should be noted while inspecting the thyroid swelling.

goiter) or pigmentation on the skin or pulsation over the swelling (toxicity, malignancy) are noted. In retrosternal goiter, there are dilated veins over the chest also. Occasionally carcinoma thyroid may get adherent to skin or can fungate **(Figs. 16-27 to 16-31)**.

Thyroglossal fistula presents on inspection as a withdrawn opening in the *midline* below the hyoid bone having a *crescentic* fold of skin with concavity downwards **(Fig. 16-32)**.

Pizzillo's method of inspection is done in short neck and obese individuals whereby the head is pushed backwards against. The resistance offered by clasped hands placed over the occiput.

Any other swelling in the neck should be seen like for lymph nodes. Lymph nodes are commonly involved in papillary carcinoma of thyroid and occasionally in follicular carcinoma of thyroid.

Palpation

Methods of Palpation of Thyroid Gland

Palpation of thyroid is done from behind with the patient sitting comfortably on a stool and flexing the neck. Both thumbs of the examiner are placed over the back of the neck (nape of the neck or close to the occiput) and fingers of each hand are placed on the respective lateral lobes for palpation. Isthmus should also be palpated like this. For detailed palpation of lateral lobe, patient is made to flex the neck towards that side to relax the sternomastoid muscle. But many specific tests are done with examiner standing in front. Flexing the neck prevents the tautness of the sternomastoid muscles. Occasionally palpation is carried out in extended

> **Occasions wherein thyroid swelling may not move upwards with deglutition:**
> - Anaplastic carcinoma thyroid—often
> - Carcinoma thyroid with extensive local infiltration into soft tissues, trachea/larynx and posterior muscles
> - Intrathoracic retrosternal extension with infiltration/impaction
> - Riedel's thyroiditis with encasement of trachea
> - Massive thyroid wherein movement upwards is difficult to observe and appreciate

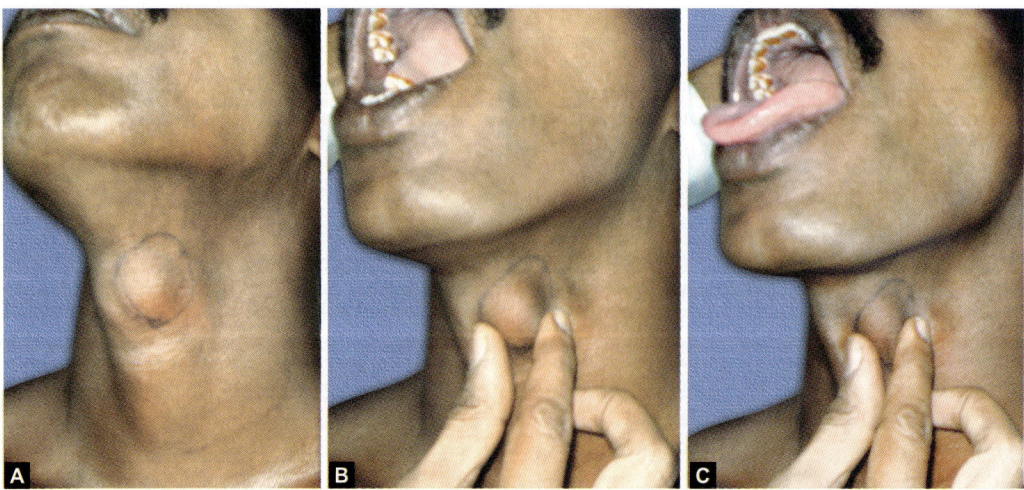

Figs. 16-26A to C Checking the *typical 'tug'* in thyroglossal cyst.

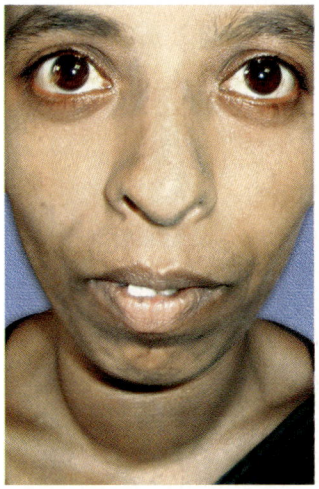

Fig. 16-28 *Diffuse toxic goiter.* Surface of thyroid here is smooth. Exophthalmos is also present.

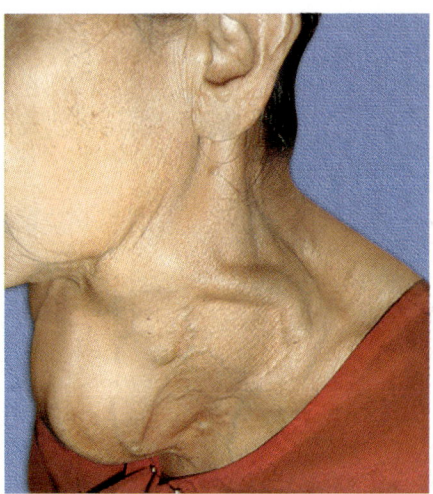

Fig. 16-29 *Large carcinoma of thyroid which is vascular.* Note the dilated veins.

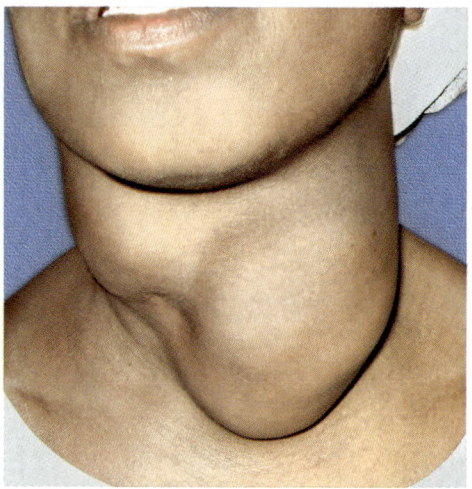

Fig. 16-30 *Recurrent nodule thyroid.* Patient has undergone thyroidectomy once earlier. Note the scar in the neck.

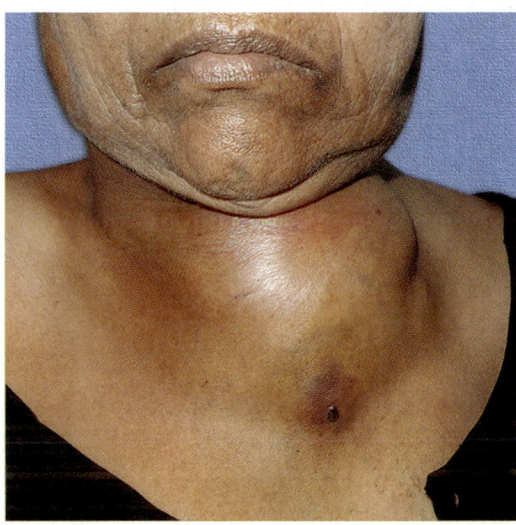

Fig. 16-31 Carcinoma thyroid— advanced. Note the size, skin involvement. *Lower margin is not visible probably extending into the retrosternum.*

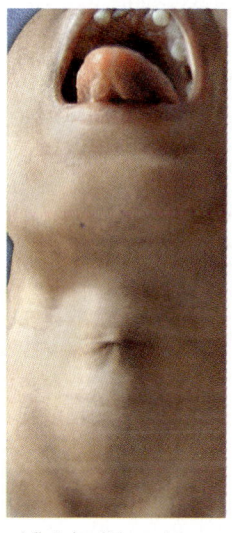

Fig. 16-32 Thyroglossal fistula. It is not a congenital one; *hood sign* (crescentic fold of skin at its lower part) is typical.

neck to make gland more prominent and accessible even though there is increased tautness of sternomastoid muscles. Isthmus is palpated over the trachea in the midline using fingers. Lateral lobes are palpated by insinuating the fingers between anterior border of sternomastoid muscle and lateral lobe or alternatively by placing the fingers along the posterior border of the sternomastoid muscle **(Figs. 16-33 and 16-34)**.

Crile's method of palpation of gland: It is the palpation of the nodule/swelling from front using the pulp of the thumb when the patient is asked to do the act of swallowing **(Figs. 16-35A and B)**.

> **WHO grading of the goiter:**
> - 0—no visible no palpable goiter
> - 1—palpable goiter but not visible with neck in normal position
> - 2—palpable and visible with neck in normal position

Pizzillo's method: It is the method used for inspection and often palpation of the thyroid gland in short necked and obese individuals. Patient is asked to keep her/his clasped hands over the occiput and head is pushed against the resisting hands. Gland becomes prominent which will be inspected or palpated from front or behind **(Fig. 16-36)**.

Lahey's method (test) of examination: It is the method used to palpate any nodules in the posterior part of the gland. It is mainly useful in solitary nodule of thyroid. Examiner should stand in front of the patient. If right lobe is needed to be palpated, left lateral lobe is pushed towards right to make posterior aspect of the right lobe more prominent as gland gets pushed and rotated towards right side. Posterior becomes posterolateral (by rotation of trachea) or lateral which is felt for any nodules. Posterior aspect of left lobe is palpated by pushing the right lobe towards left side **(Figs. 16-37A and B)**.

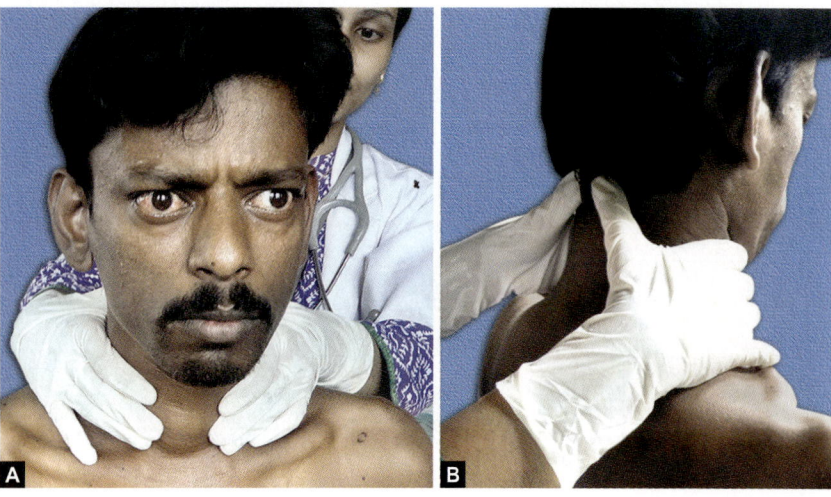

Figs. 16-33A and B *Palpation of thyroid from behind with patient is sitting in a stool comfortably and neck flexed. Careful palpation for nodules should be made.*

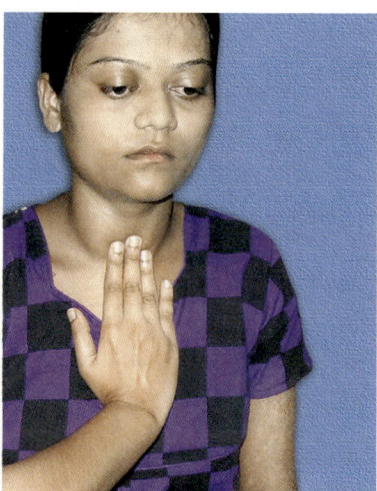

Fig. 16-34 *Palpation of isthmus is done by palpating over the tracheal rings using fingers.*

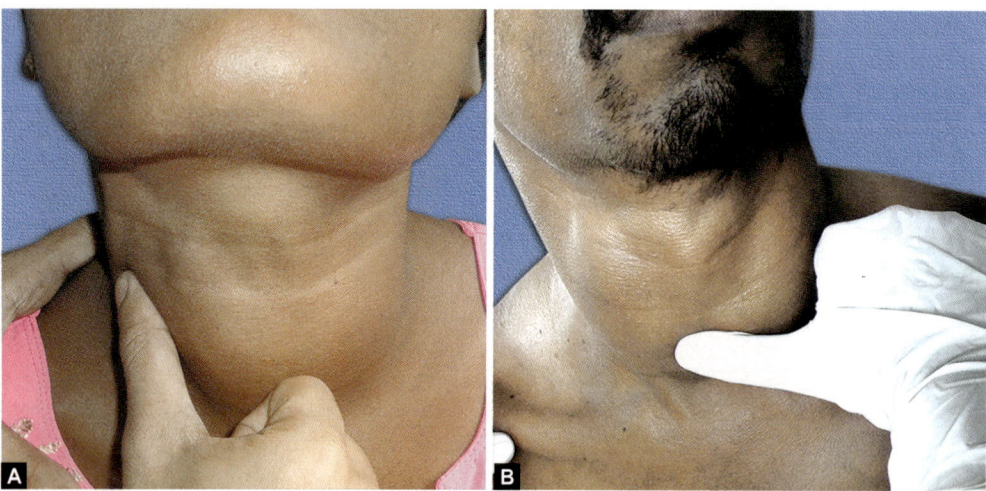

Figs. 16-35A and B *Criles method of palpation using thumb for any nodules.*

Palpatory findings of the swelling include:

Temperature over the swelling: Swelling may be warm in toxic thyroid, malignancy, thyroiditis.

Tenderness: Hemorrhage, thyroiditis, tumor necrosis can cause tenderness.

Extent/position/shape: Should be noted. Extent of each lobe including isthmus is noted.

Size: Should be measured in centimeter both vertically and horizontally.

Edge/margin: Well-defined or diffuse, lower margin which is most important should be especially mentioned; well-defined in primary thyrotoxicosis, colloid goiter, adenoma; ill-defined in carcinoma thyroid. **Lower margin of the gland/** swelling should be checked during deglutition by placing the examiner's index finger horizontally just above the sternum (**getting below the swelling**).

Surface: It is smooth in primary toxic goiter, colloid goiter, Hashimoto's thyroiditis; nodular in multinodular goiter.

Consistency: Soft or firm or hard; uniform or variable and if so different consistencies in various parts should be mentioned.

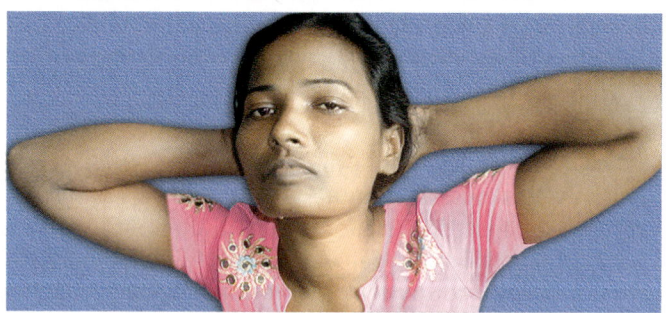

Fig. 16-36 *Pizzillo's method of examination.*

Consistency in thyroid swelling is variable in malignancy; it can be soft/firm/hard. It is hard in Riedel's thyroiditis and calcified cyst. It is firm or hard in multinodular goiter. It is soft in colloid goiter, physiological goiter and primary toxic goiter. Tensely cystic swelling can be hard; neoplastic solid swelling can be softer (due to multiplying cells)—**thyroid paradox**. Thyroid paradox is often observed in papillary carcinoma of thyroid.

Mobility of the swelling: Thyroid swelling moves upwards with deglutition.

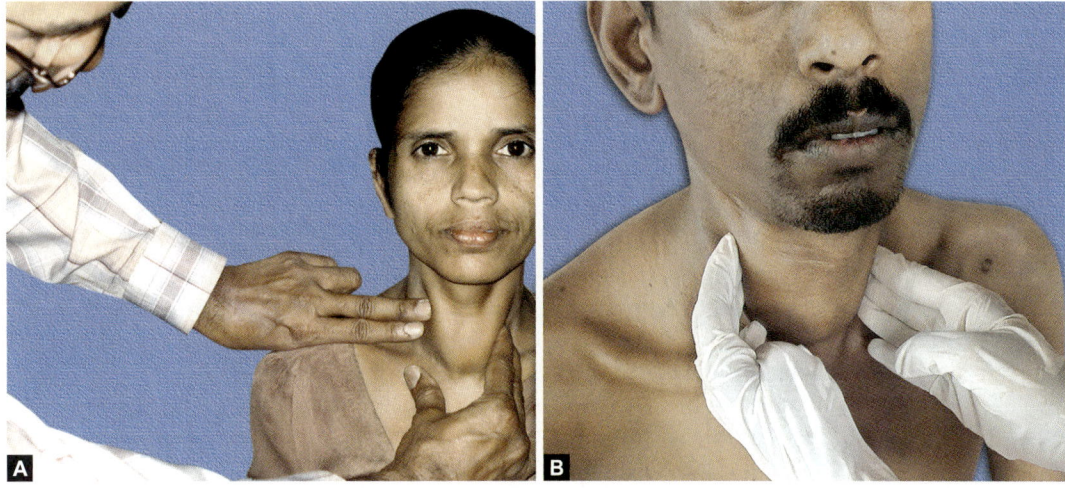

Figs. 16-37A and B *Lahey's method.*

Independent mobility: The trachea is immobilized by extending the neck. The gland is grasped and moved vertically and horizontally over the trachea. Thyroid does **not show independent upward mobility** but it shows horizontal mobility along with trachea. A small encapsulated swelling occasionally may show independent free mobility upwards. The horizontal mobility gets restricted in carcinoma thyroid **(Fig. 16-38)**.

Plane of the swelling: It is checked by asking the patient to contract the sternomastoid muscles meanwhile examiner's hand is placed under the chin of patient and patient is asked to flex the neck against the resisting hand. Relation of the single side gland to sternomastoid muscle is checked by contracting the muscle which is done by turning the chin against resistance of the examiner's hand which is placed on the opposite side. Whether *skin is free or not* is checked by pinching/rolling the skin—it is adherent in carcinoma thyroid, acute thyroiditis, or previous surgery over the thyroid. *Neck is extended to stretch the deep fascia* to check whether swelling is deep to deep fascia or not; but this is more a theoretical than a practical; its significance is doubtful **(Figs. 16-39 and 16-40)**.

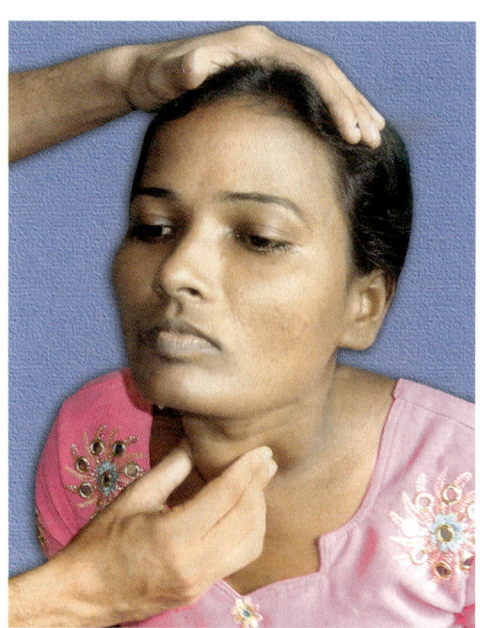

Fig. 16-38 *Mobility of thyroid* should be checked.

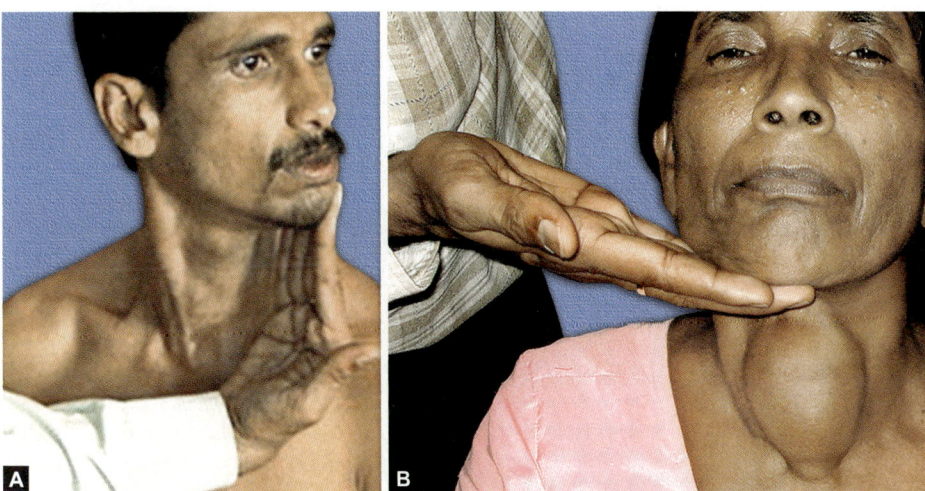

Figs. 16-39A and B *Contraction of sternomastoid one side/both sides* to confirm that thyroid is deep to deep fascia.

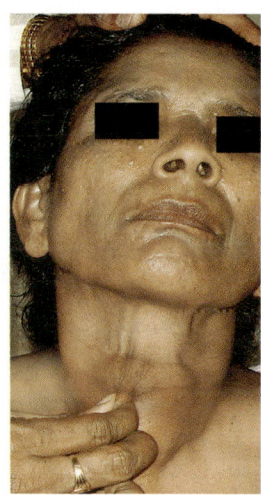

Fig. 16-40 *Skin should be pinched to confirm that swelling* is not adherent to skin.

Thrill is checked in the upper pole of the gland as superior thyroid artery is superficial and enters the gland in front at its upper pole. Thrill signifies toxicity or increased vascularity **(Fig. 16-41)**.

Kocher's test: It is the test to check for tracheal compression. Patient is asked to look straight. With fingers and thumb or with fingers of both hands, both lateral lobes of the thyroid gland are gently compressed directing posteromedially. If patient develops stridor, Kocher's test is positive (***stridor*** is harsh noise produced by the passage of air through the partially obstructed air passage usually at trachea). If patient develops no stridor it means negative. In long standing and large goiter, tracheal rings weakened because of constant pressure and trachea gets narrowed/collapsed during **compression**; but trachea is kept patent by the forward traction of the goiter itself. But after thyroidectomy, lack of support to trachea causes ***tracheomalacia***—weakening of the tracheal rings. Such patients 'need tracheostomy' after thyroidectomy. It is usually temporary tracheostomy for 2–3 weeks, as by then, the tracheal rings regain their strength to maintain the patency of the trachea. '***Scabbard trachea***' is narrowing of trachea. *Note: Scabbard* (French) means a cover for the blade of a sword or dagger or cover for a gun/tool **(Figs. 16-42A and B)**.

Confirmation of Retrosternal Extension

Lower margin of the swelling/goiter is not visible, even on deglutition. Lower margin is not palpable during deglutition. Dilated veins over neck or chest wall may be visible. Nocturnal dyspnea and dyspnea by changing the position of the neck are often observed. Normal resonant note becomes dull over the sternum on percussion **(Fig. 16-43)**.

Pemberton's sign: Patient is asked to raise both the arms above the shoulder so as to touch the ears and to keep for 3 minutes. Patient will develop dilated veins in the neck and upper chest wall, followed by puffiness and sometimes cyanosis in face and respiratory distress and rarely dysphagia. This is presumably due to narrowing of the thoracic inlet and obstruction of great veins. It means sign is positive signifying retrosternal extension of goiter. Dyspnea can occur at night during lying down or when neck is extended. Rarely recurrent nerve palsy can occur **(Fig. 16-44)**.

Position of Trachea

Position of the trachea is checked by palpation using **three fingers** from below. Middle finger is kept just above the suprasternal space and index and ring fingers are placed over sternal heads of the sternomastoid muscles on each side. Middle finger is run from above downwards along the trachea to feel the position—central or deviated **(Figs. 16-45 and 16-46)**. In solitary nodule or disease of only one lateral lobe, trachea will be usually deviated towards opposite side. Other features are absence of hollowness on the side of the deviation/prominent sternomastoid on the side of the deviation of trachea (opposite side of the enlarged gland or nodule) (***trail sign***); on auscultation, breath sounds are heard

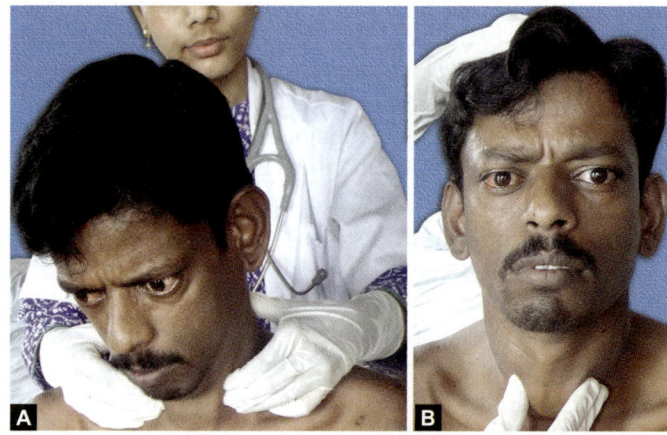

Figs. 16-42A and B *Kocher's test*. With clinician standing behind the patient, both lobes are gently compressed in posteromedial direction using fingers of both hands. Test can be done alternatively by placing thumb on one lateral lobe and fingers of the same hand on the other lateral lobe to compress the lobes posteromedially to create stridor which is a sign of compression. Stridor at rest (without compression) is a sign of infiltration; but Kocher's test is a sign of compression.

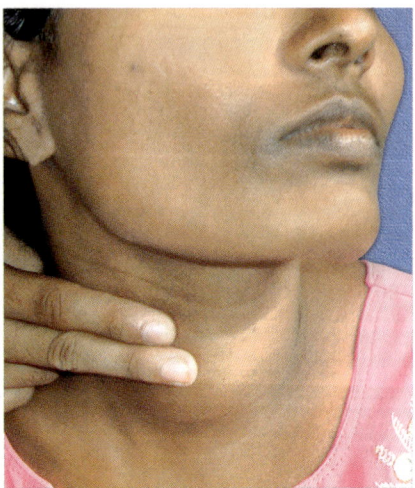

Fig. 16-41 *Superior pole of thyroid should be palpated for thrill which signifies vascularity.*

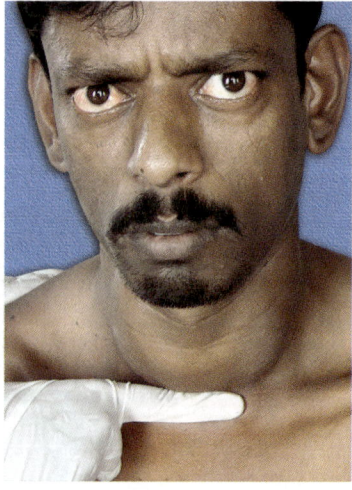

Fig. 16-43 *Lower border of the thyroid should be palpated* to confirm that there is no retrosternal extension.

Chapter 16: Clinical Approach and Examination of Thyroid

rings below. *Bare tracheal rings* are observed in ectopic thyroid (which means thyroid tissue is not present in normal location) and also in absence of isthmus (rare).

Palpation of Vessels

Carotid pulsation should be checked. It is normally felt at the level of the upper border of thyroid cartilage over medial aspect of the sternomastoid muscle on the Chassaignac tubercle (carotid tubercle) over the transverse process of C_6 vertebra. It may be deviated posteriorly/laterally in a large goiter. It may be absent in advanced carcinoma thyroid due to infiltration of the carotid sheath (encasement) by the tumor (*Berry's sign*) **(Fig. 16-47)**.

> **Possible features of suspected malignancy in solitary nodule thyroid:**
> - Any nodule can be malignant whether nodule is hard/firm/cystic/small/large/asymptomatic
> - Rapid onset/rapid recent increase in size
> - Hoarseness of voice/dysphagia/stridor/dysphagia
> - Fixity of the nodule
> - Palpable significant neck nodes

Nerve Involvement

Sympathetic chain in the neck may get involved in locally advanced carcinoma thyroid causing **Horner's syndrome**—enophthalmos due to Muller's muscle weakness; drooping of upper eyelid (ptosis); anhidrosis; miosis due to paralysis of dilator papillae; absence of ciliospinal reflex; flushing of face and nasal congestion.

Measurement of Circumference of the Neck

It has to be done at regular intervals if patient is not undergoing surgery as it is important to assess the increase in size of the thyroid (progress of the swelling).

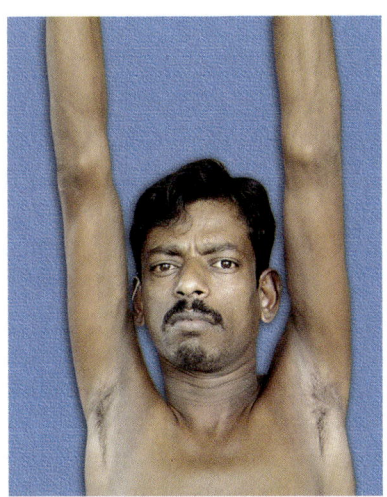

Fig. 16-44 *Pemberton's sign* for retrosternal goiter.

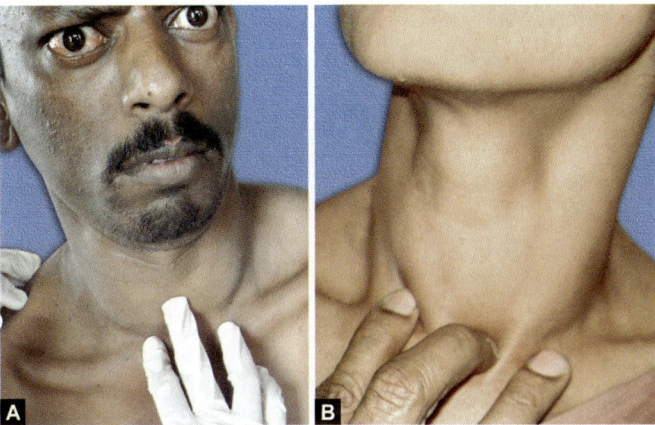

Figs. 16-45A and B *Method of examination of trachea* to find out deviation using three fingers.

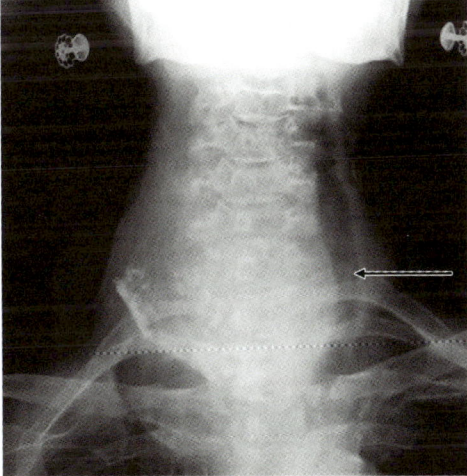

Fig. 16-46 X-ray neck showing *gross tracheal deviation* due to large solitary nodule thyroid on the opposite lobe.

well on the side of the deviation. Trachea is in central position when both lateral lobes are enlarged; here, space between trachea and sternomastoid is equal on both sides.

Superior border of the isthmus of the normal thyroid gland lies inferior to cricoid cartilage. Isthmus is felt over the tracheal

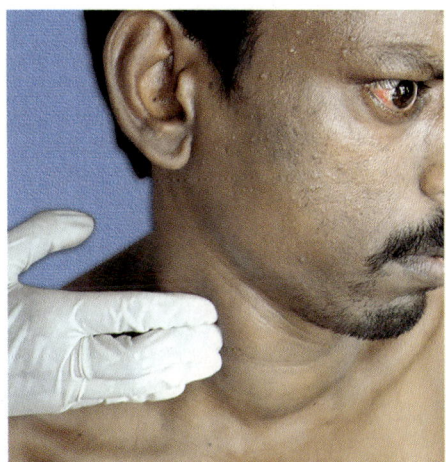

Fig. 16-47 *Palpation of carotid artery (common carotid)* at the level of thyroid cartilage on the medial border of sternomastoid muscle over Chassaignac tubercle in transverse process of C_6 vertebra. In Berry's sign, it is absent. It signifies advanced carcinoma of thyroid.

Examination of Neck Lymph Nodes

Cervical lymph nodes are looked for enlargement in secondaries from carcinoma thyroid. Extent, size, number, tenderness, surface, consistency, margin, mobility/fixity should be checked. It is commonly palpable in papillary carcinoma of thyroid. It is usually in level III and IV nodes. It could be firm, hard or cystic. It is usually brownish black in color often with papillary projections. Lymph nodes often can get enlarged in follicular carcinoma thyroid, medullary carcinoma and lymphoma. *Lateral aberrant thyroid* which was earlier thought as aberrant thyroid in lateral part of the neck is actually not so but it is secondary in lymph node with primary being papillary carcinoma of thyroid. Occult primary in thyroid wherein primary in thyroid is clinically not palpable. Primary and secondary nodes are drainage groups—primary are pretracheal nodes and prelaryngeal node (*Delphian*); secondary are deep cervical group of nodes **(Fig. 16-48)**.

Percussion

Percussion over the manubrium sterni is important. Normally it is resonant (superior mediastinum—due to trachea). Dullness signifies retrosternal extension. Tenderness may signify the secondaries in sternum from follicular carcinoma of thyroid. Direct percussion method is the usual practice. But it is often painful. Indirect method can also be used **(Figs. 16-49A and B)**.

Auscultation

Auscultation over the upper pole of the gland is done to hear bruit in patients with toxic thyroid and in very vascular tumors **(Fig. 16-50)**.

SYSTEMIC EXAMINATION

Cardiovascular system examination: It is important in thyrotoxicosis—commonly secondary type. Tachycardia, ectopic beats, pulsus paradoxus, extrasystoles, atrial fibrillation are the cardiac presentations **(Fig. 16-51)**.

Respiratory system examination: Secondaries and pleural effusion can occur in follicular carcinoma of thyroid.

Abdomen examination **(Figs. 16-52 and 16-53):** Hepatomegaly is looked for as secondaries in liver are known to occur in follicular carcinoma of thyroid. Hepatosplenomegaly can occur as part of Graves' disease or Hashimoto's disease.

Examination of skull and spine **(Figs. 16-54A and B):** Localized, warm, vascular, pulsatile secondaries can occur in skull commonly, rib and other bones occasionally as a spread from follicular carcinoma of thyroid.

Neurological: Ankle (Achilles tendon) reflex is prolonged with delayed relaxation in hypothyroidism and it is shortened and brisk in hyperthyroidism. Biceps reflex and knee jerk are also often checked **(Fig. 16-55)**.

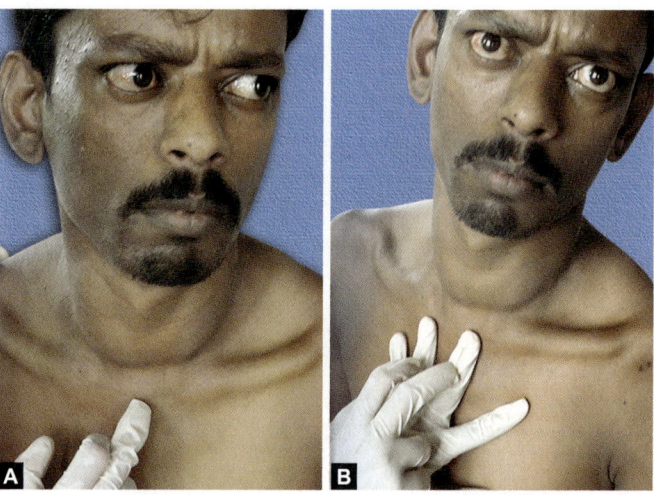

Figs. 16-49A and B *Percussion over* the *sternum* is important to rule out retrosternal extension. *Direct method* is commonly used. *Indirect method* can be used but not as sensitive as direct (percussing bone through a bone).

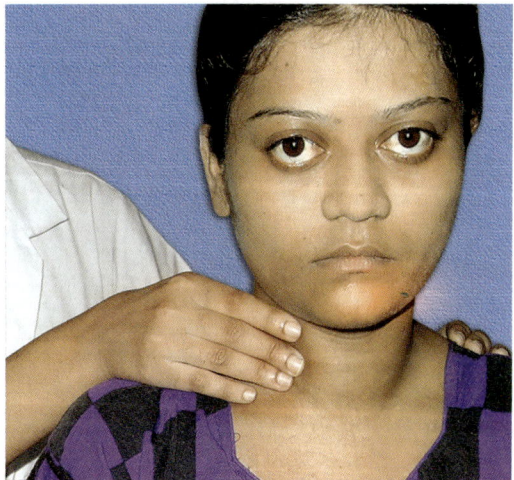

Fig. 16-48 *Cervical lymph nodes should be examined* in all thyroid swellings.

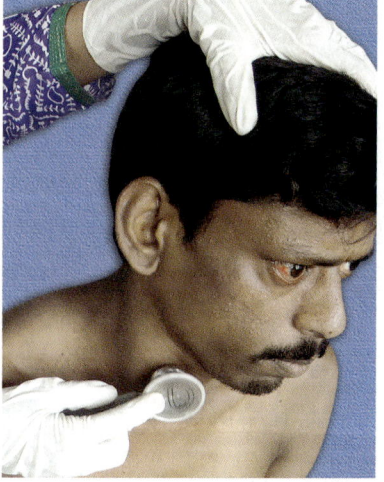

Fig. 16-50 *Bruit over thyroid* should be auscultated to find out increased vascularity over the upper pole.

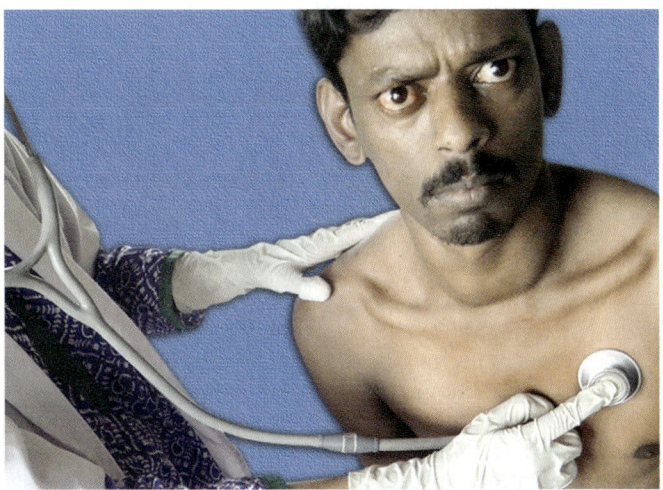

Fig. 16-51 Cardiovascular system is examined and *auscultated for cardiac problems in secondary thyrotoxicosis*.

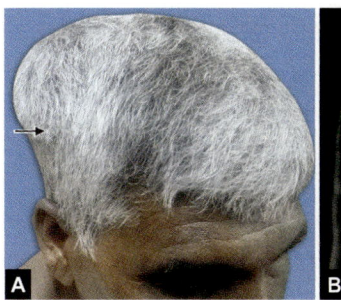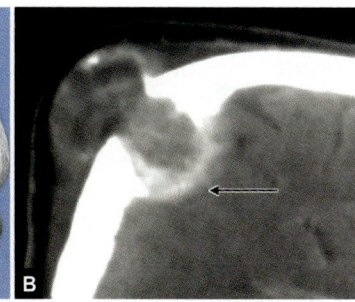

Figs. 16-54A and B Secondaries in the skull in primary follicular carcinoma of thyroid. It is *warm, soft, well localized, pulsatile, soft, not mobile, fixed swelling*. Both outer and inner tables of skull are disrupted by the tumor and its soft colloid content cause brain pulsation to be transmitted to the surface to feel the swelling as pulsatile. Note in the CT disruption of skull tables.

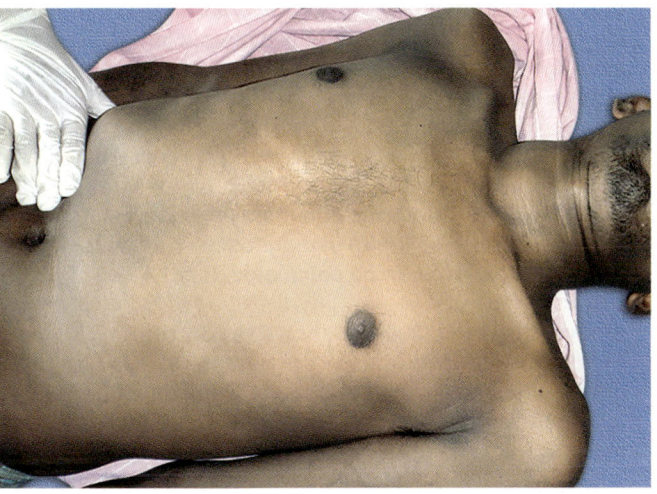

Fig. 16-52 Hepatomegaly can occur *in Graves'* and *Hashimoto's diseases* as part of the autoimmune disease.

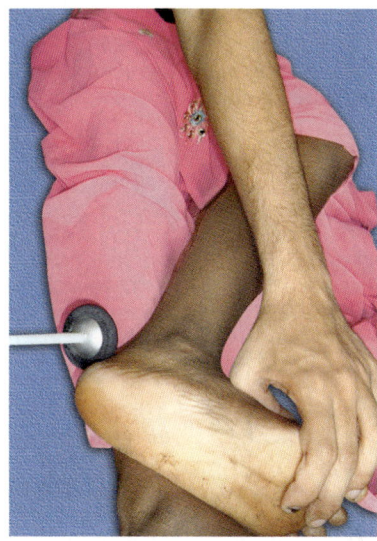

Fig. 16-55 *Ankle jerk* (reflex) is brisk in toxic thyroid and sluggish in hypothyroidism.

In a case of thyroid disease following things should be made very clear:
- *Functional status:* Hyperthyroid/euthyroid/hypothyroid
- *Compression* to trachea/recurrent nerve
- *Neck lymph nodal* status
- *Tracheal deviation, carotid* infiltration/deviation of carotid
- *Features of malignancy*
- *Retrosternal extension*
- *Cardiac, abdominal* and *respiratory* systems
- *Bony secondaries* mainly frontal bone

Recent rapid increase in thyroid swelling is due to:
- Malignant transformation in previous MNG
- Hemorrhage into a nodule
- Anaplastic carcinoma of thyroid

- **Thyroid steal:** Patient is taken to operation theatre for few days before doing surgery so as to reduce the anxiety of the patient. Eventually steal the patient for surgery.
- Condition resulting from total removal of thyroid was called **cachexia strumipriva** by Kocher.

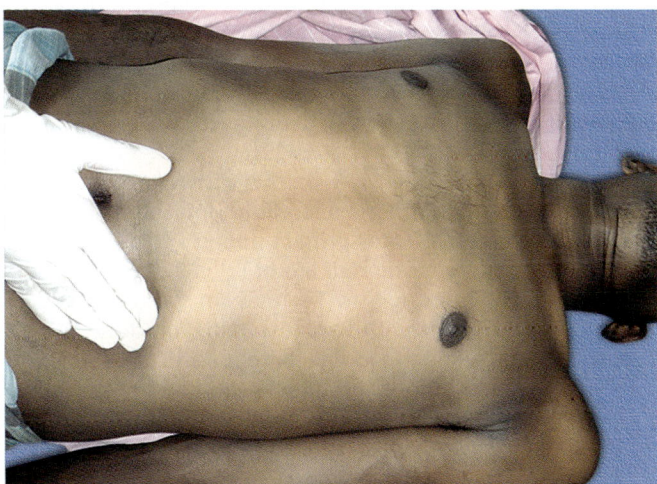

Fig. 16-53 *Palpation of spleen* in a patient with thyroid enlargement. It is seen in Graves' and Hashimoto's disease.

Case sheet writing in a patient with thyroid swelling

History
Name: Age:
Occupation: Sex: Place/residence:
Chief complaints: swelling; pain; hoarseness of voice
History of present illness
- Swelling—duration, mode of onset and progress, site of origin, number
- Pain—origin, nature, character, duration, time of starting of pain, specific features, severity, aggravating or relieving factors
- Fever—type, severity, duration
- Other lumps—when started, progress like in neck nodes, skull
- Pressure symptoms—stridor, dyspnea, hoarseness of voice, dysphagia—duration, severity
- Symptoms of toxicity; visual changes
- Symptoms of hypothyroidism

Past history
- Past history of swelling and treatment for that
- Tuberculosis, spinal diseases, diabetes, leprosy, malignancies
- **Past history of treatment and surgery; drug intake—thyroxine or antithyroid drugs or other**

Family history
- Family tree; history of tuberculosis, diabetes, malignancies; treatment history

Menstrual history

General examination: Anemia, edema, jaundice, clubbing, lymphadenopathy, **pulse, blood pressure,** temperature, attitude, nutrition, body weight. **Skin, hands, sweating, eye signs**

Local examination
Inspection
- Swelling—location/site (in relation to bony point and sternocleidomastoid muscle), size, shape, extent, color, surface of the swelling, skin over the swelling, number, edge/margin (**lower**)/border of the swelling, **movement with deglutition,** movement of the swelling, pulsation, sinus, fistula
- Pressure effects—edema, dilated veins, paralysis, deformity, wasting.

Pizzillo's method

Palpation
- Local raise of temperature, tenderness
- Size, shape and extent of the swelling, edge of the swelling, surface of the swelling, consistency
- **Crile's method of palpation, Pizillo's method, Kocher's test, Pemberton's sign, position of trachea (trail sign), lower margin, Lahey's method**
- Fluctuation, transillumination test
- Pulsatility, thrill
- Plane of the selling (should be checked in relation to sternocleidomastoid muscle by contracting it), mobility, fixity to skin or deeper structures
- Examination proximal and distal to swelling
- Examination of **sympathetic chain** and vascular systems—**carotid artery pulsation,** superficial temporal artery

Examination of oral cavity, scalp

Percussion—sternal percussion and tenderness
Auscultation—bruit over the swelling (upper pole thyroid) or carotid
Examination of cervical lymph nodes and other regional nodes
Systemic examination—abdomen, respiratory, cardiac and central nervous systems (ankle jerk), skull and spine

Thyroid Function Tests

- T_3, T_4, TSH, Free T_3, Free T_4: T_4 is transported in plasma, binding to thyroxin binding globulin and thyroxin binding prealbumin. Free T_4 is very less. Normal T_4 is 55–150 nmol/liter. T_3 is still lesser than T_4. It is 1.2–3.1 nmol/liter. Normal TSH is 0–5 IU/mL of plasma. In hyperthyroidism, T_3, T_4 are increased; TSH is decreased/undetectable. T_3, T_4 is decreased; TSH is increased in hypothyroidism. T_3 is more reliable than T_4. Free T_3 and Free T_4 are much more reliable indicators. If one investigation is to be asked, it is better to do TSH estimation. TSH increase is also seen in papillary carcinoma of thyroid. Free T_3 is 0.3% (3–9 pmol/liter). Free T_4 is 0.03% (8–26 pmol/liter). TSH is high (>40 units/liter) in primary hypothyroidism (thyroid related); it is low in secondary (pituitary related) and tertiary hypothyroidism (hypothalamus related, TRH).

- **T3 resin uptake study:** It is the most common indirect method available for the measurement of the proportion of T_4 which is unbound. Patient's serum added with radiolabeled T_3 is incubated with ion exchange resin/thyropac. It competes for unoccupied free protein binding sites of T_4. In hyperthyroidism, unoccupied free binding sites are low and so resin uptake is low; so resin uptake ratio is less than 85%. In hypothyroidism, free binding sites are more; so resin uptake is >120%. Normal range of resin uptake is 0.9–1.2 µg. 100 × total serum T_4 divided by T_3 resin uptake percentage is called as *free T_4 index*. Normal range is 55–145. Free T_4 index is commonly used; it is single best test available. It is helpful in diagnosing T_3 thyrotoxicosis. Free T_3 index also can be calculated. It is 1.4–3.5.

- **TRH stimulation test for hypothalamic-pituitary axis:** Intravenous TRH (200 µg) shows rise in serum TSH level in 20 minutes (from basal 1 µ unit/mL to 10 µ unit/mL) and reaches to normal in 2 hours. Patients with pituitary insufficiency develop a subnormal response; patient with hypothyroidism will show enhanced TSH response; in hyperthyroidism, there will be no response. This test is useful in doubtful hyperthyroidism, hypothyroidism, T_3 thyrotoxicosis, ophthalmic Graves' disease. Drugs like L-thyroxine, steroids, estrogens, levodopa interfere with the response.

- **Protein bound iodide (PBI):** It is a cheaper but nonspecific and unreliable test as it also measures nonhormonal forms of iodide. Normal value is 4–8 µg/100 mL. False positivity is seen in pregnancy, use of iodide containing cough syrups, iodide containing X-ray contrast, and oral contraceptives. False negativity is found with use of salicylates, androgens and hydantoins.

- **Radioisotope studies: Uptake study:** Thyroid traps iodine and rate reflects hormone secretion. Uptake is measured in 10–120 minutes. Later protein bound I^{131} is measured. Dose of I^{131} is 5 µ curie. Half life of I^{131} is 8 days; I^{132} is 2.3 hours; I^{123} is 13 hours. Now Technetium ^{99} is also used as it has short half-life with very less radiation dose. It gets concentrated similar to iodine isotopes and does not bind to tyrosine and so precise iodine trap can be assessed. Uptake study cannot be done after contrast X-rays like IVU. It takes 2 weeks to excrete contrast after IVU; 4 weeks after cholecystogram; many years after bronchography and myelography. *Thyroid scan:* It is done using I^{123}/I^{131} or ^{99m}Tc. It is not done in every patient with thyroid disease. It is indicated in solitary nodule; borderline toxicity; retrosternal goiter; ectopic thyroid; to study the metastases in entire body in functioning thyroid carcinomas after total thyroidectomy. ^{99m}Tc is injected intravenously. I^{123}/I^{131} is given orally. When ^{99m}Tc is used, scan is done in half an hour. When iodine radioisotopes are used, scan is done in 24 hours. Cold nodule is non-functioning nodule; hot nodule is hyperfunctioning nodule; warm nodule is normal functioning gland. In autonomous nodule, nodule is hot and rest of the gland will not show any activity. In functioning nodule which is not autonomous, nodule as well as remaining gland will show the activity.

- *Werner's T3 suppression test:* Initial isotope uptake study is done. 40 μg of T$_3$ is given to the patient orally 8th hourly for 7 days. Uptake study is repeated. In normal uptake, suppression up to 80% is noted. In toxic goiter, suppression is only 10–20%. It is used in patients with antithyroid drugs for primary thyrotoxicosis to assess the remission status, to differentiate true thyrotoxicosis from iodine avid goiter. TSH suppression will decrease iodine uptake; but in thyrotoxicosis, which is autonomous iodine, uptake is not suppressed.
- *Other tests:* BMR (increased in toxicity); serum cholesterol (decreases in toxicity); serum creatinine (increases in toxicity).

Imaging in Thyroid Diseases

X-ray imaging: Plain X-ray neck anteroposterior and lateral shows tracheal deviation and calcification (*speckled fine calcification* in papillary carcinoma of thyroid; *coarse, ring-like calcification* in MNG). X-ray bone (skull, long bones) shows lytic lesions of secondaries from follicular carcinoma of thyroid (Figs. 16-56 and 16-57).

Ultrasound neck: For thyroid and neck nodes. Solid and cystic lesions are identified. US guided FNAC can be done.

It is currently *ideal initial imaging method. Thyroid Imaging Reporting and Data System (TI-RADS)* grades thyroid swelling from TI-RADS 1 to TI RADS 5.

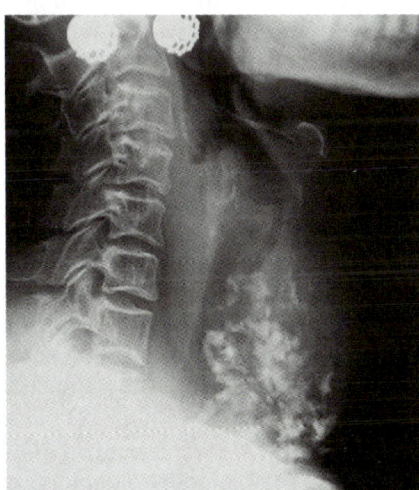

Fig. 16-56 X-ray neck lateral view showing *speckled calcification* of the thyroid.

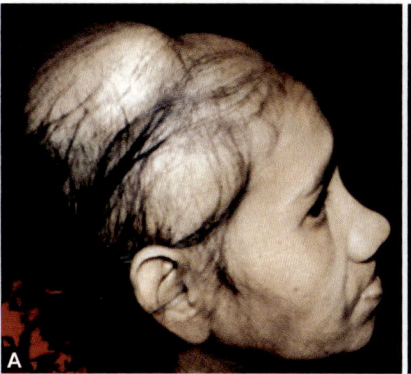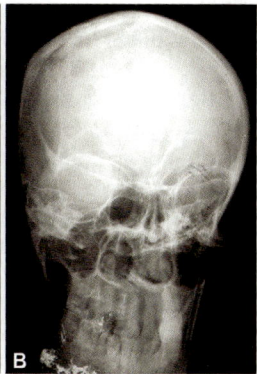

Figs. 16-57A and B X-ray skull of a patient with *secondaries in the skull*; primary is follicular carcinoma of thyroid.

CT neck in malignancies or large goiter to assess infiltration, extent, spread, etc. CT chest and abdomen is done if spread is suspected in case of malignancy. CT neck with chest is done in retrosternal extension.

Biopsy in Thyroid Diseases

1. *FNAC of thyroid* and lymph node (Fig. 16-58). *Thyroglobulin estimation of the lymph node aspiration* content is quiet significant in follicular carcinoma (Differentiated thyroid carcinoma).
2. *Frozen section biopsy* on-table and proceed may be needed. Pathologist should be available adjacent to operation theater. Its significance in thyroid surgery is a debate.

Blood Analysis

Serum thyroglobulin: Its normal value is 1–30 ng/mL (5 ng/mL). It is marker for differentiated thyroid malignancy. Repetitive titers are more reliable. Raising titers suggest disease progression. Its sensitivity and specificity is around 95%. Its half life is 30 hours. It is determined by degree of TSH receptor stimulation, total thyroid tissue normal and diseased, presence of insult to thyroid gland like thyroiditis, thyroidectomy, FNAC, radioactive iodine therapy. Its level becomes untraceable after total thyroidectomy or radioactive

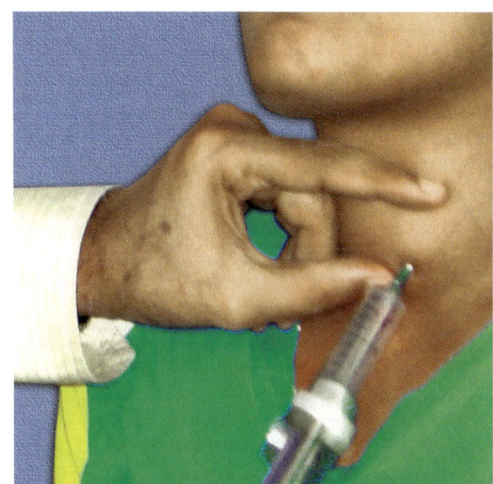

Fig. 16-58 *FNAC thyroid* is an important investigation in thyroid diseases.

ablation. It is better estimated during TSH stimulation; that is being achieved by withdrawal of intake of oral L thyroxine. In case of presence of secondaries, it is useful determinant; but depends on the volume of the metastases and type of the disease (better useful in follicular and Hurthle cell type than papillary) and site of the secondaries (more useful in bone and lung metastases). Occasionally very high levels of serum thyroglobulin level even if present fail to detect due to hook effect by anti-thyroglobulin antibodies and in such situation reassessment is done after dilution. During follow-up if patient shows higher levels of thyroglobulin, estimation that is an indication for further evaluation like USG neck/CT neck and chest, FDG PET scan, etc. for recurrence or metastases is done.

Anti-thyroglobulin antibodies: Anti-thyroglobulin antibodies following thyroidectomy or radioactive ablation become undetectable approximately for 5 years; detectable or rising level of anti-thyroglobulin antibodies suggest persistent or recurrent disease. During follow-up period if earlier undetectable anti-thyroglobulin antibodies level becomes detectable, it means there is disease recurrence even if thyroglobulin level is normal at that point of time. It is assessed always along with serum thyroglobulin estimation; if value >1:100, it is significant. But anti-thyroglobulin antibodies are present in 10% of normal population and 20% of thyroid cancers *per se*. So it is useful tool only one year after thyroid ablation in thyroid cancers. Anti-thyroglobulin antibodies also will elevate in autoimmune diseases like Hashimoto's disease.

Anti-TSH receptor antibody (TSAb/TRAbs—thyroid stimulating immunoglobulin/long acting thyroid stimulator/LATS): It is elevated in Graves' disease and exophthalmos.

Anti-thyroid peroxidase antibody also called as anti-microsomal antibody is elevated in Graves' disease and Hashimoto's disease. It is significant when it is more than 25 units/mL.

Serum calcitonin estimation: It is relevant tumor marker in evaluating medullary carcinoma of thyroid.

Hemogram is relevant as total WBC count should be available as a baseline value prior to starting the antithyroid drugs in toxic thyroid.

Other Tests

Indirect laryngoscopy (ILS) is a must in all thyroid patients who undergo thyroidectomy. Warmed ILS mirror is placed into the oropharynx and patient is asked to tell 'E' to see the abduction of the vocal cords. In 1% of the population, asymptomatic incidental vocal cord palsy is observed. Video laryngoscopy also can be done.

Exophthalmometry: It is done to assess the degree of exophthalmos in thyrotoxicosis patient. Reading of 19 mm or above is abnormal.

ECG and echocardiography are done to assess the cardiac status in thyrotoxicosis.

Solitary Thyroid Nodule

It is *a single palpable nodule* in thyroid *on clinical examination*, in an otherwise normal gland. Causes: (1) Thyroid adenomas—Follicular—common (40% of *actual single nodule* excluding solitary nodule of MNG); Hurthle cell. (2) Papillary carcinoma of thyroid—15%. (3) Only one nodule palpable in an underlying multinodular goiter—*commonest* cause *only* clinically—50% (old concept). (4) Thyroid cyst.

Types: Based on function: (1) Toxic solitary nodule. (2) Nontoxic solitary nodule. Based on radioisotope study: (1) *Hot*—means autonomous toxic nodule. (2) *Warm*—normally functioning nodule. (3) *Cold*—nonfunctioning nodule; may be malignant—20% (need not be always). Cold nodule may be due to malignancy, thyroiditis, thyroid cyst or hemorrhage. (4) *Hot or warm in Technetium-99m scan but cold in I^{123} scan*—commonly they are malignant. *Features:* Single nodule palpable in one or other lobes of the thyroid which is usually smooth, globular, firm with well-defined margin. Overlying skin is normal. *Lahey's test* does not show any other nodules in posterior part of the gland. Tracheal deviation towards opposite side is common—confirmed by trail sign, three finger test and auscultation.

Nodular Goiter

It is a slowly progressive disease with many years of history; multiple nodules of different sizes are formed in both lobes, also in isthmus, which is firm, nodular, nontender, moves with deglutition; recent increase in size signifies malignant transformation or hemorrhage (Fig. 16-56). *Complications of MNG:* Secondary thyrotoxicosis (30%); follicular carcinoma of thyroid (10%); hemorrhage in a nodule; tracheal obstruction; calcification.

Thyrotoxicosis and Hyperthyroidism

It is complex of symptoms and signs due to raised levels of thyroid hormones.

Types: (1) Diffuse toxic goiter: (*Graves' disease, Basedow's disease*, primary thyrotoxicosis). (2) Toxic multinodular goiter (Secondary thyrotoxicosis; *Plummer disease*). (3) Toxic nodule. (4) Hyperthyroidism of rarer causes: *Thyrotoxicosis factitia*. Drug-induced due to intake of L-thyroxine more than normal; *Jod–Basedow thyrotoxicosis*—because of consumption of large doses of iodides given to a hyperplastic endemic goiter; *Autoimmune thyroiditis or De' Quervain's thyroiditis*; Occasionally *carcinoma thyroid; Neonatal thyrotoxicosis*—It subsides in 3–4 weeks as TsAb titers fall in the baby's serum. It is eight times more common in females; occurs in any age group; primary type is seen commonly in younger age group; secondary is common in older age group. Graves' disease is an autoimmune disease with increased levels of specific antibodies in the blood (TSH receptor antibodies). It is often associated with vitiligo. It is often familial. Thyroid stimulating immunoglobulins (TSI)/thyroid stimulating antibodies (TsAb) and long acting thyroid stimulator (LATS) cause pathological changes in the thyroid. Histologically there is acinar cell hypertrophy and hyperplasia with absence of normal colloid in the tall columnar epithelium (normal is flat epithelium with colloid). As cells are empty, they look vacuolated. Tissues are highly vascular. Exophthalmos producing substance (EPS) causes Graves' ophthalmopathy.

Thyrotoxic crisis (thyroid storm): It occurs in a thyrotoxic patient inadequately prepared for thyroidectomy and rarely a thyrotoxic patient presents in a crisis following an unrelated operation or stress. They present in 12–24 hours with severe dehydration due to circulatory collapse, hypotension, hyperpyrexia and often cardiac failure.

Thyroid Neoplasms

Classification of thyroid neoplasm: **Benign:** Follicular adenoma; Hurthle cell adenoma; colloid adenoma—commonest; papillary adenoma—its existence is doubtful. It is invariably low-grade papillary carcinoma.

Malignant (Dunhill classification): (1) *Differentiated*—papillary carcinoma (60%); Follicular carcinoma (7%); papillofollicular carcinoma behaves like papillary carcinoma of thyroid; Hurthle cell carcinoma behaves like follicular carcinoma. (2) *Undifferentiated.* Anaplastic carcinoma (13%). (3) *Medullary carcinoma* (6%). (4) *Malignant lymphoma* (4%). (5) *Secondaries* in thyroid (rare)—from colon, kidney, melanoma.

Etiology of thyroid malignancy: (1) Radiation either external or radioiodine can cause papillary carcinoma thyroid. There was increased incidence of thyroid carcinoma among children following exposure to ionizing radiation after the Chernobyl nuclear disaster in Ukraine in 1986. Irradiation to head and neck region used to be the therapy for benign conditions like adenoids, acne vulgaris, thymus enlargement, hemangiomas which predispose papillary carcinoma of thyroid. Radiotherapy for Hodgkin's lymphoma in younger age group may later cause papillary carcinoma of thyroid. (2) Pre-existing multinodular goiter. It turns into follicular carcinoma of thyroid. (3) Medullary carcinoma of thyroid commonly and 6% of papillary carcinoma of thyroid can be familial. (4) Hashimoto's thyroiditis may predispose to papillary carcinoma of thyroid and also NHL.

Papillary carcinoma: It is 60% common; common in females (3:1) and young age group. It is called as *hormone* dependent tumor. It is a slowly progressive and less aggressive tumor. It is commonly multicentric. It spreads within the gland through intrathyroidal lymphatics to other lobe, comes out of the capsule and spreads to lymph nodes. Usually there is no blood spread. *Types:* Occult (<1.5 cmq; intrathyroidal; extrathyroidal; micropapillary carcinoma is less than 1 cm in size or clinically not detectable. *Gross:* It can be soft, firm, hard, and cystic. It can be solitary or multinodular. It contains brownish black fluid. *Microscopy:* It shows cystic spaces, papillary projections with *psammoma* bodies, malignant cells with *'Orphan Annie eye'* nuclei (intranuclear cytoplasmic inclusions, nuclear grooving). *Clinical features:* (1) Soft or hard or firm, solid or cystic, solitary or multinodular thyroid swelling. (2) Compression features are uncommon in papillary carcinoma thyroid. (3) Often discrete lymph nodes in the neck are palpable.

Psammoma bodies are seen in:
- Papillary carcinoma thyroid
- Meningioma
- Serous cystadenoma of ovary

Follicular carcinoma: It is 17% common. It is common in females. It can occur either *de novo* or in a pre-existing multinodular goiter. It is a more aggressive tumor. It spreads mainly through blood into the lung, bones, liver. Bone secondaries are typically vascular, warm, pulsatile, localized, commonly in *skull,* long bones, ribs. It can also spread to lymph nodes in the neck (10%) occasionally. *Types:* **Noninvasive:** Blood spread is not common. **Invasive:** Blood spread is common. *Typical feature: Angioinvasion and capsular invasion. Clinical features:* Swelling in the neck, firm or hard and nodular; tracheal compression/infiltration and stridor; dyspnea, hemoptysis, chest pain when there are lung secondaries; recurrent laryngeal nerve involvement causes hoarseness of voice, positive '*Berry's sign*' signifies advanced malignancy (Infiltration into the carotid and so absence of carotid pulsation); pulsatile, warm, well-localized, vascular secondaries in the skull (frontal/parietal bones), long bones. *Hurthle cell carcinoma* is a variant of follicular carcinoma of thyroid which contains abundant oxyphil cells. It spreads more commonly to regional lymph nodes than follicular carcinoma of thyroid. ^{99m}Tc *sestamibi scan* is very useful for Hurthle cell carcinoma. It does not take up I^{131} and has got poorer prognosis than follicular carcinoma.

Berry's in thyroid:
- Berry ligament
- Berry sign
- Berry picking

Anaplastic carcinoma: It is a very aggressive tumor of short duration, presents with a swelling in thyroid region which is rapidly progressive causing stridor and hoarseness of voice; dysphagia; fixity to the skin; infiltration into the carotid sheath—positive Berry's sign; swelling is hard, with involvement of isthmus and bilateral lobes; FNAC is diagnostic; tracheostomy and isthmectomy has got a role to relieve respiratory obstruction temporarily. It carries poor prognosis.

Medullary carcinoma of thyroid (MCT): It is uncommon (5%) type of thyroid malignancy. It arises from the *parafollicular 'C' cells* which are derived from the ultimobranchial body (neural crest). They are part of APUD (Amine Precursor Uptake Decarboxylation) cells. C cells are more in upper pole of the thyroid. It contains characteristic *'amyloid stroma'* wherein malignant cells are dispersed. In these patients, blood levels of *calcitonin* both basal as well as that following calcium or pentagastrin stimulation are high, a very useful tumor marker. Tumor also secretes 5-HT (serotonin), prostaglandin and vasoactive intestinal polypeptide (VIP). It spreads mainly to lymph nodes (60% common). It may be associated with MEN II syndrome and pheochromocytoma with hypertension. There may be mucosal neuromas in lips, oral cavity.

Types: (1) *Sporadic.* Usually solitary—70%. (2) *MCT with MEN II syndrome.* MCT with MEN II B with pheochromocytoma is most aggressive type. (3) *Familial MCT:* It is autosomal dominant with proto-oncogene in chromosome number 10. It is commonly multicentric (Fig. 16-59).

Malignant lymphoma: It is NHL type. Occurs in a pre-existing Hashimoto's thyroiditis (Not proved well). FNAC is useful to diagnose the condition.

Tetany

It is decreased level of calcium in blood causing its effects. *Causes:* After thyroidectomy (It is decreased level of parathormone in the blood causing hypocalcemia). It is usually temporary and lasts for 4–6 weeks. It is the commonest cause of hypoparathyroidism. Other causes of

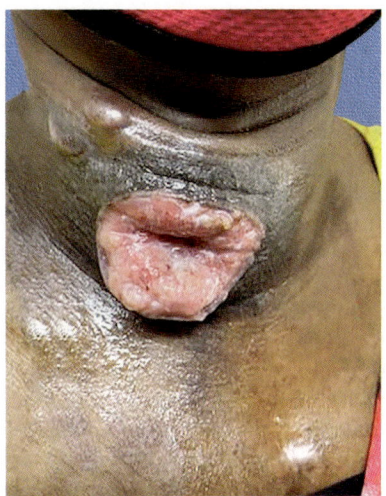

Fig. 16-59 Anaplastic carcinoma of thyroid with fungation. (*Courtesy*: Professor Gopinath Pai, KVG Medical College, Sullia, Karnataka).

hypoparathyroidism are neck dissection, hemochromatosis, Wilson's disease, Di-George's syndrome (absence of parathyroids; thymic aplasia; cardiac defects); severe vomiting, hyperventilation associated with respiratory alkalosis; metabolic alkalosis; rickets, osteomalacia; chronic renal failure; acute pancreatitis. *Clinical features:* Decreased PTH causes decrease in calcium level in the blood leading to—*circumoral paresthesia*, paresthesia of neck, fingers and toes, twitching and weakness of tongue muscles, muscles of forearm, hand, foot and digits—*carpopedal spasm*; *Chvostek-Weiss's sign*—tapping above the angle of the jaw stimulates branches of facial nerve causing the twitching of the angle of mouth and eyelids; applying the sphygmomanometer to the arm and inflating the pressure more than systolic pressure of the patient for three minutes can demonstrate carpal spasm (*Trousseau's sign*); stridor and difficulty in breathing due to paralysis of respiratory muscles; generalized weakness and twitching all over the body in severe cases mimicking *convulsions* (Fig. 16-61).

Other conditions of thyroid	Features
• **Hashimoto's thyroiditis:** *Struma lymphomatosa; diffuse non-goitrous thyroiditis*) • Common in women; is endemic along the banks of river Struma (means goiter) in Bulgaria. • It is a type of autoimmune thyroiditis; initially there is hyperplasia, then fibrosis eventually infiltration by plasma cells and lymphocytic cells with typical *Askanazy cells*.	• Painful, diffuse enlargement of usually both lobes of thyroid which is firm, tender, smooth. • Initially present with toxic features later manifest with features of hypothyroidism. • There may be hepatosplenomegaly and association of other autoimmune diseases (85%). • Significant rise in thyroid antibodies (microsomal/thyroglobulin/colloid). • May predispose to papillary carcinoma/malignant lymphoma.
deQuervain's subacute granulomatous thyroiditis Commonly seen self-limiting disease in females; viral etiology, either mumps or coxsackie causing inflammatory response with infiltration of lymphocytes, neutrophils, multinucleated giant cells.	Diffuse pain, swelling in thyroid; initially there is transient hyperthyroidism with high T3 and T4; poor radioiodine uptake
Riedel's thyroiditis (Woody thyroiditis; Ligneous thyroiditis) 0.5% common; common in males; rare benign condition often associated with mediastinal and retroperitoneal fibrosis. Thyroid tissue is replaced by fibrous tissue which extends into the capsule, to the muscle, paratracheal fascia, and carotid sheath.	• Stony hard, fixed, small swelling with stridor, Berry's sign positive (absence of carotid pulsation). Movement with deglutition is often difficult to elicit. • **Differential diagnoses:** Anaplastic carcinoma thyroid.
• **Thyroglossal cyst:** Swelling that occurs in the neck due to accumulation of fluid secreted by the unobliterated portion of thyroglossal tract/duct. It is tubulodermoid. • **Possible sites:** Beneath the foramen cecum; In the floor of the mouth; suprahyoid; subhyoid (commonest site); on the thyroid cartilage; at the cricoid cartilage level. • Thyroid may be seen in normal location or thyroid fossa may be empty in which case thyroid tissue may be present in the cyst wall. • **Note:** Thyroid cartilage is shaped like a prow of a ship and so thyroglossal tract during development sweeps towards one side. So levator glandulae thyroideae in normal people and thyroglossal cyst when develops will be towards left side.	• Swelling in the midline, towards the left, moves with deglutition as well as with protrusion of tongue ("tugging sensation" felt by the examiner when the cyst is held between thumb and forefinger) • It is smooth, soft, fluctuant, nontender, mobile, often transilluminant contains gel-like fluid. • **Complications**: Infection/abscess; malignancy—papillary carcinoma; if excision not done properly—thyroglossal fistula. • **Differential diagnosis**: Subhyoid bursa; pretracheal lymph node; dermoid cyst; solitary nodule thyroid.
Thyroglossal fistula: Not a congenital condition; following infection of thyroglossal cyst which bursts open/after inadequate removal of the cyst	• Seat of recurrent inflammation with mucus discharge; "Hood sign" characteristic. • Site—suprahyoid position/on the side of old scar.
Dyshormonogenesis: Autosomal recessive condition; familial; may be associated with congenital deafness (*Pendred syndrome);* either there is deficiency of thyroid enzymes (peroxidase/dehalogenase) or inability to concentrate or bind or retain iodine.	• Large diffuse vascular goiter involving both lobes. • Responds well to L-thyroxine.

Contd...

Contd...

Ectopic thyroid: It is ectopic thyroid tissue anywhere along the descent of thyroid during the developmental period	• Whole of the gland or some residual thyroid lies in abnormal position (posterior part of tongue; upper part of neck in midline, intrathoracic region). • Radioisotope scan, CT chest is essential to confirm
Lingual thyroid: It is a thyroid swelling in the posterior third of tongue at foramen cecum.	• It presents as round swelling, which may cause dysphagia, speech impairment, respiratory obstruction, hemorrhage. • Any disease that can occur in normal thyroid—nodules, malignancy and toxicity can occur.
Goiter in infancy: Seen in endemic areas or in mothers who were taking antithyroid drugs; untreated toxic thyroid in pregnancy can also cause toxic goiter in infant.	Presents as obvious thyroid swelling in newborn or infancy.
Retrosternal goiter: It is intrathoracic extension of the goiter; it can be substernal (goiter in the neck extending into the thorax), plunging (intrathoracic often plunges into the neck), intrathoracic only (**Fig. 16-60**).	Dyspnea, cough, stridor, lower border is not seen or felt, positive Pemberton's sign, dullness over the sternum.

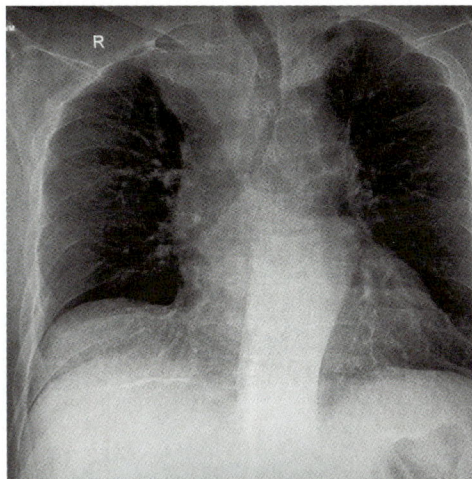

Fig. 16-60 X-ray showing retrosternal goiter with gross deviation of the trachea.

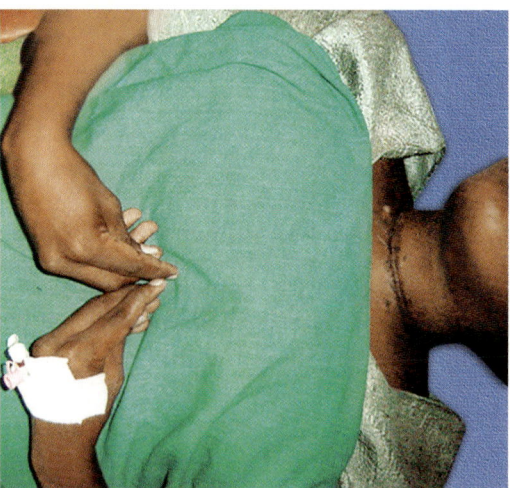

Fig. 16-61 Carpal spasm due to *tetany in post-thyroidectomy patient*. Note the thyroidectomy scar.

CASE DISCUSSION

A 30-year-old female presented with palpitation, weight loss, increased sweating, insomnia with menstrual irregularities for 8 months. Her sister noticed few days' back diffuse mild fullness in the neck in front. She also noticed that her eyes have become prominent. She had shaking of hands suggestive of tremor, diarrhea also.

What is probable diagnosis at this stage?
It is probably a case of toxic thyroid.

How you will examine this patient?
Pulse and blood pressure should be examined properly for tachycardia, ectopic or any variations. Hand and tongue tremors should be checked. Eye signs should be checked properly (in general examination usually or can be at the end in neurological examinations). Thyroid should be examined in detail for movement with deglutition, size, extent, surface, consistency, thrill, bruit and different tests should be done. Cardiovascular system should be examined. Hepatosplenomegaly may be present in primary toxic thyroid.

What type of toxicity is probably present in this patient?
It is mostly primary toxic goiter. Here symptoms appeared first, then swelling; symptoms are more severe; patient is young.

What all investigations should be done in this patient?
Thyroid function tests (T_3, T_4, TSH), US neck to check nodules, vascularity, thyroid autoantibodies, ECG, echocardiography, hematocrit.

CHAPTER 17

Clinical Approaches and Examination of Breast

Competency: SU25.1; SU25.2; SU25.3; SU25.4; SU25.5.

Pain and/or lump in the breast are the common complaints for which patient consults a surgeon or gynecologist or breast clinic. Breast cancer is one of the commonest carcinoma in females; but occasionally it can occur in males also. Breast cancer awareness programmes are common in USA with different ribbon logos (Fig. 17-1).

■ HISTORY

Age: Breast abscess is common in young feeding mothers; fibroadenoma in young women; fibroadenosis in middle-aged females; carcinoma breast is common in women in peri- and post-menopausal age group **(Fig. 17-2)**. Inflammatory carcinoma of breast occurs in younger women usually lactating. Inflammatory carcinoma is very aggressive carcinoma (IVd) with diffuse erythema, edema, Peau d'orange of the breast, usually without an underlying palpable mass, involves most of the skin over the breast due to tumor emboli within the dermal lymphatics. It often may mimic acute mastitis and surgeon may inadvertently do trial drainage of the lesion thinking it as breast abscess **(Fig. 17-3)**. Even though carcinoma breast is common in middle aged (adult), it can occur in young and elderly also.

Sex: Carcinoma female breast is 100 times more common than carcinoma male breast. But carcinoma male breast when it occurs is more aggressive. Gynecomastia is hypertrophy of male breast usually of both epithelial and stromal component. Gynecomastia only very rarely turns into carcinoma except if it is associated with Klinefelter's syndrome **(Fig. 17-4)**. Carcinoma breast is the 2nd most common malignancy in females; first one is being carcinoma cervix. Altered life style may be the cause for the same **(Fig. 17-5)**.

Address: Incidence is more in developed Western countries where nulliparity is common and diet is rich in saturated fatty acids. Incidence is more among *Parsees*, white races. Incidence is comparatively less in underdeveloped countries as the women here are multiparous. Diet rich in saturated fatty

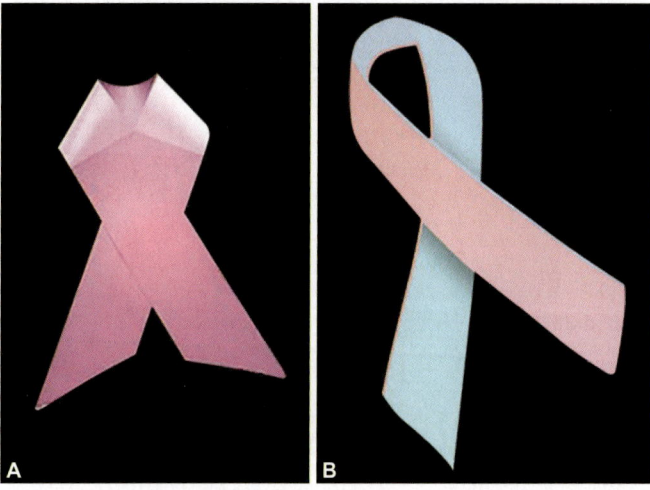

Fig. 17-1 *Pink ribbon* is the logo for female breast cancer (A); *blue pink ribbon* for male breast cancer (B).

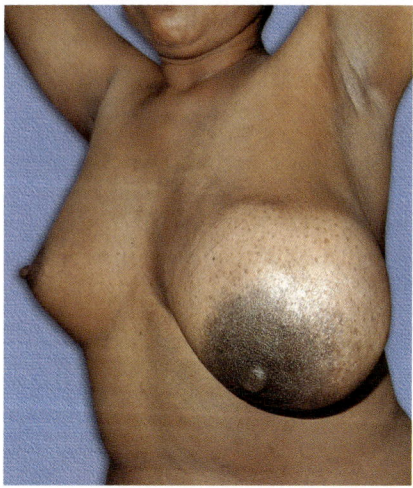

Fig. 17-2 *Left-sided breast lump.* It is the one of the commonest presentations in breast diseases.

acids used in Western society is more likely to cause carcinoma breast. It is rare in Japan. It is common in USA and England. In India incidence is one in 120 women. In Kerala it is more common with incidence of one in 60 women.

Chief Complaints

- Swelling in the right/left breast/both breasts; its time duration **(Fig. 17-6)**.
- Pain in the breast with duration; ulceration in the breast with duration.
- Discharge from nipple.
- Swelling in the breast/axilla/neck.

History of Present Illness

Swelling (lump): History of duration of swelling, its progression whether slowly increasing in size or rapidly increasing has to be asked for. Swellings of short duration are most probably due to carcinoma. But most often, once the swelling is noticed the patient immediately consults a doctor for opinion and so duration may not be clearly obtained. Condition like fibroadenoma and fibroadenosis has got long duration of history. Duration in carcinoma is usually only few weeks. History of swelling in the opposite breast is also important. In 2% of cases, breast carcinomas are bilateral; and so also fibrocystadenosis which commonly has bilateral presentation **(Fig. 17-7)**.

Pain: Duration of pain, type, timing, site and relation to menstruation has to be noted. Pain in the breast is often termed as ***mastalgia***. It is common in fibrocystadenosis and acute mastitis. There will be associated fever in mastitis. Carcinoma breast is initially painless but eventually becomes painful following infiltration or development of tumor necrosis or skin ulceration/fungation. But 10% of carcinoma breast can present with pain (***heaviness, dragging, pricking***) to begin with. Pain in fibroadenosis is more prior to menstruation

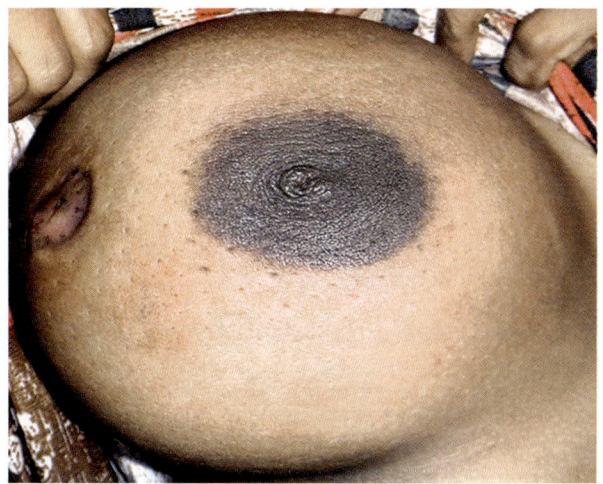

Fig. 17-3 *Inflammatory carcinoma of breast* (mastitis carcinomatosis/lactating carcinoma of breast); it is inadvertently drained thinking that it is mastitis in a lactating women.

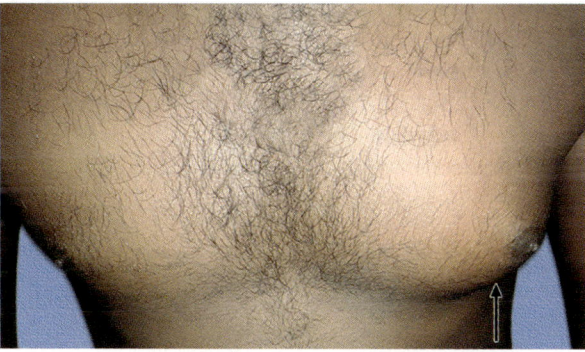

Fig. 17-4 *Gynecomastia.*

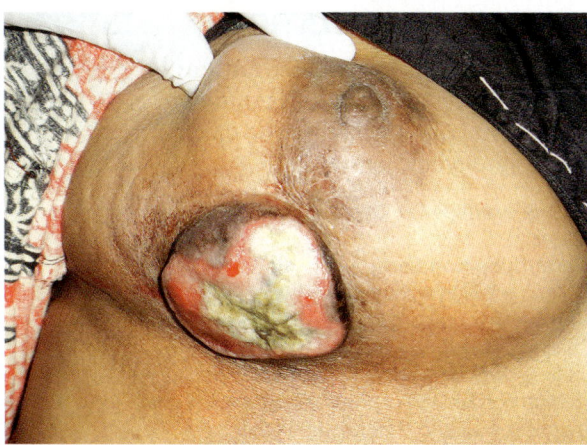

Fig. 17-5 Ulcerative carcinoma of breast.

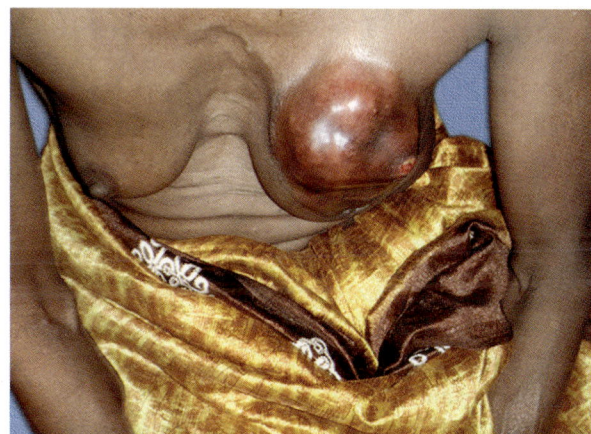

Fig. 17-6 Carcinoma breast locally *advanced with skin involvement.*

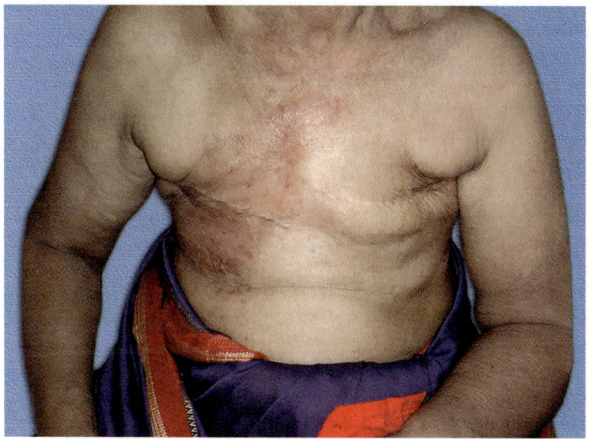

Fig. 17-7 *Bilateral mastectomy is done in this patient for carcinoma of breast.* Right side there is local recurrence.

(cyclical), and may disappear during pregnancy and after menopause. Referred pain from muscle and skeletal system (ribs) can also develop in the breast. Periductal mastitis/duct ectasia can cause pain. Patient with breast abscess will show severe excruciating pain in the breast.

Mastalgia chart is used often to assess the pain in relation to menstruation.

History of fever, duration, type of fever should be asked for. High grade fever with chills and rigors is a feature of acute mastitis or breast abscess which is commonly seen in lactation.

Nipple discharge: Duration of discharge, its type (nature, color, odor, quantity), whether it is of serous/purulent/bloody/serosanguinous/milky/greenish type has to be asked for and noted. Quantity and odor is asked. Bloody discharge is often seen in duct papilloma, carcinoma. Even though discharge is uncommon in carcinoma breast, when present it will be usually bloody or serosanguinous. Serous and greenish discharge is seen in fibroadenosis. Milky discharge is seen in galactocele/from mammary fistula due to chronic subareolar abscess; discharging pus from ruptured breast abscess. Milk is a normal discharge during lactation. Newborn can have colostrum like discharge from both breasts. Patients with prolactin secreting tumor of the anterior pituitary may present with galactorrhea. Discharge may be from the surface like from Paget's disease or from single duct or from many ducts.

History of changes in nipple: Like retraction (depression), deviation, destruction, displacement, discoloration, duplication and discharge is asked for. Recent history of changes signifies carcinoma. Often retraction may be congenital, since birth.

History of alteration in size and asymmetry of the breasts should be asked for with duration.

History of trauma: Trauma may cause hematoma in the breast and breast abscess. Direct or indirect trauma often can cause traumatic fat necrosis after few weeks. Here trauma may be forgotten or may not be noticed by the patient and swelling developed due to traumatic fat necrosis is painless, nonprogressive and nonregressive.

History related to swelling in the axilla/neck and their details like duration, progress, pain, ulceration, etc. is noted.

History related to respiratory problems like chest pain, breathlessness, cough, hemoptysis has to be asked—signifies the secondaries in lung from carcinoma breast.

History of abdominal pain, loss of appetite, decreased weight, jaundice, and abdominal distension should be asked for which signifies liver secondaries. Usually only visceral secondaries will cause loss of weight.

History related to bone secondaries—like bone pain, low back pain, altered sensation like sense of position and vibration, lower limb weakness, features of paraplegia, loss of control over urination and defecation is asked for.

History of convulsions, loss of consciousness, vomiting, limb weakness, headache, visual disturbances, behavioral changes (psychological changes) and localization changes may be seen whenever there is brain metastases.

Note: Features of secondaries can be seen many months or years after primary has treated. Bone secondaries can present as swelling or pain which will be aggravated with movements.

Past History

Past history of any surgeries of breast (recurrence can occur after excision of fibroadenoma, conservative breast surgery may cause recurrent carcinoma breast) or drug therapies like for fibroadenosis. Abscess may recur in congenital retraction of nipple; tuberculosis of breast can show recurrence; fibroadenosis may present repeatedly with long gaps of asymptomatic period.

Treatment History

Relevant history of treatment for carcinoma breast earlier and details of treatment like type of surgery, reconstruction, duration of hospital stay, adjuvant radiotherapy and chemotherapy, type and cycles of drugs used, follow-up methods should be asked in detail. History of treatment for tuberculosis (pulmonary commonly or extrapulmonary) may be relevant in tuberculosis of breast.

Menstrual History, Obstetric History and Family History

This is important in breast diseases as breast carcinoma can be familial. 10% of breast cancer patients have familial predisposition. Family history of carcinoma breast (in mother, grandmother, aunt, cousins, and 1st and 2nd degree relatives [genetic relation]), ovarian tumor or other tumors has to be noted. Often multiple tumors can occur. History of age of menarche and menopause, menstrual cycles, marital status, number of pregnancies, breastfeeding, last child birth and usage of contraceptives/postmenopausal HRT are very important. Fibroadenosis and carcinoma are more common in unmarried individuals. Carcinoma is common in urban area and higher socioeconomic groups.

Note: Pedigree chart (family tree) should be asked and placed in the case sheet.

Personal History and Treatment History

History of smoking, alcohol intake, dietary habits (high fat diet) is noted. History of any drug intake at present is important.

■ GENERAL EXAMINATION

Like for any other long case, patient should be examined for pallor, jaundice, edema feet and clubbing. Pulse and blood pressure should be checked.

> *Breast is examined in different positions to elicit different clinical features.*
> **Different positions are:**
> - Sitting position with arms by the side
> - *45° semirecumbent position* is very much convenient
> - Sitting position with leaning forward
> - Sitting position with arms over the waist
> - Sitting position with arms rising above the shoulder-to see fixity to chest wall and changes in nipple
> - Lying down position for self-examination

LOCAL EXAMINATION OF BREASTS

Normal breast should be examined first so as to appreciate what is normal to compare in a given patient. Normal breast feels granular with minimal irregularity which is more in progesterone phase of menstrual cycle. Proper exposure of both breasts from neck to waist should be done. While examining the breasts adequate privacy; and presence of a female nurse is very essential. Initially examination is carried out with the patient sitting in 45° *semirecumbent position* (lying flat makes breasts flatten and fall sideways; upright sitting position makes breasts pendulous and bulky). Later examination is done in lying down *(recumbent)* position as lump is better felt against chest wall for additional information. *Lying down position* with pillow under the shoulder blade with arm raised above the shoulder also helps breast in position to make palpation easier. During inspection, the clinician should stand in front and later on the side of the patient. *Commonly used position is sitting posture* as it is easier to examine nipples, lump and axillary nodes; and also patient will be more comfortable in that position.

All quadrants and axillary tail of Spence should be examined systematically.

Inspection

For proper inspection, *both breasts should be exposed properly including axillae*. Inspection is done in sitting position with the arms by the side of the body. Inspection is also done with the arms raised above the shoulder touching the head (with arms touching the ears) so that nipple levels, lump, dimples are seen well. Inspection is also done with the arms on the hips pressing and relaxing so that skin dimpling, nipple movements and changes become more prominent. Examination/inspection done in *bending forward* position helps to see whether breast falls forward or not; and also to see nipple retraction or failure of nipple to fall away. Carcinoma fixed to chest wall will not fall forward while bending forward. Outstretched hand pressing against a wall also helps in examining the mobility of the breast **(Figs. 17-8 to 17-12)**.

Inspection of Both Breasts

The size, shape, position and symmetry are noted on both sides. Each quadrant is inspected carefully—usually in order like upper outer, lower outer, lower inner and upper inner. Any scar of previous mastectomy/excision should be noted.

Position and extent of breast: It is noted from above downwards and side to side direction. Depending on the underlying pathology the breast may be displaced upwards/lateral and downwards. Breast may be drawn towards the growth in atrophic scirrhous carcinoma. In inflammatory carcinoma of breast, entire breast is involved with redness, edema, Peau d'orange of the skin; it is of short duration; occurs in young lactating or pregnant woman; it carries poor prognosis; there is no clear cut mass underneath. It is stage IV—locally advanced carcinoma of breast **(Fig. 17-13)**.

Size: It may be huge in giant fibroadenoma breast, small in under developed breast. Asymmetry in size can be seen in breast lumps **(Fig. 17-14)**.

Movement of the breast: Both breasts are inspected while leaning forward to see whether breasts fall forward or not.

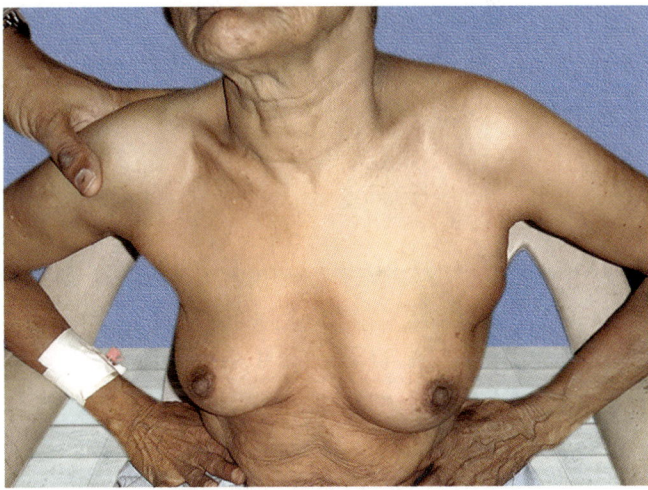

Fig. 17-9 Examination of breast *with arms over the waist.*

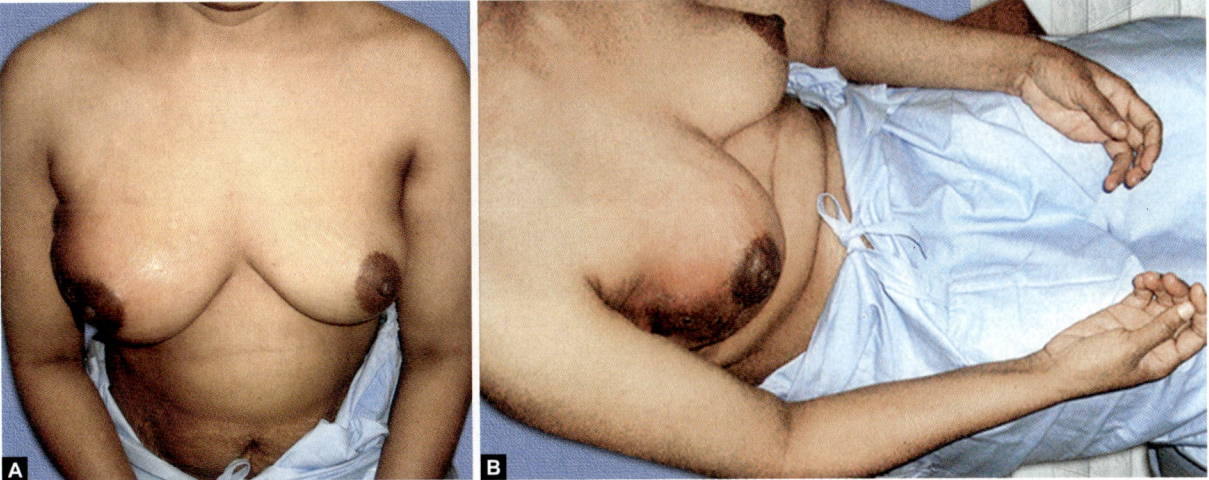

Figs. 17-8A and B Examination of breast is done in *sitting position with arms beside.*

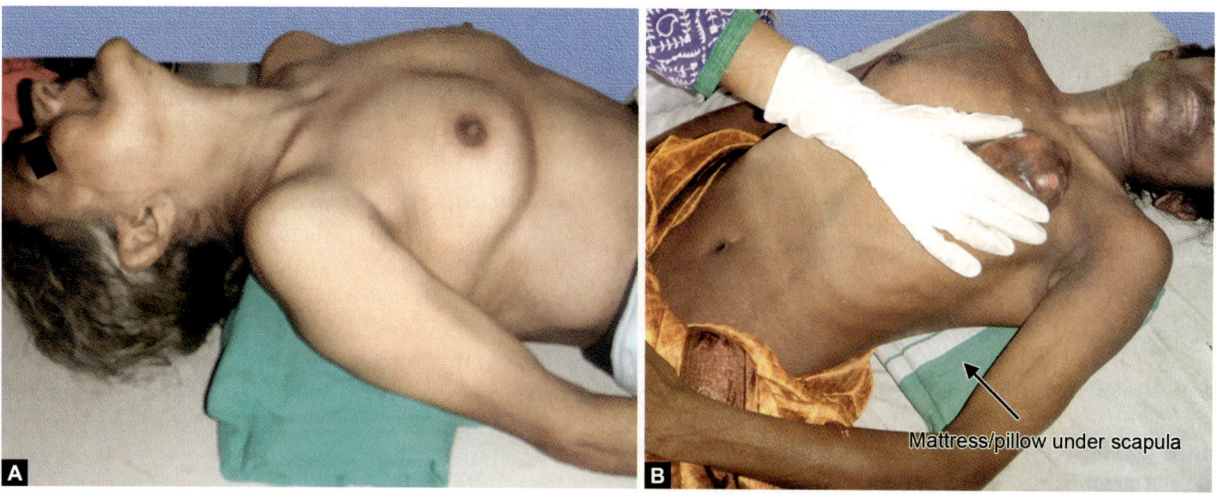

Figs. 17-10A and B *In lying down position* it is better to place a soft pillow or mattress under scapula to keep breast in position.

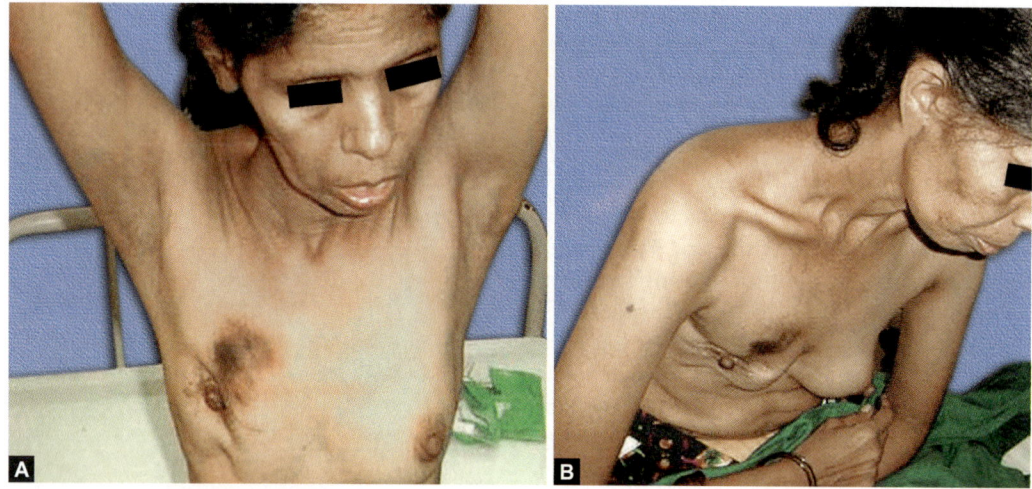

Figs. 17-11A and B Examination with both arms *raised above the shoulder and leaning forward*.

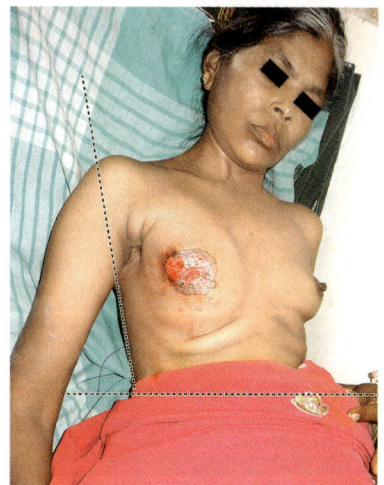

Fig. 17-12 *Examination in 45° semirecumbent position.*

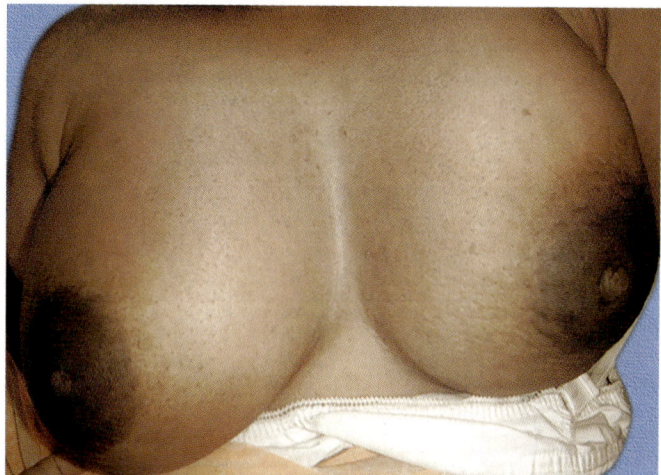

Fig. 17-13 *Inflammatory carcinoma of breast.* It is stage IV—locally advanced carcinoma breast (LACB). No clear cut mass will be felt underneath; near entire skin over the breast will be involved through dermal lymphatic spread.

Both breasts should also be inspected by asking to raise the arms above the head to see whether breast is/breasts are adherent to chest wall. Alternatively movement of the breast can be examined by asking the patient to keep the hand over the waist and keep pressing and relaxing the hand alternately. In carcinoma, if the breast lump gets fixed to underlying chest

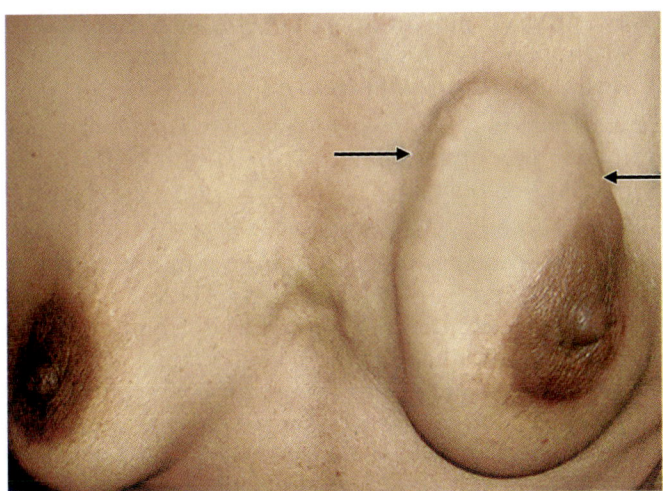

Fig. 17-14 Lump in the breast left sided. Obvious lump is *visible in the upper quadrant.*

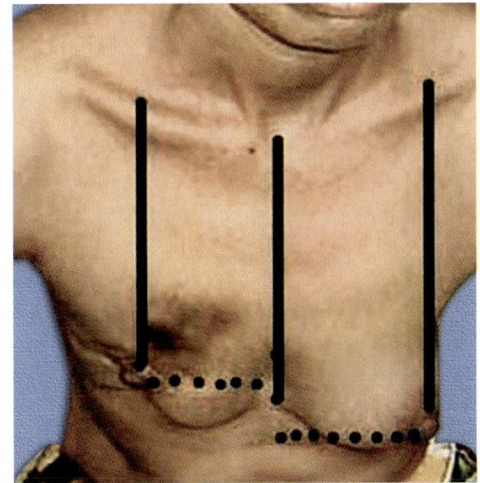

Fig. 17-15 *Nipple deviation* should be looked for in breast lumps.

wall, it will not fall forward and the puckering of the skin over the swelling becomes obvious, whereas the movement is not restricted in benign swelling.

Inspection of Nipple

Careful inspection of nipple is done for size, shape, discharge, symmetry/asymmetry, displacement (pushed up/down), retraction, ulceration, discoloration, duplication, cracks/fissures. Many of these changes occur in carcinoma.

Size and shape: Nipple retraction of recent onset may be due to infiltration of lactiferous duct by carcinoma. It is due to extension of growth along the lactiferous duct and subsequent fibrosis. Often congenital retraction may be present; so duration of nipple retraction is very important. *Retraction of nipple* can occur in duct ectasia/periductal mastitis also. Nipple retraction is *circumferential* in carcinoma; *slit like* in periductal mastitis. Nipple may become prominent when there is a swelling underneath like cyst, benign tumor, inflammatory edema. Nipple may be swollen in infection or carcinoma. *Nipple destruction* is seen Paget's disease and fungating/ulcerating carcinoma **(Figs. 17-15 and 17-16)**.

Surface: Fissuring and cracks can occur in breastfeeding mothers. Breast papilloma may begin at nipple areolar complex **(Fig. 17-17)**.

Level: Vertical distance from the clavicle and horizontal distance from the midline should be measured and compared to opposite side. Nipple may be drawn towards the lump in the affected breast. *Nipple elevation* may become prominent by raising the arm above the head; which may be due to inflammatory pathology. In fibroadenoma nipple gets displaced away from the lump.

Discharge: It is important to note the type of discharge from the nipple—blood, milk, greenish fluid, serosanguinous, purulent. Bloody discharge may be a feature of duct papilloma or carcinoma **(Fig. 17-18)**.

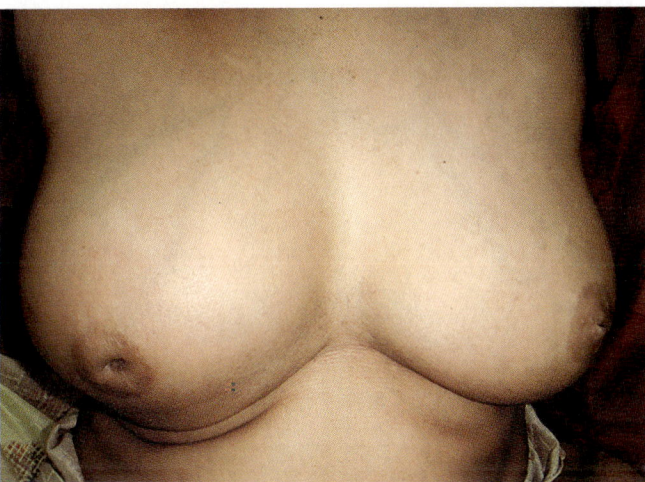

Fig. 17-16 *Retraction of the nipple*—very obvious.

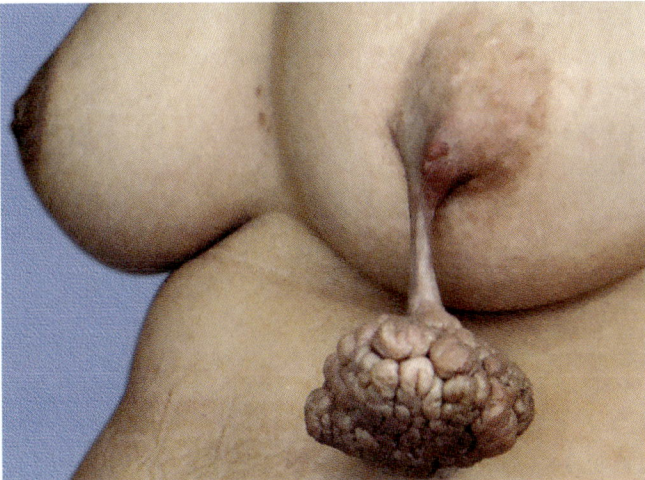

Fig. 17-17 *Papilloma* left breast.

Number: Rarely accessory nipple often may be present along the milk line from axilla to groin or in the thigh; which may show milky discharge during lactation **(Fig. 17-19)**.

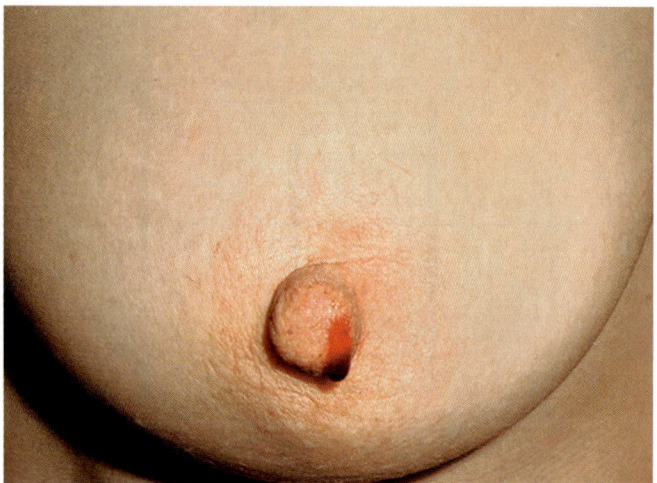

Fig. 17-18 *Bloody discharge* from the nipple. *Duct papilloma* is the commonest cause.

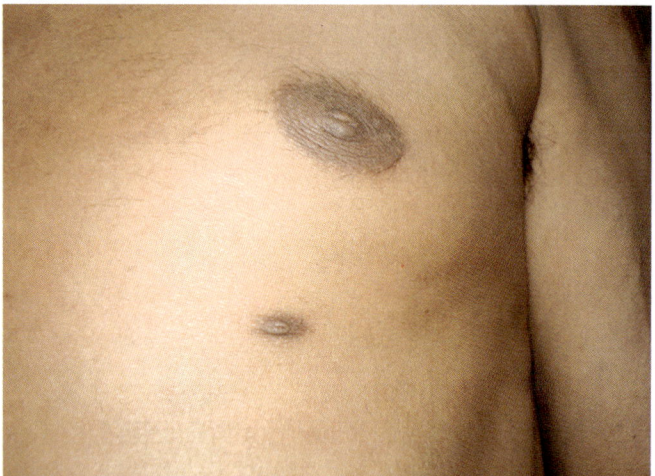

Fig. 17-19 *Accessory nipple and areola is* seen on left side.

Inspection of the Areola

Areola on both sides should be inspected for any change in color, size, ulceration, surface.

Discharges from the nipple:
Blood
- Papilloma—commonest cause
- Ectasia
- Carcinoma—5% of causes for discharge

Serous
- Fibrocystic disease
- Ectasia

Greenish
- Ectasia
- Fibrocystic disease

Purulent
- Infection
- Sometimes malignancy

Milk
- Lactation (Physiological discharge)
- Galactorrhea

Serosanguinous
- Carcinoma
- Infection

Color: Areola is pink in color in young girls, dark colored in adults, brownish during pregnancy and lactation, red in eczema and early stage of Paget's disease **(Fig. 17-20)**.

Size: Areola may increase in size significantly in large fibroadenoma or sarcoma; may be shrunken in size in scirrhous carcinoma.

Surface: Ulceration, eczema/eczema like changes over the areolar surface should be looked for. Ulceration of nipple can occur in carcinoma and **Paget's disease of breast**, a localized type of carcinoma breast. It should be differentiated from eczema. Eczema is commonly bilateral without any nodule underneath, associated with itching and vesicles, with normal nipple. It is common during lactation. Paget's disease of breast is unilateral, without vesicles and itching, with a hard lump underneath, often with destruction of nipple **(Fig. 17-21**. In normal individual, areola is slightly corrugated, with **Montgomery's glands** on it as small nodules. These glands get hypertrophied during pregnancy and lactation to form Montgomery's tubercles. Retention cyst of this gland presenting as smooth, localized soft fluctuant swelling in the areola is known to occur which often may get infected.

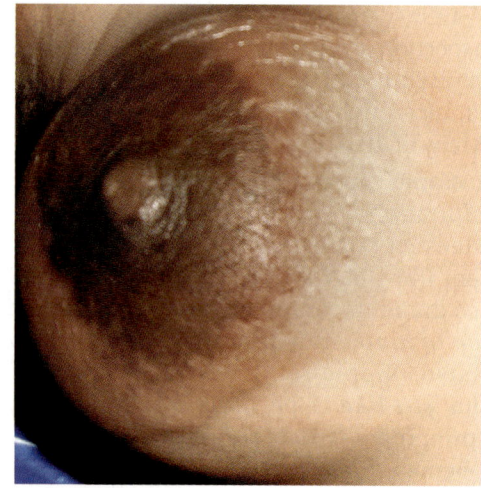

Fig. 17-20 *Typical look* of breast abscess/mastitis.

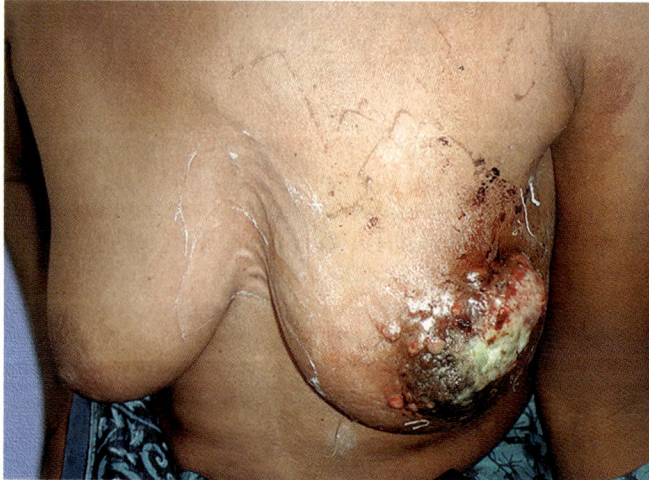

Fig. 17-21 Carcinoma breast with *skin involvement, ulceration and destruction* of areola.

Inspection of the Skin Over the Breast

Skin over the breast is inspected for retraction, pigmentation, redness/shining, dimpling, puckering, **Peau d'orange**, nodules, ulceration, fungation, and scar (**Fig. 17-22**). Any dilated veins over the skin and *cancer en cuirasse* is looked for.

Involvement/infiltration of the ligament of Cooper by carcinoma causes dimpling (is a small depression) and puckering (a small fold/wrinkle) of skin over the breast. Normal elastic ligament of Cooper becomes inelastic and shorter in carcinomatous infiltration (dimpling and puckering are inspectory findings whereas tethering is a palpatory finding). Edema of skin is due to blockade of cutaneous lymphatics causing burial of hair follicles giving the appearance of orange peel *(Peau d'orange)* (**Figs. 17-23A and B**). Peau d'orange is better visualized using *magnifying lens* (**Fig. 17-24**).

When ulcer is present, its position, size, shape, margin, floor, edge should be noted. Previous mastectomy scar, skin graft or flap coverage or scar of any breast reconstruction should be checked (**Figs. 17-25 to 17-27**).

Cancer en cuirasse is extensive involvement of the skin over the breast and chest wall with multiple nodules and ulceration by the carcinoma (**Fig. 17-28**). It looks like armor coat. Red, edematous skin is seen in acute mastitis (**Fig. 17-29**).

Dilated veins are commonly observed in cystosarcoma phyllodes, large breast abscess, and sarcoma and often in aggressive carcinomas.

Mondor's disease is superficial thrombophlebitis of veins over chest wall and breast, seen commonly in females. It is painful, tender cord-like lesion which on raising the arm above the shoulder causes puckering of skin adjacent to the dilated vein. It is a self-limiting disease.

Nodules are usually due to carcinoma; often it may be metastatic from the underlying carcinoma breast.

Ulceration is due to carcinomatous infiltration of skin. In cystosarcoma phyllodes and sarcoma, ulceration can occur as a pressure necrosis over the summit. Probing under the ulcer edge is easily possible in these conditions but not in carcinomatous infiltration (**Figs. 17-30 and 17-31**).

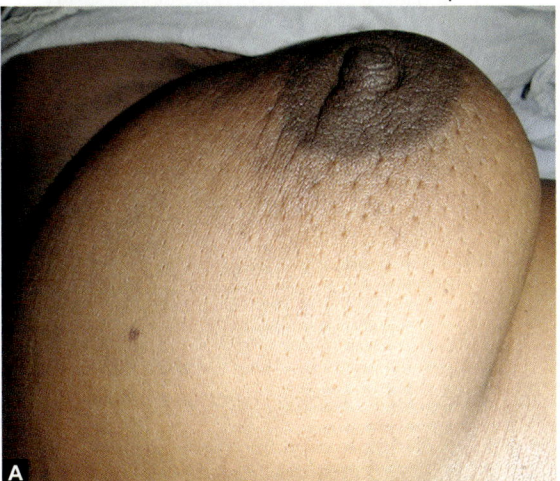

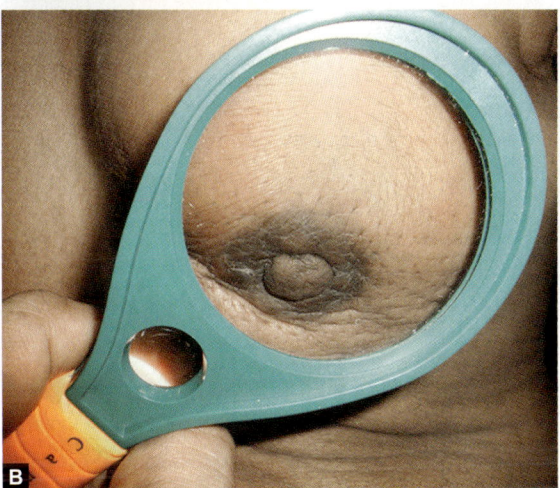

Figs. 17-23A and B *Peau d'orange.* It is due to cutaneous lymphedema following blockade of dermal lymphatics causing burial of deep-seated hair roots. It is better visualized when viewed through *magnifying lens*.

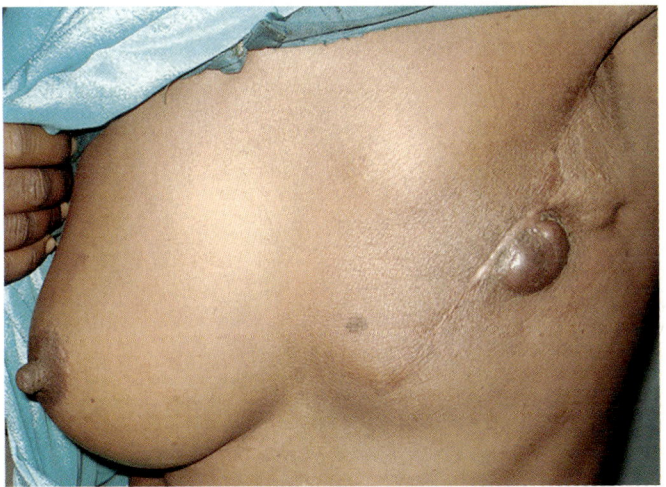

Fig. 17-22 *Recurrent carcinoma of breast.* Note the previous mastectomy scar.

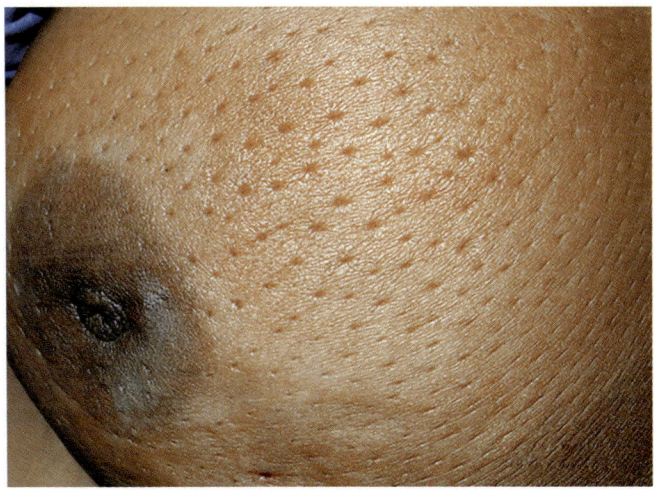

Fig. 17-24 *Typical Peau d'orange* in carcinoma breast.

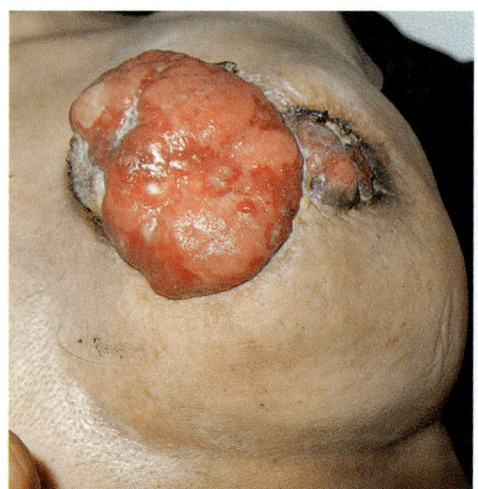

Fig. 17-25 *Fungating carcinoma* breast.

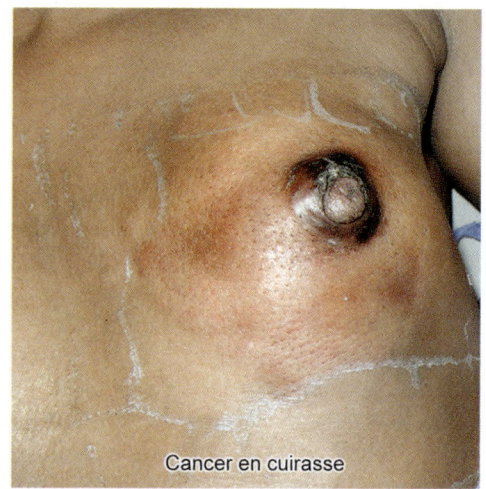

Fig. 17-28 *Cancer en cuirasse* with nodules in the chest wall and skin over the breast with carcinoma.

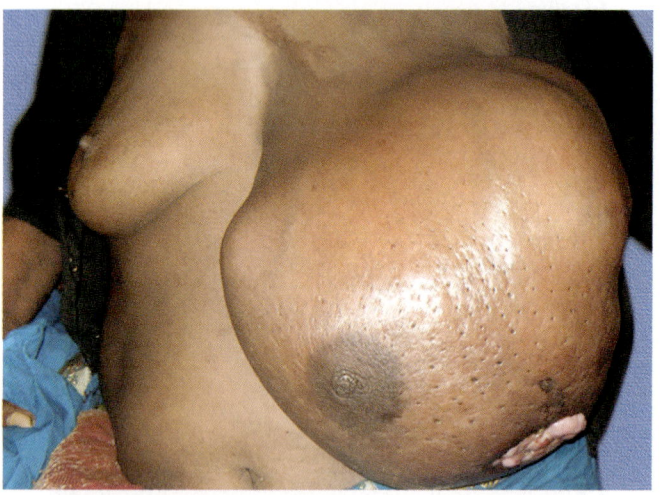

Fig. 17-26 Carcinoma breast locally advanced with skin *involvement, ulceration, Peau d'orange, dilated visible veins.*

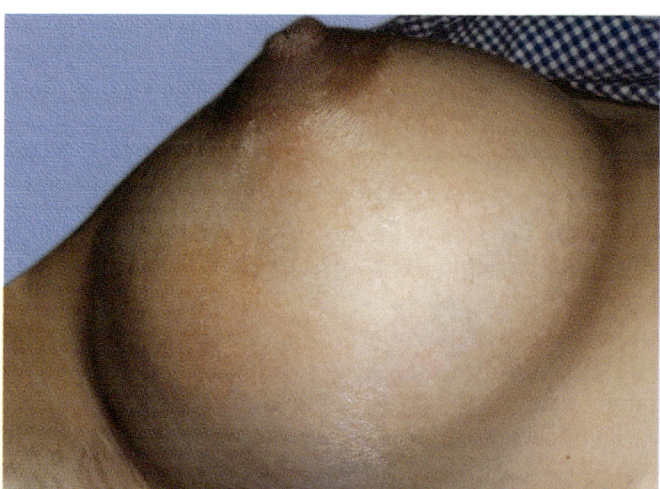

Fig. 17-29 *Acute mastitis* (breast abscess).

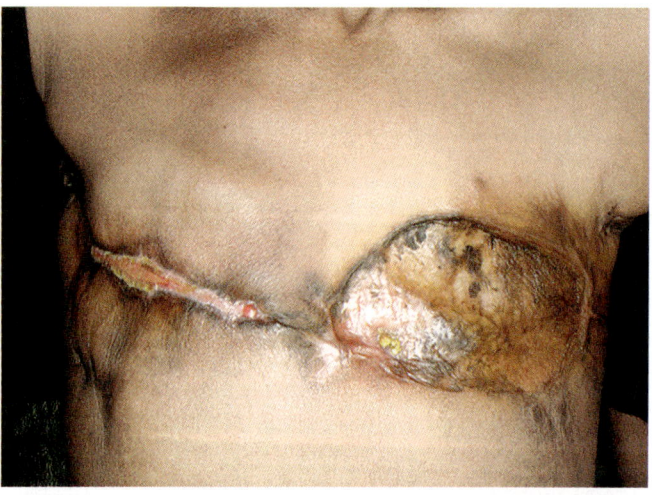

Fig. 17-27 *Bilateral mastectomy is done;* skin graft is used to cover the defect on left side.

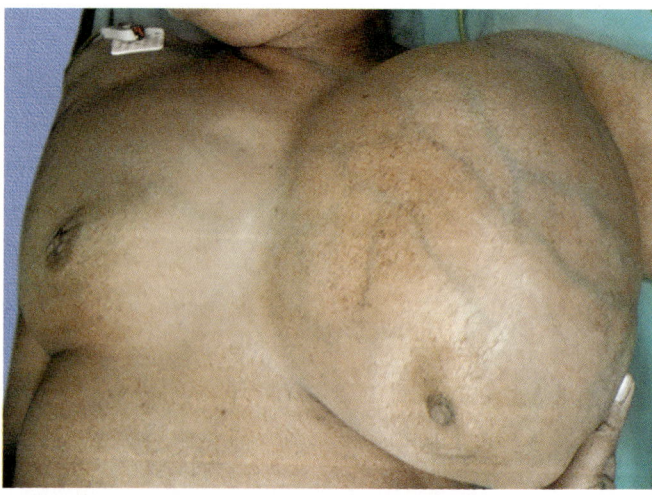

Fig. 17-30 *Cystosarcoma phyllodes.*

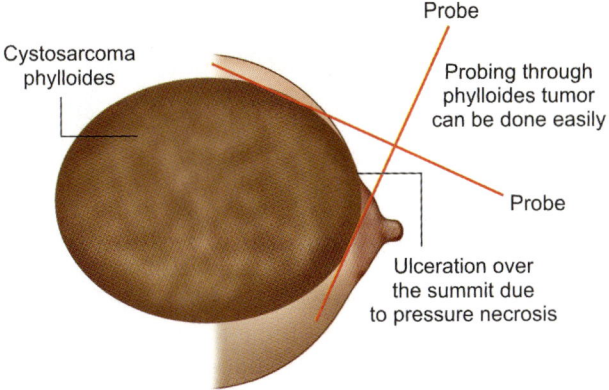

Fig. 17-31 *Pressure necrosis* of the skin over the summit can occur in cystosarcoma but tumor is not adherent to the skin. Probing can be done freely between tumor and under the skin.

Swelling (Lump) in the Breast

It is an important finding to be inspected. Its location in relation to the quadrants of the breast, number, extent, size, shape, margin, surface, overlying skin should be examined. As breast is mobile, location of the lump often cannot be ascertained in relation to bony point unless breast lump is fixed to chest wall or in post-mastectomy recurrence. Fullness is the only observation without any specified lump. It means contour is altered but borders are not well defined.

Benign swellings has smooth surface and regular margin **(Fig. 17.32)**, malignant swelling has rough surface and irregular margin. Skin over the swelling should be observed for ulcer/sinus; dimpling/puckering of the overlying skin. Upper outer quadrant is the commonest site for carcinoma breast and fibrocystadenosis (and ANDI). It is probably due to presence of more breast tissue in the upper outer quadrant. Most of the breast lumps are spherical in shape. Fibroadenoma, breast cysts have smooth surface; carcinoma has irregular surface.

Inspection of the Axilla and Supraclavicular Fossa

Arm should be raised adequately to inspect the axilla. Axilla and supraclavicular fossa should be inspected for any lymph node swelling. *Both sides should be inspected.* Accessory breast can occur in axilla which is the commonest site.

Inspection of Arm and Thorax

Edema of the arm may be due to lymphatic obstruction of axillary nodes by malignant cells spreading from carcinoma breast. Edema begins from distal to proximal and more prominent distally (***brawny edema***). Venous obstruction can also cause edema arm. Here edema is more prominent proximally in the arm and there will be bluish discoloration over the skin. It is commonly due to infiltration and often due to compression of axillary vein by lymph nodal metastatic disease. Arm edema may be seen after mastectomy also **(Fig. 17-33)**. Multiple nodules with skin thickening over the arm and chest wall due to carcinomatous infiltration is called as *'cancer en cuirasse'* as it appears like **armor coat** **(Figs. 17-28 and 17-73)**. Always both sides should be compared for any discrepancies.

Palpation

Normal breast should be palpated first **(Fig. 17-34)**. Palpation should be done using *the palmar aspect of the fingers with*

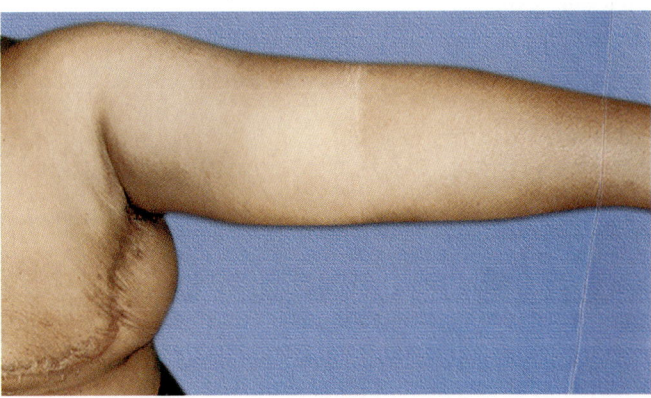

Fig. 17-33 Carcinoma of breast operated earlier with *postoperative edema arm*. Note scar of mastectomy.

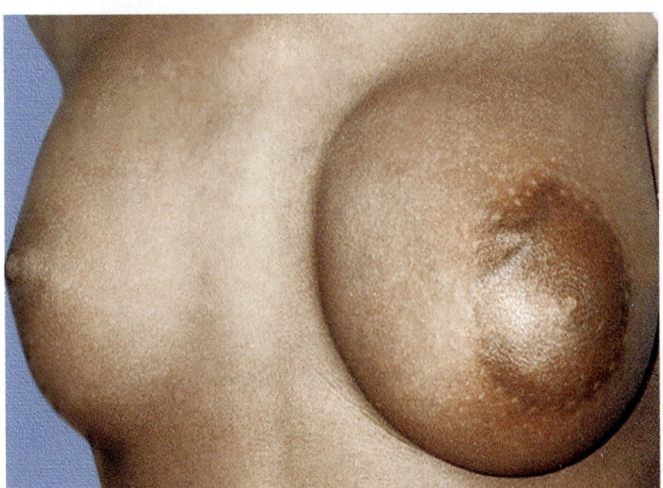

Fig. 17-32 *Fibroadenoma* left breast.

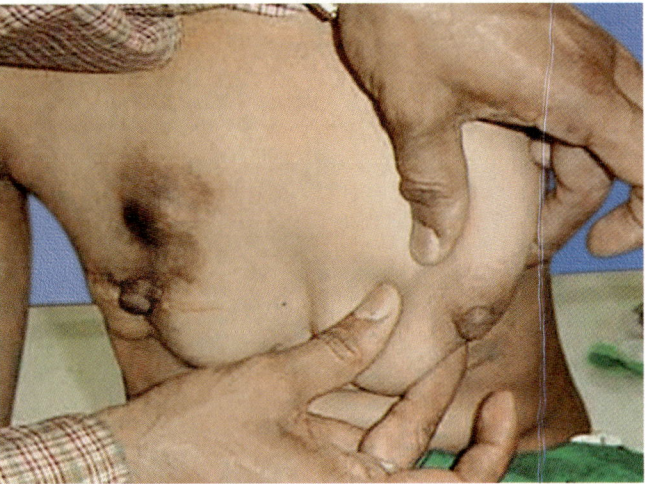

Fig. 17-34 *Normal breast should be palpated first.* Then diseased side is palpated. It should be palpated for **mass, its location, shape, size, surface, consistency, mobility and fixity.**

hand flat. Normal breast tissue is firm, lobulated with fine nodularity. Often it can be soft and smooth also. Palpation is also done between thumb and fingers. All quadrants should be palpated along with nipple areola complex and axillary tail of Spence.

> During palpation one should look for raise in temperature over the breast (observed in mastitis but also can occur in vascular tumors like medullary carcinoma and sarcoma), tenderness, nature of the swelling—its size, shape, extent, surface, margin, consistency (carcinoma is hard/stony hard and irregular), fixity to breast tissue (swelling will not have independent/differential mobility), fixity to skin (by pinching the skin), fixity to pectoral fascia (by tethering), fixity to pectoralis major muscle/serratus anterior muscle/latissimus dorsi muscle. Palpate ulcer if present—look for tenderness, its edge and base for induration, bleeding on palpation. Nipple and areola should be palpated for tenderness, eversion, induration and discharge, and mass **(Figs. 17-35A and B)**.

Local rise of temperature: It is checked with dorsum of fingers. Breast is warm in mastitis and so also sarcomas can be warmer. Aggressive carcinoma also can be warm due to increased vascularity.

Tenderness: Breast is tender to palpate in acute mastitis and abscess. Carcinoma is nontender initially but becomes tender once skin is involved or when chest wall infiltration occurs.

> **Quadrants of breast:**
> *Quadrants of breast are marked by drawing two lines, vertical and horizontal along the nipple*
> - Upper outer quadrant (includes axillary tail also)—commonest site for carcinoma—60%
> - Lower outer quadrant—10%
> - Upper inner quadrant—12%
> - Lower inner quadrant—close to mediastinum—6%
> - Central quadrant—nipple and areola region—12%

Location of lump in the breast: Fibroadenoma is common in lower quadrant; fibroadenosis and carcinoma are more common in upper outer quadrant. One should remember that it is only incidence-wise; in a given patient any disease can develop in any quadrant **(Figs. 17-36 and 17-37)**.

Number, size and shape: Carcinoma of breast is solitary; fibroadenosis can be multiple. Fibroadenoma is usually solitary but multiple fibroadenomas are known to occur occupying the entire breast tissue. Opposite breast also can

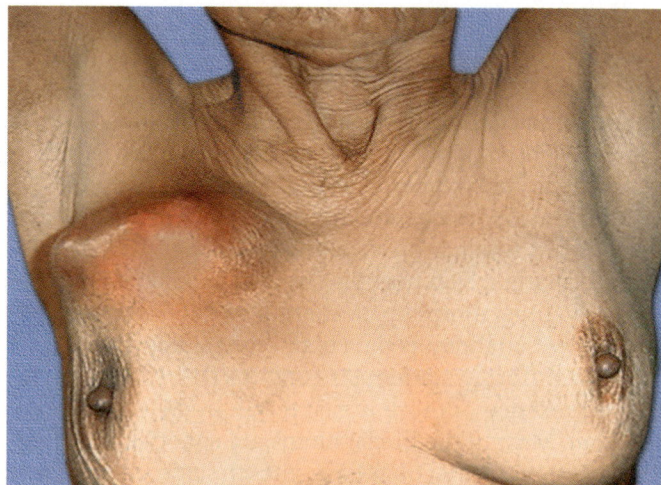

Fig. 17-36 Carcinoma breast *over the commonest site—upper outer quadrant—more visible on raising the arm.*

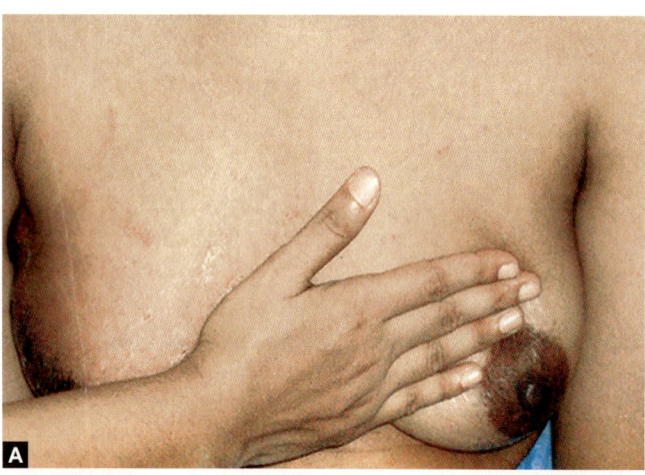

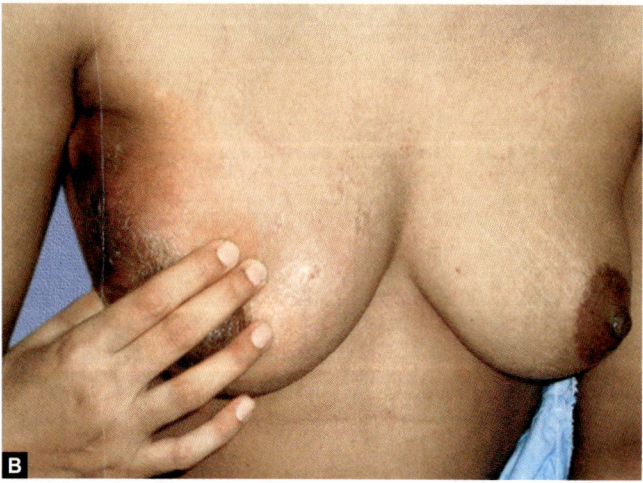

Figs. 17-35A and B Palpation of breast lump with *palmar surface of fingers*. Palpation is also done between fingers and thumb.

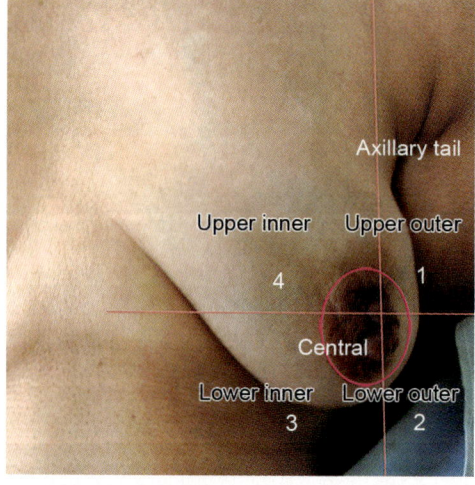

Fig. 17-37 *Quadrants of the breast*—upper outer; lower outer; lower inner; upper inner and central. Order of examining the breast quadrants is same as mentioned now. Axillary tail of Spence is part of upper outer quadrant. Carcinoma is more common in upper outer quadrant as more breast tissue by volume is present in this quadrant.

be involved especially in fibroadenosis. Size is important in staging the (T staging) carcinoma breast and so it should be measured using a tape (in cm). Ideally mass should be measured using caliper especially when breast conservative surgery is needed. Fibroadenoma more than 5 cm is called as *giant fibroadenoma*. Shape is globular in fibroadenoma; uneven in carcinoma.

Margin: Margin is well-defined and regular in fibroadenoma, breast abscess/cyst (in fibroadenoma the margins tends to slip off the palpating fingers); well-defined and irregular in carcinoma; ill-defined in fibroadenosis.

Surface: It may be nodular or granular or uneven in carcinoma. Smooth surface is seen in benign condition like fibroadenoma.

Consistency: Fibroadenoma is firm swelling; carcinoma is stony hard; fibroadenosis is firm or diffuse India rubber consistency. Sarcoma is variable with soft or firm or hard in texture. But in many occasions consistency may be variable; fibroadenoma can be hard and carcinoma may be firm. Student has to remember that cystic lesion of the breast is rare; only in such patient fluctuation is elicited from behind; transillumination is also checked in dark room using illumination source.

Fluctuation: When swelling is soft, fluctuation test is done. It is done by examiner standing or sitting behind the patient *(Victor Riddell method)* **(Fig. 17-38)**. Two hands of the examiner are placed above the shoulders of the patient. Swelling is held with one hand and with index finger of the other hand summit of the swelling is pressed/indented. Fluid displacement can be appreciated with yielding of the finger. Cystic swelling, localized abscess can be fluctuant. **Bloodgood cyst** is localized cystic swelling observed often in fibroadenosis of breast.

Transillumination test: It should be checked if there is clear fluid in the cyst. It is done using a torch placed on undersurface of breast tissue and the visibility is checked over the surface, ideally in a dark room. Rarely cystic hygroma of breast is brilliantly transilluminant. It is negative in breast abscess, cyst filled with blood. Hematoma, fibroadenoma, carcinoma are not transilluminant.

Fixity of the lump to breast tissue: It is checked by holding the breast tissue in one hand and moving the lump in other hand. If the lump is fixed to breast tissue, then breast tissue moves along with the lump. Carcinoma breast is fixed to breast tissue and moves with the breast in both directions unless it is fixed to the deeper structures and chest wall. Fibroadenoma shows free mobility (differential mobility) in all direction within the breast tissue and so is called as *'breast mouse'*/floating swelling (lump). In traumatic fat necrosis, mass is fixed to breast tissue firmly.

Skin tethering can be demonstrated by moving the lump side to side. It is due to inward puckering of the skin following involvement of the elastic Cooper's ligament which becomes inelastic. Dimpling of skin appears which can be demonstrated by raising the arms above the shoulder level. When *skin tethering occurs lump can still be moved in the arc anywhere without moving the overlying skin whereas lump cannot be moved at all without moving the skin in skin fixation* **(Fig. 17-39)**.

Fixity to skin: When tumor directly infiltrates the skin, fixity occurs. Here skin will not be moved separately over the lump. *Gliding test*—the skin overlying the tumor tissue is rolled with the flat of the hand. It is possible if skin is free. **Pinching test**—skin overlying the tumor is pinched with thumb and finger, not possible if the skin is not free **(Fig. 17-40)**. *Peau d'orange* can be better seen by pinching wider area of the skin between thumb and fingers. Whether benign or malignant, when tumor lies beneath the nipple, it is fixed to it as the main mammary duct may be travelling through the tumor tissue. But tumor beneath the areola may or may not be fixed to it as it depends on presence or absence of infiltration to areola. In advanced carcinoma breast, when the skin and chest wall gets infiltrated, a special feel of rigid coat of armor is felt—*cancer en cuirassae*.

Fixity to pectoralis major muscle: It is checked in sitting position. Patient is asked to keep her hands on her waist. Lump is moved along the direction of the muscle and also

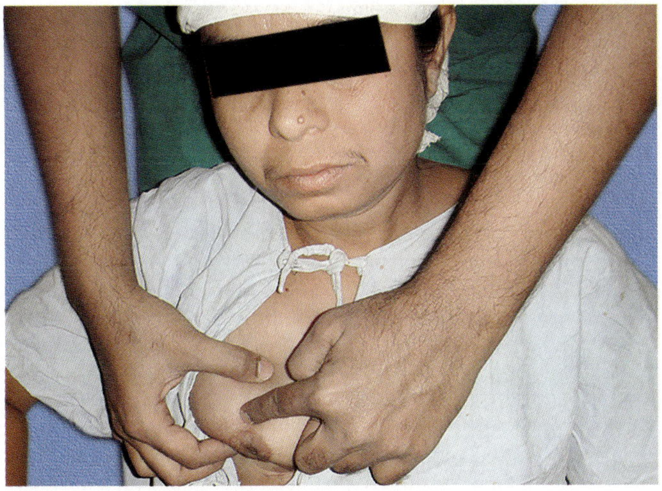

Fig. 17-38 *Victor Riddell method of eliciting fluctuation*: Fluctuation in breast lump is elicited by standing behind the patient and keeping the arms over the patient's shoulders.

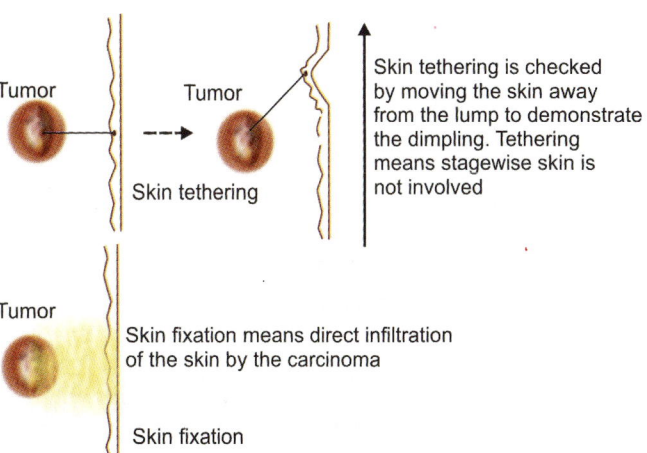

Fig. 17-39 *Demonstration of skin tethering and fixation.* Lump can be moved like an arc in skin tethering with demonstration of skin dimpling. Lump cannot be moved separately in skin fixation.

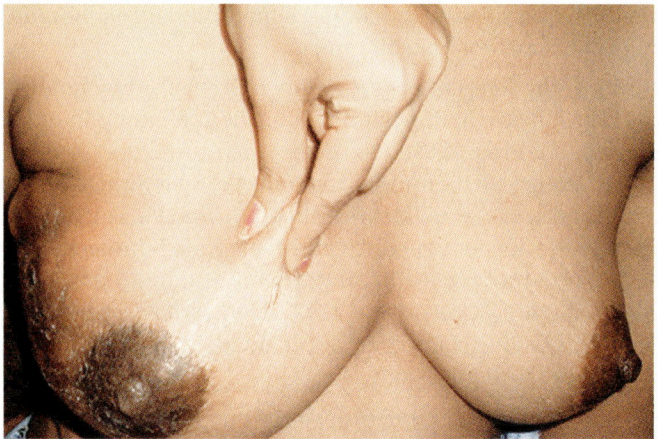

Fig. 17-40 Fixity to skin should be checked *by pinching* or *holding the skin separately* from tumor.

perpendicular to the direction of the muscle. Patient is asked to hold the hands tightly pressed over the waist to contract the pectoralis major muscle (action of the muscle is flexion of the shoulder) which is confirmed by feeling the taut muscle at anterior axillary fold. Lump is again moved *along the direction (mainly)* and perpendicular to the direction of the muscle. *Mobility along the line of muscle fibers will be restricted* totally if lump is adherent to the pectoralis major muscle. It becomes T3 stage tumor **(Figs. 17-41 and 17-42)**.

Fixity to latissimus dorsi muscle: It is checked in sitting position with examiner standing by the side of the patient. Latissimus dorsi is an extensor of the shoulder joint. Initially mobility of the lump is checked and then arm is extended against resistance with elbow flexed at 90° to contract the latissimus dorsi. If now mobility of the lump is restricted, it

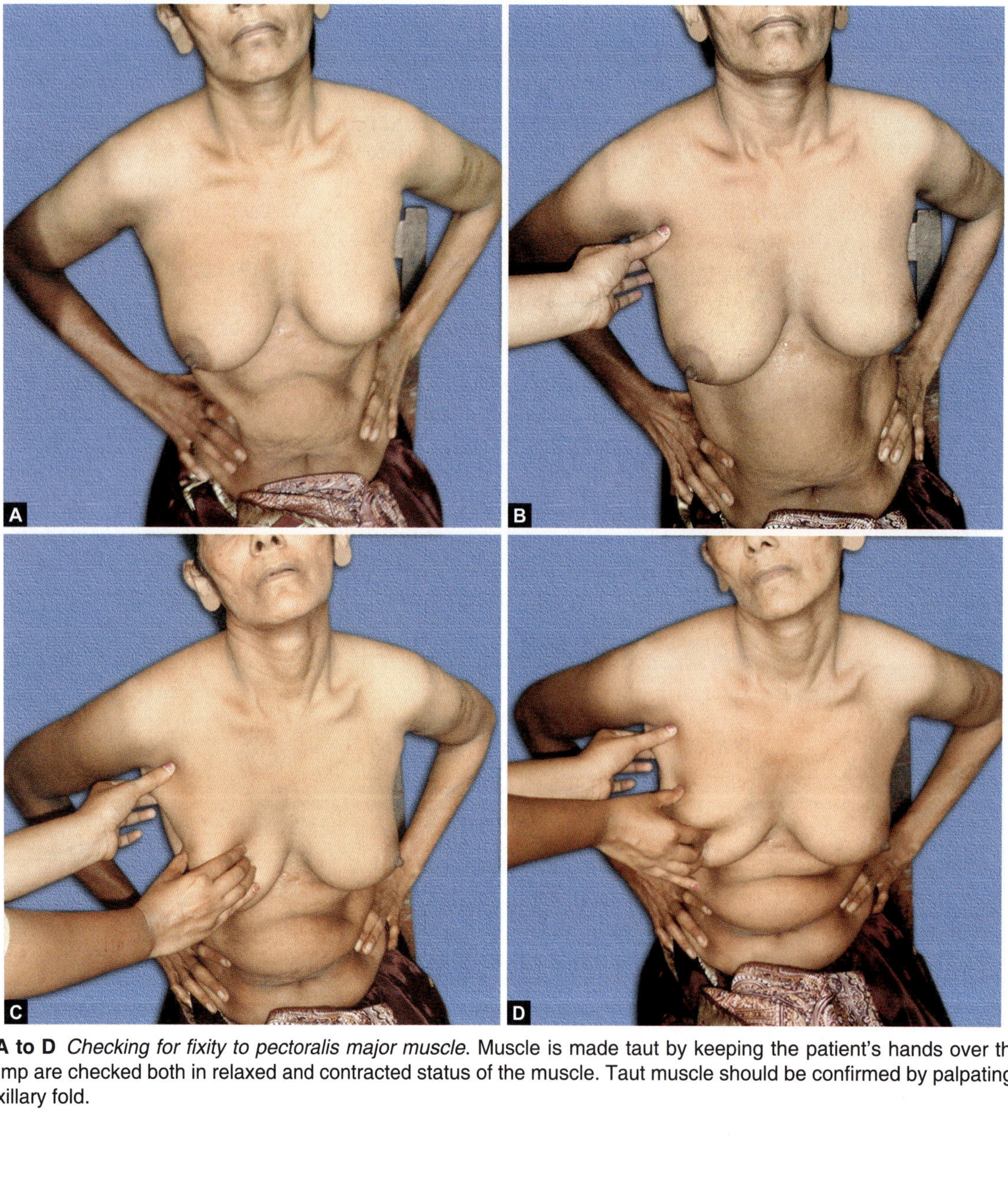

Figs. 17-41A to D *Checking for fixity to pectoralis major muscle.* Muscle is made taut by keeping the patient's hands over the waist and mobility of lump are checked both in relaxed and contracted status of the muscle. Taut muscle should be confirmed by palpating the muscle in anterior axillary fold.

Chapter 17: Clinical Approaches and Examination of Breast

confirms that lump is fixed to latissimus dorsi muscle (**Fig. 17-43**).

Fixity to serratus anterior muscle: It is assessed by checking the mobility of the lump before and after contracting the serratus anterior. Contraction of serratus anterior is achieved by pushing both the outstretched hands against resistance over a wall or over a examiner's shoulders and checking for restriction of mobility of the lump. It signifies involvement of chest wall—stage T_4 (**Figs. 17-44A to C**).

Chest wall fixity: It can be assessed by absence/presence of mobility of the mass; and breast with mass will not fall forward if it is fixed to underlying chest wall; and on raising the arm above shoulder breast with mass will not raise upward. Chest wall fixity means fixity to underlying ribs and intercostal muscles (**Figs. 17-45 and 17-46**).

Chest wall includes ribs, intercostal muscles and serratus anterior muscle but not the pectoral muscle.

Palpation of nipple: It is equally important to palpate the nipple. Tenderness, thickening, hardness, mobility should be checked. Tumor underneath nipple is usually fixed to nipple. Retraction of nipple may be confirmed by palpating it. Discharge can be better appreciated while palpating the lump in the breast or other part of breast tissue or nipple itself. Color, content (serous, blood, pus, greenish milk) of the discharge can be found. Discharge should be collected for cytology or culture or AFB staining. In retracted nipple, the base of the nipple is gently pressed to evert it. If it is due to congenital or benign cause, retracted nipple can be everted by pressing at the base. If retraction is due to carcinoma, it cannot be everted

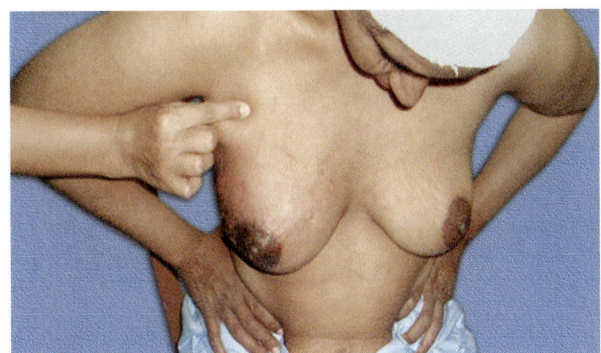

Fig. 17-42 *Proper contraction and feeling of pectoralis major muscle is important.*

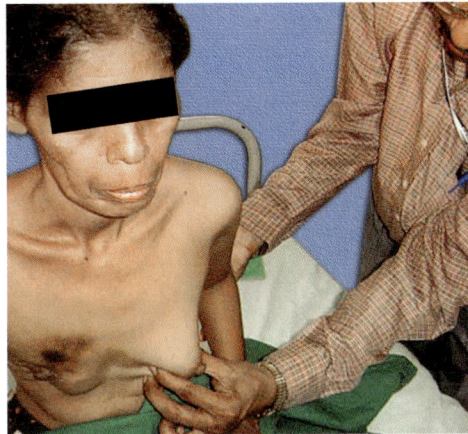

Fig. 17-43 *Fixity to latissimus dorsi muscle is checked by checking the mobility of the mass while extending the arm against resistance.*

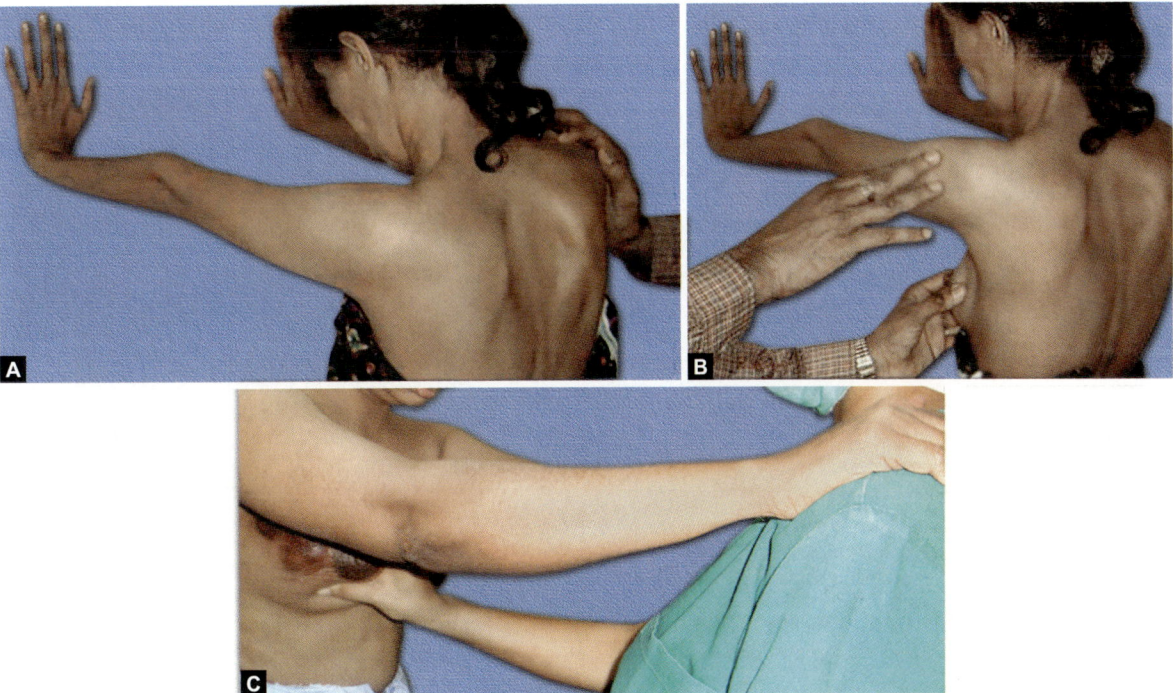

Figs. 17-44A to C *Fixity to serratus anterior is checked by checking the mobility of the lump while pushing both the outstretched hands of the patient, over the wall or over the examiner's shoulder against resistance.*

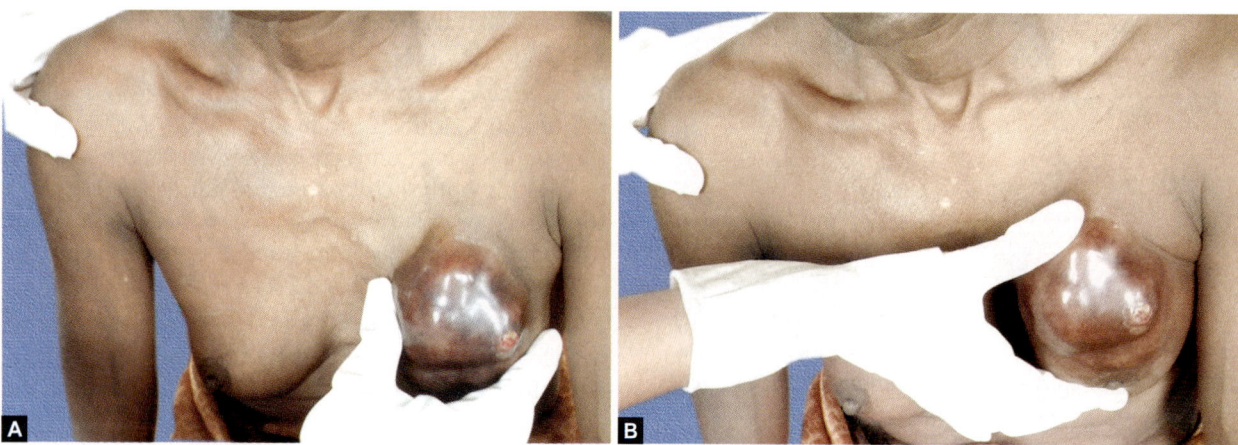

Figs. 17-45A and B *Mobility of breast lump* is checked in two directions—horizontal and vertical.

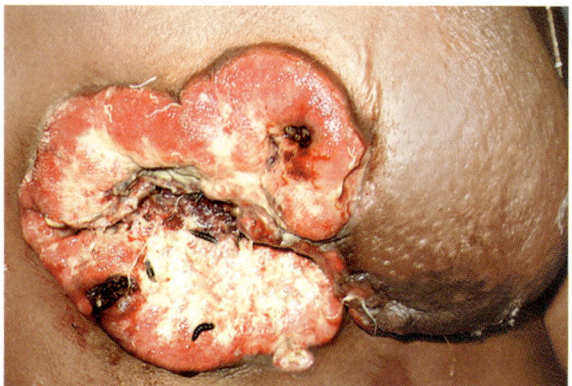

Fig. 17-46 Fungating carcinoma breast. *Note the extension of fungation into the chest wall.*

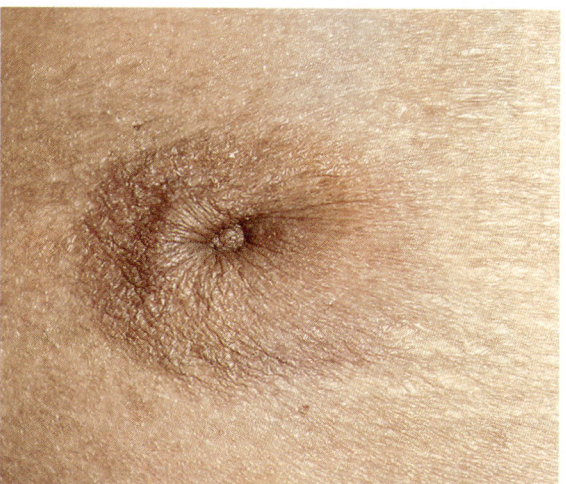

Fig. 17-47 Typical *retraction of the nipple.*

at all. Retraction is ***circumferential*** in carcinoma; ***slit like*** in duct ectasia **(Fig. 17-47)**.

> **Assessment of nipple deviation:** Nipple changes are assessed by inspection, palpation and measurement. Displacement of nipple is assessed by measuring distance between midclavicular point to the nipple. This reveals any upward/downward displacement of nipple. Outward/inward displacement is assessed by measuring the distance of nipple from midline **(Fig. 17-48)**.

> **Changes that can occur in nipple:**
> - Destruction
> - Depression (retraction)
> - Discoloration
> - Displacement
> - Deviation
> - Discharge
> - Duplication

Palpation of areola: Areola should be palpated for nodularity, thickening, ulcer. Paget's disease can cause destruction of areola.

Examination in pendulous large breast: It is better done in standing position with patient leaning forward and her outstretched hands resting on the arm of a chair or table; this

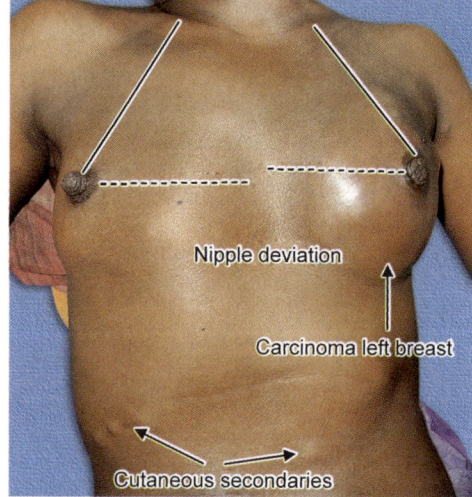

Fig. 17-48 *Nipple deviation* in carcinoma breast; note the cutaneous secondaries also (metastatic deposits).

makes the breast in hanging position which to certain extent circumvent the mammary obesity **(Fig. 17-49)**.

Examination of an ulcer over breast: Ulcer if present over the breast lump, should be examined like any ulcer with

Chapter 17: Clinical Approaches and Examination of Breast

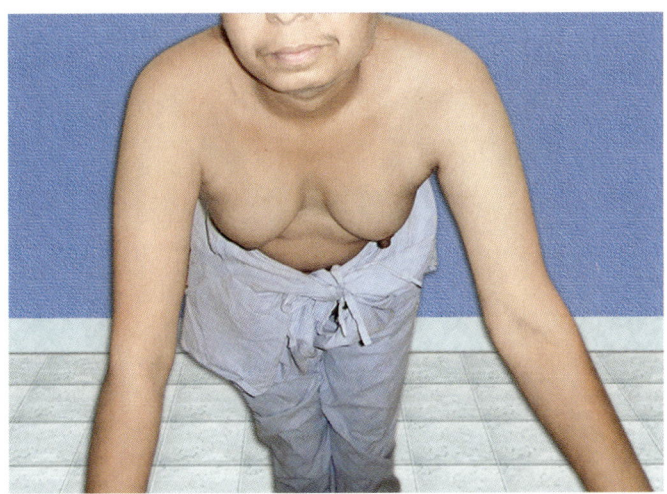

Fig. 17-49 *In pendulous breast* it is often necessary to examine after making the patient to lean by placing her hands on the arm/s of the chair.

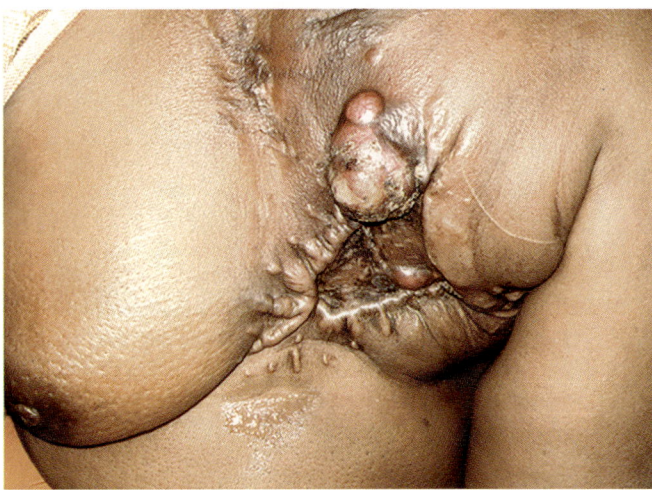

Fig. 17-51 Recurrent carcinoma breast with lesions in the scar, skin nodules, cancer en cuirasse, and Peau d'orange on the skin over opposite breast. It could be carcinoma of opposite breast probably as a spread from this side. *De novo opposite side carcinoma is also possible.*

inspection of floor, margin, edge, discharge; palpation for tenderness, induration, mobility, fixity.

Examination of ipsilateral, regional axillary lymph nodes: Anterior/pectoral, central/medial, posterior, lateral, apical lymph nodes should be examined **(Fig. 17-50)**.

Supraclavicular lymph nodes should be examined.

Examination of opposite breast and opposite axilla: Opposite axillary nodes are also examined. It may get involved through retrograde spread from internal mammary nodes or through cutaneous lymphatics **(Fig. 17-51)**.

Palpation of Axillary Lymph Nodes

It is an important step in examination of carcinoma breast **(Figs. 17-52 to 17-55)**.

Anterior, central and apical groups of lymph nodes are examined using examiners' opposite hand and lateral and

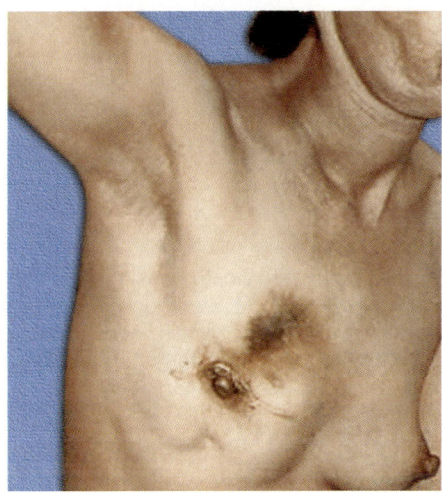

Fig. 17-52 Inspection of the axilla with *raised arm is very important clinical method.*

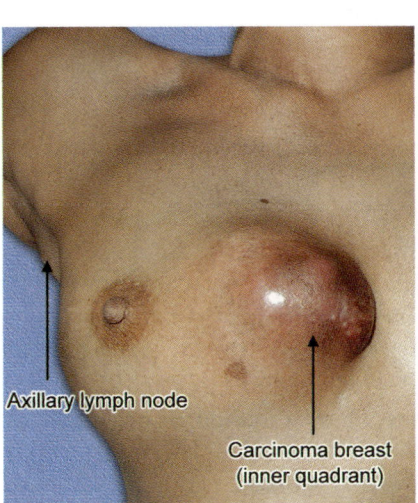

Fig. 17-50 Carcinoma right breast with *ipsilateral (same side)* axillary lymph node enlargement (spread).

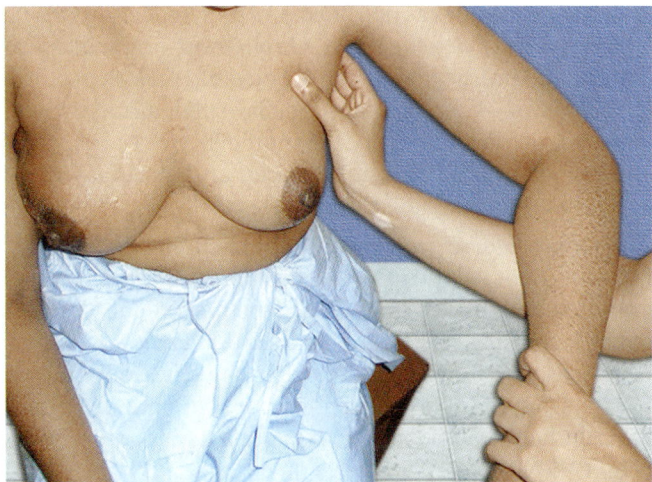

Fig. 17-53 Palpation of *left axilla using right hand.*

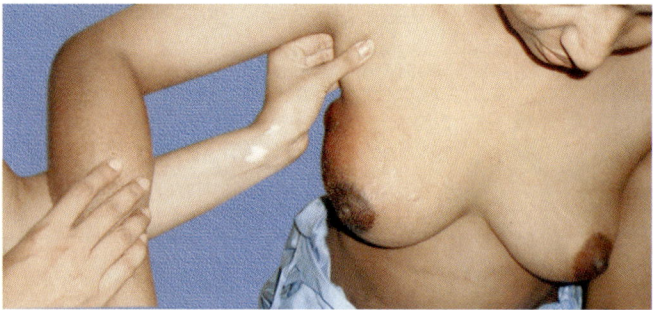

Fig. 17-54 Palpation of *right axilla using left hand*.

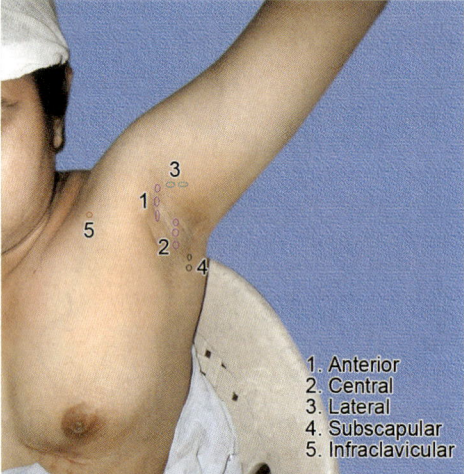

Fig. 17-55 *Location of axillary lymph nodes*—anterior, central, lateral, subscapular and infraclavicular. Even though any order of preference can be used while palpating axillary lymph nodes, usual standard order of palpating the lymph nodes are—central → lateral → pectoral → infraclavicular → subscapular (posterior).

1. Anterior
2. Central
3. Lateral
4. Subscapular
5. Infraclavicular

subscapular nodes are examined using corresponding hand of the examiner (for example, anterior, central and apical nodes of right axilla is examined by left hand of the clinician; lateral and subscapular nodes of right axilla is examined using right hand of the clinician). Even though palpation of nodes can start from any nodes as per clinician's preference, but usually it is palpated in *following orders—From front*—central; apical; brachial (lateral/near insertion of pectoralis major); pectoral. *From behind*—subscapular; supraclavicular; infraclavicular. Patient raises the arm above the shoulder; axilla is inspected and fingers of the clinician is placed on the axilla with its palmar aspect facing the chest wall medially **(Fig. 17-56)**.

Anterior/pectoral group of nodes are commonly involved nodes. Patient will be in sitting position. Raise the patient's arm high and inspect the axilla. Place the patient's forearm over examiner's forearm. Palpate the relaxed axilla over pectoralis major muscle for any lymph nodes. Examiner will use his left hand to examine the nodes (of right axilla) and his right hand will be over patient's left shoulder to support **(Fig. 17-57)**.

Interpectoral nodes (Rotter's) are also palpated similarly by insinuating the fingers between the two pectori. It signifies retrograde spread of the tumor. It is often difficult to palpate.

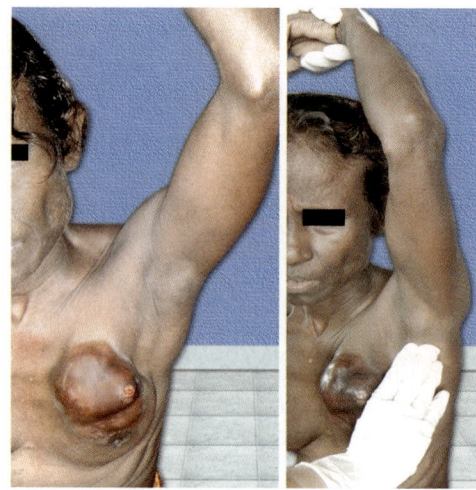

Fig. 17-56 *First step in examining the axilla* is raising the arm above the shoulder; placing the fingers high in the axilla going medially over the chest wall in the axilla.

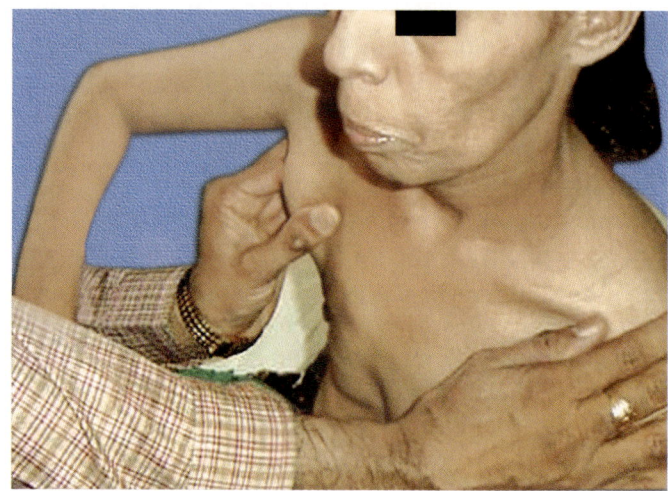

Fig. 17-57 Examination of *pectoral group* of lymph nodes.

Central group of nodes are palpated in similar way like pectoral nodes but hand in the axilla is directed medially over the lateral chest wall and with gentle rolling movements using pulp of the finger **(Fig. 17-58)**.

Lateral/humeral group of nodes are palpated with examiner's right hand (for right axilla) with left hand placed over *same side* shoulder **(Fig. 17-59)**.

Posterior/subscapular nodes are palpated with patient in sitting position and examiner standing behind the patient. By raising the arm and forearm of the patient from opposite side the posterior axillary fold is palpated between thumb and fingers **(Figs. 17-60A and B)**.

Apical nodes (Halsted nodes) are palpated (for right axilla) with left hand of the examiner placing high in the axilla with **(Herald Style's technique)** right hand supporting over the shoulder and supraclavicular region of the same side of the axilla. It is often difficult to palpate **(Fig. 17-61)**.

Supraclavicular nodes are palpated using fingers over supraclavicular fossa by standing behind the patient where the

Chapter 17: Clinical Approaches and Examination of Breast

shoulder is passively elevated thereby cervical muscles and fascia get relaxed. Two sides can be simultaneously palpated and compared **(Fig. 17-62)**.

> **Levels of the axillary nodes (Berg's levels):**
> - Level I—Below and lateral to the pectoralis minor muscle—anterior, lateral, posterior
> - Level II—Behind the pectoralis minor muscle—central
> - Level III—Above and medial to pectoralis minor muscle—apical
>
> *Note:* Total number of nodes in the axilla is around 50.

Axillary nodes on opposite side are also examined. Opposite axilla can be examined by examiner standing on the same side by leaning over the patient or can be examined by standing on the opposite side. Its involvement signifies stage IV disease. It is confirmed by FNAC.

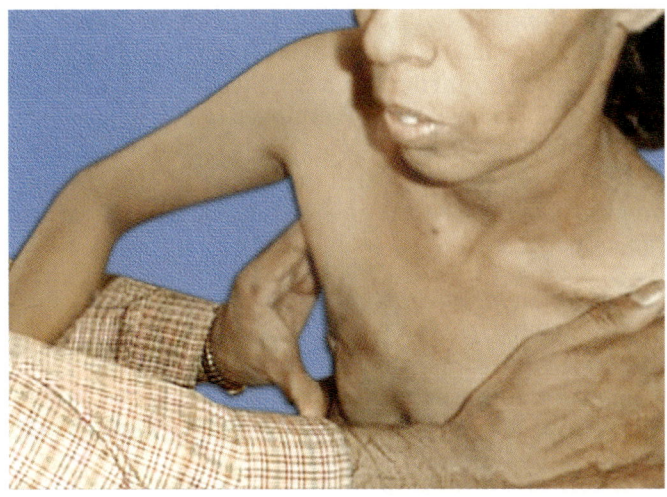

Fig. 17-58 Examination of *central group of lymph nodes*.

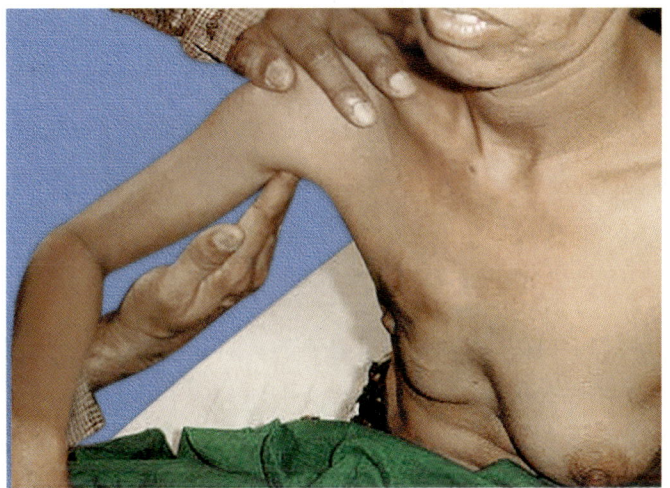

Fig. 17-59 Examination of *lateral group of lymph nodes*.

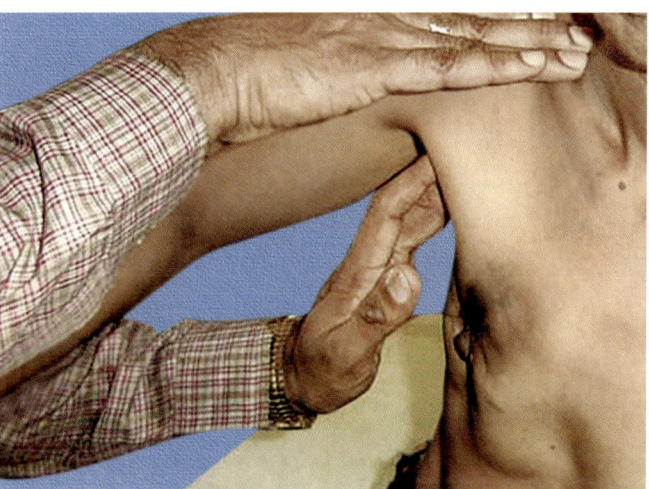

Fig. 17-61 Examination *of apical group of lymph nodes*.

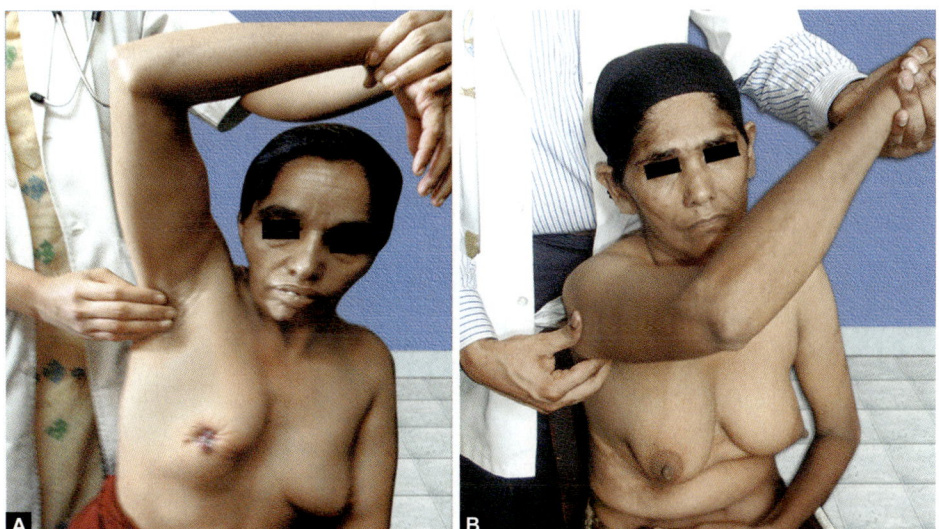

Figs. 17-60A and B Examination of *posterior group of lymph nodes*.

Axillary tail of the Spence: It is the extension of the upper outer quadrant of breast across foramen Langer deep to deep fascia. **Foramen Langer** is an opening in deep fascia over outer aspect of the breast which allows part of breast tissue to extend under deep fascia, otherwise rest all breast tissue is in subcutaneous plane. Axillary tail is located adjacent to outer border of the pectoralis major muscle. When it is involved by carcinoma it should be differentiated from pectoral node enlargement. Axillary tail will move along with main breast tissue whereas pectoral node will not move when breast is moved as it has got independent mobility. Axillary tail often extends over the lateral edge of the pectoralis major muscle up to axilla **(Figs. 17-63A and B)**.

Fixed enlarged axillary nodes can cause lymph-edema due to lymphatic block; venous thrombosis and venous edema due to venous block; and severe excruciating pain along the distribution of the median and ulnar nerves (rare in radial nerve) with often significant sensory and motor deficits due to tumor infiltration of the cords of brachial plexus (usually medial cord occasionally lateral cord).

Examination of arms for venous edema or lymphedema: Venous edema may be due to axillary vein compression by nodal mass. Lymphedema may be due to lymphatic block following nodal involvement. Lymphedema is mainly distal. It is gradual in onset and progressive. Venous edema is sudden in onset, with bluish discoloration over the skin, uniform in both distal and proximal aspect of the upper limb (forearm and arm).

Examination for mediastinal node involvement: It is done by percussion *It is not done usually as it is technically difficult.* Initially percussion for liver dullness is done. Percussion is done one space above from lateral to medial, to look for widened mediastinal border. Mediastinal nodes are common in middle mediastinum.

Note: *This method is clinically difficult to elicit.*

Examination of respiratory system: It is done to look for secondaries—altered breath sounds, features of consolidation or pleural effusion are looked for **(Fig. 17-64)**.

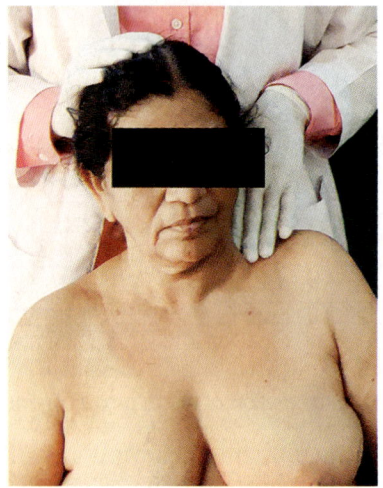

Fig. 17-62 Examination of *supraclavicular group of lymph nodes.*

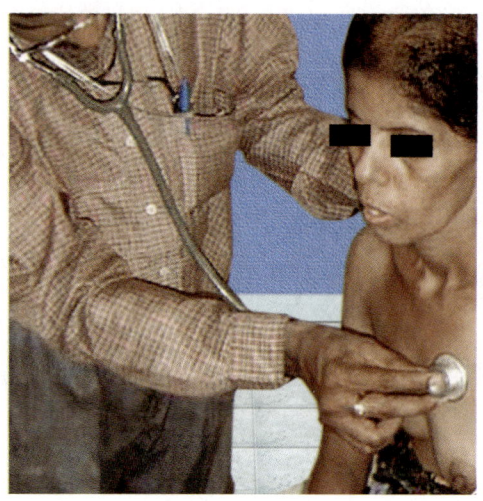

Fig. 17-64 Look for *pleural effusion and altered breath sounds* for secondaries in lungs.

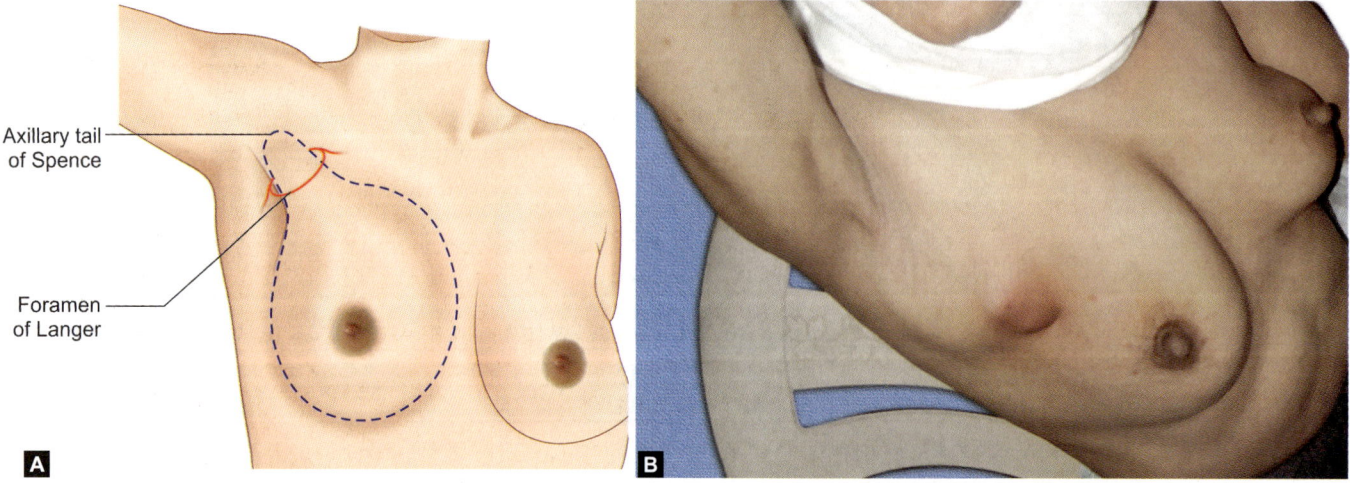

Figs. 17-63A and B *Axillary tail of Spence.* It is actually part of *upper outer quadrant.*

Examination of abdomen: To look for palpable nodular liver, Krukenberg tumors in ovaries in menstruating age group, and ascites. It is completed with digital examination of rectum (P/R), and per vaginal examination **(Fig. 17-65)**.

Examination of pelvis, spine, long bones for any swelling/tenderness/pathological fracture/restricted movements of spine, hips, etc. Spine tenderness, paraspinal spasm, spine movements should be checked. Rotation movement should be checked and is done by making the patient to sit on a stool to fix the pelvic girdle **(Fig. 17-66)**. Bones are the commonest site of secondaries (70%). Among bones, spine is the commonest (lumbar) one get involved.

Examination of central nervous system to look for any neurological deficits following metastatic disease in the brain.

Breast self-examination (BSE) has got a major role in early detection of the carcinoma breast:
Ideally done once a month, just after the menstruation, as during this time breasts are less engorged. In postmenopausal age group it is done regularly at monthly intervals (fixed day of the month).
- Examine both breasts
- American Cancer Society recommends monthly BSE after 20 years of age
- Remind the patient that 90% of breast lumps are not cancer
- Better way is in lying down position with arm raised with a mattress support behind **(Fig. 17-67)**
- Palpation is done over all quadrants of the breast using the fingers
- If any doubtful swelling is palpable, consult the surgeon
- Nursing mother should perform BSE just after feeding the baby.

Cystic swellings of the breast:
- Bloodgood cyst
- Breast abscess
- Hydatid cyst
- Galactocele
- Serocystic disease of Brodie
- Cystic necrosis in carcinoma breast
- Lymph cyst
- Hematoma in breast.

Causes of hard swellings in the breast:
- Carcinoma breast
- Antibioma breast
- Traumatic fat necrosis
- Calcified hematoma
- Fibroadenoma—hard variety.

An innovative triple ABC technique (Sribatsa Kumar Mohapatra Clinical Technique) for clinical breast examination (CBE) for breast disorders (With permission from *Prof Dr Sribatsa Kumar Mohapatra*, MS, FRCS, DNB and Dr Biswajit Mohapatra; Department of General Surgery, VSSMCH, Burla, Somalapur, Odisha).

Three sets of ABCs are used. *First ABC* stands for axilla, breast, cervical area on nonaffected side; *Second ABC* stands for axilla, breast and cervical area of the affected side and *third ABC* stands for abdomen, bones and brain, chest respectively.

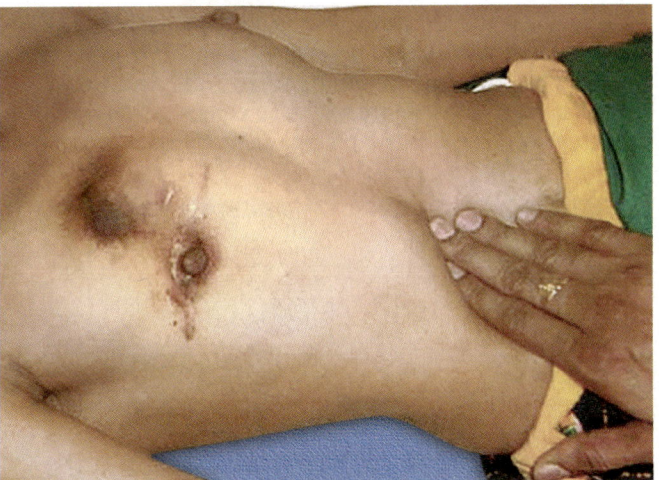

Fig. 17-65 Always examine abdomen for *liver enlargement, ascites or Krukenberg tumor* (in premenopausal age).

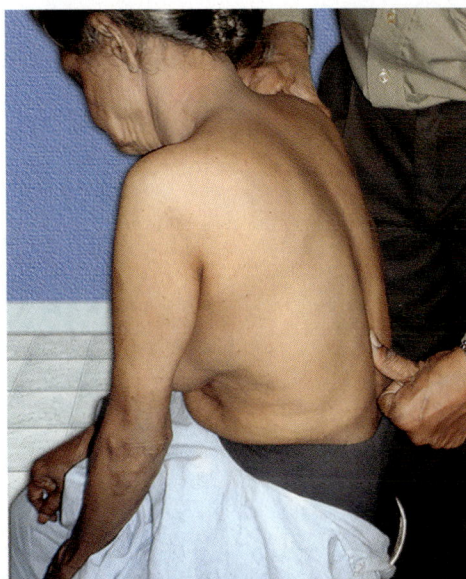

Fig. 17-66 Spine examination is a must in carcinoma breast as bone spread mainly to lumbar spines is common.

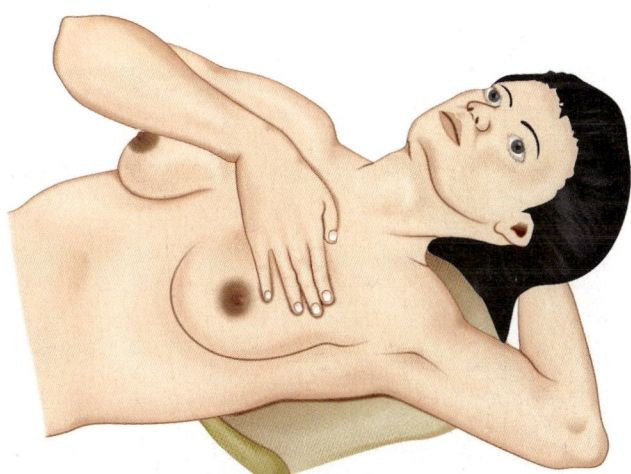

Fig. 17-67 *Self-examination* of breast is done in lying down position.

Each ABC is further given five points of importance:
- Axilla: (1) Anterior, (2) Posterior, (3) Central, (4) Apical, (5) Lateral.
- Breast (quadrants): (1) Central (nipple areola complex), (2) Upper medial, (3) Upper lateral, (4) Lower medial, (5) Lower lateral.
- Cervical area: (1) Level I, (2) Level II, (3) Level III, (4) Level IV, (5) Level V. Both sides should be checked.

For third ABC:
- Abdomen: (1) Lump (Krukenberg), (2) Liver, (3) Umbilicus, (4) Shifting dullness, (5) Digital rectal examination (DRE).
- Bones and Brain: (1) Vertebrae, (2) Ribs and sternum, (3) Proximal femur, (4) Proximal humerus, (5) Skull and brain.
- Chest: (1) Effusion, (2) Collapse, (3) Consolidation, (4) Intercostal fullness, (5) Ribs.

All findings are collectively analyzed.

INVESTIGATIONS IN CARCINOMA BREAST/BREAST LUMP

Mammography: It is plain X-ray of soft tissue of breast using low voltage and high amperage X-rays (300 MV and 40 KV). Two films are taken—*Craniocaudal* from above downward; *mediolateral* from side-to-side. Dose of radiation is 0.1 cGy, a low dose. So it is a safe and effective procedure (Fig. 17-68).

Findings to look for are—microcalcifications, contour changes, asymmetry, distortion, spiculations, changes in skin and nipple, soft tissue shadow and margins.

Breast imaging reporting and data system (BI-RADS) has got its own categories (0–6), assessment and recommendations. Mammography has got 90% sensitivity; 95% specificity.

Digital mammography is computerized electronic image of the breast with enhanced magnified pictures.

Ultrasound of Breast

It is done to look for lesion whether solid or cystic, margin of the lesion, internal echoes, retrotumor acoustic shadowing, compressibility, dimensions (Fig. 17-69). But lesions less than 1 cm may not be identified. FNAC can be done under US guidance. *Irregular margin, irregular internal echoes, irregular posterior shadowing, noncompressibility - are the features of carcinoma.* Benign lesions are smooth, rounded with well-defined margins with weak internal echoes and compressibility. It is cheaper, easily available and there is no risk of radiation. It is preferred method of screening in young females, pregnancy and early lactation.

Trucut Biopsy (Fig. 17-70)

It has become more reliable, *ideal* and efficient in diagnosing, grading, and to get receptor status (ER/PR/Her2Neu) which facilitates proper planning of the carcinoma.

Fine Needle Aspiration Cytology (FNAC) (Fig. 17-71)

It is very useful and simple; can be done under US guidance; but negative results are difficult to interpret. FNAC of opposite breast, lymph nodes, opposite axillary lymph nodes – can be done. FNNAC is Fine Needle Non-Aspirating Cytology. 23 gauge needle with special aspiration syringe is used; needle is passed into the lump and with negative pressure (40 cm of H_2O). Material is collected on a slide; a smear is made using 100% alcohol. Cytological study is done; *FNAC scoring:* C0—no epithelial cells; C1—scanty epithelial cells; C2—benign cells; C3—atypical cells; C4—suspicious cells; C5—malignant cells.

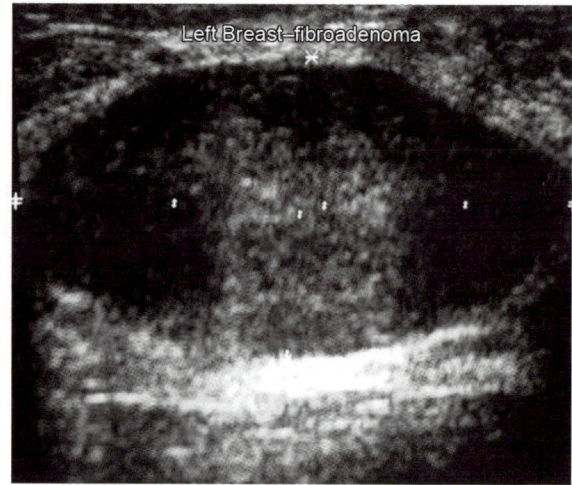

Fig. 17-69 *Ultrasound left breast* showing fibroadenoma.

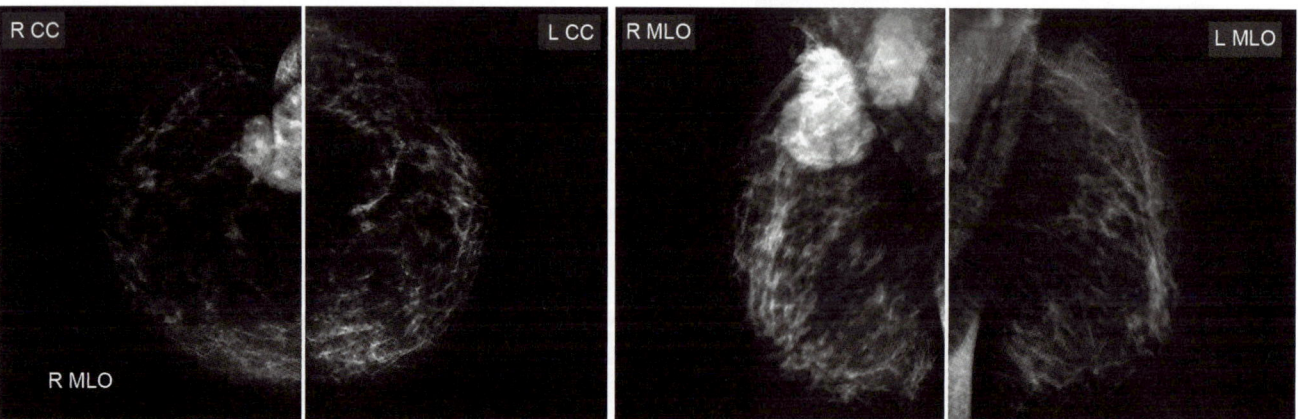

Fig. 17-68 *Mammogram of both breasts;* craniocaudal (RCC, LCC) and mediolateral (RMLO, LMLO) films are taken. Note the irregular mass lesions with spiculations in the mammogram—features of carcinoma breast.

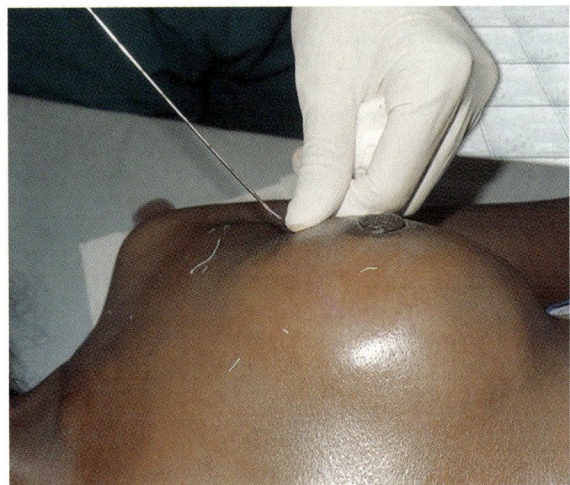

Fig. 17-70 *Trucut biopsy* is ideal investigation in carcinoma breast to confirm diagnosis, to type and to identify the receptor status.

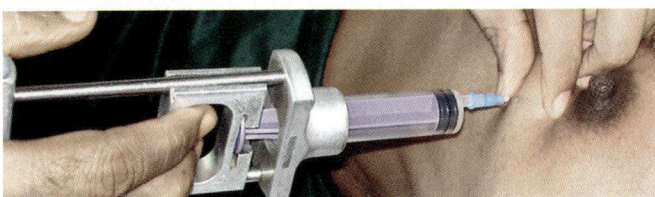

Fig. 17-71 *FNAC of breast lump.*

Advantages of FNAC: FNAC is least painful, can be done on OP basis, reliable and cheaper. Malignant deposits will not occur along FNAC track (only contraindication for FNAC is testicular tumor).

Other Investigations

Frozen section biopsy: If FNAC fails even after two trials or in cases of negative FNAC, then *on table frozen section biopsy* is done for diagnosis. It has got 20% false-negative results.

Excision biopsy is another option if FNAC and trucut becomes inconclusive; incision should be placed in such a way that it can be included in eventual mastectomy.

Chest X-ray: To look for pleural effusion, cannon ball secondaries in lungs, mediastinal lymph nodes, secondaries in rib. CT chest is *more reliable* method to see lung secondaries.

Ultrasound abdomen: To look for liver secondaries, ascites, and 'Krukenberg' tumor.

X-ray spine or MRI spine/pelvis shows osteolytic secondaries in the bone like vertebra and pelvic bones.

Radioisotope bone scan: *It is done* to look for secondaries in bone; it is not done routinely in early carcinoma of breast. Healed fractures; Paget's bone disease, osteoarthritis may show hot spots (false-positive status). Indications for whole body bone scan in carcinoma breast: T3, T4 advanced disease; advanced nodal disease; bone pain, bone swelling, pathological fracture; chest/liver secondaries.

ER (Estrogen Receptor)/PR (Progesterone Receptor)/Her2 neu Receptor *(Human epidermal growth factor receptor – 2 Neu oncogene) Assay:* Immunohistochemistry (IHC) is used to study the receptor status of the tissue (ER/PR/Her2 neu). In ER +ve status—Prognosis is good; Hormone therapy including Tamoxifen is very beneficial; response to treatment is better. Her2 neu +ve carries poor prognosis. Triple negative is basal like type – carries poor prognosis. Her2 Neu status is scored as 1 (low), 2 (borderline), 3 (high). Her2 Neu can be assessed by IHC or FISH (Fluorescent In Situ Hybridization); but FISH is costly.

Study of discharge from the nipple: To identify carcinoma cells; ductal lavage may be used to get better sample.

MRI of breast and MRI of spine *(in case of suspected spine secondaries):* It is done—to differentiate scar from recurrence; to image breasts of women with implants; to evaluate the axilla and recurrent disease.

Wedge biopsy: Wedge biopsy is done only when there is skin involvement—ulceration and fungation. Diathermy should be avoided in incision biopsy as it may distort the histology of tumor and study of hormone receptor status may not be possible.

Tumor markers: They are used mainly during follow-up period. CA 15/3 is commonly done when needed.

Sentinel lymph node biopsy (SLNB): The first axillary (SLN) node draining the breast (by direct drainage) is designated as the *sentinel node*. SLN is first node involved by tumor cells and presence or absence of its histological involvement, when assessed will give a predictive idea about the further spread of tumor to other nodes. Involvement of other nodes without SLN is less than 3% and so if SLNB is negative nodal dissection can be avoided but regular follow-up is needed. SLNB is done in all cases of early breast cancers, T1 and T2 *without clinically palpable node*. It is not done in clinically palpable axillary node. SLNB is done in: Carcinoma of breast/penis/malignant melanoma.

CT scan: CT scan of chest, abdomen and brain whenever needed. CT is said to be more useful to detect secondaries in these regions.

Biochemical analysis: Increased serum alkaline phosphatase, γ-glutamyl transaminase suggests liver secondaries. Raise in urinary hydroxyproline means collagen breakdown suggesting secondaries. A low value of urinary etiocholanolone, a metabolite of adrenal dehydroepiandrosterone in relation to total 17 hydroxycorticosteroids (in urine) is specific of breast carcinoma suggesting poor prognosis and poor response to adrenalectomy and hypophysectomy (Poor discriminants).

Newer modalities of investigations: Stereotactic core biopsy using computer mammography; vacuum assisted biopsy using 11 gauge biopsy probe; needle localized biopsy under mammographic guidance; I125 localization biopsy; *ductoscopy; gene assay* can be assessed using oncotype DX using formalin fixed paraffin tissue.

DIFFERENTIAL DIAGNOSIS

Differential diagnosis for carcinoma breast/benign diseases of breast

- Fibroadenosis
- Mastitis
- Traumatic fat necrosis
- Antibioma
- Tuberculosis of breast
- Galactocele
- Bloodgood cyst
- Mondor's disease
- Filariasis breast
- Cystosarcoma phylloides

Carcinoma Breast

Any lump in the breast can be malignant unless proved otherwise. But one has to remember that every breast lump need not be always malignant. One has to remember that differential diagnosis for carcinoma breast is same as all conditions which are benign diseases of the breast (See table above).

Incidences in carcinoma breast
- 30% of all female cancers
- 20% of cancer related deaths in females
- 2–4% bilateral; 2–5% hereditary
- Familial breast cancer—25%
- Sporadic breast cancer—70%
- Lump in the breast—commonest presentation (75%)
- 10% presents with pain (mastalgia with or without lump)
- 35–45% with mutation of *BRCA1* gene
- 70% blood spread occurs to bones

Etiology: Carcinoma breast is more common in developed Western countries. In American women, it is more aggressive. It is less common in Japan. It is second most common carcinoma in females. Incidence is 19–34%. Median age is 47 years; more common after middle age, but do can occur at any age group after 20; familial in 2–5% cases. Carcinoma in one breast increases the risk of developing carcinoma on opposite breast by 3–4 times. Incidence of bilateral carcinoma is 2%. Diet low with phytoestrogens, obesity and high alcohol intake may predispose carcinoma. It is common in nulliparous women. Early child bearing and breast feeding reduces the incidence of malignancy. Breast carcinoma is directly related to estrogen level increase. Early menarche and late menopause has got higher risk probably due to increased estrogen level. Breast cancer relative risk is qualified as relative risk (RR). RR 2.0 means risk is twice the normal population. If RR is 0.5 means risk is 50% less than normal population. In males, occasionally gynecomastia turns into carcinoma. Benign breast diseases with atypia, hyperplasia and epitheliosis have got higher risk in a patient with family history of carcinoma breast; mutation of tumor suppressor genes *BRCA 1 and BRCA 2* has also shown high-risk of carcinoma breast. *BRCA 1* has got more risk (35-45%). It is located in long arm of chromosome 17. It is also associated with ovarian carcinoma.

Classification of Carcinoma Breast
Classifications
I. Ductal carcinoma—90%
   Lobular carcinoma—10%
II. a. In situ carcinoma—Intraductal carcinoma without any invasion through basement membrane
    - DCIS (Ductal carcinoma in situ)—5–20%—papillary, cribriform, solid, comedo types
    - LCIS (Lobular carcinoma in situ)—2% [now not classified under carcinoma breast (AJCC 2018)]
   b. Invasive—invasion through basement membrane— 80%.
    - Invasive ductal carcinoma—70%
    - Invasive lobular carcinoma. It is commonly multifocal and often bilateral. It is 10–15%
III. Unilateral
   Bilateral: 2–5% common
IV. Unifocal; Multifocal. Multifocal—tumor tissues within the same quadrant. Multicentric—tumor tissues within the breast but in different quadrant.

Pathological Types
Scirrhous carcinoma (60%): It is hard, whitish, or whitish yellow, noncapsulated, irregular, with gritty, cartilaginous consistency. It contains malignant cells with fibrous stroma.
Medullary carcinoma (10%): It is also called as 'encephaloid type' because of its brain-like consistency. It contains malignant cells with dispersed lymphocytes; occurs in younger age group; associated with BRCA 1 hereditary cancers; soft and often hemorrhagic; carries better prognosis than scirrhous type.
Inflammatory carcinoma/lactating carcinoma/mastitis carcinomatosis (2%): It is common in lactating women or pregnancy; mimics acute mastitis because of its short duration, pain, warmth and tenderness. Clinically, it is rapidly progressive tumor of short duration, often involving entire breast tissue with occurrence of Peau d'orange; extending to the skin and chest wall. It rapidly metastasizes to bone and lungs. *It is always stage IVd carcinoma*. FNAC confirms the diagnosis—It contains undifferentiated cells. It mimics acute mastitis but total count is normal in inflammatory carcinoma of breast.
Colloid carcinoma (2%): It produces abundant mucin; common in elderly; presents as bulky tumor; positive for estrogen receptors.
Paget's disease of the nipple: It is superficial manifestation of an intraductal carcinoma. The malignancy spreads within the duct up to the skin of the nipple and down into the substance of the breast. It mimics eczema of nipple and areola. In Paget's disease, there will be a hard nodule just underneath the areola, which later ulcerates and also causes destruction of nipple. Histologically it contains large, ovoid, clear Paget's cells with malignant features (Fig. 17-72).
Tubular (2%), Papillary *(2%, occurs in elderly), **Cribriform*** are the other types of duct carcinomas.
Atrophic scirrhous carcinoma: It is seen in elderly females; slow growing tumor which has got better prognosis.

Note: Presently invasive breast cancer is classified as ductal and lobular. 70% are invasive breast cancers. It can be infiltrating ductal carcinoma not otherwise specified (NOS); tubular (2%); colloid (2%); medullary (basal like, triple negative means ER/PR/Her2 neu negative, aggressive, 5%).

Spread of carcinoma breast: To lymph nodes by lymphatic permeation up to axillary nodes; through lymphatic embolization from axillary nodes further. Opposite breast and axillary nodes may be involved through internal mammary nodes and dermal lymphatics. Spread through blood can occur to bone (lumbar vertebra, pelvis, and femur), liver, lungs, and brain.

Clinical features: A palpable lump which is painless initially, irregular surface, stony hard in consistency, *fixity to breast tissue*—are typical of carcinoma breast. Nipple retraction, dimpling, puckering of skin, tethering on palpation, skin fixation, ulceration, fungation, fixity to pectoralis major, latissimus dorsi and serratus anterior muscle; fixity to chest wall; palpable axillary nodes which are mobile initially but later gets fixed; palpable supraclavicular lymph nodes; palpable opposite axillary node; blood spread to bone, lungs, liver and brain—are different clinical features.

Locally advanced carcinoma of breast (LACB): It means locally advanced tumor with muscle/chest wall involvement,

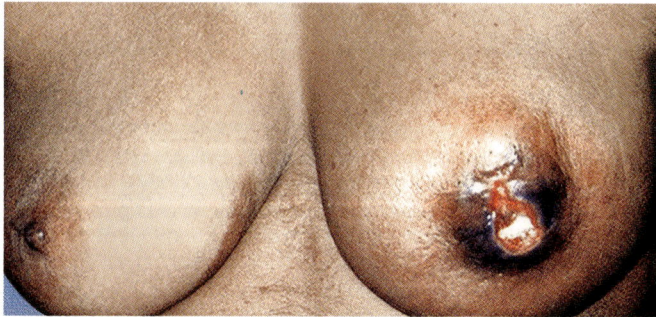

Fig. 17-72 *Subareolar carcinoma with destruction* of nipple—areolar complex

extensive skin involvement or fixed axillary nodes. It will be T3, T4a, T4b, T4c or T4d or N2 or N3. It is investigated by FNAC of tumor, mammography of opposite breast, chest CT, CT abdomen or whole body bone scan.

Metastatic carcinoma of breast: It is blood spread into different places like bone, lungs and pleura, liver, soft tissues, brain and adrenals. It is evaluated by FNAC/incision biopsy, chest CT, LFT, US abdomen, CT abdomen, whole body bone scanning, CT brain, tissue study for ER/PR/Her2 neu receptor status.

Complications after mastectomy with axillary clearance are lymphedema and eventual lymphangiosarcoma (after 3 to many years later) of the limb *(Stewart-Treves syndrome)*.

TNM staging 8th edition (2018)
T – Tumor Criteria
TX Primary tumor cannot be assessed
T0 No evidence of primary tumor
Tis (DCIS)* Ductal carcinoma in situ
Tis (Paget) Paget disease of the nipple NOT associated with invasive carcinoma and/or carcinoma in situ (DCIS) in the underlying breast parenchyma. Carcinomas in the breast parenchyma associated with Paget disease are categorized based on the size and characteristics of the parenchymal disease, although the presence of Paget disease should still be noted.
T1- Tumor ≤ 20 mm in greatest dimension; T1mi Tumor ≤ 1 mm in greatest dimension; T1a Tumor >1 mm but ≤ 5 mm in greatest dimension; T1b Tumor >5 mm but ≤ 10 mm in greatest dimension; T1c Tumor >10 mm but ≤ 20 mm in greatest dimension.
T2 Tumor >20 mm but ≤ 50 mm in greatest dimension
T3 Tumor >50 mm in greatest dimension
T4 Tumor of any size with direct extension to the chest wall and/or to the skin (ulceration or macroscopic nodules); invasion of the dermis alone does not qualify as T4; T4a Extension to the chest wall; invasion or adherence to pectoralis muscle in the absence of invasion of chest wall structures does not qualify as T4; T4b Ulceration and/or ipsilateral macroscopic satellite nodules and/or edema (including Peau d'orange) of the skin that does not meet the criteria for inflammatory carcinoma; T4c both T4a and T4b are present; T4d inflammatory carcinoma.
Note: Lobular carcinoma in situ (LCIS) is a benign entity and is removed from TNM staging in the AJCC Cancer Staging Manual, 8th Edition.

N – Node
CNx – Regional nodes cannot be assessed or previously removed.
CN0 – No regional nodes by imaging or clinical.
CN1 – Metastases with mobile ipsilateral level I and II axillary nodes.
CN1mi – Metastases larger than 0.2 mm but less than 2 mm with approximately 200 cells.
CN2 – Metastases to clinically palpable level I, II ipsilateral axillary lymph nodes that are clinically fixed or matted (CN2a); or ipsilateral internal mammary nodes in the absence of axillary nodes (CN2b).
CN3 – Metastases to ipsilateral infraclavicular (level III) nodes with or without level I and II axillary nodes (CN3a); to ipsilateral internal mammary nodes along with ipsilateral axillary nodes (CN3b); to ipsilateral supraclavicular nodes.

M – Distant metastases
M0 – No clinical or radiological evidence of distant spread
CM0 (i+) – No distant spread clinically or radiologically but presence of tumor cells less than 0.2 mm in size detected in the circulating blood or bone marrow or nonregional nodal tissues microscopy or molecular technique.
CM1 – Distant spread detected clinically and radiologically.

Staging
Stage I: T1N0M0. *Stage IIa:* T0N1M0, T1N1M0, T2N0M0. *Stage IIb:* T2N1M0, T3N0M0. *Stage IIIa:* T0N2M0, T1N2M0, T2N2M0, T3N1M0, T3N2M0. *Stage IIIb:* T4N0M0, T4N1M0, T4N2M0. *Stage IIIc:* Any TN3M0. *Stage IV:* Any T, any N, M.

■ BENIGN AND INFLAMMATORY CONDITIONS OF BREAST

Condition	Features
Fibroadenoma It is a benign encapsulated tumor; common in females (15–25 yrs) Classified under ANDI; considered as hyperplasia of single lobule of the breast **Types**: Soft/hard/giant (>5 cm size) Pericanicular/intracanalicular	Painless swelling in one of the quadrants of breast (common in lower); smooth, firm, non-tender, well-localized, and moves within the breast tissue (*"mouse in the breast"*). Axillary lymph nodes not enlarged **Investigation**: Mammography; FNAC
Fibrocystadenosis: (*Fibrocystic disease of breast/mammary dysplasia*) It is an estrogen dependent condition; common in menstruating age group. It is due to ANDI of breast causing fibrosis; cyst formation; glandular proliferation (adenosis); hyperplasia (epitheliosis)	Presents with pain and tenderness in breast during menstruation (*cyclical mastalgia*) subsides during pregnancy, lactation, and after menopause. Bilateral, painful, diffuse, granular, tender, swelling better felt by fingers than by palm, not fixed to skin, muscle, chest wall Nipple discharge if present –serous/greenish *Blood good cyst* is one of cysts get enlarged presenting as cystic swelling in the breast
Cystosarcoma phyllodes/ serocystic disease of Brodie It may be a variant of intracanalicular fibroadenoma breast; occur in premenopausal women (30–50 yrs); it is not simply giant fibroadenoma; shows wide spectrum of activity varying from almost benign condition to locally aggressive and sometimes with metastatic potential to lungs	Unilateral breast swelling grows rapidly to attain large size; swelling is smooth, nontender, soft, fluctuant, with pressure necrosis of skin over the summit (probing can be done easily between the skin and the swelling across the necrosed skin) *Gross*: Large capsulated swelling with cystic spaces and cut surface shows soft, brownish, cystic areas *Microscopy:* Cystic spaces with leaf like projections; cells show hypercellularity and pleomorphism
Traumatic fat necrosis: It may be either due to direct or indirect trauma (often forgotten). Capillary ooze following trauma causes triglycerides in the fat to dissociate into fatty acids which combines with calcium from blood resulting in saponification—causes inflammatory reaction –later presenting as nonprogressive mass in the breast	Painless swelling in the breast, smooth, hard, nontender, adherent to breast tissue; mimics carcinoma breast *Investigations*: FNAC—chalky fluid with fat globules; Mammography; Excision biopsy—confirmatory

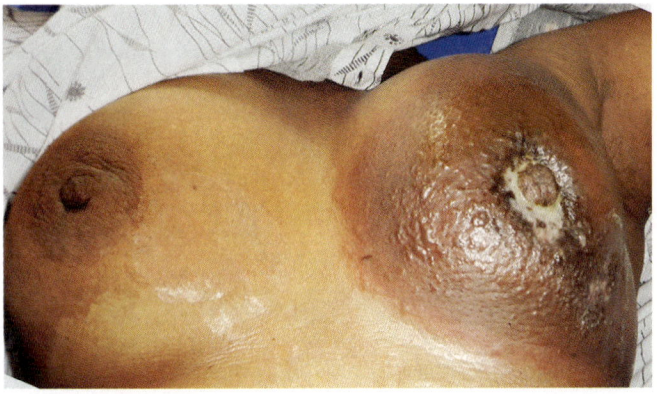

Fig. 17-73 Advanced carcinoma breast – cancer en cuirasse.

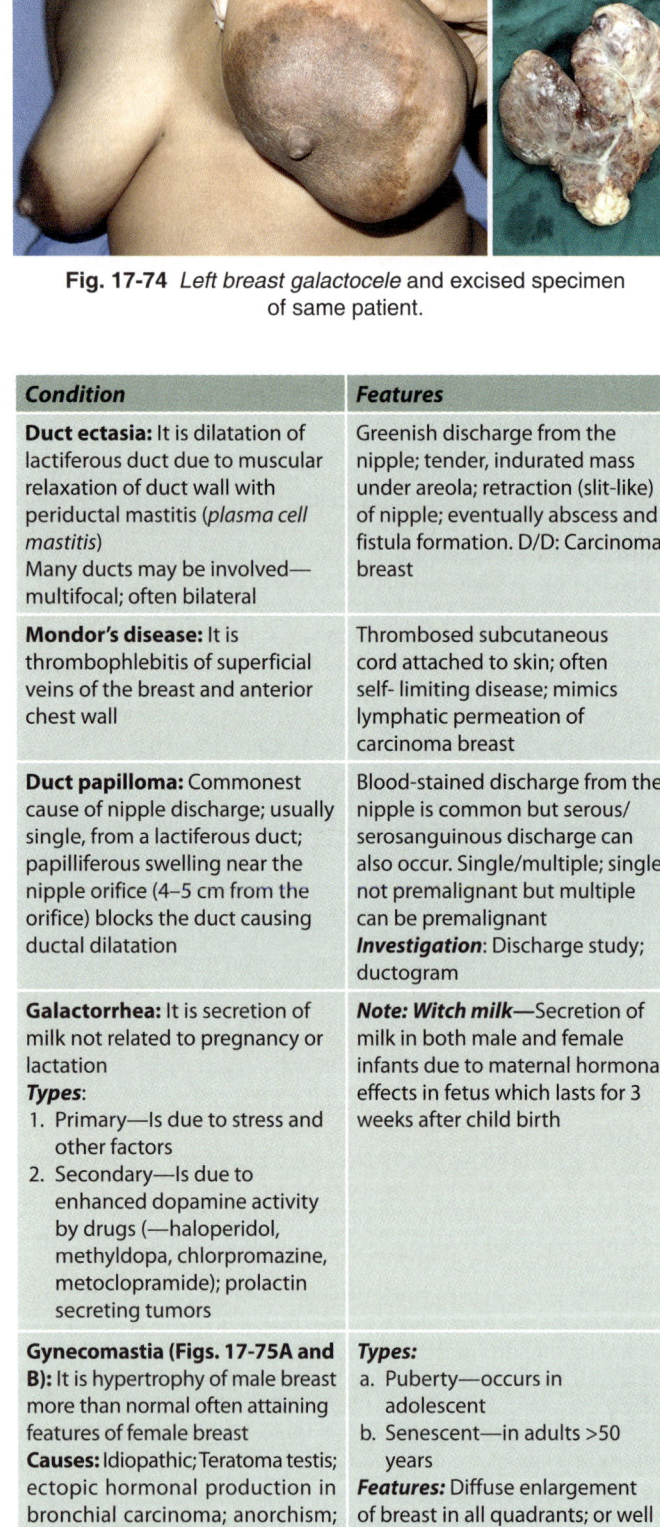

Fig. 17-74 Left breast *galactocele* and excised specimen of same patient.

Condition	Features
Galactocele: It is a *retention cyst*–sub areolar type seen in lactating women (can occur even after 6–10 months of cessation of breastfeeding)	Lump in the lower quadrant of breast, usually unilateral, large, freely mobile, soft, fluctuant, smooth surface nontender; it may get precipitated, inspissated, or get calcified; when calcified mimics carcinoma breast **Complication:** Infection—breast abscess (Fig. 17-74) **Investigation:** USG; FNAC
Mastitis: It is infection and inflammation of breast tissue **Types:** 1. **Subareolar:** Infection under the areola due to cracks in the nipple and areola 2. **Intramammary:** Infection within the breast tissue a. *Lactational abscess:* Common in lactating women; infection enters through cracked nipple or blood spread. *Staphylococcus aureus* commonest; gram negative and other bacteria also can supervene later b. *Non-lactational abscess:* Commonly occurs in duct ectasia; peri-areolar infection Bacteroides, enterococci, gram-negative, anaerobic streptococci—involved 3. **Retromammary mastitis:** It is due to tuberculosis of intercostal lymph nodes or ribs beneath or suppuration of intercostal lymph nodes	1. Red inflamed oedematous areola with tender swelling underneath. D/D: Paget's disease of the nipple 2. a. Pain in the breast; fever; diffuse redness; tenderness; induration; purulent discharge from the nipple; Initially one quadrant later whole breast may be involved. D/D: Inflammatory carcinoma of breast. **Complications:** Antibioma; sinus; recurrent infection b. Recurrent tender swelling under the areola 3. Here breast is normal
Antibioma: If inflammatory mastitis not drained but only treated with antibiotics, pus becomes sterile and localizes with thick fibrous tissue cover	Previous history of mastitis treated with antibiotics; painless swelling, smooth, nontender, hard, fixed to breast tissue, not to muscle and chest wall D/D: Scirrhous carcinoma breast

Condition	Features
Duct ectasia: It is dilatation of lactiferous duct due to muscular relaxation of duct wall with periductal mastitis (*plasma cell mastitis*) Many ducts may be involved—multifocal; often bilateral	Greenish discharge from the nipple; tender, indurated mass under areola; retraction (slit-like) of nipple; eventually abscess and fistula formation. D/D: Carcinoma breast
Mondor's disease: It is thrombophlebitis of superficial veins of the breast and anterior chest wall	Thrombosed subcutaneous cord attached to skin; often self-limiting disease; mimics lymphatic permeation of carcinoma breast
Duct papilloma: Commonest cause of nipple discharge; usually single, from a lactiferous duct; papilliferous swelling near the nipple orifice (4–5 cm from the orifice) blocks the duct causing ductal dilatation	Blood-stained discharge from the nipple is common but serous/serosanguinous discharge can also occur. Single/multiple; single not premalignant but multiple can be premalignant **Investigation:** Discharge study; ductogram
Galactorrhea: It is secretion of milk not related to pregnancy or lactation **Types:** 1. Primary—Is due to stress and other factors 2. Secondary—Is due to enhanced dopamine activity by drugs (—haloperidol, methyldopa, chlorpromazine, metoclopramide); prolactin secreting tumors	*Note: Witch milk*—Secretion of milk in both male and female infants due to maternal hormonal effects in fetus which lasts for 3 weeks after child birth
Gynecomastia (Figs. 17-75A and B): It is hypertrophy of male breast more than normal often attaining features of female breast **Causes:** Idiopathic; Teratoma testis; ectopic hormonal production in bronchial carcinoma; anorchism; after castration; adrenal and pituitary disease; leprosy; bilateral testicular atrophy; Drugs (stilbesterol, digitalis, cimetidine, spironolactone); liver disease and failure; Klinefelter's syndrome	**Types:** a. Puberty—occurs in adolescent b. Senescent—in adults >50 years **Features:** Diffuse enlargement of breast in all quadrants; or well localized, small, firm or hard nodule under the areola often painful and tender

Chapter 17: Clinical Approaches and Examination of Breast

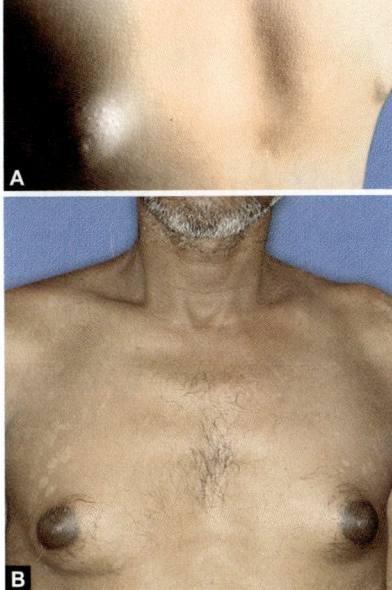

Figs. 17-75A and B *Gynecomastia*—right side breast in a young male. Compare to opposite side to note the difference in size. Bilateral gynecomastia in another old man is also shown.

Condition	Features
Tuberculosis of breast: Relatively rare but not uncommon in developing countries like India; usually associated with active pulmonary tuberculosis	Swelling in the breast with cold abscess, sinuses, typical bluish appearance of surrounding skin with matted lymph nodes in the ipsilateral axilla D/D: Carcinoma breast

Condition	Features
Mammary fistula of Atkins: Fistula from lactiferous duct to areolar skin	Recurrent abscesses beneath the areola those points through the surface causing discharging fistula
Tietze's syndrome: It is costochondritis of 2nd costal cartilage commonly seen in females, mimics mastalgia	
Congenital anomalies of breast: *Amastia* is 'absence of breast' with absence of nipple *Amazia* is 'absence of breast with presence of nipple'; it is actually 'hypoplasia of breast' Absence of breast, absence of sternal portion of pectoralis major muscle with Syndactyly of same side hand; common in males; common on right side is called as *Poland's syndrome* True polythelia is more than one nipple to one breast. Accessory nipple may be rudimentary and often looks like a mole. Diffuse hyperplasia; pendulous breasts; underdeveloped breasts are other anomalies which cause cosmetic challenge.	Accessory breasts (*Polymazia*) and nipple (*polythelia, supernumerary nipples*) can develop in axilla, groin and thigh (along the milk line). It may be unilateral or bilateral. It is due to failure of the disappearance of milk line which occurs during developmental period in normal individual. These accessory breasts may secrete milk during lactation. Accessory breast tissue is common in the axilla above the normal breast tissue

CASE DISCUSSION

A 55-year-postmenopausal woman comes with painless lump in the right breast. Duration is not clear as she noticed it only a day back to come immediately to clinician. She does not have any fever; no hemoptysis or cough; no history of back pain, headache or convulsions and abdominal fullness. She gave the history that her elder sister had similar complaint for which she was operated. On local examination, hard lump of 5 × 4 cm size is palpable in the right breast over upper outer quadrant, which is having smooth surface, hard consistency and adherent to breast tissue but not fixed to pectoralis major or latissimus dorsi muscles or to chest wall. Skin is free. Axillary lymph nodes are not palpable. Abdomen, respiratory system, spine are normal. Neurological deficits are not present.

What is the diagnosis?
Diagnosis is carcinoma right breast—$T_2N_0M_0$—Stage IIa.

Why you said it is carcinoma breast?
Postmenopausal age group with a painless lump, which is hard and adherent to breast tissue. Fibroadenoma or fibroadenosis are unlikely in this age group. Traumatic fat necrosis, antibioma of breast or tuberculosis are the other possible differential diagnoses but less likely.

How you will evaluate the patient?
Trucut biopsy for histological confirmation and for molecular staging (ER, PR, Her2 Neu) is done. Trucut biopsy is better than FNAC. US of both ipsilateral and opposite breasts are done. US axilla confirms the clinical finding. Chest X-ray, US abdomen, liver function tests are needed. CT chest and isotope bone scan may be needed only if there are symptoms or features suggestive of involvement. Mammography of the same and opposite side breasts is useful.

18 CHAPTER
Clinical Approaches and Examination of Hernia

Competency: AN15.3; AN15.4; AN44.4; AN44.5.

Hernia is an important clinical topic for undergraduates as well as postgraduate students in surgery. It is one of the commonest surgical entities that surgeons come across and so detailed knowledge of the subject is mandatory to both undergraduates and postgraduates.

Hernia means—*'to bud'* or *'to protrude'* (of sac) in Greek; *'to rupture'* (causing defect) in Latin. *It is commonly defined as protrusion of the organ entirely or partly through its containing wall*; it may be visceral hernias in groin, abdominal wall, internal hernias or hernia through thoracic wall or herniation of brain through traumatized skull or through foramen magnum into the spinal canal or muscular hernia through fascial defect. Defect is abnormal opening which may be natural or acquired and usually accompanied by the lining of the cavity from which it protrudes (sac). *In actual fact*, hernia means *defect* (defect is the hernia) and sac; protrusion of the content is not mandatory which is the eventual effect and that is why in many occasions hernia may present only with dragging pain without swelling *(occult)* or patient gives history of occasional protrusion of the swelling but not always; and when clinician examines the patient, expansile cough impulse may not be present.

Groin (inguinal, femoral) and ventral (abdominal) are commonest type of hernias; they are being discussed in this chapter. Hernia is protrusion of entire or part of the viscus through the wall that contains it. Herniation can occur from any cavities or through any defects—congenital or acquired. Inguinal, femoral, umbilical, incisional and epigastric are common hernias (Figs. 18-1 to 18-8); obturator, gluteal, lumbar or spigelian are rare hernias.

The groin even though anatomically is not a well-defined area, it includes inguinal and femoral regions; both are separated by medial part of the inguinal ligament. Clinically when hip is fully flexed inguinal and femoral regions touch each other and that area is recognized as groin. Sebaceous cyst, lipoma and neurofibroma are swellings arising from integuments; inguinal and femoral are hernias; lymphadenopathy; saphena varix and aneurysms are

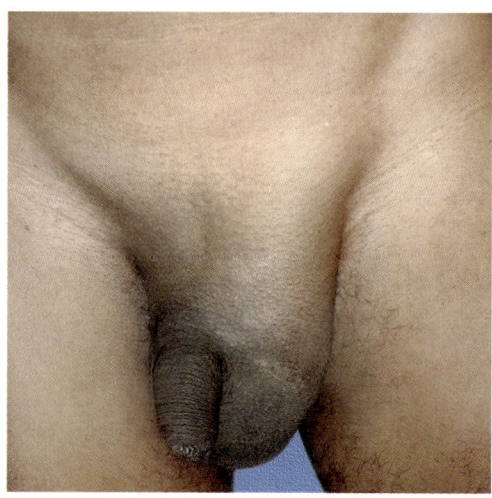

Fig. 18-1 Left sided indirect inguinal hernia; it *is common type of hernia*. It is *pyriform in shape*.

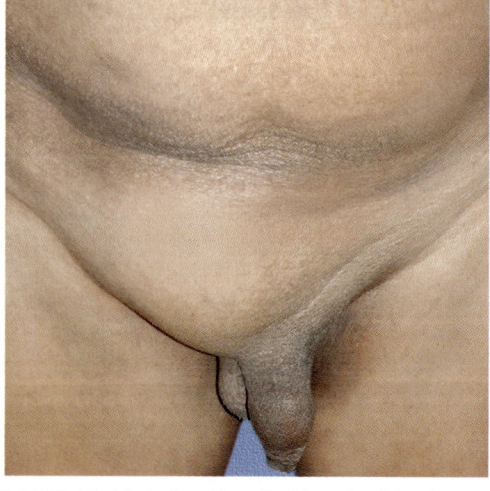

Fig. 18-2 Right sided direct inguinal hernia; it is also common variety. It is *globular in shape*.

Chapter 18: Clinical Approaches and Examination of Hernia

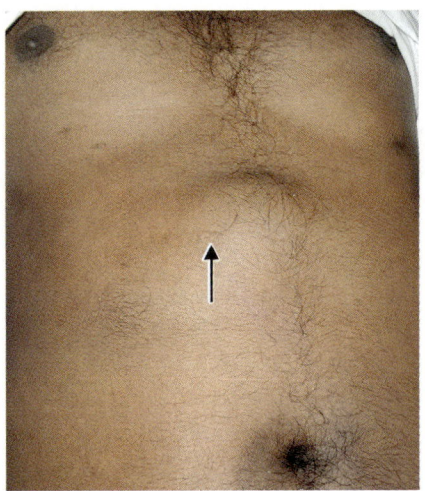

Fig. 18-3 Typical epigastric hernia. It is *herniation through linea alba*.

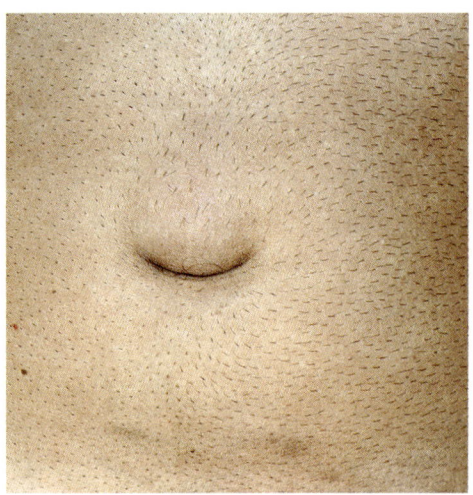

Fig. 18-6 *Paraumbilical hernia.*

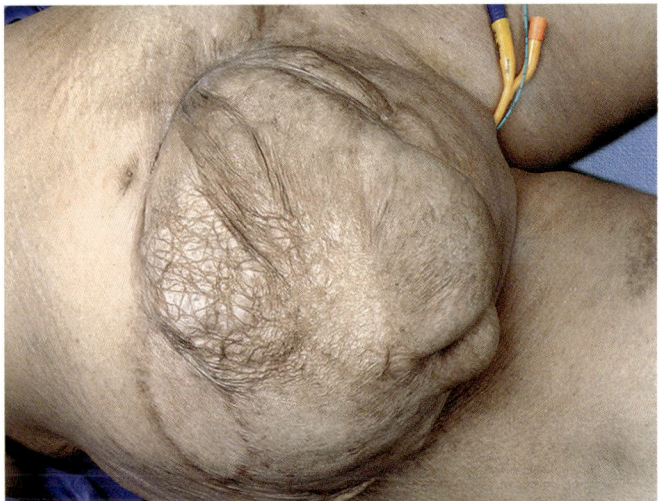

Fig. 18-4 Incisional hernia lower abdomen—*it is one of the ventral hernias.*

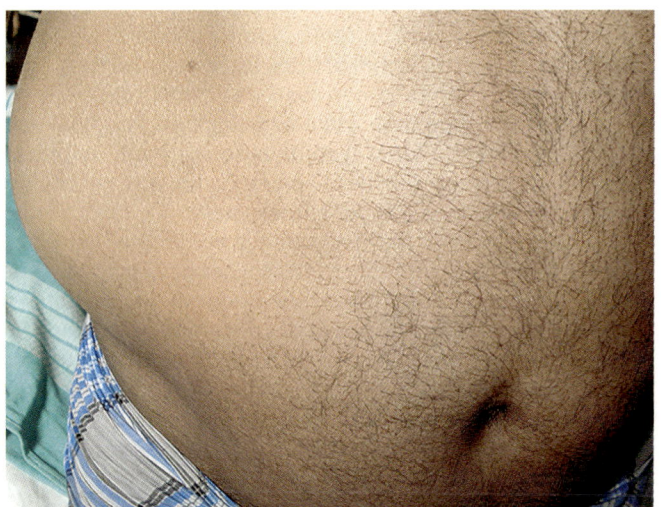

Fig. 18-7 *Lumbar hernia.*

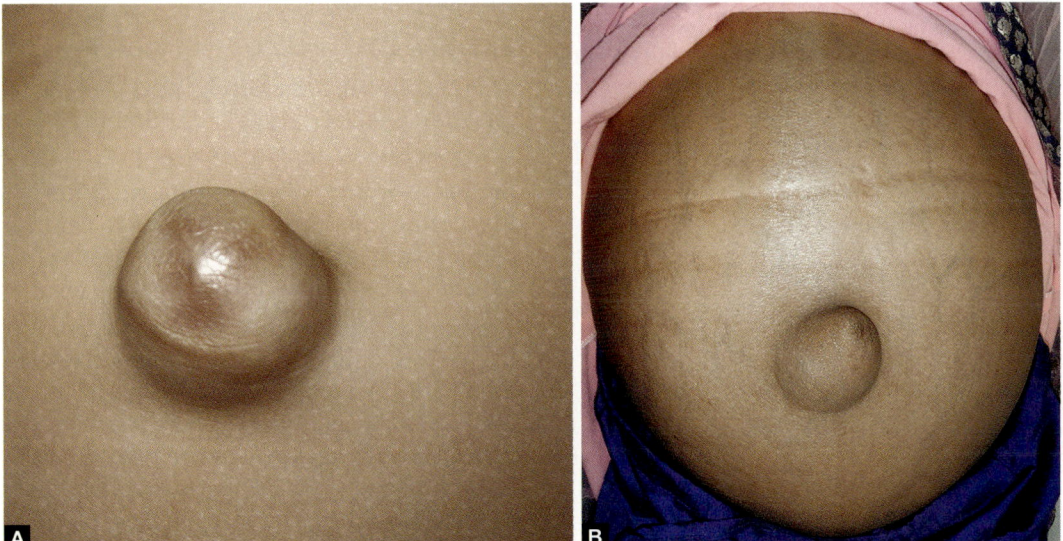

Figs. 18-5A and B (A) Umbilical hernia in a child. *It is congenital; it may regress spontaneously*; (B) *In adult umbilical hernia is acquired* often due to underlying ascites.

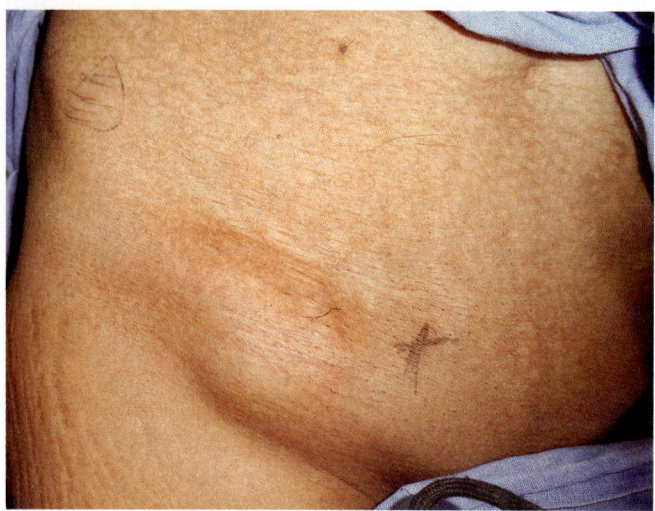

Fig. 18-8 Right sided femoral hernia; it is below and lateral to pubic tubercle; sac here is retort shaped.

vascular swellings; ectopic testis, lipoma or hydrocele of the cord, hydrocele of the canal of Nuck (in females) are inguinal canal related swellings; psoas abscess which is deeper—are groin swellings. Common groin swellings are inguinal and femoral hernias, inguinal lymphadenopathy and saphena varix. *Groin pain* may be due to hernia, funiculitis, varicocele, lymph node diseases or post surgery pain.

Inguinal hernia is the commonest abdominal hernia. It occurs through inguinal canal. Indirect hernia comes through deep ring along the cord; direct from posterior wall of inguinal canal. Usually indirect hernia is of congenital origin, occurs in a pre-existing processus vaginalis sac but often revealed later by some precipitating factors whereas direct hernia is always acquired due to weakening of posterior wall of the inguinal canal. Inguinal hernia initially is incomplete but becomes complete once it descends up to the bottom of the scrotum. *Two factors cause hernia*—one is weakness of the wall (weakness may be congenital or acquired); another is raised intra-abdominal pressure.

Parts of inguinal hernia: It consists of neck, body and fundus (Fig. 18-9). Neck is narrow in indirect sac which is obliquely placed in the inguinal canal (oblique hernia). Neck is wide in direct sac which is placed posteriorly, medially and directly. Neck is lateral to inferior epigastric artery in indirect sac; medial to inferior epigastric artery in direct sac (Fig. 18-10). Sac is opened in the fundus in indirect sac. Sac is usually not required to be opened in direct sac unless there is/are adhesions.

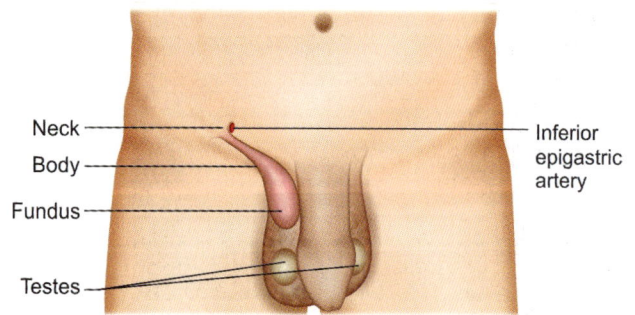

Fig. 18-9 Parts of hernia—*neck, body and fundus*.

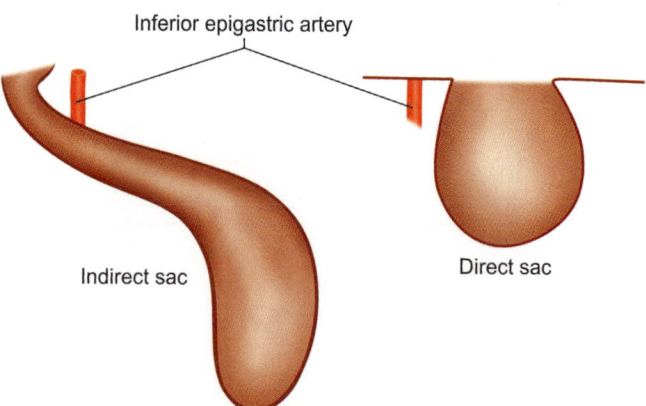

Fig. 18-10 Diagrammatic representations of *direct and indirect sacs*.

HISTORY

Name:

Age: Elderly people are more prone for direct hernia. Indirect hernia occurs in young, direct hernia occurs in old age.

Sex: Inguinal hernia is common in males (20:1, male to female ratio) and femoral hernia in females. But one should note that in females, commonest groin hernia is inguinal hernia. (Incisional hernia is also common in women).

Occupation: Men with strainfull occupation like manual laborers, sportsmen, weight lifters, gymnasts are more prone for hernia.

Chief Complaints

Swelling in the groin, right or left or both sided or swelling in the inguinoscrotal region— right/left/both sides—with duration.

Pain over the swelling—with duration. Pain in hernia may be due to adhesions, narrow neck.

History of Present Illness

Swelling

Duration of the swelling: Hernia usually has a long duration.

Mode of onset of the swelling: It may be spontaneous (hernia due to congenital defect) or on straining (coughing or lifting heavy weight) or after trauma (surgery).

Site of the first appearance of the swelling—in the groin or in the scrotum should be asked. Inguinal hernia begins in groin whereas hydrocele is purely scrotal which begins in scrotum. Femoral hernia begins below the groin crease line.

Progress and extent of the swelling: Whether it only limits to the groin or extends to the scrotum is to be asked. Congenital inguinal hernia, often seen in children but can occur at any age, the swelling reaches the bottom of the scrotum at its first appearance whereas in acquired type, the swelling is small to begin with and gradually increases in size. In femoral hernia, swelling is seen below the groin crease and gradually ascends up.

Changes in the size and extent of the swelling—on standing/walking/straining/lying down should be asked.

Reducibility of the swelling: Whether the swelling disappears on its own on lying down (direct hernia); or can be reduced by some maneuver (indirect hernia) should be also asked. If reducible then whether it completely disappears/partially/not reducible at all (irreducible hernia) has to be asked. In irreducible swelling, one should ask for the history of pain, any abdominal distension, vomiting.

History of gurgling sound in the scrotum while reducing the hernia which signifies enterocele is to be asked.

Pain

Type and severity of pain: Pain may precede the swelling in persons who are about to develop hernia and is dragging/aching type of pain in the groin more after straining, that worsens at the end of day. Pain in an existing hernia may be due to drag on omentum/mesentery, adhesions, inflammation, obstruction or strangulation. In inflamed/obstructed or strangulated hernia, pain is severe pricking type. Radiation of pain should be asked for.

Site of pain: Whether it is in the groin or in the scrotum is asked. In strangulated hernia, severe pain is present all over the abdomen.

Duration of pain—early stages of hernia are often painless but as the complication sets in, pain appears drawing the patient's attention.

Aggravating or relieving factors should be asked. Pain may be aggravated on straining/walking/weight lifting; relieved on lying down.

History suggestive of complications: Irreducibility, severe pain in the groin over the swelling, colicky abdominal pain, abdominal distension, vomiting, and constipation all suggestive of strangulation/obstruction should be asked. Frequency, character of vomitus (bilious/watery/feculent) should be asked. **Obstruction** causes abdominal distension and vomiting. **Strangulation** causes toxicity, and severe pain and tenderness. **Incarcerated hernia** is irreducible but bowel is not strangulated or obstructed; here, contents are fixed in the sac because of their size and adhesions.

History relevant to precipitating factors:
- History of chronic cough due to tuberculosis, bronchial asthma or other respiratory diseases.
- History of constipation, altered bowel habits, tenesmus, bloody stool— in relation to anorectal stricture/carcinoma.
- History of dysuria, urgency, hesitancy, altered stream, night frequency, retention of urine, burning urine, hematuria (irritative and obstructive)—in relation to benign prostatic hyperplasia/urethral stricture **(Fig. 18-11)**.

Past History

Past history of hernia surgery—same side/opposite side. Type of surgery done—whether mesh is used or repair is done; whether open or laparoscopic approach is used; whether emergency or elective hernia surgery, should be asked. Past history suggestive of irreducibility/obstruction and treatment

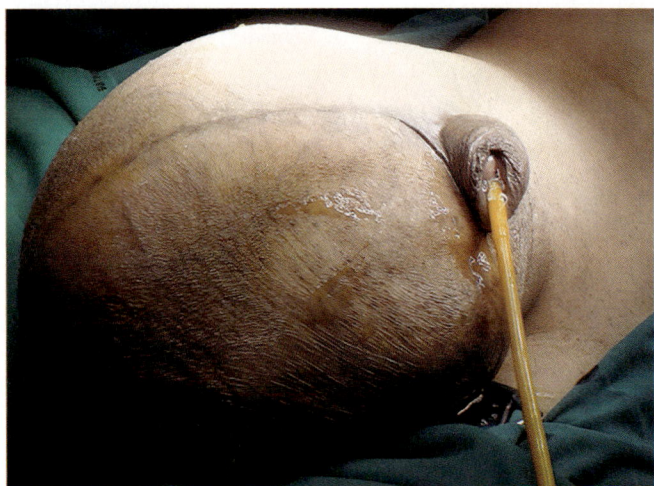

Fig. 18-11 Right-sided complete inguinal hernia in a patient with *benign prostatic hyperplasia (BPH)* who is on Foley's catheter. He needs transurethral resection of prostate (TURP) with hernioplasty.

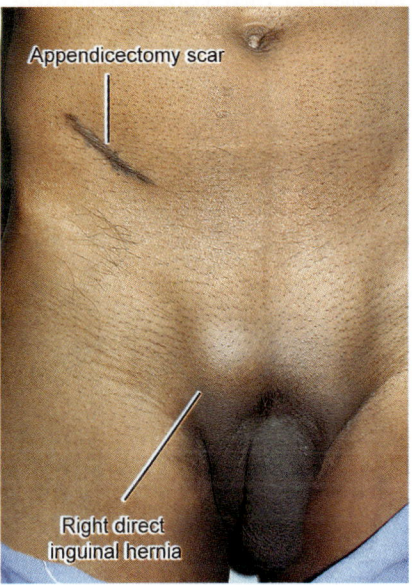

Fig. 18-12 Direct hernia (right-sided) after appendicectomy *due to injury to ilioinguinal nerve.*

received for that, whether conservative/surgical should be asked.

History of appendicectomy done earlier (ilioinguinal nerve may be injured causing right-sided direct hernia) or any *abdominal surgery* (ureterolithotomy, colostomy, lumbar sympathectomy) done and if so details about the surgery (indication—emergency/elective, details of postoperative wound, other postoperative morbidity like cough, abdominal distension, paralytic ileus) are asked **(Figs. 18-12 to 18-15)**.

History of treatment for diabetes, gonorrhea, tuberculosis, branchial asthma at present or in the past.

Personal History

History of smoking—duration and number per day, whether beedi or cigarette should be asked. ***History of pan chewing/***

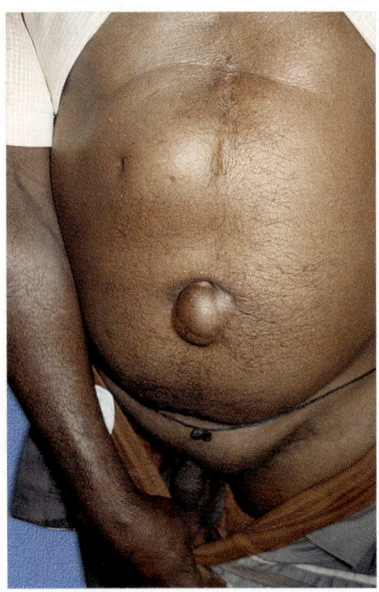

Fig. 18-13 *Multiple hernias*—incisional hernia; paraumbilical hernia; left sided inguinal hernia.

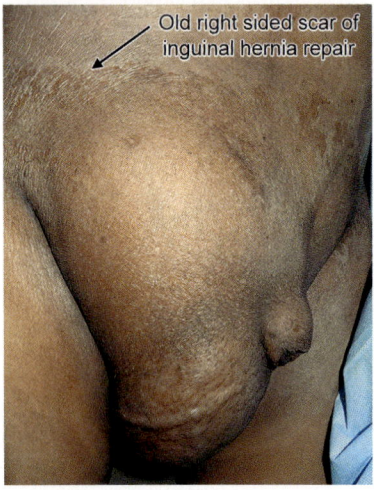

Fig. 18-14 Right sided recurrent hernia. *Note the scar of previous surgery.*

alcohol intake. Appetite and altered weight should be asked—recent history of acute loss of weight can predispose hernia. History of exposure to syphilis, gonorrhea should be asked.

GENERAL EXAMINATION

Examination is done to look for general built and nutritional status, pallor, clubbing, cyanosis, jaundice, lymphadenopathy and edema feet. Pulse and blood pressure are recorded.

LOCAL EXAMINATION

Inguinoscrotal region should be examined in standing position as swelling commonly reduces and disappears in lying down position. Area from umbilicus to mid thigh region should be exposed after taking consent for examination. Examiner sits on a stool on the right side of the patient. Later again inspection is also done in lying down supine position. Patient will be more comfortable in lying down position and reduction of the contents and examination of the abdomen are easier in lying down position.

Inspection

Inspection is always first done **in standing** straight position without bending, **later in lying** down position.

Inspection in standing position (Fig. 18-16): Both sides are observed and *side of the swelling (right/left)* should be mentioned.

Exact site and extent of the swelling—is important. Incomplete indirect inguinal hernia and usually direct inguinal hernia are located in inguinal region. Complete indirect inguinal hernia (rarely complete direct inguinal hernia) is inguinoscrotal. Swelling extends from the proximal part of the inguinal canal towards the scrotum below. Whereas direct inguinal hernia has little tendency to extend to the

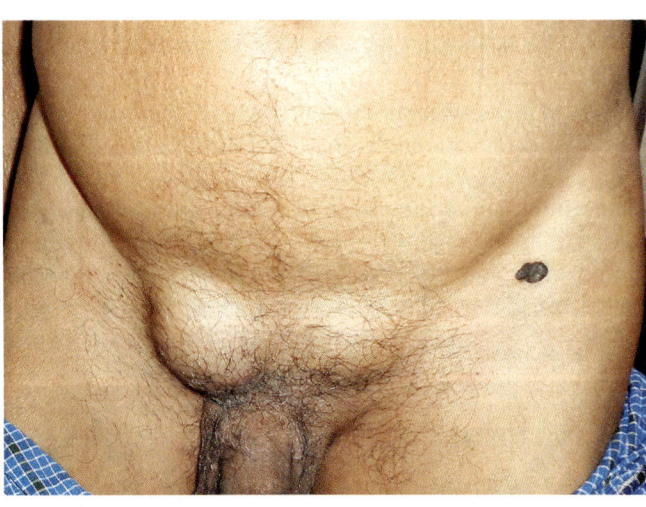

Fig. 18-15 Bilateral direct hernia. Note the medial location of the hernia. *Direct hernia occurs through Hesselbach's triangle.*

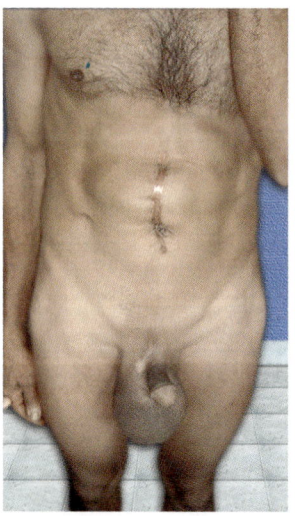

Fig. 18-16 All hernias should be inspected initially *on standing.*

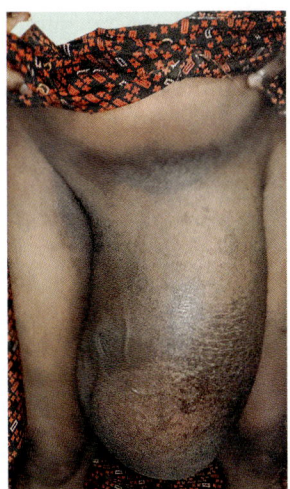

Fig. 18-17 *Giant hernia*. Note that bottom of the hernia in the scrotum is below the level of middle of the thigh (scrotal abdomen). Note also the burial of penis. Management is difficult in such patient as often the contents cannot be reduced completely into the abdomen cavity during surgery as peritoneal cavity is reduced in size; if done forcibly, it results in abdominal compartment syndrome with IVC compression and diaphragmatic elevation. (*Courtesy:* Professor Ramlingam, Kamineni Institution of Medical Sciences, Narkatpally, Telangana, India).

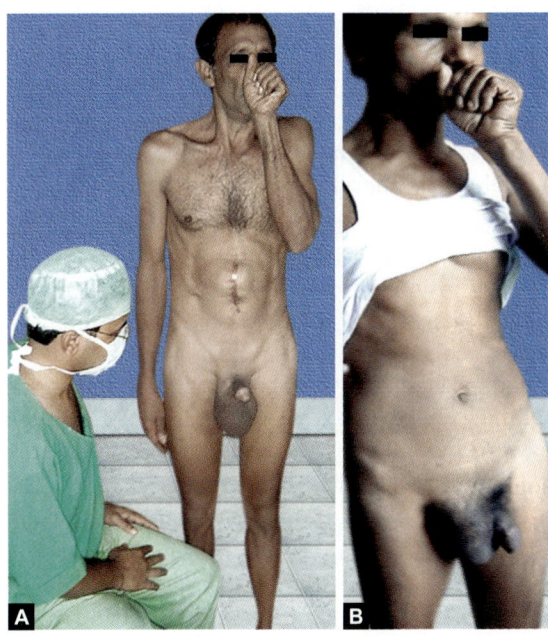

Figs. 18-18A and B *Expansile impulse on coughing is better seen than felt*. It should be inspected with patient standing and examiner sitting beside the patient.

bottom of the scrotum **(Fig. 18-17)**. Femoral hernia lies below the groin crease, below and lateral to pubic tubercle and extends upwards.

Size: Both transverse and vertical dimensions should be mentioned.

Shape of the swelling: It is **pyriform** shaped swelling in indirect inguinal hernia and **globular/hemispherical** in direct inguinal hernia or femoral hernia.

Surface: Smooth/uneven; *Margin*—well-defined/ill-defined.

Expansile impulse on coughing over the swelling is diagnostic. *It is better seen but also can be felt.* While the patient is in standing position, examiner sits beside the patient, and patient is asked to turn his face to opposite side (to prevent coughing towards examiner) and cough. Expansile impulse is visible in the groin area; or if swelling already exists, it will become much more prominent as the intestines or omentum (contents) gets driven into the hernial sac. ***Expansile impulse is momentary increase in the size of the swelling*** or appearance of the swelling during the act of coughing **(Figs. 18.18A and B)**. Often swelling appears only during act of coughing and disappears later. Absence of expansile impulse does not rule out the possibility of hernia.

> **Expansile impulse on coughing is seen in:**
> - Hernia
> - Meningocele
> - Laryngocele
> - Empyema necessitans
> - Intracranially extended dermoid
> - Saphena varix

Skin over the swelling is usually normal. Any scar/dilated veins/discoloration/redness over the swelling should be seen. Scar of recurrent hernia may be evident. Type of scar, linear or wide; healed by primary or secondary intention should be assessed. Infected wound causes wide deep puckered scar which may be the cause for recurrence. Skin may be stretched. Atrophy of skin can occur. In strangulated hernia, skin may be edematous and red. Wearing hernia truss may cause brown pigmentation of skin over the external ring due to hemosiderin deposition. Occasionally strangulated hernia may cause ulceration due to skin necrosis.

Visible peristalsis over the swelling should be noted if present (should not be mistaken for dartos muscle contraction). It means it could be enterocele. Visible peristalsis is difficult to observe or not seen in femoral hernia.

Surrounding structures: On inspection, whether testis is seen separately from the swelling or covered by the swelling all over should be noted, suggesting hernia is incomplete or complete. Penis may be pushed to opposite side in large scrotal hernia.

> **The features of hernia:**
> - Expansile impulse on coughing
> - Reducibility of the content on lying down or by direct pressure
> *Note:* These two features may be absent once hernia is strangulated.

Palpation

The landmarks at the inguinal region—pubic tubercle, inguinal ligament and anterior superior iliac spine are noted. Pubic tubercle may be reached by following the tendon of adductor longus. The patient is asked to adduct the thigh against resistance; the tendon of the adductor longus is palpated at the upper medial aspect of the thigh; tracing adductor longus upwards will reach bony pubic tubercle point. A skin crease run across the lower abdomen, convex downwards, separating the abdomen from the triangle called as mons veneris. The center of this crease on the upper edge of the pubic bones is noted; pubic tubercle lies beneath this crease 2–3 cm from the midline. Finger is placed at the center of this crease and pushed inwards to feel the pubic crest and pubic tubercle. Last bony point felt while following the iliac crest from back is anterior superior iliac spine.

Palpation should be done ideally both in standing and lying down position. In standing position, clinician either sits on a stool or stands on the same side of the hernia; one hand is placed on the back of the patient to support; examining fingers and hand are placed gently over the hernial swelling parallel to the inguinal ligament. One should not poke the fingers into the inguinal canal which will be very painful. Location, size, shape, warmness, tenderness, tension, composition (fluid, gas, solid) and reducibility should be ascertained.

Location of the swelling—*swelling is above and medial to pubic tubercle in inguinal hernia and below and lateral to pubic tubercle in femoral hernia* **(Figs. 18-19 and 18-20)**. This description actually refers to the point at which the hernia reduces into the abdominal wall, not to the position of the entire hernia. In obese patients, often it may be difficult to differentiate between inguinal and femoral hernia. Occasionally femoral hernia may ascend upwards from saphenous opening superficial to inguinal ligament to present as swelling in inguinal region which is invariably irreducible. Very rarely obturator hernia case present as swelling in the upper medial part of thigh.

When the swelling is only above the inguinal ligament, it is purely inguinal swelling. When the inguinal swelling extends into the scrotum, it is called as inguinoscrotal swelling.

To get above the swelling—whether it is possible to *get above the swelling* or not is checked: one can get above a purely scrotal swelling but not in inguinoscrotal swelling. It is checked in **standing** position. Palpation initially begins from bottom of the scrotum, between the thumb in front, index and middle fingers behind progressing upwards towards root of the scrotum which is held firmly but gently. In purely scrotal swelling like vaginal hydrocele, fingers and thumb can be approximated well without any additional structures other than cord in between (*one can get above the swelling*). In case of inguinoscrotal swelling, thumb and fingers do not meet each other properly because of the descent of hernial contents down (*one cannot get above the swelling*). It occurs in funicular and complete type of inguinal hernia but not in bubonocele **(Figs. 18-21A and B)**.

Temperature and tenderness over the swelling is noted. In strangulated/inflamed hernia, the swelling in the groin is tender and warm.

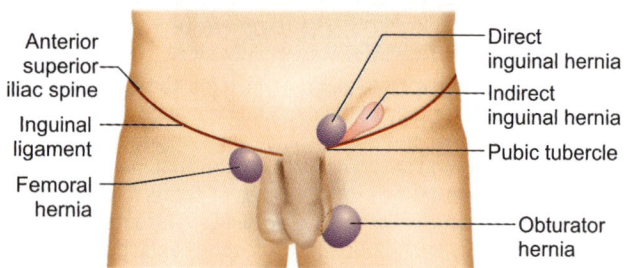

Fig. 18-20 *Anatomical location of indirect, direct, femoral and obturator hernias.* Inguinal hernia is above and medial to pubic tubercle. Femoral hernia is below and lateral to pubic tubercle. Also note the location of the obturator hernia below in Scarpa's triangle.

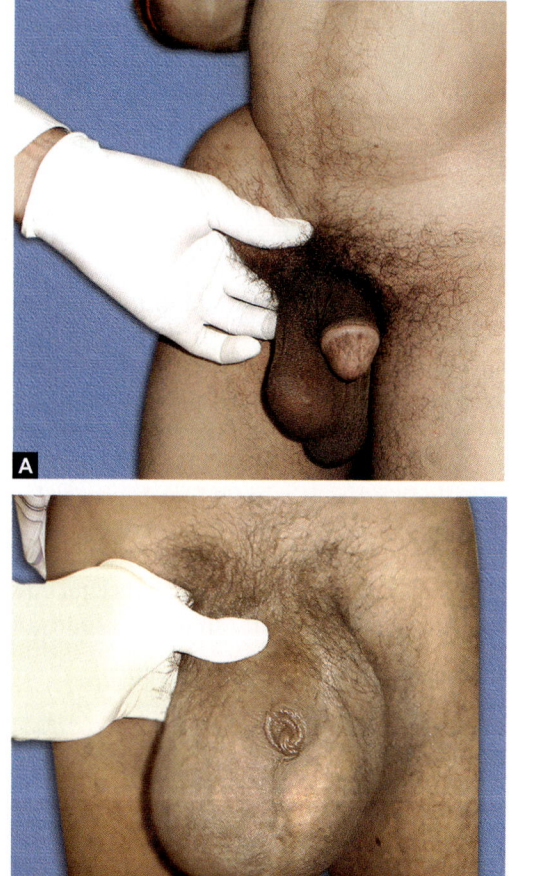

Figs. 18-21A and B In inguinoscrotal swelling *one cannot get above the swelling*. In scrotal swelling *one can get above the swelling*.

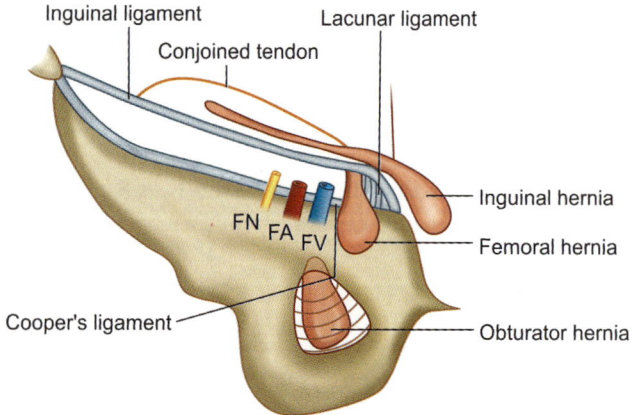

Fig. 18-19 *Diagrammatic representation of location of inguinal, femoral and obturator hernias.* Obturator hernia occurs through obturator canal, commonly presenting with features of intestinal obstruction. Often radiating pain to knee joint through geniculate branch of the obturator nerve called as Howship-Romberg sign may be the presentation. Obturator hernia is common in elderly females. FN: femoral nerve; FA: femoral artery; FV: femoral vein.

Size in vertical and transverse directions noted; *Margin*—well-defined or ill-defined; *surface* smooth/lobular/tense. Size is mentioned in centimeters as longitudinal and transverse.

Consistency—soft and *elastic in enterocele; doughy in omentocele (epiplocele)* should be noted. Obstructed hernia is tense and tender.

Reducibility of the swelling: It is checked by different methods. Reducibility is ability to return the contents of the hernia to their normal anatomical location (abdomen). Whether it reduces spontaneously on lying down (usually direct hernia) and whether it gets reduced completely or partially has to be noted. Patient himself reduces the contents easily, if asked. In enterocele, *it is difficult to reduce the first part of the content but last part gets reduced easily; and it often gets reduced with a gurgling sound. Whereas in omentocele, it is difficult to reduce the last part but first part gets reduced easily and no gurgling sound is heard.* Whether swelling needs any manipulation to get reduced like taxis is to be noted **(Figs. 18-22A and B)**. *Taxis is gradual reduction of contents of the scrotal swelling by gentle manipulation by flexion (30°), adduction (15°) and internal rotation (15°) of hip joint.* This maneuver relaxes the superficial ring and oblique (anterolateral) abdominal muscles. Fundus of the sac is held with one hand and contents are gently squeezed towards the abdomen using thumb and fingers and other hand guides the content across the superficial inguinal ring.

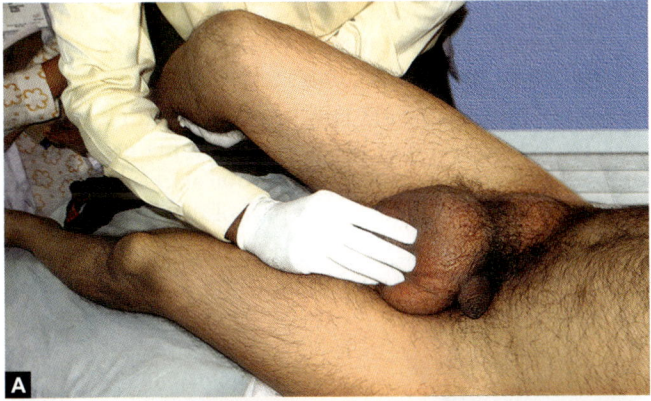

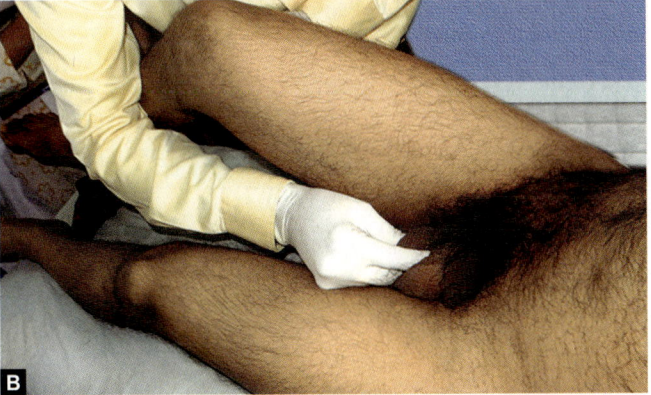

Figs. 18-22A and B Inguinal hernia is reduced in lying down position; done by elevating the scrotum and flexing, adducting and internally rotating the hip—*taxis*.

The swelling is irreducible in irreducible hernia, obstructed hernia, strangulated hernia/large hernia, sliding hernia. In initial period, hernia can get reduced in standing position. Direct hernia gets reduced directly backwards and reappears on release of fingers; indirect hernia gets reduced upwards and outwards and may not reappear on releasing the fingers but reappears on coughing.

> **Taxis** [taxis (Greek) means arrangement] is a method used to reduce a complete inguinal hernia. Hip and knee are flexed and thigh is adducted. One hand is held near the fundus of the sac in the bottom of the scrotum, other hand placed adjacent to external ring, and contents are gently reduced towards the proximal side. Often patient can himself do this technique in a better way. It is contraindicated in obstructed/strangulated hernia or femoral hernia or Maydl's hernia. Taxis should be done very gently. Forcible reduction of the hernia content which is strangulated or obstructed may cause *'reduction en masse'*. It will be dangerous as invisible gangrenous bowel inside abdominal cavity will cause peritonitis and endanger the life.

Sliding hernia is usually irreducible. Here posterior wall of the sac is formed by either bowel (usually cecum on right side or sigmoid colon on left side) or urinary bladder; it attains large size; becomes complete commonly; common on left side; usually indirect type. It is common in elderly males.

Expansile impulse on coughing—should be checked during palpation in **standing** position. After complete reduction of the contents of the swelling, either by placing finger on superficial ring or by holding the root of the scrotum between index and thumb, patient is asked to cough to feel expansile impulse on coughing. Fingers may get separated by the sudden appearance of the swelling allowing the contents to force down. Impulse will be absent in strangulated hernia, incarcerated hernia, in presence of adhesions blocking the entrance of sac. Presence of an expansile impulse on coughing is diagnostic of hernia but the absence of expansile cough impulse does not exclude the hernia because the neck of the sac may be blocked by adhesions or is very narrow and at that point of time may not allow the movement of viscera or additional viscera into the sac during the act of coughing. Cough impulse should be expansile to say hernia, otherwise it is not possible to differentiate it from swelling from spermatic cord or undescended testis.

Note: Swellings other than hernia in the groin may show transmitted impulse; that is why, *expansile* impulse which is hallmark, is important.

Using this cough impulse, *Zieman's test* is done to find out which type of hernia it could be— whether femoral/direct inguinal or indirect inguinal. This is done in standing position after reducing the hernia. Index finger is placed over the deep ring. Middle finger is placed over the superficial ring and ring finger over the saphenous opening. Patient is asked to cough. If impulse touches ***index finger it is indirect inguinal hernia; middle finger, it is direct inguinal hernia; ring finger, it is femoral hernia*** (Figs. 18-23A and B).

Deep ring occlusion test: It is the most important test in inguinal hernia. It is performed in *standing* position. Deep/

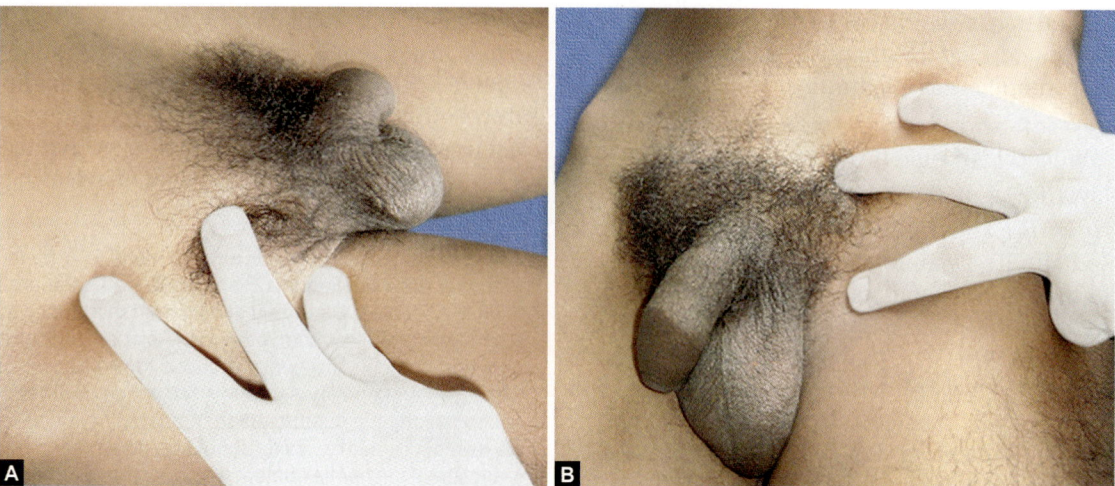

Figs. 18-23A and B *Zieman's test*—done on both sides. Three fingers are used to do Zieman's test. For right side, right hand is used; for left side, left hand is used.

internal ring is located 1.25 cm above the mid-inguinal point. Mid-inguinal point is mid-point between the anterior superior iliac spine and pubic symphysis.

(*Note:* Midpoint of the inguinal ligament is center point between anterior superior iliac spine and pubic tubercle; last bony point felt while following the crest from back is anterior superior iliac spine).

Patient is asked to lie down to reduce the hernial contents. Reduction of the contents can be done in standing position but it is often difficult as contents may reappear while releasing the fingers. It is better to place *measuring tape* between anterior superior iliac spine and pubic symphysis to exactly mark the site of mid-inguinal point. Thumb is placed over the mid-inguinal point. Patient is asked to cough. If there is expansile impulse on coughing on the medial side of the thumb, in spite after deep ring occlusion, it is then direct inguinal hernia. If there is no impulse on coughing then patient is asked to stand with thumb occluding the deep ring. Patient is once again asked to cough; impulse on the medial side of the occluded thumb is looked for to rule out the direct inguinal hernia. If there is no impulse even on standing, it is indirect inguinal hernia. The occluded thumb is removed and patient is asked to cough to show the swelling and impulse due to indirect inguinal hernia. Hernia should be reduced completely prior to deep ring occlusion test. **One cannot do deep ring occlusion test/finger invagination test/Zieman's test if hernia is irreducible** (**Figs. 18-24A to C**). **In a large indirect complete inguinal hernia,** which presents as inguinoscrotal swelling, due to widened patulous deep ring, the ring occlusion test may show impulse on the medial side of the occluded thumb making interpretation difficult.

Finger invagination test: This test is not commonly used now. Patient is asked to lie down. Contents are reduced completely. *Using the little finger,* scrotal skin is invaginated from below upwards near upper part of the testis. Finger is

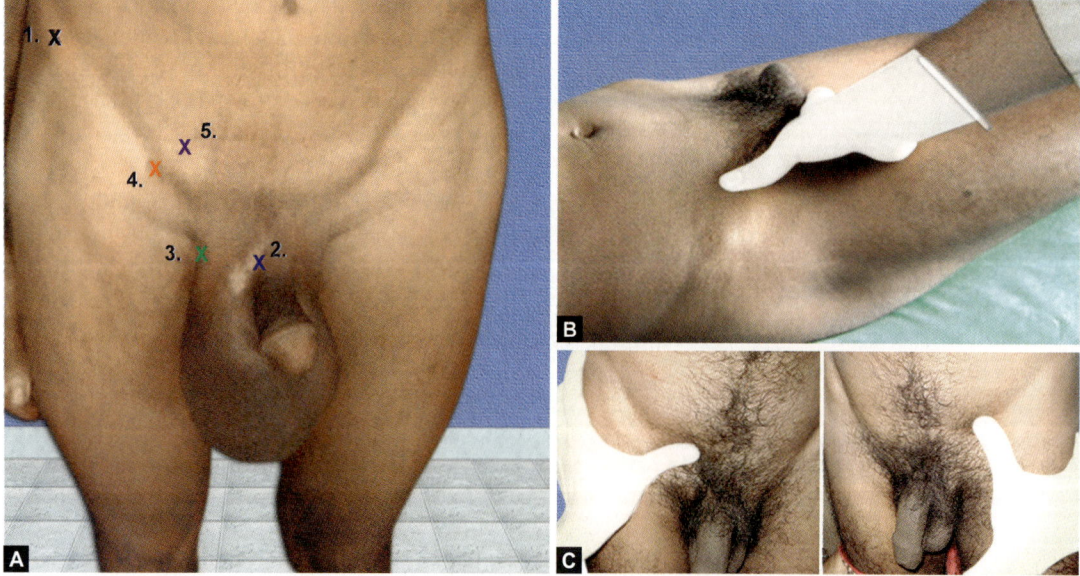

Figs. 18-24A to C *Ring occlusion test is done to find out whether hernia is direct or indirect.* If after occluding the ring swelling appears on the medial side, it is direct hernia. If swelling does not appear on occlusion and coughing it is indirect hernia. (1) Anterior superior iliac spine; (2) Mid pubic symphysis; (3) Pubic tubercle; (4) Mid inguinal point is midway between 1 and 2; (5) Internal (deep) ring point.

reached towards the superficial inguinal ring/external ring. Finger is rotated inwards so that nail is towards the cord side and pulp is towards the ring. Right hand is used for right side and left hand for left side. Normally, external ring does not or just admit the tip of the little finger. Normal superficial ring feels like a triangular slit. Patient is asked to cough. If the impulse is felt on the tip of the finger, then it is indirect inguinal hernia. If impulse is felt on the pulp then it is direct inguinal hernia. In case of complete inguinal hernia or funicular hernia, external ring is patulous which can be very well assessed by invagination test. Index finger can also be used for the test. In direct hernia, finger goes directly; in indirect hernia, finger goes upwards and outwards. One should also remember that patulous wider ring does not mean patient should have hernia always.

Invagination test should be done very gently; otherwise, it will be very painful. It cannot be done in children. This test is entirely impracticable in females **(Figs. 18-25A and B)**.

Silk glove sign: Index finger is invaginated across scrotum towards the external ring. When patient coughs, in inguinal hernia it is felt like a slit-like sensation. It is palpating the processus vaginalis over the pubic tubercle in ***standing position*** mainly to confirm whether it is patent or not and is used in children but can be useful in older age group; mainly used in identifying the presence of hernia on the contralateral side.

In femoral hernia, pressure over the femoral canal will not allow the ***contents to come out—confirmatory test***.

Palpation of testis, epididymis and spermatic cord should be done without fail. Size of the testis has to be noted. It may be atrophic/enlarged/retractile. Relation of swelling to testis also should be noted. In incomplete and funicular type as the hernia contents do not reach up to the scrotum, testis can be felt separate of the hernia contents whereas in congenital type testis cannot be felt separately as it is covered from front and sides by the hernia contents.

Opposite inguinal region, opposite testis, epididymis and spermatic cord should be examined. Presence or absence of impulse on coughing on opposite side should be mentioned.

Bulbar urethra is palpated by lifting the scrotum and feeling in the midline (to look for thickening and button-like depression—a feature of stricture urethra) **(Fig. 18-26)**.

Percussion

Percussion should be done ***in standing position.*** Without reducing contents of the swelling, percussion is done over its surface. If it is resonant, it is enterocele. If it is dull on percussion then it is omentocele **(Fig. 18-27)**.

Auscultation

Auscultation should also be done in ***standing position***. Bowel sounds may be heard over the swelling if it is enterocele.

Abdomen Examination

Abdominal muscle tone is checked in recumbent position by head and shoulder rising (without supporting the elbows) or

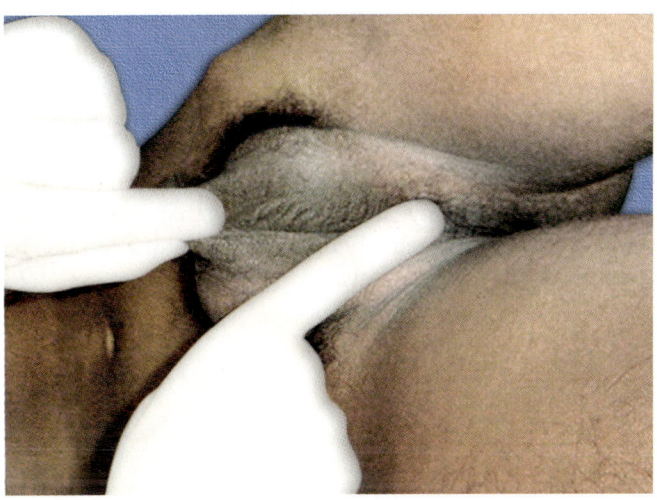

Fig. 18-26 *Bulbar urethra should be palpated* by raising the scrotum in midline posteriorly. Any stricture urethra is felt as thickening/button-like depression. Gonococcal urethritis and trauma are the commonest causes of stricture urethra. Bulbar urethra is the commonest site of stricture urethra.

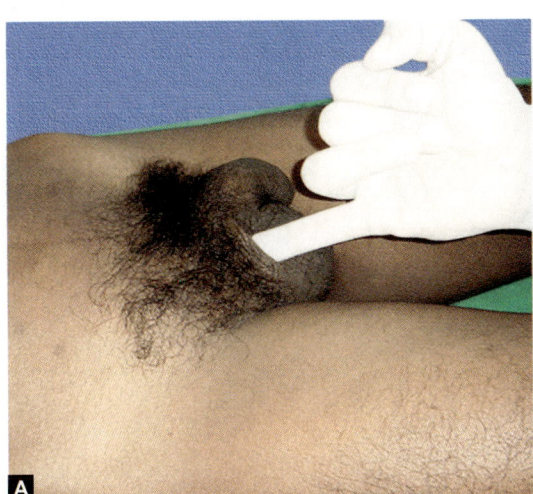
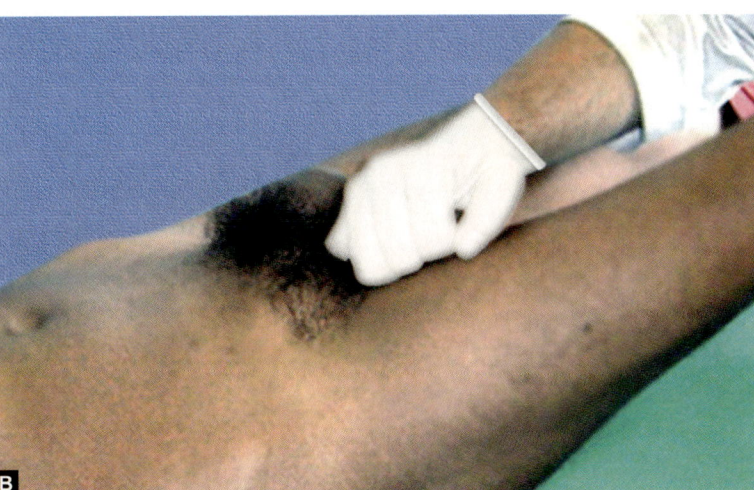

Figs. 18-25A and B *Little finger is used to do invagination test.*

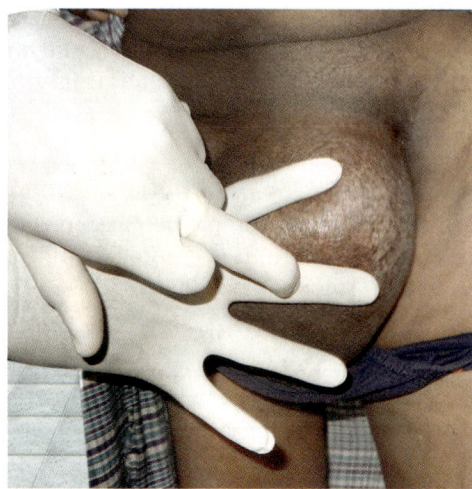

Fig. 18-27 Percussion should be done in *standing position*; resonant note suggests enterocele; dull note means omentocele.

leg rising tests **(Figs. 18.28A and B)**. It is initially inspected for any oval shaped, longitudinal, bilateral bulges in the abdominal wall *near the inguinal region* which signifies **Malgaigne bulging**. In the same position, bulging is again ascertained with the act of coughing also. It indicates poor muscle tone. Later abdomen should also be palpated for muscle tone. Firmness signifies adequate tone whereas suppleness signifies poor muscle tone. Poor muscle tone indicates that patient needs hernioplasty using mesh. Abdominal muscle tone can also be checked by Valsalva maneuver.

Any scar over the abdomen (***appendicectomy scar*** may cause right-sided direct inguinal hernia due to injury to ilioinguinal nerve); ascites or mass per abdomen should be mentioned **(Fig. 18-29)**.

> **In hernia:**
> - Inspect and palpate from front
> - Inspect and palpate from side
> - Inspect and palpate from opposite side
> - Inspect and palpate in standing and lying down positions
> - Percuss in standing
> - Auscultate in standing

Digital Examination of the Rectum (P/R)

Rectal examination is done in all hernia cases to look for prostate enlargement in elderly and rectal/anorectal strictures. Causes of rectal stricture are—recurrent proctitis, ulcerative colitis, carcinoma, previous anal surgery, LGV-induced proctitis, tuberculosis, etc. **(Figs. 18-30 and 18-31)**.

Examination of Respiratory System

Respiratory system is examined for altered breath sounds (rhonchi, bronchial breathing), effusion, etc. to find out any precipitating causes like tuberculosis, bronchitis, asthma, bronchiectasis **(Fig. 18-32)**.

Other Systems

Cardiovascular system, nervous system including spine and cranium are examined for any neurological problems for management of hernia.

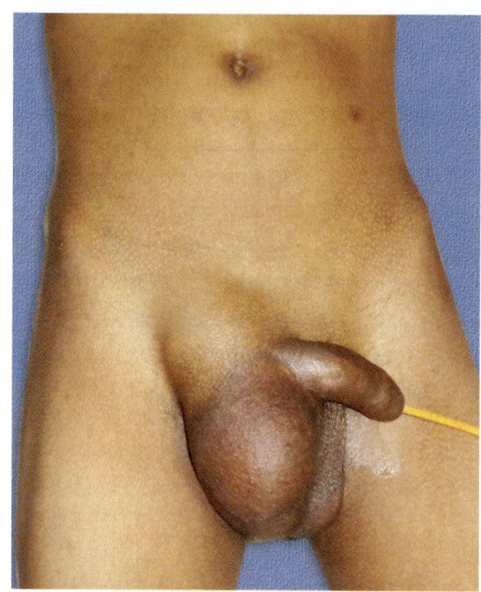

Fig. 18-29 *Right sided irreducible recurrent inguinal hernia.* Note the scar. Patient is having benign prostatic hypertrophy (BPH) which may be the cause for recurrence. Patient is on Foley's catheter.

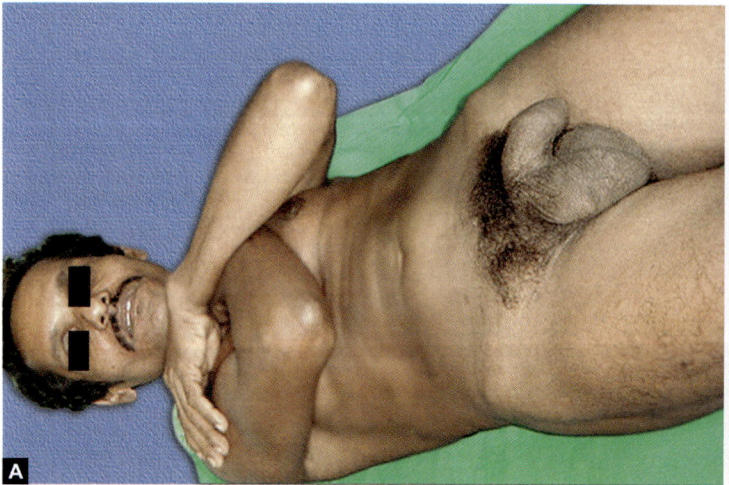

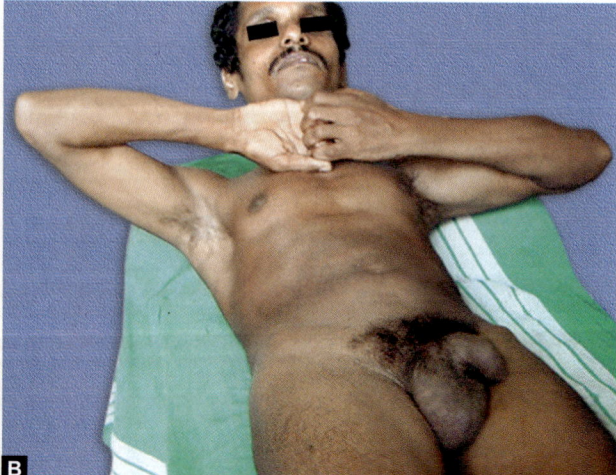

Figs. 18-28A and B *Head and shoulder raising and Valsalva maneuver tests* are needed to check the tone of abdominal muscle in hernia.

Testing Inguinal Hernia in Children

Fullness over the groin compared to opposite side is seen. In difficult small hernia, child is made to cry or jolt or jump, later superficial ring is palpated to feel the cord which will be thicker than opposite side. Rolling the contents of the inguinal canal by finger will give the sensation of finger of a rubber glove which is wet inside.

Gornall's test: Child is held from back by placing both hands of the physician over the abdomen which is pressed with fingers and child is lifted up. This raises the intra-abdominal pressure to make hernia more prominent **(Fig. 18-33)**.

Inguinal Hernia in Females

- Hernia in females is rare. Inguinal hernia is more common type of hernia in females than femoral hernia. *Expansile impulse on coughing* is diagnostic.
- Invagination test is *not possible* in females. Palpation of labium majus demonstrates **thickness** compared to opposite side indicating hernia in canal of Nuck.
- Patient should be examined properly in standing position otherwise hernia is more likely to be missed. Reducible inguinal hernia is obvious by its clinical features. But *femoral hernia* needs to be differentiated by its definitive anatomical location.
- *Differential diagnosis* for irreducible inguinal hernia in females—*A hydrocele of canal of Nuck* is smooth, fixed, fluctuant and brilliantly transilluminant swelling. *Bartholin cyst* is confined to labium majus; one can get above the swelling; it does not extend to superficial inguinal ring; it is not transilluminant. *Groin abscess* is smooth, soft, fluctuant and tender; but it is often difficult to differentiate it from strangulated hernia. Associated abdominal symptoms favour strangulated inguinal hernia.

■ INVESTIGATIONS

Relevant investigations required for inguinal hernia are chest X-ray, hematocrit, blood sugar, serum creatinine, ultrasound abdomen depending on the age/suspected cause of the hernia. Chest X-ray is done to look for bronchitis, tuberculosis and bronchiectasis. US abdomen is done to look for benign prostatic hyperplasia (BPH), residual urine, ascites, and mass lesion.

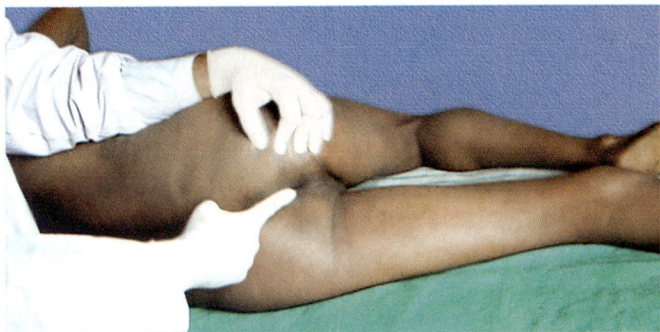

Fig. 18-30 *Clinically per-rectal examination is a must in hernia* to look for prostate enlargement, and rectal stricture which are precipitating factors.

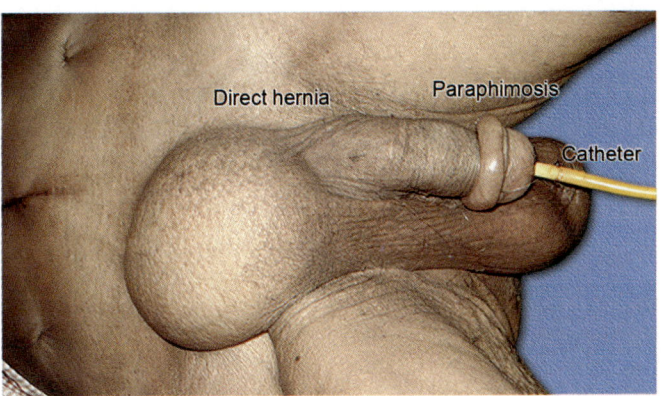

Fig. 18-31 *Inguinal hernia in a patient who is having benign prostatic hyperplasia* (BPH) with Foley's urinary catheter. He is having paraphimosis and so not able to replace back the retracted prepuce after catheterization.

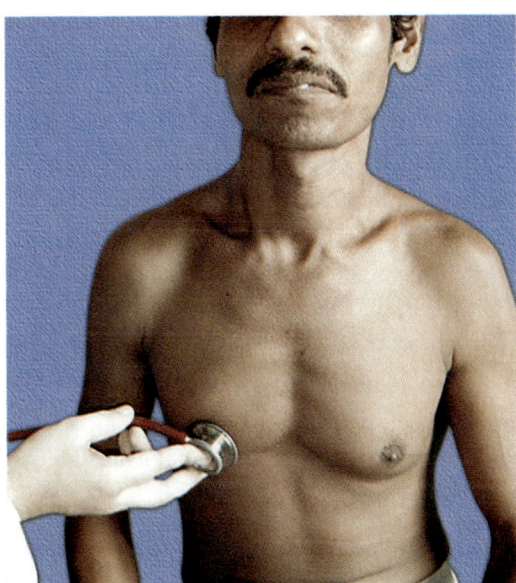

Fig. 18-32 Respiratory system should be examined to find out the precipitating causes for hernia like *bronchitis, tuberculosis or asthma*.

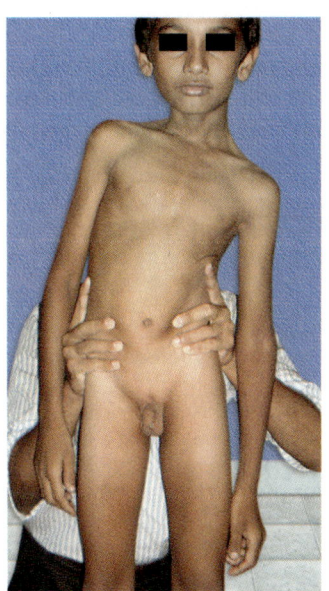

Fig. 18-33 *Gornall's test.*

Section 1: Examination in General Surgery

Case sheet writing in a patient with hernia

History
Name: Age:
Occupation: Sex: Place/residence:

History of present illness
- Swelling – duration, mode of onset and progress, site of origin, number, disappearing or reducing in size (reducibility); gurgling sound
- Pain – origin, nature, character, duration, time of starting of pain, specific features, severity, aggravating or relieving factors
- Fever – type, severity, duration
- Other lumps – site, when started, progress
- History relevant of precipitating factors – cough, constipation, urinary symptoms

Past history
- Past history of swelling and treatment for that
- Tuberculosis, spinal diseases, diabetes, leprosy, asthma, bronchitis
- Past history of treatment and surgery; history of appendectomy (open) surgery

Personal history and family history
- Smoking, chewing pan/tobacco; history of exposure (gonorrhea); family tree; treatment history

General examination
Anemia, edema, jaundice, clubbing, lymphadenopathy, pulse, blood pressure, temperature, attitude, nutrition, body weight

Local examination
Inspection – both in standing and lying down
- Swelling – location, size, shape, extent, surface of the swelling, skin over the swelling, number, edge/margin/border of the swelling, movement of the swelling, expansile impulse on coughing; visible peristalsis
- Surrounding structures – scrotum, testes, opposite side, penis (for phimosis)

Palpation
- Marking the anatomical landmarks – pubic tubercle, symphysis, anterior superior iliac spine
- Expansile impulse on coughing; reducibility
- Swelling features – local raise of temperature, tenderness, size, shape and extent of the swelling, edge of the swelling, surface of the swelling, consistency, reducibility
- Get above the swelling to differentiate from hydrocele
- Fluctuation, transillumination test
- Plane of the swelling, mobility, fixity to skin or deeper structures
- Specific tests – deep ring occlusion; finger invagination; Zieman's.
- Examination of preputial skin and bulbar urethra

Percussion – in standing position
Auscultation – for bowel sounds in standing position
Examination of regional lymph nodes
Abdomen examination – for scar, ascites, Malgaigne bulging
Digital rectal examination (P/R)
Systemic examination respiratory, cardiac and central nervous systems

---

■ HERNIA

A hernia is defined as an area of weakness or disruption of the fibromuscular tissues of the body wall. Hernia is also often defined as an actual anatomical weakness or defect.

> **'Use five fingers of the hand to complete all tests for hernia':**
> - Thumb—for deep ring occlusion test
> - Index, middle and ring fingers for Zieman's test
> - Little finger for superficial ring invagination test

> **Rules of hernia examination:**
> - Never forget to check expansile impulse on coughing and reducibility
> - Never forget to examine opposite side
> - Never forget to do per-rectal examination
> - Never forget to examine bulbar urethra
> - Never forget to check abdominal muscle tone

Groin hernia: It is hernia occurring through a myopectineal orifice. It can be indirect inguinal hernia/direct inguinal hernia or femoral hernia. 75% of abdominal wall hernias are groin hernias. 15% of males and 5% of females will develop groin hernia. Presently, all hernias in groin are grouped as *groin hernias*.

■ BOUNDARIES AND ANATOMY OF THE INGUINAL CANAL

In front: External oblique aponeurosis and conjoined muscle laterally.

Behind: Inferior epigastric artery, fascia transversalis and conjoined tendon medially.

Above: Conjoined muscle (Arched fibers of internal oblique).

Below: Inguinal ligament.

Superficial inguinal ring is a triangular opening in the external oblique aponeurosis and is 1.25 cm above the pubic tubercle. The ring is bounded by a superomedial and inferolateral crus. Normally, the ring may just admit or may not admit the tip of little finger. *Deep inguinal ring* is a U-shaped condensation of the transversalis fascia which lies 1.25 cm above the inguinal ligament midway between the symphysis pubis and the anterior superior iliac spine.

Inguinal canal: In infants, both superficial and deep rings are superimposed without any obliquity of the inguinal canal. In adults, it is 3.75 cm long, directed downwards and medially from the deep to superficial ring. In males, inguinal canal transmits the spermatic cord, ilioinguinal nerve and genital branch of the genitofemoral nerve. In females, its content is the round ligament. Inguinal canal in female is called as *canal of Nuck*.

Contents of the spermatic cord: Three arteries—testicular, cremasteric and artery of vas; three nerves—genital branch of genital nerve, nerve to cremaster, sympathetic nerve (ilioinguinal nerve is outside cord in the inguinal canal); three other structures—vas deferens, pampiniform plexus of veins and lymphatics.

In 1956, *Fruchaud* described his *myopectineal orifice* bounded medially by the lateral border of rectus abdominis, laterally by iliopsoas, superiorly by conjoined tendon and inferiorly by pectin pubis. This area is the site of groin hernia which should be covered by mesh of adequate size to strengthen the defect and to prevent the recurrence.

Classification of groin hernia

Clinical classification:
Reducible hernia: Here contents can be reduced to abdominal cavity but sac is in position
Irreducible hernia: Here contents cannot be reduced to abdominal cavity. It is due to adhesion between contents/adhesion between content and sac/adhesions between surfaces of the sac; sliding hernia; large hernia complete type; narrow neck of the sac acting as a constricting band preventing reduction of the content
Obstructed hernia: Here irreducibility causes occlusion of the lumen of the intestine but bowel remains viable
Strangulated hernia: Here irreducibility, obstruction and compromised blood supply of the bowel occurs
Inflamed hernia: Here hernial contents being Appendix/Meckel's diverticulum/Fallopian tube are inflamed or sac itself is inflamed. It is not tensed
Incarcerated hernia: Lumen of the portion of the intestine usually colon existing in a hernial sac is blocked with feces. This scybalous content of the bowel should be capable of being indented with the finger-like putty. Sac and contents are densely adherent to each other. It is always irreducible often obstructed but may not be strangulated
Occult hernia: Not detectable clinically. Dragging or severe pain is the presentation. No impulse on coughing

Gilbert classification (1987):
Type I: Hernia has got *snug internal ring* through which a peritoneal sac passes out as indirect sac
Type II: Hernia has a moderately enlarged internal ring which *admits one finger* but lesser than two finger breadth. Once reduced it protrudes during coughing or straining
Type III: Hernia has got large internal ring with defect *more than two finger breadth*. Hernia descends into the scrotum or with sliding hernia. Once reduced, it immediately protrudes out without any straining
Type IV: It is direct hernia with large full blow out of the posterior wall of the inguinal canal. The internal ring is intact
Type V: It is a direct hernia protruding out through punched out hole/defect in the transversalis fascia. The internal ring is intact
Type VI: Pantaloon/double hernia
Type VII: Femoral hernia
Type VI and VII are Robbin's modifications
Nyhus and Bendavid are other classifications

Classification of groin hernia

Classification according to contents:
Omentocele—omentum
Enterocele—intestine
Cystocele—urinary bladder
Litter's hernia—Meckel's diverticulum
Maydl's hernia
Sliding hernia
Richter's hernia—part of the bowel wall

European Hernia Society classification:
Primary; Recurrent; P or R
Lateral (indirect); Medial (direct); or Femoral; L, M or F
Defect size: — 0 = no hernia detectable; 1 = <1.5 cm (one finger); 2 = <3 cm (two fingers); 3 = >3 cm (more than two fingers); X = not investigated

TYPES OF INDIRECT INGUINAL HERNIA

It can be *incomplete* wherein sac does not reach to the bottom of the scrotum. It can be *complete* wherein sac descends completely up to the bottom of the scrotum. *Incomplete type* can be *bubonocele* where hernia limits to inguinal region without passing through the superficial inguinal ring or can *be funicular* where sac reaches up to the level of the upper part of the testis into the scrotum across the external ring.

Eighty-percent of inguinal hernias are indirect. Neck of the sac is lateral to inferior epigastric artery. All hernias (almost) in children and females are indirect type. After occluding internal ring content will not descend. It is commonly congenital occurring in a preformed (pre-existing) processus vaginalis (Figs. 18-34 to 18-38).

DIRECT HERNIA

It is 15% of all hernias; 50% are bilateral; 35% of inguinal hernias; uncommon in females; does not occur in children; always acquired due to weak posterior wall of inguinal canal. In old men, benign prostatic hyperplasia usually results in direct hernia. It occurs through Hesselbach's triangle (Figs. 18-39A and B). It is medial to inferior epigastric artery; neck is wider; sac is often thick; medial wall or content may be urinary bladder. It is globular in shape with wide neck; mainly contains extraperitoneal pad of fat; disappears spontaneously on lying down. It is usually reducible; becoming complete by descending into the bottom of the scrotum is rare but can occur. During ring occlusion test, direct sac is medial to the deep ring; during

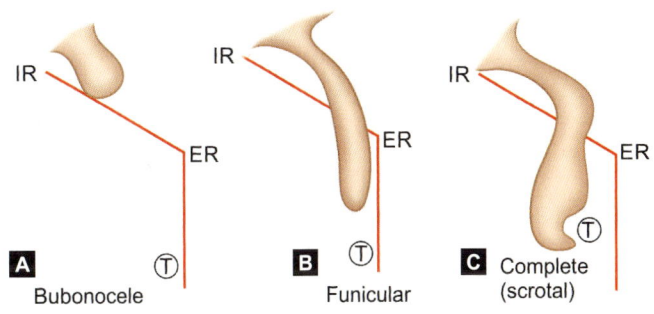

T—testis, IR—internal, ER—external ring

Figs. 18-34A to C Types of indirect inguinal hernia. *(A)* Bubonocele; *(B)* Funicular; *(C)* Complete.

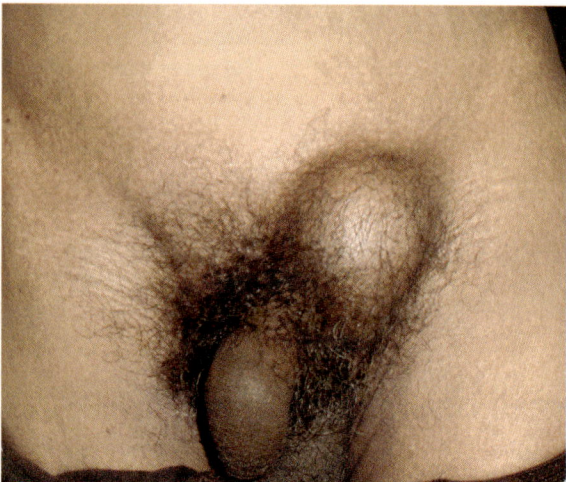

Fig. 18-35 *Bubonocele.*

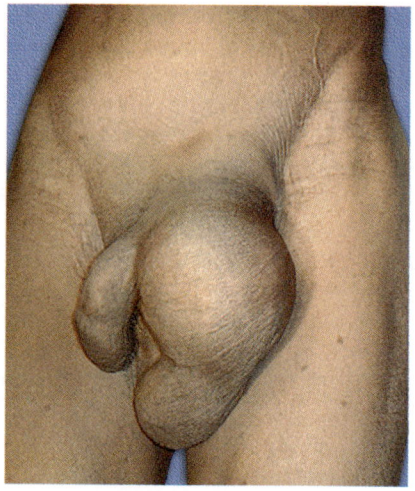

Fig. 18-36 Incomplete inguinal hernia—*funicular type*. It is probably irreducible in this patient.

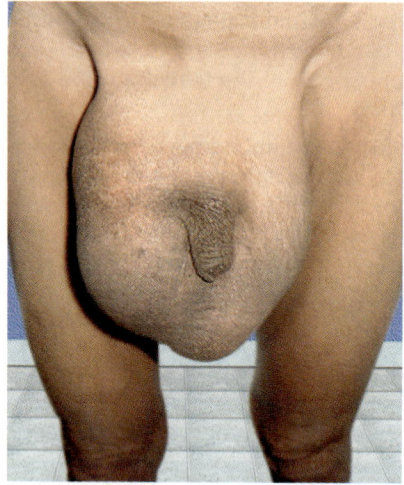

Fig. 18-37 *Complete* inguinal hernia is one where hernia descends completely into the scrotum.

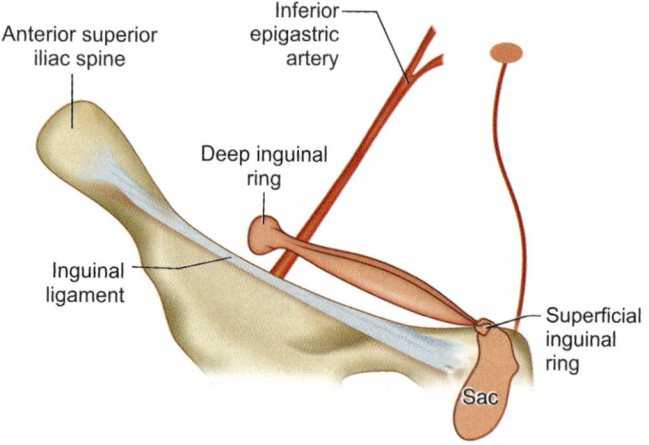

Fig. 18-38 Diagram of *indirect inguinal hernial sac*.

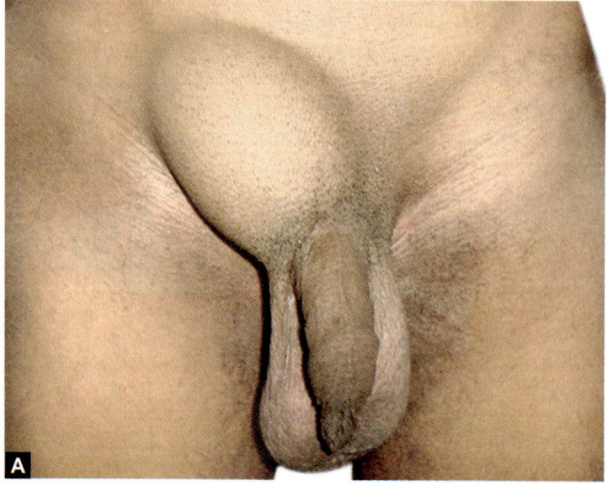

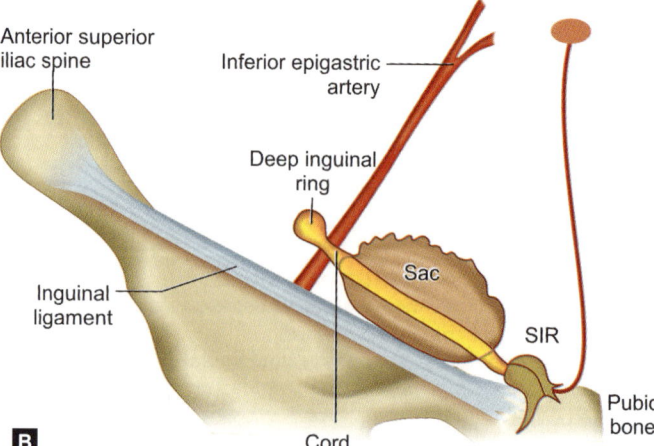

Figs. 18-39A and B *Direct hernia arises through Hesselbach's triangle.* SIR—superficial inguinal ring.

finger invagination test, impulse will be felt over the pulp of the finger. Further finger passes directly backwards into the abdomen and edge of the external ring will be felt superiorly and pubic bone inferiorly (the sign of the pubic bone). Strangulation is rare in direct hernia.

<u>**Hesselbach's triangle:**</u> It is bounded by inferior epigastric artery laterally, lateral border of rectus muscle medially and inguinal ligament below. Direct hernia protrudes out through this triangle. It is divided into medial and lateral by obliterated umbilical artery.

Precipitating Causes for Inguinal Hernia

Smoking; obesity; respiratory causes like bronchial asthma, tuberculosis, bronchitis; ascites; previous surgery like appendicectomy (injury to ilioinguinal nerve) which causes direct inguinal hernia; chronic constipation due to anorectal strictures; rectal stricture may be due to—chronic proctitis (amebic), tuberculosis of anorectum, previous anorectal surgery, rectal carcinoma or stricture due to lymphogranuloma venereum; urinary problems like benign prostatic hyperplasia (BPH), urethral stricture; straining; multiple pregnancies.

DIFFERENCES BETWEEN INDIRECT INGUINAL AND DIRECT INGUINAL HERNIAS

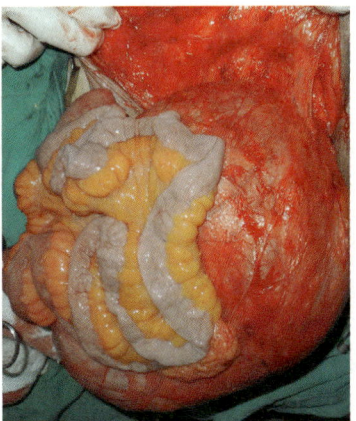

Fig. 18-40 *Enterocele* with hernia sac opened.

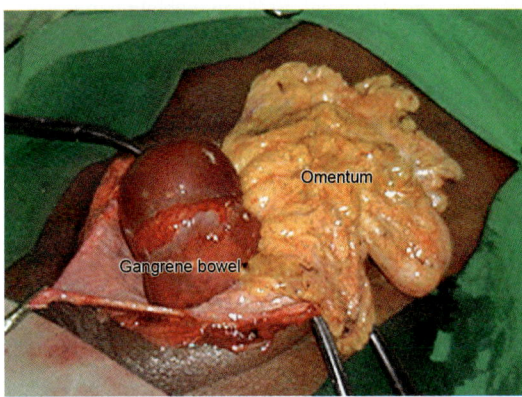

Fig. 18-41 Irreducible hernia with bowel *and omentum as contents*. Note the change in color of the bowel.

Indirect inguinal hernia	Direct inguinal hernia
Can occur from childhood to adulthood	Common in elderly
Occurs in a pre-existing sac	Always acquired
Protrusion through the deep ring; herniation occurs later	Herniation through posterior wall of the inguinal canal
Pyriform/oval in shape; descends obliquely and downwards	Globular/round in shape; descends directly forward as a bulge
Can become complete by descending down into the scrotum	Descent down into the scrotum is rare
Neck of the sac is narrow and lateral to inferior epigastric artery	Neck of the sac is wide and medial to inferior epigastric artery
Sac is anterolateral to the cord	Sac is posterior to the cord
Ring occlusion test does not show any impulse after occluding the deep ring	Test shows impulse even after occluding the deep ring
Invagination test shows impulse on the tip of the little finger	Impulse is felt over the pulp of the little finger
Zieman's test shows impulse on the index finger	Test shows impulse on the middle finger
Commonly unilateral but can be bilateral	Commonly bilateral
Obstruction/strangulation are common	Rare but can occur
Sac should be opened during surgery	Sac is not necessarily opened unless obstruction is present

In enterocele (Fig. 18-40)	In omentocele (Fig. 18-41) (epiploecele)
First part is difficult to reduce but last part is easier. There will be gurgling sound on reduction	First part is easier to reduce but last part is difficult. Has a doughy feeling
Resonant on percussion	Dull on percussion
Peristalsis is seen	No peristalsis seen
Bowel sounds may be heard	Bowel sounds not heard

Differential Diagnoses for Groin Swelling (Fig. 18-42)

Indirect/direct inguinal hernia: Swelling is above and medial to pubic tubercle; expansile impulse on coughing; reducibility are the features

Hydrocele—vaginal/encysted: One can get above the swelling; absence of expansile impulse on coughing; fluctuation is positive. **Hydrocele of the canal of the Nuck in females** which is transilluminant

Femoral hernia: Swelling is below and lateral to pubic tubercle with impulse on coughing (Fig. 18-43)

Lipoma of the cord: Swelling in the inguinal canal without any impulse on coughing. It is often observed that hernia and lipoma of the cord can coexist and is identified only on table during surgery (Fig. 18-44)

Groin abscess: Fluctuant smooth, soft, tender nonmobile swelling in the groin could be an abscess due to lymph node suppuration. It is often difficult to differentiate it from strangulated hernia

Undescended testis: It presents as firm swelling in the inguinal region; associated commonly with indirect hernia. Testicular sensation may be elicited. Empty scrotum is evident. It can be bilateral

Ectopic testis is also often located in the groin

Infantile hydrocele: It presents as swelling in the inguinal region as well as in the scrotum. Impulse on coughing will be absent as it is not communicating into the peritoneal cavity. Fluctuation and transillumination are positive

Varicocele: It appears spontaneously; may show impulse on coughing; bag of worms feeling is typical; can get reduced; left side is common

Contd...

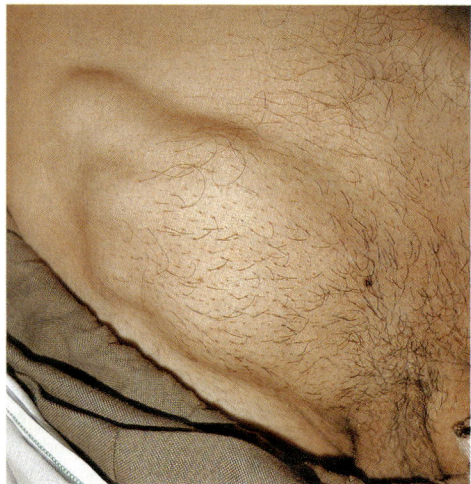

Fig. 18-42 Lymphatic swelling (*lymphangioma*) inguinal region (groin). It often mimics inguinal hernia.

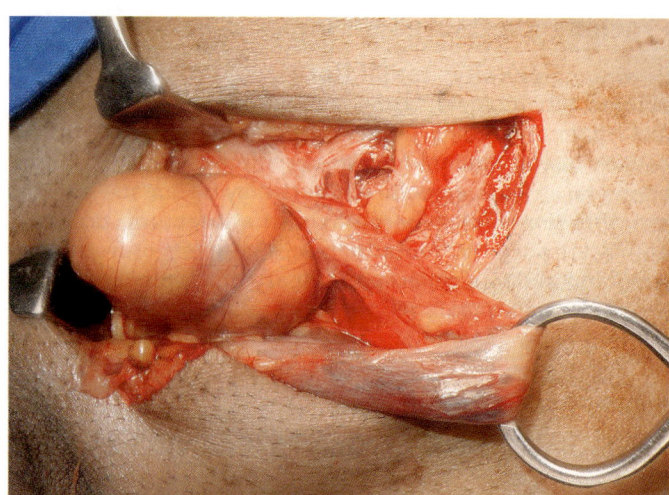

Fig. 18-44 *Lipoma of the cord.*

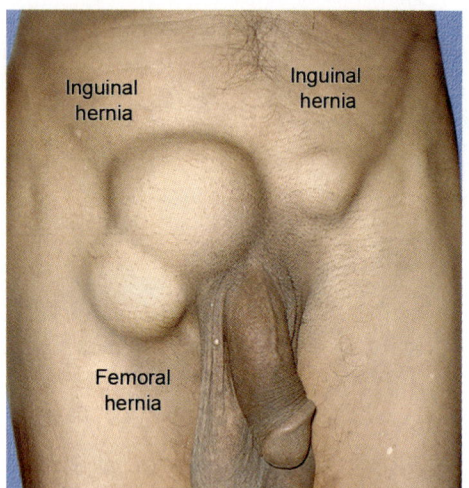

Fig. 18-43 Bilateral inguinal hernia and right-sided femoral hernia. Femoral hernia is rare in males but can occur.

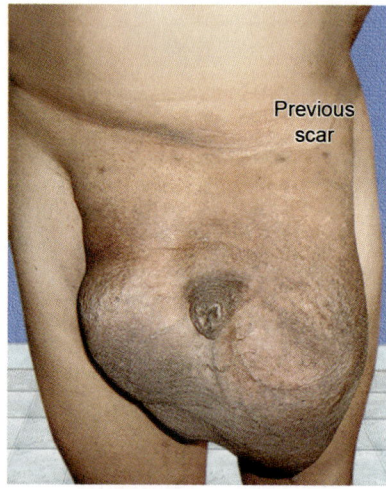

Fig. 18-45 *Recurrent hernia* left-sided. Note the scar of earlier surgery.

Contd...

Inguinal lymphadenopathy: Palpable inguinal nodes may be of vertical or horizontal group in the inguinal canal may be due to non-specific causes or filarial lymphadenitis or secondaries in inguinal nodes primary being in the limb or perineum or lymphoma	Recurrent hernia: *Causes:* Infection—most common—50%; hematoma in the wound; early straining; retained indirect sac, after repair of a direct sac (*Pantaloon hernia*); smoking, constipation, obstructive uropathy, old age, nutritional deficiencies; altered tension in repair site; altered collagen synthesis. *Clinical features:* Swelling, expansile impulse on coughing, visible scar, reducibility (Fig. 18-45)

■ INCISIONAL HERNIA

Incisional hernia is a hernia occurring through a weak scar. Writing case sheets, taking detailed history is similar to inguinal hernia.

Additional history to be collected in history of present illness: Details of surgery patient has undergone earlier. After how long incisional hernia has occurred? History of wound infection, wound dehiscence, whether surgery done was an emergency or elective, and whether tension sutures were placed or not. History of pain, irreducibility and details of precipitating factors have to be asked. Other precipitating factors similar to inguinal hernia like smoking, urinary/respiratory/abdominal symptoms should be asked (Figs. 18-46 to 18-48).

Local Examination (Abdomen)

Inspection: Scar, its extent and location, whether healed primarily or secondarily, skin over the scar and swelling is noted. Details of the swelling with expansile impulse on coughing and *examination both in lying down and standing are done.*

Palpation: Palpation is like for inguinal hernia. Size, extent, impulse on coughing must be confirmed; scar and skin should be palpated. The defect in the abdominal wall must be assessed. It is done after reducing the hernial content with patient in lying down position. Fingers are placed *horizontally* over the hernial defect and patient is asked to raise the head with arms folded over the chest (to contract the abdominal wall muscles) so that the defect is felt clearly. Its size and extent can be assessed well. Assessment can also be done

Chapter 18: Clinical Approaches and Examination of Hernia 383

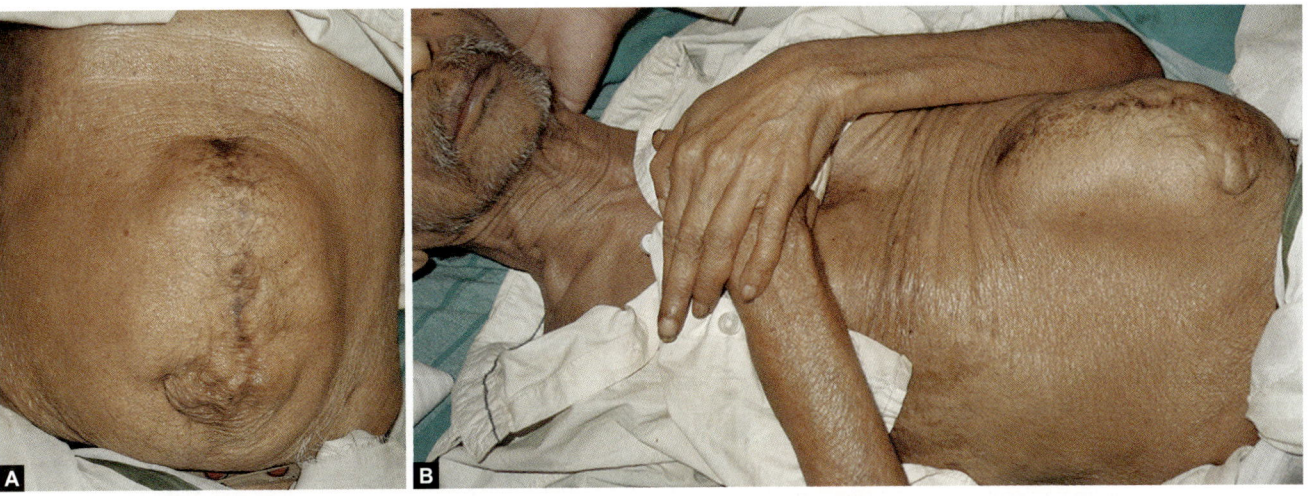

Figs. 18-46A and B *Incisional hernia—large.*

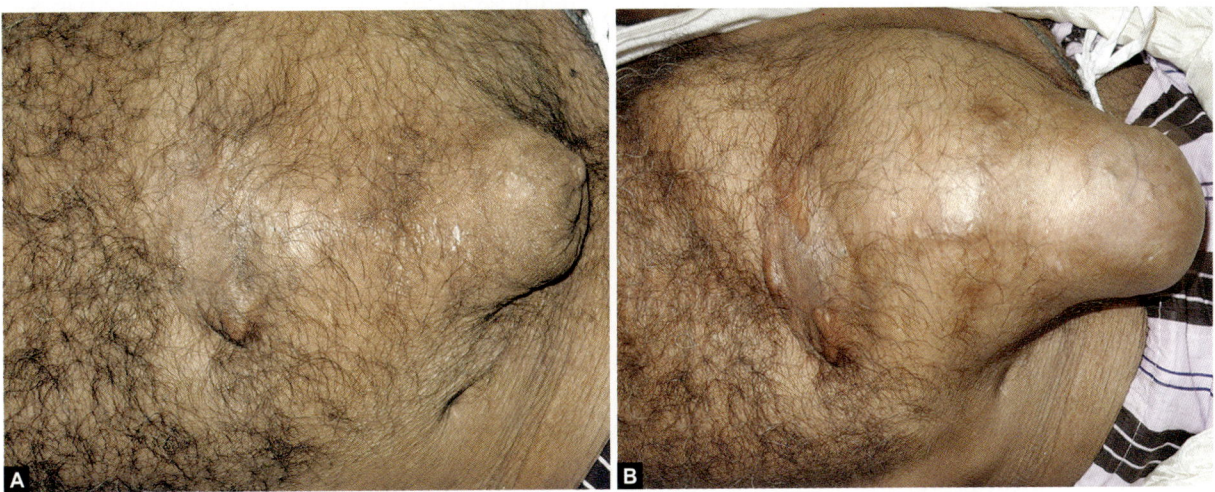

Figs. 18-47A and B Large incisional hernia with *expansile impulse on coughing*.

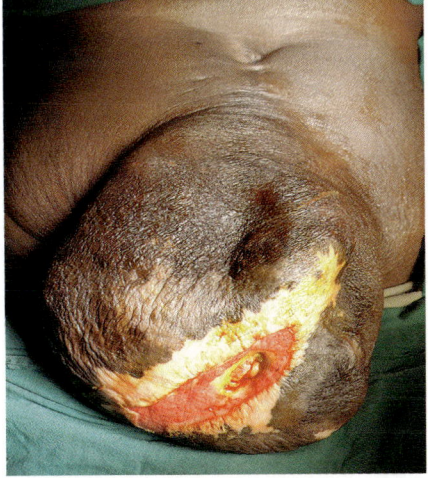

Fig. 18-48 Large incisional hernia with *ulceration over its summit*.

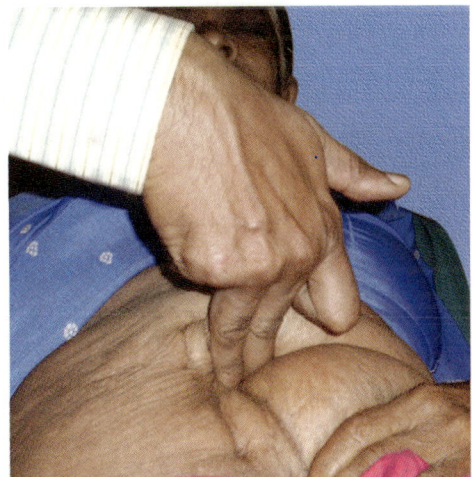

Fig. 18-49 *Defect is assessed by placing fingers* horizontally in incisional hernia.

by raising the legs instead of head (Fig. 18-49). *Gap cannot be assessed in an irreducible hernia.*

Note: Size of the defect is important to decide the type of surgical closure in incisional hernia. Midline hernia expels the content more outwards due to contraction of rectus muscles on both sides.

FEMORAL HERNIA

It is common in females. It occurs in medial most part of the femoral canal.

Surgical anatomy of femoral canal: It is the most medial compartment of the femoral sheath which extends from femoral ring above to saphenous opening below. It contains fat, lymphatics, lymph node of Cloquet. It is 1.25 cm long and 1.25 cm wide at the base. Below it is closed by cribriform fascia. Femoral ring is bounded anteriorly by inguinal ligament; posteriorly by iliopectineal ligament of Cooper, pubic bone and fascia covering the pectineus muscle; medially by concave, sharp lacunar (Gimbernat's) ligament; laterally by a thin septum separating from femoral vein.

Clinical features: Common in females (2:1), common in multiparae; rare before puberty; 20% occur bilateral, however, more common on right side; presents as a swelling in the groin *below and lateral* to the pubic tubercle (Inguinal hernia is *above* and *medial* to the pubic tubercle); swelling, impulse on coughing, reducibility, gurgling sound during reduction, dragging pain, are the usual features. When obstruction and strangulation occur which are more common (due to rigid opening of femoral canal), presents with features of obstruction—pain, tender, inflamed, irreducible swelling without any impulse. They also present with abdominal distension, vomiting, and feature of toxicity. Often femoral hernia can be associated with inguinal hernia also. *Gaur* (Surgeon, Bombay Hospital, India) *sign*: Pressure by the femoral hernial sac on the superficial epigastric and/or circumflex iliac veins causes dilatation of one or both veins in an irreducible femoral hernia (Fig. 18-50). Remember—presentations may be— No lump/expansile impulse on coughing in saphenous opening/visible impulse which gets reduced and more prominent on coughing/irreducible tender, tense swelling in femoral region often extends into inguinal region from below upwards.

Differential diagnosis for femoral hernia	
Inguinal hernia	Hydrocele of femoral hernial sac
Saphena varix	Ectopic testis in males
Enlarged Cloquet lymph node	Lipoma in femoral region
Psoas abscess	Lymph cyst in femoral region
Enlarged psoas bursa	Soft tissue tumor in femoral region
Femoral artery aneurysm	Prevescular femoral hernia

Type of hernia (other hernias)	Features
Ventral hernia Any protrusion through abdominal wall with the exception of hernia through the inguinofemoral region is defined as ventral hernia. Incisional hernia (80%) and primary defects in abdominal fascia which can cause umbilical hernia, epigastric hernia, paraumbilical hernia or Spigelian hernia are grouped under ventral hernia	Ventral hernia can be— Reducible; irreducible; obstructed; strangulated; single; multiple small defects (*Swiss cheese* hernia) (**Fig. 18.51**) *Causes:* Congenital defect; obesity; smoking; chronic cough
Epigastric hernia It is a fatty hernia of linea alba; initially, it is sacless (protrusion of extraperitoneal fat) but later develops true epigastric hernia with sac containing contents. It occurs through decussation of the linea alba above the umbilicus. It is 10% common; 20% are multiple *Swiss cheese pattern*	Often symptomless but later can cause pain, obstruction and strangulation. It is better seen and palpated in standing position as a firm nodule which is relatively non-mobile. Abdominal wall lipoma which mimics epigastric hernia is freely mobile. Often associated with peptic ulcer and so pain may be due to peptic ulcer, hence gastroscopy should be done in doubtful patients (**Fig. 18-52**)
Paraumbilical hernia It is midline herniation above or below the umbilicus through a defect adjacent to umbilicus; common above; often attains large size and sags downwards. Neck may be narrow with omentum/small bowel as contents	Obstruction/strangulation tend to occur. Commonly associated with obesity and multiple pregnancies; common in females; obese; middle or old aged. Swelling, impulse on coughing, dragging pain and reducibility are usual presentations. After reduction firm ring-like fibrous edge is felt (**Fig. 18-53**)
Umbilical hernia It is herniation through a weak umbilical cicatrix; common in infants and children; common	Ninety-five percent of umbilical hernias disappear in 2 years. If persists beyond 2 years, and if defect is more than 2 cm in size

Contd...

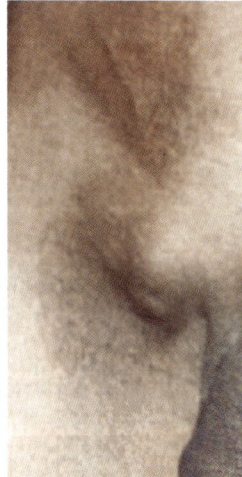

Fig. 18-50 *Gaur sign* (dilated superficial epigastric vein) in a patient with femoral hernia (Gaur, Mumbai, India).

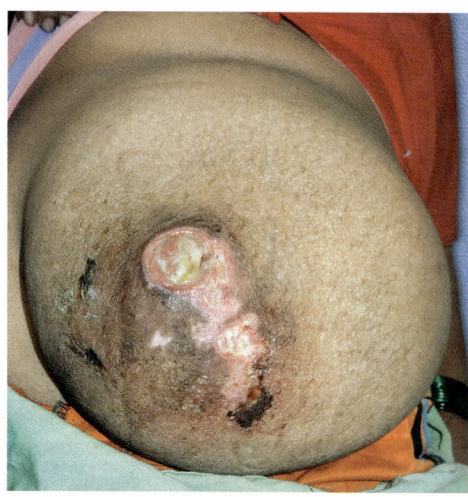

Fig. 18-51 *Large ventral hernia* with ulceration over its summit.

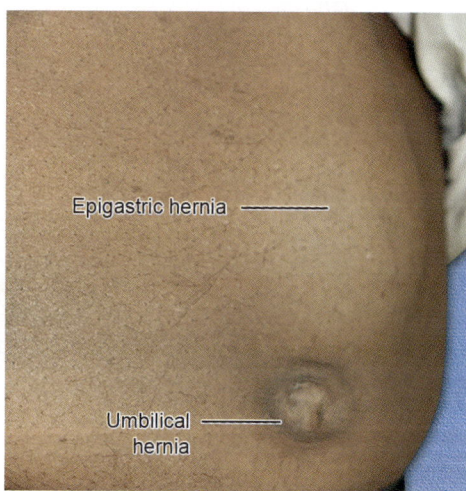

Fig. 18-52 *Epigastric hernia* and *umbilical hernia.*

Chapter 18: Clinical Approaches and Examination of Hernia

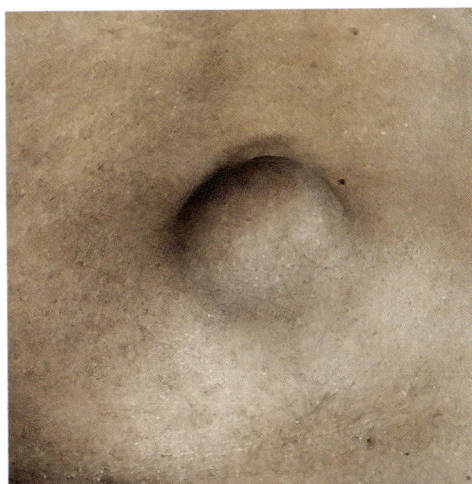

Fig. 18-53 *Strangulated paraumbilical hernia.*

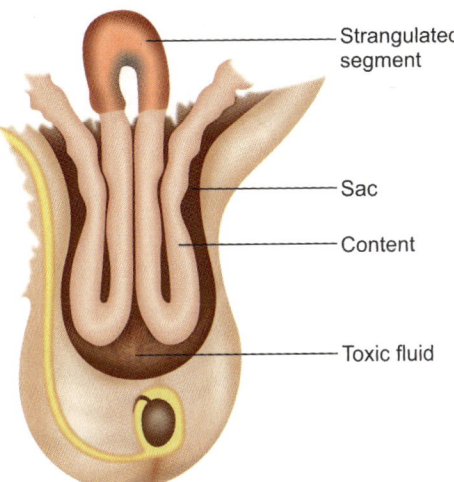

Fig. 18-54 *Maydl's 'W' hernia.*

Type of hernia (other hernias)	Features
Richter's hernia It is herniation of a portion of circumference of intestine usually small bowel leading into gangrenous change	Here patient presents with features mimicking gastroenteritis without any signs of intestinal obstruction which eventually, leads to perforation and peritonitis. It is common in femoral hernia
Sliding hernia (2%) It is always an acquired hernia with posterior wall of the sac is formed by parietal peritoneum and also by sigmoid colon/cecum/urinary bladder. It occurs exclusively in males and is common on left side; attains large size and its content is usually small bowel	Usually irreducible large hernia; often with obstruction or strangulation During surgery, posterior wall should not be separated from the sac; only partially excised and then pushed into peritoneal cavity followed by mesh repair
Pantaloon hernia It is inguinal hernia containing both direct and indirect sacs but presents as direct hernia. It is also called as *double hernia, saddle hernia* or *Romberg hernia*	So, in all cases of direct hernia, indirect sac should be looked for. Condition is one of the causes for recurrence
Strangulated hernia It is due to compromised blood supply of the contents of the hernia like bowel/omentum causing toxicity, tenderness at the site. Features of intestinal obstruction are present if the content is bowel. Narrow neck and adhesions are the causes of strangulation. It is treated by emergency surgery. In strangulated omentum, features of obstruction are not present. **Maydl's hernia:** Here bowel loop in the form of 'W' lies in the hernial sac and centre portion of the W is strangulated. It may get reduced 'en-masse'. Strangulation of centre part is common **(Fig. 18-54)**	It presents with sudden severe pain, initially over a pre-existing hernia which later becomes generalized over the abdomen; persistent vomiting, constipation and distension of the abdomen; hernia is tense, severely tender, and irreducible, without any expansile impulse on coughing. Rebound tenderness is diagnostic. Features of toxicity and dehydration; electrolyte imbalance; abdominal distension with guarding and rigidity oliguria are other features *Taxis* has no role in femoral hernia and strangulated hernia. If tried, contusion, reduction en masse and rupture of the sac can occur

Contd...

Type of hernia (other hernias)	Features
in Negroes. It is hemispherical in shape with defect felt during crying. As the content is commonly small intestine, it can cause obstruction and strangulation	or if associated with complications, surgery is indicated. Acquired umbilical hernia occurs in adult life due to massive ascites, old age

Rare Hernias

Obturator hernia is herniation through obturator canal; mainly presents as intestinal obstruction; often pain in knee joint (referred through obturator nerve [Howship Romberg sign]); rarely as a swelling in the medial side of the thigh

Funicular hernia: It is prevesical direct hernia, is herniation of prevesical fat, bladder, or intestine through a small defect in the medial part of the conjoint tendon just above the pubic tubercle; which is prone for strangulation

Spigelian hernia: It is an interparietal hernia occurring at the level of arcuate line through Spigelian point with sac lying deep to internal oblique or between internal oblique or external oblique muscles

Sportsman's hernia: Common in football/rugby players; sudden pain in groin, scrotum and thigh with swelling, soft tissue injury and adductor spasm often with muscle tear **(Gilmore's hernia)**

Lumbar hernia: It is herniation through either superior lumbar triangle bounded by sacrospinalis, 12th rib, posterior border of internal oblique–(*Grynfeltt-Lesshaft's triangle*) or inferior lumbar triangle bounded by latissimus dorsi, external oblique and iliac crest (*Petit's triangle*). It is common through inferior triangle. It should be differentiated from lipoma, cold abscess, and lumbar phantom hernia

Phantom hernia is a muscular bulge as a result of local muscular paralysis due to interference with nerve supply of the affected muscles like in poliomyelitis. It is common in lumbar region. It is often seen in lower abdomen

Infantile hernia: It is clinically difficult to diagnose; often it is diagnosed on table. Processus vaginalis is closed at internal ring and hernial sac either invaginates processus vaginalis as *'inverted umbrella'* or comes behind processus vaginalis

CASE DISCUSSION

A 65-year-old man who is a smoker presents with bilateral groin swelling of 8 months duration. He has got chronic cough and increased night urinary frequency. Dragging pain over the swelling is present. He is not hypertensive or diabetic. On examination, globular swelling of 3 × 3 cm sized is present in both groins, inguinal region which shows expansile impulse on coughing in standing position. Swelling is reducible, smooth, soft and nontender; it gets reduced with gurgling. Swelling does not extend downwards to the scrotum. Zieman's and ring occlusion tests confirmed it as direct hernia. Percussion on standing position showed resonant note. Scrotum is normal. Abdominal muscle tone was reduced on head raising test. Digital examination of the rectum showed prostatic enlargement. Respiratory system on examination showed features of bronchitis with rhonchi.

What is your complete diagnosis?
Diagnosis is bilateral incomplete direct reducible uncomplicated inguinal hernia (enterocele) due to benign prostatic hyperplasia and smoking induced chronic bronchitis.

Why it is hernia?
Because there is expansile impulse on coughing and reducibility it is hernia.

Why it is called as direct hernia?
As it is globular, reducible, ring occlusion test shows swelling on the medial side of the inferior epigastric artery it is direct hernia.

Why it is enterocele?
As swelling gets reduced by gurgling and on percussion it is resonant.

How you will investigate?
Ultrasound abdomen is done to find out prostate enlargement. Size of the prostate, lobes and residual urine should be assessed. Chest X-ray is done to confirm bronchitis. Hemoglobin, ESR, blood sugar, serum creatinine, ECG, echocardiography should be done for preparing the patient for surgery as he is old man.

CLINICAL PEARLS

- Hernia is one of the commonest surgical conditions.
- Examination in standing is very important.
- Use five fingers during examination.
- Ring occlusion test is the most important test.
- Muscle tone should be checked.
- Digital rectal examination, examination of respiratory system is a must.
- Early indirect hernias may present only as dragging pain in the groin without swelling or impulse on coughing.

CHAPTER 19

Clinical Approaches and Examination of Inguinoscrotal and Scrotal Swelling

Competency: SU30.2; SU30.3; SU30.4; SU30.5; SU30.6. AN46.4.

In this chapter inguinoscrotal and scrotal swellings other than inguinal and femoral hernias are discussed. Hydrocele and other differential diagnosis of groin swellings are discussed here. Groin is the area which covers inguinal and femoral area. Swellings in inguinoscrotal area could be purely inguinal or purely scrotal or inguinoscrotal. In inguinoscrotal swelling one cannot get above the swelling. Femoral swelling is below and lateral to the pubic tubercle.

■ HISTORY

Name:

Age: Funiculitis occurs in young age. Testicular tumor occurs in early adult age (seminoma) but can occur in young (teratoma). Varicocele presents in adolescents and young. Carcinoma of scrotal skin is seen in elderly. Torsion testis is seen in adolescents. Hydrocele is common in adult. Epididymal cyst, spermatocele are seen in adult. Tuberculous orchitis is seen in young individuals.

Address: Filarial funiculitis, orchitis, lymph varix is common in Odisha, West Bengal, coastal regions.

Occupation: Carcinoma of scrotal skin is often occupation related—those who come in contact with soot (**Chimney sweep's cancer**); tar or oil (**Mule spinner's disease**). Prolonged standing may cause varicocele (**Figs. 19-1 to 19-3**).

Inguinoscrotal and scrotal swellings:
- Encysted hydrocele of the cord
- Varicocele
- Lymph varix
- Funiculitis
- Diffuse lipoma of the cord
- Ectopic testis
- Undescended testis
- Retractile testis
- Torsion testis
- Testicular tumor
- Inguinal or iliac lymphadenopathy
- Abscess in the groin—inguinal region
- External iliac artery aneurysm
- Scrotal edema
- Epididymal cyst
- Spermatocele
- Extravasation of urine

Femoral swellings:
- Inguinal lymph nodes
- Saphena varix
- Psoas abscess
- Psoas bursa enlargement
- Lipoma in femoral triangle
- Femoral artery aneurysm
- Hydrocele of femoral hernia
- Ectopic testis

History of Present Illness

Swelling

Like any other swelling detailed history should be asked—mode of onset, progress, regress, history of trauma.

Exact site of occurrence should be asked. Inguinal hernia begins in groin; *hydrocele* (Greek word hydros means water; kele means mass), testicular tumor begins in scrotum; varicocele begins in root of the scrotum. Lipoma of cord, encysted hydrocele of the cord appears in groin or near root of the scrotum. Undescended testis presents with swelling in the groin with empty scrotum. The commonest site of ectopic testis is superficial inguinal pouch. In bilateral swellings the side on which it appeared first and after how long has it appeared on opposite side should be asked. Hydrocele can be bilateral; varicocele is more common on left side but can be bilateral (**Figs. 19-4 and 19-5**).

Mode of onset: It may be insidious/traumatic/ infective in origin. Swellings of insidious onset may be (funiculitis, scrotal abscess) or may not be (congenital hydrocele, varicocele) associated with pain. Trauma may precipitate hematocele or

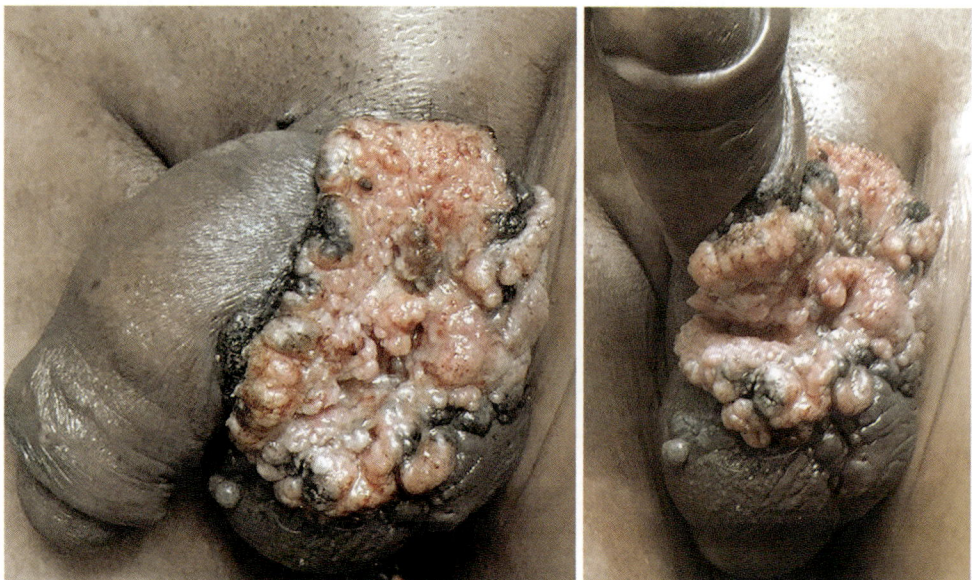

Fig. 19-1 *Carcinoma scrotum*.
(*Courtesy:* Dr Nanda Kishore MS MCh, Urologist; Father Muller's Medical College, Mangaluru.)

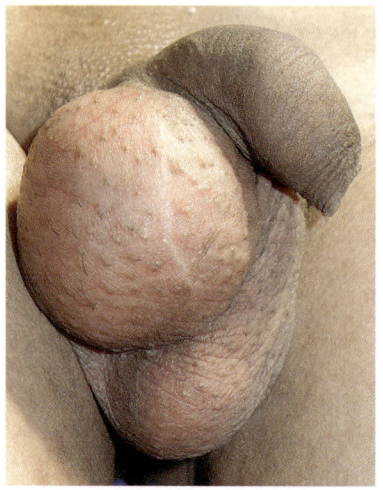

Fig. 19-2 Right-sided *hydrocele*.

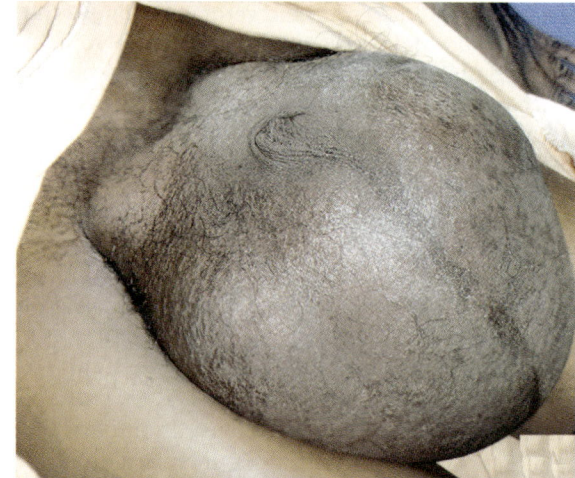

Fig. 19-4 *Bilateral hydrocele*; note the buried penis.

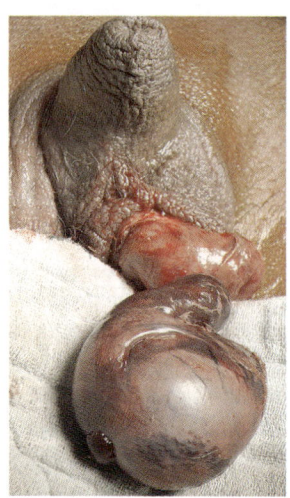

Fig. 19-3 *Torsion testis*; right testis towards right side; left side towards left side.

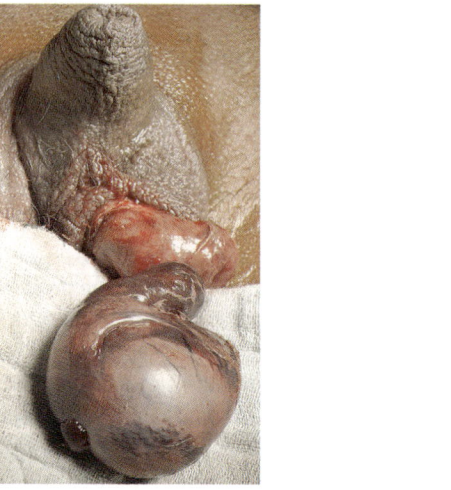

Fig. 19-5 Left-sided *varicocele*.

hydrocele. Sudden pain and swelling in scrotum is probably due to acute epididymo-orchitis or pyocele. History of trauma is coincidental in testicular tumor. Primary hydrocele is insidious in onset gets noticed only when big. Swelling due to scrotal edema may be part of generalized anasarca or due to filariasis. Trauma on bulb of urethra may cause urinary extravasation and swelling in the scrotum. Gonococcal urethritis with stricture also can cause extravasation and scrotal swelling—*watering can perineum*.

Duration: They may be of short duration (torsion testis, hematocele), or long duration (primary hydrocele, chronic inflammatory swelling, tumors of testis and scrotum).

Progress of the swelling: Inguinoscrotal swelling **(Fig. 19-6)** extend downwards towards bottom of the scrotum whereas pure scrotal swelling extends upwards towards root. Progress is very rapid in hematocele, which later becomes stationary; Rapid increase in size occurs in testicular tumors and inflammatory swelling but very slow in hydrocele **(Fig. 19-7)**.

Behavior of the swelling: Whether swelling ***disappears on lying down*** (reducible hernia will disappear on lying down, hydrocele will not disappear) to be asked. Congenital hydrocele increases in size in evening and becomes smaller in the morning.

> **Swellings which reduce on lying down in the groin:**
> - Reducible inguinal hernia—reduces rapidly
> - Varicocele—reduces spontaneously with elevation of scrotum
> - Lymph varix reduces slowly **(Fig. 19-8)**

Other swellings: In epigastric region of the abdomen (due to palpable enlarged para-aortic lymph nodes)/in the supraclavicular region due to enlarged lymph nodes may be often elicited in history.

Swelling with heaviness in the scrotum may be initial presentation of testicular tumor.

Pain

Epididymo-orchitis, funiculitis presents with pain and often fever. History of severity of pain, onset, progress, whether initially painless later become painful (in testicular tumor) should be asked. Hematocele, pyocele can be severely painful. Torsion testis presents with pain often precipitated by straining due to sudden violent contraction of the cremaster. Severe pain in scrotum and groin with fever, redness and swelling may be features of acute epididymo-orchitis. Periodic mild fever with pain, discomfort and swelling in the scrotum and spermatic cord are the features of filarial epididymo-orchitis. Pain in tuberculous orchitis and gummatous orchitis will be in the form of mild discomfort; vague dragging pain especially on long hours of standing, is seen in varicocele.

Presence of Fever

Fever often with chills should be asked for. Fever is due to infection, filarial orchitis, pyocele, etc. Evening rise of temperature may be feature of tuberculous epididymitis or funiculitis. History of cough and hemoptysis suggests associated pulmonary tuberculosis.

Trauma

History of trauma is important as scrotum being entirely outside is prone for it. Hematocele, urinary extravasation in urethral injury, hematoma scrotum in perineal injury—are important conditions to be remembered. Existing disease may be obvious after trauma.

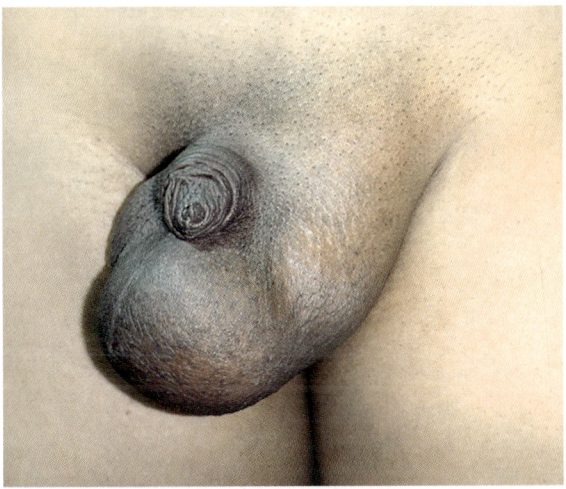

Fig. 19-6 *Inguinoscrotal swelling* progresses from inguinal region towards scrotum; inguinal hernia—funicular (in this figure) and complete types are inguinoscrotal.

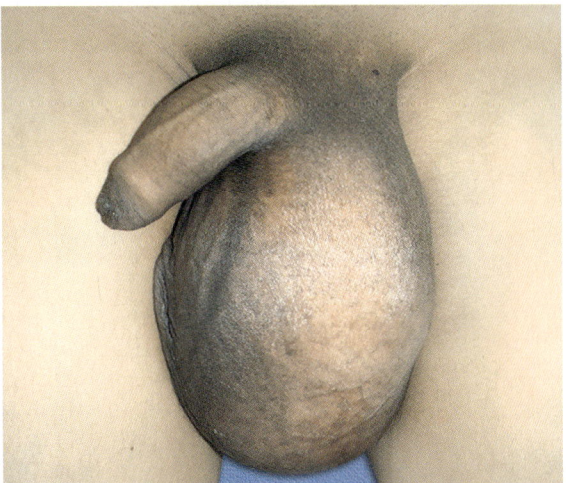

Fig. 19-7 Hydrocele is purely *scrotal swelling*.

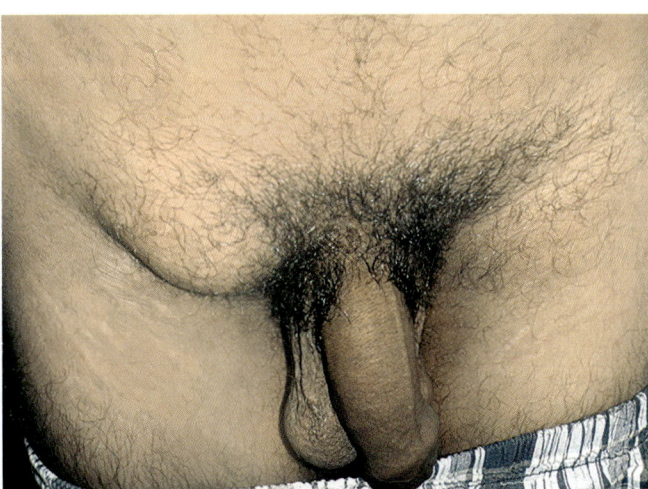

Fig. 19-8 *Lymph varix* right inguinal region (groin). It reduces only slowly; it is often compressible.

Infertility

It may be the presenting complaint in varicocele or cryptorchidism.

Past History

History of tuberculosis; old trauma; sexual exposure (in gonococcal urethritis or syphilitic orchitis) earlier are important. Patient might have undergone surgery for inguinal hernia (post-herniorrhaphy hydrocele) or hydrocele surgery. Any biopsy done in the past is to be asked.

Personal History

History of sexual contact earlier should be elicited.

■ GENERAL EXAMINATION

Pallor, nutrition, edema, jaundice should be checked; pulse and blood pressure should be recorded. Anemia and malnutrition may be features in tuberculosis or advanced malignancy.

■ LOCAL EXAMINATION

It is done under proper illumination and good exposure from nipple to mid thigh. Opposite scrotum should be examined simultaneously for comparison/to confirm the presence or absence of testis/to rule out any other pathology.

Always patient should be first examined in *standing position* (straight erect without bending) later in lying down position.

Inspection

Swelling

Swelling in the scrotum may be due to hydrocele, epididymal cyst, spermatocele, scrotal edema, and varicocele.

Site: Hydrocele is purely scrotal swelling; but large or bilocular hydrocele may extend across external ring. In encysted hydrocele of the cord and lipoma of the cord swelling may be in the groin or root of the scrotum. Swelling in the groin or superficial inguinal pouch may be due to undescended testis or ectopic testis. Here empty scrotum is obvious on inspection. Swelling due to scrotal edema may be associated with penile edema. It may be due to scrotal cellulitis, cardiac/renal/hepatic causes, filariasis, advanced secondaries in the inguinal lymph nodes blocking cutaneous lymphatic drainage, and extravasation of urine. Extravasation may be due to gonococcal urethritis or urethral trauma.

Number: It can be bilateral in hydrocele, varicocele, ectopic testis, undescended testis; multiple in sebaceous cyst. *Spermatocele* is a unilocular acquired retention cyst situated on the head of the epididymis, occurs due to blockage in sperm conduction tubes, contains **barley water** like fluid. It is a soft cystic swelling, often called as **third testis** (Fig. 19-9).

Surface: Regular and smooth in hydrocele, irregular and rough in tumor testis and scrotum, and tuberculous epididymitis.
Size: Hydrocele causes obvious swelling often very large.

Skin over the Scrotum/Swelling/Groin

It is red and edematous in funiculitis, and orchitis. Acutely inflamed skin with redness is often also a feature of **torsion testis** (Figs. 19-10A and B). Strangulated hernia also shows

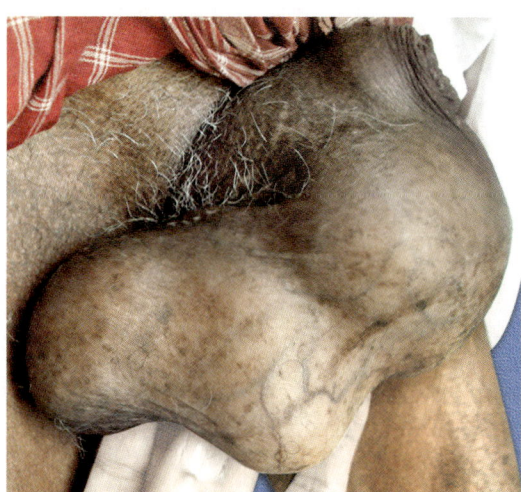

Fig. 19-9 *Spermatocele.*

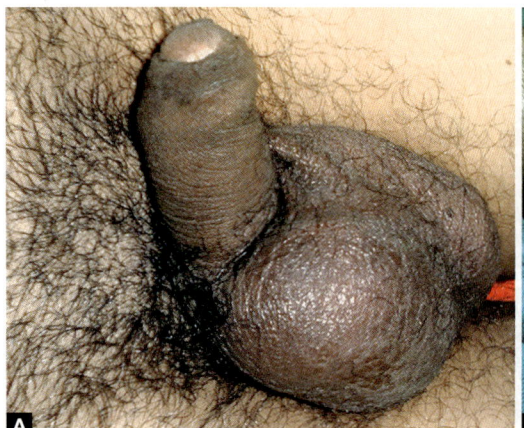
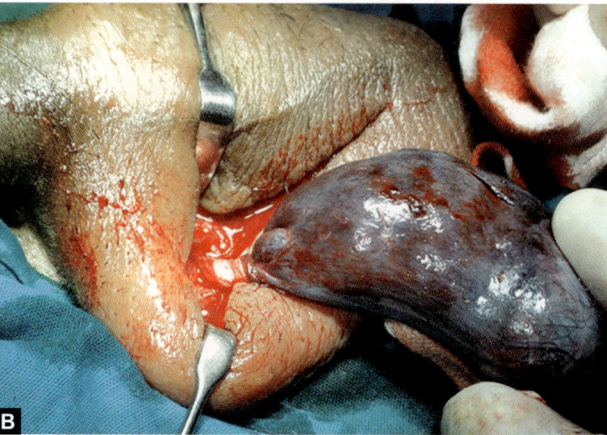

Figs. 19-10A and B *Typical look of torsion testis*—left sided.

signs of inflammation over the skin. Its extent is from scrotum to groin. Skin over the swelling may be stretched with **loss of rugosity** in long standing hydrocele. Rugosity will also be lost in syphilitic orchitis, tuberculous epididymitis and testicular tumors. Skin may be stretched often in **scrotal edema (Fig. 19-11)**. Filarial scrotal edema is non-pitting whereas scrotal edema due to other causes is pitting in nature. One has to remember that common cause of the secondary hydrocele is filarial. Clinician should be able to differentiate hydrocele from scrotal edema.

In undescended testis scrotum is not fully developed **(Figs. 19-12A and B)**. Ulcer in the scrotal skin may be due to **scrotal carcinoma** which will be having raised and everted edge, slough in the floor. All features of an ulcer explained in **Chapter 3: Examination and Clinical Approach of an Ulcer** should be mentioned. **Testicular tumor** occasionally can fungate through scrotal skin (can be anywhere but **usually anterolateral**) and present as an ulcer **(Fig. 19-13)**. **Syphilitic gummatous ulcer** is located always *on front (anterior)* of the scrotum, adherent to testis due to syphilitic orchitis. It is punched out with wash leather slough. **Tuberculous epididymitis** causes ulceration on the *posterior aspect* of the scrotum with an undermined edge. Only in anteverted testis, positions are reversed. Testis may protrude out as a granulating mass in severe infection called as **hernia testis**. Hydrocele fluid may protrude out of the tunica vaginalis testis through dartos as **hernia of the hydrocele**. Scrotal skin gangrene is a feature of **Fournier's gangrene**. **Multiple sebaceous cysts** are common in scrotum. Scrotum may show whitish vesicle containing lymph due to filariasis (**lymph scrotum**), which may rupture causing *lymphorrhagia*. Multiple ulcers in the scrotum can also occur **(Figs. 19-14 to 19-16)**.

Sinus in the scrotum can develop due to infection, postoperative cause or tuberculosis. *Urinary fistulas* in the scrotum can occur **(Fig. 19-17)**. Multiple discharging sinuses in the scrotal skin are the features of the gonococcal urethritis with discharging urine—*watering can perineum*.

Examination of Penis

Penis may be buried in large hydrocele, large inguinoscrotal hernia, and scrotal edema. Position has to be noted—it may be pushed to opposite side in large unilateral scrotal swelling. Due to extensive thickening and fibrosis caused by filariasis, it gives a typical look to the penis—**Ram's horn penis**.

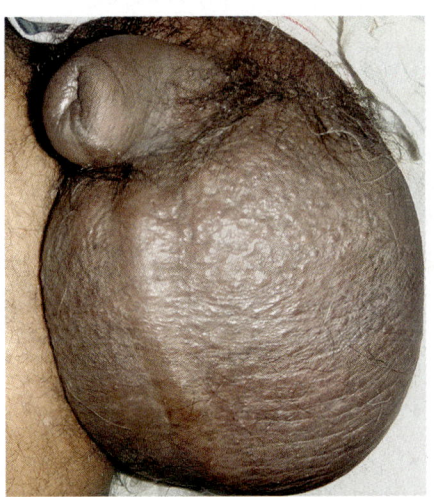

Fig. 19-11 *Scrotal and penile edema.*

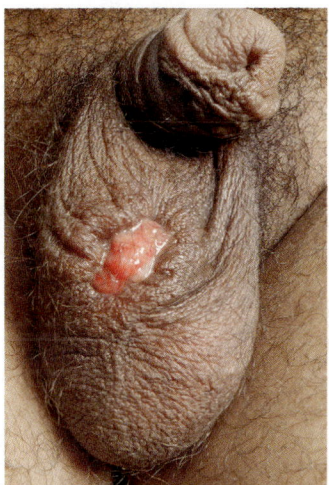

Fig. 19-13 *Scrotal ulcer; it could be nonspecific or specific.*

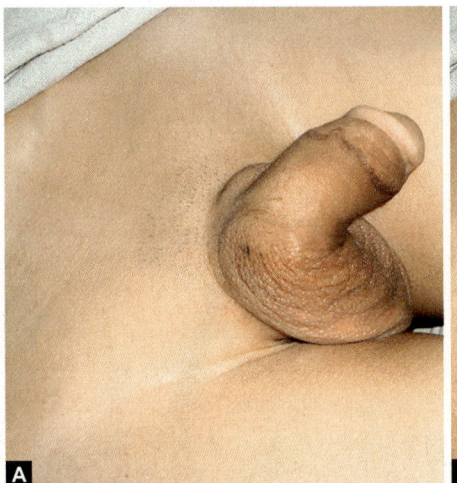
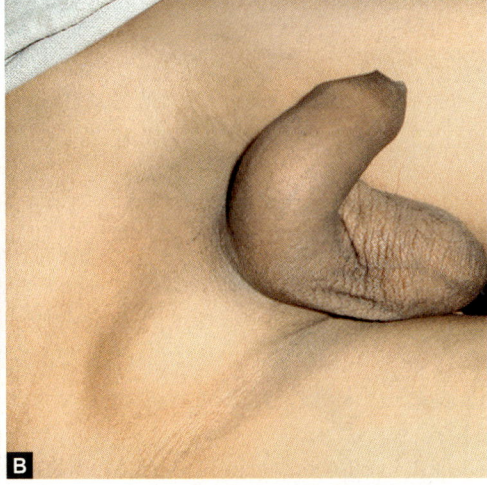

Figs. 19-12A and B *Undescended testis* in two patients. First one is bilateral and testes are not present even in groin—cryptorchidism. Note the underdeveloped empty scrotum. In second photograph it is unilateral (right sided) with visible testis (swelling) in the inguinal region.

Section 1: Examination in General Surgery

Impulse on Coughing

Inguinal hernia shows expansile impulse on coughing. Varicocele and lymph varix also show impulse on coughing but with fluid thrill. Pure scrotal swellings do not show impulse on coughing **(Fig. 19-18)**.

Groin should be inspected for swelling (inguinal nodes), ulceration, and fungation. Ulceration can occur in groin due to secondaries in the lymph nodes, bubo, tuberculosis, etc.

Palpation

Palpation of the swelling

Note: Like any other swelling **temperature, tenderness, size, shape, surface, consistency** should be checked.

Position and Extent

Exact location of swelling on palpation is important whether it is in the inguinal/inguinoscrotal/scrotal. Encysted hydrocele of the cord is located usually in the middle of the cord near the root of the scrotum occasionally in the groin. It will not extend proximally above. Lipoma of the cord, funiculitis (inflammation of vas deferens), (filarial —common), ectopic testis in superficial inguinal pouch are other groin swellings to be considered. Skin should be held to see the fixity **(Fig. 19-19)**.

Get above the Swelling

In standing position, cord is palpated for structures by placing thumb in front and fingers behind on the root of the scrotum. In hydrocele one can get above the swelling—means only cord

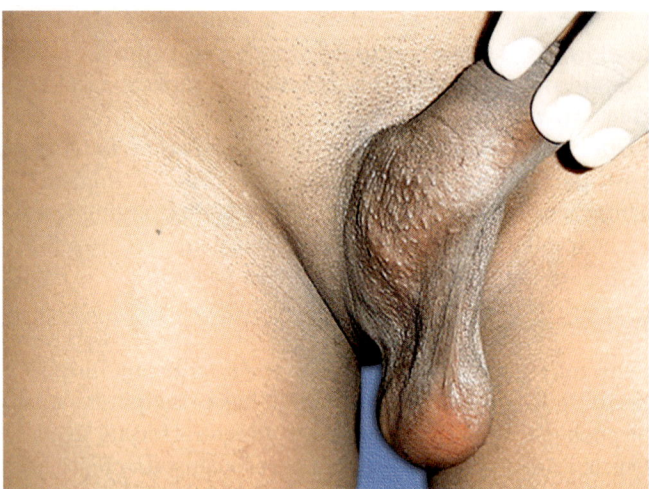

Fig. 19-14 Undescended testis with *underdeveloped scrotum on the right side*.

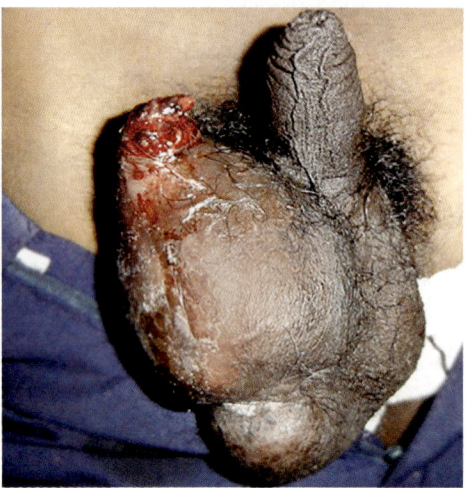

Fig. 19-15 *Testicular tumor* fungating through the skin.

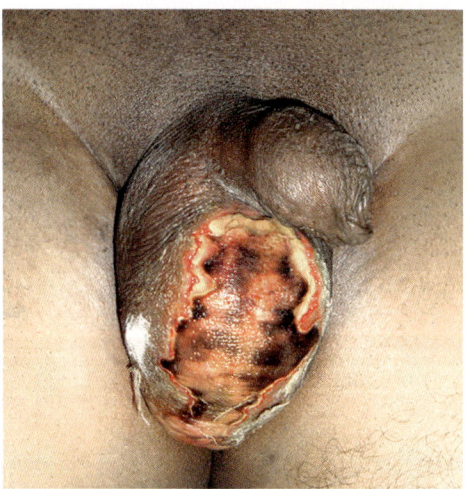

Fig. 19-16 *Fournier's gangrene.*

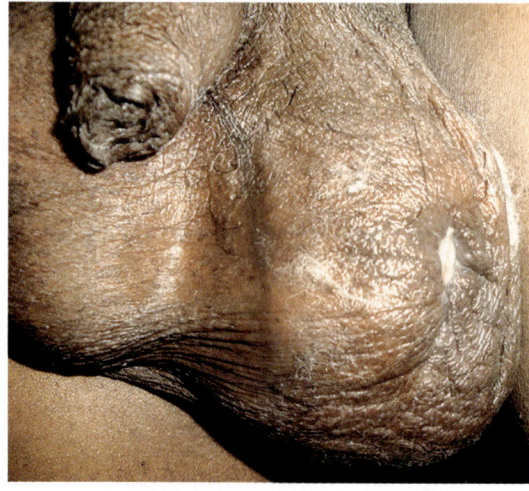

Fig. 19-17 *Discharging sinus* in the scrotum.

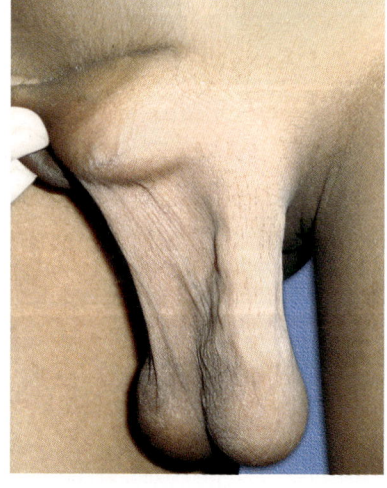

Fig. 19-18 *Varicocele* shows impulse on coughing with fluid thrill.

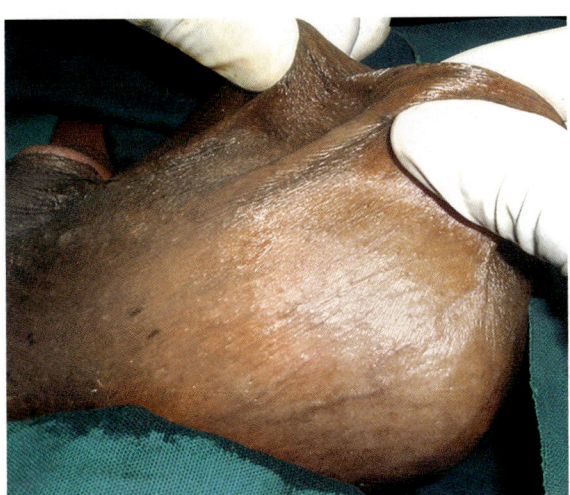

Fig. 19-19 *Skin should be held* to find out the skin fixation.

structures are felt nothing else. In inguinoscrotal hernia, one can not get above the swelling. Cord with additional structures are also felt. This is important test to confirm scrotal swelling **(Figs. 19-20A and B)**.

Consistency

Encysted hydrocele is fluctuant, cystic (Paget's test is positive), transilluminant. ***Lymph varix*** is soft, cystic and doughy. ***Varicocele*** is soft, with typical feel of 'bag of worms'. ***Hydrocele*** is smooth and soft (firm if it is tensely cystic). ***Testicular tumors*** are more solid and heavier.

Indentation Test

Pitting edema over the scrotum is seen in cellulitis, extravasation of urine, non-pitting edema in filariasis.

Fluctuation

This test is essential test for hydrocele. Upper part of the scrotum is held between thumb and fingers of one hand to steady the swelling; thumb and fingers of other hand are held at lower pole. Intermittent pressure from lower fingers will push apart the fingers over upper part and vice versa. Test is repeated in opposite direction. It is important to elicit fluctuation in two directions. It is also important to fix the swelling prior to eliciting of fluctuation. In a small swelling Paget's test is used. In bilocular hydrocele, i.e where there is swelling in the groin and hydrocele with band like narrowing near external ring, fluctuation can be elicited across the external ring above and below—***cross fluctuation*** (Other swellings which are cross fluctuant are—***psoas abscess, ranula, and compound palmar ganglion***). Hydrocele, encysted hydrocele, epididymal cyst, spermatocele, abscess are fluctuant swellings in the scrotum **(Figs. 19-21A to C)**.

Transillumination/Translucency (Figs. 19-22 to 19-28)

It is done in a dark room using a pen torch. Pen torch is placed laterally in the anterior part of the scrotum. Never place it posteriorly as testis will interfere with proper illumination. Red glow of translucency is seen in the scrotum which is better appreciated using roll of thick paper or X-ray sheet (***transilluminoscope***) placed on the opposite side (medially) especially with day light. Hydrocele becomes non-transilluminant due to thick dartos, thick unclear fluid, thick sac, hematocele, chylocele, pyocele. In epididymal cyst, it is **brilliantly transilluminant**.

> **Swellings which are brilliantly transilluminant:**
> 1. Vaginal hydrocele
> 2. Epididymal cyst
> 3. Cystic hygroma
> 4. Ranula
> 5. Meningocele

Reducibility

It is done by raising and compressing the scrotum gently. Uncomplicated inguinal and inguinoscrotal hernia are reducible. By taxis, hernial contents are gently reduced and emptied into the abdominal cavity. Hernia gets reduced abruptly and rapidly. Hydrocele is not reducible. Exception is

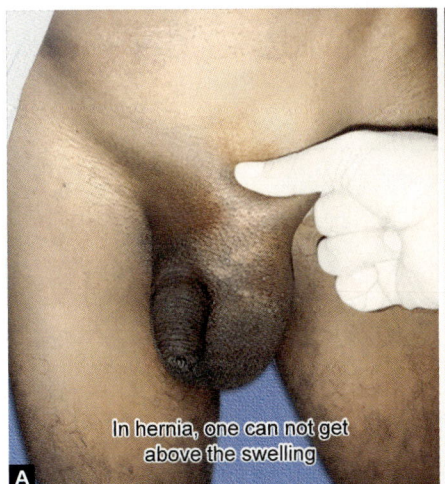
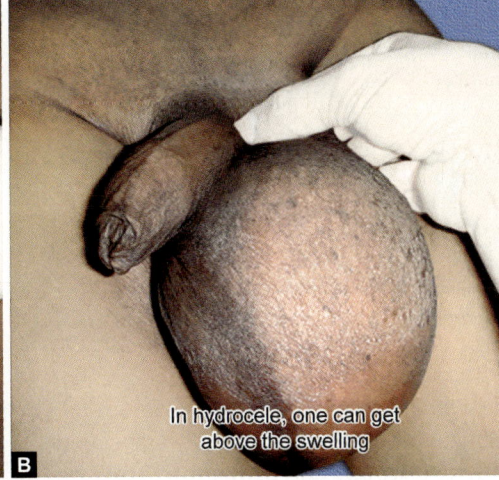

Figs. 19-20A and B In inguinoscrotal swelling *getting above the swelling is not possible*. One *can get above the swelling* in hydrocele.

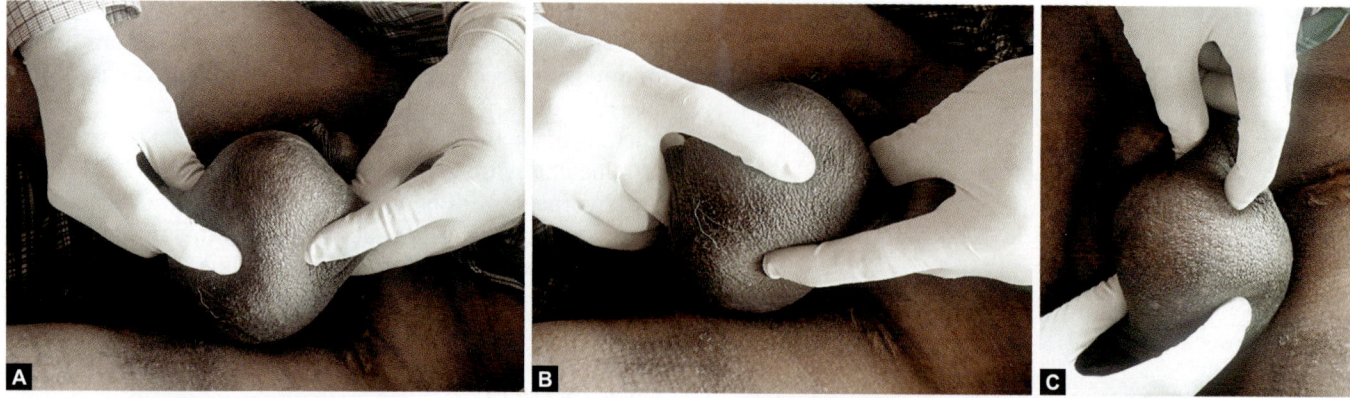

Figs. 19-21A to C *Fluctuation should be elicited in two directions* in hydrocele after fixing the swelling using fingers.

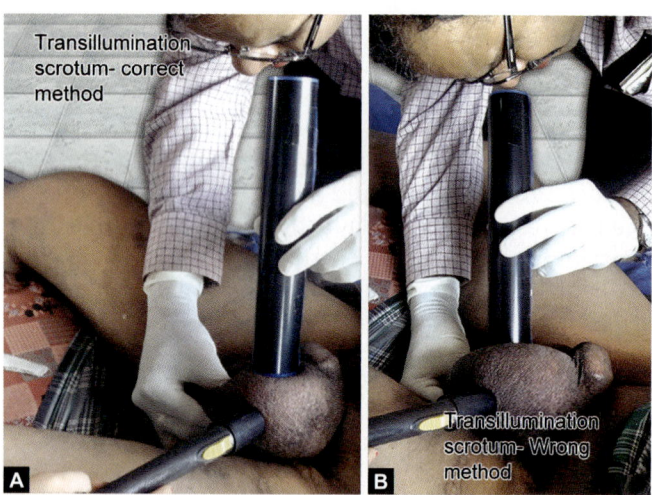

Figs. 19-22A and B Hydrocele which is transilluminant. It is checked using transilluminoscope. *It is checked transversely in the anterior aspect of the scrotum.* It should not be done on the posterior aspect as testis will interfere with the light transmission.

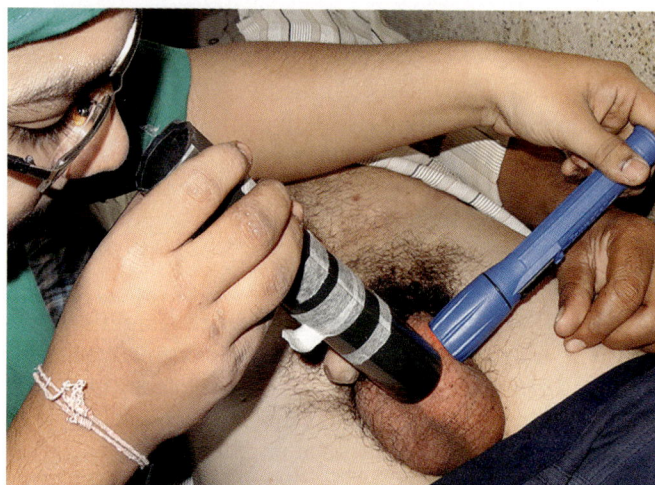

Fig. 19-24 Technique of doing transillumination test *using transillumination scope*.

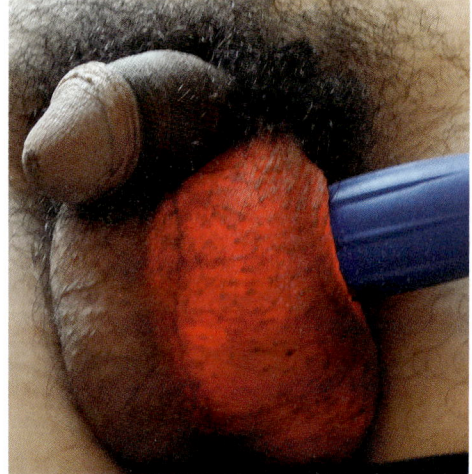

Fig. 19-23 Hydrocele is *usually transilluminant*.

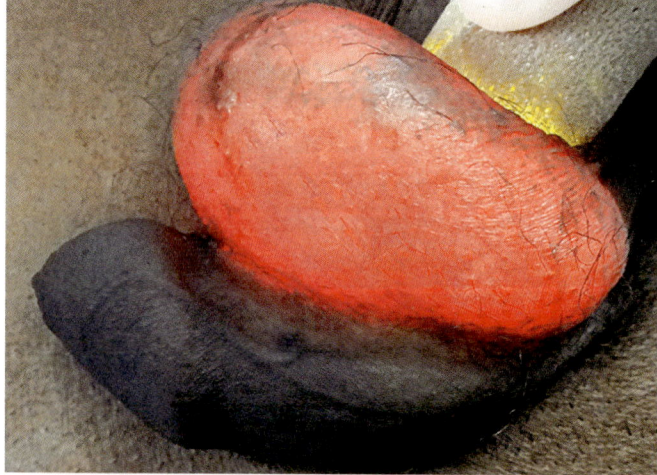

Fig. 19-25 Hydrocele which is transilluminant; *it is checked in darkroom*.

congenital hydrocele, which communicates with abdominal cavity is reducible. Congenital hydrocele is usually associated with tuberculous ascites. Varicocele and lymph varix also gets reduced while lying down but slowly and gradually.

Impulse in Coughing

The examiner holds the root of the scrotum between thumb and fingers and the patient is asked to cough. Hernia shows

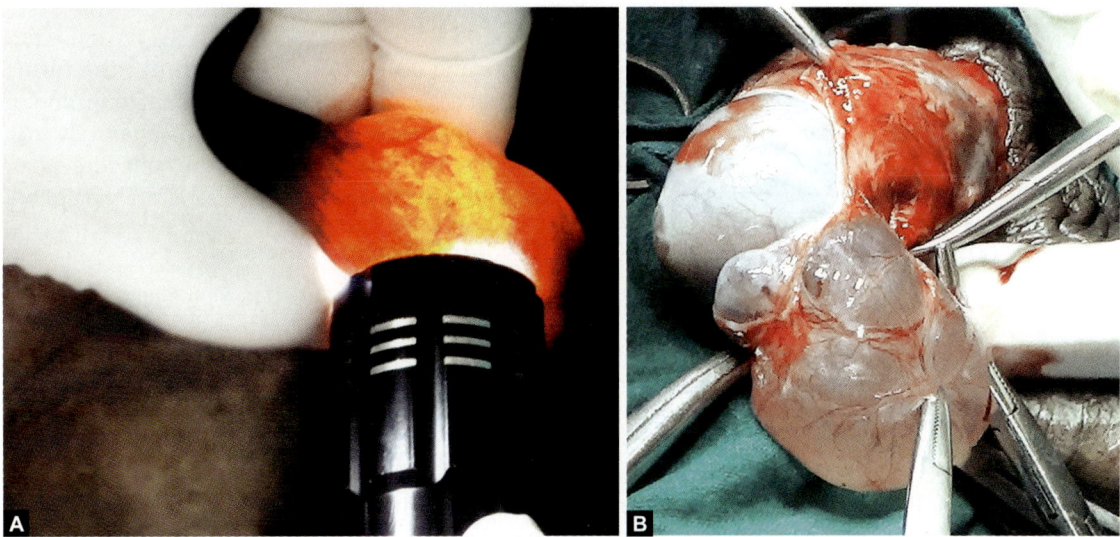

Figs. 19-26A and B Epididymal cyst is *brilliantly transilluminant* like *'Chinese lantern'* pattern.

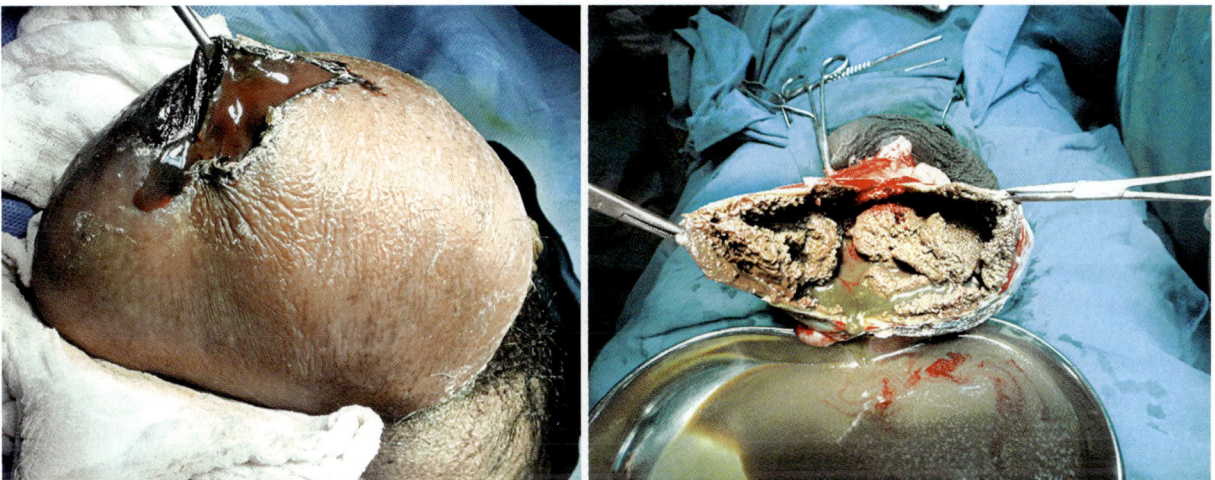

Figs. 19-27A and B *Hematocele is not transilluminant* as it contains brown or brownish red thick fluid.

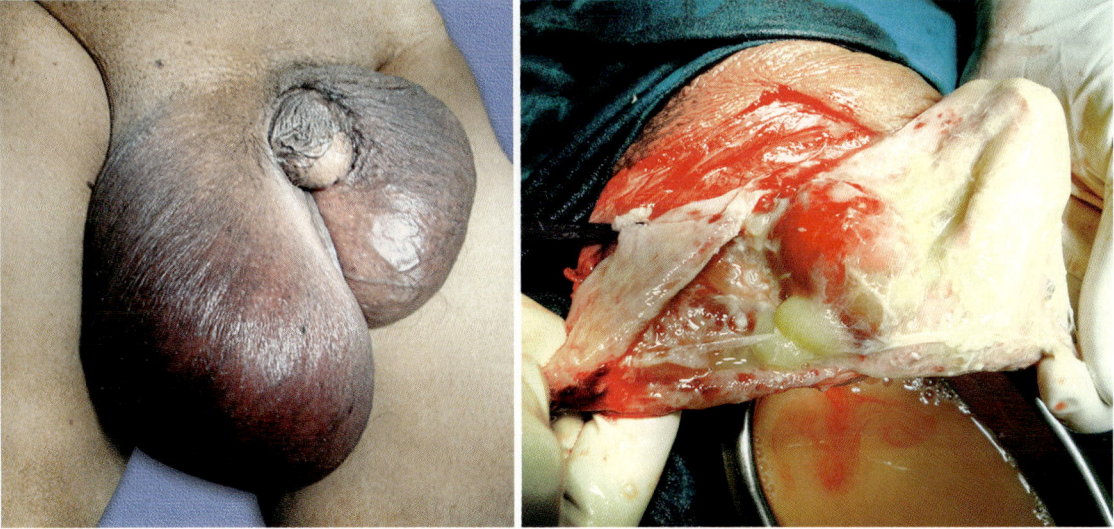

Figs. 19-28A and B *Pyocele is not transilluminant* as it contains pus.

expansile impulse on coughing. Varicocele and lymph varix also give impulse on coughing like a fluid thrill but it is not expansile.

Traction Test

It is the **test for *encysted hydrocele of the cord***. Swelling is located above the testis, which is mobile but becomes immobile once testis is pulled down from the swelling. It is used to differentiate it from epididymal cyst.

Palpation of Testis

Position

Testis may be in normal position in front with epididymis behind and globus major upwards. In ***anteverted testis,*** epididymis lies anteriorly and body posteriorly. In ***inverted testis***, testis lies upside down with globus major inferiorly. ***In incompletely inverted testis,*** testis lies horizontally. Inverted or incompletely inverted testis precipitates torsion testis. Often these changes are bilateral.

Size

Normal size is 3.75 cm above downwards; 2.5 cm from anterior to posterior; 1.8 cm side to side. It weighs 10–15 gram. Atrophied testis is smaller in size. It may be due to undescended testis or due to earlier mumps attack or developmental defect. Atrophy may be unilateral or bilateral. Larger testis may be due to tumor or filarial orchitis or syphilitic gumma. **Weight of the organ in relation to size should be assessed**. It is done by balancing the testis on the palm of the hand. Testis is **heavier in testicular tumor and hematocele**. It is lighter in gummatous testis even though size is large.

Tenderness

Testis is **tender** in orchitis. Pyocele is also tender.

Testicular Sensation

It is ***sickening sensation***/pain felt in the abdomen (at the level of umbilicus—T10) by the patient when a mild pressure is applied (*gentle* squeezing) over the testis. ***It is absent in testicular tumor, syphilis (Gumma), leprosy, chronic hematocele.*** Both side testes should be palpated. ***True testicular pain*** is located in the lower abdomen at the level of internal ring in accordance with ***Brown's law***. In suspected malignancy of testis, it should be avoided or should be gentle while eliciting to prevent the *possible spread* by squeezing into veins and lymphatics.

Note: *Testicular sensation can be elicited in vaginal hydrocele by transmitting the pressure sensation through the fluid.*

Mobility/Fixity of the Testis

Normally testis is freely mobile, but movement is restricted in chronic inflammation (orchitis, epididymo-orchitis).

Presence of Fluid

Abnormal collection of fluid within the tunica vaginalis (hydrocele) can occur—small amount in secondary hydrocele where the testis can be palpated separately from the fluid, whereas in primary hydrocele the collection is sometimes so large that the testis cannot be separately palpable.

Test for Retractile Testis

Child is made to sit on a chair with feet kept on the chair; knees fully flexed and brought over to chest wall; causing pressure on the inguinal canal downwards pushing retractile testis down into the scrotum—*Orr Chair test* (**Fig. 19-29**).

Palpation of Epididymis

It is firm uniform structure along the posterior aspect of the testis with upper head—*globus major*, middle body, lower tail—*globus minor*. **Tuberculosis** commonly involves epididymis *mainly globus minor (tail)* initially (due to retrograde spread along vas deferens). Head is involved by hematogenous spread. Epididymis tail is thickened, nodular and often tender. Later when entire epididymis is involved, epididymis will be enlarged, *craggy*, firm. Eventually coagulation necrosis → softening → cold abscess occurs on the posterior aspect of the scrotum → sinus/ulcer formation behind. Firm, irregular enlarged epididymis is common in filariasis. **Acute epididymo-orchitis** is smooth, soft tender swelling posteriorly due to bacterial or viral (mumps) causes. After prostatectomy retrograde bacterial infection can cause acute infection.

Filarial	*Epididymo-orchitis*—both testis and epididymis involved; thickened tender vas
Tuberculosis	*Epididymitis*—involving epididymis only; rather late, testis is involved only rarely; beaded vas
Syphilis	*Orchitis*—only testis is involved, rather late epididymis rarely may get involved; vas deferens not involved

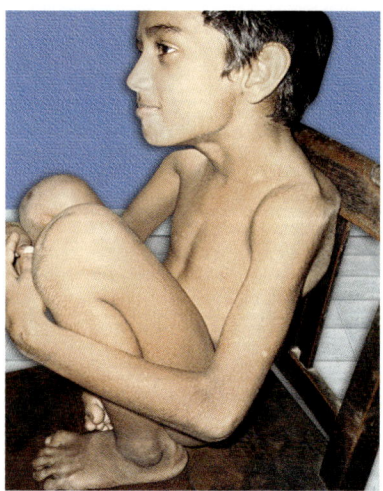

Fig. 19-29 *Orr chair test.*

Palpation of Spermatic Cord

Cord is palpated for vas deferens at the root of the scrotum between thumb and index finger **together on both sides (Fig. 19-30)**. Vas deferens normally is string like structure that slips between fingers. Vas is thickened and tender in epididymo-orchitis—acute or chronic due to funiculitis. It is thickened and beaded in tuberculosis of vas. It is thickened and tender in filariasis. Soft, doughy feel is felt in lymph varix; like '**bag of worms**' due to pampiniform plexus of spermatic cord in varicocele. Rarely testicular tumor spreads along the spermatic cord making it feel nodular and hard.

Vas deferens sign: Helps in differentiating hematocele from testicular tumor. The vas deferens in the cord is identified, palpated and followed all the way down towards, in testicular tumor it can be traced up to the upper border of the tumor, whereas in hematocele it can be traced all the way down to its lower limit.

Percussion

In inguinoscrotal swelling, tympanic note is felt if it is a enterocele, and all other swelling are dull on percussion.

Palpation of Lymph Nodes

Scrotal skin drains into horizontal group of inguinal lymph nodes; testis and epididymis drains into pre- and para-aortic lymph nodes at the level of origin of testicular artery—transpyloric nodes. Inguinal and iliac nodes may be enlarged in scrotal skin conditions and also testicular tumor that infiltrates the tunica and scrotal skin. Testicular tumor spreads to para aortic nodes and then to left side supraclavicular nodes.

Per-rectal Examination

Craggy, nodular seminal vesicles can be palpable in late stages of tuberculous epididymo-orchitis. **Picker position** is needed to palpate the seminal vesicles; patient stands and leans forward, grasping a low chair or a stool. Other conditions where seminal vesicles are palpable are tumors of the seminal vesicles and trichomonas vaginalis infection.

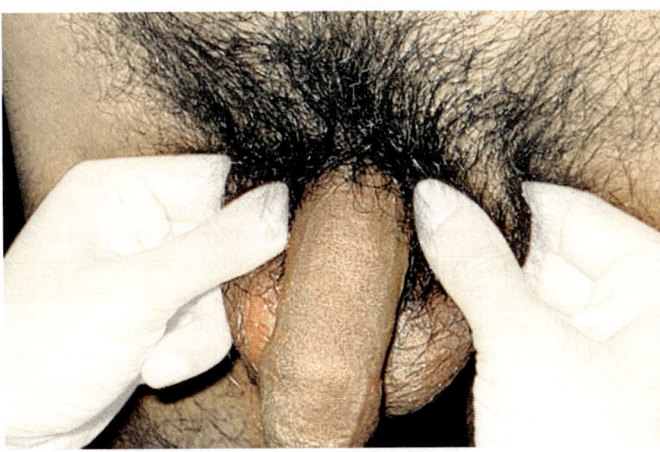

Fig. 19-30 Method of *palpation of vas*.

Systemic Examinations

Abdomen examination—Any intra-abdominal mass should be looked for in varicocele, any evidence of abdominal tuberculosis, which often co-exist with tuberculous epididymo-orchitis is looked for.

Respiratory system examination is important as secondaries can occur in testicular tumors. In tuberculosis primary focus may be in lungs.

■ INVESTIGATIONS

Blood—smear for microfilariae; VDRL for syphilis; ESR is raised in tuberculosis.

Urine for culture, AFB (early morning specimen).

Chest X-ray to see lung secondaries from testicular tumor as *'cannon ball'* type; to see pulmonary tuberculosis.

Tumor markers in testicular tumor—alpha fetoprotein (AFP); β-hCG.

US of scrotum to see hematocele, pyocele, secondary hydrocele, varicocele, testicular tumor. It is very useful in all scrotal diseases (FNAC is contraindicated in testicular tumor. Scrotal approach is also contraindicated).

CT abdomen to see nodal metastases, liver and chest secondaries.

Hydrocele

- It is the collection of fluid between the two layers of tunica vaginalis of the testis.
- *Types (Fig. 19-31):* (1) Congenital; (2) Acquired: (a) Primary, and (b) Secondary.

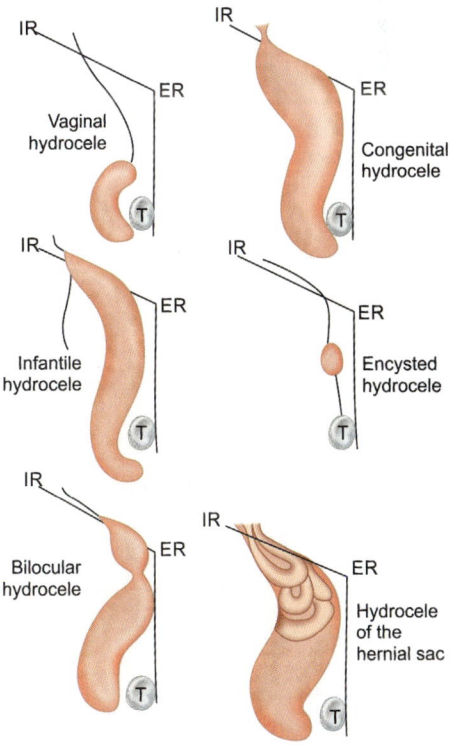

IR- Internal ring; ER- External ring

Fig. 19-31 *Types of hydrocele.*

- *Etiology:* (1) *Defective absorption* of fluid by the tunica vaginalis, probably due to damage to the endothelial wall by low grade infection; (2) *Excessive production* of fluid—as in secondary hydrocele; (3) *Interference with drainage* of the fluid by lymphatic vessels of the cord; (4) *Communication into the peritoneal cavity* are other causes.
- *Hydrocele fluid* is amber colored with specific gravity of 1.022 to 1.024. It contains water, salts, albumin, and fibrinogen. Per se hydrocele fluid does not clot, but gets activated if it comes in contact with the blood, fibrinogen and clots firmly. Often fluid contains cholesterol and tyrosine crystals (Fig. 19-33).

> **Cysts which contains cholesterol crystals:** (1) Vaginal hydrocele; (2) Branchial cyst; (3) Dentigerous cyst.

- Primary vaginal hydrocele: It occurs in middle aged, common in tropical countries. Testis is not palpable, usually attains a large size (unlike secondary hydrocele which are small except in filarial hydrocele); *fluctuant; transilluminant (initially)*.

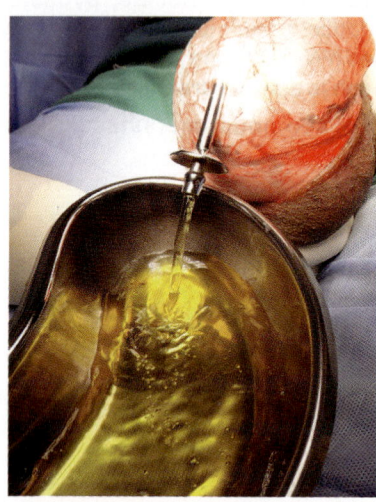

Fig. 19-32 Hydrocele fluid is *amber colored*. It does not clot usually; but once it comes into contact with blood will clot due to calcium.

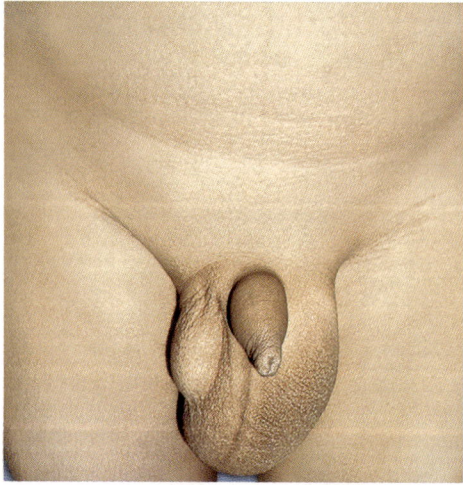

Fig. 19-33 Hydrocele in a child. *It mimics hernia. It is due to patent processus vaginalis*. Treatment is like hernia—herniotomy only through inguinal approach.

- Infantile hydrocele: Here tunica and processus vaginalis (hydrocele) are distended up to internal ring, but sac has no connection with the general peritoneal cavity.
- Congenital hydrocele: Here processus vaginalis communicates with the peritoneal cavity. As this communicating orifice is too small, bowel and/or omentum do not descend and so hernia usually will not develop. While lying down, fluid disappears gradually and while standing fluid recollects. Hydrocele cannot be emptied by digital pressure due to *'inverted ink bottle'* effect. Ascites, tuberculous peritonitis are the etiologies for the same in an adult (Fig. 19-33).
- Encysted hydrocele of the cord: It is a smooth, soft, oval, fluctuant, transilluminant swelling associated with the spermatic cord in inguinal or inguinoscrotal region. Impulse on coughing, reducibility are absent; testis is felt normal. It is due to persistent patent small portion of the tunica vaginalis in the cord but is closed above and below. On gentle traction to the testis, the swelling becomes less mobile (*traction test*).
- *Differential diagnosis:* Epididymal cyst, inguinal hernia.
- Hydrocele En Bisac (Bilocular hydrocele): Hydrocele has got two intercommunicating sacs, one above and one below the neck of the scrotum. Upper one lies superficial or in the inguinal canal or may insinuate itself in between the muscle layers—*cross fluctuant*.
- Hydrocele of the canal of the nuck: It occurs in females, in relation to the round ligament, always in the inguinal canal.
- Hydrocele of the hernial sac (5% of inguinal hernias): It is due to adhesions of the content; fluid secreted will collect in the hernial sac and forms hydrocele of the hernial sac.
- Secondary hydrocele: *Causes:* Infection: filariasis; tuberculosis of epididymis; syphilis; injury: trauma, post-herniorrhaphy hydrocele; tumor. Secondary hydrocele rarely attains large size. It is usually small, lax and testis is usually palpable (unlike primary hydrocele). Exception is secondary hydrocele due to filariasis.
- Post-herniorrhaphy hydrocele: It is a secondary hydrocele occurring after the surgery for inguinal hernia. It is due to the damage to lymphatic vessels of the tunica vaginalis and is 0.2% common. It is treated like any hydrocele but usually after about 6 months.
- Filarial hydrocele and chylocele: It occurs commonly in coastal region and in around the Equator; occurs after repeated attacks of filarial epididymitis; attains large size and the sac is thickened. Fluid contains fat, rich in cholesterol, derived from ruptured lymph varix into the tunica. It is often difficult to differentiate from primary hydrocele. In chylocele, chylous fluid collects in tunica vaginalis which may show microfilaria.
- Complications of hydrocele: Infection; pyocele (suppurated hydrocele); hematocele; atrophy of testis; infertility; rupture; hernia of the hydrocele sac through dartos.
- *Differential diagnosis*: Inguinal hernia; epididymal cyst; spermatocele; testicular tumor; scrotal edema.
- Hematocele: It is collection of blood/clot in the tunica vaginalis testis. It may be due to trauma or bleeding in an existing hydrocele. Blood gets clotted, organized and later may be calcified. Eventually, it causes testicular atrophy. *Types: Recent hematocele*—it is due to traumatic or spontaneous rupture of one of the vessels in the

tunica causing bleeding into the sac. *Features:* Sudden onset of pain, swelling after a history of trauma; tender, warm, fluctuant, but non-transilluminant; occasionally aggressive testicular tumor mimics presentation of acute recent hematocele. US of scrotum is done to rule out neoplasm and also to find out the viability of testis. Chronic or old clotted hematocele: It is usually due to slow, spontaneous hemorrhage into the tunica vaginalis without any proper history of trauma. It is painless, hard, nontender, nonfluctuant, often calcified swelling, with loss of testicular sensation. Because of the constant pressure testicular function and so testicular sensation is lost. It mimics testicular tumor.

- *Pyocele:* It is collection of pus in the layers of tunica vaginalis. It is often suppurative hydrocele. It can occur in a previously normal tunica or in a pre-existing hematocele or hydrocele which gets infected. Features: Fever, toxicity, tender swelling in the scrotum, with scrotal wall edema; often in young individuals, it may be difficult to differentiate this from the torsion testis; pus under tension eventually causes infective thrombosis of testicular vessels, leading to nonviability of the testis or testicular gangrene.

Undescended Testis

- It results from arrest of descent of the testis in some parts of its path to the scrotum. Bilateral undescended testis is called *cryptorchidism* (means hidden testis). *Anorchism:* There is complete agenesis of testis. These two can be differentiated by HCG test.
- *Embryology:* Normally kidney ascends, testis descends during development. Primitive testis develops from the genital fold which descends by a peritoneal fold called as gubernaculums; Wolffian duct develops into epididymis and vas deferens. During 9th month of gestation testis reaches deep inguinal ring. Later just before or after delivery it descends into the scrotum.
- *Incidence:* In premature infants—30%. In full term infants—4%. In later childhood—2%. Right testis is involved more commonly in 50% cases, left alone in 30% cases, bilateral in 20% cases. It is due to gubernacular dysfunction, lack of hCG, *Prune Belly* syndrome, familial.
- *Pathology: After the age of six,* testis gradually atrophies, reduces its external as well as internal secretory activity. Eventually grossly immature epithelial elements with irreversible destructive changes of the germinal epithelium occur.
- *Different location of testis:* In the abdomen just above the internal ring, extraperitoneally; in the inguinal canal; in the superficial inguinal pouch. Bilateral undescended testes which are clinically impalpable is called *as cryptorchidism.* Scrotum is *not fully developed* and testis cannot be brought down manually to the bottom of the scrotum in undescended testis.
- *Differential diagnosis:* Retractile testis; *Torsion of the undescended testis in inguinal region is difficult to differentiate from strangulated inguinal hernia;* empty scrotum may be a crucial clinical sign.
- *Complications of undescended testis:* Sterility; trauma and pain; an associated indirect inguinal hernia (70%); torsion testis; epididymo-orchitis (as the pain will be high up, it mimics acute appendicitis); testicular atrophy;

Malignant transformation in undescended testis is 20 times more common than in normally descended testis. It is higher in abdominal than in inguinally located testis. *Seminoma is* the commonest malignancy in undescended testis. The testis which has normally descended on other side (in case of unilateral undescended testis) is also more prone for malignant transformation than normal individual.

Testicular Tumors

It accounts for 1% of all malignant tumors; 99% of testicular tumors are malignant.

Predisposing factors: Undescended testis, Klinefelter's syndrome and testicular atrophy.

Classification: (1) Seminoma—40%. (2) Teratoma—32%. (3) Seminoma + teratoma—14%.(4) Interstitial tumors—1.5% (Leydig cell tumor (musculinises; Sertoli cell tumor feminises). (5) Lymphomas—7%. (6) Others.

Histological classification: (1) *Germ cell tumor*— Seminomatous: classic/spermatocytic/anaplastic. Non-seminomatous: embryonal carcinoma/teratoma/choriocarcinoma/yolk sac tumor. (2) *Sex cord tumors:* Leydig cell tumor; Sertoli cell tumor. (3) *Combined germ cell and gonadal stromal tumor.* (4) *Adnexal and paratesticular tumor.* (5) *Others*—Carcinoids, lymphomas, secondaries.

Seminoma testis: It starts in the mediastinum of the testis. Grossly it is lobulated, fleshy, homogenous, creamy or pinkish in color and it compresses adjacent testicular tissues. Histologically, malignant cells resemble spermatocytes which are *clear cells, with lymphocytic* infiltration. It spreads through testicular lymphatics into the para-aortic lymph nodes and then to left supraclavicular lymph node. Through blood, it spreads to lungs, bone, brain, liver. Seminoma is further classified as typical (classic) which is commonest; spermatocytic (in old age); anaplastic; atypical.

Teratoma: It arises from totipotent cells, i.e. ecto, meso, endoderms. Grossly tumor surface is irregular, cut section shows solid and cystic spaces with areas of hemorrhage. It often contains gelatinous fluid and cartilaginous nodules. Histologically there are four types: (1) *Teratoma differentiated*—(1%); (2) *Teratoma intermediate*—30% common—Two subtypes are A and B (more malignant); (3) *Teratoma anaplastic*—15%—secretes alpha feto protein (AFP); (4) *Teratoma trophoblastic*—1%—It shows high levels of βhCG (normal level is 100 IU).

Interstitial cell tumor: Leydig cell tumor (2%) musculinises; Prepubertal tumor shows excessive output of androgens causing sexual precocity, extreme muscular development and may mimic infant hercules.

Sertoli cell tumor (1%) feminises; Post-pubertal tumor commonly arising from Sertoli cells causes feminising effect with gynecomastia, loss of libido and aspermia.

Clinical features: Enlargement of testis; fullness and heaviness in the scrotum; pain in the testis (30%); testis will be enlarged, firm, heavy, with loss of testicular sensation; secondary hydrocele is common. Cremaster is hypertrophied and thickened. Vas, prostate and seminal vesicles are normal. It can spread to cord tissues making it nodular and hard. Often in epigastric region para-aortic lymph nodes may be palpable as hard, nodular, nontender, nonmobile, vertically placed, resonant mass (not moving with respiration). There may be hemoptysis, altered breath sounds and pleural effusion due to lung secondaries; Bone pain and tenderness due to secondaries in bone; Nodular secondaries in the liver. Occasionally it may mimic acute epididymo-orchitis or acute hematocele. Gynecomastia may be present in few teratomas.

Hurricane type is very aggressive, highly malignant testicular tumor which is more often fatal in few weeks. Rarely, if tumor comes out of the tunica albuginea (tunica albuginea is resistant for malignant cell infiltration), then scrotum gets infiltrated and spread can occur to inguinal lymph nodes.

Differential diagnosis: Acute and chronic hematocele; acute epididymo-orchitis; syphilitic orchitis; Lepra orchitis.

Other Conditions	Features
Fournier's gangrene (*Idiopathic gangrene of scrotum*): It is a vascular gangrene of infective origin caused by Hemolytic streptococci, microaerophilic streptococci, staphylococci, E. coli, *Clostridium welchii* There will be fulminant inflammation of the scrotal skin and subcutaneous tissues resulting in *obliterative arteritis of arterioles of scrotal skin leading to cutaneous gangrene*	Common in old age; minor perineal injury, infected anal fissure, drainage of periurethral abscess may precipitate the condition **(Fig. 19-34)** Sudden severe pain, redness, blackening of scrotum, fever, severe toxicity; fast spreading cellulitis extending to groin and anterior abdominal wall, *extensive sloughing of skin exposing normal testis*. **Complications**: Renal failure, septicemia, death
Funiculitis: Inflammation of vas deferens Commonly due to filariasis; but can be gonococcal/tuberculous etiology Tuberculous funiculitis associated with tuberculous epididymitis—thickened, craggy, beaded feel	Filarial funiculitis present with mild pain in the inguinal canal and cord, with fever, red, edematous, shiny skin. Sometimes edema may be severe to be mistaken for strangulated hernia (here no hernial contents felt when palpated above the deep inguinal ring). Pain may mimic pain of ureteric stone
Orchitis: It is inflammation of the testis. It is commonly associated with inflammation of the epididymis. Hence called as *epididymo*-orchitis. Orchitis is due to infection through blood, lymphatics or epididymis **Causes**: Viral infection—mumps; filarial disease; leprosy; bacterial; brucellosis; infectious mononucleosis. It can be precipitated by retrograde spread due to stricture urethra, after prostate or bladder surgery, after instrumentation. Syphilis involves testis—causing formation of gummatous ulcer on the front of the scrotum	Pain in the testis often radiates to groin due to associated funiculitis; Fever, tenderness in the testis; *Secondary hydrocele* common; Often urinary infection is noticed **Differential diagnosis**: Torsion testis; Testicular tumor (enlarged hard testis with loss of testicular sensation)
Syphilitic orchitis: Syphilis involves only testis; never vas deferens. It can be—bilateral *interstitial orchitis* seen in congenital syphilis (causing *pigeon-egg* testes in infants); if infant becomes syphilitic boy then he becomes lame (*Clutton's joints*), deaf (neurolabyrinthitis), blind (interstitial keratitis), impotent (atrophy of testes); interstitial fibrosis is bilateral causing gradual destruction of the seminiferous tubules with loss of testicular sensation without any enlarged testis	Testis is dense, rounded hard and mobile—'*billiard testis*'; *Gumma of testis* is commonest type with unilateral painless slowly enlarged hard testis with *loss of testicular sensation*. Testis is adherent to anterior part of the scrotal skin leading into softening and gummatous ulcer formation. Shotty groin, epitrochlear and popliteal lymph nodes may be palpable
Epididymitis: Inflammation of epididymis is commonly associated with orchitis—**epididymo-orchitis** **Causes**: Nonspecific, viral like mumps; bacterial; filarial; tuberculosis (It involves mainly epididymis not testis and so ulcer/sinus occurs over the posterior aspect of the scrotum not in front); gonococcal; schistosomiasis	It can be acute or subacute or chronic. Acute when it occurs from retrograde spread involves globus minor first later entire epididymis and testis. Severe pain, edema scrotum, thickened tender epididymis, secondary hydrocele are common. There may be associated prostatitis, urethritis, and cystitis also. Blood born infection involves globus major first. Retrograde spread can occur after prostatectomy, catheterization, and cystitis
Tuberculous epididymitis: It is commonly due to retrograde spread from tuberculous cystitis; *involves globus minor* (tail) first and later entire epididymis and testis in very late cases. Blood spread from lungs directly involves globus major first. *Secondary hydrocele* develops in 30% cases. 60% will be having renal tuberculosis. Digital examination of rectum (P/R) shows tender thickened palpable seminal vesicles and irregular prostate. Pulmonary tuberculosis is evident in 50% of cases	*Thickened, craggy, firm nodular epididymis* is common. Cold abscess, sinus or undermined ulcer may be present on the posterior aspect of the scrotum. Scrotal skin loses its normal rugosity with wasting of the tissue under the skin. There is *restricted mobility* (upward and downward) of testis; *thickened beaded vas* (due to tubercles) is typical
Torsion testis: It is an *emergency condition* of the testis, wherein the testis twists (rotates) in its axis compromising its blood supply. If not intervened and rectified within 12–24 hours, testis will become gangrenous. *Right testis rotates in clockwise direction whereas left rotates in anticlockwise*. Secondary hydrocele of the torsion testis is serosanguineous **Predisposing factors**: (1) Inversion of the testis. (2) High investment of the tunica vaginalis which acts like a mesentery through which testis rotates. Here testis hangs like a *clapper in bell*. (3) Presence of gap between the body of the testis and epididymis as a result of which testis twists over epididymis. (4) Heavy straining often precipitates torsion due to vigorous contraction of the cremaster, which is attached spirally	Occurs in children and adolescents; presents with sudden onset of pain in the scrotum, groin and lower abdomen. Vomiting due to pylorospasm; tenderness, redness, and edema of the scrotal skin with testis adherent to scrotal wall – are features. Torsion occurring in an imperfectly descended testis is impossible to differentiate it from strangulated hernia. Absence of testis in the scrotum may give a clue. *Deming's sign*: Affected testis is positioned high because of twisting of cord and spasm of cremaster muscle. *Angel's sign*: Opposite testis lies horizontally because of the mesorchium between testis and epididymis and is usually bilateral **Differential diagnosis**: (1) Acute epididymo-orchitis—elevation of the scrotum relieves the pain of acute epididymo-orchitis but aggravates in case of torsion testis (*Prehn's sign*). (2) Strangulated inguinal hernia. (3) Other structure in scrotum which can undergo torsion is '*Appendage of testis*'

Contd...

Contd...

Retractile testis: It is due to overaction of cremaster, as a result testis is pulled up to stay near the external ring and often mistaken for undescended testis. Testis is normally developed, can be pulled down to the scrotum. Scrotum is fully developed	*Orr chair test*— Child is made to sit with feet kept on the chair; knees fully flexed and brought close to chest wall; causing pressure on the inguinal canal downwards pushing retractile testis down into the scrotum
Ectopic testis: During developmental period of fetus, scrotal tail of gubernaculum ruptures or weakens and so other accessory tails will become stronger and pulls the testis accordingly to their site **Testis is found in ectopic sites—** a. Superficial inguinal pouch (commonest) b. Perineum c. Root of the penis d. Femoral triangle (thigh)	Testis is functioning normally, normal size, more prone for trauma, can cause psychological problem. Scrotum not fully developed
Spermatocele: Unilocular, acquired retention cyst of epididymis. Derived from blockage of some portions of the sperm conducting mechanism of the epididymis	Swelling situated in the head of the epididymis, above and behind the body of the testis; contains *barley water like fluid with* spermatozoa; soft, cystic, transilluminant; often considered by the patient having additional testis –*third testis*. Aspiration cytology confirms diagnosis
Cyst of the epididymis: Congenital in origin; Occurs in middle age. It is due to cystic degeneration of a. Paradidymis (organ of *Giraides*)—commonest b. Appendix of epididymis (hydatid of *Morgagni*) c. Appendix of testis—Vas aberrans of Haller	Tensely cystic swelling, contains clear fluid, often bilateral. As they are aggregation of many cysts, so multiloculated—brilliantly transilluminant —"*chinese lantern pattern*". Feel like "*bunch of tiny grapes*" situated behind the body of testis *Cyst of appendage of testis*—unilateral, globular rare cystic swelling on the superior pole of testis—may develop torsion
Varicocele: It is dilatation and tortuosity of pampiniform plexus of veins and also the testicular veins **Types**— *Primary/idiopathic*—95% No cause found; incompetence of valves of testicular vein; common on left side as left testicular vein joins left renal vein at right angle and is liable to get compressed by loaded sigmoid colon *Secondary*—due to specific cause like left sided renal cell carcinoma with a tumor thrombus in left renal vein causing obstruction to venous flow of testicular vein (*irreducible*) *Grading*: 1—small; 2—moderate; 3—large; 4—severely tortuous	Presents with swelling in the root of scrotum; dragging pain in groin and scrotum; "*Bag of worms*" feeling; impulse on coughing (thrill feel); on lying down reduces slowly and spontaneously **Bow sign:** After holding the varicocele between thumb and fingers patient is asked to bow—varicocele gets reduced in size as bowing reduces blood flow in testicular vein and pampiniform plexus Varicocele causes *subfertility / infertility*—as there is increased temperature in the scrotum which depresses spermatogenesis
Lymph scrotum / elephantiasis scrotum: It is dilatation and tortuosity of cutaneous lymphatics of scrotum. Excess rugosity and vesicles in scrotal skin containing clear fluid; these vesicles may rupture causing *lymphorrhagia*. Secondary infection later fibrosis of skin—leading to *elephantiasis of scrotum* **(Fig. 19-35)**	Initial pitting edema becomes nonpitting, firm, thick skin, progressing upwards gradually. Testis becomes atrophic due to lack of nutrition
Lymph varix: Here lymphatic vessels of cord become dilated and tortuous. It is due to obstruction by filarial worm. *Dancing filarial worm in USG—diagnostic*	Previous history of fever, pain, discomfort; presents with soft, cystic, elongated boggy, multiloculated swelling in the inguinal/inguinoscrotal region, thrill like impulse on coughing, gets reduced slowly, and spontaneously on lying down; groin lymph nodes enlarged.
Extravasation of urine: *It may be superficial or deep* **Superficial:** It is either due to bulbar urethral injury or due to bursting of periurethral abscess after urethral stricture. Once urine extravasates due to disruption of full thickness of the urethra anteriorly, it collects in superficial perineal space **(Fig. 19-36)** Entire scrotum, penis and often lower abdominal wall are swollen containing urine. It is painful; patient cannot pass urine through urethra; Has severe pain and shock due to pelvic injury. Often sepsis occurs and skin sloughs of leading into urinary fistulas	**Deep:** Urine spreads upwards into the extraperitoneal space of the pelvis around the bladder and prostate into the anterior abdominal wall causing deep extravasation of the urine. Here rupture of urethra is at membranous part of the urethra much more proximal than superficial type

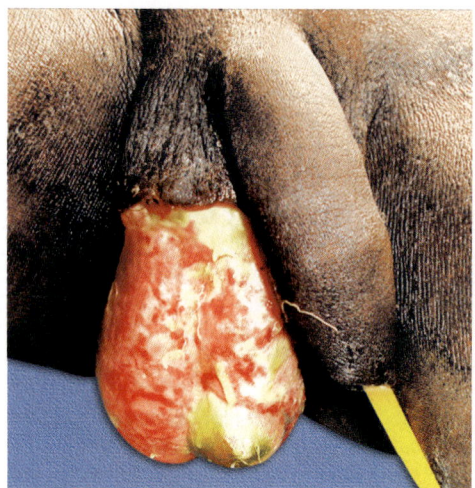
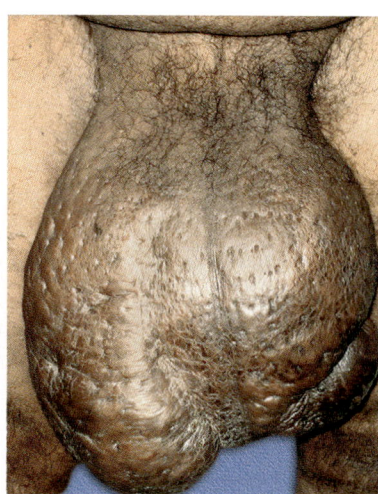
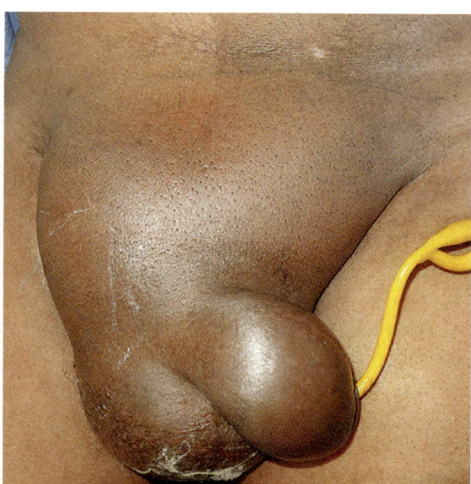

Figs. 19-34 *Fournier's gangrene.*   **Fig. 19-35** *Scrotal elephantiasis—filarial cause.*   **Fig. 19-36** *Superficial extravasation of urine.*

CASE DISCUSSION

A 30-year-old male presents with history of swelling in the right side of the scrotum of 3 years duration. It started insidiously, progressed gradually to reach the present size of 15 × 15 cm. There is no history of pain or fever. On examination in standing expansile impulse on coughing is not present; one can get above the swelling confirming it as purely scrotal. Swelling is nontender, smooth, soft, fluctuant and nontransilluminating. Skin is free. Right testis is not felt. Testicular sensation is present. Inguinal nodes are absent. Opposite side is normal. Abdomen is normal; there are no palpable para-aortic lymph nodes. Left supraclavicular region and lungs are normal.

What is your diagnosis?
It is right sided primary vaginal hydrocele.

What are the reasons?
There is no expansile impulse on coughing; one can get above the swelling; it is fluctuant. Since it has attained large size it is primary; since right testis is not palpable it is vaginal hydrocele.

Can secondary hydrocele attain large size?
Yes, it is possible; mainly secondary filarial hydrocele; otherwise all other secondary hydroceles are usually smaller in size.

What other scrotal swellings you will think of?
They are—epididymal cyst, encysted hydrocele of the cord, spermatocele, varicocele, testicular tumor.

Can testicular tumor mimic hydrocele?
It can. It causes loss of testicular sensation; firm or hard swelling in the scrotum; secondary hydrocele may be present. Patient may present only with para-aortic lymph node enlargement.

What investigation you will do in hydrocele?
Ultrasound scrotum and abdomen should be done. It confirms fluid and nature of the testis. Aspiration should not be done even FNAC is contraindicated. In suspected testicular tumors, tumor markers like β–hCG, AFP should be done.

What are the complications of hydrocele?
Pyocele, hematocele, testicular atrophy.

CHAPTER 20
Approaches and Examination of Male External Genitalia

Competency: SU30.1; AN46.5; PA29.2; PE21.14.

HISTORY

Age: Phimosis, hypospadias are seen in infants and children. Carcinoma of penis is seen in adults and old age.

Race: Muslims and Jews undergo early circumcision and so they are immune from developing carcinoma penis.

Complaints

Micturition disorders: Inability to retract foreskin in a child as history given by mother or ballooning of the prepuce during urination is seen in *phimosis*. In elderly, it is due to posthitis/subpreputial ulcer.

Visible pinhole meatus is common, which may be congenital (commonly) or acquired due to balanoposthitis or meatal ulcer. Patient may have to strain during micturition or may take a long time for the act; the flow may be in the form of drops or narrow stream.

History of increased frequency of micturition is seen in urethritis.

History of inability to place back the retracted prepuce is seen in *paraphimosis*. It may be precipitated in a patient with mild phimosis by act of intercourse. Paraphimosis may be very painful **(Figs. 20-1 to 20-3)**.

Ulcer: Ulcer in the penis, when present, the history should be asked in detail. Its location, duration, progress, pain, discharge, bleeding, urinary symptoms, associated change in the stream of urine are important. *Chancroid* (*soft sore*) is due to *Haemophilus ducreyi* develops in 4 days after exposure as a painful, tender ulcer. Syphilitic **Hunterian hard chancre** appears 4 weeks after exposure. Small painless ulcer often disappears unnoticed in lymphogranuloma inguinale (LGV). Painless vesicle or papule later forms a granulomatous ulcer in granuloma inguinale (*Donovan ulcer*) with lymph nodes involved. History of sexual contacts is very important in all these ulcers. ***Progressive painless ulcer may be carcinomatous ulcer*** (Fig. 20-4).

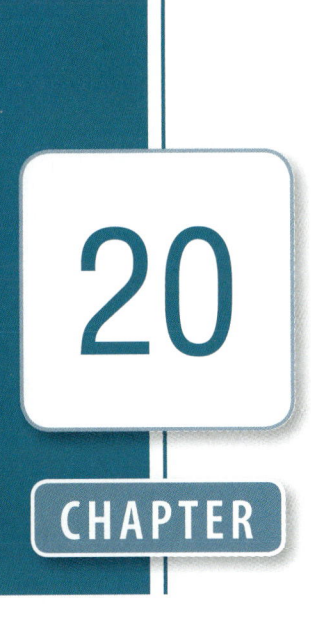

Fig. 20-1 Hypospadias; urethra opens more proximally than at the tip.

Discharge: History of discharge, its duration, site of discharge, color, quantity, smell (foul-smelling or not) should be asked. It may be serous/purulent/blood-stained.

Pain: Pain may be in the glans/in the ulcer/in the urethra. It may be during micturition (urethritis, stone, acute prostatitis, prostatic abscess, foreign body) or may be independent of act of micturition (herpes, carcinoma, balanoposthitis, paraphimosis) or after micturition (vesical calculus, acute/chronic cystitis, bladder tumor). In bladder calculus, the pain is referred to tip of glans, hence the patient will pull the tip of the glans before the micturition. Nature of pain should be asked (burning/scalding).

404 Section 1: Examination in General Surgery

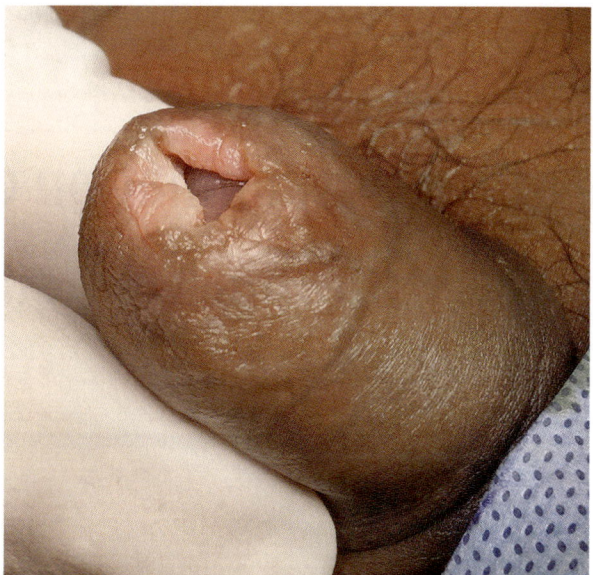

Fig. 20-2 *Phimosis*.

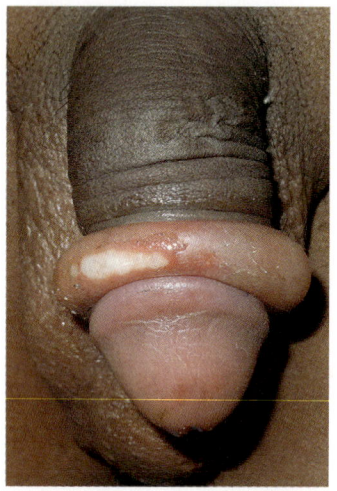

Fig. 20-3 *Paraphimosis*.

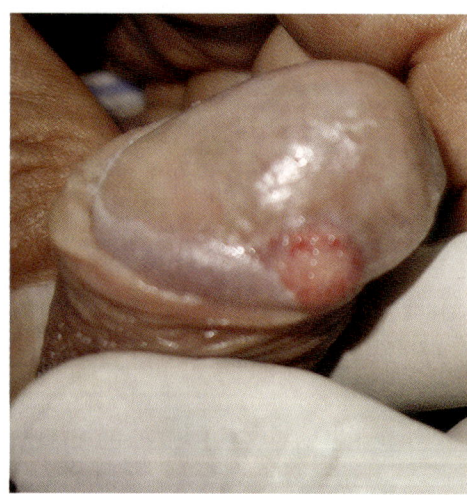

Fig. 20-4 *Ulcer over the glans penis*. It needs biopsy; it could be malignant.

History of fever may be due to infection.

Swelling: History of swelling in the groin should be asked. Carcinoma of penis can spread into the inguinal lymph nodes causing secondaries. Lymph nodes also can be involved in syphilis, lymphogranuloma inguinale. Often there will be pain, suppuration, ulceration or fungation in the groin which should be asked in detail in history.

History of *erectile dysfunction* is obtained in impotency/infertility.

Past History

History of syphilis, gonorrhea, diabetes, hypertension, tuberculosis is asked. History of surgery to the genital region is asked. History of previous penile surgery like circumcision, partial or total penectomy or inguinal block dissection should be asked (**Figs. 20-5A and B**).

GENERAL EXAMINATION

Anemia, clubbing, jaundice, nutrition should be assessed. Pulse, blood pressure should be recorded.

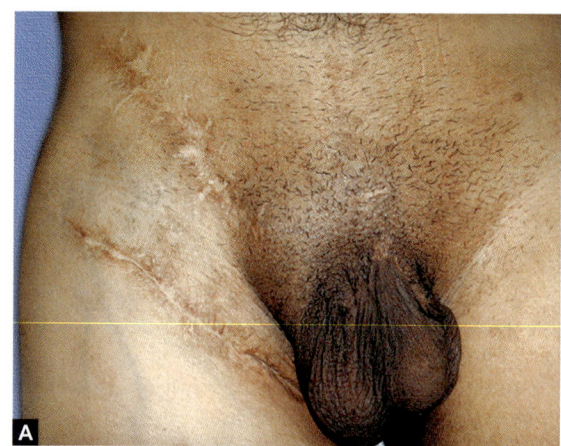

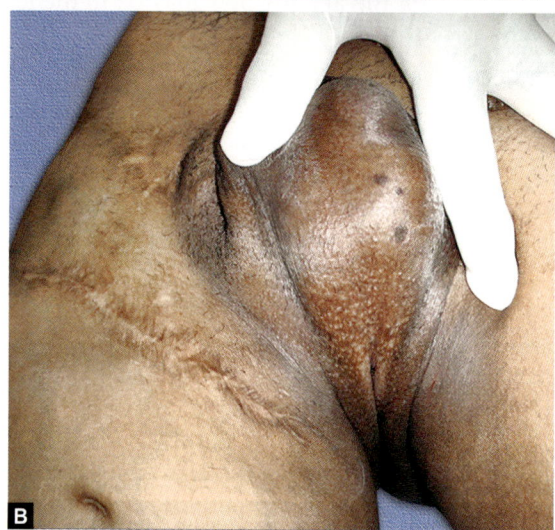

Figs. 20-5A and B *Perineal urethrostomy* developing stricture with old operated scar of ilioinguinal block dissection.

LOCAL EXAMINATION

Inspection

Inspection of Penis (Figs. 20-6A and B)

Body of the penis: Length of the penis is noted—normal/underdeveloped; girth—normal/enlarged [elephantiasis—***Ram's horn penis*** (Fig. 20-7)]; curvature—normal/abnormal (chordee); skin—color, ulcer, growth, sinus. Fournier's gangrene may extend to penis causing extensive penile skin necrosis **(Fig. 20-8)**.

Prepuce of the penis: With gloved hand, the prepuce is retracted over the glans as far as the corona. ***Phimosis*** (inability to retract the prepuce), ***paraphimosis*** (the prepuce can be retracted but tight round the corona with swelling of the glans) should be looked for. Prepuceal swelling or ulceration, edema, growth should be observed.

Glans: After retracting the prepuce whole of glans is observed for ulcer/growth. Posthitis (inflammation of prepuce) or balanoposthitis (inflammation of prepuce along with glans) with discharge is obvious on inspection.

Urethral meatus: Urethra should be examined for congenital anomaly. If urethral meatus opens more proximally along the ventral aspect, it is called as **hypospadias**. If it opens proximally over the dorsal aspect it is called **epispadias** **(Fig. 20-9)**. Based on position, hypospadias is categorized as *glandular* (glans*); coronal; penile; perineal* with bifid scrotum. Urethral meatus may not be visible in carcinoma of the glans which is close to the meatus—abnormal opening of urethra. Any *pinhole meatus* should be observed **(Fig. 20-10)**. Urethral papilloma from fossa navicularis may protrude from external urethral meatus causing hematuria and pain. Often *urethral stone* extruding just at the external meatus may be observed **(Fig. 20-11)**.

Ballooning of prepuce while micturition is obvious on inspection. Altered urinary stream occurs in carcinoma penis which is close to the meatus or rarely involving the urethra.

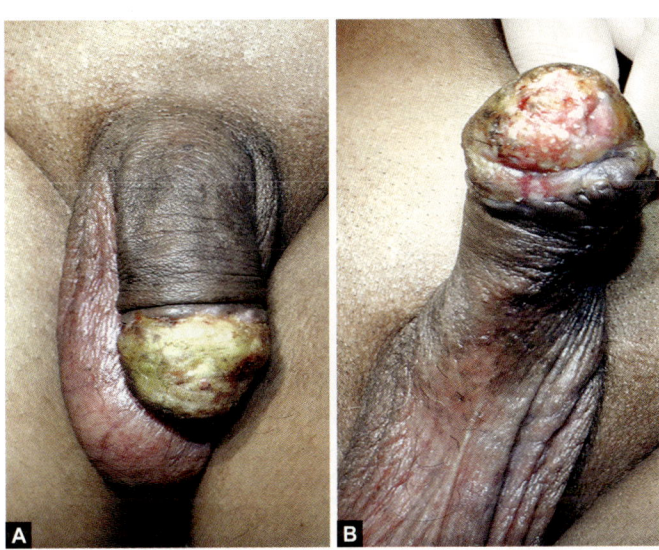

Figs. 20-6A and B Penis should be inspected *both on ventral* and *dorsal aspects*.

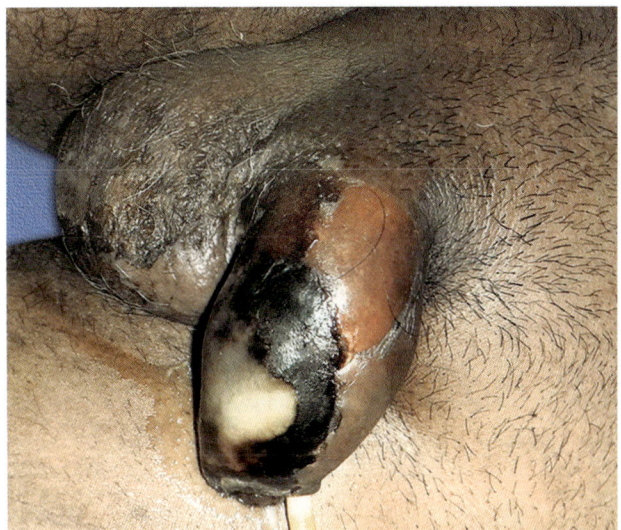

Fig. 20-8 *Fournier's gangrene* extending into the skin over the body of the penis.

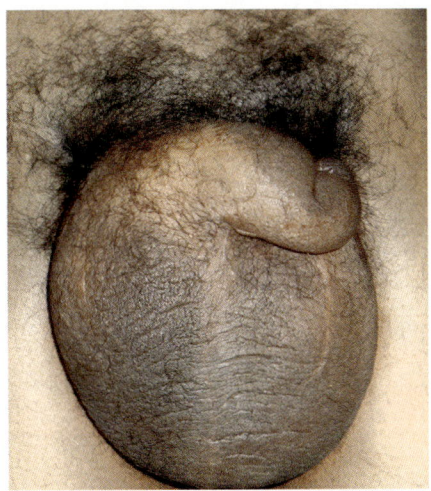

Fig. 20-7 *Ram's horn penis*—penile edema.

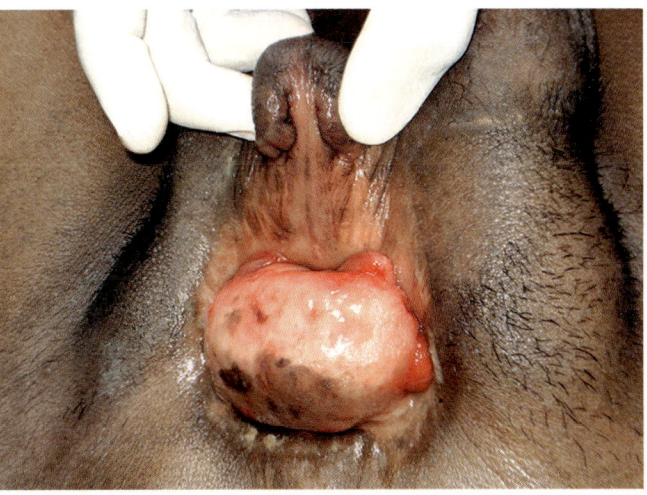

Fig. 20-9 Epispadias. *It is associated with extrophy of bladder;* one can note the visible urinary bladder surface.

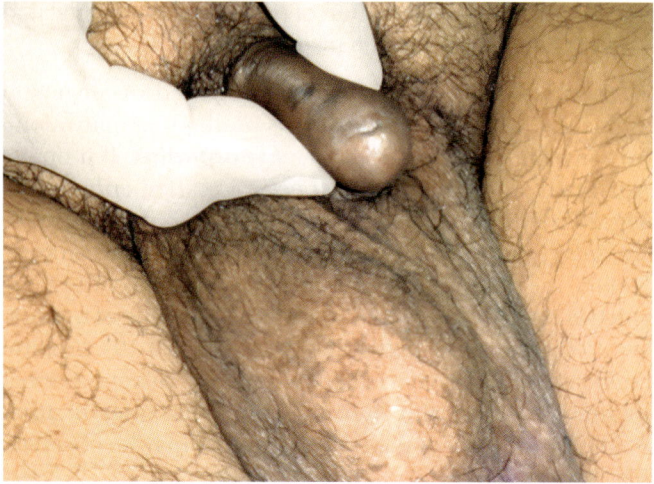

Fig. 20-10 *Pinhole meatus* causing phimosis. Ballooning of prepuce is common.

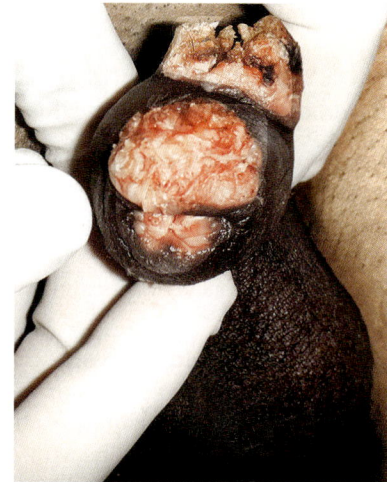

Fig. 20-12 Carcinoma penis involving *glans and prepuce*.

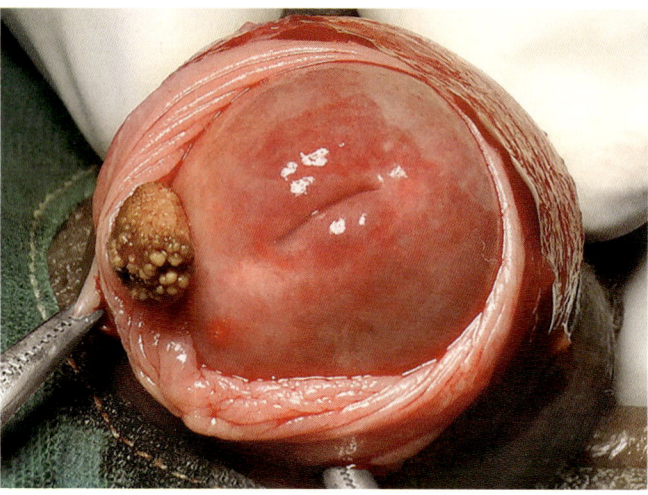

Fig. 20-11 *Stone in the meatus* which has come out.

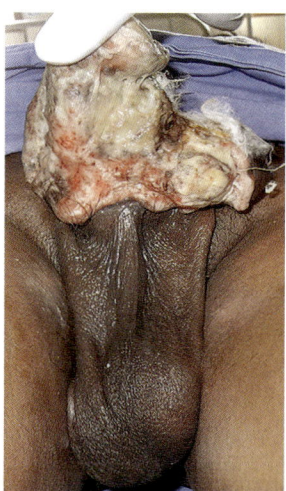

Fig. 20-13 Carcinoma penis—*involving extensively extending into the scrotum*.

Ulcer if present, its location, size, shape, edge, floor, discharge, number should be noted. It can be due to syphilitic chancre or chancroid or granuloma inguinale or epithelioma. Raised everted edge with necrotic floor is a feature of carcinoma often seen in skin of prepuce or glans **(Fig. 20-12)**. Epithelioma can also be cauliflower-like tumor **(Fig. 20-13)**.

Premalignant conditions: Leukoplakia, ***Paget's disease***—eczema like lesions in glans or inside the prepuce, ***Erythroplasia of Queyrat*** which is a red flat area in glans or inner aspect of the prepuce should be looked for.

Multiple warty-like projections may be ***condyloma acuminata***. Venereal warts are moist with foul smelling discharge **(Fig. 20-14)**.

Inspect the groin for visible swelling due to enlarged lymph nodes **(Fig. 20-15)**.

Palpation

Palpation should be done by ***wearing gloves***.

Penis is palpated for tenderness, warmness (inflammation), induration (Peyronie's disease). Ulcer, if present, is palpated

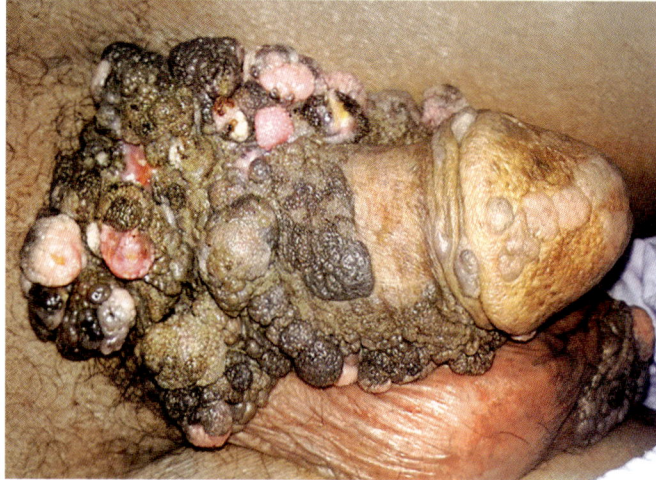

Fig. 20-14 *Condyloma acuminata* involving penile skin mainly and partly scrotal skin.

for edge and base to feel for induration, extent of induration, bleeding on touch. Prepuce may not be retraced if there is an underlying carcinoma. Prepuce and glans are carefully palpated together to appreciate the indurated swelling under

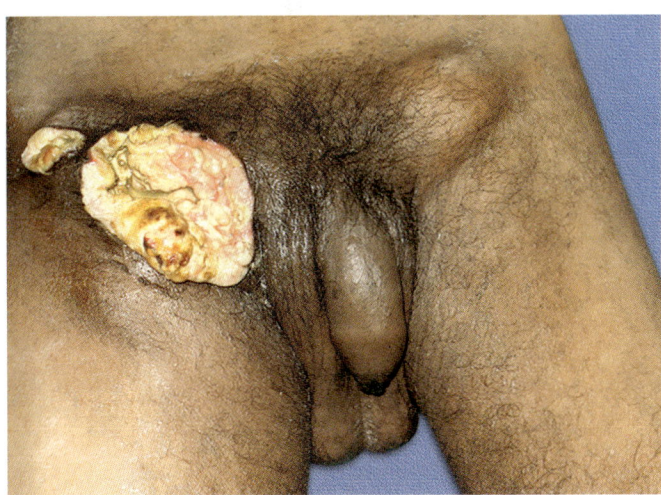

Fig. 20-15 Carcinoma of penis causing phimosis; *bilateral inguinal lymph node* secondaries; right side nodes have fungated.

the prepuce. Such patient may require circumcision or dorsal slit to visualize the lesion. Urethral discharge can be collected by milking the penis and collected discharge should be sent for culture and cytology.

Urethra should be palpated for thickening (stricture/stone) **(Figs. 20-16A to G)**.

Palpation of Lymph Nodes

Bilateral horizontal group of inguinal lymph nodes or **Cloquet's deep node** (from glans) may be enlarged. Its size, number, surface, consistency, tenderness, mobility, fixity should be checked. Iliac nodes above the inguinal ligament may be involved due to spread from inguinal nodes.

Involvement of urethra also can cause enlargement of iliac node. In 50% cases, initially the enlargement may be due to only infection. Urethral involvement is probably due to infection or tumor. External iliac group lymph nodes should also be palpated above and medial to the inguinal ligament; both sides should be examined **(Figs. 20-17A and B)**.

Rectal Examination

Digital examination of the rectum should be performed routinely to palpate the prostate.

Investigations

Wedge biopsy of ulcer; discharge study for microscopy, culture, cytology; FNAC of inguinal lymph nodes; US abdomen; chest X-ray; hematocrit; relevant investigations depending on the clinical diagnosis.

■ DISORDERS OF PENIS

Carcinoma Penis

It is commonly *squamous cell carcinoma*, but melanoma, adenocarcinoma from Tyson's gland, basal cell carcinoma and secondaries may also occur.

Etiology: **Chronic balanoposthitis, phimosis; sexually transmitted diseases; leukoplakia of glans; long standing genital warts; *Paget's disease* of penis (*Erythroplasia of Queyrat* is persistent rawness of glans penis); condyloma acuminata (human papilloma virus); balanitis xerotica obliterans; HIV infection. *Circumcision during infancy confers total immunity against carcinoma penis*. It is common in Asia and Africa.**

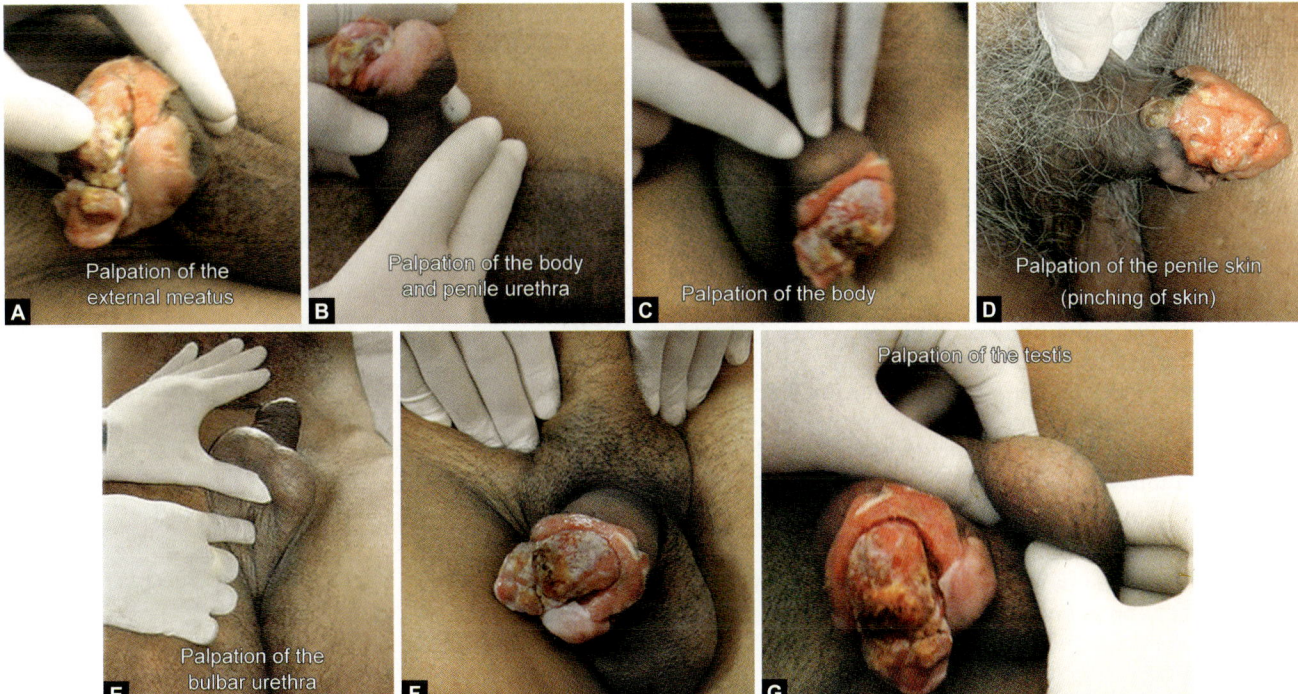

Figs. 20-16A to G *Examination in case of carcinoma of penis.*

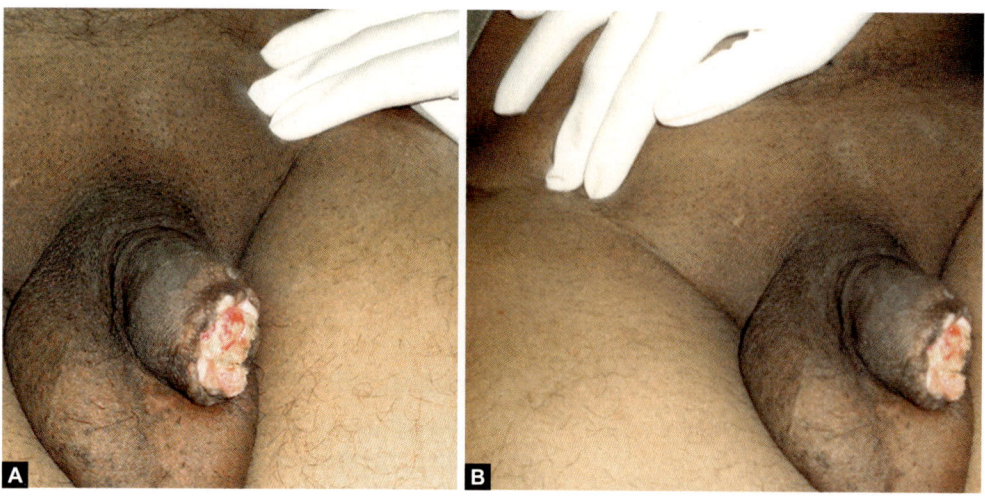

Figs. 20-17A and B Carcinoma of penis—*palpation of inguinal lymph nodes both sides.*

Pathology: *Infiltrating type* occurs in a preexisting leukoplakia; *Papilliferous type* eventually attains a large size forming fungating foul smelling lesion which often gets infected. Glans penis is the commonest site (coronal sulcus for basal cell carcinoma).

Spread: Through lymphatics to the horizontal group of inguinal lymph nodes which become nodular and hard. Lymph nodes on both sides can get involved. Later external iliac groups are involved (above and on medial aspect of the inguinal ligament). Once inguinal lymph nodes are fixed, it causes severe excruciating pain and lymphedema. *Fixed lymph node status indicates the advancement of the disease.* It may erode into the femoral vessels causing torrential hemorrhage and death. Carcinoma from penis and glans spread to inguinal lymph nodes and then to external iliac lymph nodes. From glans it also spreads to Cloquet lymph node which is located in femoral canal. Carcinoma from shaft of penis can spread directly to the external iliac lymph nodes. It spreads proximally to the body of penis causing induration. Urethral meatus may get involved causing alteration in urinary stream. *It is a locoregional malignant disease. Blood spread is rare.*

Clinical features: In an adult, recent onset of phimosis should give suspicion of carcinoma penis. Lesion is painless initially but later becomes painful due to secondary infection often accompanied by discharge which is foul smelling, purulent and irritating. Altered urinary stream; everted edge, ulcer, fungation and induration, often extending into the body of penis are other features (*see* Fig. 20-18A to G). Palpable hard, nodular inguinal lymph nodes on both sides may be present. External iliac lymph nodes may be palpable. Pain, edema, tenderness, redness develop once infection occurs. Incidence is less than 1% of male carcinomas; glans—65%; prepuce—20%; corona, shaft—10–15%. Buck's fascia is resistant for initial infiltration; urethral involvement occurs only in late cases.

Cabana sentinel node is located above and medial to the junction of saphenous and femoral vein. It is the first node to get involved in carcinoma penis (SLNB).

Diseases of penis	Features
Phimosis (*Greek—stooping up/a closure*)	
It is an inability to retract the prepuce over the glans as the end of the prepuce is narrow, like pinhole (*pinhole meatus*) **Causes:** Congenital—child has pinhole meatus with ballooning of prepuce occurs when child urinates; Balanitis (inflammation of glans)/ balanoposthitis (inflammation of glans, sac, prepuce)—common in diabetics	**Problems:** Recurrent balanoposthitis; paraphimosis; retention of urine; formation of preputial calculi due to smegma collection in preputial sac; later carcinoma penis
Paraphimosis	
It is inability to place the retracted preputial skin over the glans, which forms a tight constriction ring proximal to corona thereby blocking the venous flow leading to congestion and edema of glans **(Figs. 20-18A and B)**. It is often precipitated by sexual intercourse or iatrogenically by urethral catheterization	**Complication:** Glans may undergo necrosis or gangrenous if not treated immediately
Balanoposthitis	
It is the inflammation of glans (balanitis) and prepuce (posthitis). **Causes:** Diabetes mellitus; candidiasis; venereal diseases (syphilis, herpes genitalis; drug induced. *In adults there may be underlying carcinoma penis. It can cause phimosis*	Pain, swelling, discharge, discomfort; itching creamy, intolerable smell, difficulty to retract prepuce, multiple fissuring in the tip; itchy vesicles, with shallow painful erosions in case of herpes
Chordee	
It is fixed bending of penis, more obvious during erection	**Types:** *Ventral*—associated with hypospadias; or if excess skin on ventral aspect is excised during circumcision *Dorsal*—rare; associated with epispadias

Contd...

Contd...

Priapism	
It is persistent, painful erection of penis. Corpora cavernosa is filled with blood due to defective venous drainage; glans and corpora spongiosum not involved	**Causes:** Idiopathic thrombosis of corpora; thrombosis of prostatic venous plexus; sickle cell disease; leukemia; secondary deposits in corpora cavernosa; spinal injury or diseases and organic diseases of central nervous system
Peyronie's disease (Induratio penis plastica)	
It is development of fibrous tissue plaque on the covering of corpus cavernosum and later involving its full extent resulting in induration of corpus **Causes:** Slowly progressive disease of unknown etiology; may be due to old trauma. Often associated with Dupuytren's contracture, retroperitoneal fibrosis and plantar fasciitis	*Initial active phase*—painful erection with deformity of penis; *Quiescent phase*—Disappearance of painful erection with deformity of penis which is painless. Later indurated plaque is noticed with penile shortening and erectile dysfunction
Ram's horn penis	
It is elephantiasis of penis; usually due to filariasis	Penis becomes thick, distorted resembling horn of a ram
Hypospadias	
It is the commonest congenital malformation of urethra wherein external meatus is situated proximal than normal, over the ventral (under) aspect of penis **Classification**: a. Glandular—meatal opening in glans (commonest); b. Coronal; c. Penile; d. Penoscrotal; e. Perineal—with split scrotum and meatus is 3 cm in front of scrotum. This is associated with bilateral undescended testis	Absence of urethra and corpus spongiosum distal to abnormal orifice; Bowing / bending of penis distal to abnormal urethral orifice with poorly developed prepuce over inferior aspect; urine soakage over the scrotum with dermatitis and infection; associated with other congenital anomalies *Circumcision is contraindicated as preputial skin is required for future urethroplasty*
Epispadias	
Here urethra opens on the dorsum of the penis proximal to the glans. *Abdomino-penile is the commonest type.* Occasionally it can be glandular or penile	It is associated with dorsal chordee, ectopia vesicae, urinary incontinence and separated pubic bones
Buschke–Lowenstein tumor	
It is verrucous carcinoma of penis (5–15% common). It is a curable malignancy; locally destructive; locally invasive, HPV 6/11 viral etiology is proposed	Presents as—large exophytic, dry, verrucae-like growth. It neither spreads through lymphatics nor through blood

Venereal warts/papillomas (Fig. 20-19)	
It is the commonest benign lesion which can occur in uncircumcised or circumcised individuals; sexually transmitted disease where trauma occurs during intercourse	*Sites* are glans, corona, frenulum, and urethral meatus. Human papilloma virus is the cause. These warts are moist, multiple, with serous discharge. Intraepithelial neoplasia and carcinoma of penis may develop in these lesions at later period
Morgagni follicles infection	
These are pair of follicles which open laterally behind the lips of external urethral meatus	Once it gets infected, these openings are seen exuding pus. Often it is seen in urethritis
Tyson's gland infection	
Tyson glands are pair of sebaceous glands which secrete smegma located on either side of the frenum and ducts open into the preputial sac	When infected, present as tender firm swellings on the under surface of the glans on lateral aspect, usually as a complication of gonococcal urethritis

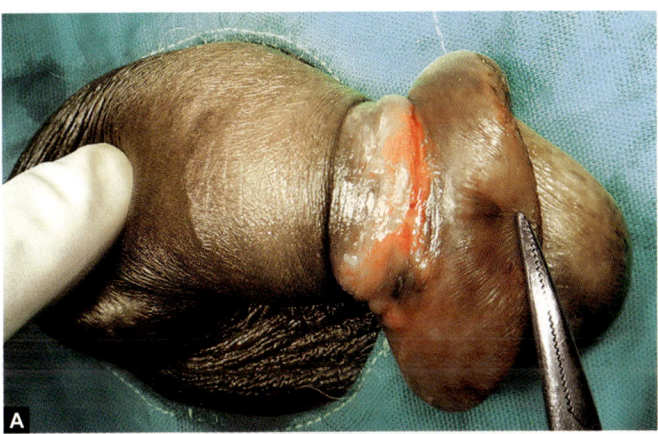

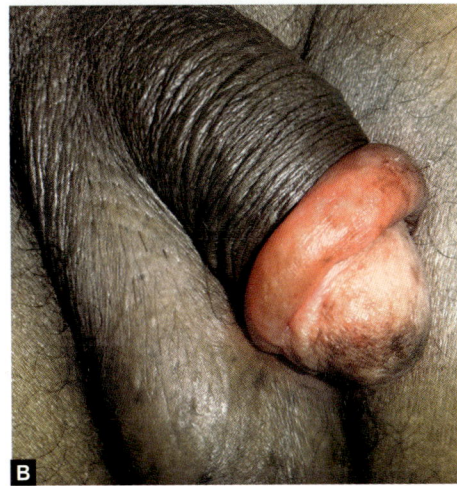

Figs. 20-18A and B *Paraphimosis.* Note the constriction band and edema.

Contd...

Meatal ulcer	
It is seen in young boys usually 1½ years after circumcision. Abrasions over the exposed unprotected meatal mucosa by napkins cause ulceration and scabbing	It causes small red ulcer in the meatus which often heals eventually causing meatal stenosis that often leads into retention of urine. Shortened anteroposterior diameter of meatus causes an acquired pinhole meatus. Secondary urinary infection is common

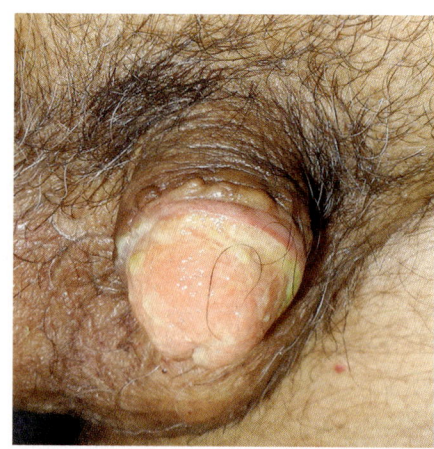

Fig. 20-19: Recurrent infection of glans – could be histoplasmosis (fungal); or venereal.

CASE DISCUSSION

A 60-year-old man comes with inability to retract his prepuce of one month duration with ulceration over the right side of the distal penis. Urination is normal. Mild pain is present. He never had fever in last one month. On local examination, prepuce cannot be retracted. There is an ulcerative lesion of 2 cm sized on the right side of the penis extending from distal part to corona line; it has raised and everted edge, with foul smelled discharge. Urethral meatus is seen away from the ulcer margin. On palpation, ulcer has indurated edge and base, base is fixed to glans underneath. Induration extends into the middle of the body of the right side of the penis. Scrotum and testes are normal. Horizontal inguinal lymph nodes on the right side are palpable – two in number; mobile, discrete, nontender, smooth and hard in consistency. Opposite side inguinal region is clinically normal. External iliac nodes are not palpable. Liver is not enlarged. Lungs are normal.

What is your diagnosis?
It is carcinoma penis—squamous cell carcinoma. Reasons are—raised everted edge of ulcer with induration; short duration; recent onset phimosis.

What is the stage?
T2, N1, M0. T2 because there is minimal deeper invasion.

What other lesions can mimic carcinoma penis?
Adenocarcinoma from Tyson's gland, melanoma, basal cell carcinoma (lymph nodes will not be palpable), verrucous cell carcinoma (lymph nodes will not be palpable), urethral carcinoma, soft tissue tumors. All these conditions rare but can occur.

What are the investigations?
Dorsal slit of the prepuce (if needed) and wedge biopsy; ultrasound abdomen; fine needle aspiration cytology (FNAC) of the lymph node are essential specific investigations.

Section 2:
Examination in Abdominal and Related Conditions

Approaches and Examinations in Chronic Abdominal Conditions

Competency: SU24.1; SU24.2; SU24.3; SU28.7; SU28.8; SU28.9; SU28.10; SU28.12; SU28.13; AN47.1; AN47.2; AN47.5; AN47.7; AN47.10; AN52.6; AN55.2; PA19.6; PA24.4; PA24.5; PA24.6; PA24.7; PA25.2; PA25.4; PA25.5.

Chronic abdominal conditions comprise vast number of diseases. Often diagnosing and managing, many of them is a clinical challenge to a surgeon. Exact clinical approach and a brief outline of different conditions are discussed here. Detailed discussion is beyond the scope of this book.

HISTORY

History taking begins with:

Name:

Age: Congenital pyloric stenosis occurs in newborn. Duodenal ulcer usually occurs before the age of 35 years. Gastric ulcer occurs after 35 years. Carcinoma stomach occurs in old age. Chronic pancreatitis, gallstone diseases and hiatus hernia occur in middle aged.

Sex: Congenital pyloric stenosis is common in male infants. Peptic ulcer, carcinoma stomach is common in males. Gallstone disease, hiatus hernia is common in females.

Occupation: Peptic ulcer is more common in professionals and executives. Old dictum '*Hurry, Worry, Curry*' is probable cause for peptic ulcer in India.

Residence: Gallbladder disease is more seen in North East India like Bihar. Peptic ulcer is more common in South India. Carcinoma esophagus and stomach are more common in South India (Karnataka). Hydatid cyst of liver is common in Central Tamil Nadu.

Complaints with History

Pain

Pain in chronic abdominal condition may be the one to which patient comes for consultation to a surgeon.

Site: Patient should be asked to point out the site of pain with one finger. It may give clue about the origin of the pain. Often pain is vague and diffuse in nature; it may not be possible to pinpoint the site of pain. Duodenal ulcer pain is pointed at **duodenal point**, 2.5 cm right and above the umbilicus. Pain in gastric ulcer is in epigastrium in midline or left-side. Pain in chronic cholecystitis is towards right side, lateral to right rectus muscle in right hypochondrium. Pain from the liver, subphrenic space, hepatic flexure of colon may be seen in right hypochondrium. Pain in hypogastrium may be from bladder, uterus, ovary, sometimes small intestine. Pain in left iliac fossa may be from sigmoid colon. Pain in right iliac fossa may be from appendix or cecum.

Duration: Duration of pain commonly suggests the duration of the disease but not always. Chronic diseases are usually of long duration. Pain of peptic ulcer disease, chronic cholecystitis, chronic pancreatitis has history of long duration. *Periodicity* of pain is important. It is seen in peptic ulcer disease. Patient develops pain for certain period of time like for few weeks or months followed by symptom-free period of few weeks or months. Pain in peptic ulcer may be seasonal. History of remission and exacerbation is asked; total number of episodes of pain, and duration of each episode and whether it was pain-free in between the episodes should be asked.

Type/nature of pain: It may be sudden colicky type (those arising from hollow viscera—intestine, biliary, ureteric); severe gripping type as in intestinal obstruction; continuous pain and discomfort from those arising from solid organ like in liver diseases; burning type of pain due to hyperacidity or reflux esophagitis. It may be mild, moderate, and severe in intensity. It may be progressive/regressive/stationary.

One should ask for any change in nature of pain. Initial periodicity of pain in peptic ulcer may change to continuous type if complication sets in—duodenal ulcer causes pyloric stenosis or gastric ulcer causes teapot or hourglass contracture.

Mode of onset and progression: Pain may be of sudden onset type in acute conditions like perforation of bowel which progresses rapidly; in chronic abdominal conditions, usually pain is of insidious onset and gradually progressive.

Radiation of pain: It is extension of pain to another site whose character is same as original pain and the original pain persists at the initial site. In posterior penetrated peptic ulcer pain radiates from epigastrium to back. Patient with chronic pancreatitis also develops radiating pain to the back. Pain in anastomotic ulcer is on left of the umbilicus (as stoma is towards left side) which radiates to left iliac fossa or to back.

Referred pain: Here the pain is felt in area distant from the site of origin, and sometimes pain may be totally absent at the site of origin, e.g. pain at the shoulder tip in subphrenic abscess; pain due to irritation of diaphragm by amoebic liver abscess is referred to tip of shoulder.

Relation with intake of food: In duodenal ulcer, pain is relieved by food intake probably due to neutralization of acid in the stomach. In gastric ulcer, pain increases after taking food. Pain appears early within half an hour after food intake in gastric ulcer, in 3 hours after food intake in duodenal ulcer, immediately after food intake in reflux esophagitis and hiatus hernia. Pain on empty stomach is called as *'hunger pain'*. It is a feature of chronic duodenal ulcer. It usually occurs in early morning. Here the patient gets up in early morning due to pain. Pain of carcinoma stomach is continuous type without any relation to food.

Aggravating factor: Hot spicy food aggravates the pain of gastritis; ingestion of fatty meal aggravates pain in gall bladder disease. Pain in ureteric colic is aggravated by jolting movements whereas stooping forwards aggravates pain in hiatus hernia.

Relieving factor: Pain is relieved by taking food in duodenal ulcer. In gastric ulcer, pain is relieved after vomiting, so patient induces vomiting by putting fingers into the pharynx to get relieved of pain. Sitting posture brings more comfort in pain due to hiatus hernia and pancreatitis. In colonic lesions, pain decreases after defecation.

Nausea and Vomiting

*Feeling (sensation) imminent desire of vomiting is called as **nausea**.* It may or may not proceed into vomiting; it is impending need to vomit. It is observed in chronic diseases like pancreatitis, carcinoma of stomach, peptic ulcer with complications, hepatitis and chronic cholecystitis. It can occur in carcinoma of pancreas, small bowel diseases, and subacute obstruction by diseases like abdominal tuberculosis. Vomiting is a feature of pyloric obstruction, gastrointestinal irritation.
Vomiting is forceful oral expulsion of gastric contents.

Regurgitation is appearance of previously swallowed food in the mouth.

Mode of onset: Whether following ingestion of food/drug/injury should be asked.

Duration: It may be in hours/days/weeks/months. History of exacerbation and remission should be asked.

Nature and quantity of vomitus: It is important to ask content, color, quantity, smell of vomitus. Vomitus may contain undigested/semidigested food particles, blood, coffee ground colored material. High GI obstruction like pyloric stenosis causes projectile vomiting containing undigested food particles. Vomitus may contain fecal material in low intestinal obstruction or gastrocolic fistulas. In paralytic ileus, vomitus contain gastric and bile juice. Effortless vomiting or regurgitation is seen in esophageal obstruction. Bleeding peptic ulcer, esophageal varices, carcinoma and sometimes leiomyoma, stomach, gastric polyp can cause hematemesis. Large quantity, rapid bleed causes frank blood in the vomitus (esophageal varices). Small quantity and slow ooze of blood mixes with acid of stomach to form acid hematin presenting as *'coffee ground'* vomitus.

Frequency: It may be continuous/intermittent. Repeated persistent vomiting is observed in pyloric stenosis, gastric ulcer. Vomiting is not a feature in duodenal ulcer.

Relation to food and pain: Vomiting after taking food is a feature in gastric ulcer (in 2 hours). Recurrent late vomiting (evening or 6–8 hours after food intake) is a feature of pyloric stenosis. Vomiting is not related to food intake in cholecystitis and pancreatitis. Vomiting or inducing vomiting relieves the pain in gastric ulcer. Vomiting will not relieve pain in cholecystitis, pancreatitis, and carcinoma of stomach.

> *Causes of vomiting are*: mechanical obstruction, gastric paresis due to pancreatitis, diabetes, postoperative, retroperitoneal tumors, appendicitis, cholecystitis, renal/biliary colic, food poisoning, sepsis, peritonitis, morning sickness in pregnancy, drug-induced (chemotherapy, opiates, NSAIDs, steroids, malaria, pyrexia, psychiatric diseases, etc).

Hematemesis

Vomiting blood is called as **hematemesis**. Chronic peptic ulcer is the commonest cause (65%).

> *Other causes of hematemesis*—are acute ulcers, acute erosive gastritis, esophageal varices
> Mallory–Weiss syndrome, carcinoma of stomach, gastric polyps, lymphomas, leiomyomas, portal gastropathy, bleeding disorders, pernicious anemia, thrombocytopenia
> **Gastric antral vascular ectasia** is a rare endoscopically confirmed condition which shows segmented dilated vessel meshes in the antral mucosa (watermelon/tiger stripe stomach). It is often associated with achlorhydria and hypergastrinemia; Osler–Weber–Rendu syndrome, aortoduodenal fistula, crest syndrome are rare causes
> **Dieulafoy's disease** is gastric arteriovenous malformation which is covered by apparently normal mucosa which occurs in proximal stomach along the lesser curve. It occurs in proximal stomach near OG junction (within 6 cm) along lesser curve (80% of the cases)

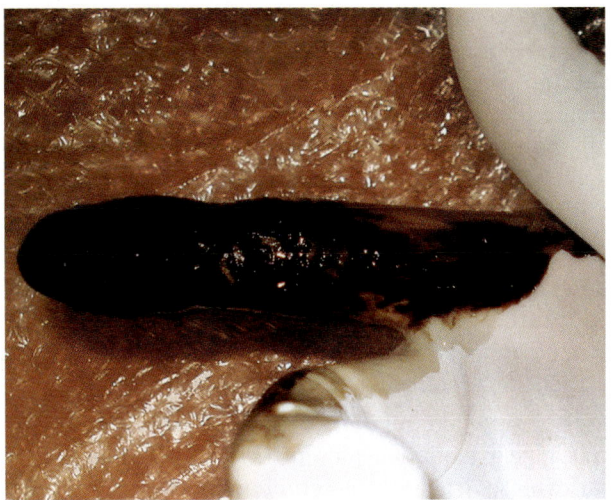

Fig. 21-1 Typical melena—*black tarry stool*.

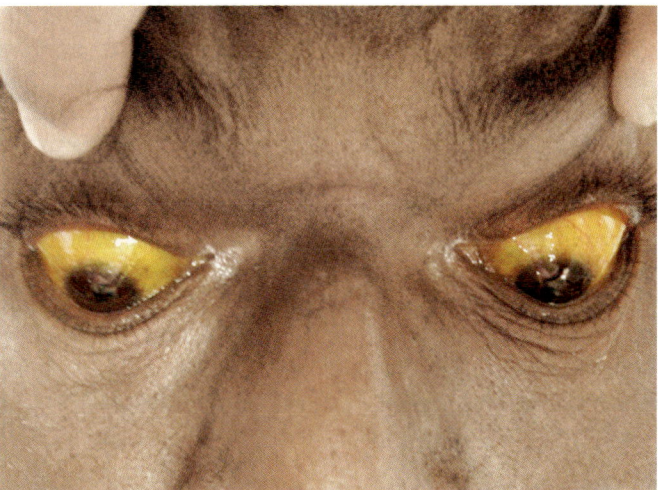

Fig. 21-2 Obstructive jaundice *(icterus)*.

Bleeding often may be severe and torrential. Profuse rapid bleeding causes hematemesis with frank red blood; slow small bleed causes coffee ground vomitus. Hematemesis should be differentiated from hemoptysis. Hemoptysis is blood in the sputum during coughing. Its content, color should be asked to differentiate properly. Gastric ulcer more often causes hematemesis. **In pseudohematemesis,** patient initially swallows the blood coming from upper respiratory tract and then vomits it out.

Melena

It is passing dark, tarry, foul smelling stool per anum. It is a feature of upper gastrointestinal bleed. Common cause is peptic ulcer bleed. Duodenal ulcer more often causes melena **(Fig. 21-1)**.

Flatulent Dyspepsia

Dyspepsia is a vague terminology which includes feeling of fullness in the abdomen after food, belching, heart burn *(pyrosis)*. It may be a feature of gallbladder disease, hiatus hernia, and pancreatitis. Precipitating factors like food/drink; relieving factors like antacids/ vomiting/defecation should be asked. **Heart burn** is sensation of warmth or burning situated substernally or high epigastrium radiating to neck or arms (peptic ulcer, reflux esophagitis, hiatus hernia). **Belching** is repetitive eructations, often seen in hiatus hernia, chronic cholecystitis, reflux esophagitis, sometimes psychogenic. Qualitative dyspepsia is dislike to fatty foods often seen in gallbladder stone and diseases.

> **Non-ulcer dyspepsia:**
> - Symptom complex with pain and discomfort in the upper abdomen
> - It occurs in 25% of population—large number
> - Anatomical or biochemical abnormalities are not discovered in this condition
> - *H. pylori* is not associated with this condition
> - Often it lasts for long time decreasing the quality of life

Jaundice/Icterus

Yellowish discoloration of sclera and mucous membrane is called as icterus (*jaundice* is biochemical evidence of raised serum bilirubin; *icterus* is the clinical word; but commonly both are used synonymously). It may be due to neoplasia like carcinoma head of pancreas, periampullary carcinoma, Klatskin tumor, cholangiocarcinoma, nodes compressing porta hepatis, carcinoma of gallbladder, hepatocellular carcinoma, secondaries in liver, biliary stone disease, hepatitis, cirrhosis, pancreatitis, pseudocyst or due to hemolytic causes. In broad daylight, jaundice is confirmed by examining sclera, skin, nail bed, under surface of the tongue, soft palate. Its duration, progression, whether persistent or intermittent, whether painful jaundice (in biliary stone) or painless jaundice (carcinoma) should be asked. History of fever (inflammatory), trauma (operative or accidental) or drugs taken should be asked. Progressive jaundice is a feature of carcinoma head of pancreas, nodes compressing porta hepatis, Klatskin tumor; intermittent jaundice is a feature of periampullary carcinoma (due to sloughing of the ampulla), stone in common bile duct. Presence of itch marks on the dorsal aspect of the hands, forearms and back suggests obstructive jaundice **(Fig. 21-2)**.

Bowel Habit

It is very important to ask history regarding proper bowel habit in chronic abdomen patients. History of diarrhea, constipation, blood in the stool, painful defecation, tenesmus, alternate constipation and diarrhea, clay colored stool (seen in chronic pancreatitis, obstructive jaundice where fat is not digested due to deficiency of pancreatic enzymes), silvery stool (seen in periampullary carcinoma where blood from the tumor necrosed area gets altered as hematin which mixes with fat). Large, loose, fatty offensive stool may be seen in chronic pancreatitis. Inflammatory bowel disease, carcinoma colon, small bowel diseases, colonic polyps, colonic tuberculosis can cause diarrhea or diarrhea alternating with constipation. Dark tarry colored melena is also typical.

Diarrhea is an increase in daily stool weight more than 200 g. There may be increased stool liquidity and frequency more than 3 times per day. Stool may be semiformed. Diarrhea is called as *acute* if it has abrupt onset with duration of 1–2 weeks; *chronic* if it is for more than 2 weeks. Mechanism may be osmotic, secretory, exudation of mucus, blood and protein from the inflamed mucosa, increased intestinal motility. ***Pseudodiarrhea*** is increased frequency without increase in stool weight which is seen in irritable bowel syndrome (IBS), hyperthyroidism, proctitis. But for all practical purpose, increased frequency may be considered as diarrhea. History of mode of onset—food intake/drug/surgery is to be asked.

Constipation is frequency of defecation less than 3 times a week often with hard stool or with difficultly to pass.

Appetite

Loss of appetite is an important feature of gastrointestinal malignancy whether it is stomach, small bowel, colon, and rectum. Appetite is increased in peptic ulcer. Appetite is normal in gastric ulcer but patient fears to take food due to pain. Aversion to fatty food is a feature of gall bladder disease (gall-bladder dyspepsia). Loss of appetite occurs in early gastric cancers and tuberculosis. Loss of appetite is progressive and significant in malignancy. Feeling of adequateness/***satisfaction*** after meal is called as ***satiety***. ***Early satiety*** is a feature of GI malignancy especially in carcinoma of stomach. ***Anorexia*** is lack of desire to eat. ***Sitophobia*** is fear of eating due to anticipated abdominal discomfort seen in IBS, chronic mesenteric ischemia.

Loss of Weight

Progressive loss of weight is seen in GI carcinomas, obstructive lesions of stomach like pyloric stenosis, malabsorption syndrome, chronic dysentery, tuberculosis. More than 10 kg weight loss in 6 months is called as ***significant weight loss*** which needs proper evaluation. Often earlier patient might not have measured his weight. Then it is better to ask how much muscle mass is reduced or loosening of clothes occurred. Often it is better to ask relatives about their observation of the changes in the patient earlier and now.

Fever

Abdominal tuberculosis may present with evening rise of temperature. Fever may be due to malnutrition, secondary infection. Cholangitis, pancreatitis, cholecystitis, and ulcerative colitis can cause recurrent episodes of fever. Even malignancy can cause fever due to pyrogenic response or tumor necrosis.

Past History

Past history of typhoid, tuberculosis, jaundice is important. Previous history of any surgery or abdominal surgery—indication, duration of hospital stay, whether it was an emergency or elective procedure, postoperative recovery, drain placed or not, any biopsy reports revealed or not, recovery period. Long-term treatment for abdominal tuberculosis may be present. Patient might be taking drugs related to peptic ulcer for long time. Whether patient was evaluated prior to therapy or surgery by X-rays, investigations, endoscopies or not should be asked. History of blood transfusions for surgery earlier is also significant.

Personal History

History of smoking (*bidis*/cigarettes/*hookahs* with frequency and duration), tobacco/*supari*, alcohol intake should be asked. ***Alcohol*** and smoking may lead into cirrhosis and portal hypertension, peptic ulcer disease, carcinoma, etc.

Dietary habits like regularity, interval between each food intake, type of food (hot spicy food is very important in peptic ulcer disease, fried food in cholecystitis) intake should be asked.

Family History

Certain gastrointestinal malignancies, ulcerative colitis, Crohn's disease often run in family.

GENERAL EXAMINATION

Built: Built is normal in duodenal ulcer; poor in gastric ulcer; emaciated in pyloric stenosis or carcinoma.

Nourishment: Anemia/hypoproteinemia/cachexia in abdominal tuberculosis, GI malignancies, liver and intestinal diseases.

Jaundice is looked for in sclera, nail bed, undersurface of tongue, soft palate.

Nails are examined for clubbing, cracks and fissuring.

Oral cavity, teeth are examined for glossitis, stomatitis, pyorrhea, ulceration.

Skin texture: poor in severe degree malnutrition, cachexia.

Respiration, pulse, blood pressure are checked.

Generalized lymphadenopathy looked for.

Overall look of the patient should be checked. ***Malignant cachexia*** is emaciated skeletonized look seen in gastrointestinal malignancy.

LOCAL EXAMINATION

Abdominal examination is essential part of chronic abdominal conditions. ***Examination is done with patient in supine position on bed exposing the abdomen from upper chest to knee level*** (Fig. 21-3). Both hands should be on the sides of the patient. It is better to ask the patient to turn to one side (towards left as examination is done from right side always), breathe comfortably and relax. It is also important to explain the patient about what you are going to examine. Often consent may be needed. When a male doctor examines a female patient, it is better to have a female nursing staff beside the doctor. Quite room and good day light is needed to examine the patient. It is ideal to have some conversation

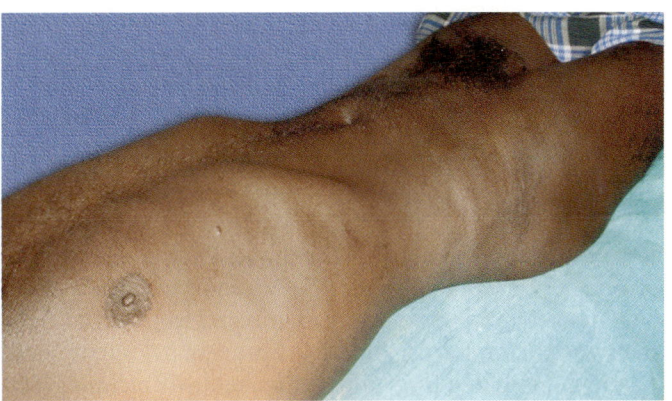

Fig. 21-3 Examination of abdomen is done with proper exposure.

with the patient while examining to ease and relax the patient. Legs may be slightly flexed at knee and hip joints.

Inspection

Inspection of abdomen is done from all the directions, including from *foot-end,* often from *head-end and side* of the patient with *eyes kept at the level of the abdomen* (**Figs. 21-4A and B**).

Shape/Contour of the Abdomen

Normally abdomen is flat or only slightly scaphoid; neither full nor retracted. It may be scaphoid in thin people, starvation, and in advanced malignancy. Fat, fluid, flatus, feces, and fetus cause symmetrical distension. Distension due to obesity causes inverted umbilicus. Umbilicus is everted in intra-abdominal causes. Localized area of fullness (due to enlargement of viscera/neoplasm) causing asymmetrical enlargement may be evident depending on where the cause lies, upper/lower abdomen. Fullness in right hypochondrium is seen in hepatomegaly, left hypochondrium in splenomegaly. Distension is more central in small bowel obstruction, peripheral in large bowel obstruction. In sigmoid volvulus, huge distension is evident on left side. In patient with visceroptosis, lower abdomen becomes more prominent on standing. Whole abdomen is distended in massive ascites or ovarian neoplasm where fullness of flanks is observed in former, not evident in latter.

Srinivasan costal sign*

"*Srinivasan costal sign*" is an inspectory finding to assess the acute distended abdomen secondary to surgical or postoperative status or medical causes under treatment. The bilateral costal margin is visualized tangentially on either side of the abdomen in supine position to appreciate this costal sign.

"*Prominence of costal margins will be lost in distended abdomen. During therapy, once distension reduces, prominence of costal margins will be visible (during recovery)*".

*(Professor Narayanaswamy Srinivasan MS, FRCS, who has earlier worked as HOD, General Surgery, Bangalore Medical College; Director of Sanjay Gandhi Accident Hospital and Research Institute, Byrasandra, Bengaluru; Dean and Director of Bangalore Medical College and Research Institute, Bengaluru; Joint Director of Medical Education, Govt of Karnataka, India)

Umbilicus

Umbilicus is normally inverted and situated midway between xiphoid process and pubic symphysis. It is displaced downwards in ascites; upwards in pelvic mass—***Tanyol's sign***. It is everted or transversely stretched in ascites; bulged out in umbilical hernia; inverted in obesity; pushed towards opposite side by one-sided mass (normal equidistant line from anterior superior iliac spine to umbilicus is deviated to one side). Vertical slit in umbilicus occurs in ovarian tumor; horizontal slit in ascites.

Movements with Respiration

Normally abdominal wall bulges out during inspiration, and falls back during expiration. In peritonitis, movement of the abdominal wall with respiration is absent. Patient will have more thoracic type of respiration. In localized inflammation, there is localized limitation of abdominal wall movement with respiration, e.g. movement looks restricted in right hypochondrium in acute cholecystitis, right iliac fossa in acute appendicitis.

Skin over the Abdomen

Skin over the abdomen is looked for:
1. **Scar:** Its length, width, margin, position, linear or wide scar should be checked. Linear scar means wound has healed by primary intention.

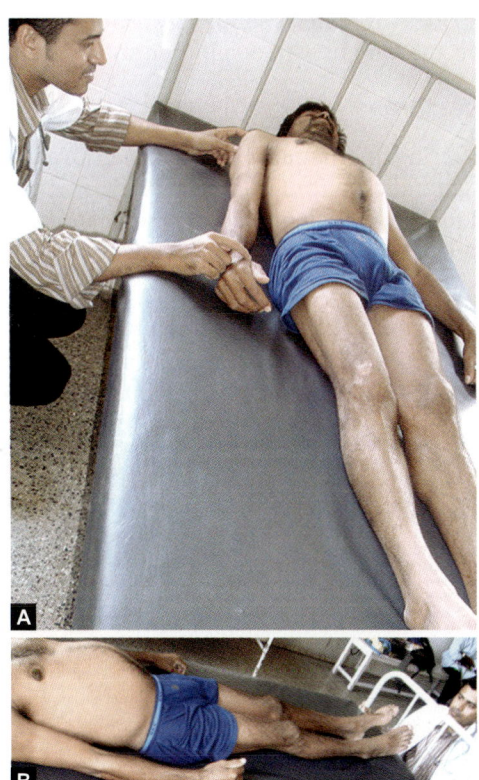

Figs. 21-4A and B Inspection of the abdomen should be done from *side as well as from foot end*.

2. ***Color:*** Redness in erythema, pigmentation (Peutz–Jeghers syndrome). Striae atrophica or gravidarum are linear marks seen over the skin of the abdomen which is due to significant stretching of the abdominal skin leading into rupture of elastic fibers. Purple striae are seen in Cushing's syndrome; linea nigra pigmentation below the umbilicus is seen in pregnancy, bluish discoloration of **Grey Turner's sign** is seen hemorrhagic pancreatitis.
3. ***Texture:*** Smooth and glossy in distension/wrinkled in abdomen with recently relieved distension.
4. ***Dilated veins:*** Dilated veins are looked for in standing position **(Fig. 21-5)**. Normally blood flow is upwards (to SVC) above the umbilicus and downwards (to IVC) below the umbilicus. Dilated veins around the umbilicus with normal pattern of flow (away from the umbilicus) are due to portal hypertension—**caput medusae**. In inferior vena caval obstruction, direction of blood flow is from below upwards. Superficial epigastric vein and superficial circumflex veins in the groin anastomose with lateral thoracic veins which drain into the axillary vein; In **IVC obstruction**, venous drainage occurs through these veins, i.e. long saphenous vein → superficial epigastric circumflex iliac veins → lateral thoracic veins → axillary vein; dilated veins are seen in paraspinal and lateral wall of the abdomen with upward direction of blood flow. If IVC obstruction is below the renal vein level, there will be bilateral lower limb edema with dilatation of superficial veins of the lower limbs and abdomen; block at the level of renal veins, there will be lumbar pain, hematuria, proteinuria; block above the level of renal veins, there will be hepatic venous flow obstruction causing acute and chronic Budd-Chiari syndrome. In **SVC obstruction**, venous blood flow is from above downwards. Method to know the direction of blood flow—two fingers are kept very closely over the vein; fingers are swept away with pressure to empty the vein; one finger is released and flow is observed; if it is empty, other finger is also released later to see the flow. It is repeated again to confirm the flow in opposite direction.
5. ***Swelling:*** Benign (papilloma); malignant [**Sister Mary Joseph's nodules** which indicates intra-abdominal advanced malignancy (colon, ovary, stomach)].
6. ***Sinus/ulcer/fistula:*** If present are noted with respect to size, location, etc.

Visible Peristalsis

Peristalsis may be visible in very thin individual even in the absence of intestinal obstruction. Visible gastric peristalsis (VGP) is seen in the epigastrium moving from left to right towards right lumbar region. It is a feature of pyloric stenosis. It can be stimulated by giving the patient to drink water (500 mL) or by rubbing the abdomen **(Figs. 21-6A and B)**. In small intestinal obstruction, peristalsis (VIP) is seen around the umbilicus in *'step ladder pattern'*. In obstruction of transverse colon, slow and periodic peristalsis is seen moving from right to left.

Visible Pulsation

Normal aortic pulsation may be visible in thin individuals. Aortic aneurysm causes visible pulsation which is *'expansile'* and is confirmed in knee-elbow position or lateral position. *'Transmitted'* pulsation may be seen over a mass in front of the aorta like pseudocyst of pancreas, retroperitoneal mass, etc. These pulsations disappear in knee-elbow position as the mass falls away from the aorta. Pulsation from congested liver may be seen in epigastrium or right hypochondrium.

Mass Per Abdomen

Any visible mass or fullness should be inspected. Its location, size, shape, movement with respiration should be inspected.

Other Sites/Areas

Hernia sites (inguinal/femoral) are observed for any swellings. External genitalia (scrotum, penis, vulva, and vagina) are observed for any visible pathology. **Supraclavicular fossa** is observed for any fullness due to lymph node enlargement.

Palpation

Palpation should be done from right side of the patient. Patient should lie down flat supine, breathing through

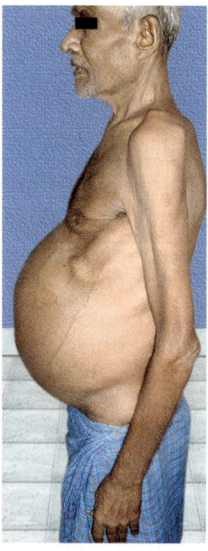

Fig. 21-5 Ascites on inspection. For *dilated veins, examination should be done on standing.*

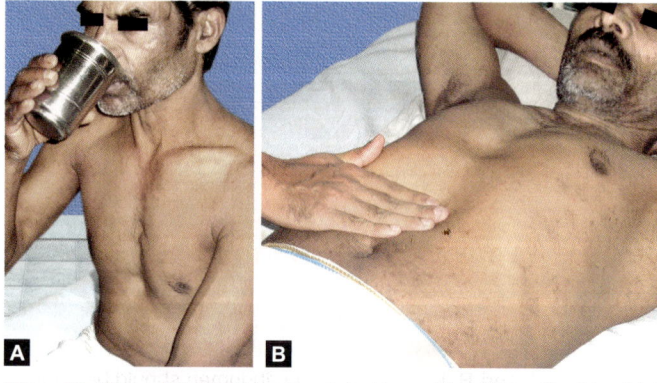

Figs. 21-6A and B VGP is stimulated by asking the patient *to drink water* or by rubbing the epigastric region.

mouth in relaxed state with head turned to opposite side. Examiner may have to sit in a chair or lean on the patient to do a proper palpation. Clinician should warm his examining hand by rubbing it with other hand or dipping in warm water. Palpation is done with flat of the hand using fingers; forearm should be in horizontal plane. Poking with the fingers placed vertically over the abdomen should be avoided. Slight flexion of hips and knees help in relaxing the abdominal muscles and prevent patient from keeping it tight and rigid. Keeping a pillow under the knees may be useful. Continuous conversation with the patient during palpation is important to console and relax the patient **(Fig. 21-7)**. Palpation should be gentle; rough, hurried and jerky palpation should be avoided as it may cause distress to the patient.

Standard Method of Palpation (Palpation of the Abdomen)

Initially palpation should be done to have a clear idea where exactly disease is suspected; is started away from the location of suspected disease, usually diagonally opposite to the site of the disease, e.g. for pain in right iliac fossa palpation, it is started from left hypochondrium; all other quadrants are examined initially and then the needed quadrant is examined carefully. Often two hands placed one over the other may be used to palpate the patient's abdomen. Palpation should be done first over nontender area then over tender area. During palpation, one should mentally visualize the structures beneath the palpating hand. Initial standard palpation is done to have a clear idea where exactly disease is suspected. Usually palpation begins from suprapubic area towards left iliac fossa then in anticlockwise direction all round to reach back to suprapubic region. During palpation, one has to assess the feel of the abdomen; normal feel is soft and elastic which yields on pressure and recoils back on release of pressure. *Muscle guarding* is the resistance offered when trying to yield the abdomen whereas in *rigidity*, the abdomen cannot be yielded at all.

Deep Palpation

It is later done gently and slowly, asking the patient to do deep inspiration so as to have complete relaxation of abdominal wall. Deep palpation is done using flexor surface of palpating fingers sinking deeper into the abdomen during each expiration. *Two hands method* is better for deeper palpation when more pressure is required especially in obese individuals **(Figs. 21-8A and B)**. Here the deeper hand is passive and superficial hand is active providing pressure on the deep hand which is engaged in feeling the tone of the muscle and lump. Muscle guarding and rigidity is better appreciated by this method.

Neville J Nicholson Maneuver

Lower end of the sternum is pressed using base of the palm of left hand progressively so that patient breathes through the abdomen, relaxing it and right hand is used to palpate the abdomen during expiration. This helps to overcome the voluntary muscle guarding.

Grainger's Method

It is very useful in uncooperative crying child. Here *child's hand is placed* over the abdomen and examiner's hand is placed over the child's hand and is palpated. When point of maximum tenderness is reached, the child withdraws the hand (due to tenderness) **(Fig. 21-9)**.

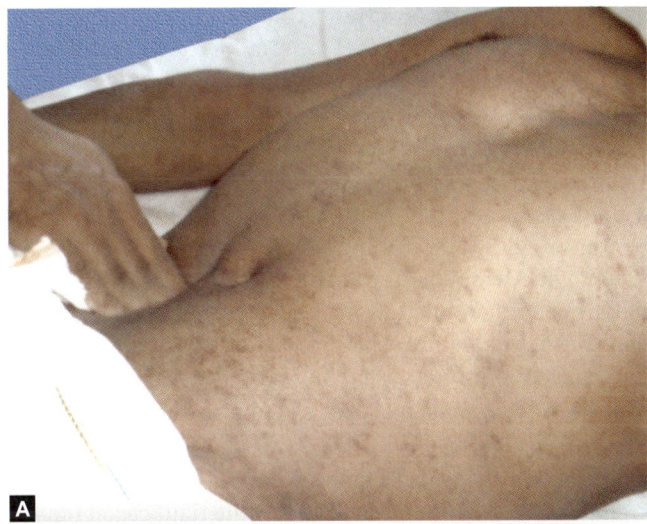

A

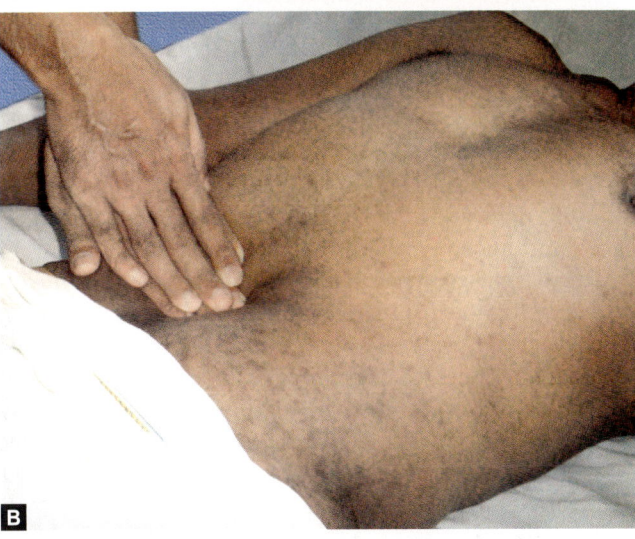

B

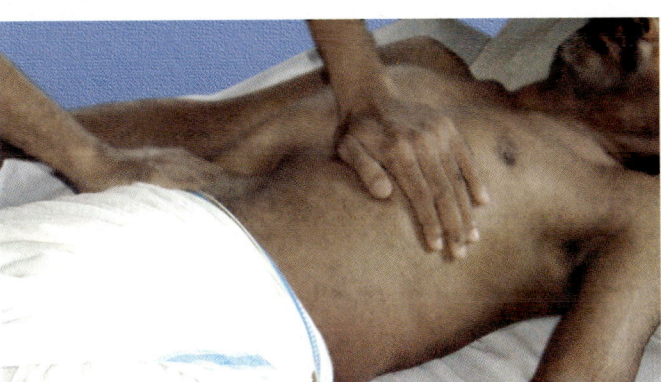

Fig. 21-7 *Palpation of the abdomen.*

Figs. 21-8A and B Methods of deep palpation of the abdomen: (A) *One hand method*; (B) *Two hands method.*

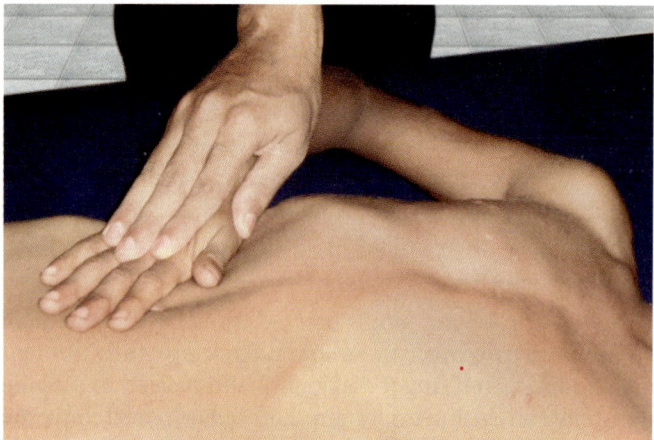

Fig. 21-9 Palpation in child/children is done using child's hand—*Grainger's method*.

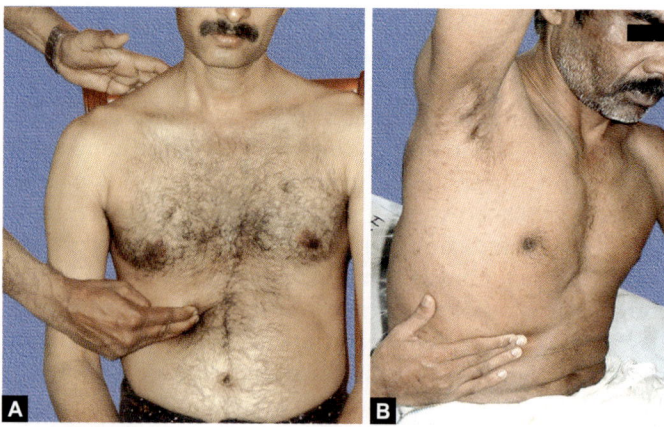

Figs. 21-10A and B *Murphy's (Naunyn's) sign* is elicited in sitting (upright) position using examiner's curled or flat upper margin of right hand fingers. It is used in cholecystitis. Original Murphy's hammer stroke method is not practiced now.

Dipping Method

When there is large quantity of fluid in the abdominal cavity, palpation of different organs is done by dipping the fingers so that fluid is displaced away from that place. It is used to palpate liver, spleen, tumors or other organs; sudden displacement of fluid makes fingers to feel tapping of the organ or mass underneath. Hand is placed flat on the abdomen and quick dipping movements are made to displace fluid.

Tenderness

While palpating, tenderness is checked by looking at the face of the patient and feel of the abdomen. When tenderness is mild, patient tolerates but winces; when it is moderate, patient winces and tightens the abdomen; when it is severe, patient winces and makes the abdomen rigid and does not allow further palpation. The site of localized tenderness is of diagnostic importance as it denotes the site of lesion.

Deep tenderness is elicited with one finger. Point of maximum tenderness (*tender spot*) should be elicited. In duodenal ulcer, it is in transpyloric plane 2.5 cm right of the umbilicus. In cholecystitis, tender point is below the right costal margin at the junction of tip of right 9th costal cartilage and lateral margin of the right rectus muscle. Here tenderness is elicited from the fundus of gallbladder.

Murphy's sign (John Benjamin Murphy, 1900) for chronic/acute on chronic cholecystitis is elicited in sitting position with patient lifting his right arm above the shoulder; examiner stands on right side of the patient and right hand fingers are placed and hooked under right costal margin lateral to the right rectus muscle. When patient is asked to take deep breath, at the zenith of the inspiration patient winces with pain as the inflamed gallbladder descends during inspiration and touches the examiner's fingers—*inspiratory arrest (catch in breath)*. Sign is also called as *Naunyn's sign* (Figs. 21-10A and B). Same tenderness if elicited in lying down position, is called *Moynihan's method/sign* (Fig. 21-11). Cartilage of 8th rib will be tender in cholecystitis.

Intercostal tenderness may be elicited in liver abscess. It is done using thumb or index finger; deep pressure over the intercostal

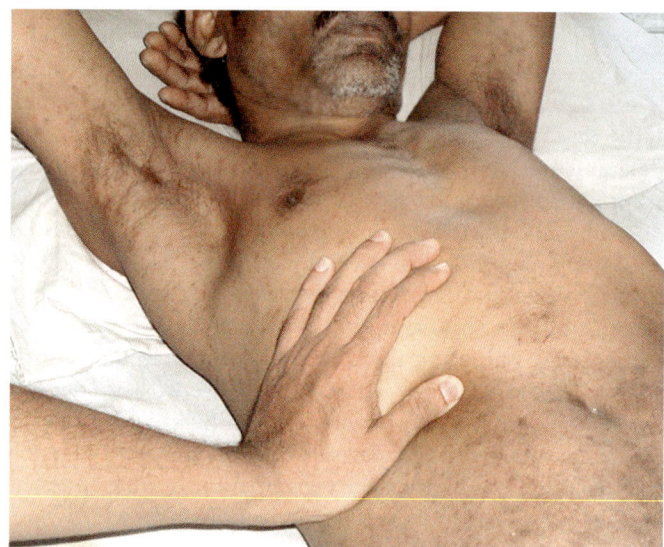

Fig. 21-11 *Moynihan's test* is done in lying down position for chronic cholecystitis.

space in midclavicular line towards laterally in the right side will cause tenderness; it is especially useful in amoebic liver abscess.

McBurney's point: A point on the right spinoumbilical line at the junction of medial 2/3rd and lateral 1/3rd; similarly *amebic point* (Sir Philip Manson Bahr point) lies on the left spinoumbilical line at the junction of medial 2/3rd and lateral 1/3rd.

Local Raise of Temperature

It is useful mainly if mass or swelling is present on the abdominal wall. Abdominal wall edema may be evident in large liver abscess, abdominal wall inflammation or suppuration.

Palpation of Different Organs

Stomach

Normally stomach is not palpable. It becomes palpable when it becomes dilated as in pyloric stenosis due to chronic duodenal ulcer (cicatrized), pyloric growth, trichobezoar, acute dilatation of stomach. Dilated stomach will be below the level of umbilicus (greater curvature). *Visible gastric peristalsis (VGP),* positive succussion splash, positive auscultopercussion test is significant. VGP may be absent if gastric paresis has occurred due to atony of stomach wall. Stomach mass is usually due to carcinoma, occasionally leiomyoma or sarcoma. Here the mass moves with respiration, freely mobile, all borders well made out, irregular surface, hard in consistency, resonant or impaired resonant on percussion. It becomes immobile once it gets fixed posteriorly. Absence of stomach mass will not exclude carcinoma of stomach.

Liver

In infants, it is palpable up to 3 years. In adults it is usually not palpable. Any palpable liver is considered as pathological. Liver is palpated using right hand. Palpation should begin well below from right iliac fossa otherwise it may be missed. Right fingers are laid flat with outer margin of the index finger held facing upwards and inwards. Fingers are pointed towards left axilla parallel to right costal margin. During deep inspiration, fingers are pressed firmly to feel; during expiration, fingers are moved upwards towards right costal margin. Patient is asked to breathe deeply and adequately. During full inspiration as fingers are moving upwards, lower margin of descended liver will come and touch the outer edge of the index finger. One should not place fingers over the rectus abdominis muscle and also not very close to costal margin. The fingers are kept there for further confirmation of the liver and also to look for other features of the liver like presence of tenderness or not; extent in cms or fingerbreadth below right costal margin; edge type—sharp or rounded; surface—smooth, irregular, granular, nodular, umbilications; consistency—soft, firm, hard. Smooth tender liver may be seen in amebic liver abscess or viral hepatitis. Nodular hard liver is a feature of secondaries in liver. Umbilication is seen in liver secondaries due to central necrosis. Hepatocellular carcinoma may be smooth/nodular; soft/firm or hard. Soft, smooth liver is felt in congestive conditions. In obstructive jaundice, liver may be enlarged due to obstruction causing dilated intrabiliary radicals—*hydrohepatosis* where liver is soft and smooth; or it may be due to secondaries (nodular, hard) from carcinoma of head or periampullary region.

Surface marking of the liver: Upper border of right lobe is at the level of 5th rib 2.5 cm medial to right midclavicular line; upper border of left lobe is at left midclavicular line at the level of 6th rib. In males it corresponds to a line joining a point 1 cm below the right nipple to a point about 2 cm below the left nipple; lower border runs obliquely from right 9th costal cartilage to left 8th costal cartilage crossing midline obliquely halfway between xiphoid and umbilicus.

Spleen

Spleen is only occasionally palpable in normal person (1–3% of normal people—in New Guinea commonly). Normal spleen is 12 × 7 cm in size. It is enlarged if it is more than 14 cm. Spleen should get enlarged three times to become palpable.

Method 1: Right hand fingers are used to palpate the spleen from right iliac fossa. Index finger is placed like palpation for liver. Fingers are moved towards left hypochondrium and upwards in each phase of respiration. Spleen is palpated under the tip of 10th rib.

Method 2: Left hand may be kept under the left lower chest wall and skin is moved downwards so that more lax skin is available to insinuate the right hand fingers under left costal margin.

Method 3: While right hand is palpating, left hand is placed under the left rib cage to lift it upwards so that spleen comes forward to facilitate the palpation by right hand.

Method 4: Spleen can be palpated from above—left side of the patient with two hands arching below the left costal margin, and during phases of respiration spleen will come down and touch the examiner's fingers. Often *tilting the patient with left side up* during palpation makes spleen to be palpated in easier way.

Method 5—Hook sign: Hooking the left costal margin with fingers is not possible in splenic enlargement.

Method 6—Middleton's maneuver: Examiner stands on left side of the patient facing towards foot-end, keeps his left hand fingers hooked under left costal margin and exerts pressure over the posterolateral aspect of the lower thorax using his right hand and spleen is felt at the end of deep inspiration **(Figs. 21-12A and B)**.

Surface marking of spleen: It is situated behind 9th, 10th, and 11th ribs with its long axis along the line of 10th rib; anteriorly it extends 4 cm from the midline (medial end) towards midaxillary line (lateral end) while posteriorly its superior angle is 4 cm lateral to 10th thoracic spine. It makes 45° angle to horizontal plane. **Its superior border is notched near its anterior end**. It is separated from these ribs by diaphragm.

Gallbladder

Gallbladder when enlarged is visible on inspection in the right hypochondrium as globular mass directed downwards and forwards below right costal margin or below the lower margin of the palpable liver just lateral to the lateral border of the right rectus muscle along the tip of the 9th rib. The mass moves with respiration, mobile horizontally, dull on percussion, soft, and smooth. It may be tender if it is empyema. Gallbladder otherwise is nontender (mucocele of gallbladder). It is palpably enlarged in condition obstructing the drainage of the gallbladder— in carcinoma head of pancreas or periampullary carcinoma. It is hard in carcinoma of gallbladder.

Courvoisier's law: Palpable enlarged gallbladder in a patient with jaundice is usually not due to stone in common bile duct because the gallbladder will become small and shrunken due to repeated attacks of inflammation. Exception: Obstructive pathology can still cause palpable gallbladder in stone in both CBD and cystic duct, pancreatic calculus at ampulla of Vater, mucocele of gallbladder due to stone in cystic duct.

Surface marking of gallbladder: It is situated at the junction of 9th costal cartilage and outer border of right rectus

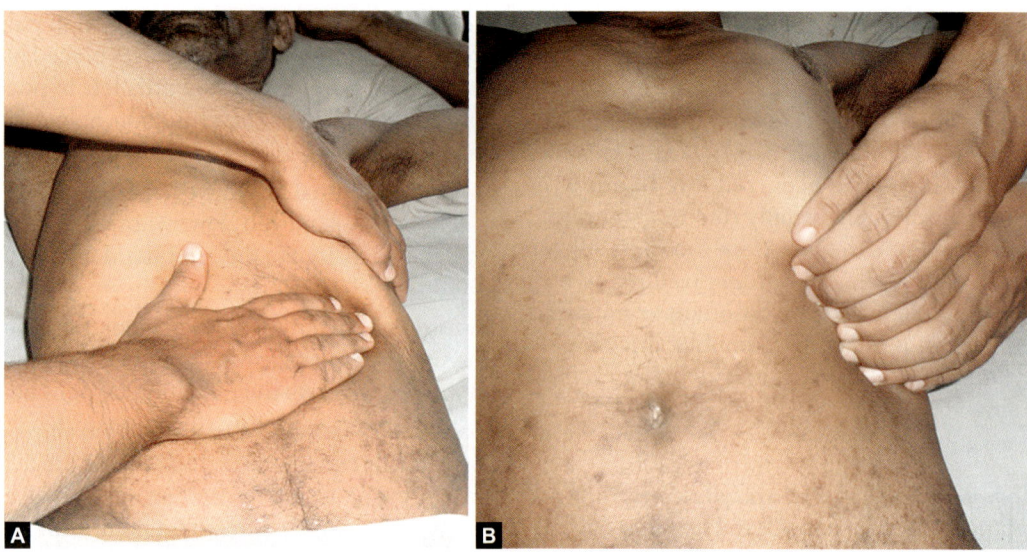

Figs. 21-12A and B Palpation of spleen—*different methods.*

abdominis. ***Grey Turner's method:*** A line is drawn from left anterior superior iliac spine through the umbilicus extending across towards right costal margin; at the junction of this line at right costal margin is the site of gallbladder.

> **Causes of splenomegaly:** Congestive cardiac failure, malaria, portal hypertension, hemolytic anemias, idiopathic thrombocytopenic purpura, kala-azar, lymphomas, chronic myeloid leukemia (massive spleen), polycythemia rubra vera, sarcoidosis myelofibrosis, typhoid fever, autoimmune diseases, splenic abscess, splenic cyst, tuberculosis.
> *Hypersplenism* is overactivity of the splenic function which has nothing to do with splenic size with typical features of splenomegaly; pancytopenia; hypercellular or normal bone marrow; reversible by splenectomy. Causes for hypersplenism are: lymphoma, cirrhosis, myeloproliferative diseases, and connective tissue diseases

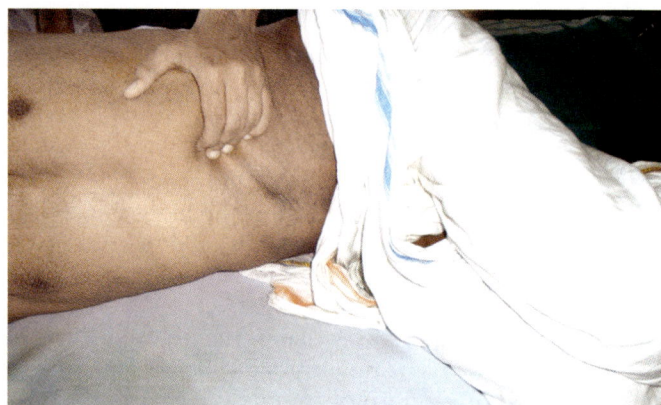

Fig. 21-13 *Eliciting Mallet–Guy sign in chronic pancreatitis.*

Pancreas

It is being a retroperitoneal organ is only felt if at all on deep palpation. It is felt if there is pseudocyst of pancreas or mass due to cystadenocarcinoma or cystadenoma of pancreas. Carcinoma of head of pancreas is usually not palpable (gallbladder is palpable here with obstructive jaundice). Pancreas in chronic pancreatitis or pancreatic cyst is better felt in lateral position from left side with patient turned towards right side with hip and knees flexed. Left subcostal and epigastric regions are deeply palpated. In this position-bowel in front will be displaced making pancreas better palpable. Tenderness elicited in this position in chronic pancreatitis is called as ***Mallet–Guy sign* (Fig. 21-13)**.

Colon

Fecal mass may be felt like a colonic mass. Fecal mass yields/moulds (indents) on pressure. It subsides or reduces in size after giving enema. Distended cecum is better seen than felt as fullness in the right iliac fossa. Colonic mass is located along the anatomical line of the colon depending on the site of pathology. It is mobile but does not move with respiration, nodular, hard, well localized mass. Anemia, diarrhea, constipation and distension are other features.

Kidney

Kidney is palpated by bimanual palpation; ballotability. In sitting position, renal angle tenderness should be checked **(Figs. 21-14A to C) (Discussed in detail in Chapter 26: Approaches and Examination of Urinary Diseases)**.

Swelling (Mass)

Any swelling in the abdomen is palpated in similar way:

Skin over the swelling is examined for raise in temperature, and tenderness. Swelling is palpated to note its edge, surface, shape, extent and location.

Consistency is known by soft/firm/hard; whether it shows pitting/indentation on pressure; fluctuation absent or present.

Compressibility and reducibility; impulse on coughing, vascularity; mobility/fixity; palpation of surrounding area to know the extent of infiltration or spread are checked.

Head raising or leg raising test (Carnett's) is done to confirm the plane of the mass if present is intra-abdominal

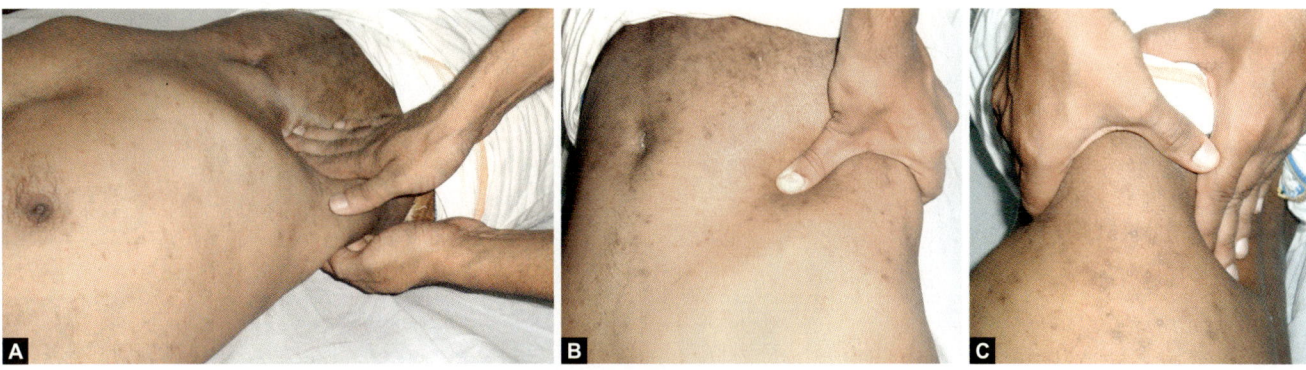

Figs. 21-14A to C Different methods of *kidney palpation*.

or not. If mass becomes less prominent during these tests, it is intra-abdominal; if mass becomes more prominent, it means it is in the abdominal wall **(Figs. 21-15 and 21-16)**.

Fluid Thrill

Fluid thrill is elicited when large amount of fluid (>2000 mL; fluid under tension) is present in the peritoneal cavity (ascites). Hand of patient or assistant is placed vertically in the midline of abdomen pressing firmly to prevent the transmission of vibration wave towards opposite side along the skin and subcutaneous plane and also to increase fluid tension inside the peritoneal cavity. Abdominal flanks on one side are tapped with fingers, vibration of fluid thrill is felt with the other hand placed on other side flank. Often such fluid thrill is positive in large ovarian cyst also **(Figs. 21-17A and B)**. But it can be differentiated by shifting dullness and **Blaxland ruler test**. Shifting dullness is done during percussion. Ascites may be due to congestive cardiac failure, portal hypertension, abdominal tuberculosis, peritoneal carcinoma and advanced malignancies.

Blaxland Ruler Test

Urinary bladder is emptied. A flat ruler is laid upon the abdomen just above the anterior superior iliac spines. With the fingers of both the hands, the ruler is pushed firmly and steadily towards lumbar spine. Abdominal aortic pulsation is felt in ovarian cyst. It is not felt in ascites **(Figs. 21-18A and B)**.

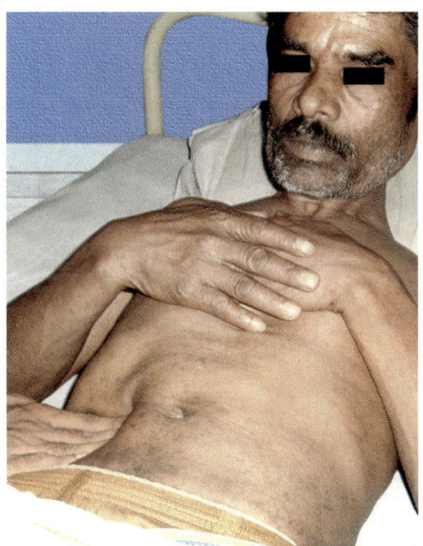

Fig. 21-15 *Head raising test.*

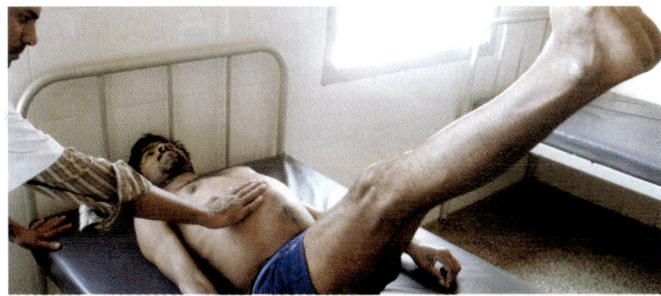

Fig. 21-16 *Carnett's leg raising test.* Both legs are raised above with knees straight and abdomen is inspected and palpated.

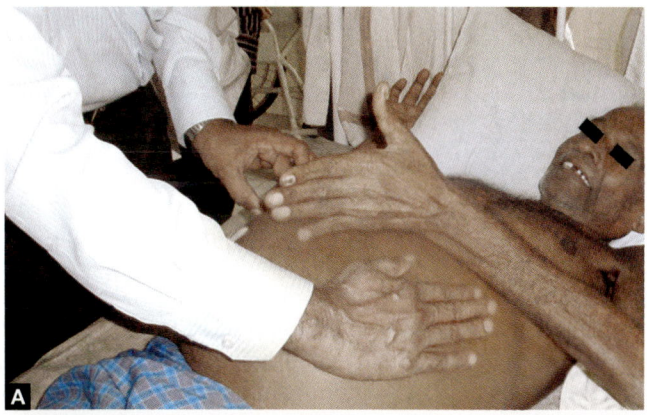

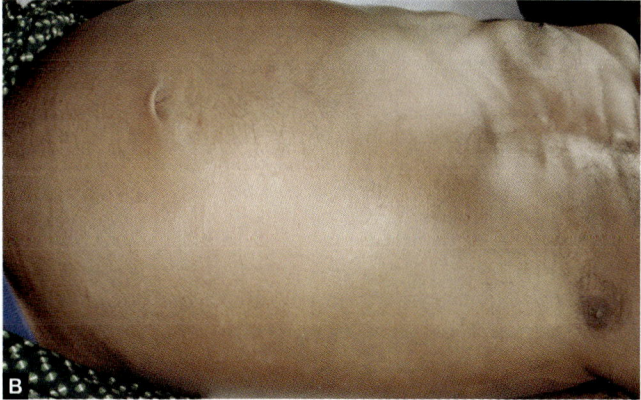

Figs. 21-17A and B Demonstration of *fluid thrill*.

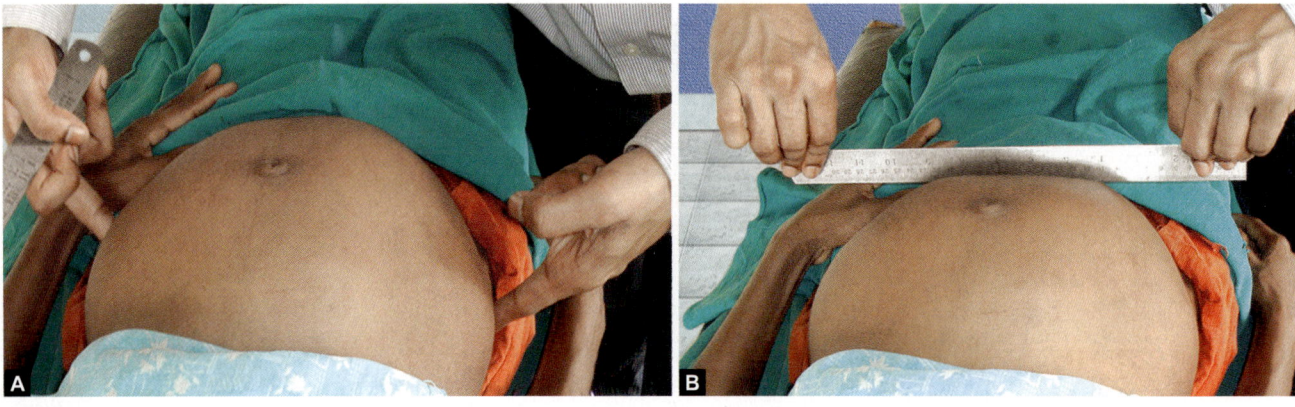

Figs. 21-18A and B *Blaxland ruler test.* First ascertain the line of anterior superior iliac spine.

Measurements

Abdominal girth measurement: It is done at umbilical level. Periodic measurement is done to assess the progress of the disease.

Measurement of the position of the umbilicus: Distance between lower end of xiphisternum to umbilicus and from the umbilicus to the pubic symphysis is equal normally. But it is displaced downwards in ascites; upwards in ovarian or pelvic tumors—**Tanyol sign.**

Bilateral spinoumbilical length measurements: Distance between anterior superior iliac spine and umbilicus is equal in both sides normally. It may be altered (decreased) in one side in case of mass in opposite side of the abdomen (usually lower abdomen or pelvis mass).

Other Sites

Palpation of hernial sites and external genitalia has to be done to exclude any pathology in that areas.

Percussion

Liver dullness is elicited in the 5th intercostal space in midclavicular line on right side. Liver span is assessed at midclavicular line from upper border to the right costal margin or palpable lower border of the liver. It is 12–15 cm in adult. Percussion is started from right 4th space downwards until dullness is reached and continued up to the lower margin of the dullness. Liver dullness is reduced in severe emphysema, right sided pneumothorax. It is obliterated in perforation of viscus causing gas under diaphragm.

> **Note:** Ultrasound may detect 30 mL of fluid in abdomen.
> *Grading of ascites:*
> Grade 1 – Detectable only by careful examination
> Grade 2 – Easily detectable small volume
> Grade 3 – Obvious ascites but not tense
> Grade 4 – Tense ascites

Percussion over the mass is important to locate the anatomical plane. Abdominal wall masses, masses in front of the bowel like liver, spleen, gallbladder are dull on percussion. Mass arising from bowel has impaired resonant note. Retroperitoneal mass is resonant (as bowel is present in front) on percussion like pancreatic mass, renal mass, aortic aneurysm, para-aortic lymph node mass, retroperitoneal tumors or cyst. Mass in the upper abdomen if dull on percussion should be confirmed whether it continues with liver dullness or not.

Shifting dullness for free fluid should be checked (1000 mL of fluid should be present). **Puddle sign** is assessing small quantity of free-fluid in the abdominal cavity in knee-elbow position- (120 mL). It is checked in same position often by auscultopercussion also **(Discussed in detail in 'Chapter 22—Examination of Mass Abdomen')**.

In ascites, it is dull in the flanks but resonant on the summit (center) whereas in ovarian cyst it is resonant in periphery but dull in the center.

Traube's area: It is bounded above by lung resonance; below by left costal margin; on the right side by left border of the liver and on the left side normal splenic dullness. Surface marking is—left anterior axillary line, 6th rib and costal margin. It lies in left lower chest behind 9th, 10th and 11th ribs. Normally it is resonant as it is occupied by stomach. It becomes dull in left-sided pleural effusion, *splenomegaly*, and *stomach (fundus) with solid tumor or fluid*, enlarged left lobe of the liver, massive pericardial effusion. It is shifted upwards in left lower lobe collapse/left lung fibrosis/left side diaphragm paralysis **(Fig. 21-19)**.

Percussion for splenic dullness: **Method 1 (Nixon's):** Patient is turned towards right side (left up; left lateral decubitus) and percussion is started at posterior axillary line proceeding perpendicularly towards anterior costal margin. Upper border of dullness is 8 cm above the costal margin in normal people. Dullness more than 8 cm signifies splenic enlargement. **Method 2 (Castell's):** Resonant note normally felt while percussing in supine position along the lowest intercostal space in anterior axillary line (left) becomes **dull** on *full inspiration* in case of splenomegaly.

Percussion over the renal angle: Normally renal angle (angle of erector spinae and 12th rib) is resonant due to colon underneath. In kidney enlargement, angle is occupied by enlarged kidney in deeper plane reflecting the colon to front and medially making it dull on percussion. Renal angle percussion is done in sitting position **(Fig. 21-20)**.

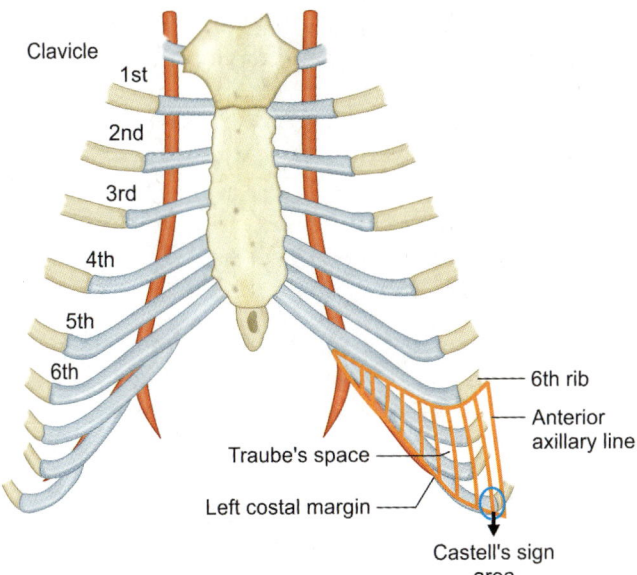

Fig. 21-19 Boundaries of Traube's space and area of percussion for Castell's sign.

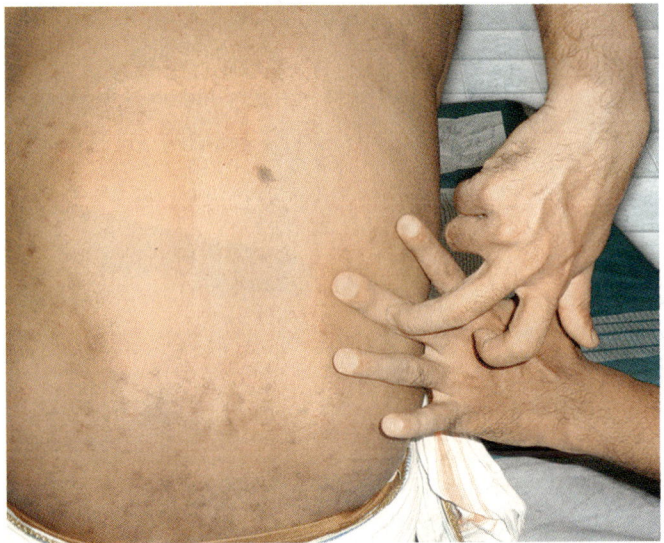

Fig. 21-20 Percussion over the renal angle in sitting position. It is *normally resonant*.

Auscultation

Bowel sounds: Normal bowel sounds (Borborygmi) are 2–4 in number per minute. It is small bowel peristalsis which is heard. Bowel sounds are checked with bell of the stethoscope in umbilical region, 2 cm to the right of umbilicus as it is the midpoint of mesentery. Usually 2–3 points over the abdomen is auscultated for at least one minute. Bowel sounds are of two types—(1) active intestinal peristaltic sound of low tone, gurgling in character, progresses to moderate intensity and stops abruptly, (2) passive intestinal sounds, heard in peritonitis and late paralytic ileus due to movement of fluid and gas in dilated bowel/ spill of contents from one loop to another. It is synchronous with the movement of the patient, loud, high pitched tinkling sound of constant intensity described as '***bells at evening pealing'***. If bowel sounds are heard more than 5 per minute, it is ***hyperperistaltic***—feature of early obstruction, enteritis, carcinoid syndrome. Absence of bowel sounds is called as ***silent abdomen*** where the heart sounds can be heard which otherwise are not heard. It is observed in paralytic ileus, late intestinal obstruction, acute peritonitis, acute pancreatitis and acute mesenteric ischemia.

Bruit around umbilicus may be due to renal artery stenosis. Bruit above the umbilicus may be due to aortic aneurysm. ***Bruit over liver*** may be due to increased vascularity—hemangioma, hepatocellular carcinoma (HCC), hepatic artery aneurysm. Hepatic rub suggests perihepatitis.

Kenawy's sign: By placing stethoscope beneath the xiphoid process, a venous hum is heard in portal hypertension which is louder during inspiration. It is due to engorgement of the splenic vein and during inspiration spleen is compressed making it louder.

Cruveilhier–Baumgarten syndrome is *venous hum* heard between xiphisternum and umbilicus in portal hypertension due to patent congenital umbilical vein draining portal vein.

Splenic rub suggests splenic infarction, chronic myeloid leukemia, endocarditis, sickle cell disease. *Bruit* in this region may be due to splenic artery aneurysm.

Auscultopercussion test for stomach dilatation: Stethoscope is placed below and to the left of xiphisternum. With the finger, gentle strokings are done from epigastrium, adjacent to stethoscope, in radial fashion. It is repeated from above downwards on left side. Change in the sound at the margin of greater curvature is obvious. All points from above downwards are marked and joined to get the level of greater curvature of the stomach. It is above the level of the umbilicus in normal individuals. It lies below in gastric outlet obstruction like pyloric stenosis, carcinoma pylorus. Only greater curvature of the stomach can be assessed as dilatation takes place at greater curvature.

Succussion splash: Stethoscope is placed over the epigastrium. Using thumb and fingers of both hands, which are placed on each side of lower chest wall, patient is held firmly and shaken to hear splashing sounds of fluid in the stomach. Note that the patient is empty stomach or had not taken any fluid for at least 4 hours, as succussion splash can be heard even in normal person giving false positive result. Positive succussion splash suggests gastric outlet obstruction.

Examination of Left Supraclavicular Lymph Nodes

It is enlarged when there is spread from gastrointestinal malignancies through thoracic duct. It is located deep to deep fascia in the supraclavicular fossa. This ***Virchow's node*** enlargement is called as ***Troisier's sign*** (Figs. 21-21A and B). It suggests advanced malignancy. FNAC of this node will give the histological diagnosis of adenocarcinoma. It is felt using finger dipping deep above the clavicle close to the sternomastoid muscle.

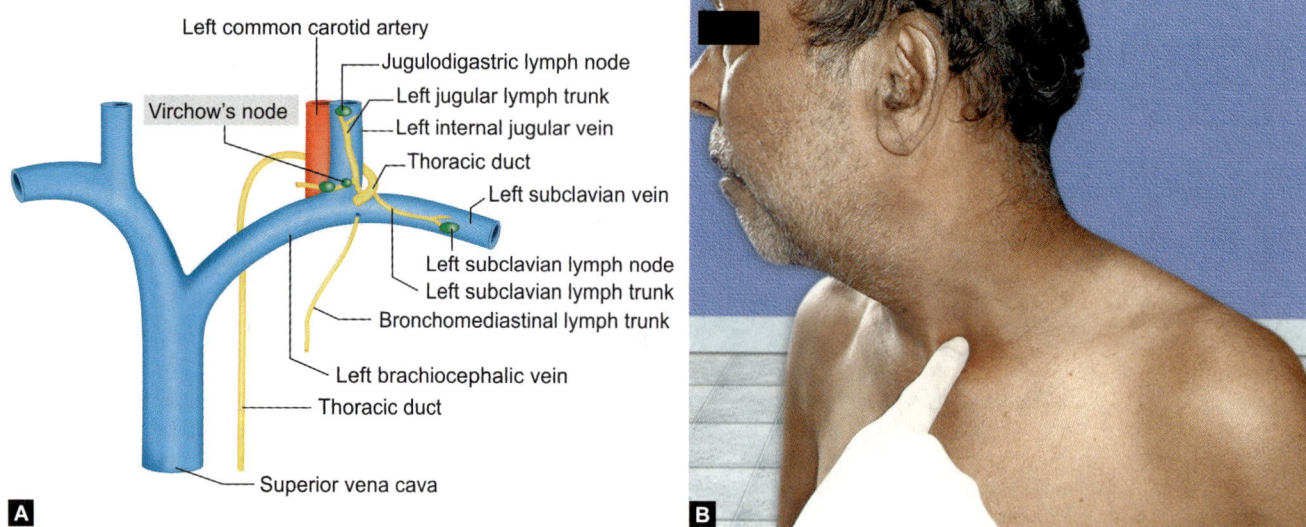

Fig. 21-21 A and B (A) *Anatomy of Virchow's node*. It is located under the lateral head or in between two heads of the left sternocleidomastoid muscle just above the sternal angle of the clavicle; (B) Palpation of left supraclavicular lymph node (Level IV; lower deep cervical)—*Troisier's sign*.

Digital Examination of Rectum

It is done to look for secondaries (***Blumer's shelf***) in anterior aspect above the prostate level. It is nodular hard with free mucosa (not adherent). It suggests advanced malignancy. It is due to peritoneal spread. It is useful in Crohn's disease (fissure-in-ano or fistula-in-ano), and other chronic conditions.

> **Virchow's node:**
> Rudolf Ludwig Karl Virchow, in 1849, noted the involvement left supraclavicular node in relation to the junction of the thoracic duct adjacent to medial part of IJV; this end node drains through few lymphatics into the left jugular trunk and to thoracic duct. Reflux from thoracic duct into this node occurs easily in abdominal malignancy. After 40 years, Troisier reported many abdominal cancers presenting with left supraclavicular lymph node involvement as external indicator and so coined the term Virchow's node and sign is called as Troisier sign. On left at C7 transverse process level, thoracic duct arches behind the carotid sheath and IJV and joins the junction of IJV and left subclavian vein; this Virchow's (end node along the thoracic duct) is located medial to this junction behind the muscular lateral head of the left sternocleidomastoid muscle or in between the two heads. Virchow's node is also called as 'signal node' or seat of the devil' node. Virchow's node is actually part of the lower deep cervical node. Its surface marking almost corresponds to end of the thoracic duct i.e. just above the sternal angle of the clavicle 1.5 cm left of the midline. Node is just medial to this point.

Pervaginal Examination

It is very essential in females especially in lower abdomen masses and when ***Krukenberg tumor*** (Carcinoma stomach) of ovary is suspected.

■ SYSTEMIC EXAMINATIONS

Examinations of respiratory system (pleurisy, effusion, tuberculosis, pneumonia), spine (for secondaries or tuberculosis), cardiovascular (congestive cardiac failure and pericardial effusion), central nervous system is essential **(Figs. 21-22 and 21-23)**.

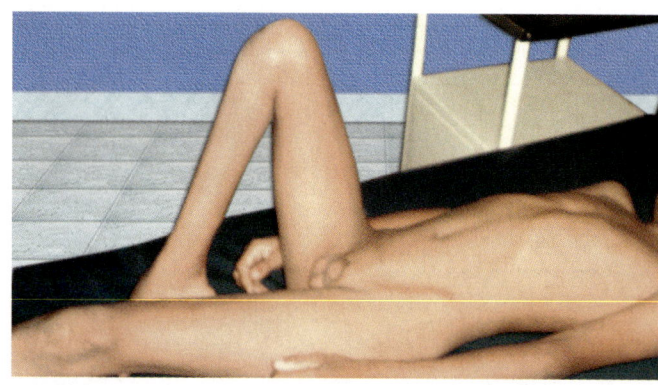

Fig. 21-22 Psoas spasm causing *hip in flexion due to psoas abscess*.

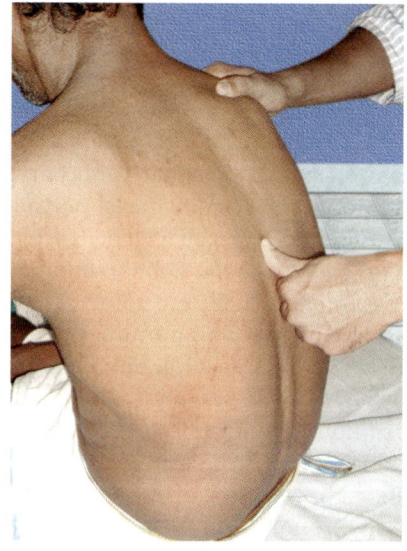

Fig. 21-23 Examination of *spine is essential* in patients.

INVESTIGATIONS

Detailed investigations and discussions of different conditions are beyond the scope of this book. Students should refer *SRBs Manual of Surgery,* and *Bedside Clinics in Surgery* for in detail discussions.

Blood: Hb%, ESR, relevant tumor markers.

Stool examination: Occult blood, steatorrhea (fat), creatorrhea (muscle fibers seen in chronic pancreatitis), mucus in stool, microscopy and culture.

A cricketing approach to the abdomen (Fig. 21-24) *(Courtesy: Professor Dr Sribatsa Kumar Mohapatra, MS, FRCS; VSSMC, Burla, Sambalpur, Odisha, India)*
- Abdomen is called as a *Pandora's box* (Greek: Box of evils; a process once begun creates many problems). Here unexpected findings may come out instead of expected ones
- In surgical/clinical point, abdomen may be considered as four areas instead of one anatomical abdomen, i.e. (1) Upper thoracic; (2) Central; (3) Pelvic; (4) Retroperitoneal
- Metaphorically abdomen is compared to cricket field; surgeon plays cricket over the abdomen for a winning championship by scoring runs
- Abdomen is compared to imaginary cricket ground with stumps; one end of the stumps is xiphoid process and other end of stumps is pubic symphysis. The pitch connecting the both stumps are the pararectal lines of both sides. Two crease lines are transpyloric (TPL) and transtubercular (TTL) lines. TPL connects the tips of the costal cartilages (CC) of both sides; 10th CC is last CC as 11th and 12th are floating ribs without any CC connecting to costal cartilage. TTL connects highest point of iliac crests which is 5 cm behind the anterior superior iliac spine. The boundary extends from supraclavicular area above to groin crease below and flanks on both sides including vertebral column on the back
- Our objective clinical finding is the ball. When ball crosses the boundary without touching the field and boundary line score is six; when it crosses boundary line through the field (touching), score is four; ball in the field either gets no score or one or two
- In surgeon's point of view, when he plays clinical cricketing, he wants to score six at the earliest. So this six runs are scored by a surgeon by palpating—(1) Supraclavicular lymph node (positive Troisier's sign); (2) External hernias; (3) Examination of spine for deformity, tenderness which may be the cause for abdominal pain; (4) Femoral pulse if bilateral symmetrical or unilateral weak indicates vascular pathology; (5) Digital rectal examination even if comes in the periphery of the field, it is very important clinical method (if you are hesitating to put your finger into the rectum, you will put your foot on it); (6) External genitalia with testicular examination in males (as originally testes are abdominal organs and drains into para-aortic lymph nodes and testicular pain is referred to the T10 segment)
- The other runs four, three, two and one are scored by examining the LUMPS (L +U+M+P+S) on the abdomen. L—liver enlargement is present or not = one score; U—status umbilicus is also important for umbilical hernia tumors/fistula/hernia/ infection of the umbilicus will give many scores; M—moving dullness indicates free fluid in the abdomen, its presence or absence carries one score; P—palpating further for guarding, rigidity, tenderness, rebound tenderness and local rise of temperature—scores/runs; S—splenic examination whether palpable or not scores one run
- Final important scoring comes from finding a lump in any of the nine segments/regions

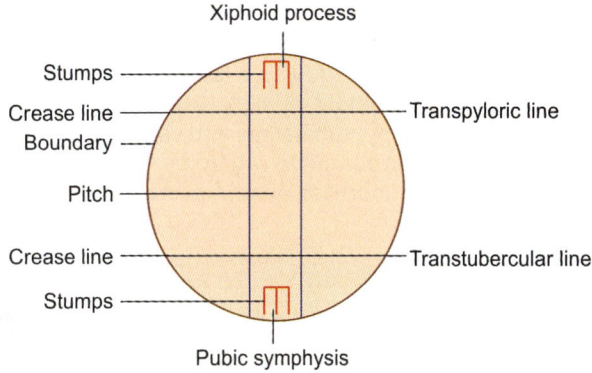

Fig. 21-24 *A cricketing approach* to the clinical examination of abdomen.

- A good surgeon who scores all the runs can win the match to reach the diagnosis of the disease. Thus, cricketing approach to abdomen may help some of our best brains who are not only best at cricket but also at the field of surgery

Gastric Function Tests

Patient is overnight fasting; should not take any antacids and anticholinergics for 24 hours. Nasogastric tube is passed early morning and gastric juice is aspirated under fluoroscopy after confirming the tip of tube is at mid stomach level. Normally it is around 70 mL. If it is more, it suggests pyloric stenosis or hypersecretion. Tube now is connected to low pressure 5 cm Hg suction to have continuous aspiration. Later one hour aspiration is collected. It is called as *morning basal secretion*. Free acid level means only HCl level; total acid level means HCl plus other acids in the stomach.

Dragstedt test: Gastric content is aspirated through continuous low pressure suction for 12 hours from 9 pm to 9 am and the juice is collected. Normal volume is 400 mL. It is increased in duodenal ulcer due to vagal hyperactivity; increased very much, more than a liter in Zollinger–Ellison syndrome. Normal HCl level in this is 10–20 mEq. It is 40–80 mEq in duodenal ulcer (↑); 100–300 mEq in ZE syndrome (↑↑); 5–15 mEq in gastric ulcer (↓). Basal secretion is the secretion from the parietal cell mass *in resting* condition. It is <5 mEq/hour normally; >5 mEq in duodenal ulcer; 1–2 mEq in gastric ulcer. Peak/maximal secretion is secretion in one hour after stimulation. Stimulation may be using pentagastrin (now used)/Kay's augmented histamine/Hollander's insulin. It gives *maximal/peak acid output*.

Pentagastrin test: Initial basal secretion is collected. 6 μg of pentagastrin is injected IM/SC and 15 minutes gastric samples are taken for one hour. Peak/maximum acid output is assessed. Normal is 25–27 mEq; in gastric ulcer, it is upto 15 mEq; in duodenal ulcer, it is 35–38 mEq; in ZE syndrome, it is >60 mEq, very high; in carcinoma stomach, it is very low.

Kay's augmented histamine test: After collection of basal fasting sample, mepyramine maleate 100 mg IM is injected to neutralize histamine side effects without interfering gastric effects. After 30 minutes, histamine acid phosphate 0.04 mg/kg is injected SC. Free acid level (only HCl) is assessed. In stomal ulcer, it is 30–35 mEq; in duodenal ulcer, it is 30–40 mEq; in gastric ulcer, it is less than 15 mEq.

Hollander's insulin test: It is useful to assess postoperatively and confirm the completeness of vagotomy. 0.2 units/kg weight of insulin is injected IV to a fasting patient so as to create hypoglycemia below 35 mg% which stimulates the parietal cells through hypothalamus and vagus causing acid secretion. Patient with complete vagotomy will not show the increased acid level. Increase in acid secretion in first one hour is called *early response* and if it is more than 30 mmols/L suggests incomplete vagotomy. *Delayed response* is between 1st and 2nd hours and is due to delayed gastrin release.

Chew and spit test: Nasogastric tube is passed. Patient chews a meal and spits it out to stimulate acid production through vagus. Gastric contents are aspirated and studied for acid level.

Other evaluation methods	Findings and features
Barium meal X-ray (Fig. 21-25) It is done using *barium sulfate (95% w/v) solution* of which 400–600 mL is given orally. *Gastrograffin* also often used. Microcrystalized barium sulfate solution is better. Procedure should be done in empty stomach under fluoroscopic guidance. Buscopan injection is given to the patient to delay the gastric emptying. Glucagon also can be used. Effervescent tablet (calcium carbonate and antifoaming agent) is given to the patient. Further X-rays are taken to get double contrast barium meal X-rays **Barium meal follow through X-ray** is done as late films often after giving prokinetic agents like metoclopramide Contrast studies are also used in gastric fistulas, trichobezoars, etc. Hypotonic duodenography: It is same as barium meal X-ray but duodenal hypotonia is achieved by giving injection glucagon or buscopan so that air contrast hypotonic barium X-ray study shows better picture	• Duodenal ulcer—shows absent/deformed duodenal cap • Benign gastric ulcer—shows *niche* (due to ulcer) and *notch* (due to spasm) • Gastric outlet obstruction—dilated greater curvature below iliac crest level, mottled look, duodenal obstruction • Carcinoma stomach—irregular filling defect • Carcinoma head of pancreas—pad sign; periampullary carcinoma— *Frostberg* reverse '3' sign • Chronic duodenal ileus—obstruction at mid-third part of the duodenum • Stomal ulcer—ulcer crater at stoma • Duodenal diverticula—trifoliate duodenum • Pseudocyst of pancreas—widened vertebro-gastric angle
Enteroclysis: It is visualization of entire length of small intestine to assess anatomical problems. **Indications:** Small bowel diseases/ileocecal tuberculosis, stricture, small bowel tumors, partial obstruction and Crohn's disease. **Technique**: Patient is prepared overnight with empty stomach and laxatives. Nasojejunal tube is passed. Prokinetic drug like metoclopramide given. Micro barium sulfate solution (50% w/v) or gastrograffin or water-soluble iodine dye solution is (500–800 mL) passed through the tube. Under fluoroscopic guidance, X-rays are taken as required	**Features** such as narrowing, smooth/irregular filling defect, localized dilatation, obstruction or features of specific conditions are looked for. In conditions like ileocecal tuberculosis, enteroclysis and barium enema X-rays are combined **Problems:** Poor patient acceptance and technical difficulty. Capsule endoscopy or enteroscopes are better options to visualize the small bowel. When nasojejunal tube is not able to be passed, barium meal follow through X-ray is done by taking late films of barium meal

Barium enema X-ray (Fig. 21-26):
Required preparations—24 hours liquid diet, laxatives for two nights and enema on previous night
About one liter of barium sulphate/micro barium sulphate solution (25% w/v) is infused per anally into the colorectum using an enema tube from an enema can. Patient will be initially in left lateral position and later in prone position. In children, a Foley's catheter with inflation is used to maintain the retention of enema. Procedure is often observed under fluoroscopy. Injection buscopan is injected (20 mg IV) to relax the colon. X-ray film is taken after complete filling. Patient is asked to evacuate the barium and later post-evacuation film is taken. Air is insufflated into the colon to get air contrast film. Additional different view films are taken to see the suspected area properly
Indications: Carcinoma colon; ileocecal tuberculosis (combined with enteroclysis); ulcerative colitis; Crohn's disease; ischemic colitis; colonic polyps; intussusception; congenital megacolon; gastrojejunocolic fistula; congenital diaphragmatic hernia (Bochdalek)
1. *Hirschsprung's disease:* Foley's catheter should not be used while doing barium enema in case of Hirschsprung's disease. Here barium is used in dilute saline but not in water. It is done to look for the extent of disease and three zones
   i. Distal immobile spastic segment, i.e. aganglionic zone
   ii. A proximal, middle transitional zone of about 1–5 cm length with less, sparse number of ganglions (Cone)
   iii. A still more proximal, hypertrophied dilated segment is actually the normal ganglionic area
	2. *Carcinoma colon:* Irregular filling defect; apple core lesion especially on left side; metachronous growths (growths in different parts of the colon) should be looked for—5% common; narrowing of left-sided lesion
	3. *Ulcerative colitis:* Loss of haustrations; contracted smooth colon; presence of pseudopolyps; *Collar button ulcers*—contiguous mucosal involvement; hose pipe/pipe stem lesions; increased presacral, space more than normal (normal <1 cm)
	4. *Ileocecal tuberculosis:* Pulled up cecum due to fibrosis and contraction; obtuse ileocecal angle (normal angle is acute); hurrying of barium due to rapid flow—*Stierlin sign*; narrow ileum with thickened ileocecal valve, *Fleischner*—inverted umbrella sign; incompetent ileocecal valve; ulcers and strictures in terminal ileum—napkin lesions; *Gooseneck appearance*—ileum hanging from fibrosed; pulled up cecum
	5. *Crohn's disease*: Aphthoid ulceration; skip lesions; rectum is not commonly involved; *string sign of Kantor*; Cobble stone appearance—pseudo-sacculations; raspberry/rose thorn appearance; fistula or strictures
	6. *Sigmoid diverticula*: Saw teeth appearance of sigmoid colon—concertina like—serrated appearance; champagne glass sign—partial filling of barium with stercolith inside the diverticula; fistula to adjacent structures
	7. *Intussusception*: Claw sign—coiled spring sign: pincer end; empty right iliac fossa—mainly in plain X-ray abdomen with multiple air fluid levels (on ultrasound—target sign/pseudo kidney sign/bull's eye sign)
	8. *Ischemic colitis*: Thumb print sign in splenic flexure

Contd...

Contd...

Other evaluation methods	Findings and features
Oral cholecystography: Patient is advised to have fat-free diet for 3 days. On previous night, 6 tablets of *iopanoic acid (Telepaque)* are given orally. Next morning, plain X-ray abdomen is taken to visualize the gallbladder. Later fatty meal is given and X-rays are taken at 10, 15, 30 and 60 minutes to see the change in the size of the gallbladder (which should be less in size compared to the earlier film, as the gallbladder contracts on stimulation if it is functioning normally) **(Fig. 21-27)**	Smooth filling defect signifies non-opaque stone **Contraindications**: Patients with serum bilirubin >3 mg%, acute cholecystitis. OCG is not done nowadays **Note: Inravenous cholangiogram:** It is done to visualize bile ducts and biliary tree by injecting *IV meglumine ioglycamate (Biligram)* and taking X-ray abdomen. It can be combined with OCG. **Problems**: Poor visualization and drug reaction. It is not very useful if serum bilirubin is >3 mg%. This is also not done nowadays
Endoscopic retrograde cholangiopancreatography (ERCP): It is done under C-arm guidance; under sedation like midazolam or propofol anesthesia. Patient is placed in prone position with the head turned to right. After passing side viewing gastroduodenoscope, sphincter of Oddi is identified and cannulated. Under visualization, 3 mL water soluble iodine contrast is injected into the bile duct and pancreatic duct. When cannula goes upwards beside vertebra, it is in bile duct; and if cannula goes across the vertebra, it is in pancreatic duct **(Fig. 21-28)** **Therapeutic uses:** Extraction of biliary duct stone; nasobiliary drainage; stenting of tumor in the CBD or in the pancreas; dilatation of the biliary stricture; endoscopic papillotomy	**Indications**: Malignancy—irregular filling defect; chronic pancreatitis—*chain-of-lakes* appearance; congenital anomalies, stones; stricture of biliary tree; choledochal cyst; for sampling of biliary and pancreatic juices for analysis and cytology; brush biopsy from tumor site **Complications**: Pancreatitis; duodenal injury; cholangitis; bleeding **Relative contraindications**: Acute pancreatitis; previous gastrectomy; altered prothrombin time (corrected by injection Vitamin K, FFP); bleeding disorders
Percutaneous transhepatic cholangiography (PTC): It is done in case of severe obstructive jaundice under coverage of appropriate antibiotics and after control of any bleeding tendency. With the help of fluoroscopy, *Chiba (university) or Okuda needle* which is long, flexible, thin, blunt, without bevelled end, is passed into the liver through right 8th intercostal space in midaxillary line. Once needle is in the dilated biliary radicle, bile is aspirated (sent for culture, cytology, analysis); and then water-soluble iodine dye is injected into the same so as to visualize the dilated biliary radicles, also the site and extent of any obstruction, (i.e., tumor, stricture)	Procedure can be used for therapeutic stenting across the biliary tree through any obstruction either in the hepatic ducts or in the CBD into the duodenum **Complications**: Bleeding, biliary leak, biliary peritonitis and septicemia **Magnetic resonance cholangiopancreatography (MRCP):** MRCP is a non-contrast imaging method, better than ERCP as diagnostic tool in biliary and pancreatic diseases. T2 images are used
Gastroscopy: It is visualization of interior of stomach, duodenum and esophagus; used for diagnosing any pathology—gastric ulcer; duodenal ulcer; gastritis; stomal ulcer; carcinoma stomach; esophagitis; esophageal varices. Biopsies from the suspected cases of malignancy or for *Helicobacter pylori* can be taken **(Fig. 21-29)** *Endosonography* can be done to assess the staging, operability of carcinoma stomach or esophagus. *Fiberoptic flexible gastroduodenoscopy* also can be used. *Videoendoscopy* is used not only for diagnosis but also mainly for therapeutic procedures. Both *end viewing and side viewing* gastroscopes are available For therapeutic procedures—variceal injection or ligation; stenting of pseudocyst of pancreas through gastroscopy; polyp removal; submucosal resection; for ERCP—diagnostic, side viewing gastroscope is required	**Procedure:** Gastroscopy is done following eight hours of fasting. After lignocaine spray into the oral cavity, gastroscope is passed gently down the esophagus when the patient does the swallowing action. Once the scope is inside the stomach, air is inflated and different parts of the stomach are visualized. Fundus is visualized by retropulsion. Scope is passed through the pylorus to see first and second parts of the duodenum. Looked for any pathology and if required biopsy is taken. Often midazolam sedation is beneficial to have an easy passage. **Complications**: Bleeding, aspiration, perforation (rarely)

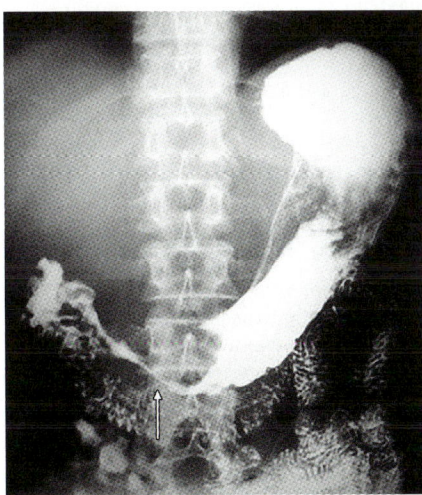

Fig. 21-25 *Barium meal X-ray* showing polypoid growth.

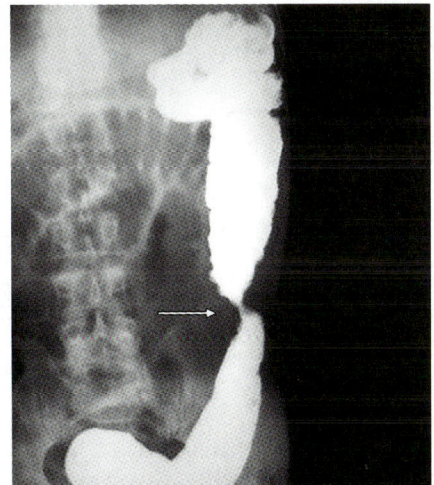

Fig. 21-26 Barium enema X-ray showing growth *with stricture in the descending colon.*

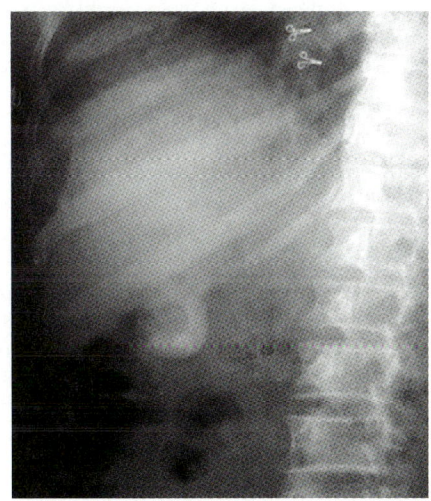

Fig. 21-27 *Oral cholecystogram* done to see the function of the gallbladder.

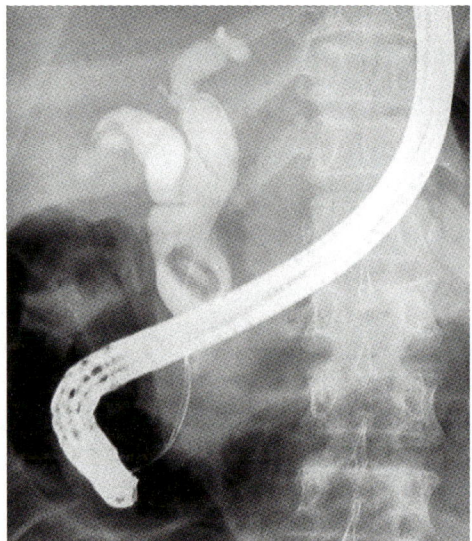
Fig. 21-28 *ERCP* showing stone in common bile duct.

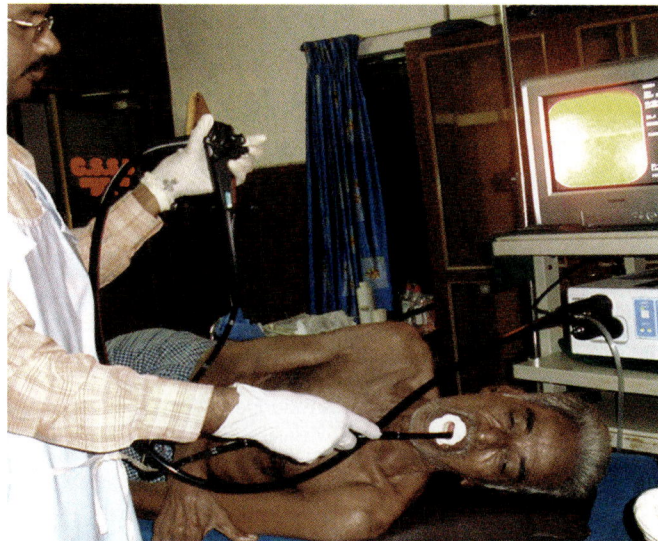
Fig. 21-29 *Gastroscopy* is being done.

Other evaluation methods	Findings and features
Ultrasound abdomen: It is very useful to identify gallstones and liver pathology. But not a good method for assessing pancreas *Endosonography (EUS)* is very useful to detect the lesion, deeper extent, invasion, nodal status; guided aspiration is also can be done	**Radioisotope scanning:** Inorganic iodide is given orally 2 days prior to block the thyroid. I^{131} labeled serum albumin or technetium-99m is administered. 10 minutes later, scanning is done in supine position. It is useful to find out focal and diffuse diseases; abscess like in liver or subphrenic space; inflammatory pathology. ^{75}Selabeled methionine is used to scan pancreatic lesions. It is also useful in GI bleeding. Blood loss is measured with help of RBCs labeled with Cr^{51} which is injected intravenously **Selective angiography** of superior mesenteric artery and inferior mesenteric artery is often helpful in detecting the site of bleed. Once identified, therapeutic embolization can be used to control the bleeding. Bleeding of 0.5 mL/minute can be detected **Diagnostic laparoscopy; and laparoscopic ultrasound** are also useful

DIFFERENT CHRONIC ABDOMINAL CONDITIONS

Conditions	Features
Chronic Benign Gastric Ulcer	
Etiological factors: Atrophic gastritis, smoking, alcohol consumption. Giant gastric ulcer is benign gastric ulcer more than 3 cm in size Lesser curve ulcer is usually benign; greater curve ulcer is commonly malignant **Complications:** Hourglass contracture, teapot deformity, erosion into left gastric/splenic arteries, perforation and malignant transformation. Risk of carcinoma is 6–23% **Barium meal X-ray** shows niche (ulcer crater) and notch on opposite side (due to spasm of circular muscle)	Typical pain is more after taking food and is relieved by inducing vomiting. Vomiting per se as a symptom is seen in 15% cases. Appetite is normal but patient avoids food in order to avoid pain and so loses weight. Deep tenderness in midepigastrium; periodicity, hematemesis/melena (25%) are other features **Daintry Johnson classification:** Type I—near lesser curve in the antrum; Type II—proximal gastric ulcer with duodenal ulcer; Type III—pre-pyloric ulcer; Type IV—proximal gastric ulcer or in cardia
Duodenal Ulcer	
Etiological factors: 'Hurry, worry, curry'—stress, anxiety are the basic etiological factors; common in blood group O positive; *Helicobacter pylori* infection is seen in more than 90% of duodenal ulcers. Other causes—NSAIDs, steroids, alcohol, smoking and hyperparathyroidism. **Complications:** Pyloric stenosis, bleeding, perforation and penetration into pancreas. Chronic duodenal ulcer will never turn into malignancy	Anterior ulcer perforates (2%); posterior ulcer bleeds (5%). Pain is typically in duodenal point. Hematemesis and melena is more common. Patient has more appetite and eats more to relieve pain and so gains weight. Hunger pain, early morning pain, periodicity, water brash, melena are other features **Investigations**: Gastroscopy, biopsy for *Helicobacter pylori* is needed. Barium meal X-ray shows deformed or absent duodenal cap

Contd...

Contd...

Conditions	Features
Gastric Outlet Obstruction **Etiology**: Pyloric stenosis is due to congenital/chronic duodenal ulcer/carcinoma pylorus **Features**: *Hypochloremic, hyponatremic, hypokalemic, hypocalcemic, hypomagnesemic metabolic alkalosis* with *paradoxical aciduria* is typical. Persistent pain, vomiting, decreased appetite and loss of weight, without any periodicity, visible gastric peristalsis, positive succussion splash, positive auscultopercussion test are the special features	**Barium meal X-ray**— shows absent duodenal cap, if it is due to cicatrised chronic duodenal ulcer; greater curvature is below the level of iliac crest; mottled stomach due to retained food particles which gives coated/mosaic appearance; barium will not pass into the duodenum; dilated stomach **Goldstein saline load test**: Half an hour after 750 mL of saline instillation into the stomach, if retained saline/content is more than 250 mL, it suggests gastric outlet obstruction
Carcinoma Stomach It is the *"captain of men of death"* **Etiological factors**: More common in Japan; can be familial (Napoleon family). *H. pylori* is the main causative agent. Diet (smoked fish), gastric polyp, pernicious anemia, gastric remnant, smoking, alcohol, benign gastric ulcer, chronic gastritis—are the other causes **Classifications**: *Lauren's*—intestinal and diffused. *Japanese* (for early gastric cancer—involvement of mucosa or submucosa with or without lymph nodes): protruded, superficial elevated or flat or depressed, excavated. *Borrmann's* (for advanced cancer—involvement muscularis or serosa with or without lymph node spread): polypoid; ulcerated with or without clear margin; diffused; unclassified **Leather bottle stomach** (*Linitis plastica*) is diffuse type of carcinoma of stomach with mother of pearl look with enormous proliferation of fibrous tissue in submucosa	**Clinical features**: Recent onset of loss of appetite and weight; upper abdominal pain; vomiting with features of gastric outlet obstruction, i.e. (VGP, +ve auscultopercussion test, +ve succussion splash) **Mass abdomen**: Mass in pylorus lies above the umbilicus, nodular, hard, with impaired resonance, mobile, moves with respiration, all border well made out; dysphagia when mass is in upper epigastrium; when it arises from the body of stomach, it may present as only mass abdomen. Along with jaundice, liver may be palpable with secondaries which are hard, nodular (50%) with umbilication Ascites; *positive Troisier's sign* (Virchow's node in neck); positive rectovesical secondaries (*Blumer shelf*); migrating thrombophlebitis, (also seen in carcinoma pancreas); anemia, cachexia; hematemesis, malaena; occasionally carcinoma stomach can present as perforation to begin with. Rarely present as secondaries in the liver with silent primary in stomach. Secondaries in umbilicus, as *sister Joseph's nodules*
Gallstones **Types**: (1) Cholesterol stones are 6% common, often solitary. (2) Mixed stones are 90% common. It contains cholesterol, calcium salts of phosphate, carbonate, palmitate, proteins and are multiple, faceted. (3) Pigment stones are small, black or greenish black, multiple, often they can be sludge-like Common in 'fat, fertile, forty, flatulent, female'. Common in Western countries and in North East India **Effects of the gallstones**: (i) *In the gallbladder*—silent asymptomatic stones; acute cholecystitis; chronic cholecystitis; empyema gallbladder; perforation causing biliary peritonitis or pericholecystitic abscess; mucocele of gallbladder; Limey gallbladder; carcinoma gallbladder. (ii) *In the CBD*—secondary CBD stones; cholangitis; pancreatitis; Mirizzi syndrome (compression of CBD by stone from cystic duct or cholecystocholedochal fistula). (iii) *In the intestine*—cholecystoduodenal fistula causing gallstone ileus and so intestinal obstruction	**Chronic cholecystitis**: It is chronically inflamed, thickened gallbladder, which is non-functioning and nondistending **Causes**: Gallstones, cholecystoses, chronic acalculous cholecystitis. **Clinical features**: (1) Pain in right hypochondrium may be colicky, or persistent. (2) Positive Murphy's sign—in sitting position during deep inspiration, patient winces with pain at the summit of the respiration while palpating in right hypochondrium. (3) Flatulent dyspepsia
Trichobezoar (Rapunzel Syndrome) It is hair-ball commonly seen in a stomach of females with psychiatric illness who swallow hair regularly. It forms a ball like mass occupying the full stomach	**Clinical features**: Hematemesis; gastritis; loss of appetite; perforation; occasionally mass in the epigastrium which can be moulded. Barium meal is confirmative
Chronic Pancreatitis It is persistent progressive irreversible damage of the pancreas due to chronic inflammation **Types**: Chronic relapsing pancreatitis or chronic pancreatitis. It can be chronic non-calcifying or calcifying pancreatitis. Stones may be in the duct or in the parenchyma. **Etiology**: Alcohol; stones in biliary tree; malnutrition, diet; hyperparathyroidism; hereditary (familial hereditary pancreatitis); idiopathic; trauma; congenital anomaly, etc. (pancreatic divisum). Chronic pancreatitis is more common in males, common in Kerala, South India (Induced by diet rich in Tapioca) **Pathology**: It shows atrophy of acini, hyperplasia of duct epithelium, interlobular fibrosis, calcifications, ductal dilatation, with strictures in the duct	**Clinical features**: (1) *Pain* in epigastric region, persistent and severe, which radiates to back. This pain is due to irritation of retropancreatic nerves, or due to ductal dilatation and stasis, or due to chronic inflammation itself. (2) *Exocrine dysfunction*: Diarrhea, asthenia, loss of weight and appetite, steatorrhea (signifies severe pancreatic insufficiency), malabsorption, etc. (3) *Endocrine dysfunction*: Diabetes mellitus. (4) *Mild jaundice* is due to narrowing of retropancreatic bile duct and cholangitis. (5) *Mass per abdomen*, just above the umbilicus, tender, nodular, hard, felt on deep palpation, not moving with respiration, nonmobile, resonant on percussion. Chronic pancreatitis can lead to carcinoma pancreas **Complications of chronic pancreatitis**: Pseudocyst of pancreas, pancreatic ascites, CBD stricture, duodenal stenosis, portal or splenic vein thrombosis, peptic ulcer, carcinoma pancreas

Contd...

Contd...

Conditions	Features
Pancreatic Tumors **Classification** (1) **Exocrine tumors**: *Benign*: Benign cystadenoma; is rare. *Malignant*: (i) Adenocarcinoma in ampulla or periampullary region or head of pancreas. *Periampullary carcinoma* may consist any of the components—duodenal mucosa, CBD, pancreatic duct component or all. Occasionally squamous cell carcinoma or combination of adenosquamous can occur. (ii) Cystadenocarcinoma of pancreas occurs commonly in body and tail of the pancreas, which usually attains a large size (5%). (2) **Endocrine tumors**. (3) **Lymphomas** **Exocrine pancreatic tumors**: *Etiology*: Smoking; alcohol; high energy diet rich in fat; chronic pancreatitis; familial pancreatitis. *Sites*: Head and neck region; ampullary and periampullary region; body and tail *Pathology*: (1) 75% are adenocarcinomas, common in elderly people. Arising from primitive cells or acinar cells or duct cells. It is common in head, neck and ampullary region. Most often it begins as carcinoma in situ (2) Cystadenocarcinomas occur 1% of all pancreatic malignancies. They are large cystic tumors, which are slow growing, occurring in the body and tail of the pancreas. They are commonly papillary—cystic tumors. Occasionally mucinous cystic tumors are also seen **Clinical features**: Ampullary tumors mainly present with jaundice and weight loss. Carcinoma head and neck tumors present with weight loss and jaundice. Cystadenocarcinoma of pancreas presents with pain, weight loss and mass *Jaundice* is of obstructive nature which is of short duration, severe, progressive, associated with pruritus (due to deposition of bile salts in the skin which releases histamine) *Painless jaundice* is seen in ampullary malignancies. In periampullary carcinoma, necrosis of tumor occurs sometimes, as a result of which jaundice may reduce temporarily thus becoming *intermittent*	*Pain* presents in the right hypochondriac, epigastric, or left hypochondriac region depending on location of the tumour. *Back pain*, when it is present is due to involvement of retropancreatic nerves, or pancreatic duct. Diarrhea, steatorrhea, *silvery stool* (due to undigested fat mixing with metabolized blood which is derived from the ooze of periampullary growth); loss of appetite and weight; scratch marks on the back. *Migratory superficial thrombophlebitis*: *Trousseau's sign* (10%) is due to release of platelet aggregating factors from the tumor or its necrotic material (Trousseau himself died of carcinoma pancreas who had migrating thrombophlebitis). Ascites; left supraclavicular palpable lymph node; secondaries in rectovesical pouch (Blumer's shelf) *Gallbladder may be palpable* which is nontender, soft, globular, smooth, moving with respiration, mobile horizontally, dull on percussion *Courvoisier law* favors gallbladder enlargement. Liver is enlarged, smooth, firm, nontender due to dilated bile filled biliary radicles—*hydrohepatosis*. Liver can show multiple hard nodules due to secondaries. Cystadenocarcinoma of pancreas can present with mass in epigastric region, which is nonmobile, not moving with respiration, smooth, soft, nontender. Splenic vein thrombosis with splenomegaly (10%) can occur **Pancreatic endocrine tumors**: 1. Insulinoma—Whipple's triad 2. Gastrinoma—peptic ulcer 3. Glucagonoma—diabetes, necrolytic migratory erythema 4. Vipoma (Verner–Morrison syndrome)—watery diarrhea hypokalemia syndrome 5. Somatostatinoma—diabetes, steatorrhea
Hirschsprung's Disease	
It is a congenital, familial condition occurring in newborn due to the absence of ganglion cells—Auerbach and Meissner plexus in anorectum, which may extend proximally either a part or full length of the colon It has got **three zones**: (1) Distal immobile spastic segment, i.e. aganglionic zone; (2) A proximal, middle transitional zone of about 1–5 cm length with less, sparse number of ganglions (cone); (3) A still more proximal, hypertrophied dilated segment is actually the normal ganglionic area **Types**: 1. Ultra-short segment HD—only anal canal and terminal rectum is aganglionic 2. Short-segment HD—anal canal and rectum is completely involved 3. Long-segment HD—anal canal, rectum and part of the colon is involved 4. Total colonic HD—anal canal, rectum and full length of the colon is involved	**Clinical features**: Common in males. In 90% of cases, symptoms appear in early neonatal period, i.e. within three days of birth. Present with complaints of *failure to pass meconium*. After introducing finger into the rectum, child passes *toothpaste like stool*, with evidence of straining. Distension of the abdomen with features of intestinal obstruction is seen. Constipation with history of passing stools once in 3–4 days with straining is seen throughout the childhood and also in adolescent period. Occasionally condition can cause intestinal obstruction **Investigations**: *Plain X-ray* abdomen shows intestinal obstruction. *Biopsy* from all three zones is taken to study the ganglions and hypertrophic nerve terminals in spasmodic segment. *Barium enema* is done to look for the extent of disease and three zones. Foley's catheter should not be used while doing barium enema in case of Hirschsprung's disease. *Anorectal manometry* shows the absence of rectoanal reflex which is diagnostic **Complications**: Colitis, intestinal obstruction; growth retardation, constipation **Differential diagnosis**: Total neuronal dysplasia; acquired megacolon, anorectal malformation
Ulcerative Colitis	
An inflammatory condition of rectum and colon of unknown etiology perhaps related to stress, westernized diet, autoimmune factor, familial tendency, allergic factor Disease commonly starts in the rectum, spreads proximally to the colon and often into the ileum as *backwash ileitis* **Pathology**: Multiple minute ulcers occur initially, with proctitis and colitis → These ulcers extends into the deeper layer → Spasm of the bowel → Stricture of the colon → Permanently contracted colon → In between ulcers, epithelial thickening occurs which appears like polyps → *Pseudopolyposis*	**Two types of presentations**: 1. *Fulminant type*—5% common. It is a severe form, with continuous diarrhea with passage of blood, mucus and pus. Patient is ill and dehydrated; mimics fulminant amoebic colitis, severe typhoid and dysentery. Later abdominal distension occurs. May go for *acute toxic dilatation (1.5%) of transverse colon* wherein the diameter of transverse colon >6 cm. It has high mortality and requires emergency surgery, i.e., either colostomy or resection with ileostomy and later ileoanal anastomosis

Contd...

Contd...

Conditions	Features
Clinical features: More common in females, begins in third decade. Watery diarrhea, mucus or blood-stained discharge per rectum; colicky pain, spasms; decreased appetite and loss of weight; relapses and remissions at regular intervals **Complications**: Pseudopolyposis; turning into malignancy; stricture formation commonly in rectosigmoid and anal canal; toxic megacolon in transverse colon; massive hemorrhage; fistula-in-ano; *Associated with* liver cirrhosis (50%); skin lesions; arthritis; iritis, ankylosing spondylitis; sclerosing cholangitis, carcinoma of gallbladder	2. *Chronic type (95%)—lasts* for months and years with diarrhea, blood loss, anemia, invalidism, abdominal discomfort and pain **Investigations**: (1) Barium enema—shows loss of haustrations, narrow contracted colon (hose pipe colon), mucosal changes, pseudopolyps. It is avoided in fulminant cases. (2) Sigmoidoscopy and biopsy Colonoscopy also is required. Due to very high incidence of malignant transformation—in ulcerative colitis (10–20%), multiple biopsies should be taken from suspected areas of the colon. Risk increases with age of the patient and duration of the disease (20%)
Familial Adenomatous Polyp (FAP)	
It is inherited as an autosomal dominant neoplastic condition (chromosome No. 5). Incidence is equal in both sexes, involving commonly the large intestine but can also occur in stomach, duodenum and small intestine. It is familial with a high potential for malignant transformation. It can be associated with duodenal or ampullary carcinomas, *Gardner's syndrome* [Desmoid tumor in the abdomen, osteomas (75%) and epidermoid cysts] and also *Turcot's syndrome* [FAP + brain tumor (medulloblastoma or gliomas)]	It presents in younger age group—15–20 years; usually multiple (over 100); presents with lower abdominal pain, loose stools with blood and mucus, weight loss. If there is no adenoma at the age of 30 years, it is not FAP of colon
Carcinoma Colon	
It is commonly adenocarcinoma; very rarely adenosquamous, squamous carcinoma can occur. *Adenocarcinoma*: Sigmoid colon (21%) is the commonest site of malignancy after rectum (38%). In cecum it is 12% common **Etiology**: *Diet*: Red meat and saturated fat increase the incidence of colonic cancer. Cholesterol increases the bile acid concentration in the intestinal lumen which acts as cocarcinogen. High fiber diet protects the colon against cancer *Genetic*: Carcinoma colon is more common in individuals with *adenoma colon* or with *familial adenomatous polyposis—FAP* or with long standing ulcerative colitis. Alcohol and cigarette smoking increase the risk. Aspirin and other NSAIDs protect against colonic cancer **Types**: Patient can have de novo multiple primary carcinomas in different parts of the colon at same time, i.e. *synchronous* (5%), or can present with growth in different parts of the colon in different periods, i.e. *metachronous* (2–5%) *Gross types*: *Annular* (stenosing)—it is more common on left side. *Tubular*; *ulcerative* (common on right side); *cauliflower-like*. Here the growth spreads round the internal wall and so it often presents with intestinal obstruction **Spread**: Locally to the bladder, obstruct ureter and so cause hydronephrosis. It can perforate and cause peritonitis/pericolic abscess/fecal fistula. Growth may get adherent to psoas muscle posteriorly. Growth through lymphatics spreads to pericolic, epicolic, intermediate and principal group of lymph nodes	40% of carcinoma colon spread to liver via portal veins—secondaries may be either solitary or multiple, present as enlarged liver with hard, umbilicated nodules. Rarely it spreads to bone, lung, skin **Features**: It occurs usually after 50 years of age. Familial type can present in younger age group. Commonly presents with loss of appetite and weight, anemia, abdominal discomfort and mass per abdomen. 20% of cases are present as acute intestinal obstruction. Right sided growth commonly presents with anemia, palpable mass in the right iliac fossa, which is not moving with respiration, mobile, nontender, hard, well-localized with impaired resonant note. Carcinoma cecum occasionally can present like acute appendicitis or intussusception with intestinal obstruction. Left-sided growth presents with colicky pain, altered bowel habits (alternating constipation and diarrhea), palpable lump, and distension of abdomen due to subacute/chronic obstruction. Later may present like complete colonic obstruction. Tenesmus, with passage of blood and mucus, with alternate constipation and diarrhea, is common. Bladder symptoms may warn colo-vesical fistula. Enlarged liver with multiple umbilicated hard secondaries, ascites, rectovesical secondaries, palpable left supraclavicular lymph nodes are other presentations. *Fecal strength of Streptococcus bovis bacteria increases many folds in colonic cancer patients compared to individuals without colonic cancer*

Approaches and Examination of Acute Abdomen

CHAPTER 22

Competency: SU24.1; SU24.3; SU28.9; SU28.10; SU28.15; SU28.18; AN47.3; AN47.4; IM5.8; IM15.5.

It is sudden severe attack of abdominal pain to such an extent that patient is in severe agony and often in shock. Many of the conditions causing acute abdomen may be life threatening like perforation of intestine. Proper clinical examination is the essential step in these patients to conclude the diagnosis and to plan the therapy.

Note: Acute abdomen may not be a *cute abdomen* to surgeons.

CAUSES OF ACUTE ABDOMEN

Intra-abdominal causes:
Inflammation: Acute appendicitis, acute cholecystitis, acute salpingitis, acute diverticulitis, acute Crohn's, acute mesenteric adenitis, primary acute peritonitis
Perforation of bowel
Acute intestinal obstruction: In the lumen (roundworm, gallstones), in the wall (stricture, intussusception, tumor), outside wall (hernia, bands, adhesions, volvulus)
Mesenteric vessel occlusion by thrombosis or embolism
Hemorrhage: Ruptured ectopic gestation, ruptured tropical spleen like malarial, ruptured aortic aneurysm
Torsions: Twisted ovarian cyst, twisted splenic pedicle
Colicky causes: Ureteric, biliary, intestinal, appendicular

Extra-abdominal causes:
In the abdominal wall: Abdominal wall abscess, Meleney's spreading gangrene, rupture of abdominal wall muscles, inferior epigastric artery tear and hematoma formation. **In thorax:** Lobar pneumonia, diaphragmatic pleurisy, pericarditis, angina pectoris, coronary disease.
Retroperitoneal causes: Acute pyelonephritis, retroperitoneal lymphadenitis and lymphangitis, ruptured aortic aneurysm
Diseases of spine, spinal cord and intercostal nerves: Pott's tuberculous spine, gastric crisis of Tabes dorsalis, herpes zoster of intercostal nerves with neuralgia.
Other causes: Malaria, typhoid, porphyria, diabetic crisis, sickle cell disease, purpura, hemophilia, etc.

Common causes of acute abdomen in children:
- Acute appendicitis
- Intussusception
- Intestinal obstruction due to roundworms, bands and adhesions
- Acute nonspecific mesenteric lymphadenitis—below 6 years
- Meckel's diverticulitis
- Primary acute peritonitis

Causes in females other than causes which are seen in both sexes:
- Ruptured ectopic gestation
- Ruptured ovarian cyst
- Torsion of ovarian cyst
- Acute salpingitis
- Tubo-ovarian abscess
- Torsion or degeneration of uterine fibroid

■ HISTORY

Age: Sigmoid volvulus, carcinoma colon causing obstruction, diverticulitis are common in old people. Acute pancreatitis, acute cholecystitis, perforation are common in adults. Appendicitis is common in young adults. Roundworm obstruction is common in children. Midgut volvulus, intussusception, congenital hypertrophic pyloric stenosis are common in infants. Intestinal atresia, meconium ileus, anorectal malformation are common in newborn.

Sex: Ruptured ectopic gestation, twisted ovarian cyst are seen in females. Acute cholecystitis, primary peritonitis are common in females. Volvulus, intussusception, perforated peptic ulcer are common in males.

Residence: Perforation is more common in India where diet is rich with spicy foods. Acute cholecystitis is common in Bihar and north east India. Pancreatitis is common in Kerala and in Western countries.

Socioeconomic group: Perforation, roundworm obstruction is more common in lower socioeconomic group; appendicitis is more common in higher socioeconomic group due to high protein low fiber diet intake.

History of Present Illness

Pain

Pain is the most common presentation of acute abdomen.

Site of pain should be confirmed by asking the patient to point at one place using his finger—***pointing test*** (Fig. 22-1). Pain is in right hypochondrium in acute cholecystitis; in right iliac fossa at McBurney's point in acute appendicitis; in the loin in urinary stone; in epigastrium in acute pancreatitis. In case of diffuse pain or deep seated pain, patient use his whole hand instead of finger to show the area of pain.

Mode of onset of pain: It may be sudden or insidious in onset. It is sudden, dramatic in onset in perforation, stones, torsion whereas in acute intestinal obstruction, it is initially less severe gradually progresses and becomes more. Pain in acute appendicitis starts in early morning, initially boring and vague but later becomes severe and localized. Pain in duodenal ulcer perforation follows the afternoon food and becomes severe stabbing in nature in the evening or night. History of straining is present preceding the pain in perforation and torsion; movements or jolting precipitates the colicky pain of ureteric stone. Sudden severe pain with pallor and features of shock in a female, one should suspect ruptured ectopic pregnancy; here menstrual history and last menstrual period should be asked; ultrasound, urine pregnancy test, raised serum βHCG confirms the diagnosis; patient needs emergency surgery (open or laparoscopic).

Type of pain: It may be ***continuous*** type (as in perforation, torsion, hemorrhage, inflammation) or ***intermittent***, colicky type. ***Colicky pain*** is gripping in nature which appears suddenly and disappears suddenly due to spasm of hollow viscus like intestine (intestinal colic), ureter (ureteric colic), and common bile duct (biliary colic). Throbbing pain of cholecystitis, severe agonizing pain of acute pancreatitis, twisting pain of torsion, continuous burning pain of peritonitis and duodenal ulcer perforation are other types of pain. Pain is severe at the onset, in perforation of viscus, torsion, acute pancreatitis, mesenteric/splenic artery embolism.

> **Colicky pain:**
> It is gripping pain for certain period, subsides for some time and suddenly reappears again in similar fashion. Associated with nausea, vomiting, belching, retching, tachycardia, but abdomen is soft, guarding and tenderness is less compared to severity of pain.
> **It can be:**
> - *Ureteric colic* due to ureter stone.
> - *Biliary colic* (gallbladder colic due to spasm of gallbladder to force the stone).
> - *Intestinal colic* due to toxic enteritis, infection, lead colic in painters.
> - *Appendicular colic* in obstructive appendicitis.

Change in character of pain: Pain may be initially colicky type in intestinal obstruction but later becomes severe and continuous when peritonitis sets in; whereas the initial appendicular colic becomes persistent pain of obstructive appendicitis which diminishes suddenly when perforation occurs. In 2nd stage of peptic ulcer perforation, the initial severe pain diminishes for some time due to dilution of gastric contents by the peritoneal fluid. This situation of feeling better after the initial phase of severe pain is termed as *'fool's paradise'* which is not a good sign.

Change in position of pain or spread of pain: In acute appendicitis, pain initially begins at umbilicus but later shifts to right iliac fossa. Initial visceral pain occurs in and around umbilicus due to same segmental nerve supply (T_{10}), later pain in right iliac fossa is due to parietal peritonitis.

Migration of pain: In duodenal ulcer perforation pain initially begins in epigastrium but with spread of peritonitis so also the pain migrates down when once gastric contents spills over into the right paracolic gutter.

Radiation of pain: In acute pancreatitis, pain begins in epigastrium and radiates to back. In posterior penetration of duodenal ulcer pain is felt at epigastrium as well as at the back.

Referred pain: Pain is said to be referred if it occurs at the same segmental cutaneous distribution of the nerve. Visceral part is sympathetic supply of the segment whereas the cutaneous part is somatic. Examples are—diaphragmatic irritation due to subphrenic abscess, inflammation, clot causes pain over the skin over shoulder through C3, C4 of phrenic nerve and supraclavicular nerve. Head down position will aggravate the pain. Gastroduodenal and jejunal diseases have referred pain to epigastrium (T_{5-8}); ileum and appendix to umbilical region (T_9, T_{10}); colon to hypogastrium ($T_{11,12}$, $L_{1,2}$); ureteric colic pain is referred from loin to groin to scrotum and inner part of upper thigh through genitofemoral nerve ($L_{1,2}$). Gallstone colic refers from right hypochondrium to inferior angle of scapula (T_{7-9}). Pleuritis, hemothorax, pneumothorax causes referred pain to the abdominal wall mimicking acute abdomen.

Aggravating and relieving factors: Colicky pain is *relieved by* local pressure; inflammatory pain gets *aggravated by* pressure.

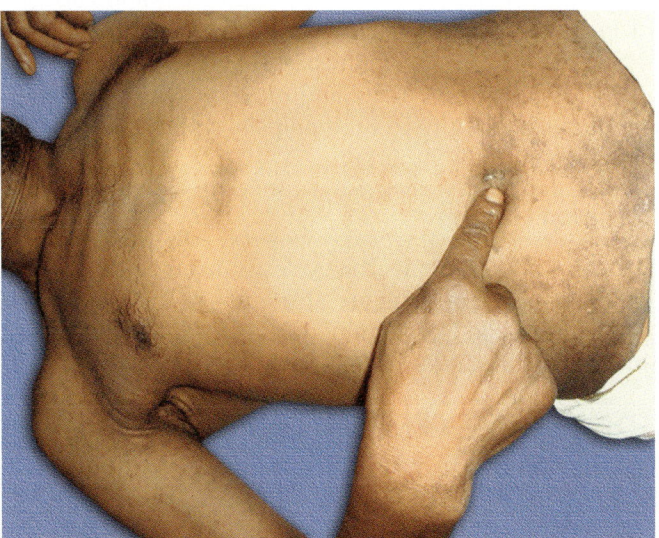

Fig. 22-1 Patient is asked to point out the site of pain at one point—*pointing test*.

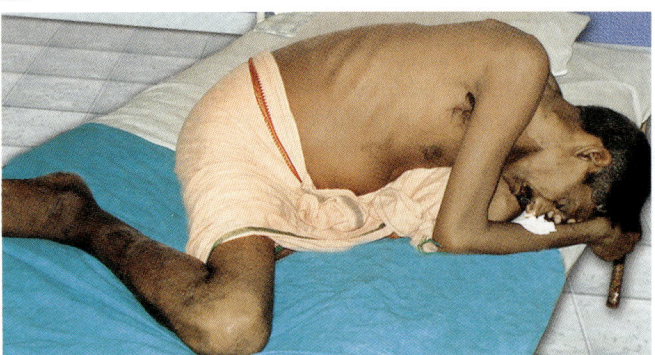

Fig. 22-2 Patient leans forward in acute pancreatitis to relieve pain.

In cholecystitis, appendicitis, ureteric stone, pain aggravates by movements and jolting. Pain of diaphragmatic irritation aggravates on coughing, and deep breathing. Pain in acute peritonitis is relieved if patient avoids any movements and stay still and aggravates on movement. Pain is aggravated by spicy food in gastric ulcer; fatty meal aggravates the pain of cholecystitis; vomiting relieves the pain of gastric ulcer and colicky pain of ureteric stone. Pain of acute pancreatitis is relieved by sitting and leaning forward (**Fig. 22-2**).

Vomiting

Character of vomiting whether projectile (as in high intestinal obstruction or pyloric stenosis) or effortless, regurgitation (paralytic ileus, peritonitis).

Frequency of vomiting—repetitive and profuse in acute pancreatitis and acute intestinal obstruction; periodical and infrequent in duodenal ulcer perforation and acute appendicitis.

Quantity of vomitus and nature of the vomitus should be asked—***vomitus*** may be gastric, bilious, intestinal, feculent (very rare unless there is gastrocolic fistula) or blood stained. In intestinal obstruction, initially the gastric contents and bile come out, later the foul smelling form lower intestinal contents come out. Bilious vomiting occurs in colic. Bile may be absent when there is CBD obstruction or in congenital hypertrophic pyloric stenosis.

Relation of vomiting with pain: Vomiting develops ***after*** feeling of pain in acute appendicitis, pancreatitis, colic (biliary, renal). Pain and vomiting appears simultaneously in high intestinal obstruction. *Pain first; nausea and vomiting next; with fever (last)—Murphy's triad*. There will be *increased abdominal sensitiveness (hyperaesthesia) on right side* with tenderness.

Duration of onset: Vomiting is the ***early*** feature in proximal intestinal obstruction (jejunal); it is ***late*** feature in distal obstruction (terminal ileum); ***absent*** in large bowel obstruction.

History of ***hematemesis*** is seen in erosive gastritis, esophageal varices, bleeding peptic ulcer—fresh blood/coffee brown colored due to mixing of blood with acid of stomach.

Bowel Habits

Quantity, nature, frequency, odor, color, blood staining, passing mucus is enquired. Appendicitis can cause diarrhea if pelvic appendix irritates the rectum. Appendicitis also may cause colonic spasm leading into constipation. Absolute constipation occurs in acute intestinal obstruction and generalized peritonitis which means neither feces nor flatus is passed. Bloody putrid stool is seen in mesenteric ischemia. Diarrhea may be a feature of acute ulcerative colitis, enteritis, regional ileitis. Frequent passing blood and mucus with distension is a feature of acute intussusception. ***Tenesmus*** (painful, futile straining on stool with passage of mucus and blood in stool) is seen in pelvic appendicitis, pelvic abscess.

Abdominal Distension

Patient often presents with fullness of abdomen which is gradually progressive and is associated with constipation and vomiting.

Urinary Symptoms

Burning urine, frequency, strangury (passage of few blood stained urine after frequent painful attempts of micturition) can occur in retrocecal/pelvic appendicitis, pelvic peritonitis due to irritation of lower end of ureter or bladder.

Other History

History of ***fever, chills and rigors*** are important in acute abdomen. High temperature is seen in inflammatory condition (appendicular abscess, subphrenic abscess) and peritonitis. Fever with rigors is seen in portal pyemia, septicemia and cholangitis. ***History of jaundice*** may be significant in acute cholecystitis, pancreatitis. ***History of melena*** is important in bleeding peptic ulcer. ***History of fainting attacks*** is important in ectopic pregnancy in females; rupture spleen, torsion, hemorrhage.

Past History

Past history of laparotomy is important in intestinal obstruction. Earlier history of renal stone disease, appendicitis treated with drugs, biliary colic, jaundice, pancreatitis is asked. History of periodicity of pain in duodenal/gastric ulcer, hematemesis or melena in the past should be asked for. Past history suggestive of acute abdomen and hospitalization is important. History of tuberculosis, typhoid, dysentery, diabetes mellitus is important.

Personal History

History of missed menstrual cycles is taken which suggest ectopic pregnancy in acute abdomen in females. Urine pregnancy test and US abdomen may confirm the diagnosis. Smoking, alcohol intake, diet history are important.

■ GENERAL EXAMINATION

General look
Facies: Typical ***facies hippocratica*** of terminal stage of peritonitis is described as anxious look, sunken bright eyes, pinched face, and cold sweat. In severe ***dehydration*** signs like sunken eyes, dry tongue, and drawn cheeks are noted.

Anxious look of face is seen in perforation, intra-abdominal hemorrhage, torsion, acute intestinal obstruction.

Pallor: Severe sudden pallor with shock in a female may be due to ruptured ectopic gestation. Other causes of extreme pallor are intra-abdominal hemorrhages like rupture spleen should be suspected where there is history of trauma. There is a typical cyanotic hue with prostration in face of patients with hemorrhagic pancreatitis.

Attitude: Patient stays in the bed in supine position *still* without moving in case of acute peritonitis as movements will increase the pain. Whereas in late stages of peritonitis when patient develops septic shock he becomes restless, irritable, grumbling. Patient rolls/tosses in the bed with agony in colicky pain. Patient with acute pancreatitis is found sitting and leaning forwards as this position gives comfort (**Fig. 22-2**).

Pulse: Pulse rate is of prognostic importance not diagnostic. In initial period of acute peritonitis, acute appendicitis, and acute pancreatitis pulse remains normal but once sepsis develops and disease progresses tachycardia develops gradually. In ruptured ectopic there is only tachycardia to begin with. In acute intestinal obstruction, pulse is initially normal but soon becomes rapid due to dehydration. Tachycardia with extreme pallor signifies internal hemorrhage.

Blood pressure: It remains normal initially in many acute conditions other than in internal hemorrhage and hemorrhagic pancreatitis. Hypotension develops in late stage of peritonitis and septicemia.

Respiration: In acute abdomen initially **respiration** is normal but later tachypnea may develop. That is due to septic shock, peritonitis or pleural effusion (in acute pancreatitis).

Temperature: *Fever* is a common feature of acute appendicitis or acute cholecystitis. Fever may not be present in many acute abdominal conditions. In some conditions like acute appendicitis fever suggests the severity of the disease. Once patient develops septicemia (***cold shock***) fever may not be present.

Tongue—may be moist, dry (dehydration) or coated (toxemia). Brown coated tongue suggests toxemia. *Cyanosis* may be evident. Pallor and ***jaundice*** may be evident.

Eyes: Sunken in severe dehydration due to vomiting and diarrhea.

Skin—appears dry wrinkled in severe dehydration.

Urine output—is important indicator in acute abdomen. 50 mL/hour urine is the required output. Hourly estimation is needed.

LOCAL EXAMINATION OF ABDOMEN

Inspection

Expose the abdomen from nipples to middle of the thighs for proper inspection.

Contour of the Abdomen

Distension of the abdomen is gradually progressive in acute intestinal obstruction. It is minimal or absent in proximal

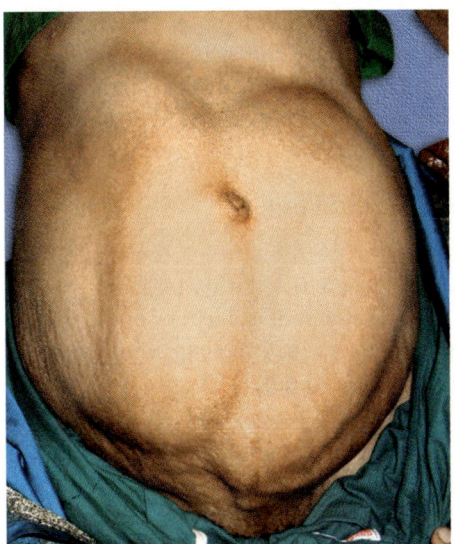

Fig. 22-3 *Distension of abdomen due to dilated colon—could be due to sigmoid volvulus.*

small bowel obstruction; it is central in distal small bowel obstruction in umbilical region; it is peripheral in large bowel obstruction; asymmetrical, more to the left in sigmoid volvulus. It is not obvious in acute appendicitis, acute cholecystitis. Distension is gradually progressive in acute peritonitis. It is not observed and abdomen remains scaphoid in biliary or ureteric colic. Generalized distension occurs in intestinal obstruction, internal hemorrhages, late stage of peritonitis, paralytic ileus. Abdominal girth should be measured in acute abdomen cases (at the level of umbilicus) and should be repeated at regular intervals (2nd hourly) to check the progression. Flank fullness should be observed (**Fig. 22-3**).

Umbilicus

Normal umbilicus is situated midway between xiphisternum and symphysis pubis. The position may be displaced due to any distension or intra-abdominal mass. Normally it is inverted. Umbilicus may be everted or transversely stretched due to in abdominal distension following excessive fluid accumulation in peritonitis, or hemorrhage. Bluish discoloration and edema around umbilicus (***Cullen's sign***) may be a feature of acute hemorrhagic pancreatitis, or ruptured ectopic pregnancy.

Movements with Respiration

It should be observed by sitting by the side of the patient with eyes at the level of the abdomen. Restricted movement of the abdomen with respiration is seen in peritonitis where all quadrants show restrictions. Localized limitation of the movement with respiration is seen in localized diseases like appendicitis or cholecystitis.

Visible Peristalsis and Pulsation

Patient is asked to take deep breath and hold it at the end of expiration as long as he can. Now the abdomen is observed for peristaltic movements. ***Step ladder*** peristalsis is typical of small bowel obstruction seen around umbilicus in central abdomen. In large bowel obstruction, waves are seen along the line of colon from right to left in right hypochondrium, umbilical, and left hypochondrium. Visible pulsations are seen in aortic aneurysm.

Skin over the Abdomen

Discoloration or patches of ecchymosis of flank (***Grey Turner's sign***) is seen in acute hemorrhagic pancreatitis. Skin stretch marks, scratch marks, blisters, edema of skin are other features to be observed. Old scar of laparotomy if present should be inspected in detail.

Hernial Orifices

Hernial orifices should be inspected for impulse on coughing. One of the common causes of intestinal obstruction is obstructed inguinal hernia. Impulse on coughing may be absent in obstructed hernia but swelling will be obvious. Even femoral, umbilical or incisional hernia can cause intestinal obstruction **(Fig. 22-4)**.

External Genitalia

Examination is done to look for pin-hole meatus/phimosis that may lead to urinary retention with bladder distension. In torsion testis there may be pain in iliac fossa mimicking appendicitis or diverticulitis.

Palpation

Patient is made to relax by making him lie comfortably over a couch with a pillow under the head and hand by the side of the body and legs flexed 45° at hip and knee at 90°. He is asked to take slow deep breathe along with conversation so as to relax him. Examiner should keep his **hands warm**. *Fingers should be kept flat over the abdomen to palpate from ventral surface of the fingers not from the tip of fingers.*

Hyperesthesia

Inflamed abdominal organ causes cutaneous hyperesthesia, which can be confirmed by scratching the skin or gently holding the fold of skin. **Sherren's triangle (Fig. 22-5)** is formed by lines joining umbilicus, anterior superior iliac spine and pubic symphysis, which show hyperesthesia in acute gangrenous appendicitis. Once this appendix bursts hyperesthesia disappears. In acute cholecystitis an area of hyperesthesia is often evident between 9th to 11th ribs behind on right side—**Boas's sign.** Irritation in the under surface of diaphragm by internal hemorrhage causes hyperesthesia over the shoulder region.

Muscle Guarding and Rigidity

Muscle guarding signifies the inflammation of visceral peritoneum whereas rigidity signifies the inflammation of even parietal peritoneum. Respiratory movements are absent in the area where there is rigidity. It is ***very important sign*** of parietal peritonitis. It is involuntary abdominal wall muscle contraction as a protective phenomenon which is present both during inspiration and expiration. Voluntary guarding brought by the patient due to fear/apprehension for examination or shyness for exposure will disappear during expiration. Patient is asked to do deep slow breathing through his mouth. With fingers kept flat over the abdomen rigidity is checked in both phases of respiration. Guarding is checked all over the abdomen. It is also checked using both hands kept one over the other **(Fig. 22-6)**. Deeper hand passively feels the rigidity; outer hand presses the abdomen through deeper hand. Localized rigidity is observed often in right upper abdomen in case of perforated duodenal ulcer in initial period; in right iliac fossa in acute appendicitis; in the loin, in retrocecal appendicitis. Rigidity is absent in pelvic appendicitis, ureteric/biliary colic, in early acute intestinal obstruction without bowel gangrene.

Tenderness

It is elicited by touch or pressure over the inflamed organ **(Fig. 22-7)**. Diffuse tenderness is seen in generalized peritonitis.

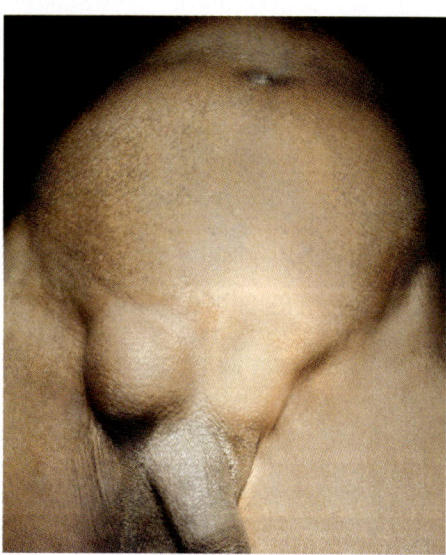

Fig. 22-4 *Right side obstructed inguinal hernia* with distension of the abdomen. Left side hernia is also present but is not causing obstruction in this patient.

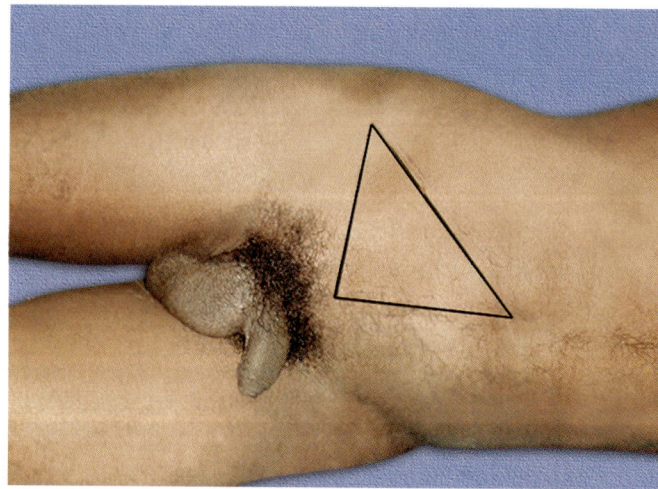

Fig. 22-5 *Sherren's triangle*—hyperesthesia zone. Also note the McBurney's point.

Chapter 22: Approaches and Examination of Acute Abdomen

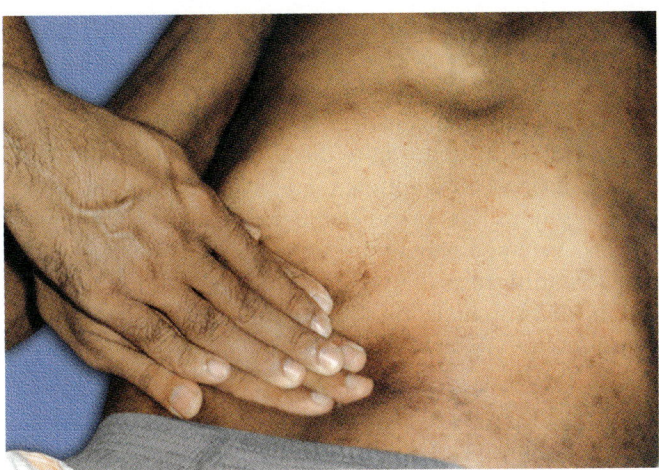

Fig. 22-6 *Both hands are used* to palpate to overcome the rigidity.

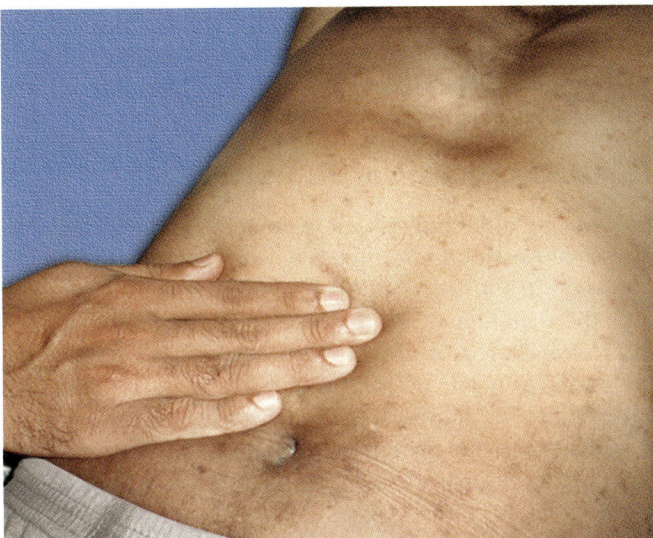

Fig. 22-7 Palpation of abdomen using *flat of the fingers gently*. First tenderness is elicited.

Point tenderness is elicited using one finger while palpating directly over the site of the organ. ***McBurney's tenderness*** is typical of acute appendicitis which is in right spinoumbilical line at junction of medial 2/3rd and lateral 1/3rd. Tenderness in acute cholecystitis is located at the tip of 9th costal cartilage near the lateral margin of the right rectus muscle (***Murphy's point***). Tenderness is present in loin in acute pyelitis. Tender area wil l be more clear if patient coughs. Extent and severity of tenderness should be elicited. Tenderness can also be elicited by percussion over the location. Appendicular tenderness will be better elicited in lateral position as intestines will be shifted towards left side and abdomen will be relaxed.

Rebound Tenderness/Release Sign/Blumberg's Sign

Abdomen is gently palpated and pressed down deeply with each expiration. When the hand is abruptly released to spring back the abdominal muscles to its original position, patient winces with pain. It is due to inflammation of parietal peritoneum over the inflamed organ which also springs back along with the muscles. ***Springing back of the peritoneum is very painful***. It is useful in acute appendicitis (denotes gangrenous or perforation), acute peritonitis, and intestinal obstruction (denotes bowel becoming gangrenous) (Fig. 22-8).

Special Tests to Elicit Tenderness in Acute Appendicitis

- **Rovsing's sign:** When pressed in the left iliac fossa intestine gets pushed towards right iliac fossa pressing the inflamed appendix causing tenderness in right iliac fossa which is a definitive feature of acute appendicitis (Fig. 22-9).
- **Cope's psoas test:** Retrocecal appendicitis irritates psoas major muscle causing flexion of right hip joint. Patient develops pain when this muscle is stretched by hyperextending the hip joint with patient turning towards his left side (Fig. 22-10).
- **Cope's obturator test:** Stretching of the obturator internus muscle by flexing and internally rotating the hip joint will cause pain if inflamed appendix is in pelvic position and gets irritated by the obturator internus muscle (Fig. 22-11).

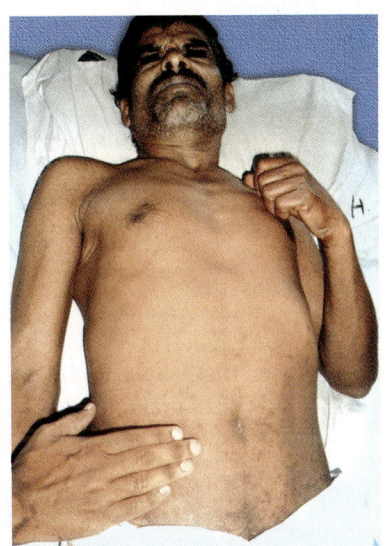

Fig. 22-8 Rebound tenderness.

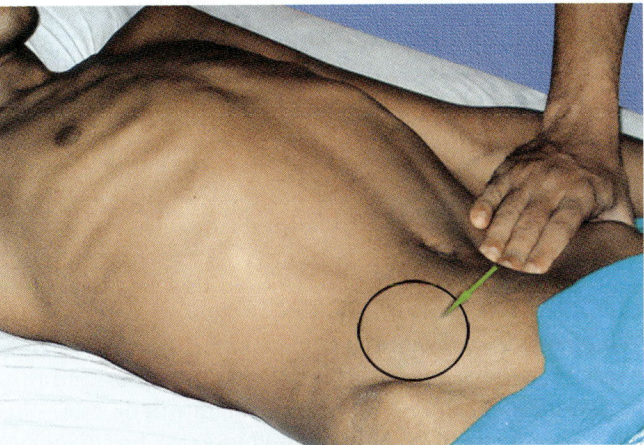

Fig. 22-9 Rovsing's sign.

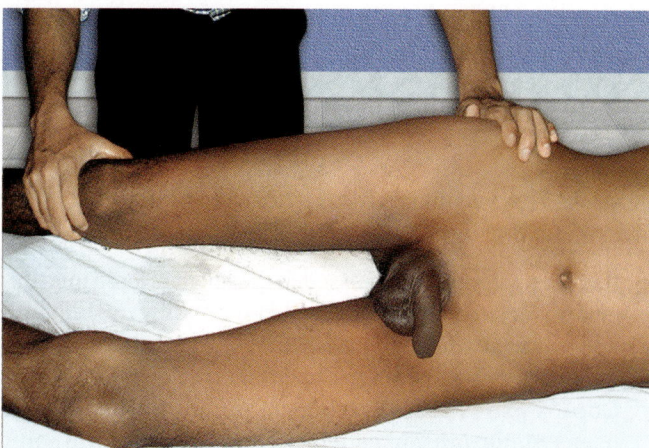

Fig. 22-10 *Cope's psoas test.*

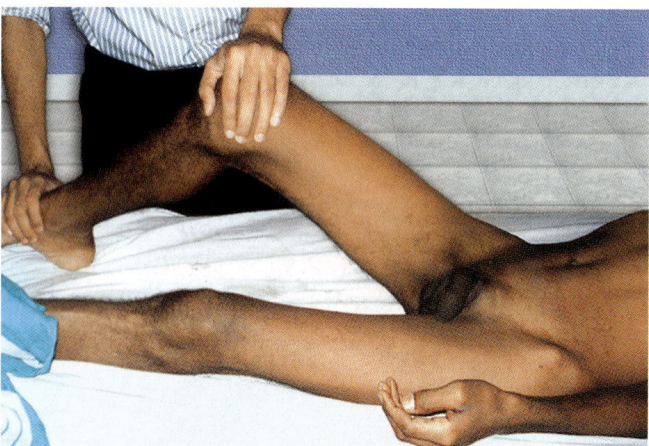

Fig. 22-11 *Cope's obturator test.*

- **Baldwing's test/sign:** Flank is pressed with hand and with knee extended patient raises his right hip from the bed to cause contraction of psoas major muscle which irritates inflamed retrocecal appendix to develop pain.

Mass Abdomen

Detailed features of the mass should be assessed – examples like appendicular mass, colonic mass.
All viscera including liver, spleen, kidney are palpated. In case of intestinal obstruction, dilated loops of intestines can be palpated with the flat of the hand which softens and hardens intermittently. Sausage shaped mass around umbilicus may be felt in intussusception.

Other Palpation

Palpation for distension of abdomen, hernial sites are important.

Percussion

Tenderness may be elicited by percussion. Free fluid can be checked by same methods like shifting dullness, fluid thrill in peritonitis. It should be gentle as pain will be more. Just percussion in the flanks to elicit dullness may be sufficient if patient is in agony.

Obliteration of liver dullness should be specifically checked in acute abdomen. It is the definitive sign of bowel perforation. Upper border of liver is checked by percussing in right midaxillary line from above downwards. Obliteration of liver dullness with resonant note throughout is due to presence of gas/air between diaphragm and liver. It is present in 70% of perforations. Gas under diaphragm may not be evident if gas leak is less; if patient has undergone laparotomy earlier causing adhesions above liver, if perforation is in ileum. Interposition of colon/intestines between liver and diaphragm causes obliteration of liver dullness.

Auscultation

Absence of bowel sounds causing **silent abdomen** is typical pathognomonic sign of diffuse peritonitis, paralytic ileus. Bowel sounds are increased in early phase of intestinal obstruction with metallic tinkles or borborygmi; diminished bowel sounds is seen in internal hemorrhage. Bowel sounds are normal in biliary/ureteric colics. Normal bowel sounds are called as **'clicks or gurgles'** (Fig. 22-12).

Digital Examination of the Rectum

Ballooning of rectum which is empty is a feature of acute intestinal obstruction or acute peritonitis. It is probably of neuronal origin but exact cause is not clear. Tenderness over the right side is felt in acute appendicitis. Tenderness in retrovesical/retrouterine pouch is a feature of diffuse peritonitis or pelvic peritonitis. Pelvic abscess often may be felt in front as a boggy swelling which is soft, and tender. Rectal examination is done in left lateral position usually but dorsal position may be used if patient is severely ill. Red currant jelly in the stool may be seen in intussusception. Annular growth in rectum may be palpable.

Pervaginal Examination

It is important in acute salpingitis, ruptured ectopic gestation, twisted ovarian cyst, etc.

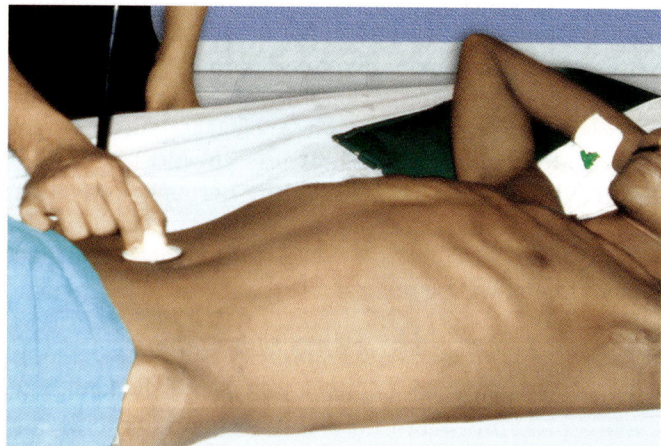

Fig. 22-12 Auscultation of the abdomen for bowel sounds is important. *Silent abdomen is a feature of acute peritonitis.* In early intestinal obstruction bowel sounds are increased.

Examination of External Genitalia

Scrotum, testes, cord and vas deferens should be examined as inflammation in these organs mimics acute abdominal condition especially acute appendicitis and ureteric colic.

SYSTEMIC EXAMINATION

Examination of respiratory and cardiac system is done to look for pneumonia, pleurisy, basal pneumonia, myocardial infarction or angina pectoris. Pain from lesion of lower and middle lobe of lung on right side is referred to right hypochondrium mimicking cholecystitis. All these conditions are known to present as pain abdomen but abdomen will be soft without distension and other features of specific diseases are evident.

Herpes zoster infection may present like acute abdomen pain (acute cholecystitis) due to hyperesthesia.

Tuberculosis of spine (Pott's) may present like acute abdomen in children and so spine should be examined **(Fig. 22-13)**.

Neurological examination (Central and peripheral nervous system). Many neurological conditions mimic acute abdomen. Tabes dorsalis with gastric crisis is a known entity presenting as acute pain in the abdomen and vomiting. Lightning pain in legs, papillary changes (Argyll Robertson), absence of knee and ankle jerks are obvious in tabes dorsalis.

INVESTIGATIONS

1. **Blood: Leukocytosis is common in peritonitis. In septicemia count may be decreasing so serial estimation is needed.**
   Blood urea, serum creatinine and electrolytes are estimated to confirm uremia and electrolyte imbalance due to dehydration or sepsis.
   Liver function tests, platelet count, prothrombin time estimation, serum calcium, amylase, lipase are done in acute pancreatitis.
   Plasma fibrinogen, C reactive protein (normal is 6 mg/L), serum methemoglobin are often specific in inflammatory conditions.
   Urinary lipase, diastase (normal is 10–30 units) are relevant in acute pancreatitis. Urine analysis is a must for pus cells and red cells.
2. **Plain X-ray abdomen is simple and very relevant investigation.**
   It is taken in erect posture or lateral decubitus position in severely ill patients. Gas under diaphragm (perforation), multiple air fluid levels of intestinal obstruction, calcified areas in the pancreatitis (stones) are looked for. Jejunum shows volvulae conniventis; ileum is characterless; colon shows haustrations. More the number of air fluid levels, distal is the obstruction. Normal X-ray shows 2 or 3 air fluid levels—fundus, duodenum, occasionally cecum. Ground glass appearance is a feature of acute peritonitis (Figs. 22-14 to 22-16).

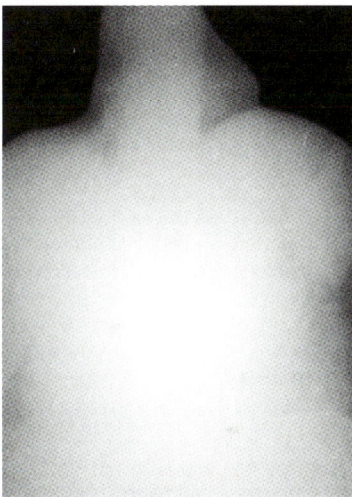

Fig. 22-14 Plain X-ray abdomen showing *ground glass appearance*—a feature of acute peritonitis.

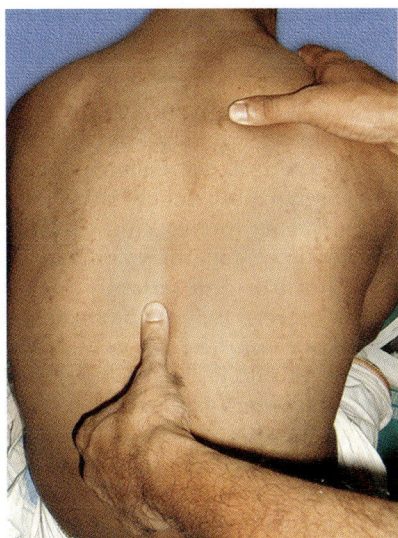

Fig. 22-13 *Spine should be examined* in acute abdomen cases.

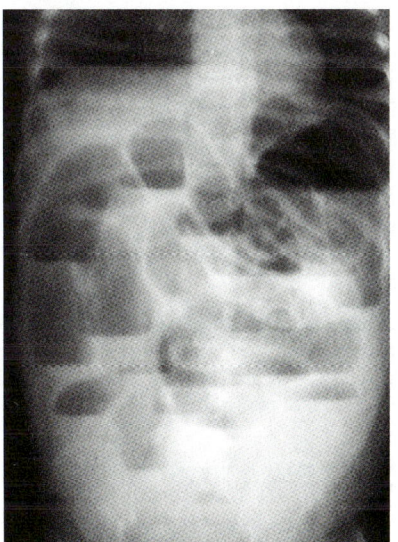

Fig. 22-15 Plain X-ray abdomen showing *multiple air fluid levels*—a feature of intestinal obstruction.

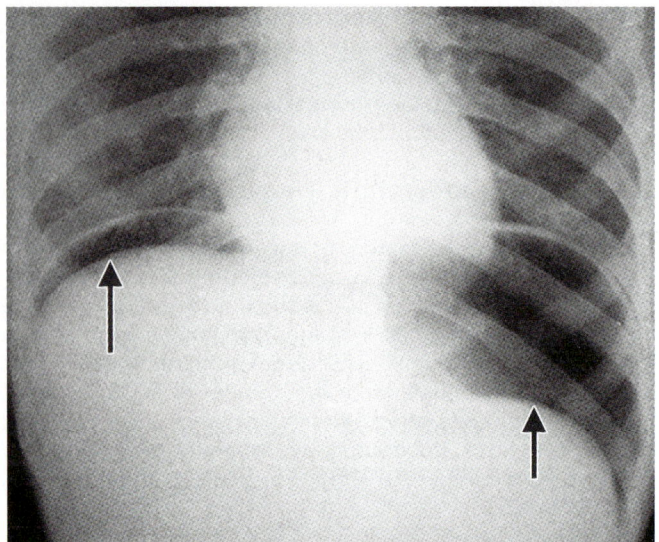

Fig. 22-16 X-ray abdomen in erect posture showing *gas under diaphragm*. In severely ill patient, X-ray *left lateral decubitus is taken*.

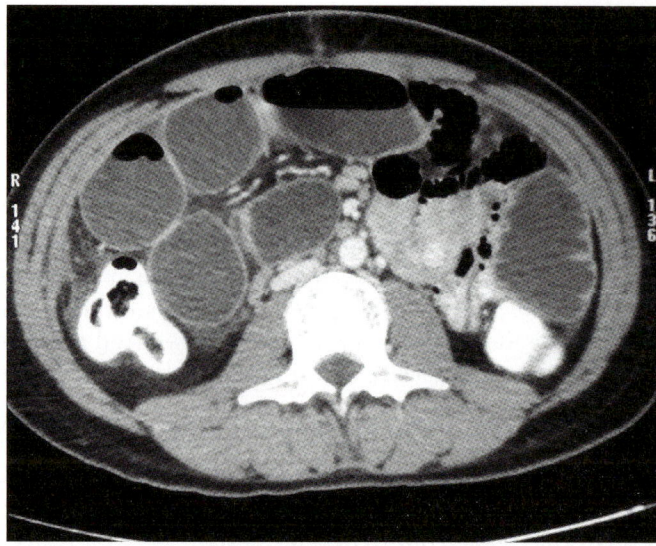

Fig. 22-17 CT scan showing intestinal obstruction. *CT is the ideal investigation for intestinal obstruction.*

Different signs in X-ray in perforation:	Conditions which mimic pneumoperitoneum (pseudopneumoperitoneum):
• *Cupola sign:* Crescent-shaped radiolucency under the diaphragm • *Rigler's sign:* Visualization of both aspects of the bowel wall being outlined by gas on either side • *Inverted V sign:* Gas on either sides of the falciform ligament • *Football sign:* Collection of gas in the center of the abdomen like a football • *Triangle sign:* Gas between bowel loops	• Subpulmonary pneumothorax • Chilaiditi syndrome • Subphrenic abscess due to infections by gas forming organism like *Clostridium Welchii* • Subdiaphramatic fat or omental fat under the diaphragm may rarely mimic gas under the diaphragm

3. US abdomen will show air in the peritoneal cavity. Poor window due to dilated bowel makes it difficult to identify the cause.
4. CT abdomen is very relevant investigation in intestinal obstruction, acute peritonitis and acute pancreatitis. In intestinal obstruction CT is useful but contrast into the bowel (orally) cannot be given (IV contrast can be given) (Fig. 22.17).
5. Cholescintigraphy using HIDA—hippuric immunodiacetic acid or I^{131} Rose Bengal radioisotope scan has got 100% accuracy in diagnosing acute cholecystitis.
   Laparoscopy is newer modality to identify the pathology. If perforation is identified it can be closed through laparoscopy.

Note: Gastrointestinal contrast studies (barium) or endoscopy is not done in acute abdomen. Occasionally dilute gastrograffin contrast study can be done with care. Barium will leak into the peritoneal cavity causing chemical peritonitis.

■ ACUTE APPENDICITIS

Etiology: (1) Altered diet. (2) Familial susceptibility. (3) Obstruction of the lumen of appendix causing obstructive appendicitis. *Blockage* may be due to Fecoliths, stricture, foreign body, roundworm or threadworm. *Adhesions and kinking*—Carcinoma cecum near the base, ileocecal Crohn's disease. (4) Distal colonic obstruction. (5) Abuse of purgatives. Fecolith is the commonest cause.

Organisms: E. coli (85%), enterococci (30%), streptococci, anaerobic streptococci, *Cl. welchii, Bacteroides*.

Types: (1) *Acute non-obstructive appendicitis:* Inflammation of mucous membrane with redness, edema and hemorrhages which may go for following courses: Resolution; Ulceration; Fibrosis; Suppuration; Recurrent appendicitis; Gangrene; Peritonitis. (2) *Acute obstructive appendicitis*: Here pus collects in the blocked lumen of the appendix which has become blackish, gangrenous, edematous and rapidly progresses leading to perforation either at the tip or at the base of the appendix. This will lead to peritonitis, formation of appendicular abscess or pelvic abscess. Most often there will be thrombosis of the appendicular artery. (3) *Recurrent appendicitis:* Repeated attacks of non-obstructive appendicitis leads to fibrosis, adhesions causing recurrent appendicitis. (4) *Subacute appendicitis* is milder form of acute appendicitis.

Clinical features: It is rare before the age of two, common in children and other age groups. *Pain*: Visceral pain starts around the umbilicus due to distension of the appendix, later after few hours somatic pain occurs in right iliac fossa due to irritation of parietal peritoneum by the inflamed appendix. Pain eventually becomes severe and diffuse which signifies spread of infection into the general peritoneal cavity. *Vomiting:* Due to reflex pylorospasm. *Constipation* is the usual feature *but diarrhea* can occur if appendix is in post-ileal or pelvic positions. *Fever, tachycardia, fetor oris* are other features. *Urinary frequency:* Inflamed appendix may come in contact with bladder and can cause bladder irritation. *Tenderness and rebound tenderness* in right iliac fossa (*release sign—Blumberg's sign*) are typical. *Rovsing's sign:* On pressing left iliac fossa, pain occurs in right iliac fossa which is due to shift of bowel loops which irritates the parietal peritoneum. Hyperextension (in case of retrocecal appendix—*Cope's psoas test*) or internal rotation (in case of pelvic appendix—*obturator test*) of right hip causes pain in right iliac fossa due to irritation of psoas muscle and obturator internus muscle respectively. *Baldwing's test* is positive in retrocecal appendix—when legs lifted-off the bed with knee extended, the patient complains of pain while pressing over the flanks. P/R examination shows tenderness in right side of the rectum. Often infection gets localized by omentum, dilated ileum and parietal peritoneum leading to *appendicular mass*. Most often suppuration occurs in the localized area resulting in *appendicular abscess*.

Stethoscope sign in acute appendicitis: By placing the bell of the stethoscope at McBurney's point to hear bowel sounds and later deeply pressed during each phase of expiration to elicit tenderness; by sudden release of stethoscope patient winces with pain. Absent bowel sounds, tenderness and rebound tenderness are typical signs of acute appendicitis. If bowel sounds are exaggerated then either gastroenteritis or early intestinal obstruction is a possibility. (*Courtesy:* Professor Dr SK Mohapatra MS, FRCS (Edin), DNB, FAIS, FICS, FIMSA; and Dr Dharbind Kumar Jha, Department of General Surgery, VIMSAR, Burla, Odisha).

Differential diagnosis for acute appendicitis

- Perforated peptic ulcer.
- Acute cholecystitis.
- Enterocolitis.
- Mesenteric lymphadenitis.
- Crohn's disease.
- Meckel's diverticulitis.
- Salpingitis.
- Ectopic gestation—ruptured.
- Ruptured or twisted ovarian cyst.
- Right ureteric colic.
- Right acute pyelonephritis.
- Lobar pneumonia.
- Acute pancreatitis.
- Acute crisis of porphyria.
- Diabetic abdomen, etc.

Alvarado scoring for appendicitis:	Score:
Migrating pain.	1
Anorexia.	1
Nausea and vomiting.	1
Tenderness in right iliac fossa.	2
Rebound tenderness.	1
Elevated temperature.	1
Leukocytosis with count more than 10,000.	2
Shift to left with neutrophilia in peripheral smear	1
Total score:	10

Score less than 5: Not sure.
Score between 5–6: Compatible.
Score between 6–9: Probable.
Score more than 9: Confirmed.

Acute Cholecystitis

Commonly occurs in a patient with pre-existing chronic cholecystitis but often also can occur as a first presentation. Usual cause is impacted gallstone in the Hartmann's pouch obstructing cystic duct.
Clostridium Welchii can cause gas in the gallbladder and also septicemia which can be life-threatening—*emphysematous cholecystitis*.
Classification: *Acute calculous cholecystitis and acute acalculous cholecystitis*. Acute cholecystitis can lead to perforation, which usually occurs in the fundus or in the neck (*Hartmann's*). It can cause cholecystoduodenal, cholecystointestinal or cholecystobiliary fistula, peritonitis, pericholecystitic abscess, cholangitis and septicemia.
Bacteria in acute cholecystitis: E. coli; Klebsiella; Strep. faecalis; Salmonella; Clostridium welchii.
Clinical features: Sudden onset of pain in the right hypochondrium, with tenderness, guarding, and rigidity. Palpable, tender, smooth, soft gallbladder is evident. Area of hyperesthesia between 9th and 11th ribs posteriorly on the right side (*Boas's sign*). Jaundice may be present.
Differential diagnosis for acute cholecystitis: Duodenal ulcer perforation; acute pancreatitis; acute appendicitis; acute pyelonephritis; lobar pneumonia; ruptured ectopic pregnancy. Cardiac conditions and right-sided pneumonia may mimic sometimes.

Acute Pancreatitis

Acute pancreatitis is an acute inflammation of the prior normal gland parenchyma which is usually reversible or an acute attack in a pre-existing chronic pancreatitis. It causes series of enzyme activation leading to its dangerous pancreatitis effects. It may lead into pancreatic necrosis, sepsis, acute respiratory distress syndrome (ARDS), acute renal failure, septicemia, hypocalcemia, pneumonia, disseminated intravascular coagulation (DIC). It causes hemorrhagic and ecchymotic patches at various places due to enzymatic degradation—in flanks (*Grey Turner's sign*), around umbilicus [*Cullen's* (*Grunwald's* is more severe) sign], below the inguinal ligament (*Fox sign*), around axilla (*Pandiaraja'a sign*). Pain and resistance over the head of the pancreas 7 cm above the umbilicus is called as *Korte's sign*. Pain on pressure under the xiphoid process (*Kamenchik's sign*); pain while pressing lateral to left erector spine and below the left 12th rib (*Mayo Robson's sign*)—are other signs.
Trapnell's etiological classification of acute pancreatitis:
Major causes: Biliary tract disease 50%; alcoholism 25%.
Other causes: Trauma; after biliary, gastric, splenic surgery; hyperparathyroidism; hypercalcemia; diabetes; porphyria; drugs: steroids, INH, diuretics, septran, azathioprine; viral infections (mumps, coxsackie); autoimmune diseases; vascular diseases; idiopathic.
Clinical features: Presents with sudden onset of upper abdominal pain, which is referred to back, vomiting, high fever, often mild jaundice (due to cholangitis). Clinical signs include tachypnea with cyanosis, tenderness, rebound tenderness, guarding, rigidity and abdominal distension, features of shock and dehydration, oliguria. Grey turner's sign, Cullen's sign, Fox sign.
Differential diagnosis for acute pancreatitis: Perforated duodenal ulcer; cholecystitis; mesenteric ischemia; ruptured aortic aneurysm; ectopic pregnancy; salpingitis; intestinal obstruction; diabetic ketoacidosis.

Acute Peritonitis

Types:
1. *Primary peritonitis* is commonly due to *Pneumococcus* and seen in young girls between 3–6 years; Infection spreads from lower genitals through Fallopian tubes, from upper respiratory tract infection or from middle ear in males; uncommon after 10 years of age; common in malnourished child and child with nephritis. Child is toxic, severely ill and will go into septicemia very early. TC is very high >30,000.
2. *Secondary peritonitis* is secondary (commonest type) to any bowel or other visceral pathology, e.g. perforation, appendicitis.
3. *Tertiary peritonitis* occurs after the treatment for any abdominal surgeries, which is usually severe and may go in for SIRS or MODS early. Mortality for diffuse peritonitis is 10%.

Contd...

Contd...

Bacteria causing peritonitis: (a) *Bacteria from GIT—E. coli*, anaerobic streptococci, anaerobes (bacteroides), *Klebsiellla, Cl. Welchii*. (b) *Bacteria not from GIT—Gonococcus, Pneumococcus, Streptococcus* are from fallopian tubes—occurs in young females, commonly. Most common bacteria during peritonitis phase is *E. coli* and during abscess formation is *B. fragilis*.

Mode of infection: Perforation of the GIT; penetrating or blunt trauma; surgery; drains; dialysis; foreign body; appendicitis, cholecystitis; intestinal obstruction with strangulation; via Fallopian tubes; through blood spread.

Factors affecting the spread of the infection in peritonitis: Rapidity by which the pus is gushed into the peritoneal cavity (e.g. burst appendix, perforations). Amount of peristalsis (more the peristalsis more the spread); virulence of the organism; localizing action of the omentum (in children localization is poor as omentum is small); immunosuppression; anatomical nature of the peritoneal cavity, etc.

Clinical features: Sudden onset of pain; fever, vomiting, tenderness initially localized later becomes diffuse; rebound tenderness; guarding and rigidity; tachycardia, tachypnea; tenderness on P/R examination; distension with silent abdomen; eventually leading to, septicemic shock, *Hippocrates facies* and loss of consciousness.

Amoebic Liver Abscess

It is common in India and other tropical countries; caused by a parasite *Entamoeba histolytica*. More common in alcoholics and cirrhotic patients.

Pathology: Initially from infected rectosigmoid or ileocecal region, amoebic trophozoites reach the liver through portal veins causing amoebic hepatitis may be in the form of microabscesses all over the liver. This might resolve on its own or with antiamoebic drugs, but many times lead to a localized amoebic liver abscess. In 70% of cases it is single large abscess, in 30% it is multiple, and that may involve both lobes. In addition to poor prognosis, problems and difficulties in treating is more common in multiple abscesses.

Amoebic liver abscess is *more common in right posterior-superior region because of streamline effect* (i.e. the portal vein is in direct continuation with the right branch); can be multiloculated; pus is chocolate-colored, classically called as anchovy sauce, contains dead liver cells, RBCs, necrotic material. Pus may be green due to bile admixture.

Complications: (a) Rupture into lungs leading to expectoration of chocolate-colored sputum resulting in natural regression of abscess; (b) Rupture into the peritoneum causing peritonitis which requires emergency laparotomy; (c) Rupture into pleural cavity leading to empyema which is the commonest complication; (d) Rupture into bare-area causing retroperitoneal abscess; (e) Rupture into the intestines, or to the skin (*Amoebiasis cutis*); (f) Most dangerous is rupture into pericardial cavity (cardiac tamponade) which has got very high mortality requiring emergency thoracotomy and pericardial decompression; (g) Septicemia and liver failure can occur in a patient with amoebic liver abscess with cirrhosis.

Features: Common in males, may be after an attack of amoebic dysentery, or many months after the attack or history of dysentery may not be there at all. They present with fever, loss of weight, chills and rigors, pain in the right hypochondrium, soft, tender, smooth, liver with increased liver span. *Intercostal tenderness* is elicited which is a useful clinical sign. Right-sided pleural effusion may be evident. Mild jaundice is not uncommon especially in cirrhotic patient and multiple abscesses which may signify poor prognosis. Tenderness, rigidity and skin edema in right hypochondriac region may be present in acute cases. In *chronic* amoebic liver abscess, smooth, firm/hard, nontender liver may be palpable.

Differential diagnosis: *For acute type:* (1) Acute cholecystitis; (2) Acute presentation of hepatocellular carcinoma (HCC) due to hemorrhage or necrosis. *Chronic abscess* will mimic hepatoma in every respect.

Perforated Duodenal Ulcer (Incidence 5%)

It is common in males (8:1); *anterior ulcer* perforates. In 80% of cases there is a history of chronic DU. In 20% cases it is silent perforation. Perforation can occur in acute ulcers or in acute presentation of a preexisting chronic ulcer.

Perforation may be precipitated by steroids, analgesics (NSAIDs), alcohol, antimalarials.

Stages of perforation:

I: Stage of chemical peritonitis: Once perforation occurs, stomach contents escapes into the peritoneal cavity. The acid from the stomach causes chemical peritonitis leading to severe pain in epigastric region, vomiting, tenderness, guarding, rigidity, tachycardia, sweating.

II: Stage of reaction (Stage of illusion): Peritoneum secretes lot of fluid to neutralize the escaped content and so temporarily the pain reduces, and the patient feels better. It lasts for about 6 hours.

III. Stage of diffuse bacterial peritonitis: After about 6 hours, bacteria from GIT (escape) migrate from the site of perforation causing diffuse peritonitis. Patient is toxic, with tachycardia, hypotension, tachypnea, vomiting, fever, dehydration, oliguria; tenderness and rebound tenderness all over the abdomen; guarding and rigidity, initially in the epigastrium but later all over the abdomen; dullness over the flank because of fluid; obliteration of liver dullness because escaped gas gets collected under the diaphragm; silent abdomen with absence of bowel sounds; tenderness felt on per rectal examination. Sometimes fluid from supracolic region slowly trickles down along the right paracolic gutter, collects in right iliac region causing pain and tenderness in right iliac fossa mimicking appendicitis. Often slow, small perforation presents with subacute features, but diffuse peritonitis sets in eventually in 24–48 hours.

Terminal stage: Patient may have oliguria, septicemia, shock, *Hippocratic facies* (sunken eyes, rapid breathing, ill look), with multi-organ dysfunction syndrome (MODS). *Investigations:* Plain X-ray erect abdomen: Shows gas under diaphragm in 70% of cases. In 30% of cases, there will be no gas under diaphragm. It may be due to either the gas leak is less than 1 mL or due to previous surgery causing adhesions between liver and diaphragm. *Chilaiditi's syndrome* is the interposition of the colon in front and above the liver. It is common in children and elderly. It may be mistaken for gas under diaphragm in plain X-ray abdomen. US abdomen shows free fluid and often gas.

Subphrenic Abscess (Fig. 22-18)

There are four intraperitoneal and three extraperitoneal spaces.

Intraperitoneal spaces

Right anterior intraperitoneal space: It is bounded by right lobe of the liver and diaphragm, coronary and right triangular ligament, and to the left by falciform ligament. Abscess here occurs due to cholecystitis, perforated duodenal ulcer, postoperative, appendicitis, duodenal cap blow out.

Right posterior intraperitoneal space (Rutherford Morrison's kidney pouch): It is bounded in front by the liver and gallbladder, above by the liver, behind by the right, kidney and diaphragm, below by the transverse colon and hepatic flexure, to the left by foramen of Winslow and duodenum. It is large and deepest space of all. *It is the commonest site for subphrenic abscess. Causes:* Appendicitis, cholecystitis, postoperative, perforated duodenal ulcer, intestinal obstruction.

Contd...

Contd...

Left anterior intraperitoneal space: It is bounded above by the diaphragm, behind by left lobe of liver and left triangular ligament, gastrohepatic ligament and anterior surface of the stomach, to the right is the falciform ligament. *Causes* for abscess here are surgeries of the stomach, tail of the pancreas, spleen, colon (splenic flexure) and diverticulitis.

Left posterior intraperitoneal space: It is bounded by stomach, pancreas, greater omentum, liver, transverse colon (lesser sac). Commonest cause here is pseudocyst of pancreas. Rarely perforated gastric ulcer.

Extraperitoneal spaces

Right extraperitoneal space is right perinephric space and *left extraperitoneal space* is left perinephric space. *Causes:* Abscess here is due to tuberculosis, trauma and hematoma. *Midline extraperitoneal* space is bare area of the liver. Pus collects here commonly due to amoebic liver abscess and pyogenic abscess of the liver.

Clinical features of subphrenic abscess:

Pus somewhere, pus nowhere else, pus under diaphragm—Bernard's aphorism.

History relevant to the specific causes, history of previous surgery. Fever with chills and rigors; pain in right hypochondrium; tenderness in right hypochondrium; sympathetic right-sided pleural effusion due to congestion and hyperemia of the diaphragm; pain in the right shoulder due to irritation of phrenic nerve; Hiccough, tachycardia and tachypnea.

Differential diagnosis: Amebic abscess; pylephlebitis; empyema; pulmonary collapse.

Investigations: Plain X-ray chest and abdomen shows soft tissue shadow, pleural effusion, tenting of diaphragm, collapse of the lung. US abdomen confirms the diagnosis. TC is high. CT chest is diagnostic.

Complications: Empyema; respiratory arrest; septicemia.

Perforation of Typhoid Ulcer

Perforation usually occurs in 3rd week of the infection. Ulcers are multiple, arranged in parallel and in anti-mesenteric border of the ileum. One or more ulcers may perforate and many ulcers may be on impending perforation.

Features: Patient is toxic presents with, severe diarrhea, relative bradycardia, soft abdomen, obliterated liver dullness, abdomen without guarding and rigidity (because of Zenker's degeneration).

Investigations: Possibility of missing typhoid perforation is very high. *X-ray in erect posture* will show gas under diaphragm. *Widal test* is positive. *Blood culture* and *stool cultures* are often required as other methods for diagnosis.

Meckel's Diverticulum

It is 2% common; 2 feet from the ileocecal valve; 2 inch in length. It is congenital, results from incomplete closure of vitellointestinal duct; arises from the antimesenteric border of the ileum, contains all three layers of the bowel with independent blood supply; may be connected to, or communicate with the umbilicus through a band or fistula.

Investigation: Technetium Tc^{99} radioisotope scan; X-ray abdomen to look for complications like obstruction, perforation, etc; laparoscopy is very useful.

Presentation: *Severe hemorrhage*—most common presentation, seen in children aged 2 years or younger; intestinal obstruction, perforation, intussusception, peptic ulceration, diverticulitis (In 20% of cases mucosa contains heterotopic epithelium like gastric, colonic and/or pancreatic tissues)—features will mimic acute appendicitis; Littre's hernia; silent Meckel's diverticulum found during laparotomy or laparoscopy or by radioisotope study.

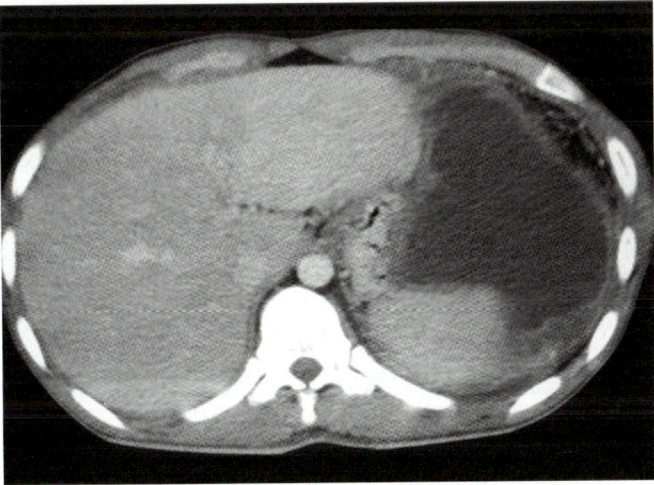

Fig. 22-18 CT scan showing left *subphrenic abscess*.

INTESTINAL OBSTRUCTION

Classification: Congenital, Acquired.

Classification of intestinal obstruction	
Congenital	**Acquired**
• Anorectal malformations	Hernia (commonest)
• Congenital megacolon	Postoperative
• Adhesions	Intussusception
• Duodenal atresia	Roundworm
• Intestinal atresia (ileal)	Gallstones
• Bands and adhesions	Tuberculosis
• Malrotation	Malignancy
• Volvulus neonatorum	Internal hernias

Pathology

Changes proximal to the bowel obstruction: Intestinal obstruction → Increased peristalsis → Becomes vigorous → Obstruction not relieved → Peristalsis ceases → Flaccid paralyzed dilated bowel. Fluid collects just proximal to the obstruction which is derived from saliva, stomach, pancreas and intestine. Because of edema and inflammation absorption decreases, sequestration of fluid from the circulation into the lumen occurs and bacteria (*E. coli, Klebsiella,* anaerobes, bacteroids and other organisms) multiply, toxins are released—*toxemia* occurs. This leads to severe dehydration, electrolyte imbalance. Proximal to the collected fluid, air accumulates [derived from swallowed air (70%), diffusion from blood into the lumen (20%), from digested product and bacterial action (10%)], in which main component is nitrogen (90%) and also hydrogen sulfide. During vigorous peristalsis air enters the distal fluid, results in *churning*, is the reason to cause *multiple air-fluid levels in plain X-ray abdomen.*

Changes at the site of the obstruction: Initially venous return is impaired → Congestion, edema of bowel wall which turns purple → later this jeopardizes the arterial supply → Loss of shineness, black color, loss of peristalsis → *Gangrene and perforation* occurs → Bacteria and toxins migrate into the peritoneum → *peritonitis.*

Closed loop obstruction: When there is obstruction in the large bowel, with ileocecal valve competence, pressure increases in the cecum → Stercoral ulcer form in the cecum → Gangrene → Perforation → Peritonitis (Fecal). Perforation also can occur at the site of obstruction due to the malignant growth.

Bowel distal to the obstruction is inactive and collapsed.

Clinical features: *Abdominal pain:* Initially colicky and intermittent; later continuous and severe. *Vomiting:* In *jejunal* obstruction it is early and persistent. In *ileal* obstruction, it is recurrent occurring at an interval; initially bilious later feculent. In *large bowel* obstruction, vomiting is a late feature. *Distension:* It is absent or minimal in case of *jejunal* obstruction; obvious with visible intestinal peristalsis (VIP) and borborygmi sounds in case of ileal obstruction. It is enormous in case of large bowel obstruction. *Constipation:* It is *absolute*, i.e. neither faeces nor flatus is passed. *Exceptions* where constipation may not be there Richter's hernia obstruction; Gallstone obstruction; Mesenteric vascular occlusion; Intestinal obstruction with a pelvic abscess. It causes *dehydration* → Oliguria → Renal failure. *Features of toxemia and septicemia:* Tachycardia, tachypnea, fever, sunken eyes, cold periphery. *Features of strangulation:* Shock, tenderness, rebound tenderness, guarding and rigidity, absence of bowel sounds. In case of strangulated hernia, a swelling which is tense, tender, rigid, irreducible, no expansile impulse on coughing and history of (H/o) recent increase in size is seen. *Per-rectal examination:* Shows *empty, dilated rectum*, often with tenderness. If rectal growth is the cause for obstruction, it may be palpable. *Plain X-ray abdomen:* Multiple air-fluid levels. Proximal the obstruction lesser is the air fluid level; distal the obstruction more is the fluid level. Normally, three fluid levels can be seen in plain X-ray film—at fundus of stomach, at duodenum and often at cecum. *Jejunum* shows concertina effect due to *valvulae conniventes*. Ileum is smooth and characterless. Large bowel shows *haustration.*

Note: Barium enema and meal is contraindicated in acute intestinal obstruction.

Different Conditions Causing Intestinal Obstruction

Adhesions and Bands

Adhesions and bands are the commonest cause of intestinal obstruction in Western countries.

Causes: *Infection* due to peritonitis, appendicitis, post-laparotomy, and other acute infective abdominal conditions; *materials used during surgery*—suture materials like silk, thread, and foreign body, mop, and gauze, talc powder can cause dense inflammatory reactions; *drugs* like sulphonamides and penicillin's; *ischemia of bowel* due to poor blood supply, sepsis; *gynecological conditions, bowel injury, radiation-induced enteritis, Crohn's disease,* other inflammatory bowel diseases; *specific conditions* like tuberculosis, malignancy.

Clinical features: Pain abdomen—colicky type: recurrent and episodic. Distension, vomiting; constipation; reduced bowel sounds on auscultation; previous surgical scars commonly observed; dehydration, tachycardia, hypotension are other features **(Figs. 22-22-19 and 22-20).**

Types: Type I—*fibrinous adhesions* occur during 5–10th post-surgical period; usually gets resolved completely. It is avascular and flimsy. Type II—*fibrous adhesions*—dense vascular adhesion that occur because of lack/poor blood supply due to which bowel gets attached to part of peritoneum or omentum or other part of the bowel to maintain blood supply. It will persist and precipitate intestinal obstruction, often-subacute and recurrent type. Adhesions due to tuberculosis are severe, dense and difficult to separate.

Acute Intussusception

It is *telescoping of one segment of bowel to adjacent* bowel. Ileocolic is the commonest type.

Causes: Common in infants during weaning period between 6–12 months, where the *Peyer's* patches of the ileum gets hypertrophied and act as point for intussusception. Polyp, submucosal tumors are other causes.

Features: Pain, distension, features of obstruction, constipation; *sausage-shaped mass* palpable in the abdomen usually towards left side with concavity towards umbilicus which is smooth, firm, contracts under palpating fingers, intermittently appears and disappears, mobile, does not move with respiration, resonant or impaired resonant on percussion; often recurrent. Empty right iliac fossa is observed (*Sign de Dance*). *Red currant jelly stool* is common. Microbarium enema X-ray shows *claw sign.* US is diagnostic.

Volvulus (Figs. 22-21A and B)

Volvulus *is twist of loop of the bowel.* It could be gastric, midgut, cecal or sigmoid.

Sigmoid volvulus is commonest type; common in elderly males, rotates in *anticlockwise rotation* and has to rotate more than 1½ turn to cause volvulus. *Cecal volvulus* is more common in young people, common in females, rotates in clockwise direction. It is common in pregnancy.

Predisposing factors are adhesions, peridiverticulitis, loaded pelvic colon, long pelvic mesocolon, narrow attachment of sigmoid mesentery.

Features: Sudden pain, absolute constipation, enormous distension of abdomen, tympanic abdomen, dehydration, late feculent vomiting, perforation and gangrene colon causing peritonitis. Abdomen feels like a tyre. X-ray abdomen shows *omega sign or coffee bean sign.*

Bolus Obstruction

Causes: *Roundworms* cause bolus obstruction in ileum; can perforate inflamed ulcerated bowel causing peritonitis. *Gallstone ileus* is due to cholecystoduodenal fistula wherein gallstones roll down towards ileum causing bolus obstruction. *Food bolus* formed by dry fruits, coconut, orange pulp, undigested vegetables obstruct at 24 cm proximal to ileocecal valve (narrowest part).

Meconium pellets, stercoliths, foreign body, trichobezoars are other causes of bolus obstruction.

Features: Pain, distension, vomiting. Occasionally bolus mass may be felt in the right iliac fossa

Chapter 22: Approaches and Examination of Acute Abdomen

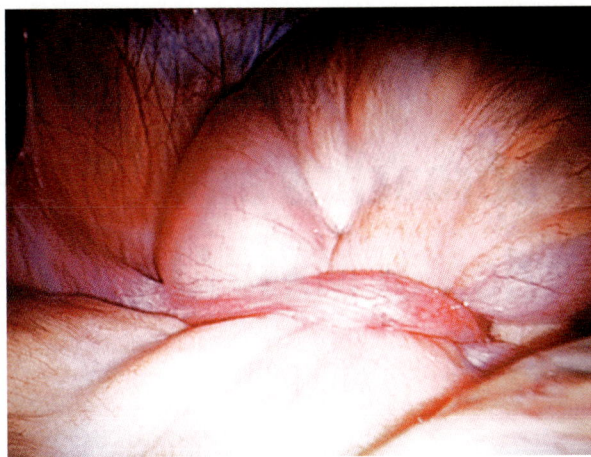

Fig. 22-19 Laparoscopic *view of band* in the right iliac fossa causing intestinal obstruction.

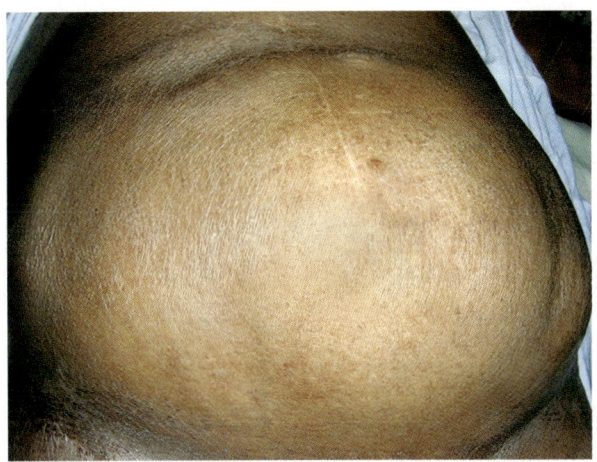

Fig. 22-20 *Postoperative adhesive obstruction* causing lower abdomen distension.

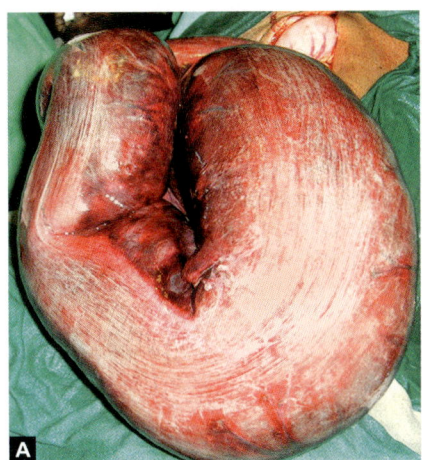
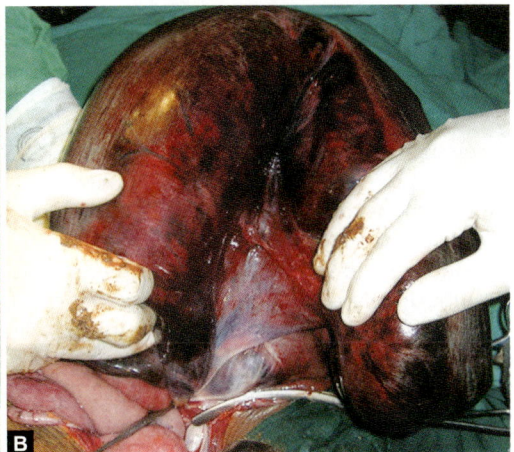

Figs. 22-21A and B *Sigmoid volvulus*—gangrenous.

■ OTHER ACUTE ABDOMEN CONDITIONS

Acute Salpingitis	Munchausen's Syndrome
It is the inflammation of Fallopian tubes. **Features:** Pain begins at hypochondrium later spreads to iliac fossa. Scalding pain in the urethra, fever, tenderness in iliac fossa, mass, vaginal discharge, tender cervix on per vaginal examination.	It is abdominal malingering wherein patient tells long history of his disease like a story. His abdomen shows several scars of earlier surgeries. It may be abdominal, bleeding or with faints, fits, palsies, etc. Appendicectomy is the common initial operation which patient undergoes.
Ruptured Ectopic Gestation	**Ruptured Aortic Aneurysm**
Sudden severe pain in the abdomen, distension, marked pallor, tachycardia, tachypnea, missed menstrual period, discoloration around the umbilicus, tenderness in iliac fossa, shifting dullness, rebound tenderness, soft tender cervix, drop in hemoglobin, positive urine pregnancy test. US confirms the diagnosis.	It may be intraperitoneal or extraperitoneal (retroperitoneal). Retroperitoneal rupture causes sudden severe pain in the abdomen, back pain, pallor, shock, tenderness, rigidity of abdomen. Blood clot may be felt like a mass in the iliac fossa. Condition often mimics acute pancreatitis, perforation of bowel, myocardial infarction.
Acute Nonspecific Mesenteric Lymphadenitis	**Medical Conditions Causing Abdominal Crisis**
Occurs in children below the age of 6 years occasionally can occur up to 14 years. **Features:** Pain in right iliac fossa and umbilicus; fever, vomiting, tenderness in right iliac fossa; guarding not obvious; tenderness elicited in supine position will shift towards left once patient is kept in left side position—*Klein's sign*; rebound tenderness is absent; occasionally on deep palpation tender lymph nodes may be felt.	**Diabetic crisis** presenting as acute abdominal pain which occurs just prior to development of diabetic coma due to very severe hyperglycemia. Patient will be ketotic. **Porphyria crisis** present as violent intestinal colic with constipation, precipitated by barbiturates and sulphonamides (idiosyncrasy); distended abdomen without rigidity is the feature. Urine kept overnight shows dark red color. **Hyperlipidemia crisis** causes left sided abdominal pain and is familial. **Other causes:** Malaria, sickle cell crisis (splenic destruction—autosplenectomy; mesenteric vessel occlusion), hemophilia, acholuric jaundice, tabetic crisis (gastric crisis).

23

Approaches and Clinical Examination of Mass Abdomen

CHAPTER

Competency: SU28.18; AN44.1; AN44.6; AN47.5; AN48.8; AN55.1; AN55.2; PA19.6; PA24.4; PA24.7; PA25.4; PA32.6; IM5.8.

'*Mass abdomen*' often called as 'abdominal lump' but both are synonymous. Abdominal swelling is not commonly used in mass abdomen; but if it is from abdominal wall then word 'abdominal wall swelling' can be used. Examination of mass abdomen is important and should be methodical. It needs eliciting all findings methodically and carefully along with the detail history to analyze and conclude finally. Examining mass abdomen is a clinical challenge which requires through anatomical knowledge and applications. Mass may be from the abdominal wall or intra-abdominal compartment or retroperitoneal compartment. Mass may also be from pelvis.

Abdomen is divided into nine regions by four lines (Fig. 23-1).

Upper horizontal or *transpyloric line* is midway between the suprasternal notch and symphysis pubis or line between tips of ninth costal cartilages on each side. It is often midway between xiphisternum and umbilicus.

Lower horizontal line is transtubercular line at the level of two tubercles (5 cm behind the anterior superior iliac spine along the iliac crest) on the iliac crest.

Regions in the abdomen:
- Right hypochondrium
- Epigastrium
- Left hypochondrium
- Right lumbar region
- Umbilical region
- Left lumbar region
- Right iliac fossa
- Hypogastrium
- Left iliac fossa

Right vertical line is the line through the midpoint of right anterior superior iliac spine and pubic symphysis. It is usually a line joining right midclavicular and right midinguinal points.

Left vertical line is the line through the midpoint of left anterior superior iliac spine and pubic symphysis. It is usually a line joining left midclavicular and left midinguinal points.

Quadrants in the abdomen are four in number formed by two lines—one is vertical midline through the umbilicus; another is horizontal line passing through the umbilicus. Quadrants are—right upper, right lower, left upper and left lower (Figs. 23-2 and 23-3).

■ HISTORY

Chief Complaints

- ***Mass per abdomen***—ask for duration, progress, site, mass appearing/disappearing (like in intussusception, Dietl's crisis of hydronephrosis kidney, and choledochal cyst)
- ***Pain in the abdomen***—region of pain; duration of pain to be mentioned
- ***Vomiting***—duration
- ***Hematemesis, malena***—duration
- ***Satiety***
- ***Jaundice***—yellowish discoloration of sclera—duration

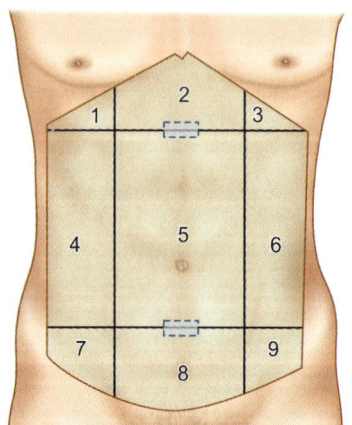

1. Right hypochondrium
2. Epigastrium
3. Left hypochondrium
4. Right lumbar region
5. Umbilical region
6. Left lumbar region
7. Right iliac fossa
8. Hypogastrium
9. Left iliac fossa

Fig. 23-1 *Different regions* in the abdomen.

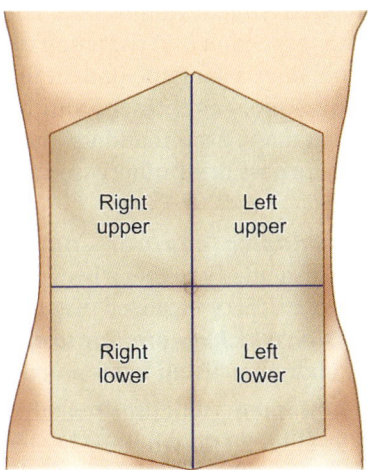

Fig. 23-2 *Different quadrants in the abdomen.* They are four in number formed by two lines—one is vertical midline through the umbilicus; another is horizontal line passing through the umbilicus. Quadrants are—right upper, right lower, left upper and left lower.

- *Loss of appetite and decreased weight*
- *Altered bowel habits*—constipation/diarrhea
- *Fever*

History of Present Illness

Mass per abdomen: Duration, progress, site, mass appearing/disappearing (like intussusception, Dietl's crisis of hydronephrosis kidney, and choledochal cyst) should be asked.

Pain abdomen: Site of origin of pain; onset (sudden/insidious); duration; radiation of pain/referred pain; type of pain—intermittent/persistent; dull constant/severe pricking/colicky; periodicity with an interval of free period—ulcer pain often has periodicity unless it is complicated; relation to food intake—becomes more/less/not related to meals; relation to vomiting/induced vomiting; aggravating/relieving factors; pain in relation to bowel habits/urinary habits.

Vomiting: Duration, frequency, relation to food, type (projectile/effortless).

Vomitus: Content (food/blood/bile); quantity; smell; color—coffee ground/bloody/yellow; taste; relation to pain; details of hematemesis if present. It is better to ask the patient to collect and keep the vomitus and clinician should personally observe it.

Satiety: Sensation of fullness after taking food (early satiety) signifies gastrointestinal pathology like carcinomas.

Jaundice: Duration, color (greenish yellow suggests obstruction), severity, progress (progressive/intermittent/static/reducing). Presence of fever with jaundice—cholangitis; association with **pruritus** (usually on the dorsum of the hand forearm, back), clay colored stool / silvery stool is important. It is an important factor in relation to liver, gall bladder or pancreatic masses.

Loss of appetite and decreased weight: Weight loss more than 10 Kg in short period/6 months is significant.

Bowel habits: Constipation, diarrhea, bloody diarrhea, spurious diarrhea, melena, tenesmus with duration, type, and distension of abdomen. Clay colored stool suggests obstructive jaundice. History of incomplete evacuation, change in bowel habits should be asked.

Fever: Its character is important to be noted in abdominal tuberculosis, amebic liver abscess, cholangitis, malignancy with tumor necrosis, infected pseudocyst of pancreas.

Altered urinary symptoms: History of frequency, urgency, hematuria, pyuria, oliguria, painful urination, burning urine, difficulty in passing urine, hesitancy, hiccough, edema feet or face; relation of urinary symptoms to pain, mass in abdomen should be asked for.

Other relevant history: Cough and hemoptysis, bone pain, etc.—suggestive of metastases.

Past History

Earlier history of abdominal surgery—reason for surgery, how long ago it was done, whether earlier symptoms are relieved or not, whether the symptoms are now similar or different, whether it was an emergency or an elective surgery, whether it was earlier properly investigated or not, whether drain was placed or not—if placed when it was removed; what content was coming through the drain, whether blood transfusion was done during surgery or in postoperative period.

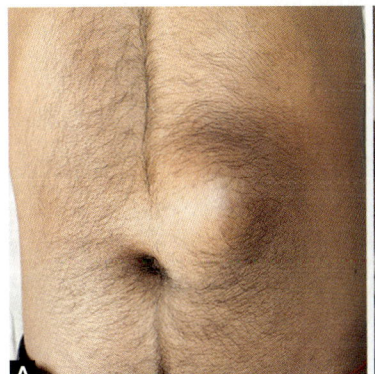 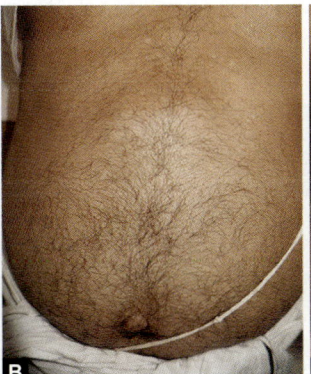 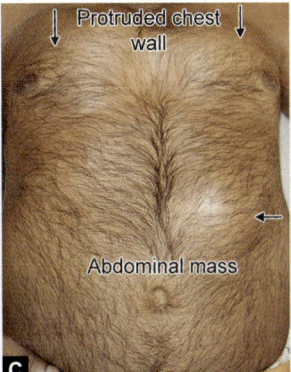 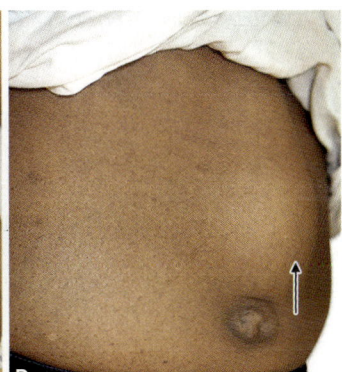

Figs. 23-3A to D *Different masses in different regions* in the abdomen.

Personal History

History of alcohol intake, diet, smoking, etc. has to be noted.

Treatment History

Any relevant history of surgery in the past, chemotherapy for malignancies, abdominal tuberculosis treated, and so on.

Family History

Any relevant history in the family should be taken as some GI malignancies run in families.

GENERAL EXAMINATION

Pallor, jaundice, clubbing, edema feet, cachexia are noted. **Scratch marks** on the dorsum of hand, forearm, back is seen in obstructive jaundice due to pruritus (often intractable) **(Fig. 23-4)**. Pulse/blood pressure is recorded. Genitalia, respiratory and cardiovascular system should be examined.

LOCAL ABDOMINAL EXAMINATION

Inspection

Inspection of the abdomen is done with patient lying in supine position exposed from midchest to midthigh region with arms extended and laid by the side of the body. Inspection is done from side of the bed as well as from head and foot end with eye kept at the level of the abdomen **(Figs. 23-5 and 23-6)**.

After examination in lying down position, it is often needed to examine (both inspection and palpation) the abdomen in standing position, after asking the patient to walk few steps which makes mass more prominent and better palpable. In lower abdomen mass, examination should be done after asking the patient to pass urine otherwise catheter should be passed to empty it.

Shape of the abdomen/contour—normal/scaphoid/distended. When distended whether it is symmetrical uniform distension/asymmetrical or localized distension is noted. *In localized distension which may be due to abdominal mass,* the quadrant of abdomen distended is noted.

Skin over the abdomen—whether stretched/pigmented; presence of scar **(Fig. 23-7)** whether healed primarily or secondarily; site of scar, length and width of scar fungating lesion **(Fig. 23-8)**; whether there is any incisional hernia or not.

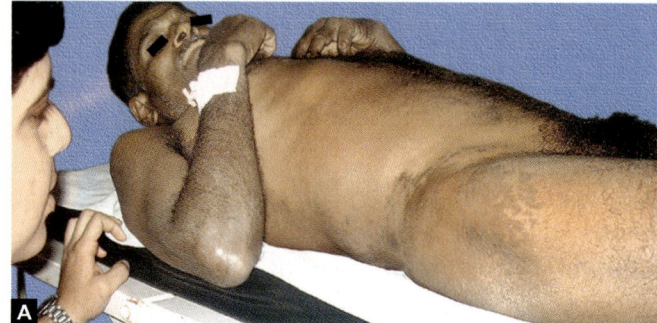

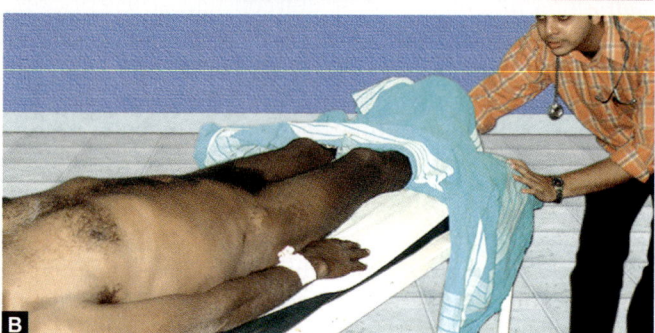

Figs. 23-6A and B Inspection of the abdomen should be done *at the level of the patient's abdomen both from right side as well as from foot end.*

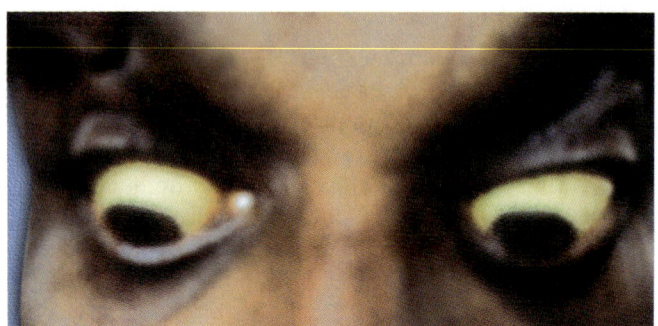

Fig. 23-4 *Obstructive jaundice* in a patient with carcinoma head of pancreas. Note the sclera for discoloration. Severe itching is common in these patients.

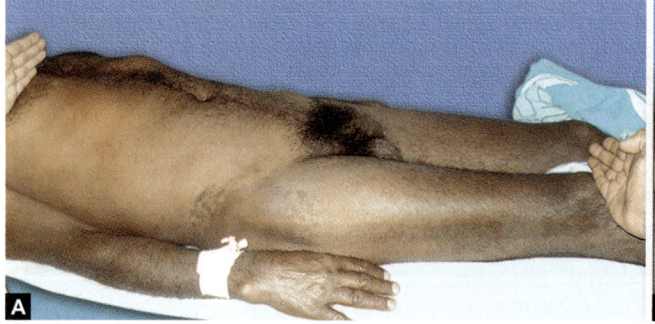

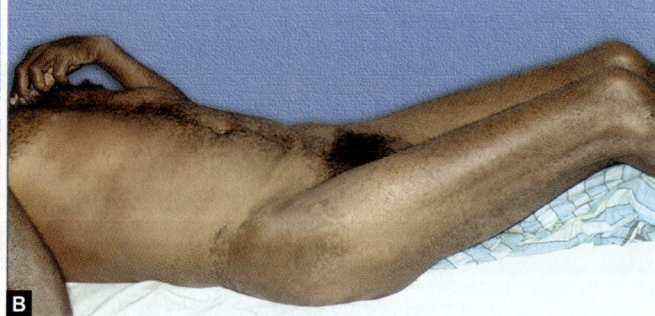

Figs. 23-5A and B *Proper exposure of the abdomen* from midchest to midthigh and position of the patient is important for proper abdominal examination.

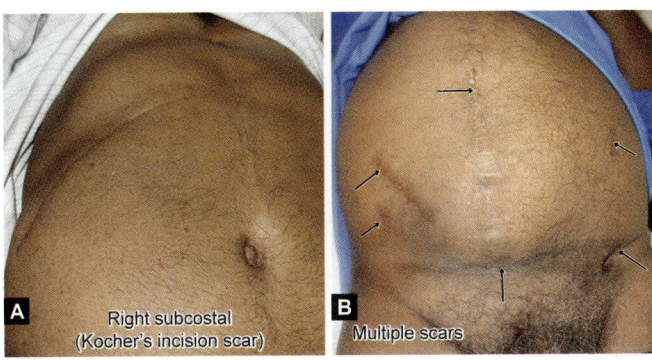

Figs. 23-7A and B *Presence scar/scars may give the idea* about the indication for the earlier surgery. Depending on the anatomical location, presence of drain marks will give often fair idea about the old surgery.

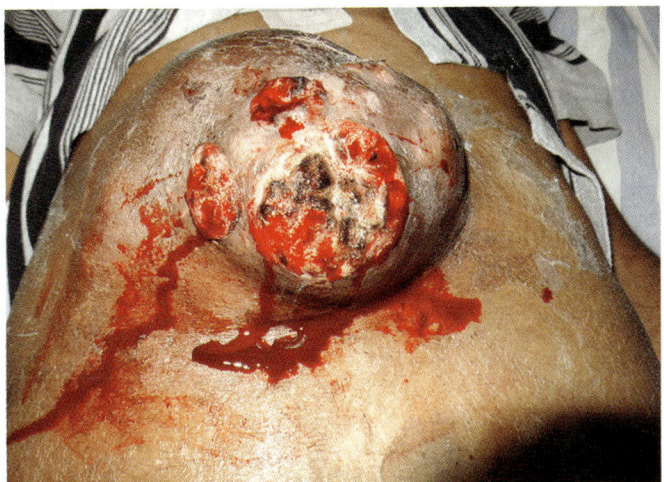

Fig. 23-8 *Large mass abdomen which is fungating* through the abdomen. It could be fungating abdominal wall mass or rarely intra-abdominal mass getting adherent to abdominal wall causing fungation.

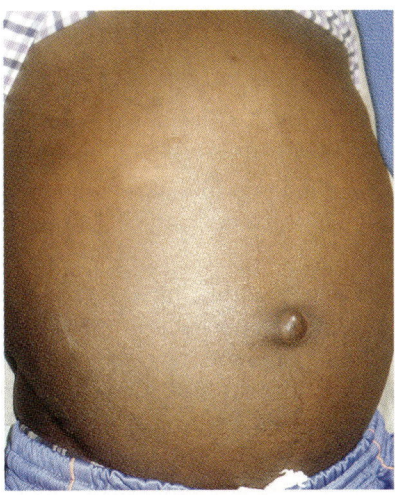

Fig. 23-9 Ascites showing everted umbilicus which is shifted downwards *(Tanyol sign)*.

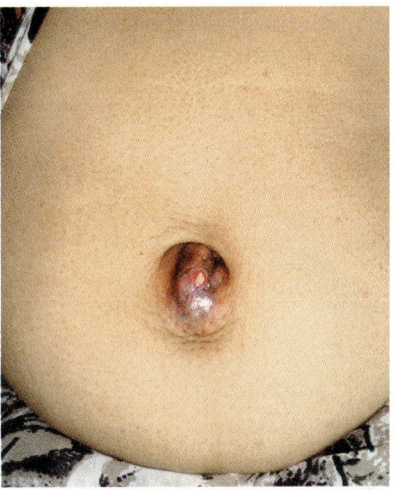

Fig. 23-10 *Sister Joseph secondary nodule in the umbilicus.*

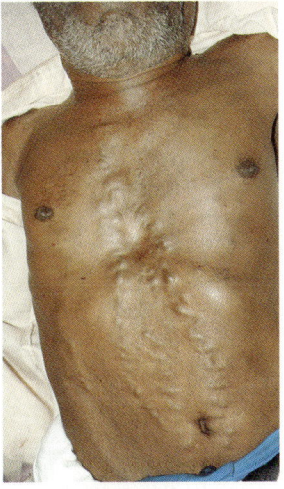

Fig. 23-11 *Dilated veins in the abdominal wall extending into the chest wall.*

Umbilicus: Position is noted. It may be everted/inverted. *Tanyol sign:* Umbilicus is shifted upwards in pelvic/ovarian mass and downwards in ascites **(Fig. 23-9)**. *Sister Joseph nodules* can occur in the umbilicus as secondaries from abdominal GI malignancies through ligamentum teres **(Fig. 23-10)**. Umbilical black eye is *Cullen's sign* of discoloration of umbilicus seen in acute pancreatitis. Umbilical concretions, umbilical discharge (sinus/fistula), bluish tinge in ruptured ectopic gestation (*Cullen's*), yellow tinge around umbilicus in acute pancreatitis in women (*Johnston*)—should be observed.

Movements of regions with respiration should be noted. Any restriction of movement in any region is noted.

Dilated veins over the abdomen should be looked for **(Fig. 23-11)**—*caput medusae* is dilated veins radiating from the umbilicus—seen in portal hypertension. In *inferior vena caval obstruction* (lateral abdominal wall) dilated veins are visible with their flow of blood from below upwards towards superior vena cava. In *superior vena caval obstruction* dilated veins are visible with blood flow from above downwards. Dilated veins should be inspected in standing position. Direction of flow should be checked by placing two fingers closely over the vein and a portion of vein is emptied by milking the vein. Now the fingers are released one by one to see the direction of blood flow. Normally abdominal wall drains to superior vena cava above the umbilicus and to inferior vena cava below the umbilicus—*water shed area* (**Figs. 23-12 and 23-13**). Dilated veins are also seen in cachexic patient due to loss of subcutaneous fat.

Pulsations over the mass or any region should be noted. Patient should hold the breath after full expiration to see for pulsations.

Visible peristalsis should be looked for—*Visible gastric peristalsis* (*VGP*) is seen in epigastrium region with waves beginning from left upper abdomen directed downwards and towards right to umbilical region. It is stimulated by drinking a glass of water or by massaging the epigastrium. It signifies gastric outlet obstruction. But visible gastric peristalsis may be absent when gastric paresis develops when stomach becomes dilated in gastric outlet obstruction, where it is silent without any motility. *Visible intestinal peristalsis* (*VIP*) occurs in **step ladder** pattern in central abdomen from left to right or vice versa. Visible colonic peristalsis may be obvious from right to left along the line of colon.

Inspection of the mass: Its location (exact location should be mentioned as in which region it is located and then its extension into the other region should be mentioned later); extent; approximate size; well defined or ill defined (often mass is not clearly seen but fullness is visible); margins whether clear or not or which part is clear and which part is not; presence of movement of mass with respiration or not (upper abdomen mass which comes in close contact with diaphragm like liver, stomach, spleen, gallbladder, omental mass, kidney mass moves with respiration). Mass which was initially mobile may not be mobile later once it gets fixed to retroperitoneum or deeper plane. But occasionally mass which was initially not mobile, may start moving with respiration once gets attached to structures like omentum. Lower abdominal mass, retroperitoneal mass will not usually move with respiration. Composite mass may move with respiration because of its component like omentum, lymph nodes, bowel, etc. (**Figs. 23-14 and 23-15**).

Loin should be inspected from behind in sitting position (**Fig. 23-16**).

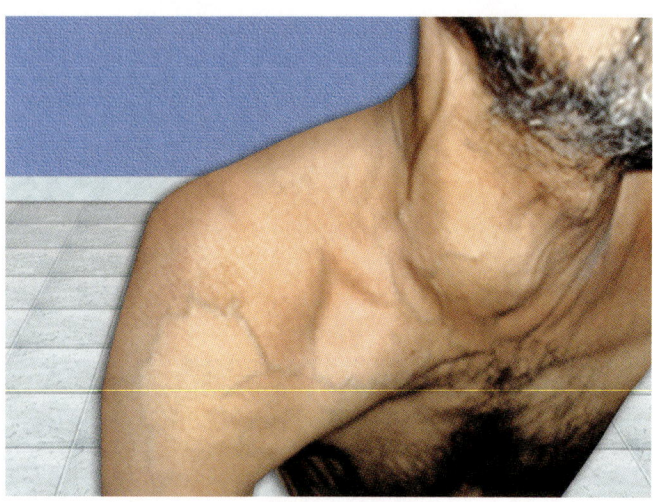

Fig. 23-12 Superior vena caval obstruction causing *dilated veins in the neck chest wall and shoulder*. Note the neck swelling extending into the mediastinum.

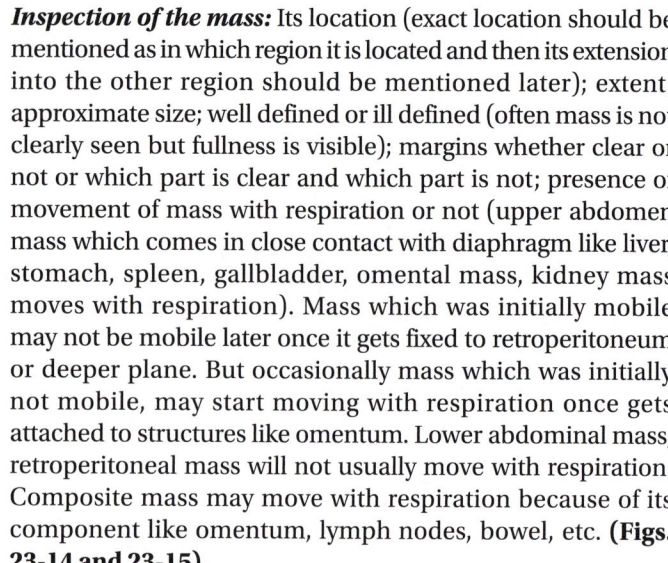

Fig. 23-14 *Visible large upper abdomen mass*—could be enlarged liver/pseudocyst of pancreas/retroperitoneal mass.

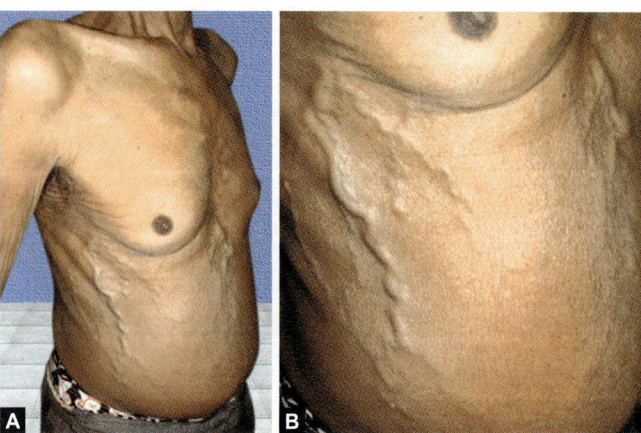

Figs. 23-13A and B Inferior vena caval obstruction causing *dilated veins over the lateral aspect of the flank with flow of blood upwards*.

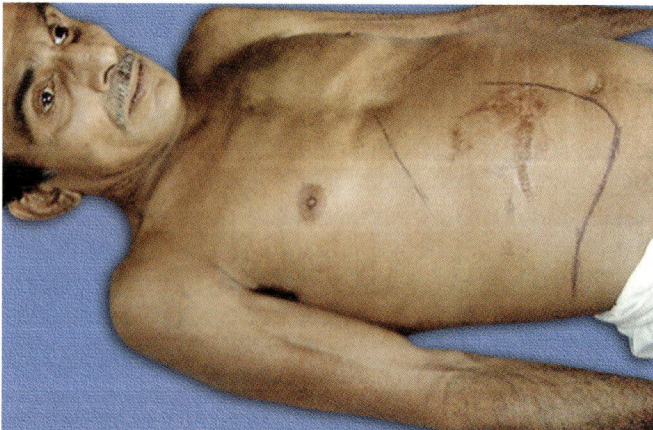

Fig. 23-15 Large secondaries in liver. *Patient has undergone enucleation of left eye (with artificial eye) for primary melanoma choroids*—15 years ago. Now he has presented with late large liver secondaries.

Chapter 23: Approaches and Clinical Examination of Mass Abdomen

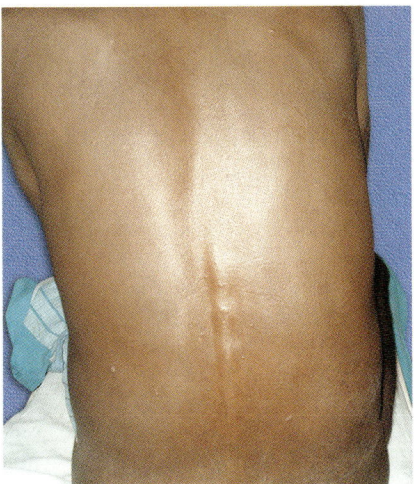

Fig. 23-16 *Loin should be inspected* from behind for fullness and edema.

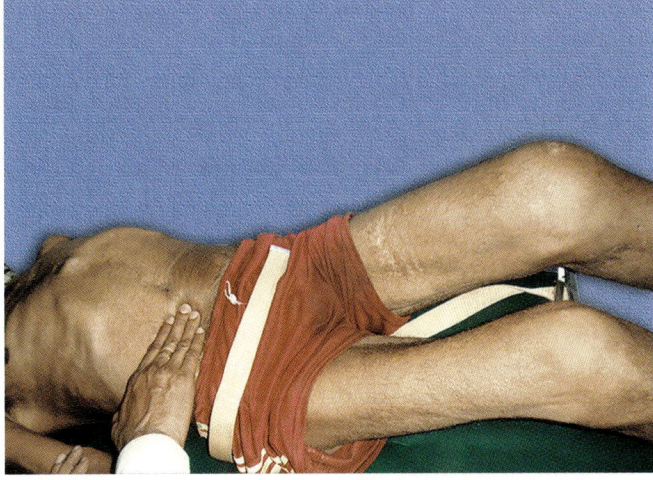

Fig. 23-18 *Palpation of abdominal mass using fingers.*

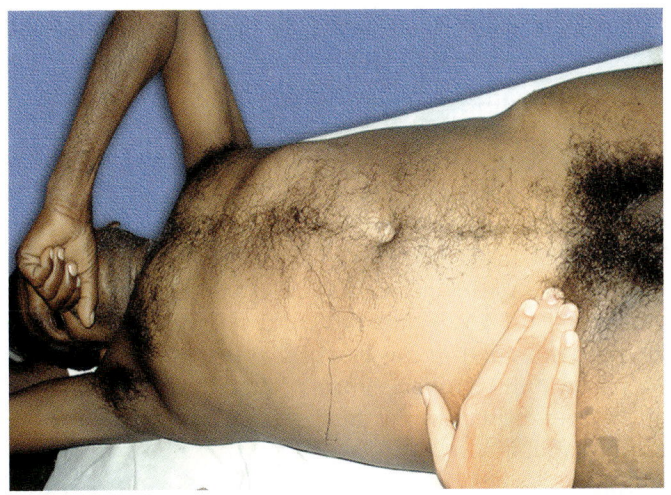

Fig. 23-17 *Impulse on coughing should be seen* and also felt to confirm associated hernia (better elicited in standing position).

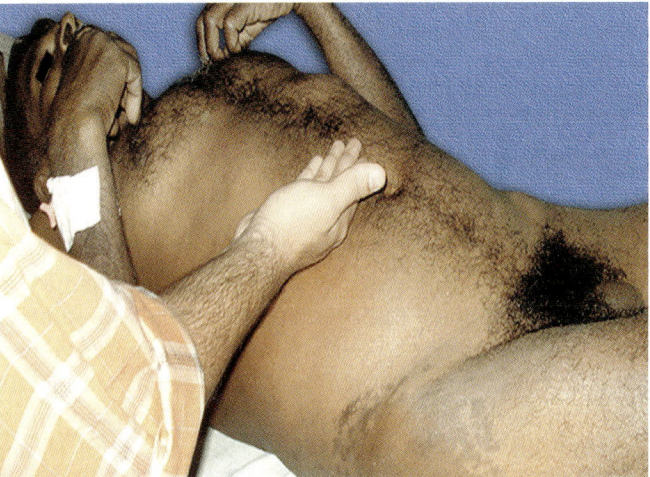

Fig. 23-19 *Checking the temperature of the abdomen* using dorsum of the hand.

Inspection of hernial orifices and genitalia—is very essential. Scrotum should be examined for testicular tumor which may present as epigastric mass due to secondaries in para-aortic lymph nodes **(Fig. 23-17)**.

Palpation

While palpating the abdomen patient should relax and breathe deeply with mouth open to relax the abdomen otherwise the rigidity of the abdominal muscle come in way of proper palpation. Hands should be warm and forearm should be horizontal at the same level as patient's abdomen. Palpation is done with ventral aspect of the fingers, gently without hurry. Legs should be partially flexed at hips and knees **(Fig. 23-18)**.

Local Rise of Temperature (Fig. 23-19)

It is checked on the skin overlying mass using back of hand. It suggests inflammatory pathology. ***It is difficult to elicit*** local rise of temperature in intra-abdominal masses unless it is adherent to abdominal wall or if it is an abdominal wall mass.

Tenderness

Tenderness over the abdomen or over the mass must be noted. It may be due to inflammatory pathology. Often malignant condition may cause tenderness either due to secondary infection or due to tumor necrosis.

Position of the Mass

Anatomical location of the mass is important; it suggests the possible origin of the mass from where it arises. For example, mass in the right hypochondrium could be liver or gallbladder or kidney; mass in lower abdomen may be arising from pelvis. Position is mentioned with corresponding regions of the abdomen.

Size and Shape of the Mass

Size of the mass is measured longitudinal versus transverse and is mentioned in centimeters. If multiple masses are present, though ideally all masses should be measured, it is of usual practice to mention the size of the largest mass then of the smallest mass. Size of the mass arising from individual organs like stomach, liver or spleen should be mentioned separately (carcinoma stomach with liver secondaries; hepatosplenomegaly of portal hypertension). Gallbladder mass is globular; liver mass is horizontal; spleen mass is obliquely placed; it may suggest the origin of the mass. Shape is initially inspected and confirmed by palpation.

Surface and Consistency of Mass

Surface may be **smooth** like in liver abscess, hydrohepatosis, hydatid cyst, spleen enlargement; may be **nodular** like in cirrhosis of liver, secondaries in liver, neoplastic conditions; may be **granular** like in omental mass. **Consistency** of abdomen mass may be **soft** like in hydatid cyst, liver abscess; **firm** like in spleen enlargement, polycystic disease of liver or kidney; **hard** like in hepatoma of liver, secondaries in liver or other neoplastic masses in the abdomen from stomach/colon/small bowel /kidney etc.

Note: One cannot elicit fluctuation in an intra-abdominal mass as mass cannot be fixed which is a prerequisite condition to check fluctuation; so it is uncommon to mention fluctuation in intra-abdominal masses and usually masses are termed as soft (not cystic). (Hydatid thrill can be elicited in hydatid cyst during percussion but not by palpation).

Margin

Well-defined margin which is distinct may be a feature of neoplasm. Ill-defined margin may be seen in inflammatory or traumatic pathology. Which margin is indistinct whether upper or lower should be confirmed. In the upper abdomen, palpating the upper margin is important. In liver mass upper margin is not felt whereas it is felt in stomach mass. Upper margin of the mass may be difficult to feel in mass from fundus of stomach. Feeling the lower margin is important in the lower abdomen mass. If lower margin is not clear one has to find out whether mass is extending into pelvis or not. Rectal or per vaginal examination confirms the pelvic mass. Often full bladder may interfere or mimic the mass and so mass should be palpated again after emptying the bladder, if needed after passing a urinary catheter. Margin may be better felt with change in position either sitting, standing, or lateral position **(Fig. 23-20)**.

Mobility of Mass

Movement of mass with respiration: Masses, arising from the organs which have direct/indirect contact with diaphragm move with respiration. Mobility of the mass with respiration is checked by keeping the fingers near the lower margin of the mass. During inspiration (on deep breathing) mass moves down to touch the hand of the examiner and during expiration it moves back to its original position. Liver, gallbladder, stomach, spleen, kidney (even though retroperitoneal it shows slight significant movement with respiration vertically), omental mass, occasionally mass from flexures of colon move with respiration. Mass arising from pancreas, adrenals, small bowel, colon, retroperitoneum will not move with respiration.

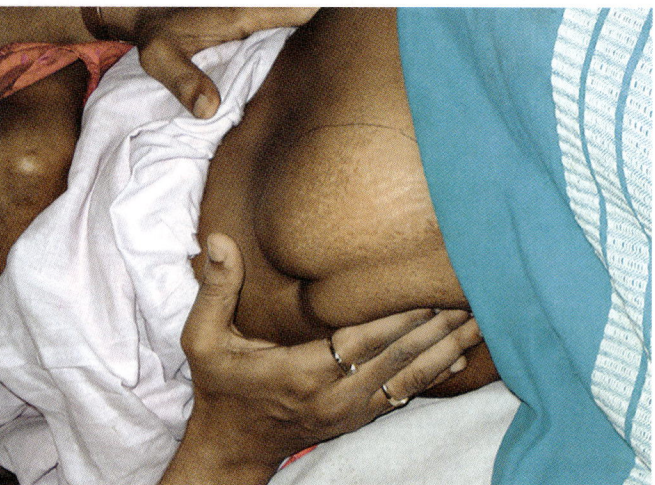

Fig. 23-20 Often abdominal mass should also be examined *in lateral position to get better feeling* and findings.

Intrinsic mobility of mass: Mass is held between thumb and fingers and moved in vertical and horizontal directions. If there is restriction in movement, which movement is restricted should be checked **(Figs. 23-21A and B)**. Totally fixed mass will not be mobile at all. Some masses move in both directions like mass from stomach, colon, small bowel; some masses move only in one direction like mesenteric cyst moves only from left upper to right lower quadrant direction i.e. perpendicular to the line of mesentery; some masses may show only transverse intrinsic mobility like gallbladder mass. Liver mass moves with respiration but difficult to have intrinsic mobility.

Pulsatile mass: Swellings arising from (aneurysm) or in front of abdominal aorta are pulsatile. Aneurysms show expansile pulsation, here change in position either lateral or knee elbow position will not alter the intensity of the pulsation. Whereas in transmitted pulsation like in pseudocyst of pancreas (masses in front of the aorta), pulsation will become less or non pulsatile with change in position as the mass in front of the aorta will fall away from it and becomes nonpulsatile.

Note: Two finger test is difficult to elicit in the intra-abdominal pulsatile mass—the two index fingers placed over the swelling will divert apart with each pulsation. Whereas the swellings in front of abdominal aorta show transmitted pulsation (two fingers will not divert apart).

Plane of the Swelling

Head raising test or leg raising test (Carnett's test): It is done to confirm whether mass is in the abdominal wall or intra-abdominal **(Fig. 23-22)**. Mass seen initially is palpated and patient is asked to raise his head along with shoulders with arms folded over the chest. If mass disappears or becomes smaller, it is intra-abdominal mass; if it becomes more prominent or remains same it is in the abdominal wall. This maneuver is done to make the abdominal muscle taut. Raising

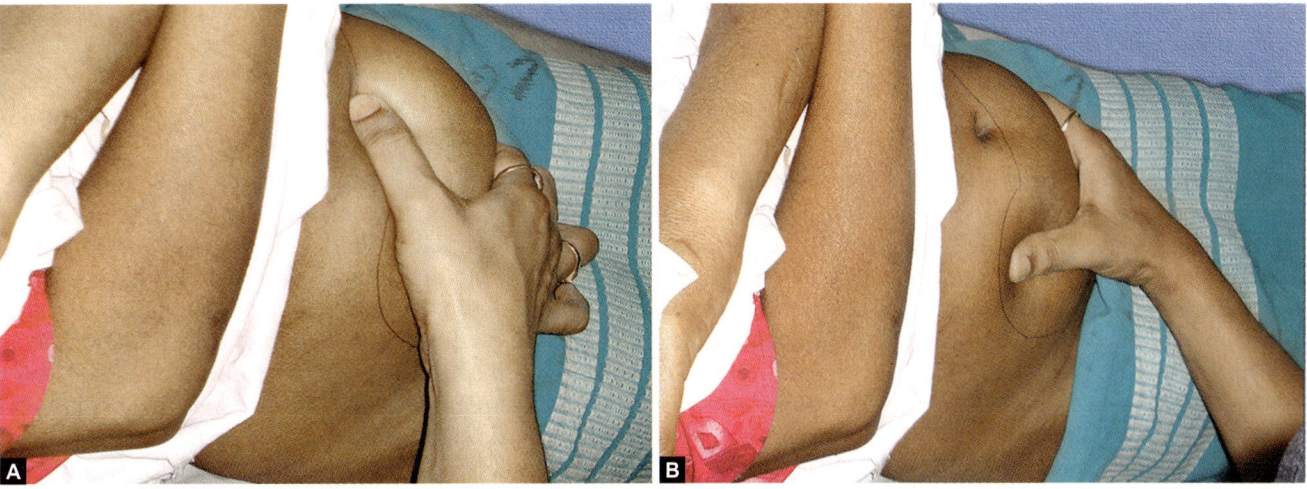

Figs. 23-21A and B *Intrinsic mobility of the mass* should be checked in all abdominal masses.

both legs straight above the bed (**Carnett's test**) and blowing out air by holding the nose tightly with fingers and mouth shut—**Valsalva maneuver** can also be used for the same. Abdominal wall mass will become prominent and immobile during these maneuver. The mass superficial to the muscles (lipoma, sebaceous cyst, neurofibroma) will still have mobility even when the abdominal muscles are made taut. Mass arising from or adherent to muscle will not move when the muscle are made taut (*recurrent fibroid of Paget's*).

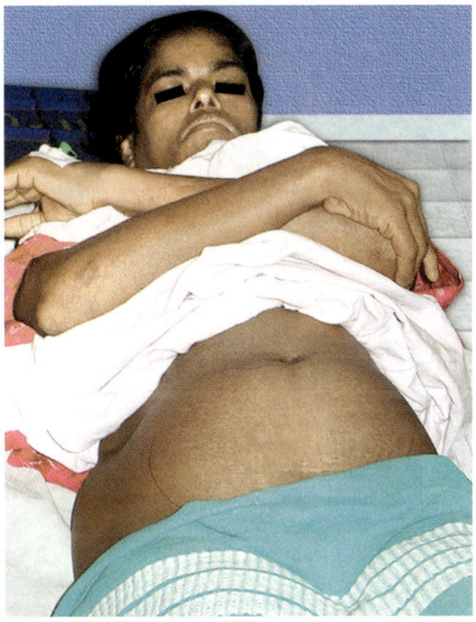

Palpation of Liver

Liver is palpated by placing flat of the hand parallel to the right costal margin—initially near right iliac fossa with fingers directed upwards up to the margin of the right rectus. Slowly with each phase of respiration fingers should move upwards towards right hypochondrium to feel the lower margin of the liver. The surface of the liver is then felt for tenderness, nodularity, round/sharp margin. Level of lower margin should be measured in centimeters from right costal margin. In children below 3 years, liver is palpable 3 cm below the right costal margin. Liver is not palpable or just palpable in normal adult. Whenever there is ascites liver is palpated by '**dip method**'—(dipping fingers quickly so as to displace the fluid). Liver may be enlarged *upwards* in hydatid cyst, and liver abscess (**Figs. 23-23A to C**).

Normal liver span in adult is (vertical height) 12–15 cm. Liver span in infant is 2.4–2.8 cm. At the age of 14 years it is 5.5–7.5 cm.

Palpation of Gallbladder

Normally it is not palpable. When enlarged its lower margin may be in right side of umbilical region/right lumbar region/

Fig. 23-22 Head raising test should be done to find out whether mass is intra-abdominal or in the abdominal wall.

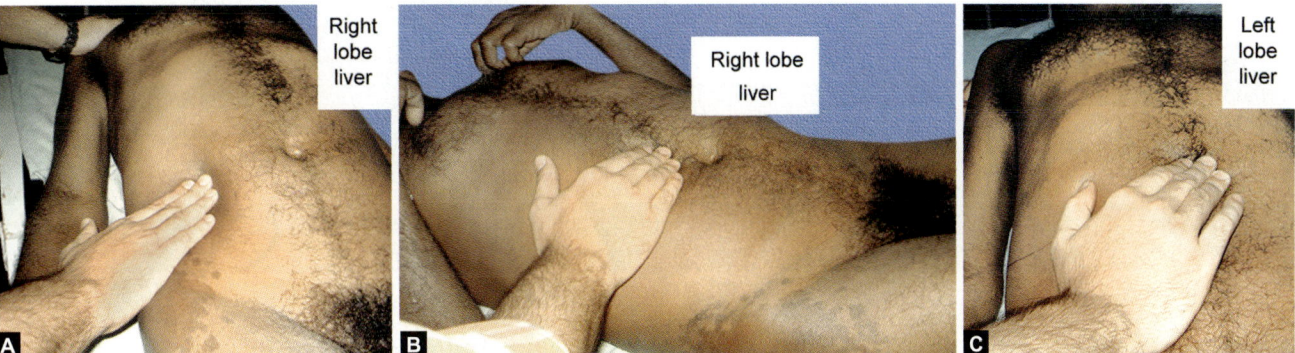

Figs. 23-23A to C *Method of palpating the liver* right lobe and left lobe.

right iliac fossa. It moves with respiration, globular in shape, smooth and soft, may be horizontally mobile but not vertically, upper margin merges under the liver when liver is enlarged or under the right costal margin. It is usually in right hypochondrium, just right of the right rectus muscle.

Murphy's sign is elicited in sitting position. Patient winces with pain at the summit of inspiration while palpating in gallbladder area. During deep inspiration, inflamed gallbladder comes down and touches the palpating finger causing tenderness. It is observed in chronic cholecystitis. When it is elicited in lying down position it is called as ***Moynihan's sign (test)***.

Stomach

Stomach is palpated in the epigastrium. Entire stomach may be dilated and palpable due to gastric outlet obstruction. Succussion splash and auscultopercussion tests should be elicited in such occasion.

Succussion splash: Patient should not take anything orally for 4 hours as gastric emptying time for liquid is 4 hours. If patient drinks fluid succussion splash may be positive even when stomach is not dilated. Bell of the stethoscope is placed in the epigastrium. Two thumbs of the two hands are placed over the bell and fingers of each hand are placed on costal area on each side and patient is shaken well to hear the splashing sound. This can be occasionally elicited by dipping the hand over the dilated stomach also **(Fig. 23-24)**.

Auscultopercussion test: It is positive in gastric outlet obstruction. Bell of the stethoscope is placed over the epigastrium. Abdominal wall is scratched using pencil or fingertip by radiating strokes from bell area towards left hypochondrium, left lumbar, epigastrium and later towards right part of the umbilical regions. Change in the note of the sound is marked at each stroke line. All these points are joined to mark the greater curvature of the stomach. By this procedure only greater curvature is assessed. This is because—only greater curvature dilates significantly when there is obstruction not lesser curvature, and greater curvature is more towards surface whereas lesser curvature is in deeper plane. Normally, greater curvature is above the level of umbilicus on surface marking. In gastric outlet obstruction it shifts below the level of umbilicus **(Figs. 23-25A to C)**.

Stomach mass is commonly due to carcinoma stomach but occasionally it can be due to gastric lymphoma or leiomyoma of stomach. Mass of carcinoma stomach is in the epigastrium or upper part of umbilical region—which moves with respiration; all borders are well made out; mobile in all directions; nodular and hard; upper border is well made out; with impaired resonant *note* on percussion. If mass is close to the fundus of stomach then upper border may not be clearly felt. Often patient should be examined in lateral position or after making the patient to walk for few minutes so as to allow the mass to come down to make it easily palpable. When mass arises from the pylorus it will be just above right of the umbilicus presenting with features of gastric outlet obstruction. Mass from the body of the stomach is horizontally placed extending towards the left hypochondrium, commonly without features of obstruction. Often a composite mass of carcinoma, lymph nodes, omentum and part of the liver may

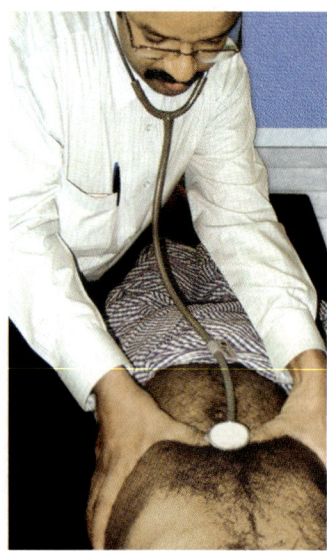

Fig. 23-24 *Succussion splash.*

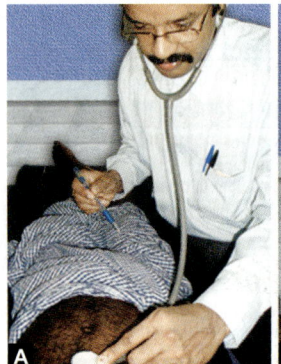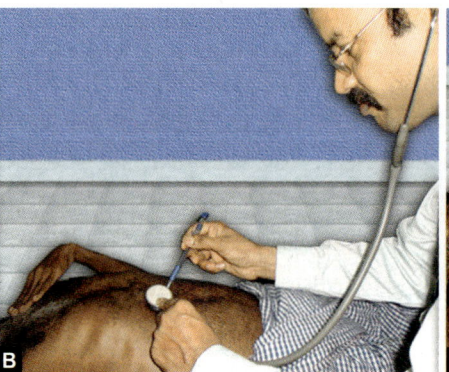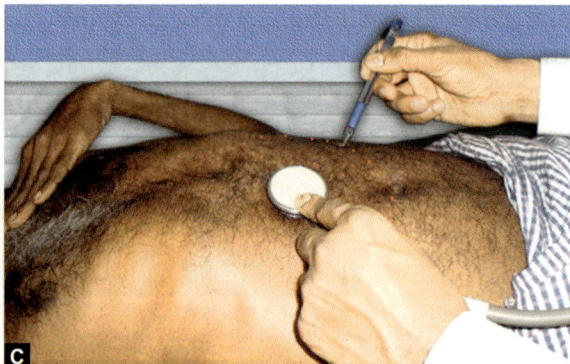

Figs. 23-25A to C *Auscultopercussion test.*

be palpable and attains a large size also. Carcinoma stomach when fixed may not move with respiration and may find it difficult to differentiate from pancreatic mass (Even though carcinoma pancreas is rarely palpable, one should suspect carcinoma pancreas in case of palpable gallbladder and progressive severe jaundice.). Often carcinoma stomach can also cause jaundice when there are extensive secondaries in liver in both lobes. In such occasion along with stomach mass nodular secondaries in liver with ascites is also evident. Patient with mass near the esophago-gastric junction presents with dysphagia. **Linitis plastica** (diffuse type of carcinoma stomach in submucosal plane) usually presents with loss of appetite and decreased weight with reduced stomach capacity. It usually does not present as mass abdomen. When mass is palpably present, it is a composite mass of nodes, omentum and stomach. It carries poor prognosis. Clinically palpable carcinoma stomach (as mass) is considered as advanced carcinoma stomach as involvement of serosa means 'advanced' as per the definition. Without serosal breach it is difficult to palpate clinically. But it could be still surgically resectable **(Fig. 23-26)**.

In infants pyloric mass of congenital pyloric stenosis is palpated from *left side* of the patient.

Pancreatic Mass

It is palpable in the epigastrium. It is deep, nonmobile, not moving with respiration, with bowel in front. It is felt on deep palpation. Pseudocyst mass has rounded lower margin with transmitted pulsation. Pancreatic masses are usually resonant.

Palpation of Spleen

Spleen is normally not palpable. It becomes clinically palpable when it enlarges more than three times. Nonpalpable spleen still could be enlarged. Spleen enlarges towards right iliac fossa across umbilical region directing obliquely—downwards, forwards, inwards. It is palpated by placing fingers of right hand over right iliac fossa with left hand under left costal margin for support. Fingers of right hand are gradually and gently moved towards left hypochondrium during phases of respiration to feel the splenic upper margin near anterior end often with **a notch** (notch need not be present always). Fingers cannot be insinuated under the left costal margin. Spleen is smooth, firm in consistency, moves with respiration, and usually nontender unless massively enlarged. Often patient need to be tilted towards right side to palpate the spleen easily. It can be palpated from left side by hooking the left costal

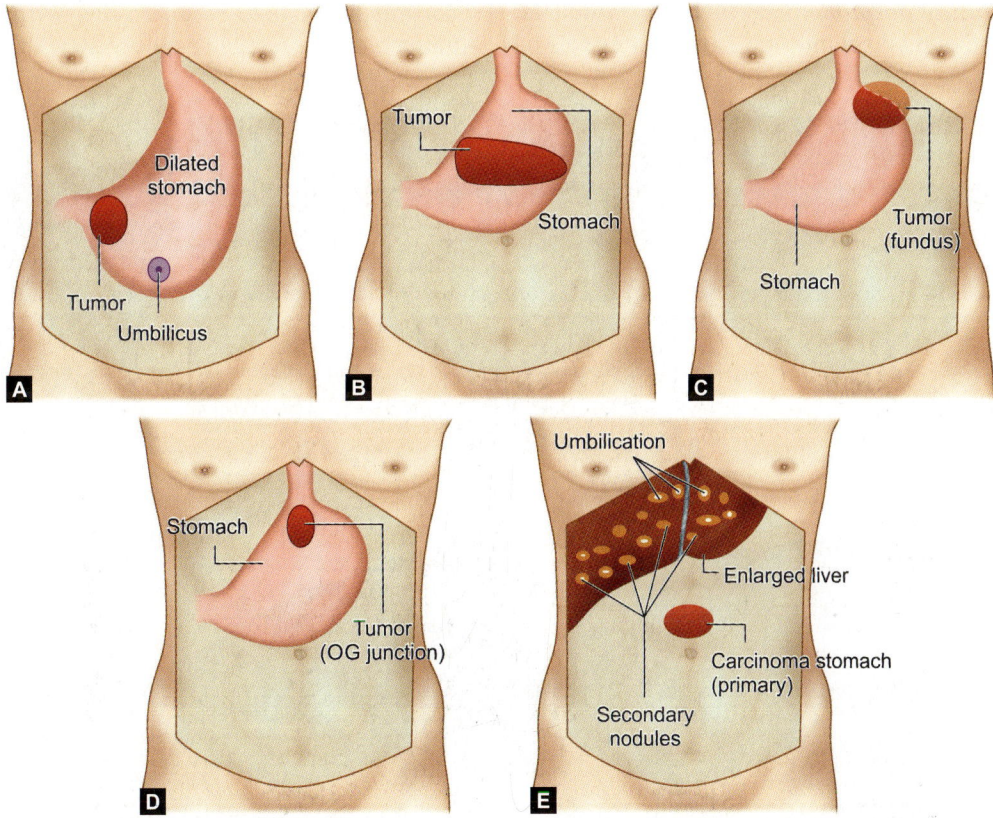

Figs. 23-26A to E *Carcinoma pylorus causes gastric outlet obstruction with palpable mass above the umbilicus.* Carcinoma body of stomach mainly presents as loss of appetite and decreased weight with horizontally placed stomach mass. Carcinoma from fundus of the stomach presents as mass abdomen with loss of appetite and weight. Carcinoma OG junction presents as dysphagia. Carcinoma stomach is one of the common causes of secondaries in liver.

margin—**hook sign** (refer Chapter 21, page 461) (Spleen is dull on percussion) **(Figs. 23-27A to E)**.

Palpation of Kidney/Loin Mass

If loin mass is present, it should be checked by **bimanual palpation**. Patient in lying down position, right kidney is examined from right side; left kidney from left side. Right hand is placed over the abdomen in front of lumbar region; left hand is placed behind the region. Fingers of both front and back hands are approximated to compress the loin. Mass if present is felt properly. Its size, shape, tenderness, surface, consistency, movement with respiration, mobility, medial extent should be checked.

Ballottability: It is again done for loin mass. Right hand fingers are placed in front; left hand fingers are placed behind. Left hand fingers are pushed forward from behind so as to push the loin mass forward. Examiner can appreciate that mass is moving forward and touching his fingers in front. Ballottability of kidney is due to soft perinephric pad of fat and pedicle on the medial side on which kidney moves/rotates. Kidney mass is bimanually palpable and ballottable. If there is adhesions due to perinephric inflammation or renal cell carcinoma infiltrating the perinephric tissues, kidney will be only bimanually palpable but not ballottable.

Kidneys are normally not palpable. When kidney is enlarged, it will be **bimanually palpable, may be ballottable** (left hand from behind is pushed anteriorly and kidney can be felt moving forward and touching/ pushing the right hand in front), moves with respiration (as it is related to diaphragm), vertically placed with resonant colonic band in front because of medial and anterior push of the colon by enlarged kidney. It is smooth and soft in hydronephrosis; hard and nodular in carcinoma kidney; firm, nodular and bilateral in polycystic kidney disease. Hand can be insinuated between upper part of the mass and right costal margin. It usually does not cross the midline (to opposite side).

Murphy's kidney punch is eliciting tenderness in renal angle in *sitting position* from behind. In sitting position from behind loin should be inspected for any fullness. **Renal angle** tenderness is elicited using thumb pressing at the angle (renal angle is between erector spinae muscle and 12th rib). Renal angle also should be percussed to look for any change in note. Normally it is resonant on percussion because of the ascending/descending colon, which the enlarged kidney displace it making it dull on percussion **(Figs. 23-28 to 23-30)**.

Note: Renal mass looses all its features once it is fixed and advanced. Intraperitoneal mass once adherent posteriorly to retroperitoneum behaves clinically like a retroperitoneal mass.

Small Bowel Mass

It is felt as mobile, localized mass with resonant or impaired resonant note. It does not move with respiration. In intussusception sausage-shaped mass with concavity towards

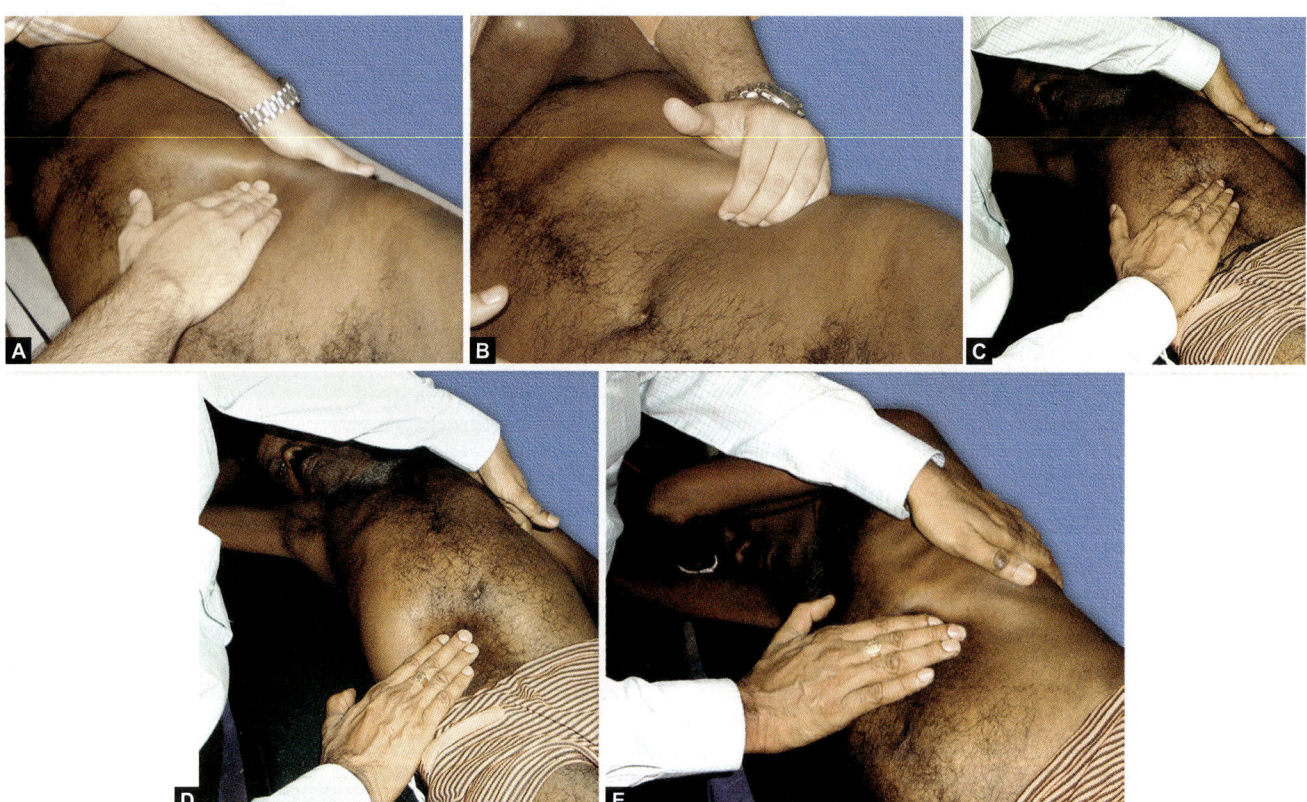

Figs. 23-27 to E Method of palpating spleen and also eliciting hook sign.

Chapter 23: Approaches and Clinical Examination of Mass Abdomen

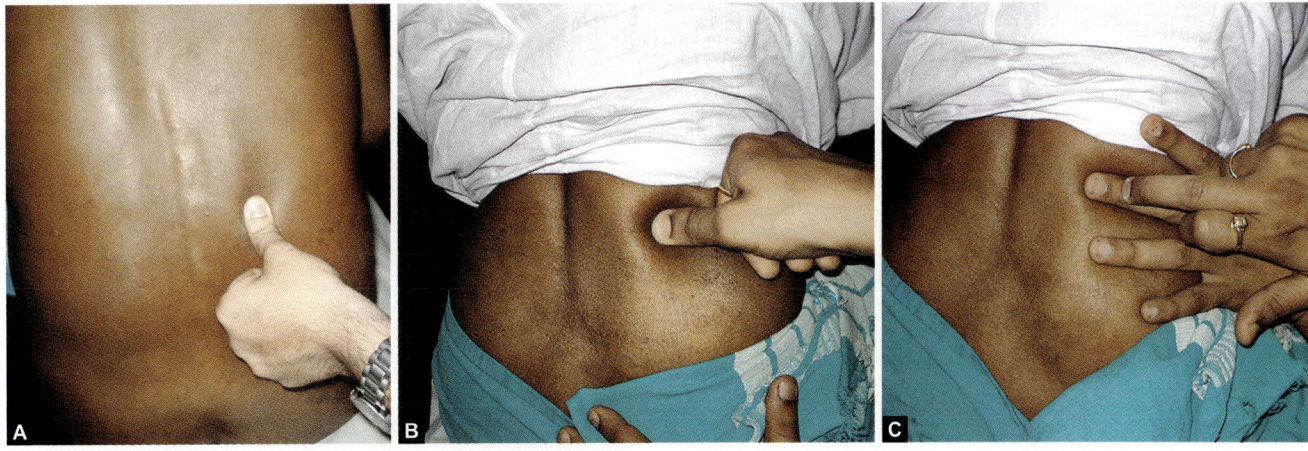

Figs. 23-28A to C Renal angle should be palpated and percussed in a kidney mass—*in sitting position.*

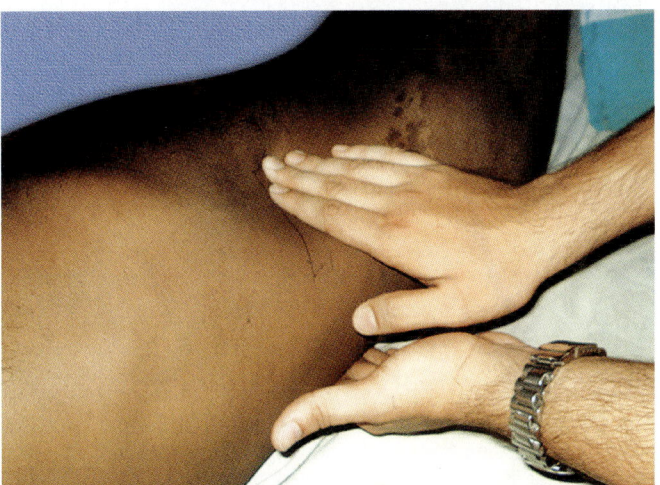

Fig. 23-29 Palpation for kidney mass—*for ballottability and bimanual palpation.*

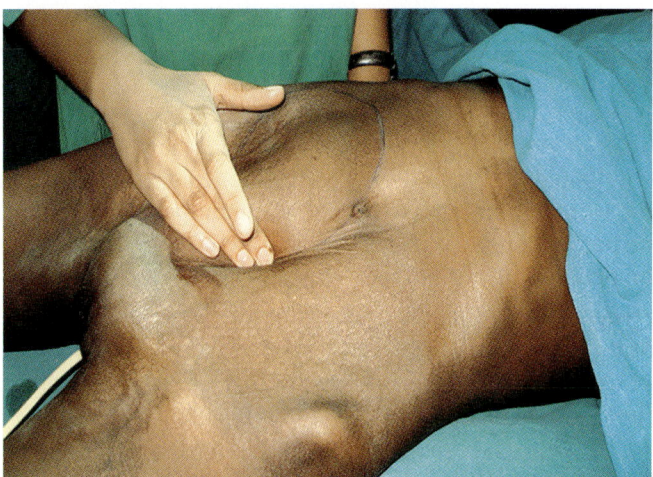

Fig. 23-31 Palpating the lower border of the mass is very important in lower abdominal masses. *Bladder should be emptied or catheterized before palpation.*

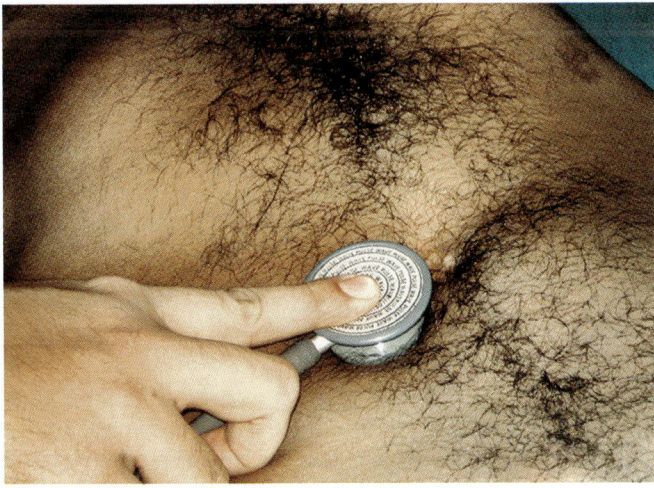

Fig. 23-30 *Renal bruit* should be auscultated.

umbilicus is palpable. It appears and disappears and contracts under the palpating finger.

Note: *All masses in the lower quadrants should be palpated after emptying bladder or passing a urinary catheter.* Upper border is clearly felt but not lower border which merges into the pelvis. Mass also should be *bimanually palpable* by placing fingers in rectum or vagina (**Fig. 23-31**).

Examination of External Genitalia

External genitalia should be examined for any swelling or loss of testicular sensation or secondary hydrocele. Hernia orifices should be examined for cough impulse and any swellings.

Often there may be more than one mass in the abdomen. So when one mass is felt always look for **other relevant masses.**

Retroperitoneal Masses

Retroperitoneal masses and pulsatile mass like aneurysms should be examined in knee-elbow/knee-chest position. Retroperitoneal mass will not fall forward whereas intra-abdominal mass will fall forward. **Aortic aneurysm** with **expansile pulsation** will retain its pulsation whereas mass with **transmitted pulsation** will show reduced/absent pulsation in knee elbow position (**Figs. 23-32A to C**).

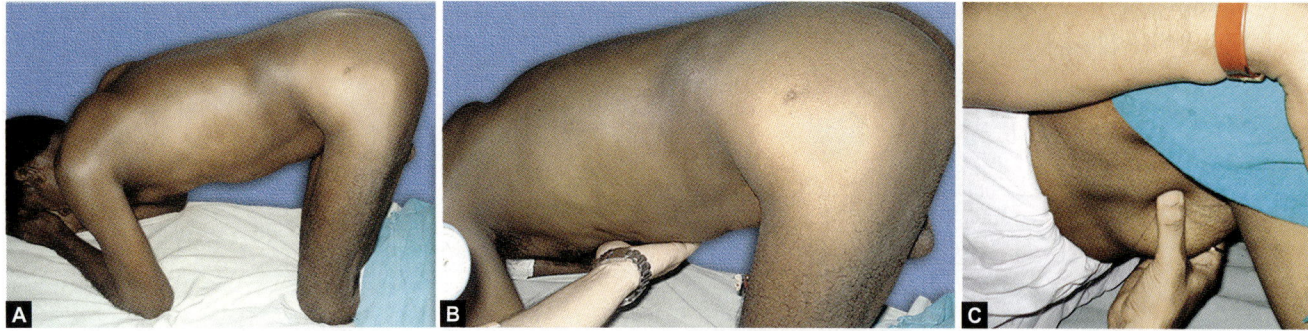

Figs. 23-32A to C *Knee elbow position*—palpation of retroperitoneal mass. Mass can be held to check mobility, relations.

Percussion

Liver dullness should be assessed by percussion. It is done by percussing from above downwards over right intercostal spaces in midclavicular line. Liver span also can be assessed by this **(Fig. 23-33)**.

Percussion over the mass is very important **(Fig. 23-34)**. Mass in front of the bowel is dull on percussion like parietal/abdominal wall mass, liver, spleen, gallbladder, etc. Mass from the stomach/small bowel/colon shows impaired resonance on percussion. Mass from retroperitoneum shows resonance on percussion.

Hydatid thrill is elicited using three fingers. Index, middle and ring fingers are placed over the liver mass with gaps between each fingers. Percussion is done over the middle finger to feel the fluid thrill over other two fingers.

Percussion for free fluid: Shifting dullness—with patient in supine position, percussion is done over the epigastrium initially to confirm resonant note. The percussion is then continued towards symphysis pubis; then from center of abdomen towards one side flank till the dull note is heard. Patient is tilted towards opposite side to make area of percussion directed upwards and also to displace any fluid from that side. After 1-2 minutes (time to allow fluid to shift towards opposite side) without removing the fingers same area is percussed to get resonant note which confirms the presence of fluid. The percussion is repeated by turning the patient to opposite side **(Figs. 23-35A to D)**. At least 1 liter of free fluid must be present in the abdomen to get positive shifting dullness. In massive ascites, fluid is confirmed by ***eliciting fluid thrill***. Patient is asked to place his hand over the epigastrium with ulnar side of the hand pressed firmly in midline. Examiner should keep his one hand over one lumbar region of the patient and with fingers of other hand, opposite lumbar region is tapped to elicit fluid movement as ***fluid thrill***. Very small quantity of fluid can be detected in knee elbow position. In this position, umbilical site is percussed to elicit dullness which signifies positive ***puddle sign***—*signifying minimal ascites*. At least 100 ml of free fluid need to be present for the puddle sign to be positive **(Figs. 23-36 and 23-37)**.

Percussion over renal angle is done to look for resonance (normal) or dullness (abnormal). Normal renal angle is occupied by ascending (right) or descending (left) colon and

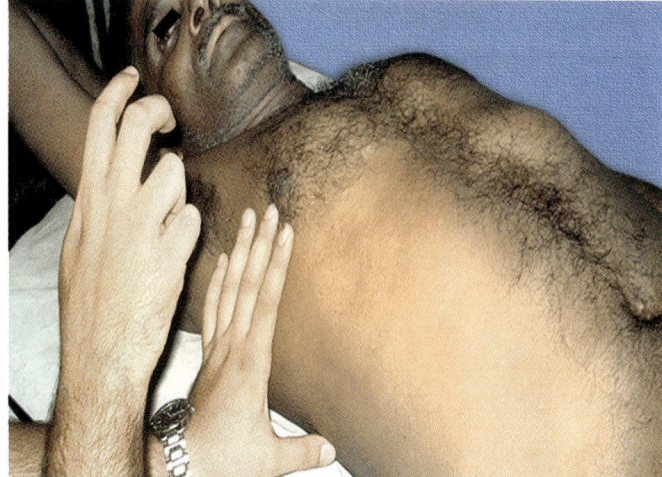

Fig. 23-33 *Liver dullness should be assessed* (upper border of liver) by percussing from above downwards in intercostal spaces in midclavicular line and space is marked.

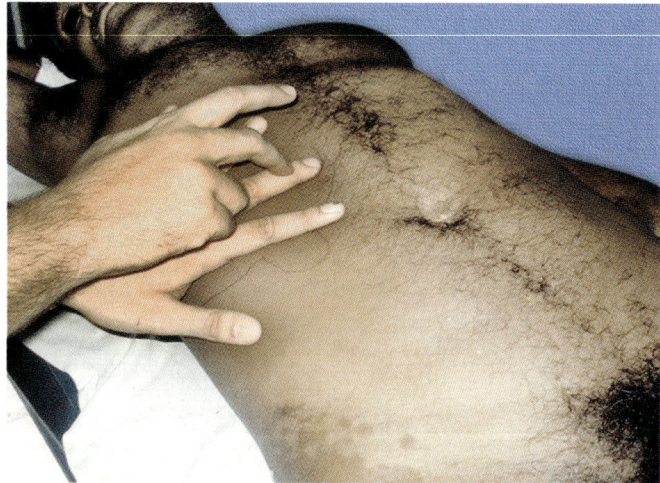

Fig. 23-34 *Percussion over the mass is essential* to say whether mass is anterior to bowel (dull); from the bowel (impaired resonant) or behind the bowel (resonant).

is resonant. When kidney is enlarged, it pushes the colon in front and medially thereby replacing it and so becomes dull on percussion. Renal angle is examined in sitting position between 12th rib and erector spinae muscle (Renal angle should be examined for fullness, tenderness, percussion note).

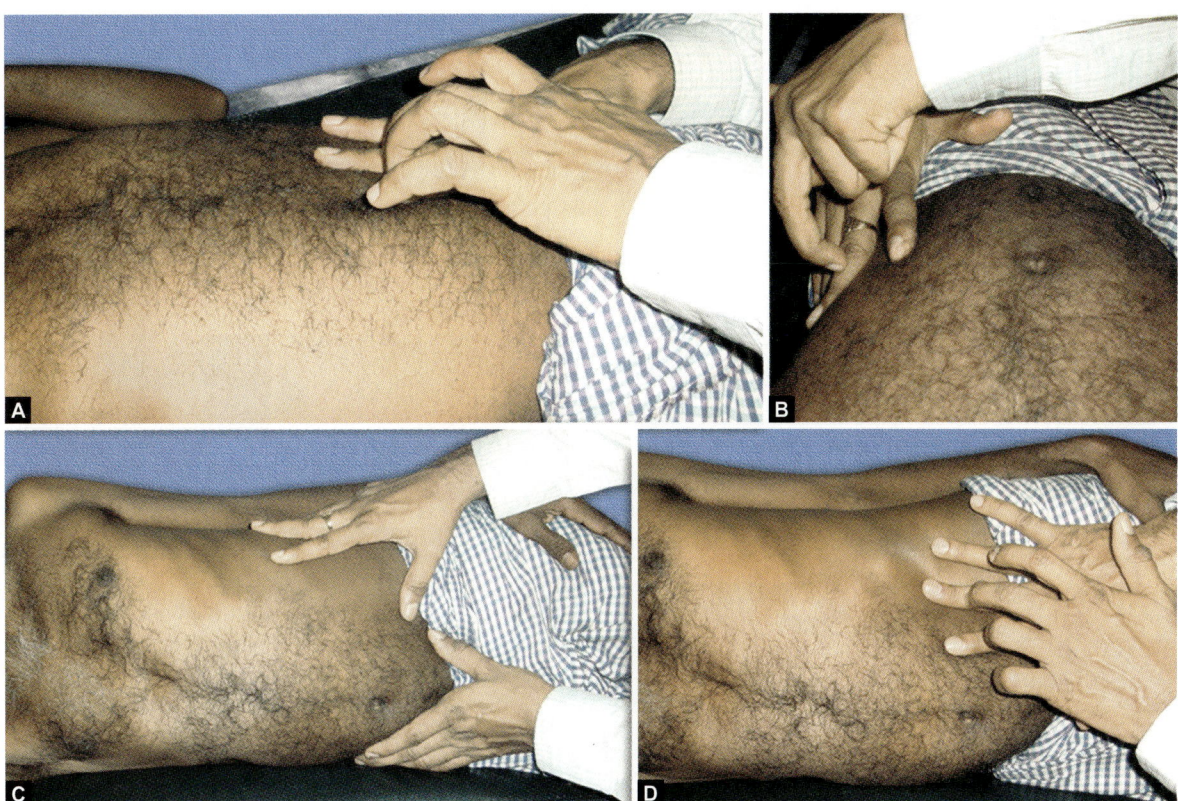

Figs. 23-35A to D Confirming ascites/free fluid in the peritoneal cavity by percussion—*classical method.*

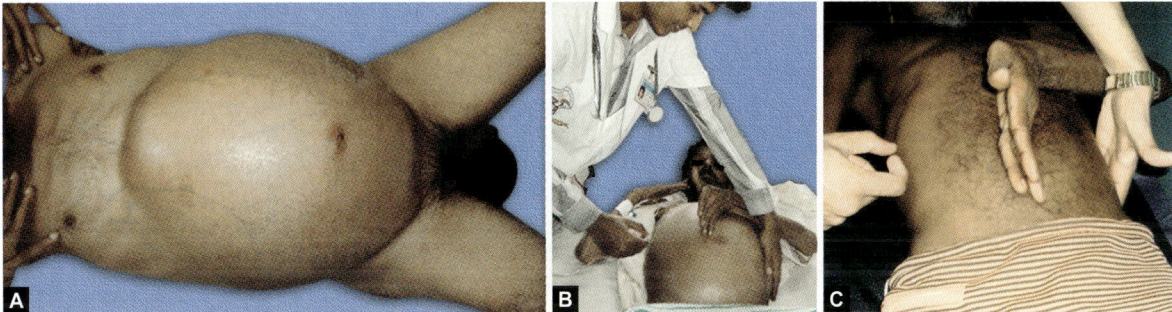

Figs. 23-36A to C Massive ascites. *Eliciting fluid thrill in massive ascites.*

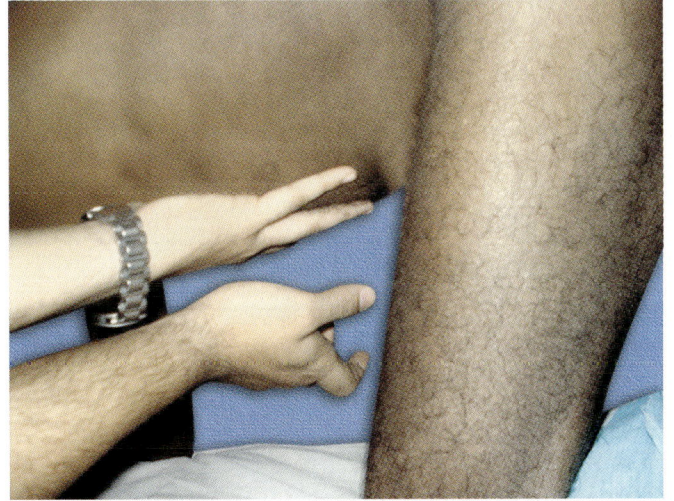

Fig. 23-37 Looking for minimal ascites in knee—elbow position—*Puddle sign.*

Auscultation

It is done to hear bowel sounds, bruit over the renal artery just to the side of the umbilicus, over the mass like liver which signifies vascularity, bruit over aneurysm.

Other Relevant Examination

Examination of hernial orifices and external genitalia: To rule out hernia; testis is palpated for enlargement and loss of testicular sensation (in testicular tumors) (**Fig. 23-38**).

Left supraclavicular fossa should be palpated for Virchow's node enlargement—*Troisier's sign*—as secondary deposits.

Axillary group of lymph nodes are examined as they drain the upper part of anterior abdominal wall and umbilicus. *Inguinal group of lymph nodes* are to be examined as they drain the lower part of the anterior abdominal wall and umbilicus.

Examination of respiratory system for effusion, altered breath sounds suggestive of metastases.

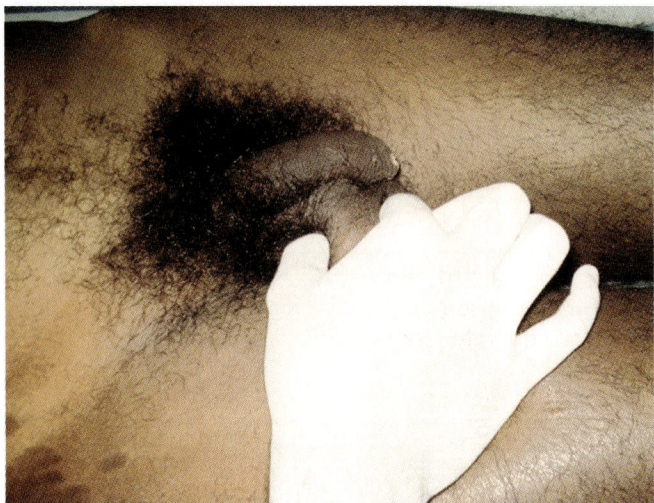

Fig. 23-38 External genitalia should be *palpated for mass/hydrocele*.

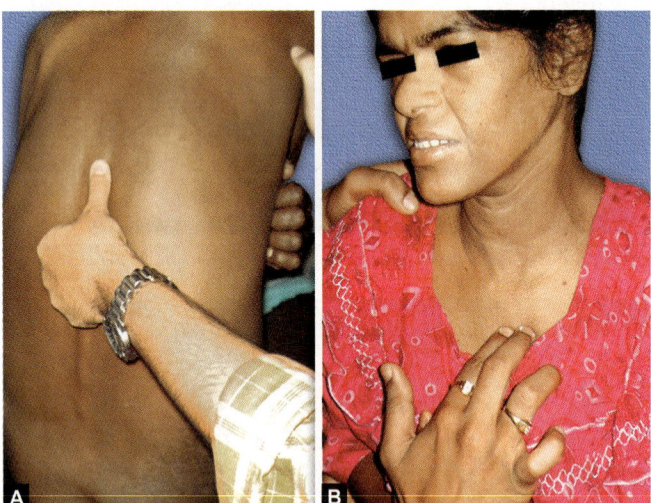

Figs. 23-39A and B *Spine and other skeletal system* should be examined in patient with mass abdomen.

Examination of skeletal system—sternum, spine, skull and other bones for tenderness, swelling, pathological fracture, neurological deficits (**Figs. 23-39A and B**).

Digital Examination of Rectum (Per Rectal Examination)

Per rectal examination (P/R) must be done in all cases of abdominal mass. It is done with patient in left lateral position with right leg flexed completely and left leg kept straight. Procedure is done after informing patient about the technique and taking consent. Xylocaine jelly is applied over the anus. It is inspected for discharge, opening, skin changes and swelling. Pulp of the gloved right index finger is gently pushed into the anorectum in the direction of the umbilicus. Sphincter tone is assessed. Posteriorly sacral curvature, rectal mucosa are assessed. Finger is turned towards front. Prostate, its texture, size, median groove are felt. Rectum is palpated for any growth, stricture or secondary nodule in front above (as a hard nodule with free rectal mucosa—*Blumer shelf*). Gently finger is removed and fingertip should be inspected for content staining—blood/mucous/pus, etc. (**Figs. 23-40A to C**). P/R is contraindicated in acute fissure in ano.

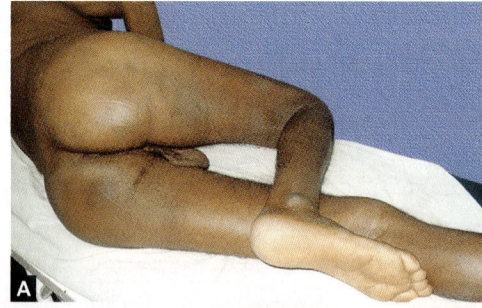

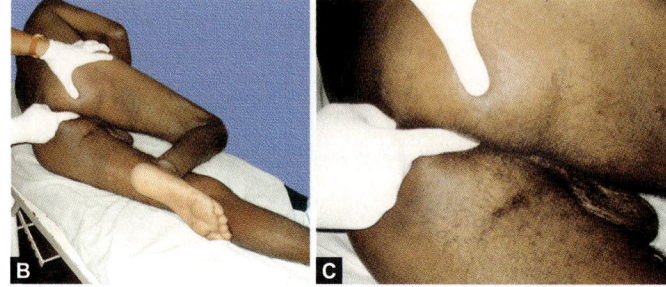

Figs. 23-40A to C Digital examination of the rectum is important (P/R; Per rectal examination).

Per Vaginal Examination

It is done whenever pelvic mass is suspected with lower margin of the mass merging into the pelvis. Bimanual palpation is often done under general anesthesia in lower abdominal masses.

■ DIFFERENTIAL DIAGNOSIS

Mass in any quadrant should be assessed first whether it is in the abdominal wall or intra-abdominal or retroperitoneal. From which specific organ mass is arising should be ascertained. Pathological nature of the mass must be assessed. So, initially *anatomical diagnosis* is made and later *pathological diagnosis* is thought of, finally the *final diagnosis is concluded.*

MASS IN THE RIGHT HYPOCHONDRIUM	
Parietal swellings	*Intra-abdominal swellings*
• Sebaceous cyst, lipoma, neurofibroma, cold abscess (from ribs or spine, presents as soft, fluctuant nontender well-localized swelling), liver abscess or subphrenic abscess rupturing into the abdominal wall presenting as parietal wall abscess	• Liver: Congenital Riedel's lobe; amoebic hepatitis or liver abscess, portal pyemia or pyogenic liver abscess, gumma of liver (large smooth hard hepatomegaly), hydatid cyst of the liver, hepatocellular carcinoma (HCC), secondaries in liver, early cirrhosis of liver or macronodular type. • **Gallbladder:** Mucocele, empyema, carcinoma, due to malignant CBD obstruction. • **Subphrenic** abscess • **Pylorus** of the stomach and duodenum • **Hepatic flexure** of the colon: Carcinoma; inflammatory mass • **Right kidney:** RCC, hydronephrosis • **Right adrenal gland**

Palpable Liver Mass as Mass in Right Hypochondrium

It is horizontally placed; usually moves with respiration; upper border is not felt; it is dull on percussion; (this dullness continuous over liver dullness above); fingers cannot be insinuated under right costal margin.

Conditions where liver gets enlarged:
1. *Soft, smooth, nontender liver:*
   a. Hydrohepatosis: It is due to obstruction of CBD causing dilatation of intrahepatic biliary radicles (usually malignant CBD obstruction but can occur in obstruction due to stones).
   b. Congestive cardiac failure.
   c. Hydatid cyst of the liver: Here mass is well localized in the liver with typical hydatid thrill (Three fingers are placed over the mass widely. When central finger is tapped fluid movement elicited is felt in lateral two fingers) (Figs. 23-41A and B).
   d. Congenital Riedel's lobe is a tongue shaped projection from the lower border of the right lobe of the liver. It is often mistaken for enlarged gallbladder but is wider, flat and not spherical.
2. *Soft, smooth, tender liver:*
   a. Amoebic liver abscess: Here liver often gets adherent to the anterior abdominal wall and will not move with respiration. Intercostal tenderness and right sided pleural effusion is common. History of amoebic dysentery few months before may or may not be there. Fevers, referred pain in right shoulder, pallor, mild jaundice, elevation of upper border of the liver are the features. Subcutaneous pitting edema in right hypochondrium is often very significant. X-ray will reveal the elevated diaphragm with pleural effusion. Amoebic hepatitis: Liver will be tender, smooth, soft or firm (Fig. 23.42).
   b. Viral hepatitis also causes smooth, soft, tender liver. Patient develops multiple joint pains in viral hepatitis.
   c. Portal pyemia: It causes tender soft liver with toxemia, jaundice.
3. *Hard, smooth liver:*
   a. Hepatoma (HCC): Here a large, single, hard nodule is palpable in the liver. But occasionally there can be multiple nodules when it is multicentric. Rapidly growing tumor can also be soft. Hepatoma often can also be tender due to tumor necrosis or stretching of the liver capsule. Vascular bruit may be heard over the liver during auscultation. It mimics amoebic liver abscess in every respect.
   b. Solitary secondary in liver: It is not common but can occur (when primary is in colon); features of primary tumor may be present.
4. *Hard liver with multiple nodules:*
   a. Multiple secondaries in liver: Hard nodules here have umbilication which is due to central necrosis.
   b. Macronodular cirrhotic liver or early cirrhosis.

Causes for massive liver enlargement: Gummatous liver (*Hepar lobatum*); secondaries in liver from melanoma; often large hepatoma. Melanoma especially primary from choroids can cause secondaries in liver as late as 15 years after therapy (surgery) for primary.

Palpable Gallbladder in Right Hypochondrium

It is smooth and soft (except in carcinoma gallbladder); mobile horizontally (side-to-side); moves with respiration; located in lateral margin of the right rectus muscle, below the right costal margin or below the lower margin of the palpable liver; dull on percussion.

Conditions where gallbladder is palpable.
1. *Soft, nontender gallbladder*:
   a. Mucocele of the gallbladder.
   b. Enlarged gallbladder in obstructive jaundice due to carcinoma head of the pancreas or periampullary carcinoma or growth in the CBD.

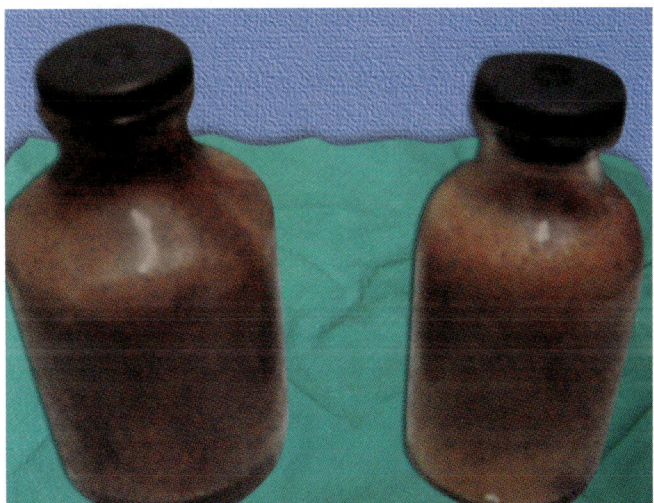

Fig. 23-42 *Anchovy sauce pus* in amoebic liver abscess.

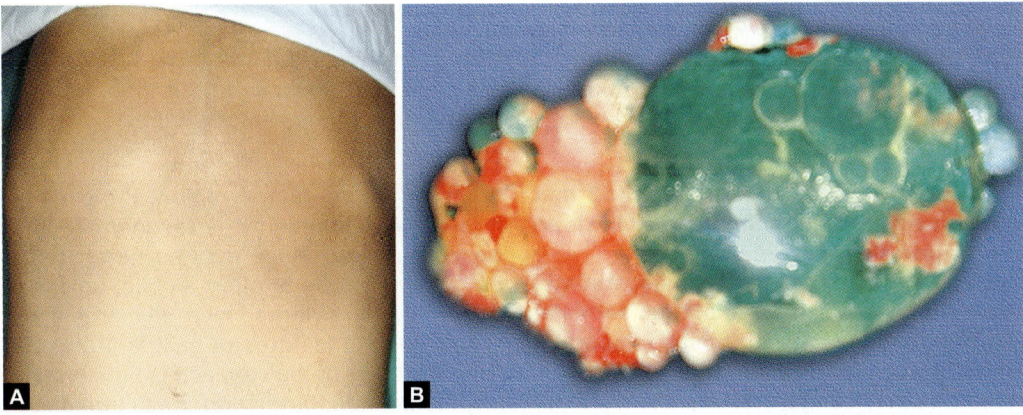

Figs. 23-41A and B *Hydatid cyst of liver*—fullness in right hypochondrium. Operated specimen of hydatid in same patient.

2. *Hard gallbladder:* Carcinoma gallbladder.
3. *Smooth, tender, soft or firm gallbladder mass:* Empyema gallbladder, acute cholecystitis mass.

Other Masses in the Right Hypochondrium

a. Pericholecystic inflammatory mass: It is tender, smooth, firm or soft, not mobile, intra-abdominal mass often with guarding.
b. Mass arising from upper pole of the kidney: It may be due to renal cell carcinoma or hydronephrosis.
c. Adrenal tumor may be pheochromocytoma or adrenocortical carcinoma. It is nonmobile; does not move with respiration; extends medially; often crosses midline; fluctuating hypertension is common. Renal angle is normal and resonant. In children, it could be neuroblastoma. Such neuroblastoma may cause secondaries in skull.

Surgical Jaundice

Causes: Biliary atresia; choledochal cyst; CBD stones; ascending cholangitis; biliary strictures; sclerosing cholangitis; carcinoma of head and periampullary region of the pancreas; cholangiocarcinoma; Klat skin tumor (Carcinoma at the confluence of hepatic ducts above the level of the cystic duct and so will cause hydrohepatosis without GB enlargement); extrinsic compression of CBD by lymph nodes or tumors; parasitic infestations.

> **Courvoisier's Law:**
> 'In a patient with jaundice if there is palpable gallbladder, it is not due to stones'.
>
> In obstruction due to CBD stone, gallbladder does not distend because it is chronically inflamed, thickened and fibrotic.
>
> In malignancy, like carcinoma of head of the pancreas or periampullary carcinoma, gallbladder will be distended and palpable to the right of rectus muscle in the right hypochondrium, as nontender, globular, smooth, soft, dull mass which moves with respiration and with horizontal mobility. *Exceptions for the rule are*—absence of gallbladder; intrahepatic gallbladder; previous cholecystectomy; double impacted stone; large stone in Hartman's pouch.

Classification of Causes of Obstructive Jaundice

Congenital: Biliary atresia, choledochal cyst
Inflammatory: Ascending cholangitis, sclerosing cholangitis.
Obstructive: CBD stones.
Neoplastic: Carcinoma of head or periampullary region of pancreas, cholangiocarcinomas, Klat skin tumor.
Extrinsic compression of CBD by lymph nodes or tumors.

Portal Hypertension

Sustained raise of portal pressure more than 12 mm Hg. Isolated splenic vein thrombosis causes left sided sinistral/segmental portal hypertension. Causes are: (a) Prehepatic—portal/splenic vein thrombosis, trauma, periportal inflammation, hypercoagulable status, neonatal umbilical sepsis. (b) Hepatic (80%)—cirrhosis, idiopathic, primary biliary cirrhosis, hepatitis, schistosomiasis, Wilson's disease, hemochromatosis, congenital hepatic fibrosis. (c) Post-hepatic—Budd-Chiari syndrome, constrictive pericarditis, veno-occlusive disease, congestive cardiac failure. Presentations: Esophageal varices (hematemesis/melena), splenomegaly, ascites, jaundice, features of encephalopathy. Investigations: Gastroscopy, LFT, splenoportography, US abdomen, CT abdomen, prothrombin time, liver biopsy.

Pugh's modification of Child's Grading

	Child A	**B**	**C**
Bilirubin	<2.0 mg	2.0–3.0 mg	>3.0 mg
Albumin	>3.5	3.0–3.5	<3.0
Ascites	None	Controlled	Uncontrollable
Mental status	Normal	Disoriented	Coma
Nutrition	Very good	Good	Poor
Score	5–6	7–9	10–15
Prothrombin time	Increased up to 3	Increased between 3–6	Increased >6

MASS IN THE EPIGASTRIUM

Parietal swellings	Intra-abdominal mass (Fig. 23-43)
• Sebaceous cyst, lipoma, neurofibroma, cold abscess (from ribs or spine, presents as soft, fluctuant nontender well-localized swelling), liver abscess or subphenic abscess rupturing into the abdominal wall presenting as parietal wall abscess. Abscess in left lobe of liver rupturing into parietal wall • **Epigastric hernia**—specific	• Left lobe of the liver—abscess, hepatoma, secondaries • Stomach—congenital pyloric stenosis, carcinoma, gastric ulcer perforation forming an abscess in the lesser sac, carcinoma of stomach, leiomyoma of stomach • Transverse colon mass • Omental mass • Pancreatic mass • Lymph nodal mass • Aortic aneurysm • Retroperitoneal swellings like cyst, sarcoma, teratoma

Palpable Left Lobe of the Liver

It lies in the epigastric region; its upper border cannot be felt; It moves with respiration; It extends towards left hypochondriac region; It is dull on percussion. When amoebic liver abscess occurs in left lobe, it gets adherent to anterior abdominal wall, mass will not move with respiration and is immobile, causes edema of the abdominal wall and is dull on percussion. Occasionally bowel may interpose between liver and abdominal wall making it resonant and feel like a retroperitoneal mass.

Conditions where left lobe of the liver is palpable. Hepatoma, amoebic liver abscess in left lobe, left lobe secondaries, hydatid cyst of the left lobe.

Features of Stomach Mass

It lies in the epigastric region; It moves with respiration; It is intra-abdominal; It is resonant or impaired resonant on percussion; Mass may be better felt on standing or on walking; Mass is often mobile, unless it gets adherent posteriorly; In pylorus mass, all margins are well felt which is mobile with features of gastric outlet obstruction; Mass from the body of the stomach is horizontally placed without any features of obstruction; Mass from the upper part of the stomach near the O-G junction causes dysphagia. Mass from

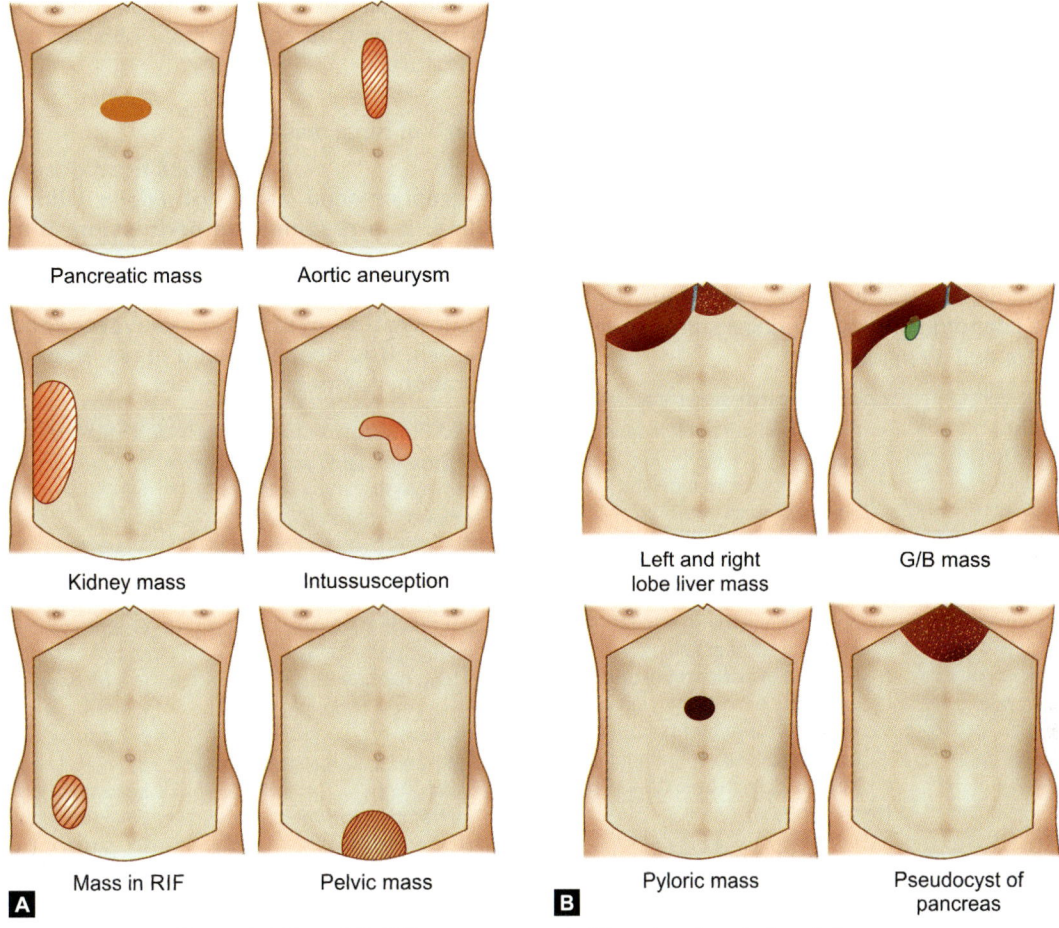

Figs. 23-43A and B Different masses at different regions in the abdomen.

the fundus of the stomach is in the upper part of the epigastric region towards left side. Carcinoma stomach is nodular and hard. It is commonest cause for stomach mass. Leiomyoma of stomach is smooth and firm.

Pseudocyst of the Pancreas

Mass lies in the epigastric region which is smooth, soft, does not move with respiration, not mobile, resonant on percussion. It can be tender if it gets infected, has got transmitted pulsation. It is confirmed by placing the patient in knee-elbow position. Lower border is well felt but upper border is not clear.

Baid test: Because stomach is pushed forwards, Ryle's tube when passed, can be felt per abdomen on palpation.

Pseudocyst of the pancreas is quite common condition. It has got a false capsule (not true capsule) as there is no epithelial lining. It usually occurs in 3 weeks after an attack of acute pancreatitis. Lesser sac is the commonest site. It also can occur in relation to duodenum, jejunum, splenic hilum and colon. It can be of communicating and noncommunicating type. It often mimics aortic aneurysm, retroperitoneal cystic tumors, cystadenocarcinoma of pancreas.

Cystadenocarcinoma of the Pancreas

Mass is smooth, firm, does not move with respiration, not mobile, resonant on percussion. Patient also has back pain.

Colonic Mass

It is commonly due to carcinoma of transverse colon but can be due to intussusception, hyperplastic tuberculosis, and diverticulitis. It is mobile, horizontally placed, nodular, hard mass which does not move with respiration; Cecum will be dilated and palpable; It is resonant or impaired resonant on percussion; Patient will be having bowel symptoms, loss of appetite and decreased weight as seen in tuberculosis, carcinoma. Ileocolic intussusception is the commonest type.

Para-aortic Lymph Node Mass

Presents as mass in the epigastric region which is deeply placed, not mobile, not moving with respiration. It is vertically placed above the *level of the umbilicus* and resonant on percussion. Causes for enlargement are: *Secondaries, lymphomas or tuberculosis.*

Aortic Aneurysm

It is smooth, soft, pulsatile (expansile pulsation which is confirmed by placing the patient in knee-elbow position or in lateral position. Pulsation persists even in knee-elbow position; whereas transmitted pulsation disappears or decreases in intensity). It is vertically placed above the level of the umbilicus, not mobile, not moving with respiration and resonant on percussion.

Omental Mass

Omentum gets thickened with nodules and irregular surface. Omental mass moves with respiration, has nodular surface, firm in consistency, dull on percussion. Often lower margin is rolled up which is a feature of tuberculosis (Rolling is due to fibrosis). Omentum may get involved in malignancy as secondaries or in inflammatory conditions as part of inflammatory mass. Omentum is the usual component of any composite mass.

Enlarged Spleen

Spleen has to enlarge three times to be palpated clinically. It enlarges towards the right iliac fossa from left costal margin. It moves with respiration, mobile, obliquely placed, smooth, soft or firm, with a notch on the superior margin near anterior end. Fingers cannot be insinuated over the upper border. It enlarges downwards, inwards and forwards. '**Hook sign' is positive**, i.e one cannot insinuate the fingers under the left costal margin. It is dull on percussion.

Intussusception	Carcinoma transverse colon
• Ileocolic type is the commonest • Red currant jelly • Mass appears and disappears • Smooth, firm sausage shaped mass around the umbilicus with concavity towards umbilicus • Empty right iliac fossa • Mass contracts under the palpating fingers	• Anemia, loss of appetite and weight • Alternate constipation and diarrhea • Palpable mass in the epigastrium or umbilical region (upper part)—nodular, hard, impaired resonant, does not move with respiration, mobile in all directions • Features of obstruction/closed loop obstruction when *ileocecal valve* is incompetent • Ascites, liver secondaries later • Colonoscopy proves the diagnosis
Colonic tuberculosis	**Inflammatory conditions like diverticulitis**
• Usually hyperplastic type • Loss of appetite and weight • Irregular mass often adherent and nonmobile • Impaired resonant • Ascites, doughy abdomen may be present • Difficult to differentiate clinically from carcinoma • Colonoscopy confirms the condition	• Pain, bowel symptoms • Mass which is tender, firm, nonmobile • Often it is a composite mass lesion comprised of small bowel, omentum • May be adherent to abdominal wall • Pericolic abscess, internal fistula may be the presentation

MASS IN THE LEFT HYPOCHONDRIUM	
Parietal swellings • Sebaceous cyst, lipoma, neurofibroma, cold abscess (from ribs or spine, presents as soft, fluctuant nontender well localized swelling), liver abscess or subphrenic abscess rupturing into the abdominal wall presenting as parietal wall abscess	**Intraabdominal and retroperitoneal mass** • Splenomegaly—malaria, kala-azar, hereditary splenomegaly, idiopathic thrombocytopenic purpura (ITP), hemolytic anemias, lymphoma, porphyria, splenic cysts (rare) • Splenic flexure of colon—carcinoma • Tail of the pancreas—pseudocyst, tumor • Left subphrenic space • Left kidney—hydronephrosis, renal cell carcinoma (RCC), polycystic disease • Left adrenal gland tumor

Left sided colonic mass (splenic flexure): It is mobile, nodular, resonant, and does not move with respiration. It is commonly due to carcinoma colon. Bowel symptoms like diarrhea, tenesmus, constipation, intestinal obstruction, may be a feature.

Left renal mass from upper pole of any cause: It has got features of renal mass.

Left sided adrenal mass: It does not move with respiration. It is deeply placed mass, not mobile. Often it crosses the midline. It is resonant on percussion. It mimics kidney mass.

Mass arising from the tail of the pancreas: It could be pseudocyst or cystadenoma/cystadenocarcinoma of pancreas. It is deeply placed mass, does not move with respiration, nonmobile, resonant.

Splenic mass	Renal mass
• Enlarges towards umbilicus and right iliac fossa— inwards, forwards, outwards • Moves with respiration—well • Splenic notch **on the superior border** anterior end • Smooth, firm, dull on percussion • Felt on palpation • Renal angle is normal and resonant • Not bimanually palpable nor ballottable • Cannot insinuate/hook under left costal margin	• Enlarges downwards towards left iliac fossa • Moves with respiration—slightly • No notch is felt • Colonic band of resonance in front • Felt on deep palpation • Renal angle is full; dull on percussion; may be tender • Bimanually palpable and ballottable • Can insinuate fingers under left costal margin

Hereditary spherocytosis: It is an autosomal dominant disease effecting males and females equally. Here there is an increase in red cell permeability to sodium. So sodium leaks into the red cells by which it becomes spherical and more fragile. This leads to greater loss of membrane phospholipid resulting in weakening of the membrane with increase in energy and oxygen requirement. So these RBC's are destroyed in spleen causing hemolytic anemia, hemolytic jaundice, unconjugated hyperbilirubinemia, pigmented gallstones, cholangitis. Clinical features: Pallor, jaundice, recurrent fever, pain abdomen, splenomegaly, hepatomegaly, chronic leg ulcer. Gallstones are seen in 60% cases. Acute hemolytic crisis can occur. Investigations: Fragility test: Here increased fragility of the erythrocytes is the typical feature. Hemolysis occurs in 0.6% or in even stronger solutions. Reticulocyte count is increased significantly. Fecal urobilinogen is increased. Labeled radioactive chromium shows faster red cell destruction. US abdomen is done to look for gallstones, spleen, liver, CBD. Peripheral smear, hematocrit and LFT. Direct Coomb's test is negative.

Idiopathic thrombocytopenic purpura (ITP): It is development of *antiplatelet antibodies*, which damage patient's own platelets. *Clinical features:* Purpuric patches in skin (buttocks and limbs), mucous membrane (most common presenting sign); epistaxis; menorrhagia, hematuria; GIT bleeding; intracranial hemorrhage (most dangerous); splenomagaly (25%); *Hess tourniquet test* is positive (By applying sphygmomanometer and inflating for 10 minutes just below the systolic pressure causes more than 20 petechiae in cubital fossa in 3 cm circled area). *Differential diagnosis:* Other causes for purpura; increased capillary fragility; bone marrow suppression due to aplastic anemia; chemotherapy;

DIC; autoimmune diseases. *Investigations:* Bleeding time is increased; Clotting and prothrombin time are normal; Platelet count is decreased; Bone marrow biopsy reveals increased megakaryocytes; US shows splenomegaly only in 25% cases. *Types: Acute* is common in children. *Chronic* is common in adult. In children, spontaneous regression occurs in 75% of cases after one attack.

<u>Felty's syndrome:</u> Chronic rheumatoid arthritis; leucopenia; splenomegaly, recurrent infections, ulcers in leg and ankles, anorexia, lymphadenopathy are the features.

Palpable Kidney Mass

There will be fullness in the loin which is better observed in sitting position. Mass moves with respiration. It is vertically placed, bimanually palpable, and ballottable. Renal angle is dull on percussion (normally it is resonant due to colon). There is a band of resonance in front due to reflected colon. It does not cross the midline.

MASS IN THE LUMBAR REGION	
Parietal wall swellings	**Intra-abdominal swellings**
• Cold abscess in lumbar region may be due to Pott's disease • Lumbar hernia—impulse on coughing • Soft tissue tumors like anywhere	• Renal mass • Liver mass right side; splenic mass left side • Colonic mass • Gallbladder mass right side • Retroperitoneal masses

Conditions where kidney gets enlarged

<u>Hydronephrosis:</u> It is smooth, soft, lobulated, nontender mass.

<u>Pyonephrosis:</u> History of throbbing pain in the loin, pyuria and fever with chills. It is smooth, soft and tender kidney mass which is nonmobile due to inflammatory adhesion.

<u>Perinephric abscess:</u> Bulge in the loin; dullness on percussion; bending the trunk away from the side of the lesion; fever, tachycardia. *Mathe's sign*: In Intravenous Urography (IVU) imaging in standing and lying down positions show kidney to be in same position whereas in normal individual kidney will be lower in standing position than in lying down position.

<u>Polycystic kidney:</u> History of loin pain and hematuria. Present with hypertension, anemia and features of renal failure. Usually bilateral but one side presents early than the other side. It has lobulated, smooth surface.

<u>Renal cell carcinoma:</u> History of mass in the loin, hematuria, fever and dull pain. Mass is nodular and hard. It does not cross the midline.

Mass from the Ascending Colon on Right Side or Descending Colon on Left Side

History of altered bowel habits with decreased appetite and weight. Mass is nodular, hard which does not move with respiration and is not ballottable. It is resonant or impaired resonant on percussion. Renal angle is resonant. Proximal dilated bowel may be palpable.

Adrenal Mass

It is nodular and hard, does not move with respiration, not mobile and often crosses the midline. It is felt on deep palpation, resonant in front and not ballottable.

Retroperitoneal Tumors

They are not mobile, resonant and do not fall forward in knee-elbow position. They are deeply placed mass which are usually smooth and hard. They may be retroperitoneal sarcomas or teratomas, etc. Often retroperitoneal tumors attain large size. Inferior vena cava (IVC) compression is often seen causing dilated veins in the lateral abdominal wall with direction of blood flow upwards. They occupy many regions in the abdomen. Obstruction of ureters can cause hydronephrosis (Fig. 23-44).

Retroperitoneal Cysts

They are *smooth and soft* with the same features as retroperitoneal tumors. They often attain large size.

MASS IN THE UMBILICAL REGION	
Parietal swellings	**Intraabdominal and retroperitoneal mass**
• Umbilical adenoma • Umbilical hernia rectus sheath hematoma, abdominal wall abscess common in this region • Desmoid tumor	• Stomach and duodenum • Small intestine—tumor, intussusception, inflammatory • Mesenteric mass—cyst, tumor, nodal mass • Transverse colon • Omentum • Pancreas • Para-aortic nodes • Aorta and iliac arteries • Retroperitoneal swellings

> **Usual masses are:**
> Mesenteric cyst; Omental cyst; Ovarian cyst (Pedunculated); Small bowel tumors; Extension of masses from other region.

<u>Mesenteric Cyst:</u> Causes: Chylolymphatic; enterogenous; cysts of urogenital remnant; teratomatous dermoid cysts; Other causes: Traumatic hematoma and cyst formation, Tuberculous cold abscess of mesentery, Hydatid cyst of mesentery. *Chylolymphatic cysts* are the commonest one. It arises from congenitally misplaced lymphatic system. Common in ileum, is a thin walled cyst with flat endothelium, containing lymph or chyle which is either milky or cream colored. It is solitary and commonly unilocular with loop of the bowel in front. It has got independent blood supply, i.e. not from the adjacent bowel loop. So enucleation is done

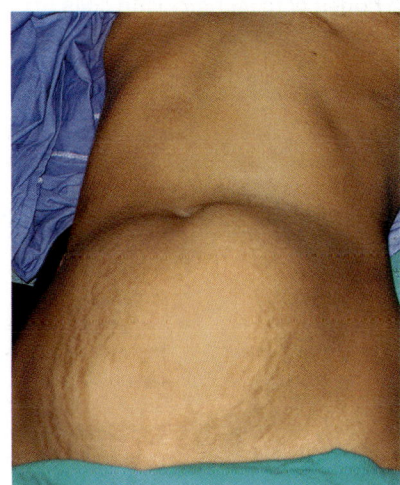

Fig. 23-44 Retroperitoneal tumor.

without resecting bowel. *Enterogenous type* arises as a diverticulum or duplication from the adjacent bowel. Hence, it is a thick walled cyst (contains all layers of the bowel) and receives its blood supply from the adjacent bowel (not independent). So resection of the adjacent bowel along with the cyst is essential. Enucleation is contraindicated. Clinical features: It is common in 2nd decade, often in childhood. It presents as painless abdominal swelling in umbilical region, smooth, fluctuant, not moving with respiration. It is mobile freely in the direction perpendicular to the line of mesentery. Line of attachment of the mesentery is an oblique line starting from a point 2.5 cm left of the midline and 1.0 cm below the transpyloric line extending downwards to the right iliac fossa at the junction of right lateral and transtubercular plane. There is a band of resonance in front of the cyst. Complications of mesenteric cysts: *Torsion of cyst* can lead to *volvulus* of the adjacent bowel; *Rupture of the cyst; Hemorrhage* into the cyst; *Infection:* Patient presents with acute painful swelling in umbilical region. *Differential diagnosis:* Hydronephrosis; omental cysts; tuberculosis.

> **Tillaux's triad:**
> - Soft fluctuant umbilical swelling
> - Freely mobile in a direction perpendicular to mesentery
> - Zone of resonance all around

Omental cyst: It is smooth, soft and nontender, moves with respiration, mobile in all directions, dull on percussion. Omentum may also get involved by tuberculosis (rolled up omentum), secondary deposits (irregular and hard), may form a composite mass.

Small bowel swellings: Small bowel lymphomas; Small bowel tumors/carcinomas; Intussusception.

Intussusception: Present as a mass in umbilical region usually towards left and above the umbilicus; occasionally towards right side. Mass is intra-abdominal, *sausage shaped*, well defined, smooth, firm and mobile. Mass does not move with respiration, contracts under palpating fingers. Often mass disappears and later reappears. Mass is resonant or impaired resonant on percussion. *'Red currant jelly'* stool with features of intestinal obstruction may be present.

Tuberculous mesenteric lymphadenitis (Tabes mesenterica): Matted lymph nodes of mesentery with coils of intestines can present as mass in umbilical region.

MASS IN THE RIGHT ILIAC FOSSA	
Parietal swellings	**Intraabdominal and retroperitoneal mass**
• Abdominal wall tumor • Abdominal wall abscess • Iliac abscess, appendicular abscess extending into the abdominal wall • Actinomycosis in right iliac fossa often extending into the abdominal wall and may form discharging sinuses with sulphur granules	• Appendicular mass or abscess • Carcinoma cecum • Ileocecal tuberculosis • Amoeboma • Psoas abscess • Lymph node mass either mesenteric or external iliac lymph nodes • Bony swellings • Ectopic kidney • Undescended testis (abdominal) • Actinomycosis

Appendicular Mass: It *is smooth or granular, firm, tender* mass in the right iliac fossa. It is formed by dilated ileum, omentum, inflammatory fluid and inflamed appendix which is often adherent to the abdominal wall. It is not mobile. It does not move with respiration. It is *resonant on percussion* (Fig. 23-45). It is well localized mass with distinct borders. It develops 3–4 days after an attack of acute appendicitis. Commonly with conservative treatment (*Ochsner Sherren*) regime) mass gradually reduces in size. Size of the mass should be marked out to observe the daily response. Occasionally if they don't respond for therapy, sepsis may progress leading to peritonitis or suppuration may occur causing appendicular abscess.

Appendicular abscess: It is smooth, *soft, tender and dull mass* in the right iliac fossa with indistinct borders. It is located on lower and outer aspect of the right iliac fossa. As pus has got tendency to come to surface in dependent position, it reflects the bowel towards periphery and so it is dull on percussion. Redness and abdominal wall edema is evident. Appendicular abscess need to be drained surgically.

Carcinoma cecum: It is nodular, hard mass in the right iliac fossa. It does not move with respiration. It is mobile but mobility may be restricted once it gets adherent to psoas major muscle behind. Mass is resonant or impaired resonant on percussion. Anemia, anorexia, loss of weight is common. Occasionally features of intestinal obstruction may be present. Carcinoma with pericolic abscess may present as tender firm smooth mass in the right iliac fossa. Fever, tachycardia are also the features. Barium enema X-ray/colonoscopy/carcinoembryonic antigen (CEA)/US abdomen are the investigations.

Ileocecal tuberculosis: Mass in the right iliac fossa which is smooth, hard, resonant and nontender; does not move with respiration and has restricted mobility; Cecum may be *pulled up* to lumbar region due to fibrosis. It is often clinically difficult to differentiate from carcinoma and ileocecal tuberculosis. Bowel symptoms, anemia with loss of appetite and weight is common. Barium studies, colonoscopy, CT abdomen are the investigations needed. Obstruction may be the presenting feature. Usually hyperplastic type of ileocecal tuberculosis present as mass in right iliac fossa.

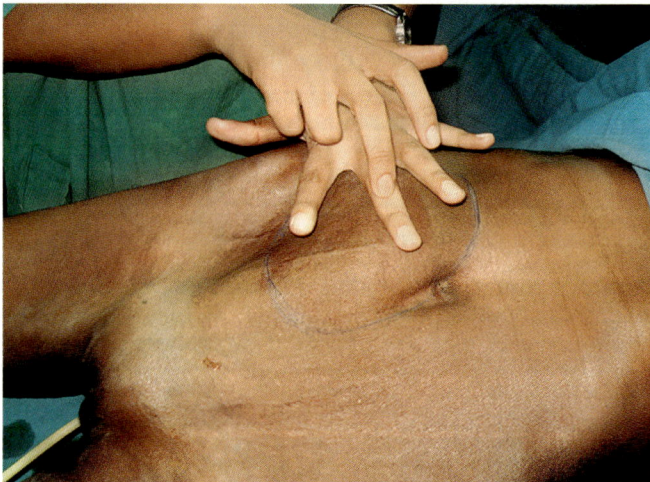

Fig. 23-45 *Percussion over the mass in right iliac fossa.* Retroperitoneal mass is resonant. Bowel mass is impaired resonant. Mass from abdominal wall is dull on percussion.

Amoeboma: History of dysentery with pain in the right iliac fossa may be present. Well defined palpable mass in the right iliac fossa which is smooth, hard, not mobile, may or may not be tender. It slowly increases in size and after certain period it stops progression. Initially features of ameobic typhlitis may be present. *Amoebic typhlitis* is inflammation of cecum due to *Entamoeba histolytica* infection. Tenderness over both iliac regions with thickening of colon is common. Amoebic typhlitis is usually associated with sigmoid amoebic colitis. Perforation, bleeding, stricture, paracolic abscess formation, ischiorectal abscess and fistula formation are the complications.

Crohn's disease or regional ileitis: It is a *granulomatous, noncaseating inflammatory condition of the ileum commonly* and *of the colon often.* Etiology: Unknown, but a familial and infective nature is thought of. Diet, food allergy, mycobacterium paratuberculosis are thought of. Pathology: Inflammation → Granuloma formation → Cicatrization → Thickening of the bowel wall → Adhesions → Fistula formation. Mesentery is thickened, edematous, with enlarged lymph glands which will never break nor calcify. Rarely jejunum, stomach and other parts of GIT are involved. In colon, it is commonly observed in cecum and ascending colon. Anal fissure is very common association. Clinical features: (a) *Acute presentations* (5%) of Crohn's disease mimics acute appendicitis with severe diarrhea. Often there will be localized or diffuse peritonitis. (b) *Chronic Crohn's: First stage*: Mild diarrhea, colicky pain, fever and tender, firm, nonmobile mass in right iliac fossa with recurrent perianal abscess. Anemia and diarrhea is usual. *Second stage:* is either acute or chronic intestinal obstruction due to cicatrization with narrowing. Steatorrhea, colitis, anemia, fissure in ano, fistula in ano is common. *Third stage:* Fistula formation—enterocolic, enteroenteric, enterovesical, enterocutaneous, etc. Crohn's disease is independent of age, sex, social and economic status and geographic area. It is familial. It is *precancerous condition but not as much as ulcerative colitis.* Investigations: *Barium meal follow through* shows: Straightening of valvulae conniventes; Multiple defects (*cobblestone* appearance); Cicatrisation of ileum (*string sign of Kantor*); Rose thorn appearance of the bowel wall. Radiologically Crohn's disease is classified as *nonstenosing type or stenosing type.*

Actinomycosis of right iliac fossa: Disease begins in cecum, inflammatory mass develops which gets adherent to abdominal wall in right iliac fossa. Mass will be nonmobile irregular hard, often tender due to secondary infection. Later induration of abdominal wall develops followed by suppuration and multiple discharging sinus formation discharging sulphur granules. Disease process is often triggered by appendicectomy.

Roundworm bolus mass in right iliac fossa: It presets as smooth, soft or firm, yielding rounded mass in the right iliac fossa which is mobile and tender due to adjacent enteritis. Features of intestinal obstruction—distension, vomiting, constipation, ill health, malnutrition are evident. It is common in children; common in developing countries.

Iliac lymph node mass: Iliac nodes are located in the right iliac fossa on medial aspect above the inguinal ligament. It is deeply seated mass which is smooth/nodular, firm or hard. If it is of inflammatory origin it may be smooth and firm or soft and tender. In lymphoma it is smooth and firm; nodular and hard in secondaries.

Mesenteric lymph node mass in right iliac fossa: It may be due to tuberculosis, lymphoma, secondaries or composite mass.

Iliopsoas abscess: It is localized; smooth, soft, nonmobile mass in the right/left iliac fossa. *Psoas spasm* (flexion of the hip joint) is typical. Spine may show *gibbus, tenderness, paraspinal spasm*. Spinal movements will be restricted. Tuberculosis of sacroiliac joint also can cause cold abscess. Often psoas abscess extends below the inguinal ligament lateral to the femoral artery. Such patient develops swellings on either sides of the inguinal ligament which is cross fluctuant.

Ectopic kidney: It is a developmental abnormality wherein kidney does not ascend to its normal position. Ectopic kidney may be in the pelvis or in the right iliac fossa. It is deeply placed firm nonmobile mass in the right iliac fossa which does not move with respiration. It is resonant on percussion. Usually when it is pathological it is palpable like hydronephrosis, pyonephrosis, polycystic kidney disease, or neoplastic disease. IVU is diagnostic. Radioisotope scan is done to see the function. CT is also needed.

Undescended testis: Testis from lumbar region descends to scrotum along the inguinal canal. Failure of descent makes it imperfectly/undescended testis. It may be abdominal or inguinal in location. Abdominal testis may be in right iliac fossa. It is often difficult to palpate and identify as it is usually atrophied. These undescended testes are 20 times more prone for malignant transformation and when it develops, it may be clinically palpable as mass in right iliac fossa (left iliac fossa in left side) which is nodular, hard, nonmobile.

Mobile kidney: It is usually normal kidney which attains undue mobility probably having peritoneal covering also which can be brought down as far below as to right iliac fossa in right side type. But kidney can be replaced back to normal location.

Hydrops gallbladder: Enormously distended gallbladder can descend down and may palpable in right iliac fossa.

Pelvic masses: Ovarian tumor/cyst; tubo-ovarian mass; uterine fibroid; pyosalpinx; broad ligament cyst can present as mass in iliac fossa. Lower border of such mass merges into the pelvis and so is not felt; on per vaginal examination mass is well felt. It is bimanually palpable often done under general anesthesia. Emptying the bladder is important while examining the pelvic masses.

Urinary bladder diverticulum: It can be felt as a soft, tender, and mobile mass in the iliac fossa which may get emptied partially after catheterization. Cystogram, cystoscopy and CT abdomen confirms the diagnosis.

Mass in the Left Iliac Fossa

All conditions are same as in right iliac fossa. Appendicular mass and abscess will not occur here. Sigmoid pathology—diverticulitis and carcinoma are left iliac fossa diseases.

Diverticular disease of the colon: They are *acquired herniations* of colonic mucosa through circular muscles at the points where blood vessels penetrate. It is commonly localized to sigmoid colon (90%) but occasionally seen in full length of the colon. It is a *false diverticulum* with only *mucosal* herniation. Rectum is *not* affected. *Saint's triad* (5%) diverticulitis; hiatus hernia; gallstones. It is rare in Asian and

African countries because of the high fiber diet. It is common in Western countries. *Diverticulosis* is the initial primary stage of the disease wherein there is hypertrophy, muscular in coordination leading to increased segmentation and increased intraluminal pressure. At this stage they are often asymptomatic, but very often get severe spasmodic pains due to colonic segmentation, fullness of abdomen, bloating and flatulent dyspepsia called as *painful diverticular disease*. *Diverticulitis* is the second stage due to inflammation of one or more diverticula with pericolitis. It presents with persistent pain in left iliac fossa, lower abdomen distension, bleeding per anum, fever, loose stool, recurrent constipation, tenderness in right iliac fossa, palpable and thickened sigmoid colon. Mass may be palpable in the left iliac fossa which is smooth, soft, tender, nonmobile because of inflammatory adhesions. Often abdominal wall edema with redness may be present. P/R may reveal a tender mass. It is the *commonest cause of lower GI bleed in Western countries*. Complications of diverticulitis: Perforation and pericolic abscess or peritonitis; progressive stenosis and intestinal obstruction; Profuse colonic hemorrhage (17–20%); Fistula formation (5%)—colovesical (commonest type with pneumaturia occasionally passing feces); colovaginal; coloenteric; colocutaneous. *Note:* Diverticulitis is not a pre-cancerous condition.

<u>Carcinoma of sigmoid colon:</u> It presents as discomfort, fullness in left iliac fossa with diarrhea, constipation, tenesmus, bleeding per anum, colonic obstruction. Often a hard, nodular mass may be felt in the left iliac fossa, initially mobile but later becomes immobile once it is fixed. It can often be soft and tender if there is complication of pericolic abscess. In such occasion, it may be adherent to anterior abdominal wall.

Mass in the Hypogastrium

<u>Bladder mass:</u> It is in the lower midline. Lower abdomen is distended which is more obvious on standing. It is dull on percussion. Lower border is not felt. It can be mobile in horizontal direction. Mass reduces in size after emptying the bladder. It can be felt on per-rectal examination. All causes of retention of urine cause palpable bladder. It also can be neoplastic either carcinoma bladder (common) or leiomyoma or sarcoma bladder.

MASS IN THE HYPOGASTRIUM	
Parietal swellings	**Intraabdominal and retroperitoneal mass**
• Urachal cyst • Abdominal wall abscess • Abdominal wall tumors like in other regions	• From urinary bladder • From uterus, Fallopian tube and ovaries—fibroid, ovarian cyst, tubo-ovarian mass • Pelvic abscess • Tumors of pelvic bone—chondrosarcoma • Pelvic soft tissue mass

<u>Uterine mass:</u> It is midline mass which is smooth or hard. Lower border extends into the pelvis and is not felt. Pregnancy with history of amenorrhea has to be cited. History of last menstrual period is important (LMP); history of vomiting, lower abdominal discomfort is common; urine pregnancy test and US confirms pregnancy. Uterine fibroid is the commonest tumor which is felt per abdomen in the midline or often extending into iliac fossae. It is slowly progressive, vertically placed, horizontally mobile, firm nodular mass, lower border is not felt as it is merging into pelvis, dull on percussion, ascites is not a feature. It is felt on pervaginal examination. Occasionally leiomyosarcoma or endometrial sarcoma may be the cause of uterine mass. They are smooth, firm often soft, rapidly progressive mass in the hypochondrium.

<u>Ovarian mass:</u> It is smooth, soft, tensely cystic, mobile mass merging into the pelvis, felt per vaginally. It should be differentiated from ascites. Ascites is dull in the flank, resonant in the center/summit of the abdomen; ovarian cyst is dull in the center, resonant in the flanks as intestines are pushed towards periphery. *Blaxland (Athelstan Blaxland) ruler test* shows pulsation in ovarian cyst not in ascites. In all lower abdomen masses P/R and/or P/V is must. Bladder should be emptied using a catheter prior to palpation (Fig. 23-46).

Investigations for Mass Abdomen

Hematocrit, Liver function tests, renal function tests, stool/urine examination.

Ultrasound abdomen.

Endoscopies—Gastroscopy-Colonoscopy-ERCP-MRCP.

Barium studies—Barium meal-Barium enema-Barium meal follow through.

CT scan—contrast CT is ideal for mass abdomen as it clearly gives idea about the origin of mass, its extent and operability, vascularity, relation to major vessels. Intravenous as well as oral water soluble iodine contrast agent should be given (Fig. 23-47).
- MRI.
- Endosonography.
- Ascitic tap.
- Diagnostic laparoscopy.
- Ultrasound guided/CT-guided biopsy.
- Intravenous urogram (IVU)/retrograde pyelogram (RGP)/cystoscopy/isotope renogram.
- Exploratory laparotomy.

> In all regions parietal masses can occur:
> - Benign and malignant soft tissue tumors. Commonest is lipoma
> - Fatty hernia of linea alba, interstitial hernia
> - Desmoid tumor
> - Parietal wall abscess

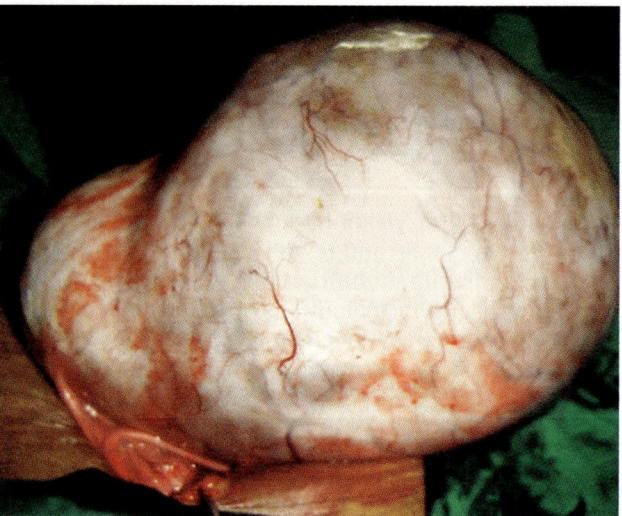

Fig. 23-46 *Ovarian cyst*—large tumor on table finding.

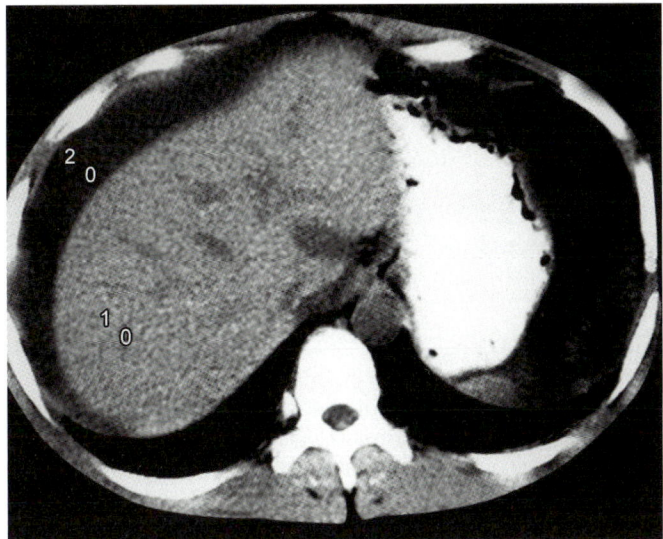

Fig. 23-47 *CT scan abdomen* showing ascites and secondaries in liver.

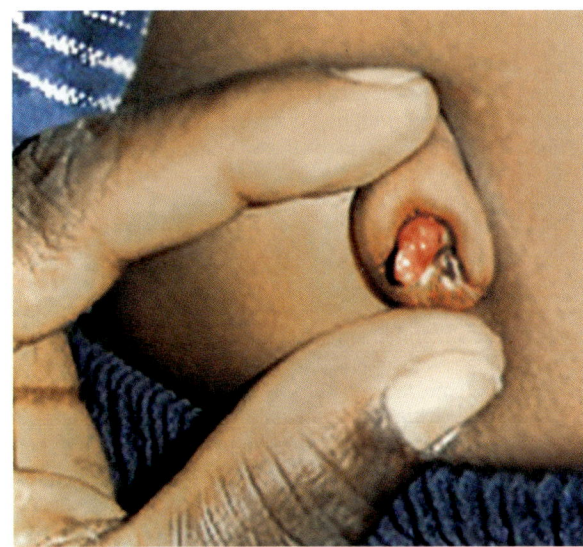

Fig. 23-48 *Umbilical granuloma.*

DISEASES OF THE UMBILICUS AND ABDOMINAL WALL

Diseases of the umbilicus and abdominal wall	*Anomalies of vitellointestinal duct*

1. **Inflammations**: Omphalitis; umbilical granuloma; pilonidal sinus.
2. **Fistulas**: (a) Fecal—patent vitellointestinal duct, neoplastic ulceration; tuberculosis of peritoneum. (b) Urinary— patent urachus.
3. Umbilical hernias.
4. Umbilical calculus (**Umbolith**).
5. **Neoplasms**:
  a. *Benign*—adenoma (*Raspberry tumor*); endometrioma.
  b. *Malignant*—primary (rare); secondary carcinoma— *Sister Joseph's nodule* through lymphatics of the round ligament, primary being in the stomach, colon, ovary, uterus, breast (often blood spread).
	1. It may remain completely patent, forming an *intestinal fistula*.
	2. Only a small portion near the umbilicus may remain patent causing discharging *umbilical sinus*. Often the mucosa of this retained portion (epithelial lining) protrudes or everts to form *umbilical adenoma*.
	3. Duct is closed on either side, but the intervening portion may remain as an *intra-abdominal cyst*.
	4. *Vitellointestinal duct* which is obliterated can remain as band which may be a seat for intestinal obstruction, volvulus, internal herniation.
	5. *Meckel's diverticulum* itself can cause diverticulitis, obstruction.
	Note: Fistulogram is useful. MRI delineates track well.

Umbilical Granuloma (Fig. 23-48)	*Umbilical Sinus (Fig. 23-49)*
It is due to chronic infection of the umbilical cicatrix, causing sprouting of granulation tissue, leading to the formation of umbilical granuloma. It occurs in any age group, but common in infants and children. Presents as umbilical discharge with tender, red swelling protruding from the umbilicus which bleeds on touch. It has to be differentiated from the anomalies of vitellointestinal duct. It also mimics umbilical adenoma.	It is discharging sinus through umbilicus. It is common condition. **Causes:** Persistent vitellointestinal duct towards umbilical side; persistent urachus; tuberculosis; umbilical infection or umbolith; pilonidal sinus of umbilicus; urachal malignancy. **Features:** Pain, swelling, discharge and tenderness over the umbilicus. **Investigations:** Discharge study—culture, cytology, AFB; sinusogram; CT abdomen; chest X-ray—needed.
Umbilical Adenoma (Raspberry Tumor)	*Umbilical Fistula*
Commonly seen in infants; due to partially obliterated vitellointestinal duct towards umbilical side causing prolapse of the mucosa giving rise to *Raspberry tumor;* which protrudes out as a red swelling which is moist with mucus and tends to bleed on touch. It often gets infected, discharging pus through the umbilicus. Histologically, it consists of columnar epithelium rich in goblet cells. **Differential diagnosis:** Umbilical granuloma.	It is fistulous communication between umbilicus and organs in the abdomen either intestine or urinary bladder. **Causes:** Patent vitellointestinal duct discharging fecal matter through umbilicus; patent urachus discharging urine; post-laparotomy; tuberculosis of abdomen either intestine or urinary bladder. Along with discharge, pain, tenderness, excoriation is common.
Patent Urachus	*Abdominal Wall Tumors (Not Uncommon)*
Allantoic duct/stalk which is remnant of cranial part of ventral urogenital sinus forms urachus. It gets fibrosed and forms median umbilical ligament. When urachus is patent it can form—*Patent urachus* (Urachal fistula) between umbilicus and dome of the urinary bladder. *Urachal sinus* occurs when only umbilical side of the urachus remains patent. *Urachal cyst* occurs if only middle portion of the urachus remain patent with lining and fluid content. *Urachal diverticulum* occurs when bladder side of the urachus is patent.	*Benign*: Common tumors are lipoma, fibromas, neurofibromas, and fibromatosis. *Malignant tumors* occasionally when occurs, are either from skin or soft tissues. They may be desmoid tumor, soft tissue sarcoma like fibrosarcoma, dermatofibrosarcoma, liposarcoma, umbilical secondaries (*Sister Joseph Mary tumor*). **Features:** Painless (symptomatic) progressive swelling; Often with ulceration; may attain large size; dull to percuss; on contracting the abdominal wall muscles swelling becomes prominent and less mobile.

Contd...

Contd...

Features: Persistent discharge from the umbilicus often stained with urine if it is fistula; Recurrent infection and bleeding; Pain in the umbilicus and below; Recurrent urinary infection.
Investigations: Fistulogram to see the extent; US abdomen; Discharge analysis and culture; Urine analysis.

Differential diagnoses —abdominal wall abscess, hematoma, intra-abdominal tumors (adherent to abdominal wall).
Investigations: US abdomen, CT abdomen is diagnostic. Biopsy is essential.

Desmoid Tumor

It is a slow growing tumor involving muscle and soft tissue of the abdominal wall, below the level of the umbilicus. 80% of cases occur in women, commonly after deliveries; common over old abdominal surgical scars (lower abdomen) may be due to old hematomas; often associated with the familial adenomatous polyposis of colon (FAP), osteomas, odontomes, epidermal cysts (Gardner's syndrome). It is unencapsulated, hard, fibroma, presently classified under *aggressive fibromatosis;* locally spreading, often undergoes myxomatous changes. Recurrence rate is high.

Rectus Sheath Hematoma

It is due to injury to superior and inferior (more common) epigastric arteries that supply rectus abdominis muscle.
Causes: Trauma; surgery; spontaneous hematoma; blood dyscrasias; severe straining and exercises; tetanus and other convulsions; patients on anticoagulants; puerperium.
Features: Common in females; Sudden onset of swelling in lower abdomen, which is tender, warm, firm on one side of the abdomen; does not cross the midline; with bluish discoloration of skin over the swelling. US and aspiration confirms the diagnosis; should be differentiated from other masses and parietal hernias.

Exomphalos (Omphalocele)

It is the failure of all or a part of the gut to return to the coelomic cavity during early fetal life as coelomic cavity has not developed properly. Sac covering the content is very thin, consists of three layers—outer amniotic membrane, middle Wharton's jelly and inner peritoneal layer. Sac may get ruptured during birth.
Types:
Exomphalos minor: Here the sac is small and umbilical cord is attached to the summit, with small bowel as the content.
Exomphalos major: A large defect is present with contents lying completely outside. Umbilical cord is attached to the inferior aspect of the sac. Contents are small bowel, large bowel and liver. Often the sac will rupture during delivery, which in turn leads to severe infection and high mortality.
Omphalocele is often associated with the congenital anomalies of the cardiac and genitourinary system.

Gastroschisis (Belly Cleft) (Fig. 23-50)

It is a defect of the anterior abdominal wall just lateral to the umbilicus; common in premature babies; almost always to the right of an intact umbilical cord. Umbilicus is normal. Evisceration of the bowel develops through the defect during intrauterine life. There is no peritoneal sac and irritating effect of amniotic fluid causes chemical peritonitis with formation of thick, edematous membrane. Non-rotation and intestinal atresia are common associations. Cardiac anomaly is not common as in omphalocele. After delivery, these infants are more prone for fluid loss, hypothermia, hypovolemia, sepsis, metabolic acidosis. Necrotizing enterocolitis is also common in such infants (20%).

Abdominal Wall Abscess

Causes: Infected hematoma; Umbilical sepsis spreading into the abdominal layers causing the abscess; Blood spread from distant focus.
Features: Tender, soft/firm, nonmobile swelling which is well localized, adherent to skin and underlying abdominal muscles. Aspiration will show pus. It should be ruled out from intra-abdominal mass, cold abscess, parietal hernia. US is diagnostic.

Meleney's Progressive Synergistic Bacterial Gangrene of the Abdominal Wall

It is due to infection by microaerophilic streptococci, staphylococci and other anaerobes of the postoperative abdominal or thoracic wounds; common in HIV, diabetic and immunosuppressed people.
Features: Sudden pain, redness, blackening and gangrene of the skin of the abdomen with abdominal wall necrosis. Toxicity, septicemia, renal failure can occur.

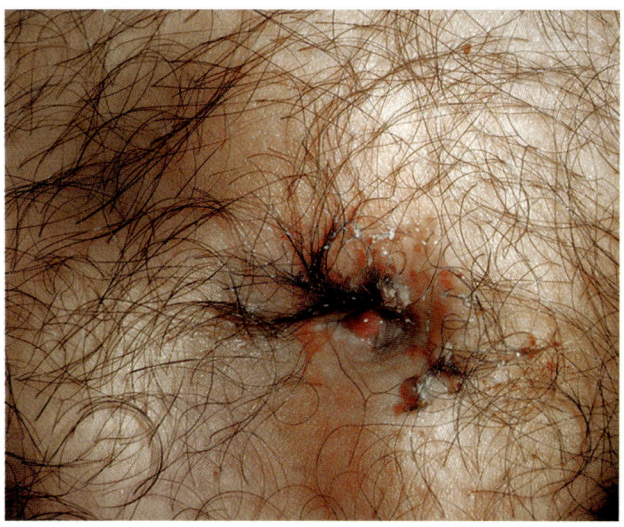

Fig. 23-49 Discharging *umbilical sinus.*

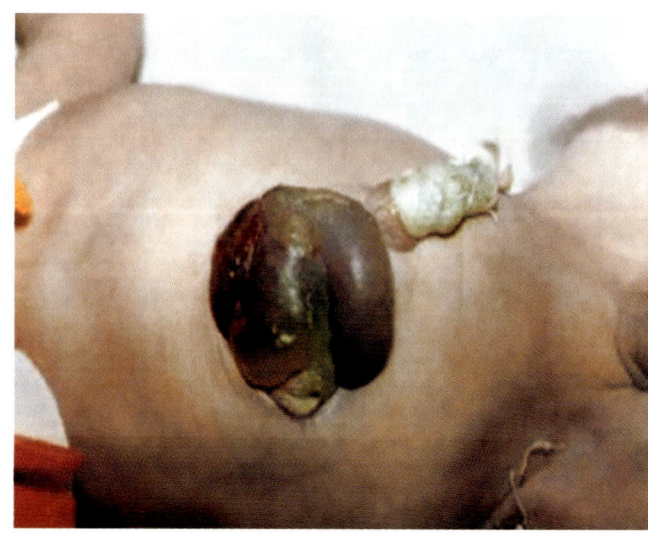

Fig. 23-50 Gastroschisis.

CASE DISCUSSION

A 60-year-old man comes with the history of decreased appetite, early satiety, vomiting and loss of weight in last 3 months. He does not give any history of jaundice, melena, hematemesis. Vague abdominal discomfort in the upper abdomen is present. On examination, he is anemic, jaundice is not present. On inspection of the abdomen, there is no distension; no visible mass but visible gastric peristalsis is present. On palpation, mass is palpable in the epigastric region just above the umbilicus which is 3 × 3 cm in size, mobile, smooth surface, hard in consistency which also moves with respiration. Stomach is dilated on auscultopercussion test. Liver is not palpable, free fluid in the peritoneal cavity is absent. Left supraclavicular lymph node is not palpable. Digital examination of the rectum (P/R) does not show any nodules. Other systems are normal.

What is your diagnosis and why?
It is carcinoma of stomach. Patient presents with vomiting, presence of visible gastric peristalsis, dilated stomach, palpable mass suggestive of stomach.

Whether it is early or advanced?
It is advanced. Reason is—palpable mass is considered advanced because serosa will be invariably involved once it is palpable making it advanced.

What are the differential diagnoses?
Lymphoma and GIST of stomach involving the antrum are the differential diagnoses.

Why PR should be done?
To check rectovesical secondaries (Blumer shelf) which are hard nodules in the anterior aspect of the rectum and mucosa will be free.

What does the supraclavicular lymph node suggests?
It suggests advanced abdominal malignancy commonly gastric. It is actually an external indicator of the abdominal malignancy. It is located just above the sternal end of the clavicle in between the two heads of the sternocleidomastoid muscle (Virchow's node; Troisier's sign).

What investigations are done?
Ultrasound of the abdomen; gastroscopy and biopsy (minimum 10), serum electrolytes, hematocrit, CT scan of the abdomen.

24

Approaches and Examination in Rectal and Vaginal Problems

Competency: SU28.16; SU28.17; AN48.8.

Rectal examination is an essential part of the surgical field without which clinical methods in surgery is incomplete.

■ HISTORY

History of Present Illness

Bleeding Per Rectum

This is the most important history and commonest history to which patient attends surgical clinic.

Quantity of blood loss—mild in drops or severe, jet like.

Mode of onset—traumatic/following hard stool; acute bleed/or chronic, intermittent bleed.

Duration of blood loss, number of times in a day bleed occurs is important.

Nature of blood (color)—whether frank blood or not. Bright red means bleeding is from rectum and anal canal; dark red means it is from the colon proximal to rectum; black or altered blood means from small bowel; melena means from upper gastrointestinal bleed.

Relation with feces—in bleeding from proximal colon blood mixes well with soft feces of proximal colon. Bleeding from the anorectum causes blood on the surface of the stool. Blood separate from feces occurs when blood collects in the rectum, irritates it causing urge to defecate and patient will pass blood with mucus; which is seen in carcinoma of rectum, diverticulitis, polyps, and ulcerative colitis. Fresh blood in the pan or toilet paper at the end of defecation is due to bleeding from piles or fissure. Mucus discharge is common in complete prolapse. Bleeding occur independent of defecation in prolapsed piles, rectal polyp, fistula in ano.

Note: Bleeding in children is due usually to rectal polyp (**Figs. 24-1 to 24-8**).

History of Discharge

Discharge may be purulent, mucus or blood mixed. It can be due to ruptured perianal abscess, fistula in ano, piles, colitis, carcinoma, Crohn's disease. There may be foul smelling, severe discharge as seen in carcinoma of rectum.

Causes for bleeding per anum	
Piles	Carcinoma rectum
Fissure in ano	Carcinoma colon
Polyps	Diverticulitis
Ulcerative colitis	Intussusception
Amoebic colitis	Vascular anomaly of the colorectum
Fistula in ano	Mesenteric ischemia

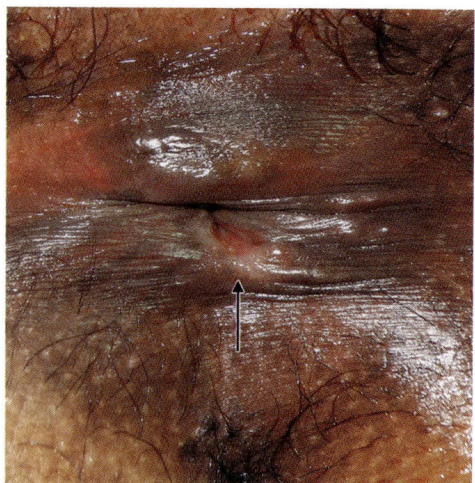

Fig. 24-1 Fissure in ano (*canoe shaped*).

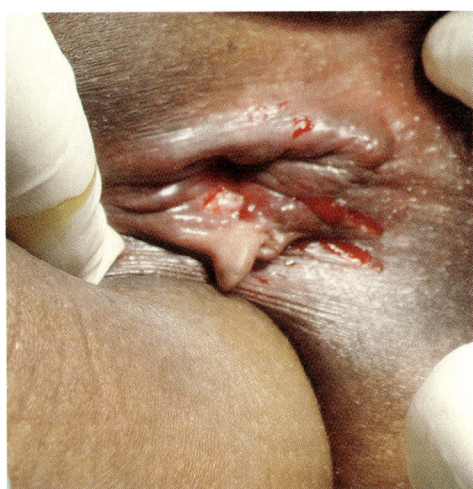

Fig. 24-2 *Fissure in ano* with external tag and also fissures are multiple.

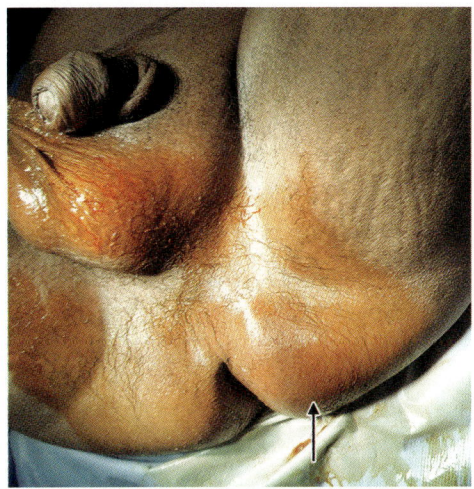

Fig. 24-5 Left-sided *ischiorectal abscess* (perianal). Note the swollen inflamed area.

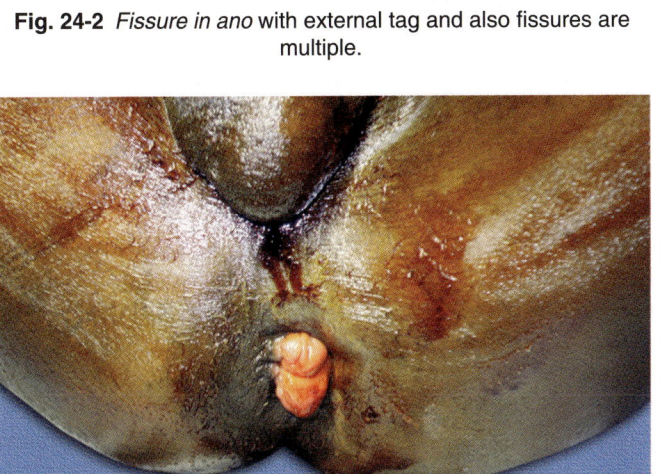

Fig. 24-3 *Prolapsed piles*. Note the internal and external parts.

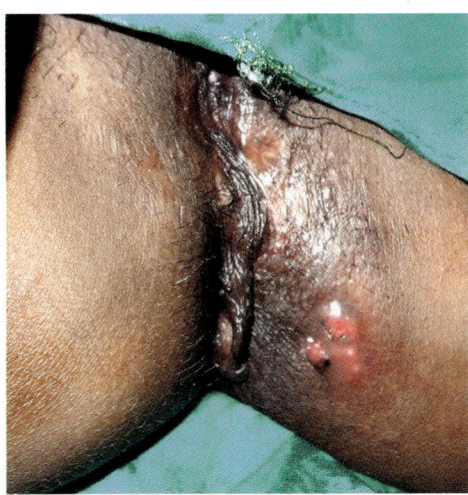

Fig. 24-6 *Fistula* in ano.

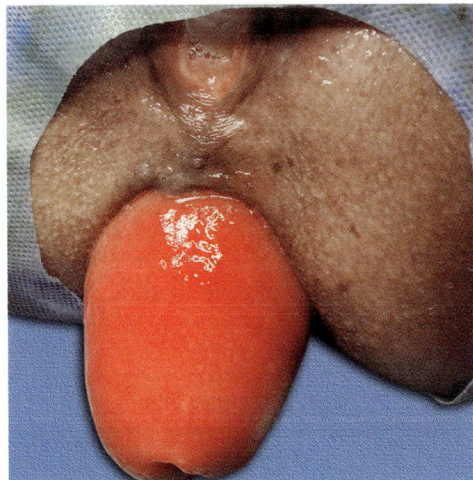

Fig. 24-4 Complete *rectal prolapse*.

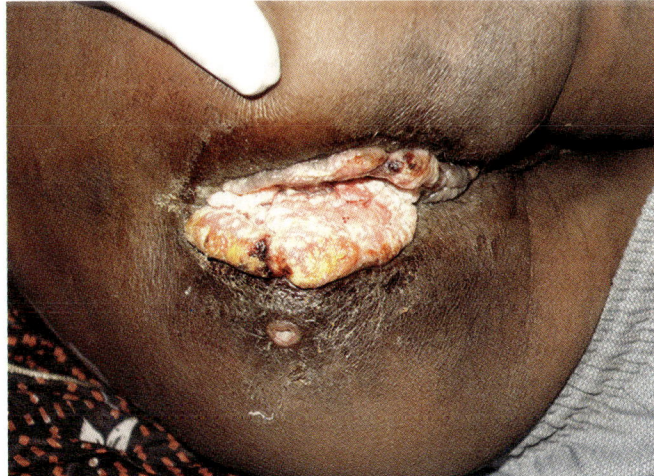

Fig. 24-7 *Carcinoma anal canal*. Note the ulceroproliferative nature.

History of Pain

Pain in the anus: Disease below the dentate line is painful; above it is painless. Throbbing pain is seen in perianal abscess (with swelling); sharp severe pain is seen in acute fissure in ano; pain begins at the time of defecation and persists with burning even after some time in chronic fissure in ano. Fistula in ano presents with intermittent pain and swelling that becomes severe, and opens at the same point where it

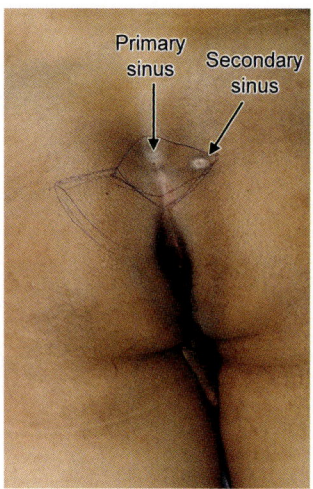

Fig. 24-8 Pilonidal sinus; note the location—in between the buttocks over the sacrum; it has got *primary sinus in midline and secondary sinus laterally*.

regularly discharges and pus come out. Such episode repeats at regular intervals and patient presumes that fistula has healed. Once discharge starts it becomes relatively painless. Piles when complicated become painful (thrombosis, prolapse, infection, strangulation). In rectal growth, patient may have tenesmus. Carcinoma of rectum is initially painless but become painful once it infiltrates pararectal tissues and nerve plexus or by spread below the dentate line.

Pain in the abdomen: It is probably due to intestinal obstruction which may be subacute or acute due to an annular type of growth. Here inflammation (colitis) causes edema and blocks the lumen completely. Spasmodic pain is common in lower abdomen in colorectal diseases like carcinoma and ulcerative colitis.

History of Altered Bowel Habits

Constipation, diarrhea, alternate constipation and diarrhea, spurious diarrhea, tenesmus are different presentation of altered bowel habits. Left sided stenosing growth causes constipation. Stasis of fecal matter causes infection and colitis leading into mucus discharge distally across stenosed area to cause diarrhea. Annular type presents rather early due to constipation and so carries good prognosis. If there is a proliferative growth in the rectal ampulla, then patient has **incomplete sense of evacuation** after defecation due to sensation of fullness in rectum. Because of this sensation of fullness, patient strains painfully and tries to empty the bowel but without succeeding which is called as **tenesmus**. In ulcerative type of carcinoma rectum, fecal matter collected overnight in the rectum which also contains blood, mucus, pus from ulcerated lesion irritates and stimulates the rectal wall, causing for the patient real urgency to pass stool once he gets up in the morning—'***morning spurious diarrhea'***. ***Tape-like/pipestem*** stool is a feature of anorectal growth due to narrowing of the passage.

History of Mass Per Anum

Mass coming out through the anus during defecation may be due to rectal polyp, hemorrhoids, rectal prolapse. Mass which has come out may retract back to original position spontaneously or by manual push (using fingers). In 4th degree piles, one cannot push the pile mass inside. In complete prolapse rectum often it cannot be pushed back inside and is called as ***procidentia***.

History of Itching/Pruritus (Latin) Ani

Itching in perianal region is common and is due to many causes. Often it is intractable. It may be due to causes in *anorectum* (piles, fissure, etc); causes in the *vagina* (*Trichomonas, Candida,* gonorrhea, cervical erosions); *perianal skin* conditions (Tinea cruris, *Candida*); *parastitic* causes (threadworm); *general* causes (psychogenic, lack of hygiene). Pruritus may be *wet* (fissure, fistula, carcinoma, over intake of liquid paraffin) or *dry* (diabetes, poor hygiene).

Causes of pruritus ani:

Poor hygiene	Allergy/dermatitis/psoriasis
Fissure/fistula/piles	Intertrigo
Warts/polyps	Cervical erosions
Trichomonas vaginalis infection in females Candidiasis, gonorrhea, tinea	Erythrasma (*Corynebacterium minutissimum*)
Parasites (threadworm)/epidermophytosis	Diabetes mellitus
Carcinoma anorectum	Psychological causes

History of Weight Loss

History of loss of weight and reduced appetite is seen in carcinoma, ulcerative colitis, diverticulitis.

Past History

Previous history of surgery for piles, fistula, anorectal abscess; history of tuberculosis, drug treatment (for ulcerative colitis, Crohn's may be the cause of fistula) are important. History of severe diarrhea/dysentery is taken in children as it may be the cause for prolapse.

Family History

Hemorrhoids, polyps, carcinoma often run in family.

Bright red color	Polyps
Red currant jelly	Intussusception
Maroon-colored stool	Meckel's diverticulum
Blood mixed with stool	Carcinoma of colon
Blood streaked on stool	Carcinoma of rectum
Blood and mucus	Colitis
Blood only	Diverticulitis, carcinoma of rectum
Blood after defecation/blood splashes in the pan	Piles
Melena	Upper GI bleed

Chapter 24: Approaches and Examination in Rectal and Vaginal Problems

Personal History

History of type of food intake is taken—spicy food, low fiber diet, inadequate water intake all are responsible factors of constipation.

EXAMINATION OF THE ANORECTUM

- 'If you do not put your finger in (to the rectum), you put your foot in it.'
- It is *criminal negligence* if digital examination of rectum is not done in an anorectal case.
- 10 cm of the anus/anorectum can be assessed by digital examination.
- First *inspection of the anal canal* is done; then *palpation of the anal canal*; later *digital examination* of the rectum is done. Then proctoscopy is done.

Different Positions Used for DRE [Digital Rectal Examination (P/R)]

Left lateral—Sims' position: Patient lies with right leg placed above the left and flexed; left leg below the right and semiflexed, buttocks projecting over the edge and trunk across the bed (not parallel) **(Figs. 24-9A and B)**.

Right lateral position: It is the position with right leg up and flexed to feel the rectosigmoid growths which will fall forward and downward **(Fig. 24-10)**.

Dorsal position: It is used in severely ill patients where changing the position of the patient is contraindicated. Patient lies on the bed supine in semi-recumbent position, with hips and knees slightly flexed. Right hand of the examiner is passed behind the right thigh of the patient and anorectum is felt using right index finger. Left hand of the examiner is kept over the suprapubic region for bimanual palpation. Rectovesical pouch and pelvis assessment can be done well in this position but anus cannot be inspected in this position **(Fig. 24-11)**.

Lithotomy position: It needs special table to position the patient. This position is suitable for bimanual examination under general anesthesia, proper inspection of the anus and palpation. Biopsy and therapeutic procedures can be carried out in this position **(Figs. 24-12A and B)**.

Knee-elbow position: It is used for palpation of prostate and seminal vesicle. Seminal vesicles are normally very soft and not palpable. It becomes palpable in tuberculous seminal

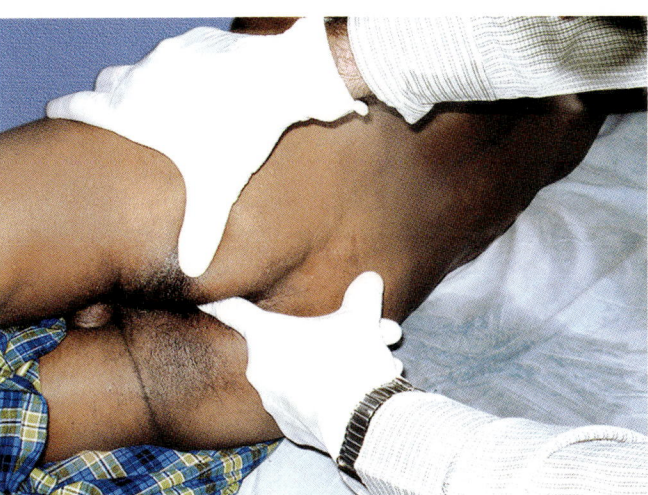

Fig. 24-10 Digital examination in *right lateral position*.

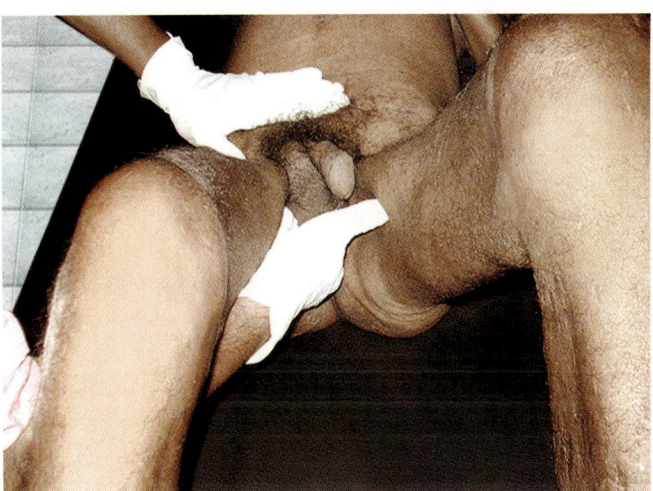

Fig. 24-11 Digital examination of the rectum in *dorsal position*.

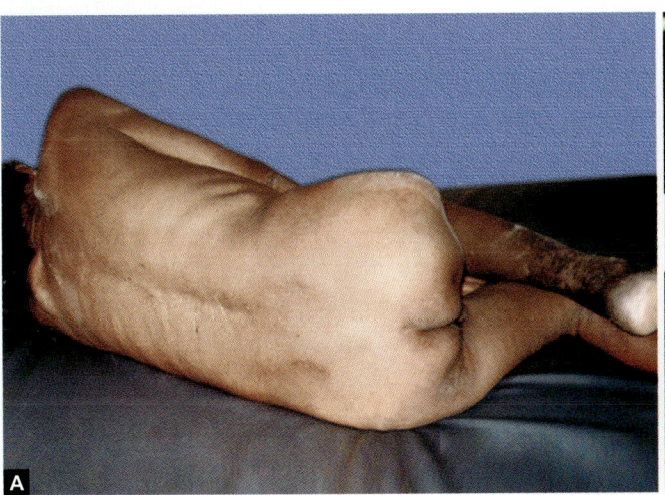

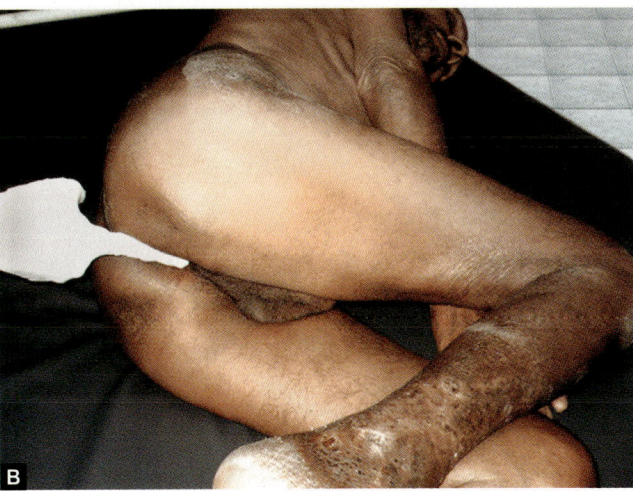

Figs. 24-9A and B *Sims' position* and doing per rectal examination.

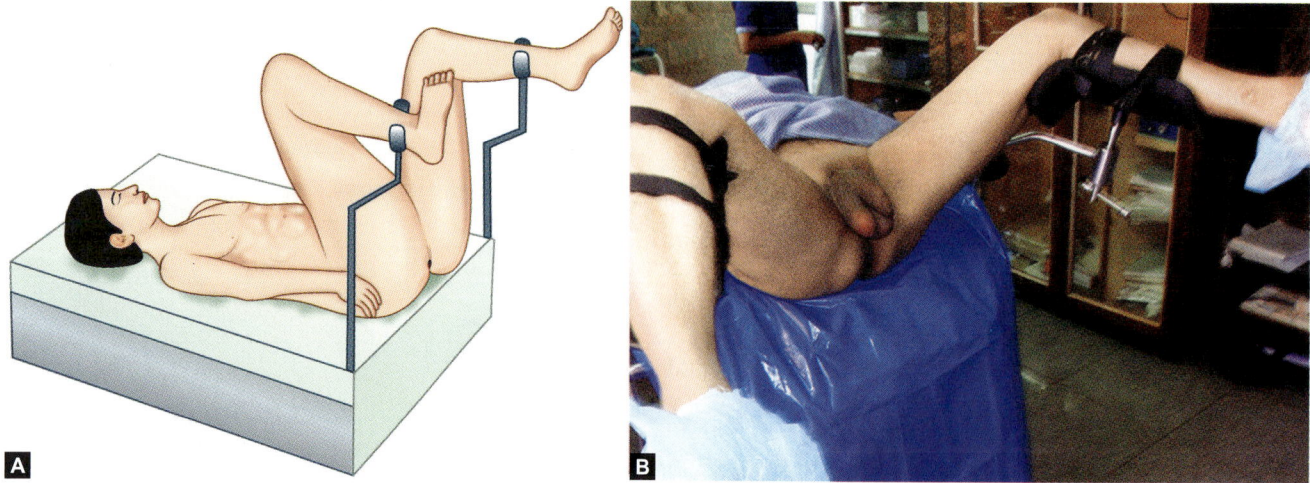

Figs. 24-12A and B *Lithotomy position* used for examination and all perineal surgery like for fissure, piles, and fistula, abdominoperineal resection for carcinoma rectum (APR).

vesiculitis, *Trichomonas vaginalis* infestation, abacterial nongonococcal urethritis **(Fig. 24-13)**.

Picker position: It is used to palpate seminal vesicles in obese patients or in patients with prostatic hyperplasia. Patient stands and leans forward grasping a low chair or stool; seminal vesicles are palpated using fingers **(Fig. 24-14)**.

Inspection of the Anal Canal and Perineal Area

Swellings (sentinel pile, external pile, papilloma, condyloma), ulcer, fissure, fistula in ano, pilonidal sinus, carcinoma, perianal inflammation abscess are looked for during inspection **(Fig. 24-15)**.

Fissure in ano is checked by retracting the buttocks laterally using fingers on each side. It is common in posterior midline position **(Fig. 24-16)**.

Fistula in ano: Location, number of openings in fistula in ano should be noted. External orifice looks like a whitish raised small point area with often redness around and discharge from the orifice. Distance of the external orifice from the anus should be noted. They are classified as anterior and posterior

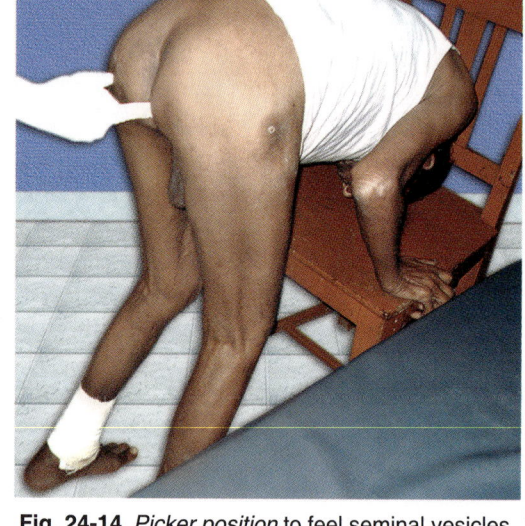

Fig. 24-14 *Picker position* to feel seminal vesicles.

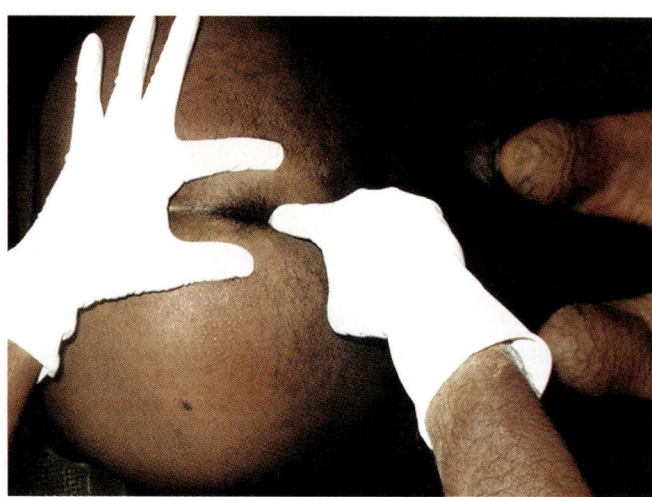

Fig. 24-13 Rectal examination in *knee-elbow* position.

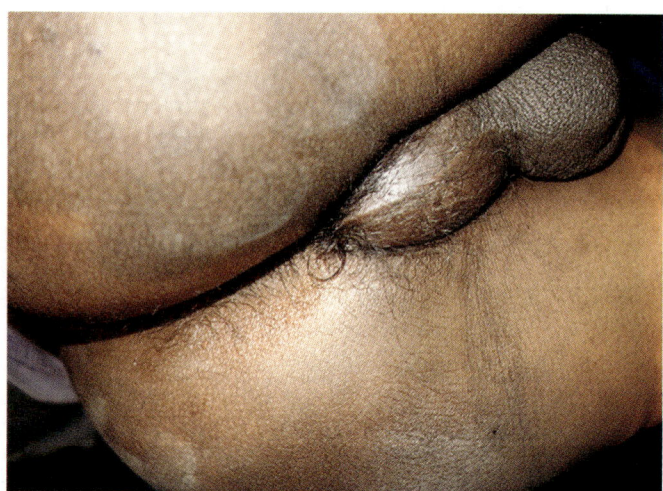

Fig. 24-15 *Periurethral abscess* often mimics perianal abscess; such abscess should be drained after urinary catheterization. In periurethral abscess, urinary symptoms are obvious.

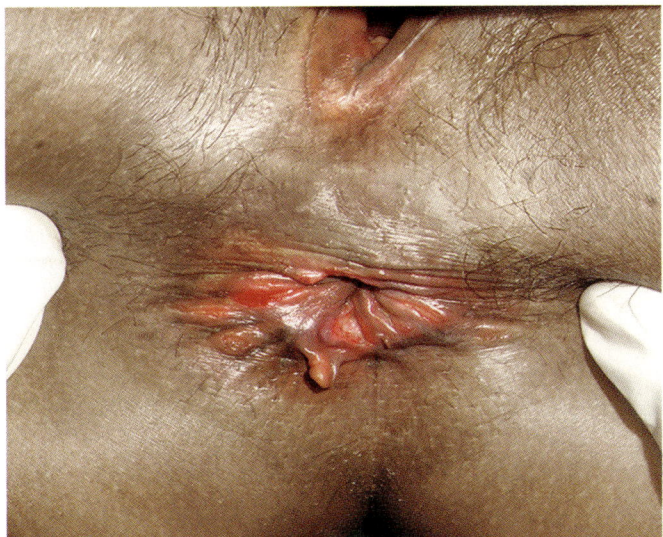

Fig. 24-16 *Multiple fissures in ano.* Note the method of retraction of the buttock. Note the prominent posterior fissure with sentinel pile.

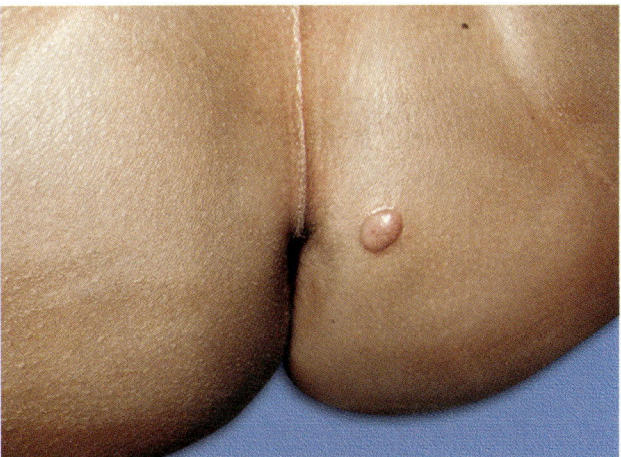

Fig. 24-17 *Fistula in ano*—with single posterior external opening (right sided; probably low type).

fistulas based on the position of external opening whether situated anterior/posterior to the imaginary transverse line passing through the midpoint of anus. The site of internal opening depends on the position of the external opening. Posterior fistulas have curved path (internal opening lies in midline in between two sphincters); and anterior fistulas have straight/direct path (internal opening lies in the same radial line) is the common rule called as **Goodsall's rule.** Often there may be multiple external openings. Fistula with single external opening, if its distance from anal margin is <5 cm it is of low variety; if the external opening is >5 cm from anal margin it is of high variety with internal opening lying above the anorectal ring **(Figs. 24-17 to 24-19)**.

Note: Causes of perineal fistulae are—Fistula in ano (commonest), urethral fistula (usually due to burst periurethral abscess in a preexisting urethral stricture); fistula due to osteomyelitis of underlying ischial bone, sacrum or coccyx.

Pilonidal sinus is confirmed in prone position retracting the buttocks properly. Small sinus opening or openings are evident in the midline and paramedian positions few centimeters proximal to the anus over the sacrum posteriorly in midline **(Figs. 24-20 and 24-21)**.

Condyloma acuminata are multiple, pedunculated papilla like lesions caused by papilloma variant virus. It is transmitted by sexual contacts. Itching, discomfort, pain, ulceration due to rubbing against clothes is common features. They may be associated with other sexually transmitted diseases like HIV, gonorrhea. It may involve wider area of the perineum, labia majora, scrotum, etc **(Fig. 24-22)**.

Anal canal carcinoma can mimic piles or fistula in ano **(Fig. 24-23)**.

Condyloma lata occurs in secondary syphilis as flat raised white hypertrophied epithelium at mucocutaneous junction. It is highly contagious.

Ulcer with everted edge with bloody discharge is feature of anal carcinoma.

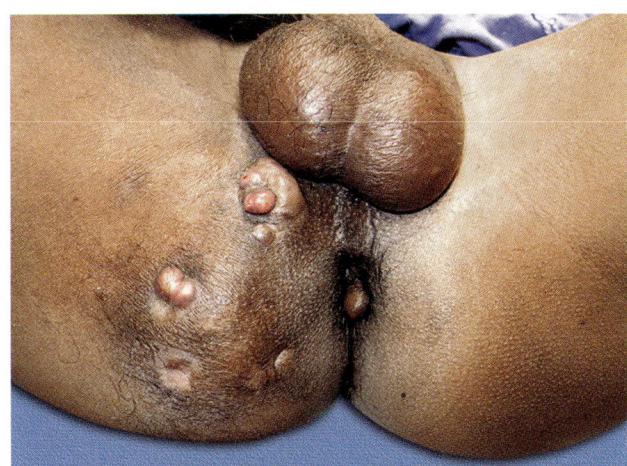

Fig. 24-18 *Multiple fistula in ano.* It may be Crohn's disease, carcinoma, HIV. MRI is essential in such fistula with specific evaluations.

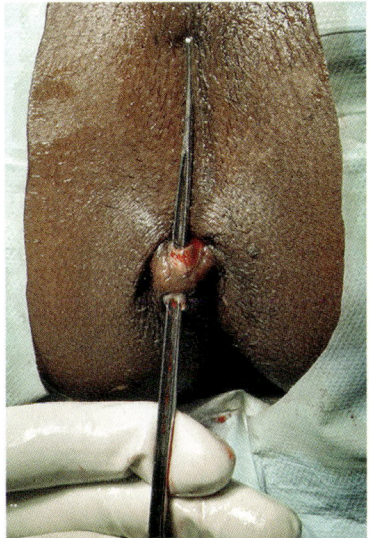

Fig. 24-19 *Low fistula in ano—probing.* Probing should be done gently in operation theater often under anesthesia. Posterior fistula in ano has got its internal opening in posterior midline whereas anterior fistula in ano is straight and its internal opening is straight corresponding to the location to the external opening *(Goodsall's rule)*.

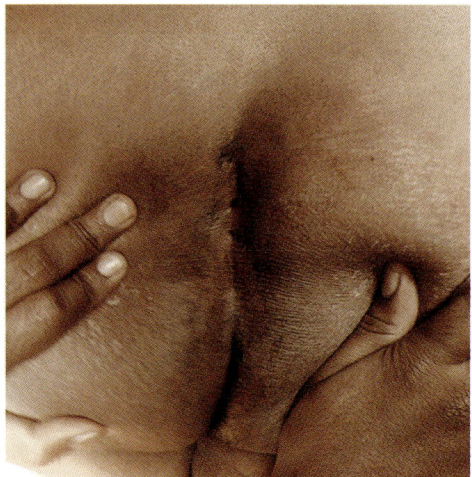

Fig. 24-20 By retracting the buttocks in prone position *pilonidal sinus* is inspected.

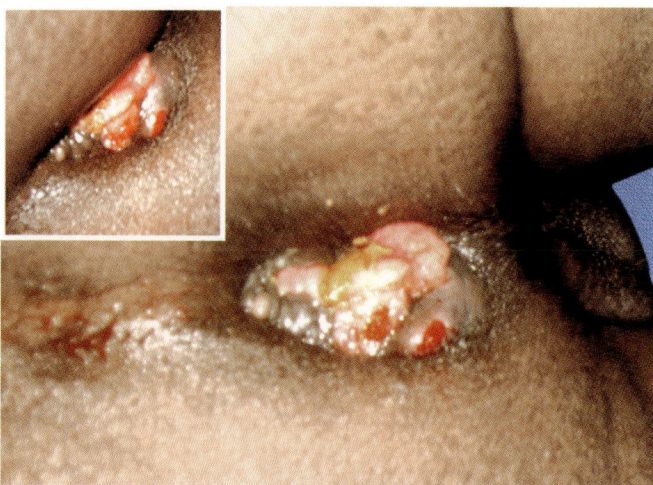

Fig. 24-23 *Anal canal carcinoma*. Squamous cell carcinoma is commonest type—80%.

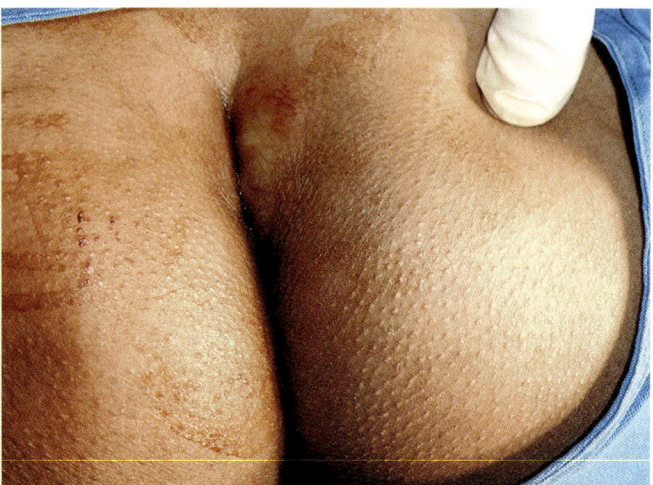

Fig. 24-21 *Pilonidal abscess*; it will form pilonidal sinus. Initial presentation is as abscess often.

Often it may be proliferative lesion. Itching marks with redness and edema around may be a feature of inflammation.

Piles	Rectal prolapse
Segmental	Circumferential
Plum colored	Red colored
Outer cover of skin with inner mucosa	Only mucosa

Prolapse rectum is examined with patient in **squatting position** and he is asked to strain as if he is passing the stool. Rectal mucosa protruding out downwards can be seen. If it is less than 3 cm it is partial prolapse; if it is more it is complete **(Figs. 24-24 to 24-26)**. **Prolapsed piles should be differentiated from prolapsed rectum.** A prolapsed pile is segmental (with 3 segment) with a skin cover over it and mucosal part on the inner aspect whereas there is anteroposterior slit in incomplete prolapse of rectum.

Rectal polyp (Fig. 24-27) *or intussusception* of the colon also rarely may protrude out through the anal canal.

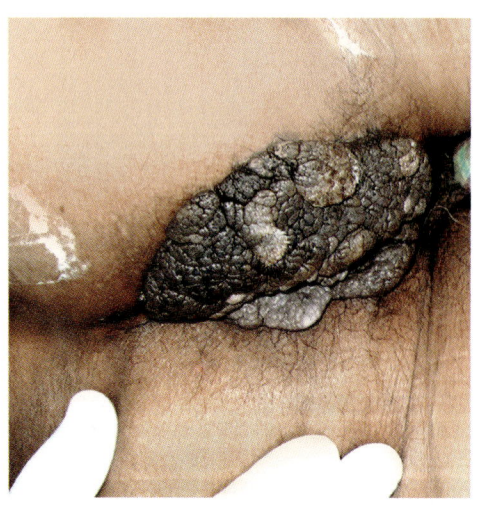

Fig. 24-22 *Anal papilloma*. It often attains very large size. It could be of viral origin. It can turn into squamous cell carcinoma.

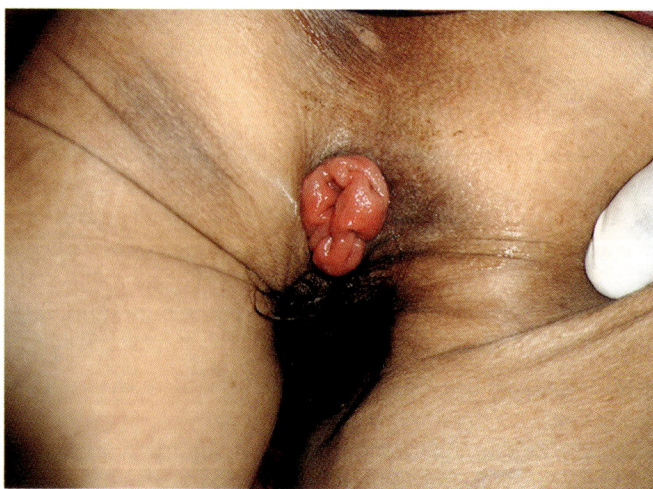

Fig. 24-24 *Partial* rectal prolapse.

Chapter 24: Approaches and Examination in Rectal and Vaginal Problems

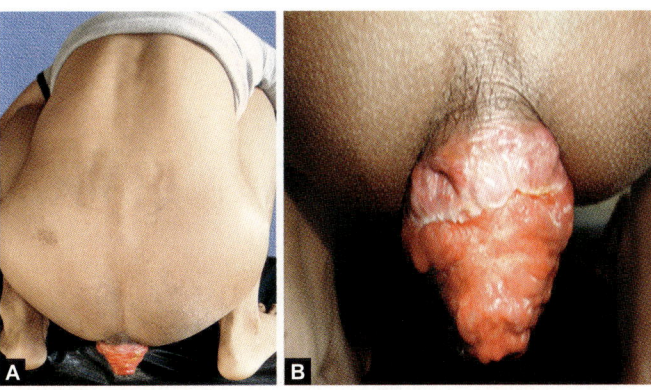

Figs. 24-25A and B Complete rectal prolapse. It should be confirmed by observing the patient *during straining in squatting position.*

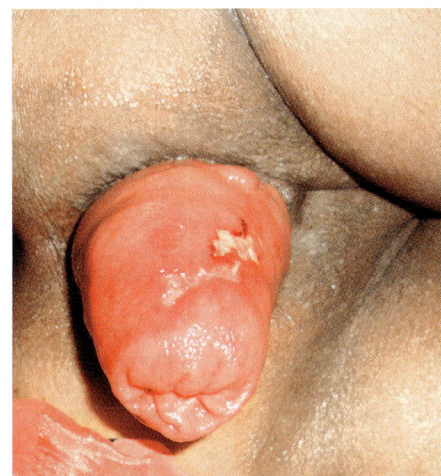

Fig. 24-26 Complete *rectal prolapse.*

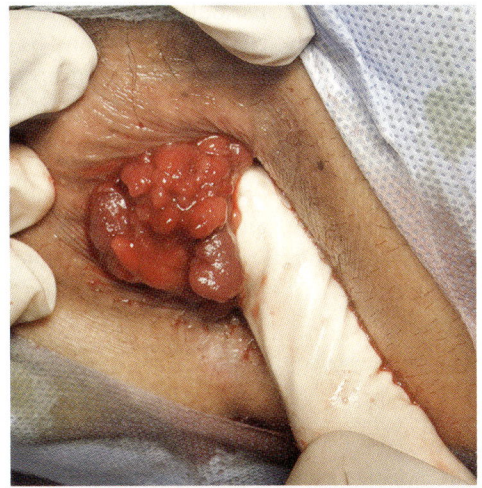

Fig. 24-27 *Rectal polyp* coming out through the anus.

Note:
- Pigmented *melanoma* lesion may be evident if carefully inspected. It may be mistaken for thrombosed piles.
- Ulcerated melanoma in the anus *may not* be black.

Palpation of the Perineum and Anal Canal

Perineum should be palpated for abscess, perianal hematoma (**Fig. 24-28**), ulcer, growth, external opening of the fistula

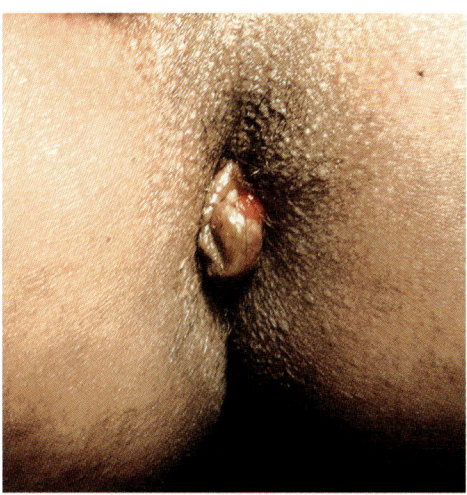

Fig. 24-28 *Perianal hematoma.*

in ano. Swelling is palpated for temperature, tenderness, induration, fluctuation, mobility/fixity to deeper structures. Palpation of the edge of an ulcer for induration (anal canal carcinoma) should be done. Ischiorectal abscess will be tender and indurated.

Rectal prolapse should be differentiated from **intussusception (sigmoidorectal)**. In intussusception, finger can be insinuated between intussusceptum and anal canal; but in rectal prolapse finger cannot be insinuated between prolapsed mucosa and skin margin.

Bidigital palpation of the anal canal with one finger inside, thumb outside and feeling the wall should be done in abscess or fistula. Fistula track may *be multiple*. Specific causes like tuberculosis, carcinoma, lymphogranuloma venereum, bilharziasis, Crohn's disease, ulcerative proctitis should be thought of. Fistula due to *tuberculosis* shows clear watery discharge, ragged margin, discolored surrounding skin *without* any protrusion or induration (**Figs. 24-29A and B**).

Digital Examination of Anorectum (DRE) (Per Rectal; P/R)

- It is **contraindicated** in acute fissure in ano as it causes severe pain.
- Often enema is necessary prior to rectal examination to clear the *loaded feces* in the rectum.

    Proper positioning is done. Disposable gloves are used. Patient should be told about the procedure and asked to breathe through mouth and relax. Anus is lubricated with lubricant or xylocaine jelly. Pulp of the index finger is used. In children little finger may be used. Pulp is kept flat over the anus. With gentle pressure finger is pushed gradually into the *anal canal* once anal sphincter relaxes and gently rotated.

Anal canal—wall of the anal canal should be assessed for thickening, tenderness, sphincter tone, swelling ulcer, fissure, etc. **Anal groove** or anal intermuscular depression is felt just inside the anal verge which is demarcation

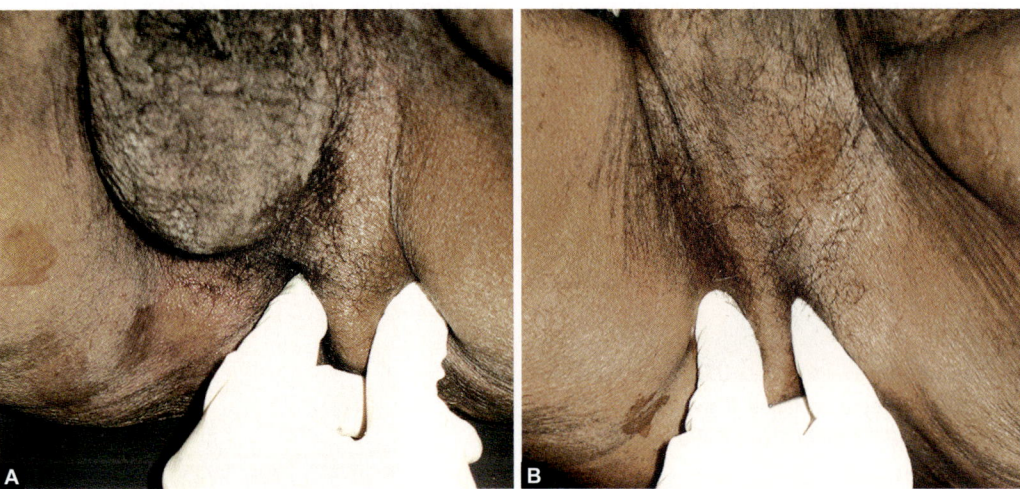

Figs. 24-29A and B *Bidigital examination* (palpation) of the anal canal.

between external and internal hemorrhoidal plexus and external and internal sphincter muscles. **Anorectal ring** is situated at the junction of anal canal and rectum. It is 2–3 cm in length. Puborectalis component of levator ani muscle is arranged like a sling and is well felt laterally and behind it. Fistula or anorectal abscess should be assessed in relation to this ring. Bidigital examination with index finger in the anal canal and thumb outside is done on both sides and compared. By this submucosal and perianal abscess are made out. Abnormal mobility and tenderness of coccyx can be made out. Sphincter tone is assessed. **Loss of sphincter tone** is confirmed by giving digital traction on the sphincter by hooking the finger around the anorectal ring, sphincter is found gaped, rectal mucosa and lumen is displayed. Vaginal deliveries, badly performed rectal surgeries, congenital, neurological diseases and *senility*/old age (most common cause) are some of the causative factors.

Rectum: Finger is pushed as high as possible to reach rectum. *First lumen is felt; then wall of the rectum; lastly deeper plane outside the rectal wall is felt* (Figs. 24-30 and 24-31).

Digital Examination of Rectum (P/R)
No abdominal examination is complete without a per rectal examination

A. It is done to palpate
  1. Carcinoma rectum
  2. Stricture rectum
  3. Polyps
  4. Thrombosed piles
  5. BPH and carcinoma prostate
  6. Secondaries in the rectovesical pouch (Blumer shelf)
  7. Sphincter tone
  8. Pelvic abscess (is felt as boggy swelling)
B. To feel internal opening in anal fistulas
C. In bimanual palpation of the bladder or pelvic tumors
D. In acute abdominal conditions—it reveals dilated empty rectum with tenderness

In the lumen:

Lumen of rectum is spacious. Ballooning of the rectum is a feature of intestinal obstruction. Mass may be felt. It is better felt during straining. Fecal matter often hard may be felt. Foreign bodies if present can be felt. Rarely, apex of intussusception may be felt.

In the wall:

- Lower valve of Houston may be felt in the mucosa like a rim. *Ulceration*, irregularity, proliferative lesion, tenderness should be felt.

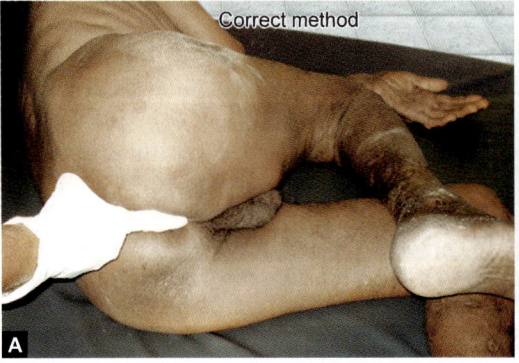
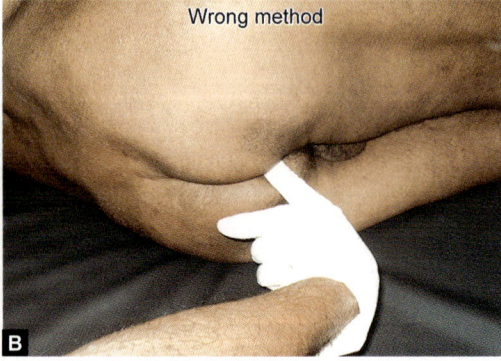

Figs. 24-30A and B *Correct method and wrong method* of doing finger examination of the rectum. Pulp should be used parallel while passing the finger into the anal canal (not perpendicularly using tip of finger).

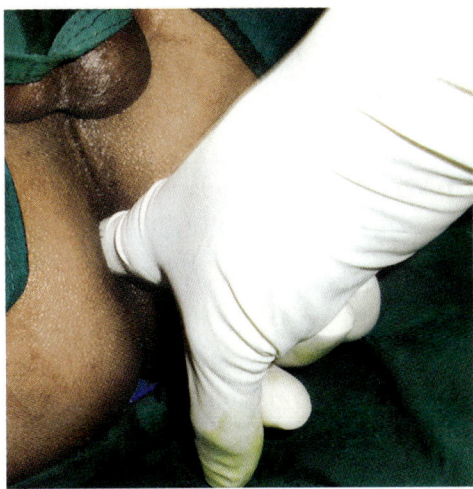

Fig. 24-31 Rectal examination in *lithotomy position*.

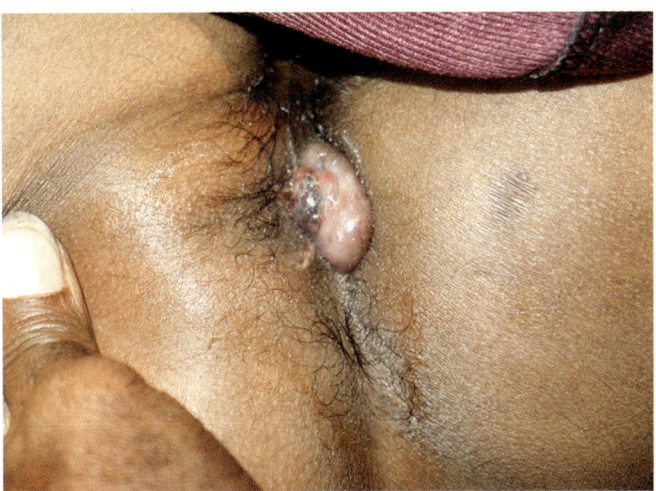

Fig. 24-32 *Thrombosed piles* with prolapse.

- In case of **ulceration, size,** shape, induration, extent, number of lesions should be felt. Whether upper limit can be reached or not should be assessed. Ulcer may be due to tuberculosis, gonorrhea, syphilis, malignancy. Malignant ulcer has everted edge and indurated base.
- **Thickening of wall** or narrowing of lumen due to *stricture* is noted. Its situation, extent, nature of mucous membrane is assessed. Stricture may be due to trauma or postoperative or carcinoma or tuberculosis or lymphogranuloma venereum or chronic proctitis of any cause, will be felt like narrowed area where finger may not be able to pass through it. Diaphragm at periphery with central hole is typical. A **narrow crescentic** circular mucosal fold felt 4 cm from anal verge in young individual is probably due to imperfect fusion of the hindgut to proctodeum causing *congenital stricture*. Postoperative, post-radiotherapy and traumatic strictures are *fibrous* type where there is smooth thickening of the wall. Malignant stricture is *hard, irregular, indurated and often ulcerated type*. Stricture of lymphogranuloma is *tubular and rubbery*. Lumen narrowing can be caused by pressure from outside due to mass lesion

  Note: Stricture may be congenital; traumatic; inflammatory; neoplastic; others (spasm of sphincter).
- **90% of rectal carcinoma** can be felt on per rectal finger examination. Often present with painless rectal bleeding; growth at rectosigmoid is constrictive type, hard in consistency; growth in ampulla is proliferative type with everted edge and indurated base. Mobility/fixity, extent of deeper infiltration should be analyzed. *Bimanual examination* with other (left) hand over the suprapubic region should be done. Extent of spread into the bladder, prostate or vagina in females should be assessed. Posterior spread into the sacrum should be confirmed.
- **Internal opening** of the *fistula in ano* can be felt as a button like indurated area in **midline** on posterior surface (commonly). Often it can be high or multiple or on anterior surface.
- **Thrombosed piles** *can be felt by finger* (usual internal piles *cannot* be felt as it is very soft; it is only seen through proctoscope) **(Fig. 24-32)**.

Polyp of rectum may be felt as a rounded soft swelling with warty irregular surface, often red in color and bleeds on touch; with finger tip its extent, base can also be determined; and by flexing the finger often it can be pulled down to the anus to properly inspect and feel.

Outside the rectal wall:

- When finger is passed high above, sacral promontory can be felt. Ischial spine can be felt laterally.
- **Prostate** is felt anteriorly deep to mucosa. Both lateral lobes are felt. Normally it is bilobed, smooth, firm, rubbery with a central/median sulcus or groove with rectal mucosa moving freely over it. It is tender in acute prostatitis and prostatic abscess. In benign prostatic hyperplasia (BPH), it is felt as smooth, firm, enlarged, upper border cannot be reached and median groove less conspicuous. In carcinoma prostate, it may be nodular and hard. Size is not a criteria for carcinoma prostate. In carcinoma it may be normal sized with central sulcus obliterated and rectal mucosa fixed in advanced lesion. Base of the bladder, rectovesical pouch, seminal vesicles are felt anteriorly. Seminal vesicles are normally not palpable. It is felt in knee-elbow position or *Picker* position. Seminal vesicles are felt in upper lateral aspect of the prostate in tuberculosis with irregular feel. Secondaries in rectovesical pouch are felt in front above the prostate as a hard mass deep to mucosa and are called as **Blumer shelf** (George Blumer—New Haven Connecticut). Pelvic abscess is felt as smooth, soft, tender, and *boggy* swelling in front of this pouch.
- **In females,** cervix, uterus, vagina and rectouterine pouch (Douglas) is felt per rectally. Cervix is felt in front like projection—*pons asinorum* (bridge of asses—Latin). Uterus also can be well felt bimanually. Retroverted uterus can be confirmed. If patient is wearing a pessary it can be felt like a mass. Blood, secondaries, pus can be felt in this pouch. Lump outside the rectal wall, subserosal fibroid, edematous Fallopian tube can be felt.
- **Lateral palpation:** Ischiorectal fossa, lateral wall of pelvis, lower end of ureters, internal iliac arteries are felt laterally. Ischiorectal abscess is felt as tender tense swelling. A

stone in the lower ureter, iliac artery aneurysm may be felt through rectal examination. Pelvic bone mass (tumor or infective), hip joint central dislocation, fracture pelvis can be felt. Pelvic appendicitis causes tenderness and often mass in the lateral wall of rectum in front. Salpingitis, ovarian cyst/tumor, ectopic gestation can be felt per rectally.

- ***Behind,*** coccyx can be palpated with index finger inside and thumb over coccyx for tenderness abnormal movements *of **coccydynia*** and fracture of coccyx. Sacrococcygeal teratoma and post-anal dermoid when present can also be felt.
- ***Bimanual examination*** is carried out in dorsal position by placing left hand over the suprapubic region and right index over the rectum. Any pelvic mass can be felt well on rectal examination and bimanual examination. Size, shape, consistency fixity, relation of the mass to other structure can be assessed **(Fig. 24-33)**.

> **Note:**
> - Mucosal lesions are better felt by downwards stroking than upward pushing of the finger
> - After finishing the rectal examination, finger should be inspected for presence of blood, feces, mucus or pus. It can be collected in gauze for proper inspection
> - Massive edema of rectal wall may be noted in sigmoid volvulus due to inferior mesenteric vein occlusion
> - Often it is difficult to find out whether lump felt is in the wall or outside. Finger is placed on one side of the lump and slid over the elevation of the lump to feel the presence or absence of continuity of the overlying mucosa
> - Pelvic masses, urinary bladder can be assessed well by bimanual rectal examination
> - In female child per vaginal examination is usually avoided; per rectal examination allows palpation of entire pelvic viscera
> - In neonates and infants up to 3 months, rectal examination is done using little finger

Examination of Lymph Nodes

Carcinoma below the dentate line spreads to horizontal group of inguinal lymph nodes; carcinoma above this line, spread to iliac nodes. Iliac nodes can be felt by deep palpation above and medial aspect of the inguinal ligament. Pelvic and para-aortic nodes are to be palpated to see for enlargement.

Abdominal Examination

It is done to look for liver secondaries (nodular hard liver); ascites, features of intestinal obstruction.

■ VAGINAL EXAMINATION

Always change the glove after doing vaginal or rectal examination. Usually vaginal examination is done first then followed by rectal examination. 'Never insult the vagina by examining the rectum first'. Even then glove should be changed after vaginal, before rectal examination.

Position: Left lateral position is used to begin with. Dorsal position is better to examine the urethral orifice. Lithotomy position is needed for proper assessment and bimanual examination. General anesthesia is preferred.

Inspection: Labia should be inspected for swelling, skin changes. Surrounding area should also be inspected. Ulcer, swellings, itch marks, introitus should be inspected. Presence or absence of hymen should be noted in introitus. Small sharp edged opening admitting only the fingertip is a virgin hymen. In pregnancy introitus looks bluish. Blood stained discharge is seen in menstruation, abortion, ectopic pregnancy, and carcinoma. White purulent discharge is seen in vaginitis, cervicitis, endometritis and pelvic infections. Profuse watery, yellow often frothy discharge with pruritus is a feature of *Trichomonas vaginalis* infestation. Thick curdy discharge is seen in *Candida* infection. Purulent discharge is seen in gonorrhea.

Palpation: Labia are separated using thumb and forefinger of the left hand. Using lubricated index and middle fingers of the right hand palpation is done. Index finger is introduced first then middle finger is passed. First cervix then anterior, lateral and posterior fornices are palpated in that order.

Chancre, lymphogranuloma venereum, granuloma inguinale, chancroid, herpes, leukoplakia, carcinoma, papillomas can occur in vulva. Sebaceous cyst also can occur in vulva. Pruritus marks may be evident. Vaginal discharge may be evident.

Bartholin glands are palpated over ***posterior part*** of the labia majora between finger and thumb. Gland is deep and posterior. Bartholin cyst is a retention cyst. It often can get infected forming an abscess. Often it is bilateral **(Fig. 24-34)**.

Straining down will make cystocele any uterine descent obvious. Cystocele is descent of bladder through anterior vaginal wall. Rectocele is descent of rectum through posterior vaginal wall.

Stress incontinence is checked in full bladder by asking the patient to cough and urine will spill out from the bladder.

Anovaginal bidigital examination: It is done by placing index finger in the rectum and thumb in the vagina or by placing right index finger in the rectum and left index finger

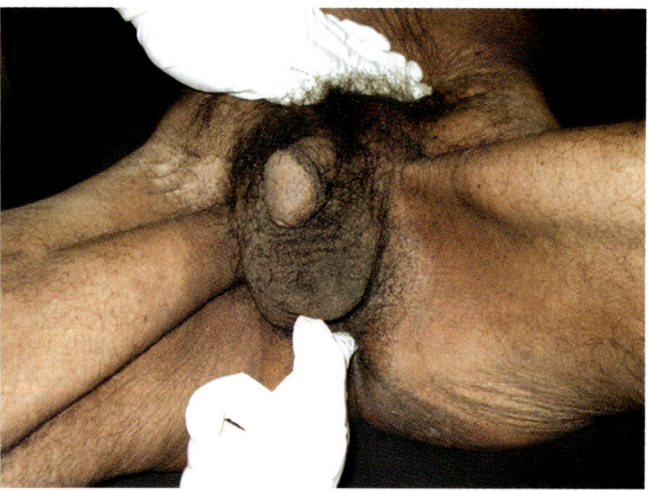

Fig. 24-33 *Bimanual palpation* of the rectum.

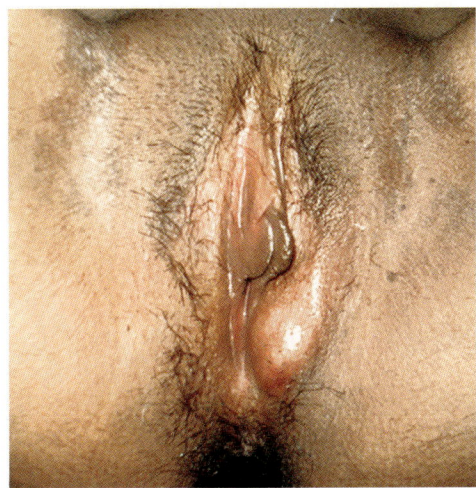

Fig. 24-34 Bartholin cyst forming an abscess.

in the vagina. It is used to palpate anterior anorectal lesion or posterior vaginal wall lesion or to check the musculature of the perineum (tone).

Bimanual examination (Nicolas Puzos, Paris): Lubricated right hand fingers are kept high in the vagina; left hand fingers placed above the pubic symphysis is pressed downwards and backwards. Size, position (ante or retroverted) of the uterus is made out; in thin females ovaries may be felt. Normal fallopian tubes are not palpable. When it is enlarged it may be palpable. Size, shape, extent, surface, consistency of the pelvic swelling is assessed. Relation of the bladder to the mass anteriorly and pouch of Douglas posteriorly is assessed.

Carcinoma cervix, carcinoma uterus, fibroid uterus, ovarian neoplasm, endometriosis should be considered in vaginal examination.

Proctoscopy (Kelly's)

Indications: Diagnostic—piles, fissure in ano, polyps, stricture, etc. *Therapeutic*—injection therapy for partial prolapse or piles, cryotherapy for piles, polypectomy, biopsy for carcinoma rectum or anorectum.

Types: **Illuminating and nonilluminating.**

Parts: Proctoscope is conical shape, with proximal diameter more than the distal, so as to illuminate the light at the required site properly. Obturator is the inner part which allows the easy insertion of the proctoscope.

Positions for proctoscopy: **Left lateral position (common), right lateral, lithotomy, knee-elbow position.**

Technique of proctoscopy: **After doing digital examination, proctoscope with the obturator is introduced inside, through the anal canal in the direction towards the umbilicus. The obturator is removed. Proctoscope is withdrawn and during the course of withdrawal, any pathology has to be looked for.** *Acute anal fissure is contraindication for proctoscopy (Figs. 24-35 to 24-38).*

Sigmoidoscopy

It is used to visualize rectum and sigmoid colon, take biopsies from suspected lesions and do therapeutic procedures (polypectomy, control of bleeding, etc). There are *two* **types: (1)** *Rigid*—**25 cm long, with illumination. (2)** *Flexible*—**60 cm long. In lateral position as in P/R examination or proctoscopy, sigmoidoscope with obturator is passed into the rectum and obturator is removed. Rectosigmoid is inflated with air and**

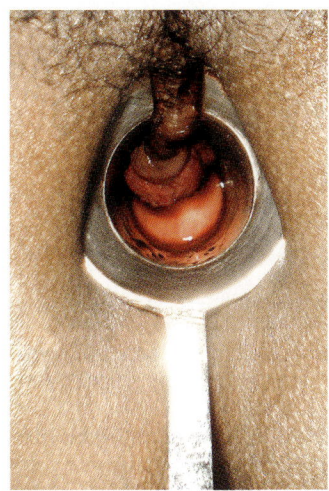

Fig. 24-35 *Proctoscopic* view of the internal pile.

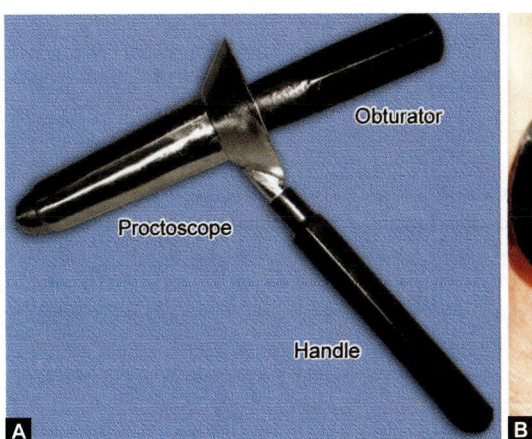
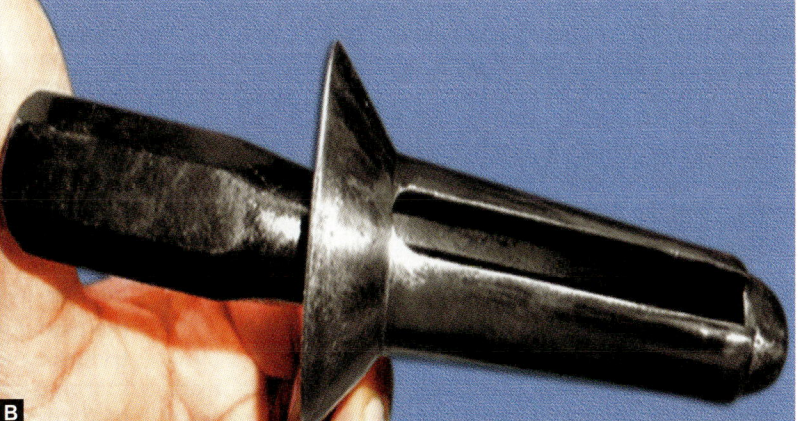

Figs. 24-36A and B *Proctoscopy and obturator.* Grooved proctoscopy is also shown which is useful for therapeutic purpose.

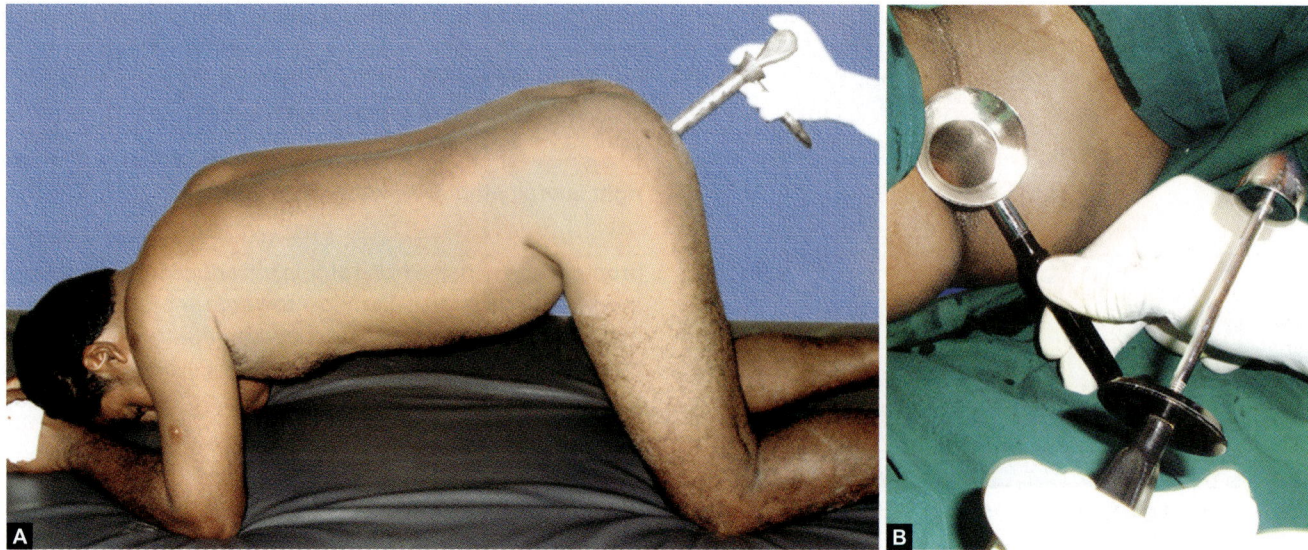

Figs. 24-37A and B Proctoscopy in *knee-elbow position*. It can be done in *left lateral*, *lithotomy* positions also.

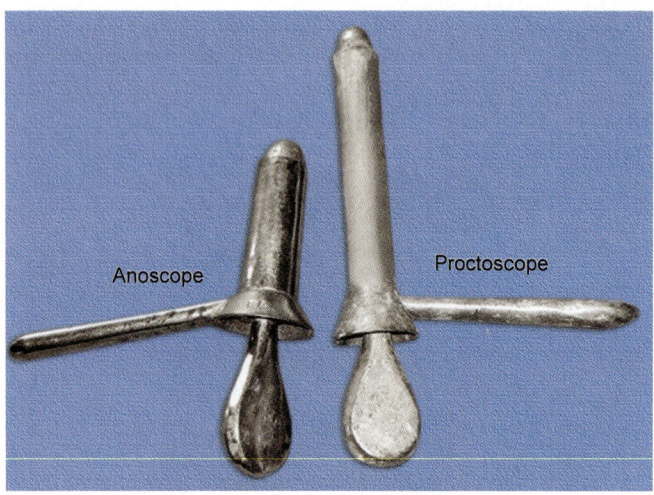

Fig. 24-38 *Anoscope and proctoscope.* Anoscope is smaller than proctoscope.

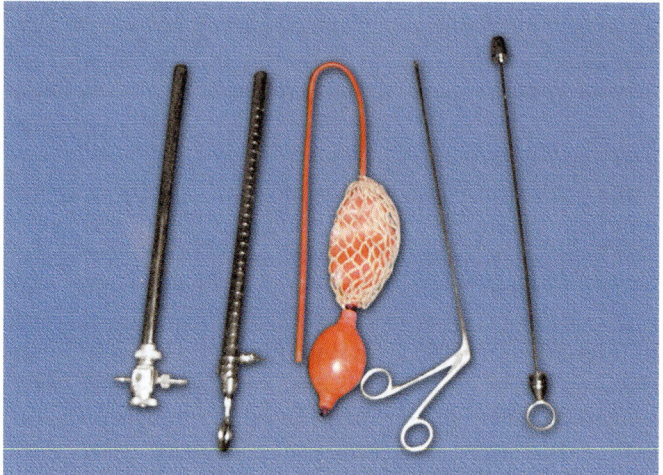

Fig. 24-39 *Rigid sigmoidoscope* with inflation balloon and biopsy forceps.

scope is negotiated into the sigmoid by *Alpha (α) maneuver*. Looked for any disease, biopsies are taken and also any required procedure is done. *Precaution:* Should be careful in acutely inflamed sigmoid colon, because chances of perforation is high (Fig. 24-39).

Colonoscopy

It is 160 cm long, flexible scope. It helps to visualize full length of the colon; to take biopsies from different parts of the bowel; to identify synchronous growths; to remove polyps. Technique is same as sigmoidoscopy, but can be passed up to the cecum. It takes a long time and requires expertise to do the same.

ANORECTAL DISEASES

Carcinoma Rectum

It is common in females. It usually originates from a pre-existing adenoma or papilloma (tubular polyp); in 3% of cases it occurs in multiple sites (synchronous).

Etiology: Red meat and saturated fatty acids increase the risk; High fiber diet reduces the risk; Alcohol and smoking increases the risk; FAP and adenomas are more prone to carcinomas. *Gross:* It can be *Ulcerative; Papilliferous; Infiltrative.* *Histologically:* It is *adenocarcinoma.* *Spread: Local spread*—initially, it spreads locally circumferentially (takes 12–18 months to complete the circumference of the bowel). Later spreads out to the muscular coat and perirectal tissue; then to prostate, bladder, seminal vesicles in males and uterus and vagina in females; posteriorly into the sacrum and sacral plexus, laterally into the ureters. *Lymphatic spread*—above the peritoneal reflection, spread occurs upwards along the colic lymph nodes. In midrectum into the pararectal and midrectal lymph nodes. Downward spread is rare, occurs when growth is close to the anal canal, into the inguinal lymph nodes. *Venous spread* occurs into the *liver, lungs, adrenals* and other areas. *Clinical Features:* Bleeding per rectum/anum (may mimic hemorrhoids); morning spurious diarrhea; tenesmus; bloody slime; sense of incomplete evacuation; altered bowel habits; urinary symptoms are due to infiltration of the bladder or prostate;

back pain due to invasion of sacral plexus; ascites, liver secondaries, urinary symptoms. *90% of rectal growths can be felt by per-rectal examination.* **Investigations:** Proctoscopy; sigmoidoscopy; biopsy using *Yeoman's* forceps; barium enema in case of FAP and synchronous growths; US abdomen; CT scan to see operability; MRI pelvis; *endorectal ultrasonography.* **Differential diagnosis:** Inflammatory stricture, amoebic granuloma, tuberculosis, carcinoid, solitary ulcer syndrome.

Rectal Prolapse

It is circumferential descent of bowel through the anal canal; commonly seen in infants, children and elderly individual; common in females (6:1).
Etiology: Decreased sacral curvature and decreased anal canal tone with diarrhea, cough, malnutrition. In adults, common in multiparous due to weakening of supporting tissue and levator ani muscle; atony of the sphincter, increased intra-abdominal pressure due to any cause (like neurological diseases, spinal injury, old age).
Types:
a. Partial prolapse wherein only mucosa and submucosa of the rectum descends, not more than 3.75 cm. There is no descent of the muscular layer. It is the commonest type of rectal prolapse.
Clinical features: There is history of mass per anum, which is observed when child is allowed to strain in *squatting position*. It is pink in color and circumferential
b. Complete prolapse: Also called as procidentia, is less common than partial prolapse. It is more common in females (6:1); due to weakened levator ani and supporting pelvic tissues. The descent is always more than 3.75 cm, contains all layers of the rectum (i.e. including muscular layer); often descends down up to 10–15 cm. It is often associated with the uterine descent (uterine prolapse). It is also thought to be as an intussusception of the rectum
Clinical features: Complete descent of the rectum which is red in color, often painful; bleeding can occur because of the congestion; sepsis, discharge, fever, anemia are other features. Per rectal examination shows lax sphincter. Anteriorly, peritoneal sac comes down as a pouch which may contain small bowel
Differential diagnosis: Rectosigmoid intussusception, third degree piles

Pilonidal Sinus (Jeep Bottom; Driver's Bottom)

It is of infective origin and occurs in sacral region between the buttocks, umbilicus and axilla. It is common in hair dressers (seen in interdigital clefts), jeep driver; common in 20–30 years of age; common in males and mostly affects hairy men.
Commonest site: Interbuttock sacral region.
Clinical features: Discharge—either serosanguinous or purulent; pain—throbbing and persistent type; tender swelling seen just above the coccyx in the midline (*primary sinus*); and on either side of the midline (*secondary sinus*). Tuft of hairs may be seen in the opening of the sinus

Pathology: Hair penetrates the skin causes dermatitis, infection, pustule and sinus formation which again sucks hair further by negative pressure forming pus and granulation tissues leading into multiple primary and secondary sinuses. *Primary sinus* occurs in the midline. *Secondary sinus* occurs laterally (paramedian)
Causes for recurrence (20%**)**: Improper removal; overlooked diverticulum of the sinus; entering of the new hairs through the scar; breaking of the scar

Piles/Hemorrhoids/Figs

(*Piles = a ball or mass, Hemorrhoids = blood to ooze, Figs = a fruit (Anjoora)*)
It is abnormal sliding downwards of anal cushions due to straining or other causes. **Types**: Internal; external; internoexternal. **Classification** *I*: *Primary hemorrhoids*: Located at 3, 7, 11 o'clock positions, related to the branches of the superior hemorrhoidal vessel which divides on the right side into two, left side into one. *Secondary hemorrhoids*: One which occurs between the primary sites. **Classification II**: *First degree hemorrhoids*: Piles within, that may bleed but do not prolapse. *Second degree hemorrhoids*: Piles that prolapse during defecation but return back spontaneously. *Third degree hemorrhoids*: Piles that prolapse during defecation but can be replaced only by manual help. *Fourth degree hemorrhoids*: Piles that are permanently prolapsed **(Fig. 24-40)**
Etiology: Hereditary; morphological—weight of the blood column without valves causes high pressure—superior rectal veins have no valves (as they are tributaries of portal vein) and so more congestion. Other causes are straining, diarrhea, constipation, overpurgation, carcinoma rectum, pregnancy; portal hypertension (rare cause)
An arterial pile: It is hemangiomatous condition of superior rectal artery entering the pedicle of internal hemorrhoid which will bleed profusely
Clinical features: Bleeding—1st symptom '*Splash in the pan*'— 'bright red and fresh'—occurs during defecation; mass per anum; discharge—a mucoid discharge; pruritus; pain—may be due to prolapse, infection or spasm, etc; anemia; on inspection, prolapsed piles will be visualized; on P/R examination only thrombosed piles can be felt
Through proctoscopy, exact position can be seen as a bulge into the proctoscope. Sigmoidoscopy or colonoscopy or barium enema should be done if there is any suspicion of associated malignancy
Complications: (1) Profuse hemorrhage which may require blood transfusion; (2) Strangulation—piles are being gripped by anal sphincter; (3) Thrombosis—piles appear dark purple/black, feels solid and tender; (4) Ulceration; (5) Gangrene; (6) Fibrosis; (7) Stenosis; (8) Suppuration leading on to perianal or submucosal abscess; (9) Pylephlebitis (portal pyemia) is rare but can occur in 3rd degree piles after surgery

Anal Fissure (Fissure in Ano)

It is an ulcer in the longitudinal axis of the **lower anal canal**; commonly occurs in the midline, posteriorly (more common in males), but can also occur in the midline anteriorly (more common in females)
Causes: Because of the curvature of the sacrum and rectum, hard fecal matter while passing down causes a tear in the anal valve leading to posterior anal fissure. Anterior anal fissure is common in females due to lack of support to pelvic floor. Other causes—hemorrhoidectomy, Crohn's disease, venereal disease, ulcerative colitis, tuberculosis, etc.
Types: Anal fissure can be acute or chronic
Acute anal fissure: It is a deep tear in the lower anal skin with severe sphincter spasm without edema or inflammation. It presents with severe pain and constipation

Contd...

Contd...

Chronic anal fissure: It has got inflamed, indurated margin with scar tissue. Ulcer at its inferior margin is having a skin tag which is edematous, acts like a guard— **Sentinel pile**. Proximally hypertrophied anal papilla is seen

Clinical features: Common in middle aged women, not in elderly. Pain is severe in nature in acute type whereas less severe in chronic. Constipation, bleeding and discharge are other features; P/R examination and proctoscopy is not possible in acute fissure in ano. General anesthesia is required for examination. In chronic fissure, ulcer is felt with button-like depression, induration and often sentinel pile

Differential diagnosis: Carcinoma anal canal; inflammatory bowel disease; venereal diseases; anal chancre (painful); tuberculous ulcer; proctalgia fugax

Complications: It can cause repeated infection—fibrosis—abscess formation—fistula formation

Anorectal Abscess

Commonest causative organism is *E. coli*. Others are *Staph. aureus, Bacteroides, Streptococcus, B. proteus*. Common origin is by infection of an anal gland (cryptoglands). Other causes: Injury to anorectum; cutaneous infection; blood-borne infections. Many anorectal abscesses are associated with anal fistulas

Classification: Perianal; ischiorectal; submucous; pelvirectal; fissure abscess (in relation to fissure in ano)

Perianal (60%): Usually results due to suppuration of anal gland or suppuration of thrombosed external pile or any infected perianal condition. It lies in the region of subcutaneous portion of external sphincter. *Clinical features*: Pain in perianal region; tender smooth swelling in the region, with difficulty in sitting

Ischiorectal abscess (30%): Commonly due to extension of low intermuscular anal abscess laterally through external sphincter; but often can be blood or lymphatic born. Fat in the fossa is more prone for infection because it is least vascularized

Fossa communicates with that of opposite side through post-sphincteric space and so horse-shoe like abscess can occur. It presents with tender, indurated, brawny swelling in the skin over the ischiorectal fossa with high fever. Well-localized swelling and fluctuation are absent in ischiorectal abscess. **Submucous abscess (5%):** It occurs above the dentate line, which can be drained with sinus forceps, through a proctoscope. **Pelvirectal abscess**: It is situated between the upper surface of levator ani and pelvic peritoneum. It is almost like a pelvic abscess, occurs secondary to appendicitis, salpingitis, diverticulitis, Crohn's. US abdomen is done to rule out the above factors

Differential diagnosis of anorectal abscess: Periurethral, Bartholin, tuberculous abscess

Problems with anorectal abscess: Recurrent abscess formation; fistula formation.

Fistula In Ano

It is a track lined by granulation tissue which connects perianal skin superficially to anal canal or rectum deeply; usually occurs in a pre-existing anorectal abscess which burst spontaneously. *Other causes are*: Tuberculosis, carcinoma, Crohn's disease, ulcerative colitis, lymphogranuloma venereum, hydradenitis suppurativa

Classifications

Based on level—(1) *Low level fistulas*—these open into the anal canal below the internal ring; (2) *High level fistulas*—these open into the anal canal at or above the internal ring

Standard classification: Subcutaneous; submucous; low anal; high anal; pelvirectal

Park's classification: Intersphincteric; transsphincteric; supralevator

Low-level fistulas: Presents with seropurulent discharge, along with skin irritation and one or more external opening may be present with induration of the surrounding skin. Often it may heal superficially but pus collects in the cavity forming an abscess which again discharges through same or new opening. In case of ischiorectal fossa most often both fossae communicate with each other from behind causing *horse-shoe fistula*

Goodsall's rule: Fistulas with an external opening in relation to the anterior half of the anus is of direct type. Fistulas with external openings in relation to posterior half of the anus, have a curved track may be of horse-shoe type, open in the midline posteriorly and may present with multiple external openings all connected to a single internal opening

Tuberculous fistulas do not have induration, will have pale granulation tissue with watery discharge and they are most often multiple

Per rectal examination shows indurated internal opening usually in the midline posteriorly. Most of the fistulas are on posterior half of anus.

Investigations: Chest X-ray, MR fistulogram (**Fig. 24-41**) ESR and barium enema X-ray. If required

High level fistulas: Its upper opening is at or above the anorectal ring. It is difficult to treat. Common causes are Crohn's disease; ulcerative colitis; trauma; carcinomas; foreign body. Incontinence may follow after lay opening of these fistulas

Malignant Tumors of Anal Canal

Types: *Squamous cell carcinoma* is the commonest type. *Predisposing causes*: Papilloma, irradiation, dermatitis, long standing fistula in ano. Usually present as a fungating or ulcerative growth, spreads to inguinal lymph nodes. Biopsy and FNAC of lymph nodes are the essential investigations

Basaloid carcinoma—it is rare, non-keratinising squamous cell carcinoma; highly malignant

Mucoepidermoid carcinoma—arises near squamocolumnar junction.

Basal cell carcinoma can occur. Melanoma—blue/black in color mistaken for thrombosed pile

Adenocarcinoma from the anal glands in a pre-existing fistula in ano

Other Conditions

Solitary Ulcer Syndrome

It is mainly thickening and disorganization of muscularis mucosa with superficial ulceration; usually 4–12 cm from the anal verge in the anterior wall of the rectum; but often can occur in sigmoid colon. In 30% cases there are multiple ulcers. Most often there will be only inflammation and induration of the area without an ulcer. Condition is commonly associated with rectal prolapse

Differential diagnoses are carcinoma, tuberculosis, ulcerative colitis

Proctalgia Fugax

It is sudden severe recurring pain in the rectum of unknown cause with segmental pubococcygeal spasm

Features: Common in young people may be due to stress, straining. Common at night, starts suddenly, lasts for few minutes and then subsides spontaneously. Pain is unbearable and severe with often constipation. Gradually subsides on its own

Contd...

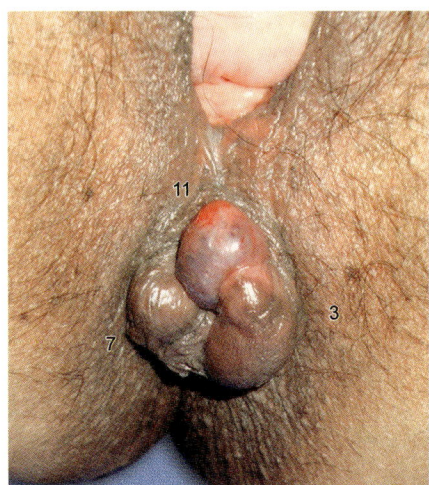

Fig. 24-40 *4th degree hemorrhoids in a female patient.* Note: 3, 7, 11 are locations of primary hemorrhoids.

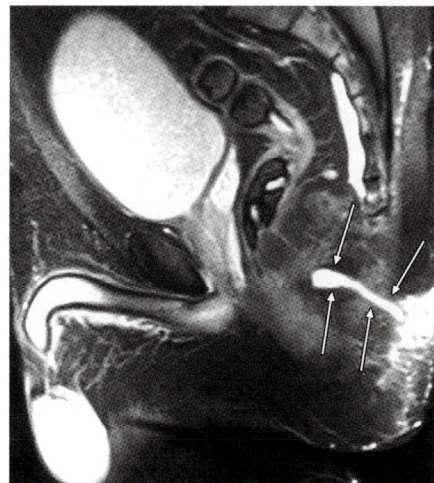

Fig. 24-41 *MR fistulogram.* It is ideal imaging method for fistula in ano; it delineates extensions very well. Endorectal ultrasound is also quiet useful.

Contd...

Proctitis	Anal Incontinence
It is inflammation of rectal mucosa often with the inflammation of colon and anal canal **Types**: Acute; chronic (A) Nonspecific—common: Ulcerative proctocolitis as part of ulcerative colitis. (B) *Specific*: Bacillary dysentery; Amoebic proctitis—common; combined amoebic and bacillary; gonococcal proctitis; lymphogranuloma inguinale (LGV); tuberculous proctitis; bilharzial proctitis due to *Schistosoma hematobium*; enema-induced proctitis especially of herbal enemas **Clinical features**: Pain per rectum and anum; tenesmus; passage of mucus and blood; frequently urge to pass stool; fever, loss of appetite; pain and tenderness in left lower abdomen; P/R is tender **Investigations**: Sigmoidoscopy is more relevant than just proctoscopy; stool study, stool culture; mucosal biopsy; serological tests; relevant investigations like ESR, blood smear, and chest X-ray	Continence of anal canal is maintained by two factors. (1) Normal rectal and colonic pressure and activity. (2) Normal pelvic floor function **Types**: (1) *Urge incontinence*—here rectal and colonic pressure and activity is increased but normal pelvic floor. (2) *True incontinence*—here rectal and colonic pressure and activity is normal but defective pelvic floor function. (3) *Full incontinence*—here rectal and colonic pressure and activity is reduced and also defective pelvic floor function. (A) Temporary—often it is seen after Lord's dilatation; treated by reassurance. (B) Permanent—needs definitive therapy. *Causes*: Irritable bowel syndrome, severe diarrhea, prolapsed piles, rectal prolapse, old age, malnutrition, debilitating illness, congenital anomalies, trauma, surgeries, injury during childbirth in females, spina bifida, spinal tumors, spinal injuries and surgeries, malignancy, post-irradiation, psychological causes **Evaluation of the patient**: For specific causes; anorectal manometry; per rectal examination; sigmoidoscopy
Anorectal Malformations (ARM)	**Wingspread classification of ARM**
It is imperfect fusion of the post-allantoic gut with the proctodeum. Incidence is one in 4500 newborns. **Clinical features**: Newborn presents with inability to pass meconium, abdominal distension, features of intestinal obstruction, improper anal dimple, sometimes with complaints of passing meconium per urethra. It can be associated with—cardiac anomaly, tracheoesophageal fistula, renal anomalies and spinal anomaly **Investigations**—*Invertogram* usually taken 6–12 hours after birth so as to allow air to reach the rectal pouch. Length between the rectal pouch and anal dimple marker is more than 2.5 cm in high anal fistula. In low fistula, rectal pouch is distal to the *Stephen's line* (pubococcygeal line). In intermediate, pouch is at the level of ischial spine (Kelly's point). In high fistula rectal pouch is proximal to the Stephen's line *Murugassu's technique*: Through visible anal dimple, meconium is aspirated by passing a needle into the rectal pouch in sitting propped up position. Water soluble iodine dye is injected. Lateral X-ray is taken to study the level through Stephen line and Kelly's point	*Low*: Covered anus; anovestibular fistula; anal stenosis; anal membrane. It is below the level of pelvic floor (puborectalis), easy to diagnose and treat, good outcome *Intermediate*: It occurs at the level of puborectalis with or without fistula *High*: It can be with or without a fistula into the bladder, urethra and uterus

25. Approaches and Examination in Dysphagia

Competency: SU28.5; SU28.6.

Dysphagia is a distressing symptom of proximal gastrointestinal diseases. It is defined as difficulty in swallowing.

Aphagia is inability to swallow.

Odynophagia is painful swallowing.

Globus pharyngeus is sensation of a lump lodged in throat.

Phagophobia is fear of swallowing.

Sitophobia is fear of eating due to subsequent anticipated abdominal discomfort seen in mesenteric vascular insufficiency and regional ileitis.

Nausea is feeling of immense desire to vomit.

Retching is labored rhythmic contraction of respiratory and abdominal muscles that may proceed into vomiting eventually.

Hiccough (Hiccup/Singultus) is sudden spasmodic involuntary contraction of diaphragm with closed glottis causing short sharp inspiratory sounds.

Regurgitation is appearance of previously swallowed food in the mouth without vomiting.

Water brash is sudden filling of mouth with saliva as a reflux response.

Heartburn/pyrosis is sensation of burning or warmness substernally or in the high epigastrium which radiates into the neck and arms.

Belching is chronic repetitive eructations.

■ HISTORY

Age: Esophageal atresia and dysphagia lusoria are seen in infants. Foreign body, diphtheria, retropharyngeal abscess are common in children. Stricture, achalasia cardia, esophageal webs are common in middle aged. Carcinoma of esophagus is common in old age. Hysteria causing dysphagia is common in young girls.

Sex: *Sideropenic dysphagia* due to esophageal webs (*Plummer–Vinson syndrome*) is seen in females. Carcinoma esophagus is common in males.

Complaints and History of Present Illness

Dysphagia: Sudden onset of dysphagia is seen in foreign body impaction (fish bone, food bolus, solid materials) in children; acute inflammation of pharynx, retropharyngeal area, and esophagus. ***Slowly progressive*** for ***long period*** is a feature of benign disease like achalasia, benign stricture. ***Rapidly progressive dysphagia of short duration*** is a feature of carcinoma of esophagus. In achalasia, to begin with dysphagia is mainly to liquids as weight of solid food opens up the area of spasm to relieve dysphagia. In carcinoma esophagus, first it is for solid, later to liquid. Food getting stuck is classical history but site of blockage is difficult to assess even though patient points out the site. In Plummer–Vinson syndrome, dysphagia may be recurrent, waxing and waning.

Pain: It is mainly discomfort but often pain may be predominant symptom. It is commonly observed in reflux esophagitis and corrosives. Pain may be under the sternum.

Vomiting: Nature of the vomitus, hematemesis, content, smell, should be asked for. Paraesophageal hernia causes post-prandial vomiting.

Regurgitation: It is common in achalasia, pharyngeal pouch and sliding hiatus hernia.

Cough: When there is obstruction in the esophagus, food, liquid, saliva may aspirate into the lungs causing aspiration, bronchopneumonia. Achalasia, pharyngeal pouch, carcinoma may cause cough. Tracheo-esophageal fistula causes severe cough after feeding.

Dyspnea and Voice Change: Mediastinal compression by mediastinal lymph nodes or other masses can cause dyspnea or stridor. Lymph node compressing the recurrent laryngeal nerve also can cause hoarseness of voice. Hoarseness of voice may be due to advanced carcinoma of pharynx where dysphagia is also main symptom.

Loss of Appetite and Weight: It is a feature of carcinoma of esophagus. Weight loss is also a feature of achalasia cardia.

Past History

Past history of surgery, chemotherapy, radiotherapy for carcinoma, neck pathology should be asked. Past history of vagotomy may be the cause for dysphagia. Treatment for hiatus hernia earlier is important.

Personal History

Smoking, alcohol and diet history is important in carcinoma esophagus.

■ GENERAL EXAMINATION

Patient will be emaciated with significant weight loss in carcinoma esophagus. Glossitis, atrophied smooth, pale tongue is common. Pulse on both wrists will be different and not equal in aneurysm of aorta. Clubbing may be evident if there is associated lung pathology. Tonsils may be the site of the primary causing dysphagia. Pharynx should be examined for retropharyngeal abscess and ulcers.

Examination of Neck

It is very important to examine the neck. Neck is examined for thyroid, lymph node mass and pharyngeal pouch. Pharyngeal pouch is a soft swelling on the left side of the neck; on pressing the swelling patient develops regurgitation. Left supraclavicular area should be examined for lymph node enlargement.

Standing behind the patient, examiner holds the cricoid cartilage with an upward traction. Downwards tug can be felt with each aortic pulsation—'*tracheal tug*' is a feature of aneurysm of arch of aorta.

Examination of Chest

Respiratory system is examined for pleural effusion, pneumonia, lung abscess, tracheal displacement, dullness over the sternum on percussion.

Abdominal Examination

Liver may be enlarged and is nodular, hard due to secondaries from lower third esophageal carcinoma. Rarely OG junction mass may be palpable in the epigastrium.

Examination of Spine

Tuberculosis of spine can cause dysphagia by abscess at retropharyngeal region or mediastinum.

■ DYSPHAGIA

Dysphagia is difficulty in swallowing. Painful swallowing is *odynophagia*. It can be *acute*—due to foreign body or acute infection or *chronic* due to causes like stricture or carcinoma, etc. Associated hoarseness of voice may be present in advanced pharyngeal or post-cricoid carcinomas. Laryngeal carcinoma at late stage also can cause dysphagia along with hoarseness of voice. Dysphagia can be *oropharyngeal* or *esophageal* depending on the cause. Dysphagia may be due to pathology in *voluntary/pharyngeal phase* of the swallowing wherein patient also develops coughing while swallowing. Dysphagia due to problem in *esophageal involuntary phase* of swallowing is specified by food getting stuck in the pathway. But site of "*food getting stuck*" feeling is not relevant. Dysphagia can be *progressive or intermittent*.

Causes of dysphagia		
Extraluminal causes	**Causes in the wall of esophagus or other area**	**Causes in the lumen**
• Mediastinal nodes— secondaries/ lymphoma/ tuberculosis • Aortic aneurysm • Rolling hiatus hernia • Thyroid enlargement— malignant • Dysphagia lusoria • Congenital anomalies • Mediastinitis/ mass	• Carcinoma esophagus • Corrosive/tubercu- lous/inflammatory/ congenital stricture esophagus • Gastroesophageal reflux disease (GERD) • Achalasia cardia • Esophageal candidi- asis • Plummer–Vinson syndrome • Esophageal diverticu- lum • Carcinoma posterior 1/3rd of tongue/ pharynx • Diffuse esophageal spasm • Congenital anomalies • Retropharyngeal abscess/peritonsillar abscess (Quinsy)/acute tonsillitis/pharyngitis	• Foreign body in the esophagus — coin/dentures/ fish or meat bone **Other causes** • Cranial causes (neurological) — bulbar palsy/ infarction/ hemiplegia • Vertebrobasilar insufficiency

Causes of Dysphagia

Common Causes

- *Gastroesophageal reflux diseases* (GORD/GERD): Hiatus hernia.
- *Carcinoma esophagus:* Here dysphagia is of short duration and progressive. 2/3rd of the lumen should be blocked by tumor to develop dysphagia.
- *Foreign body esophagus:* It may be coin/bone piece/ denture. It is common in children. It causes acute dysphagia. It may be life-threatening often.
- *Carcinoma of pharynx* or posterior 1/3rd of the tongue.
- *Corrosive strictures:* It is usually alkali stricture. Squamous mucosa has resistance to acid effect to certain extent.
- *Esophageal candidial infection:* It is becoming common due to immunosuppression in association with HIV infection; steroid therapy; cancer chemotherapy; post-transplant period, etc. Presentation is dysphagia and odynophagia. Oral candidiasis (thrush) is obvious. Endoscopy shows whitish curd-like plaques in the esophageal mucosa which can not be moved (food particles can be moved). Barium swallow shows mucosal ulceration and irregular areas. Biopsy confirms the diagnosis.

- **Plummer–Vinson syndrome,** 1924 (Paterson–Kelly syndrome, 1919): Features are superficial glossitis (smooth, pale tongue without papillae), anemia (hypochromic) and dysphagia due to esophageal webs or spasm (triad); koilonychia, brittle nails, hyperkeratotic mucosa (precancerous) are other features.
- **Mediastinal swellings:** Primary tumors/nodal mass either lymphoma or secondaries or tuberculosis.

Rare Causes

Diffuse esophageal spasm: They are in coordinated contractions of esophagus causing chest pain or dysphagia. It is common in distal 2/3rd of the esophagus. Hypertrophy of circular muscle fibers with very high persistent pressure of 400–500 mm Hg is specific.

Dysphagia lusoria: It is a congenital vascular anomaly of aortic root. In *dysphagia lusoria*, an *aberrant right subclavian artery runs* in a transposed position arising from descending aorta that courses posterior to esophagus. Often there will be a complete vascular ring around trachea and esophagus. Commonly they are asymptomatic. Presentations may be dysphagia, chest pain, stridor, wheeze and recurrent respiratory infection (usually presents after the age of 40 years).

Thyroid swelling: It is uncommon to develop dysphagia in a thyroid swelling. There will be always dyspnea when dysphagia develops. Large malignant thyroid or anaplastic thyroid can cause dysphagia with dyspnea or stridor.

Boerhaave's syndrome: It is vertical full thickness tear of lower esophagus due to vomiting with closed glottis. It is often life-threatening and emergency.

Neurological causes such as stroke, bulbar palsy, motor neuron disease, Parkinson's disease, etc.

Congenital anomalies of esophagus; mediastinal fibrosis.

Drug-induced dysphagia: Drugs like KCl, quinine, NSAID can cause dysphagia.

Other cases: Esophageal candidiasis; Chaga's disease.

Evaluation of a Patient with Dysphagia

Proper history; Hematocrit; Chest X-ray often may show mediastinal mass lesion/foreign body. *Esophagoscopy:* Once lesion is detected, it is treated accordingly. Biopsy from lesions, endotherapy, if needed, should be carried out (like F/B removal; stricture dilatation; sclerotherapy). *Rigid Negus* esophagoscope is used to remove foreign body under general anesthesia. *Fiberoptic/video flexible* esophagoscope is used for diagnosing and taking biopsy.

Barium swallow may show irregular filling defect or extrinsic compression. Water soluble contrast is used in suspected perforation or fistula. Achalasia cardia shows '*bird beak*' esophagus with proximal dilatation (Figs. 25-1A and B). *Cork screw* esophagus is a feature of diffuse esophageal spasm. Shouldering and irregular filling defect is a feature of carcinoma of esophagus.

CT scan of chest and neck is very useful method to identify the anatomical location of the cause (nodes/tumor/aorta/cardiac cause/congenital). Extent, spread, nodal status, size and operability of tumor are also well assessed. *Esophageal manometry* is done in achalasia cardia/GERD. *24 hours pH monitoring* is ideal and most accurate for GERD. Small pH probe (transnasal catheter) is passed in the distal esophagus 5 cm proximal to upper margin of LOS under manometry guidance. Probe is connected to a digital recorder worn by the patient for 24 hours. Record is analyzed using a computer. A pH less than 4 for more than 4% of total 24 hours period (more than near to one hour in 24 hours) is pathological reflux. It is often assessed by scoring system. Radio telemetry pH probes are used now without any nasal tube. It is passed and placed on the esophageal wall using endoscope.

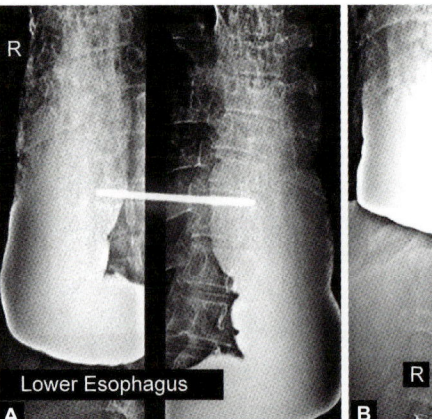
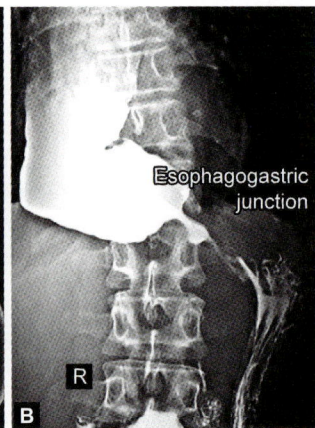

Figs. 25-1A and B Barium swallow showing dilated esophagus (*sigmoid esophagus/megaesophagus*) in achalasia cardia.

Endosonography is very useful in many conditions causing dysphagia. It can assess site, layers of the esophagus, nodes, spread, etc. properly. Different layers are seen as alternating hyperechoic and hypoechoic bands.

Ultrasound abdomen to see abdominal nodes/liver/ascites; MRI study.

Endoscopic esophageal staining using labeled iodine is used to identify early carcinoma in esophagus. Normal mucosal cells contain glycogen which takes iodine and so stains brown, whereas carcinoma cells will not take up iodine and so mucosa appears pale (not stained).

> **Esophageal motility disorders:**
> - Neurological—stroke, bulbar palsy, motor neuron disease, multiple sclerosis, Parkinson's disease
> - Muscular—myasthenia, muscular dystrophy
> - Pharyngeal pouch
> - Diffuse esophageal spasm
> - Nutcracker esophagus
> - Autoimmune disorders such as systemic sclerosis, polymyositis and CREST syndrome
> - Reflux associated
> - Idiopathic
> - Eosinophilic allergic esophagitis
> - Achalasia cardia
> - Gastroesophageal reflux disease (GERD)
> - Alcoholic neuropathy

DISEASES OF ESOPHAGUS

Foreign body in esophagus

Common foreign bodies encountered—coins, pins, dentures, fish or meat bone.
Site of impaction—Cervical constriction—C6; Broncho-aortic constriction—T4; Diaphragmatic constriction—T10; Pre-existing malignancy or inflammatory stricture site.
Features— Sudden dysphagia, chest pain, breathlessness.

Barrett's esophagus

Squamous epithelium of lower end of esophagus is replaced by diseased columnar epithelium in response to GORD (*columnar metaplasia*).
Types:
Long segment—length of metaplasia is more than 3 cm.
Short segment—if the length is less than 3 cm.
Complications:
Malignant transformation
Barrett's ulcer—ulcer at or above squamocolumnar junction; more prone for bleeding, perforation, adenocarcinoma.

Hiatus hernia

Classification – *Sliding (85%)/ Rolling (10-12%)/Combined.*
Type 1—sliding: Commonest type; It is the cephalad displacement of gastroesophageal junction through the hiatus into the mediastinum; usually small, asymptomatic reducible. It is associated with the GERD.
Type 2—rolling: It is superior migration of fundus of the stomach alongside of the GE junction and esophagus into the mediastinum with GE junction in normal intra-abdominal location; presents with pain, hiccough, regurgitation, cardiac abnormality. **Complication**: Gangrene of stomach, perforation into mediastinum/peritoneum, gastric volvulus.
Type 3: Combination of the above (1 and 2).
Type 4: Hernia containing other abdominal viscera as content like transverse colon and omentum.
Reflux esophagitis
Types: *Acute*—following burns, trauma, infection, peptic ulcer; ***Chronic*—**in sliding hernia, after gastric surgery.
Site—lower esophagus.
Pathology: There is bleeding granulation tissue in lower esophageal mucosa causing spasm of adjacent longitudinal muscle—pulls the adjacent gastric area upwards into the esophagus. **Grading:** 1—mucosal erythema; 2—mucosal erythema + superficial ulceration; 3—mucosal erythema+ superficial ulceration+submucosal fibrosis; 4—mucosal erythema+ extensive ulceration+ paramural fibrosis.
Features: Part of GORD; Pain, burning sensation in retrosternal area, referred to shoulder, neck, arm; Heartburn, dysphagia, anaemia.

Achalasia cardia

It is failure of relaxation of cardia (esophago-gastric junction) causing progressive dysphagia more to liquids than to solids; common in females (20—40 years of age). **It is *precancerous condition.*** It is due to disorganised esophageal peristalsis, as there is failure of integration of parasympathetic impulses causing *functional obstruction.*
Etiology factors: Stress, Vitamin B1 deficiency, Chagas disease.
Features: Triad: Progressive dysphagia, regurgitation, weight loss. Recurrent pneumonia, malnutrition, ill-health.
Barium swallows—*Pencil- like* smooth narrowing of esophagus; Dilatation of proximal esophagus (*sigmoid esophagus*); Absence of fundic gas bubble.
Chest X-ray—pneumonic patches; Esophageal manometry; esophagoscopy (to rule out carcinoma) should be done.

Mallory-Weiss syndrome

Superficial longitudinal tear in the mucosa of the stomach at or just below the cardia and lower esophagus (10%) at 1-o'clock position; seen in young adults suffering from migraine / vertigo with prolonged violent vomiting.
Features—Severe vomiting, hematemesis, features of shock.

Boerhaave's syndrome

It is a tear in the lower third of the esophagus which occurs when a person vomits against a closed glottis causing leaking into mediastinum, pleural cavity, peritoneum.
Features: Sudden onset of severe chest pain (crunching effect)—*Hamman's sign;* pain abdomen, shock; *Meckler's triad*—Vomiting; chest pain; subcutaneous emphysema. Chest X-ray—pneumo-mediastinum—'V" *sign of Naclerio.*
Differential diagnosis— Myocardial infarction; pancreatitis.
Complications: Mediastinitis; septicaemia.

Gastroesophageal reflux disease (GORD/GERD)

It is a pathological reflux from the stomach into the lower esophagus.
Anatomical factors: Obesity, altered length of intra-abdominal esophagus, altered obliquity of O-G junction, reduced pinching action of crus of diaphragm.
Physiological factors: Reduced lower esophageal sphincter pressure, altered transient relaxation period in LOS, reduced esophageal clearance mechanism.
Other factors: Delayed gastric emptying due to diabetes, neuromuscular block, gastroparesis, medications; increased gastric distension and gastric acid hypersecretion; alcohol, smoking, stress, lifestyle.
Types: A*symptomatic, uncomplicated symptomatic GORD and symptomatic complicated GORD.*
Features: Fatty dyspepsia; odynophagia; appearance of symptoms within seconds of ingestion of food is typical; chest pain and heartburn (pyrosis); epigastric pain, regurgitation; laryngeal symptoms; dysphagia will occur once complications begin; symptoms are more with change of position; chronic cough, shortness of breath and hoarseness.
Complications: Reflux esophagitis; sliding hiatus hernia; stricture lower end esophagus; esophageal shortening; Barrett's esophagus; carcinoma (adeno) esophagus.
Differential diagnosis: Achalasia cardia; carcinoma esophagus; peptic ulcer; gallstones; pancreatic diseases; gastritis.

Tracheo-esophageal fistula

Types:
H-type.
Lower end blind, upper end connected to trachea.
Both ends blind.
Upper end blind, lower end connected to oesophagus (85%).
Recognised within 24 hours of birth. Newborn regurgitates all feeds, continuous pouring of saliva from mouth—diagnostic.
Obstruction revealed while passing nasogastric tube. Contrast study reveals fistula and obstruction.
Associated with VACTER anomalies— V—Vertebral defects; A—Anal atresia; C—Cardiac defects (PDA/ VSD); TE—Tracheo-esophageal fistula; R—Radial hypoplasia and renal agenesis.

Contd...

Plummer-Vinson syndrome (Paterson-Kelly syndrome)	**Corrosive stricture of esophagus**
It is a premalignant condition. (1) Esophageal webs seen in uppermost portion of esophagus with spasm of circular fibers; mucosa in esophageal web is hyperkeratotic, desquamated; friable; (2) Iron deficiency anemia; (3) Superficial glossitis, Cheilitis, koilonychias; (4) Splenomegaly. **Note:** *Schatzki ring*: It is semicircular protrusion of lower esophageal mucosa located at or just above the OG junction involving only mucosa and submucosa not the muscle; presenting as dysphagia and reflux.	Mainly due to alkali—sodium hydroxide; occasionally acid (sulfuric acid, nitric acid). Causes extensive inflammation of the mucosa with periesophagitis which if not treated will lead to multiple strictures in esophagus **Complications:** Severe life-threatening necrotizing lesion requiring immediate surgical intervention.

Carcinoma esophagus

Etiology: Diet, deficiencies; mycotoxin; alcohol and tobacco; Achalasia cardia; Esophageal webs.
5% common; Common after 45 years; Common in men; Common in **China-Henan** province. Tylosis is familial, autosomal dominant condition with palmar plantar keratoderma with 60% of family members getting carcinoma esophagus. Barrett's esophagus in lower third causes adenocarcinoma.
Common in middle third—50%—Squamous cell carcinoma. Lower third—33%—Adenocarcinoma 9 (in Barett's esophagus). Upper third—7%—Squamous cell carcinoma.
Gross: Annular; ulcerative; fungating—cauliflower-like.
Spread:
Direct: In upper third, it spreads through muscular layer and gets adherent to left main bronchus, trachea, and left recurrent laryngeal nerve (causes hoarseness), aorta or its branches (causes fatal hemorrhage, but rare). It may perforate and cause mediastinitis. It may get adherent to pleura also.
Lymphatic spread: It spreads both by lymphatic permeation and lymphatic embolization. It can cause satellite nodules elsewhere in the esophagus away from the main tumor. Above in the neck, it spreads to left supraclavicular lymph nodes. In the thorax, it spreads to para esophageal, tracheobronchial lymph nodes to subdiaphragmatic lymph nodes. In the abdomen, it spreads to celiac lymph nodes.
Blood spread occurs to liver.

Features:
Recent onset of dysphagia; (dysphagia to develop two-third of the lumen should be occluded); Regurgitation; anorexia and loss of weight (severe, cachexia); Pain—substernal or in the abdomen; Liver secondaries; Bronchopneumonia; Features of broncho-esophageal fistula in carcinoma of upper third esophagus; Supraclavicular lymph nodes may be palpable.
Investigations:
Barium swallow: Shouldering sign and irregular filling defect; esophagoscopy to see the lesion, extent and type; biopsy for histological type and confirmation; chest X-ray to see pulmonary infection; bronchoscopy, to see invasion in upper third growth; *esophageal endosonography* to look for the involvement of layers of esophagus; CT scan to look for local extension and status of tracheobronchial tree in case of upper third growth; US abdomen to look for liver and lymph node status in abdomen; endoscopic esophageal staining with labeled iodine will result in normal mucosa being stained brown, but remains pale in carcinoma (as carcinoma mucosa will not take up iodine).

Section 3: Examination in Specialized Areas

CHAPTER 26: Approaches and Clinical Examination in Urinary Diseases

Competency: SU29.1 to 29.11; AN52.7; PA29.3; PA29.4; PA29.5; MI7.1.

Hematuria, retention of urine, increased frequency and burning urine are the common presentations of urinary diseases. It will cover wide range of diseases from inflammation to neoplasm from kidney to urethral end.

■ DEFINITIONS OF VARIOUS TERMS

Polyuria is urine volume above 3 liter/day. It is seen in diabetes insipidus, diabetes mellitus, diuretic phase of acute tubular necrosis, on diuretic drugs, hypercalcemia, hypokalemia, polydipsia (increased thirst), and salt losing nephritis.

Nocturia means volume of urine passed at night becomes equal or exceeds of day time. It is seen in BPH, diabetes mellitus, diabetes insipidus, cardiac failure on drugs, insomnia.

Dysuria is pain/burning during urination.

Strangury is painful desire to urinate which starts in bladder radiating down into the urethra; but pain will not be relieved; urine also will not be passed.

Frequency of urine refers to passing urine at frequent intervals even though bladder is not full but patient feels sense of fullness of bladder due to irritable bladder.

Urgency is an exaggerated sensation to urinate.

Incontinence is inability to retain the urine in the bladder.

Enuresis is involuntary passage of urine during sleep or at night. It is normal in children below 2 years of age.

Pyuria means presence of pus cells in urine >10 WBCs/cu mm of uncentrifuged midstream urine in females; >3/cu mm in males. Contamination by vaginal secretions is more in females. Pus cells >5/high power field in centrifuged urine in either male or female is also called as pyuria.

Sterile pyuria is presence of WBCs but culture is sterile— seen in treated urinary infections by antibiotics or in urinary tuberculosis/pregnancy/cyclophosphamide chemotherapy/ prostatitis.

Proteinuria: Normal adult excrete protein up to 150 mg/day of which 5–15 mg is albumin and remaining are others about 30 types proteins and Tamm–Horsfall mucoprotein (renal cell glycoprotein). Excretion of protein more than 150 mg/day is called as *proteinuria*. 150 mg to 1 g/day is called as mild proteinuria; 1–3.5 g/day is moderate; >3.5 g/day is massive.

Microalbuminuria: It is early morning urine albumin/creatinine ratio >3 or albumin excretion rate of 20–200 µg/minute or 30–300 mg/24 hours. Excretion of mainly albumin suggests glomerular disease—*selective proteinuria*.

Orthostatic proteinuria is proteinuria seen in daytime collected urine which is <1 g/day with absence of protein in urine collected at early morning. It is seen in 2–5% of adolescents.

Pneumaturia is passing air bubbles in the urine. It suggests vesicocolic/vesicointestinal fistula. Often it may be seen in emphysematous pyelonephritis due to gas producing organisms (in diabetics).

Azotemia is an increase in blood urea and serum creatinine.

Oliguria means decreased urine output which is inadequate to maintain life—less than 400 mL/day.

Anuria means absence of urine flow. It is usually referred to absence of excretion of urine in renal tubules. It is referred as less than 50 mL/day. *Anuria* due to obstructive uropathy is mechanical block.

■ HEMATURIA

It is presence of red blood cells in urine. If it is more than 3/cu mm in uncentrifuged urine, it is pathological.

Early (initial) hematuria: Urethral origin, distal to external sphincter
Terminal hematuria: Bladder neck or prostate origin
Diffuse (total) hematuria: Source in the bladder or upper urinary tract

Types

a. *Gross* (visible to unaided eye).
b. *Microscopic* (>3 RBC's/HPF)

False hematuria: Discoloration of urine from pigments such as food coloring agents and myoglobin.

Silent hematuria is due to tumors of kidney or bladder unless proved otherwise.

Hematuria may be due to lesions of *urinary tract*; *adjacent organ diseases* causing transmitted inflammation to bladder or ureter (acute appendicitis, salpingitis, pelvic abscess) or malignant infiltration of ureter or bladder (carcinoma rectum or cervix or uterus or bowel infiltrating the bladder or ureter); *general diseases* like blood dyscrasias, scurvy, malaria, bacterial endocarditis, emboli, right heart failure, renal vein thrombosis; collagen diseases; *drug-induced* like anticoagulants.

Isolated hematuria is due to bleeding from urethra to renal pelvis without any proteinuria, casts or cells.

Nephronal hematuria is due to blood entering the tubular fluid is trapped in a cylindrical mould of gelled Tamm–Horsfall protein to produce RBC casts containing degenerated RBC with clumps of hemoglobin. It suggests glomerulonephritis/tubulointerstitial injury, vasculitis. Hematuria with proteinuria carries bad prognosis.

Hemoglobinuria is presence of free hemoglobin in urine. It is due to intravascular hemolysis or strenuous exercise.

Causes for hematuria
- Renal injury
- Urinary stones
- Wilm's tumor
- Tuberculosis
- Renal cell carcinoma
- Cystitis
- Bladder tumor
- Urinary bilharziasis
- Benign prostatic hyperplasia (BPH), carcinoma prostate
- Renal infarct
- Glomerulonephritis
- Blood dyscrasias

Investigations

Urine culture and sensitivity is used to assess the infective nature of the urine.
Urine test for hematuria—*Benzidine test;* ultrasound to look for the stone, tumor in the urinary tract; cystourethroscopy to look for bladder or urethral pathology; IVU look for function of the kidneys; urinary cytology for diagnosing urothelial malignancy; CT abdomen/pelvis depending on the location of the site of the cause; renal function tests; bleeding time, clotting time, prothrombin time, platelet count.

■ RETENTION OF URINE

It is accumulation of urine in the urinary bladder. Kidneys excrete urine in normal quantity. But patient passes only small amount of urine or does not pass urine at all causing *distended bladder*. In anuria due to renal failure, patient does not pass urine as kidney does not secrete any urine and bladder is not distended (Fig. 26-1).

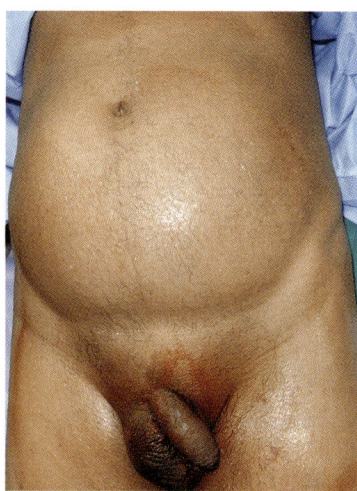

Fig. 26-1 Typical look in a man with retention of urine—distended bladder.

Causes

Urethral injury; benign prostatic hyperplasia (BPH); stricture urethra; carcinoma prostate; stone in the urethra; bladder tumor near bladder neck; phimosis with meatal stenosis; bladder neck hypertrophy; posterior urethral valve; prostatitis or urethritis; neurogenic causes like head and spinal injuries; postoperative cause; pelvic and perineal surgeries; drug-induced retention of urine—anticholinergics, antihistamine drugs, antidepressants.

Clinical Features

Pain and swelling (fullness) in the suprapubic region; inability to pass urine; smooth, soft swelling that is tender in acute/nontender in chronic, lying in hypogastric region which is dull on percussion; with increased desire to micturate on pressure in acute type but such desire will be absent in chronic type; upper border of bladder may be up to umbilicus; presence of features relevant to specific causes is seen in urethral meatus, phimosis, bulb of urethra, prostate, nervous diseases. *Digital examination of the rectum* feels backward and downward displacement of the prostate by distended bladder which feels cystic. Neurological examination is essential. *Cricket ball bladder* in infants is due to retention of urine due to posterior urethral valve.

Acute retention: It is rare. It is sudden inability to pass urine. There is painful distension of the bladder. It is seen in urethral trauma, due to anesthesia, or surgery (perineal/abdominal). There is increased desire to pass urine.

Chronic retention is gradual collection of urine in the bladder due to ineffective emptying of the bladder completely. Bladder is distended and is painless. It is common in elderly. Frequency, difficulty in urination, overflow incontinence is common. Infection in such chronic retention makes it painful.

Acute on chronic retention: Patient is having chronic obstructive condition like BPH; due to infection, acute inflammation and edema of mucosa of urethra, sudden total blockage sets in causing acute on chronic retention of urine.

Investigations: US abdomen; blood urea, serum creatinine; urine microscopy.

Note: In retention of urine prostate should not be assessed during rectal examination. It should be assessed only after catheterization and emptying the bladder.

Causes of retention of urine

Urinary causes
- Phimosis, meatal stenosis
- Stricture urethra, rupture urethra, posterior urethral valves, urethritis, stone in urethra, urethral tumors
- BPH, carcinoma of prostate, prostatic abscess, prostatitis
- Bladder stone, tumor, bladder neck contracture (Marion's disease)

Compression from outside
- Carcinoma cervix, ovarian tumors, rectal and pelvic tumors, paraphimosis, pregnancy

Neurogenic causes
- Spinal injuries
- Spinal diseases—Pott's disease
- Spinal cord diseases—disseminated sclerosis, tabes dorsalis, transverse myelitis

Other causes
- Postoperative (perineal surgeries); tetanus, hysteria, drugs like anticholinergics, muscle relaxants, tranquilizers

---

■ INCREASED URINARY FREQUENCY

Normal urinary frequency is 5–6 times a day. Increased frequency may be observed if fluid intake is more than normal; if there is increased urine formation like in diabetes mellitus or interstitial nephritis; if total quantity is normal but frequency increases due to some pathology in the urinary system. Diurnal frequency is observed in vesical stone which causes irritation of trigone of bladder during daytime. Night frequency is common in BPH. Frequency is equal during day or night time in cystitis. Increased frequency, acid urine, sterile pyuria are features of renal tuberculosis. Gonococcal urethritis also causes increased frequency.

Causes of increased frequency:

In the kidney:	Stone; tuberculosis, pyelitis
In the ureter:	Stone, ureteritis
In the urinary bladder:	Stone, cystitis, pelvic infections like salpingitis, appendicitis, compression by ovarian cyst, fibroid, retroverted uterus, malignant infiltration of bladder by carcinoma rectum/uterus
In the prostate:	Prostatitis, BPH, carcinoma
In the urethra:	Stone, gonococcal urethritis, stricture, balanitis

---

■ HISTORY

Age: Carcinoma of prostate is a disease of elderly after 60 years. Benign prostatic hyperplasia is common after 50 years. Polycystic kidney disease is common in middle-aged even though it is congenital. Renal calculi are common after 30 years. Renal cell carcinoma is common in middle-aged. Wilm's tumor is seen before the age of 4.

Sex: Stone disease and renal cell carcinoma are common in males. Cystitis is common in females.

Residence: Bladder stone is common in Punjab and Rajasthan. Schistosomiasis is common in Africa, Iraq, and Iran.

Occupation: Bladder carcinoma is common in industrial workers. Stone disease is common in manual laborers who dehydrate commonly.

History of Present Illness

Pain

Renal pain: It is dull ache in the renal angle between erector spinae and 12th rib. It is constant pain in the loin often in the upper outer quadrant of abdomen spreading along subcostal area towards umbilicus. Patient places his thumb in front pointing towards umbilicus and fingers over renal angle. It is due to stretching of renal capsule and renal pelvis. Causes of pain may be stone, infection, tuberculosis, hemorrhage in the cyst or tumor. Often opposite kidney may undergo hypertrophy and cause pain in opposite loin (renorenal reflux). When renal pain is severe, this severity may vary from time to time mimicking renal colic. But such renal colic, often named as, is a misnomer as it is never a gripping type of pain and it persists in between severity of episodes. Onset, progression, severity should be asked for.

Ureteric pain: It is typical. It is due to spasm of the muscular tube of ureter and stretching of the capsule of pelvis and ureter. It originates in the loin in renal angle radiates along the course of the ureter along the waist, towards the groin to reach the penis and scrotum in males, and labia majora in females. It also radiates to upper part of thigh through genitofemoral nerve (L_1). This is because upper ureter and testis has got common innervation (T_{11}, T_{12}) and lower ureter and upper thigh have got common innervation (L_1). This *colicky pain* is gripping in nature, becomes very severe and subsides completely with a pain-free interval, and appears again in a waxing and waning manner. Jolting movements will precipitate the pain. Pain is usually associated with nausea and vomiting due to reflex pylorospasm. Stone in the upper ureter causes pain in the loin radiating to the testis; pain in the lower ureter radiates to McBurney's point in right side mimicking acute appendicitis, to amebic point in left side mimicking amebic colitis/diverticulitis (T_{12}-L_1). Stone and clot are the common causes of ureteric obstruction **(Fig. 26-2)**.

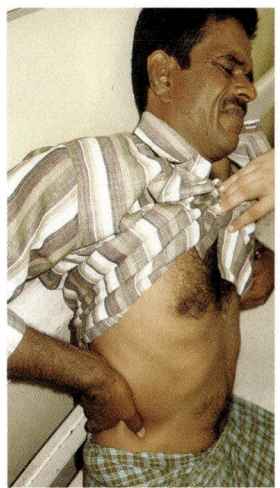

Fig. 26-2 *Renal pain.* Patient holds the pain area with thumb which is pointing towards umbilicus and winces with pain (observe wincing with pain in eyes).

Vesical pain: It is often suprapubic, midline dull ache type. Occasionally, it may be severe pain also. Causes are—acute retention of urine, bladder stone, tuberculosis, schistosomiasis of bladder. In vesical calculus, on standing, stone comes in contact with trigone of the bladder which is very sensitive and causes pain whereas it is less painful on lying down as stone moves/floats towards fundus. Pain originates in suprapubic region and gets referred to tip of the penis. Children will scream suddenly by holding and pulling the prepuce. Hematuria at the end of urination is common. Chronic retention of urine hardly produces any suprapubic pain unless it is infected. Cystitis often causes referred pain in distal urethra. Strangury is common **(Fig. 26-3)**.

Prostatic pain: It is peculiar aching discomfort or fullness in the perineum and rectal area. Referred lumbosacral pain may be the occasional symptom in prostatitis. Prostatic abscess causes throbbing pain. BPH or carcinoma prostate usually will not cause any pain. Carcinoma prostate when once becomes locally advanced can cause pain. Back pain in carcinoma prostate is probably due to secondaries in sacrum (osteosclerotic).

Urethral pain: It is scalding pain occurring at the end of the micturition usually due to urethritis.

Swelling

Duration of swelling, mode of onset, progress, one side or both sides should be asked like in any swelling. Painless swelling in the loin often with hematuria could be due to renal cell carcinoma. Painless swelling in a child below 5 years is probably due to Wilm's tumor. Swelling appearing and disappearing often with pain is probably due to **Dietl's crisis—intermittent hydronephrosis**. Bilateral renal swelling could be as a result of bilateral hydronephrosis due to congenital PUJ obstruction or polycystic kidney disease. One kidney may be involved early than the other.

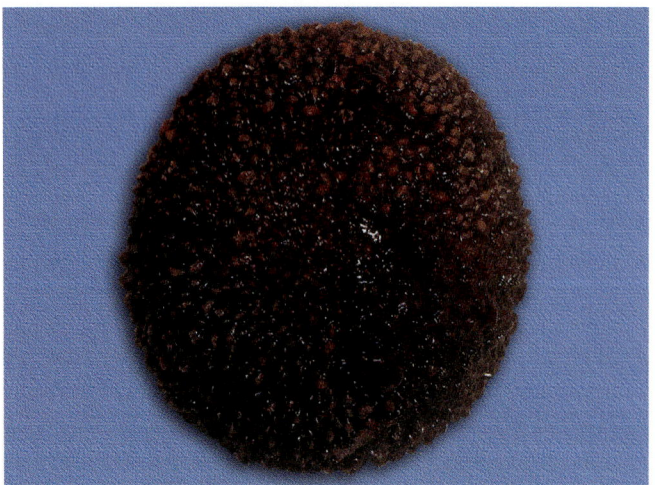

Fig. 26-3 *Oxalate type* of bladder stone. It is usually brownish black with spikes. It is one of the common causes of vesical pain.

Hematuria

Blood in the urine is an important history in the urinary system. Patient often first approaches doctor for hematuria. It may be due to many causes—stone, tumor, infection. Quantity and relation to micturition is important. **Early hematuria,** i.e. at the beginning of the urination is due to urethral cause; **terminal hematuria**, i.e. at the end is due to bladder diseases; **total hematuria** is throughout the urination and is probably due to renal or prerenal causes. Association of pain and type of pain should be asked. Red urine (without red cells) is probably due to diet (Beet root), phenolphthalein, cakes, fruit juices (rhodamine B). Hemolytic diseases can cause hemoglobinuria with red urine.

Retention of Urine

Acute retention is painful; chronic is painless. BPH, carcinoma of prostate, urethral causes to be considered. It should be differentiated from anuria.

Change in the Stream of Urine

Normal force and stream in urination is projectile. It becomes vertical and slow in old age due to BPH. Straining improves the stream in urethral stricture. In enlargement of median lobe of prostate, straining reduces the stream as median lobe comes closer to internal meatus to block it. Bladder stone or pedunculated bladder papilloma may cause sudden stoppage of stream by blocking the internal opening of the bladder. Patient can pass urine by change of posture.

Frequency of Micturition

Increased frequency of urination is observed in cystitis and BPH. There will be retention of urine or increased residual urine in these patients. Night frequency is typical feature of BPH.

Anuria or Oliguria

In anuria, bladder is empty as there is no urine formation. It is a feature of renal failure. It may be prerenal; renal or postrenal.

History of Incontinence

True—patient passes urine without warning and bladder is empty. ***False***—it is overflow incontinence in a distended full bladder. ***Urge***—when there is urgency to pass urine, few drops of urine will be passed; seen in cystitis in women, BPH in men. ***Stress***—urine comes out while straining like laughing, coughing due to weak sphincter.

Urethral Discharge

It is early morning gleet (glairy fluid) in prostatitis. Profuse and purulent in gonococcal urethritis.

History of hiccough, edema feet, thirst, vomiting, insomnia are other history to be noted.

Urinary features to look for are:
- Weak urinary stream
- Prolonged bladder emptying
- Inadequate bladder emptying
- Abdominal straining
- Hesitancy
- Urgency
- Posturination dribbling of urine
- Irritation and painful urination
- Increased urinary frequency
- Nocturia—night urination (nocturnal frequency)
- Incontinence of urine
- Bladder pain
- Dysuria (painful urination)
- Ejaculatory problems

Other Symptoms

Fever, chills, rigors are features of acute urinary infection. If associated with backache, abdominal pain and distension, then it could be due to acute pyelonephritis.

Colonic, liver or pancreatic disease like features can develop due to close proximity and irritation.

Past History

History of tuberculosis, drug intake, treatment earlier for renal failure/stone diseases/obstructive uropathy/surgeries should be asked.

Family History

Many urinary diseases may run in family. Chronic renal failure/polycystic disease of kidney may be familial.

GENERAL EXAMINATION

Anemia may be a feature of chronic renal failure. Dry tongue is a feature of renal failure. Altered respiration, edema feet and face, often anasarca are seen in renal failure. Hypertension is often seen in polycystic kidney disease, renal cell carcinoma, renal artery stenosis, and hydronephrosis.

LOCAL EXAMINATION

Kidney

Inspection

Kidney mass is inspected well in **sitting position**. It may not be obvious in lying down position. **Fullness** in the loin is seen from behind **(Fig. 26-4)**. **Renal angle** (between lateral border of sacrospinalis and 12th rib) is inspected. In perinephric abscess, **scoliosis** of lumbar spine with concavity towards affected side is typical. Here bending the trunk away from the side of the lesion causes pain. Redness, edema over the region suggests inflammation and abscess. In bilateral diseases, both loins are full. Inspection is also done from front.

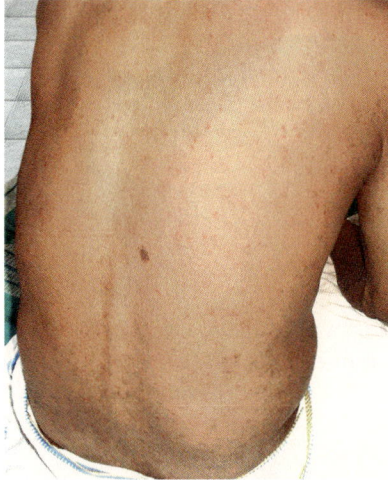

Fig. 26-4 *Loin should be inspected* from behind in sitting posture.

Palpation

Normal kidney is *not* palpable usually. Mobile kidney may be palpable if it is having mild hydronephrosis due to recurrent kinking. *Right side* kidney is palpated from *right side*; *left side* kidney is palpated from *left side*. Kidney is **bimanually palpable**. In enlarged *right* kidney, left hand fingers are placed behind loin over renal angle to lift the kidney; right hand is placed in front, below the costal margin over abdomen; patient is asked to take deep breath; during every phase of expiration when muscle is getting relaxed right hand in front is pushed posteriorly to feel the kidney. Its size, shape, surface, consistency and extent should be assessed. Movement with respiration is confirmed during deep inspiration. Usually enlarged kidney moves downwards during inspiration. In perinephric collection, pyonephrosis with inflammation around and locally advanced renal cell carcinoma kidney may not move with respiration. Hydronephrosis and cystic diseases show cystic swelling. Carcinoma, tuberculosis causes solid, hard irregular swelling. Renal mass also can be felt in *side position* (towards normal side). In newborn, kidney mass can be palpated well with fingers of the hand in renal angle and thumb of the same hand in front. Both sides are palpated together with both hands **(Figs. 26-5A and B)**.

Ballottement/ballotability: One hand is kept behind in the loin; other hand is kept in front over the abdomen. When sharp short forward pushes are made by fingers behind to displace the kidney mass front (displacing hand); bouncing impact is felt by the fingers in front (feeling/watching hand). Very large mass (large hydronephrosis), locally advanced renal cell carcinoma, mass with inflammation surround will not be ballotable.

Murphy's kidney punch: In sitting position, patient folds the hands in front to stretch the back to elicit the sign better, and using the thumb, examiner presses at renal angle to elicit tenderness **(Fig. 26-6)**.

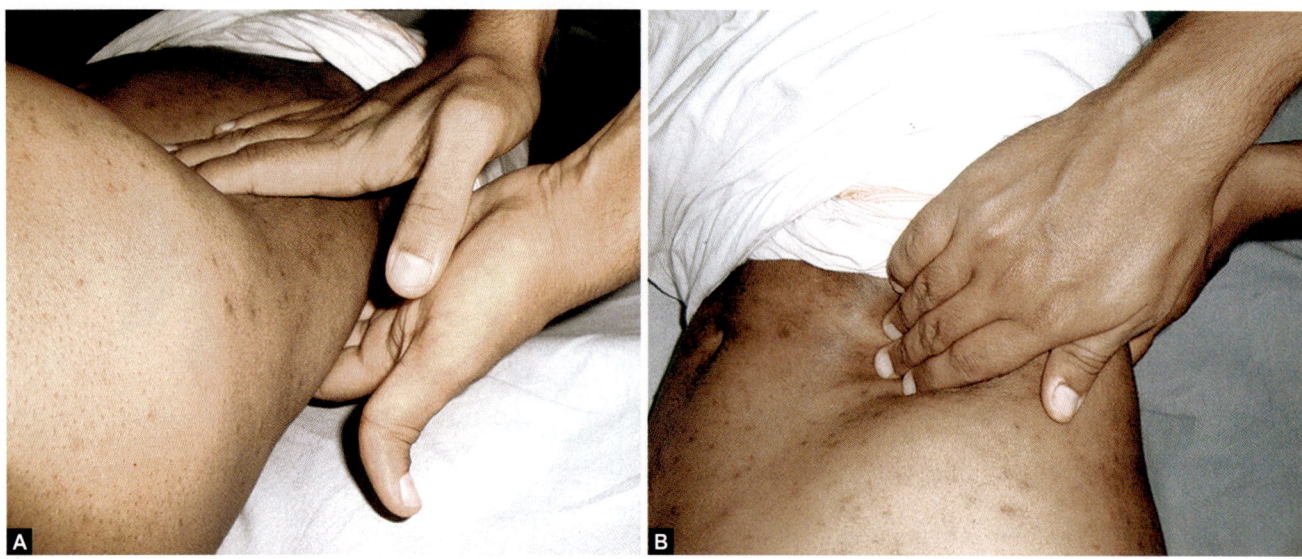

Figs. 26-5A and B *Bimanual palpation* of the kidney.

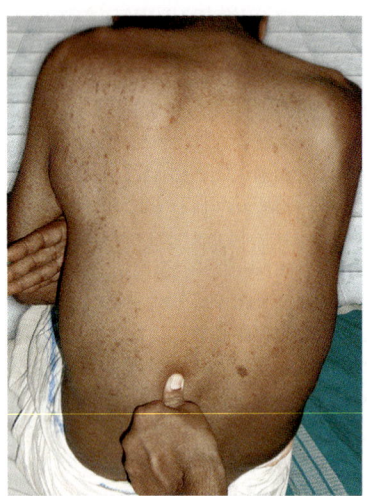

Fig. 26-6 *Murphy's kidney punch.*

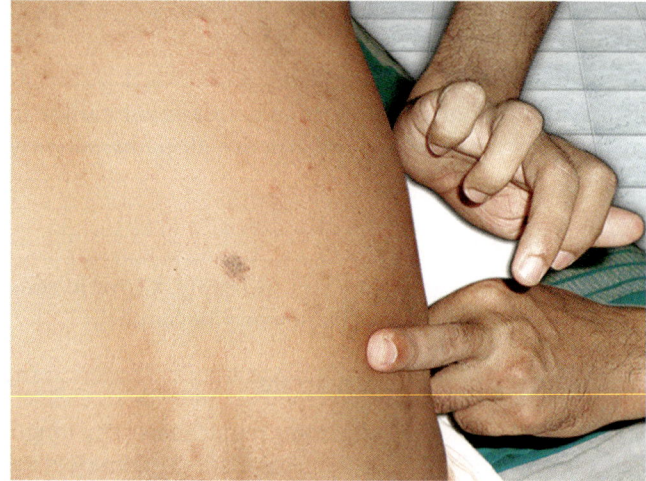

Fig. 26-7 *Percussion over renal angle* in sitting position. Renal angle is normally resonant.

Pitting edema may be evident at renal angle in perinephric abscess.

Features of renal mass:
- Reniform shape
- Mass in loin
- Moves with respiration downwards
- Bimanually palpable
- Ballotable
- Band of colonic resonance in front
- Dullness in renal angle (normally renal angle is resonant due to colon)
- Always can insinuate between costal margin and mass

Differential diagnoses for renal mass:
- Splenic mass
- Colonic mass
- Adrenal mass
- Liver mass in right side

Percussion

Renal mass is resonant *in front* due to colonic band. Renal angle is percussed *in sitting posture*. Both sides should be percussed to compare. **Normal renal angle is resonant** due to colon. Inflation of air by passing rubber catheter per rectally makes (normal) resonance of normal renal angle better on percussion (**Baldwin's method**). When kidney *enlarges,* it displaces the colon in front and medially making renal angle *dull on* percussion (**Fig. 26-7**).

Auscultation Around Umbilicus (Right or Left)

It is done to hear systolic bruit in renal artery aneurysm or renal artery stenosis.

Ureter

Usually cannot be felt. Distal part may be felt per vaginally or per rectally, occasionally in ureteric stone or tuberculosis.

Bladder

Empty bladder lies in the pelvis; once it fills with more than 150 mL of urine, it is palpable in hypogastric region, suprapubically. Fully distended bladder will reach up to umbilicus. Fullness is **visible** in suprapubic region up to umbilicus on inspection. **Soft/elastic** tender (in acute retention) mass is felt on palpation. It is **dull** on percussion. Distended bladder can be felt on *rectal* examination. **Cricket ball-like hard bladder** is typical of posterior urethral valve in children. Bimanual palpation of bladder is done under general anesthesia with index finger of one hand (right) in rectum pushing the bladder forward and other hand placed in suprapubic region to feel the bladder. It is useful in bladder tumors. Base of bladder is normally not felt. Stone in this area and tumor can be felt especially with bimanual palpation under general anesthesia. Extrophy of bladder and epispadias are two developmental conditions **(Fig. 26-8)**.

Prostate

It is palpated by digital examination of rectum in left lateral or knee-elbow position. Lithotomy position is used to palpate prostate bimanually under general anesthesia. Size, surface (smooth in BPH, nodular or irregular in carcinoma), consistency (normal is rubbery; in BPH it is firm; in carcinoma, it is stony hard), median groove (it is obliterated in carcinoma), mobility of rectal mucosa, tenderness (tender is prostatitis or prostatic abscess) in looked for. Usually median lobe is not felt per rectally but after passing a urethral bougie, median lobe can be felt. Prostatic massage is important in chronic prostatitis which often has vague symptoms.

Seminal Vesicles

Knee-elbow or *Picker position* is used to palpate seminal vesicles. Normally they are not felt. It is felt in infection as cystic tender mass; in tuberculosis as firm irregular mass.

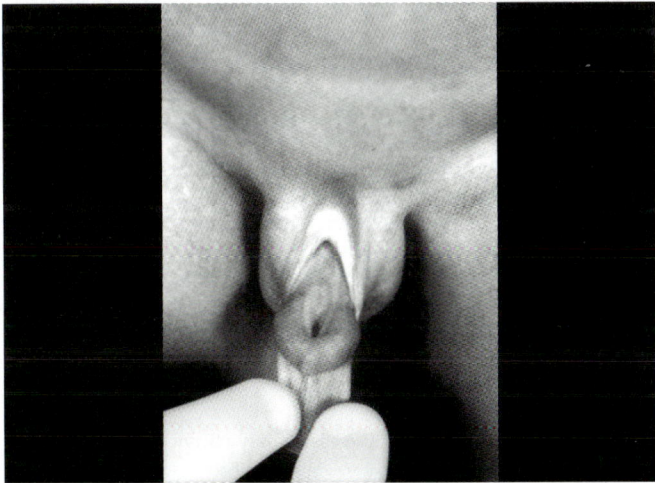

Fig. 26-8 *Epispadias.*

Urethra

Discharge, fistula, tenderness are looked for; bulbar urethra is felt by lifting the scrotum and feeling in midline (in stricture thickening of urethra and crescent-like feel will be present). Stone may be felt. Often stone may be visible near the tip of urethra.

Digital Examination of Rectum (P/R)

Rectal examination is a must in all urinary diseases. **Lax rectal sphincter tone** implies that there is laxity in urinary sphincter also. Rectal and anal diseases should be ruled out by proctoscopy examination.

Palpation of prostate is important. Its size is noted. But symptoms are not related to the size of the prostate. Severity is assessed by prostatism, retention of urine or residual urine. Surface of the normal prostate is smooth; it becomes nodular or irregular in carcinoma. Normal prostate has got rubbery consistency; it becomes spongy in congestion; firm in chronic inflammation; hard and nodular in carcinoma of prostate. Median groove is normally felt in most of the individuals (occasionally it may be absent); this groove maybe obliterated in carcinoma of prostate. In normal individual and in benign prostatic hyperplasia (BPH), rectal mucosa is freely mobile from underlying prostate; but in prostatic carcinoma rectal mucosa may be adherent to prostate with restricted mucosal mobility. Prostatic massage is important in chronic prostatitis and while doing it three bottle urine test is done but massage of prostate should be avoided in suspected carcinoma or acute prostatitis or urethritis. Usually median lobe of the prostate is not felt; but if urethral catheter is passed median lobe may be palpable.

Palpation of the seminal vesicle is done in Picker position; patient in standing position bends forward towards a chair while doing rectal examination. Normal seminal vesicles are not palpable; it is palpable in tuberculosis, tumors or other inflammatory conditions.

Palpation of bladder and bladder stone can be done by per rectal examination. In normal individual base of the bladder is not palpable. Bladder tumors may be felt by digital examination of rectum (bimanual abdominorectal palpation); but general anesthesia is preferred for that.

SYSTEMIC EXAMINATION

Lungs should be examined for secondaries from renal cell carcinoma through inferior vena cava (blood spread, lung is the commonest site of secondary in RCC) **(Fig. 26-9)**.

Parathyroid enlargement may occur in hyperparathyroidism with multiple stones in the kidney.

Cardiovascular system should be examined in relation to hypertension.

Associated congenital anomalies should be looked for in congenital conditions like polycystic kidney disease.

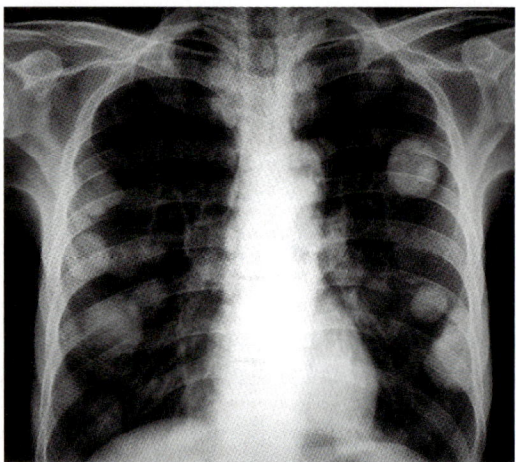

Fig. 26-9 *Secondaries in lungs* in renal cell carcinoma; lung is commonest site of spread in RCC.

EXAMINATION OF URINE

24 hours urine sample is checked. In renal tuberculosis, early morning urine sample is needed for AFB analysis. Color, clearness/cloudiness, quantity should be checked. *Midstream urine* is collected for bacterial analysis and culture. Midstream urine shows sediments if there is phosphate or pus. If after adding acetic acid sediment disappears, it is due to phosphate. Bile in the urine gives greenish brown color with yellow brown foam on shaking. It becomes greenish after sometime due to oxidation of bilirubin to biliverdin. In patient with porphyria, urine is orange colored and on exposure for few hours to air, upper part of the collected urine becomes amber colored. Cascara, senna, rhubarb turns urine brown; salicylic acid, pyridium turns to reddish yellow; sulfonal turns to pink; methylene blue to greenish in small amount and blue in large quantity. Beeturia is due to betacyanin pigment in urine after eating beetroot. Urine will be milky white in chyluria.

Two glass urine test or *three glass urine test* is often significant. First sample is from urethra and prostate, second sample is from bladder, third from kidneys. Prostatic threads may be present in first sample suggestive of chronic prostatitis. Urine should be analyzed for crystals, bacteria, pus cells, malignant cells. Sterile acid pyuria is a feature of tuberculosis. Such urine should be assessed for AFB, culture. Normal pH of urine is 4.5–7.5. In diabetic acidosis, it is below 4.5; above 7.5 in presence of urea splitting organisms. After 12 hours of overnight fluid restriction urine is collected for specific gravity. Early morning sample is used. Normal is 1.020. If it is less than 1.010, it suggests renal failure.

Selective urine sample from each kidney for specific analysis can be taken by ureteric catheterization using cystoscopy.

INVESTIGATIONS

Blood evaluation: Polycythemia may be a feature in renal cell carcinoma. Anemia is seen in renal failure. Tumor markers like CEA in RCC or AFP in bladder tumor may be raised.

Renal function tests: (1) Proteinuria. (2) Specific gravity. (3) PSP test—after passing urine, phenolsulfonphthalein is injected intravenously; patient is given 20 mL of water every half hourly; urine is collected every half hourly and assessed for PSP dye. If 50–60% of dye is present in first half an hour urine sample; 15% in next half an hour sample, it suggests adequate renal blood flow and tubular function. (4) Creatinine clearance value normally is 70–140 mL/hour. It suggests glomerular filtration rate. Chromium 51 labeled EDTA is more accurate method. (5) Blood urea is 20–40 mg/100 mL; serum creatinine is <1.3 mg%.

Plain X-ray KUB (Kidney, Ureter and Bladder)

Preparation of the patient: Enema/bowel wash/laxative is given on the previous day and the patient is asked to fast in order to reduce the bowel gas shadows in X-ray. High penetration X-ray is taken in supine position which covers from *pubic symphysis to lower two ribs*. Often films are taken in deep inspiration, after full expiration and also in standing positions.

Interpretation of the film: First bony parts are looked for, i.e. the hip, pelvis, lumbar vertebrae for fractures, scoliosis, spina bifida, secondaries in the spine. *Kidney shadow*—kidney shadow is visualized in plain X-ray KUB due to difference in the density between kidney (high vascularity) and perinephric fat (low vascularity). Findings that are looked for are size, location, calcification and stones. In congenital absence or ectopic kidney, this shadow may be absent. It may be enlarged in hydronephrosis, renal cell carcinoma. It extends normally from upper level of 1st lumbar vertebra to lower level of 3rd or middle of 4th lumbar vertebra. Right kidney shadow is lower than left due to liver in right side. In children, perinephric fat is absent and so kidney shadows are not visualized. Renal stones are radiopaque commonly (90%) and so are visualized in plain X-ray KUB. Renal stone changes its position in films taken during inspiration and expiration. In lateral view, renal stone overlaps/superimposes the vertebrae but gallstones are located in front of the vertebrae. *Psoas shadow*—It is visualized well in normal KUB. *It is obliterated* in enlarged kidney; scoliosis due to inflammatory or infiltrative causes; malignancy; tuberculous spine with cold abscess (psoas abscess); splenic injury (left-sided shadow); retroperitoneal tumors. *Ureteric line* is looked for any radiopaque oval shadow (ureteric stone). It runs along the tips of the *transverse processes of the lumbar vertebrae*, crosses the *sacroiliac joints* and heads up to a point medial to the *ischial spine*. Bladder, prostate and urethral areas are visualized for any lesion.

> **Differential diagnosis for radiopaque shadow which mimics renal stone:**
> - Calcified lumbar or mesenteric lymph node
> - Gallstone (10% are radiopaque)
> - Concretion in appendix
> - Phleboliths
> - Ossified tip of 12th rib
> - Chip fracture of transverse process of vertebra
> - Calcified renal tuberculosis
> - Calcified suprarenal gland
> - Drugs or foreign body in the alimentary canal

Ultrasound Abdomen

It is mainly of kidney, ureter, bladder and prostate area. It is commonly used imaging for most of the urinary diseases. Fort stones, hydronephrosis, carcinoma, prostate enlargement USG is the main initial screening method used (Fig. 26-10).

Intravenous Urogram (IVU)

Procedure: Renal function must be normal. Overnight fasting for 8 hours is advised. Laxatives are given to reduce bowel shadow and get a good quality film. First a plain X-ray KUB is taken (IVU should not be read without doing KUB). Then 1 mL test dose of *sodium diatrizoate (urograffin) or meglumine iothalamate* IV is injected and waited for 5–10 minutes. If no adverse reaction occurs, then full dose—1 mL/kg body weight of urograffin is given intravenously (about 40–50 mL). X-ray KUB is taken in 3–5 minutes which will show the nephrographic and secretory function of the kidneys. Later after 10, 15 minute and then 20–30 minute films are taken. Further films are taken depending on the need. Films are taken earlier in children as excretion is quicker. Film can be taken as late as 72 hours. Late films show bladder pathology as well as residual urine. In case of *renal failure* with high blood urea, dose of dye is increased to 2 mL/Kg body weight to get a better film—*infusion IVU*. Often diuretics are used in these patients to have better secretion. Lower abdominal compression can be done to have better definition of calyces but not done in children and patients with abdominal aortic aneurysm. *Minute IVU:* In case of renal artery stenosis, within first minute many films are taken to get a nephrographic shadow (where a small, concentrated kidney is seen). *Nonvisualization of kidney:* No contrast is seen in the film even after 12 hours (Fig. 26-11).

Indications for IVU	Findings
1. Hydronephrosis	Clubbing of calyces

2. Congenital anomaly
  a. Horseshoe kidney
  b. Duplex kidney and double ureter
  c. Ureterocele
  d. Polycystic kidney disease
  e. Retrocaval ureter
	Flower vase appearance
	
	Adder (cobra) head appearance
	Spider leg appearance
	Reverse 'J' sign with hydronephrosis

3. Renal cell carcinoma	Irregular filling defect
4. To see the function of the kidneys in bilateral diseases	Bilateral stones, obstructive uropathy
5. After surgery for urinary diseases	To see the function of kidneys and outcome of the surgery
6. Renal injury	To see the function of other kidney (a very specific investigation)

Contraindications:
1. Iodine sensitivity—may go for anaphylaxis. Hence, all precautions must be taken and essential drugs should be available while doing IVU.
2. Multiple myeloma and hypergammaglobulinemias (acute renal failure may be precipitated due to dehydration and also dye makes an insoluble complex with Bence-Jones proteins which blocks the renal tubules).
3. Toxic thyroid.

Retrograde Pyelography (RGP)

Indications: Failure of showing any secretions in an IVU as late as 72 hours film; urinary tuberculosis; urothelial tumors from the renal pelvis.

Procedure: Under general anesthesia, cystoscope is passed. Ureteric orifice is visualized. Ureteric catheter is passed. 3–5 mL of dye, sodium diatrizoate is injected. Patient is put in 15° head down position to allow the dye to reach upper urinary system. X-ray is taken. Often 4–6 mL of air is infused afterwards to differentiate stone in pelvis from papillary tumor—*pneumopyelography*.

Advantages: Prior to dye injection selective urine sample can be taken from each ureter. Brush biopsy from suspected urothelial tumors of upper urinary tract can be taken; Better delineation of anatomy is possible (due to more concentration of dye).

Disadvantages: Anesthesia is required and is laborious.

Antegrade Pyelogram/Urogram

Under fluoroscopy or US guidance 18 gauged 15 cm length needle is passed into the dilated renal calyx and dye is injected to delineate the pelvicalyceal system.

Renal Angiogram

Indications: Renal artery stenosis; renal artery atheroma; renal artery aneurysm; occasionally renal cell carcinoma; arterial anomalies.

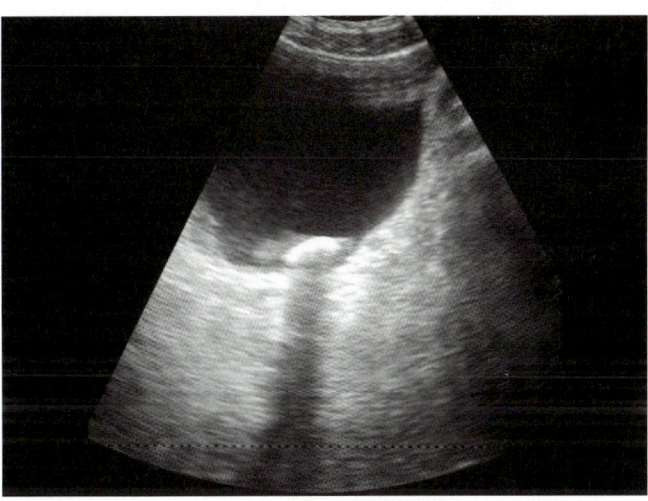

Fig. 26-10 Ultrasound showing bladder stone (*vesical calculus*).

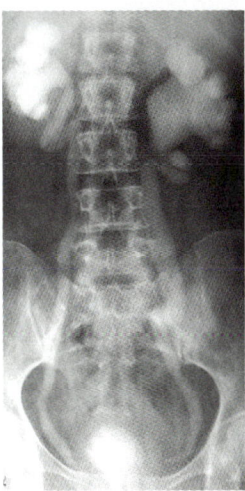

Fig. 26-11 *Bilateral hydronephrosis* with hydroureter—IVU film.

Procedure: *Retrograde Seldinger technique:* Through femoral artery, selective angiogram is done to visualize tumor vascularity, narrowing, anomalies. 10 exposures in 10 seconds are taken. Therapeutic embolization, transluminal balloon angioplasty for renal artery stenosis can also be done. Translumbar approach for angiogram (through aortogram) is also used (Fig. 25-12).

Complications: Paraplegia; embolism; dissecting aneurysm; bleeding; renal tubular necrosis.

Renal pharmacoangiogram: Noradrenaline is injected along with the dye. Normal vessels will constrict in response to noradrenaline. But since tumor is autonomous, vessels in renal cell carcinoma do not respond to noradrenaline and so *tumor blush* is seen. Digital subtraction angiography (DSA) is very useful to assess the renal tumors.

Flush Venogram

It is very useful to assess IVC and renal veins in RCC.

Micturating Cystourethrography (MCU)

Indications: Vesicoureteric reflux; Posterior urethral valve.

Procedure: Catheter is passed into the bladder. Dilute iodine dye is infused. X-ray is taken during micturition. *Free reflux* is looked for. X-ray is taken on applying pressure over the suprapubic region. *Pressure reflux* is studied. *Vesicoureteric reflux* is graded depending on the severity of the reflux: *Grade I*—ureters are seen; *II*—ureters and pelvis are seen; *III*—ureters, pelvis, calyces are seen; *IV*—with grossly distended calyces; *V*—tortuous elongated serpentine ureters. It can be unilateral or bilateral. Often it is associated with posterior urethral valve. It is often complicated by infection, pyonephrosis and renal failure.

Ascending Urethrogram

It is the investigation of choice for *stricture urethra*. Red rubber catheter is passed into the external meatus. Water soluble iodine dye is injected through the catheter. Oblique X-ray films are taken to visualize the urethra. Site, size, extent of stricture and extravasation can be found out in urethrogram. It is useful tool to see diverticulum, dilated prostatic ducts, bladder neck obstruction.

Isotope Renography

A measure of individual kidney function is obtained by this method using a gamma camera. Radio-labelled Technetium 99m DMSA (Dimercaptosuccinic acid) or DTPA (Diethylene triamine pentaacetic acid) is given intravenously. *It shows:* (a) *Early* vascular phase; (b) *Then* secretory phase; (c) *Later* excretory phase. This allows the assessment of renal plasma flow to each kidney and the efficiency and effectiveness of pelvicalyceal excretion also.

Problems: (1) Positioning of counters. (2) Often difficult to differentiate from muscle mass. It is only a supportive investigation.

Cystoscopy

Indications: To examine urethra, bladder, ureteric orifice—for any pathology (tumor, infection); To visualize any bladder fistulas; To treat—urethrotomy (in stricture urethra), TURP for BPH and carcinoma prostate, bladder tumor resection, bladder stone removal (cystolithotripsy, cystolitholapaxy), ureteric catheterization, fulguration of posterior urethral valve. Contraindication: Acute cystitis and prostatitis.

Types: *Rigid; flexible.* Procedure: Patient is placed in lithotomy position. Under G/A or spinal anesthesia after cleaning and draping, cystoscope is passed using continuous *glycine irrigation* (to avoid TURP syndrome). The parts of the urethra are visualized while passing the cystoscope—urethroscope. Once bladder is reached, it is looked for diverticula, hypertrophy and other pathologies. Ureteric orifices are visualized at 4 and 8 o'clock positions. Normal urinary efflux is noted. If 5 mL of sterile indigocarmine is injected intravenously, a blue jet of dye coming down from the ureteric orifices can be seen in 3–5 minutes—chromocystoscopy. In hematuria of suspected renal cause, cystoscopy is done during active bleed; but if suspected bleed is from bladder, cystoscopy is repeated once bleeding stops.

Complications: Urethral injury, bleeding, water intoxication.

Urethroscopy

Anterior urethroscopy is done in stricture, chronic urethritis, and foreign body using air inflation. Posterior urethroscopy is done with irrigation fluid to see prostatic urethra with verumontanum, sinus pocularis, ejaculatory ducts, prostatic ducts.

CT Scan

It is used to assess tumors, lymph node status, IVC spread, local infiltration, metastases in liver, lungs, etc. It is very useful in inflammatory condition also. CT scan is superior to MRI. PET scan is better in staging urological tumors (Fig. 26-13).

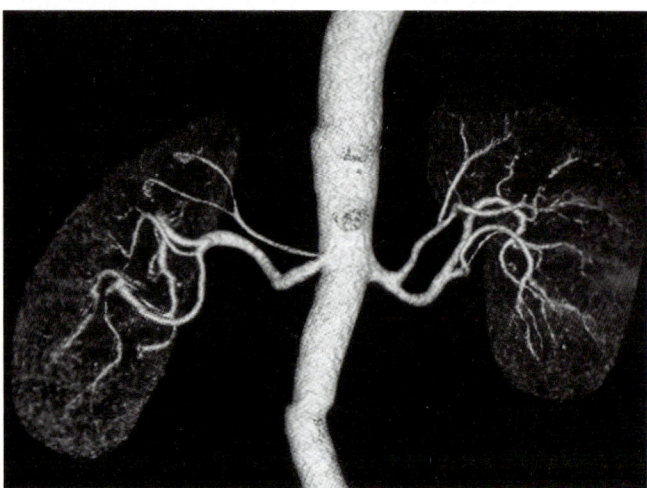

Fig. 26-12 *Renal angiogram.*

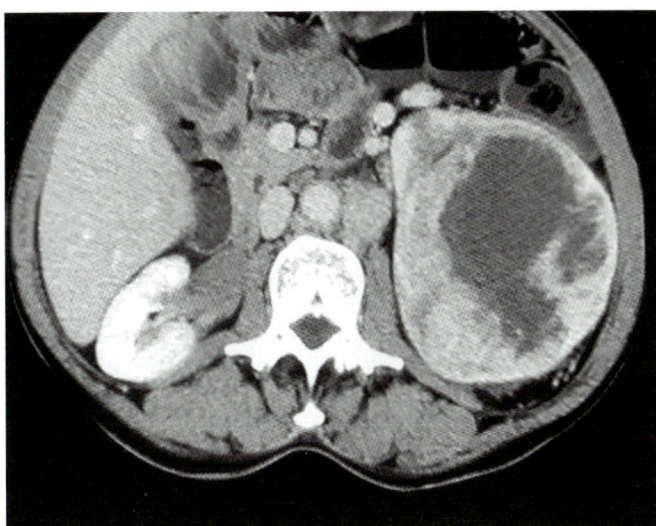

Fig. 26-13 CT showing *renal cell carcinoma*.

DISEASES OF THE KIDNEY

Hydronephrosis (HN)

It is an aseptic dilatation of pelvicalyceal system due to *partial or intermittent obstruction* to the outflow of urine.

Unilateral	Bilateral
A. Extramural: 1. Aberrant renal vessels (vein or artery) 2. Compression by growth (carcinoma cervix, carcinoma rectum) 3. Retroperitoneal fibrosis 4. Retrocaval ureter	A. Congenital: 1. Congenital stricture of external urethral meatus. Pin-hole meatus 2. Congenital posterior urethral valve
B. Intramural: 1. Congenital PUJ obstruction—commonest 2. Ureterocele 3. Neoplasm of ureter 4. Narrow ureteric orifice 5. Stricture ureter following removal of stone, pelvic surgeries or tuberculosis of ureter	
C. Intraluminal: 1. Stone in the renal pelvis or ureter 2. Sloughed papilla in papillary necrosis	

Classifications: (A) Unilateral HN; Bilateral HN without renal failure; Bilateral HN with renal failure. (B) *Intermittent HN:* Obstruction occurs; swelling and pain appear in the loin. After sometime patient passes large amount of urine following which swelling and pain disappear—*Dietl's crisis.* Persistent HN: It is due to persistent partial obstruction. (1) HN only. (2) HN with hydroureter. (C) Depending on the types of pelvis (1) Extrarenal pelvic HN (80%). (2) Intrarenal pelvic HN (20%)—destruction of kidney is earlier and severe in case of intrarenal pelvic HN as compared to extrarenal pelvic HN.

Clinical features: In unilateral cases: Congenital PUJ obstruction and calculus are the most common causes. M:F ratio 2:1. Right side kidney is affected more commonly. Presents with dull aching loin pain with dragging sensation or heaviness. Presents with mass in the loin which is smooth, mobile, ballotable, moves with respiration, dullness in renal angle with a band of colonic resonance in front. Attacks of acute renal colic dysuria, hematuria, if infected fever and tenderness in renal angle, occasionally hypertension are other features. *In bilateral cases:* Lower urinary tract obstruction presents with loin pain; features of bladder outlet obstruction—frequency, hesitancy, poor stream. Kidneys are often not palpable if renal failure develops early. Bilateral upper urinary tract obstruction presents with loin pain, mass in the loin, attacks of renal colic. In bilateral case, when severe, features of renal failure like oliguria, edema, and hiccough may be present.

Complications: Pyonephrosis, perinephric abscess, renal failure in bilateral cases.

Investigations: Blood urea and serum creatinine. Urine for microscopy. *US abdomen:* Type of pelvis, thickness of parenchyma, site of obstruction and cause of obstruction (stones) can be made out. *IVU:* To find out the function of diseased as well as opposite kidney. Normal calyx is cup-shaped. It gets *flattened* and later *club-shaped* which eventually becomes *broadened* in hydronephrosis (Figs. 26-14A and B). *Whitaker test:* Through a percutaneous fine needle into the renal pelvis saline is infused (10 mL/minute) to get a initial raise in pelvis pressure then becomes constant whereas in HN it raises persistently. *DTPA isotope renal scan* is done to assess the function of the kidney.

Pyonephrosis: It is collection of pus in pelvicalyceal system, which is converted into a multiloculated sac. It occurs due to infection of preexisting hydronephrosis; following acute pyelonephritis or as a complication of renal calculus, either pelvic stone or staghorn calculus. *Clinical features:* Triad—anemia, loin swelling, pain. Present as tender mass in the loin which is smooth, soft, not mobile, not moving with respiration. Patient may also have cystitis, pyuria, burning micturition. Features of toxicity such as fever with chills and rigors may be seen. *Investigations:* Plain X-ray KUB may show renal calculus. IVU shows HN. *Cystoscopy* reveals cystitis with *efflux of purulent pus* through the ureteric orifice. US shows dilatation.

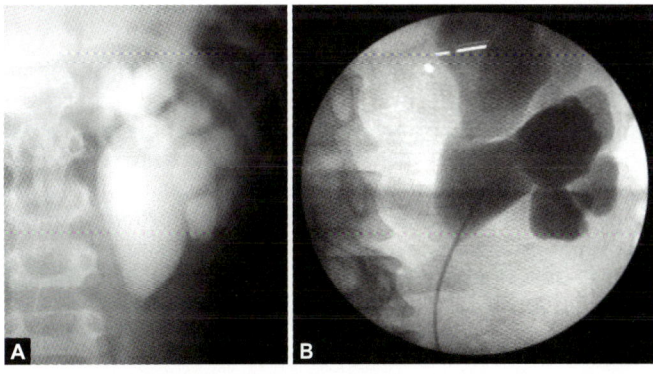

Figs. 26-14A and B (A) *IVU showing hydronephrosis.* Note the dilated renal pelvis; (B) is C-arm image.

Urinary Calculus

Renal Calculus

It is more common in males; 90% are radiopaque (Gallstones are more common in females; 90% are radiolucent).

Etiology: Vitamin A deficiency; low citrate level; infection; immobilization; hyperparathyroidism; hyperoxaluria; cystinuria; medullary sponge kidney; stasis; Randall's plaque (urinary salts deposition); microlith formation (Carr's postulates); sarcoidosis; myelomatosis, gout, hypervitaminosis D, neoplasms on treatment, hypomagnesuria; renal tubular acidosis.

Types: (1) *Oxalate stones* (75%): Also called as *mulberry stone* as it is brown in color, with sharp projections. It is invariably calcium oxalate stone, shows *envelope shaped crystals in urine*. (2) *Phosphate stones* (10–15%): It is either calcium phosphate or calcium, magnesium, ammonium phosphate stone usually occurring in an infected urine. It is smooth and dirty white in color. In alkaline urine, it enlarges rapidly, filling renal calyces taking their shape called as *staghorn calculus*. It is radiopaque and attains a large size. (3) *Uric acid stones:* are smooth, hard, yellowish, multiple and radiolucent. They are seen in gout, hyperuricosuria, and altered purine metabolism. (4) *Urate stones.* (5) *Cystine stones* occur in *cystinuria* where there is defective absorption of cystine from the renal tubules (autosomal recessive condition). It is seen in young girls, occurs *only in acid urine*. It is multiple, soft, yellow in color and the color changes to *greenish hue* on exposure. It attains large size. It is radiopaque because it contains sulfur. (6) *Xanthine stones* are very rare, smooth, brick red in color, due to altered xanthine metabolism. Here there is deficiency in xanthine oxidase enzyme. (7) *Indigo stones:* Very rare. Blue in color. (8) *Struvite stone:* It is compound of magnesium, ammonium, phosphate mixed with carbonate. It occurs in presence of ammonia and urea splitting organisms in urine.

Clinical features: (1) *Pain:* Renal pain is located over renal angle, hypochondriac and lumbar region. Often it is severe, with vomiting due to pylorospasm. Often radiating to groin and testis. (2) Hematuria is common. (3) Pyuria. (4) Fever. (5) Tenderness in renal angle, with often palpable mass in the loin which is bimanually palpable, ballotable, smooth, soft, moves with respiration. (6) As urinary tract infection. (7) Incidental finding. (8) Often hypertension. Plain X-ray KUB shows radiopaque stone; IVU is done to see the function; US is diagnostic; urine analysis and culture to identify the bacteria. CT scan is ideal investigation.

Ureteric Calculi

It is always of renal origin. Nature of stones is same as that of renal stones. They are commonly of elongated shape. They can get impacted at narrow sites at different levels—PUJ; where ureter crosses the iliac vessels; where ureter crosses vas deferens/broad ligament; where ureter penetrates outer layer of bladder muscle; in the intramural portion of ureter near the ureteric orifice. Stones less than 5–8 mm size may pass spontaneously.

Problems with ureteric stones: Obstruction, hydronephrosis, infection, impaction, ureteral stricture.

Clinical features: (1) *Pain*—colicky type, radiates from loin to groin often to the tip of the genitalia, testis. It is severe in intensity. It mimics *appendicitis, cholecystitis, ovarian or tubal pathology*. (2) Nausea, vomiting, sweating due to pain and reflex pylorospasm. (3) Hematuria, dysuria, frequency, strangury. (4) Tenderness in iliac fossa and renal angle (no rebound tenderness).

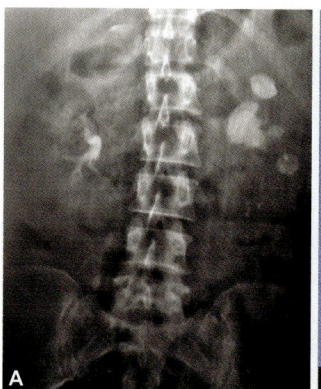 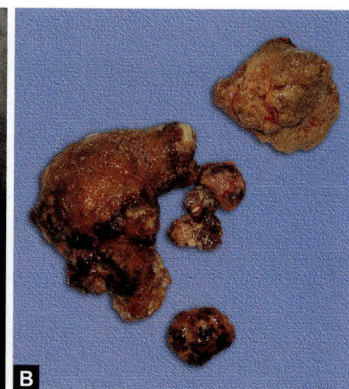

Figs. 26-15A and B *Left sided staghorn calculus* with X-ray showing the same in an IVU—plain X-ray KUB will show better picture.

Staghorn Calculus

It is the stone occupying the renal pelvis and calyces (Figs. 26-15A and B). It is usually phosphate or ammonium magnesium phosphate (*Triple phosphate*) stone. It is white in color, soft, smooth, occurs in preexisting infection (commonly *E. coli*). It can *be unilateral or bilateral*. Patient with *bilateral* stones may go in *for renal failure*. Pain, hematuria, renal failure in bilateral cases, fever with chills and rigors are the presentations.

Vesical Calculus

Types: Primary vesical calculus: It occurs in sterile urine. It usually comes down from kidney through ureter into the bladder and there it gets enlarged. It is usually *oxalate* stone. Oxalate stone is usually single, primary stone, brownish black in color (due to deposited blood pigment over the surface), hard and with spikes over the surface which irritates bladder mucosa causing hematuria (*mullberry stone*). *Secondary vesical calculus*: It occurs in the presence of infection. It is usually phosphate *stone*, occurs in bladder only. Phosphate stone is smooth, soft, ivory white in color. It is either calcium phosphate or ammonium, calcium and magnesium phosphate (*Triple phosphate stone*). *Uric acid and urate stones* are single or multiple, primary, nonradiopaque, smooth, pale yellow in color. *Cystine calculus:* Occurs in cystinuria and is radiopaque due to high sulphur content. Clinical Features: Common in males. Often occurs in children. *Frequency* is more during day time than during night, because during the day, due to ambulation stone comes in contact with the trigone of the bladder and irritates, whereas during night, stone slips towards the fundus, away from the trigone and so less frequency and pain. *Pain:* More during day which is referred to the tip of penis or labia. Also increases during jolting and movements. Suprapubic pain and tenderness may be present.

Note: Hematuria: Often terminal. Interruption of urinary stream and often acute urinary retention. Features of cystitis: Burning micturition, fever, pain. P/R or P/V: Large stone may be palpable. Stone may be identified incidentally in plain X-ray KUB or US

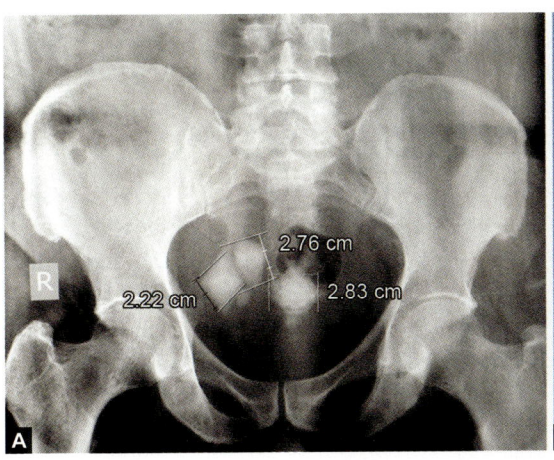
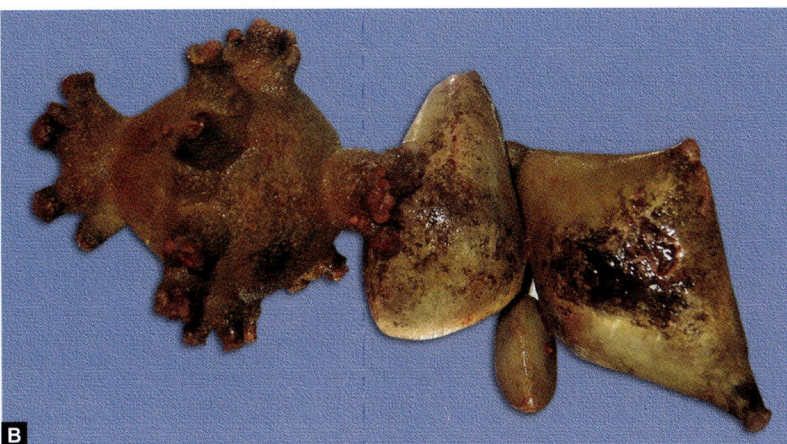

Figs. 26-16A and B Multiple urinary bladder stones; X-ray is typical.

abdomen. Investigations: Urine microscopy shows envelope crystals in oxalate stone, hexagonal type in cystine stone. Other investigations are urine culture, blood urea, serum creatinine, serum calcium, inorganic phosphate, uric acid. Plain X-ray KUB shows radiopaque stones—90%. IVU to see function of the kidney. US abdomen is diagnostic. Cystoscopy to see radiolucent stone (Figs. 26-16A and B).

Wilms' Tumor (Nephroblastoma)

It arises from embryonic connective tissue containing epithelial and connective tissue elements. It is located in one of the poles of the kidney. It is bilateral in 5% cases. It is common in first 4 years of life.

Gross: It is smooth, soft, fleshy, pinkish white in color, often with hemorrhagic areas.

Microscopy: Malignant primitive glomeruli and primitive tubules, with epithelial and connective tissue cells.

Spread: Mainly through blood into the lungs, liver and rarely to bones.

Clinical features: Triad: Mass, fever, hematuria. (1) *Mass abdomen is commonest presentation.* Mass is smooth, mobile, firm or hard, lobular, located in the loin, moves with respiration, bimanually palpable, ballotable, with dullness in renal angle and with resonant band in front. It does not cross the midline. *Differential diagnosis* is adrenal neuroblastoma which is knobby and nodular, does not move with respiration and crosses the midline. (2) *Fever:* May be due to tumor necrosis. (3) *Hematuria* is a grave sign as it signifies rupture of tumor into the renal pelvis. (4) *Hypertension* (25%). (5) 12% of cases are associated with congenital anomalies and syndromes.

Investigations: US abdomen, IVU, renal angiography, X-ray abdomen—*egg shell* peripheral calcification is diagnostic, CT abdomen.

Differential diagnosis: Adrenal tumor, retroperitoneal tumor, renal cyst, polycystic kidney disease.

Renal Cell Carcinoma (RCC)

Also known as *hypernephroma*—(it is a misnomer), Grawitz tumor, clear cell carcinoma, internist tumor.

It is an adenocarcinoma arising from renal tubular cells—most common site is proximal renal tubular cell. More common in males; more common in 5th–6th decade of life.

Etiology: It is associated with von-Hippel-Lindae disease (Cerebellar hemangioblastoma, retinal angiomatosis, tumor or cysts of pancreas). RCC here is commonly bilateral. High animal fat diet; environmental factors like asbestos, lead, cadmium and tobacco; cigarette smoking; chromosomal aberration; acquired cystic kidney disease after long-term dialysis are some of the risk factors.

Pathology: Gross: It attains a large size. Commonly located in *upper pole*, sometimes in lower pole but rare in the middle. Cut section is *yellowish* due to lipoid content with areas of hemorrhage and necrosis. This noncapsulated tumor is very vascular. *Microscopy:* Malignant cells which are cubical or polyhedral contain lipid, cholesterol and glycogen. Spread: (1) *Local:* Into the perinephric pad of fat, calyces and renal pelvis. (2) *Blood spread:* RCC enters the renal vein as *proliferating tumor thrombus* which extends into the IVC and later gets detached causing *cannon ball secondaries* in the lung which are often calcified. Once primary tumor is removed, secondaries may regress due to tumor immunity. Occasionally secondaries occur in bone, liver and brain. Left testicular vein which drains into left renal vein may get blocked by proliferating tumor thrombus resulting in *irreducible left-sided varicocele*. (3) *Lymphatic spread:* To hilar lymph nodes, para-aortic lymph nodes.

Clinical features: M:F::2:1. *Triad*—Hematuria; pain; palpable mass. Others are clot colic; dragging discomfort in the loin; mass in the loin which moves with respiration, mobile, nodular, hard, with dull renal angle and resonant band in front; left-sided *varicocele* which is *irreducible*. *Atypical presentations:* (A) Due to secondaries: Pathological fractures, persistent cough and hemoptysis. (B) *Persistent pyrexia* with no evidence of infection (*P*yrexia of *U*nknown *O*rigin). (C) Constitutional symptoms: Malaise, lethargy and severe anemia. (D) Polycythemia: 4%. (E) Hypercalcemia, hypertension (Surgical renal conditions associated with hypertension—PCKD, Renal cell carcinoma, renal artery stenosis, chronic glomerulonephritis). (F) Nephrotic syndrome (very rare). (G) Stauffer's syndrome: Non-metastatic liver dysfunction which gets corrected after nephrectomy.

Investigations: Urine microscopy shows RBCs. IVU—shows mass lesion and irregular filling defect. US abdomen—reveals the size, extension, lymph node involvement, spread to the liver, status of renal vein and IVC. CT scan is confirmatory and also helps to know the status of renal vein and IVC. Renal angiogram is done through Seldinger technique via transfemoral route, to see the vascularity. Pharmacoangiogram (Inject noradrenaline along with dye while doing angiogram)—as tumor vessels are autonomous, they will not constrict whereas adjacent normal vessels will constrict, so tumor blush is visualized. Through angiogram therapeutic embolization of tumor can be done to reduce the vascularity of tumor. Chest X-ray shows cannon ball secondaries. Often it is calcified. CT chest and bone scan are done to look for bone secondaries. Other tests are—peripheral smear, serum calcium, hematocrit and ESR.

Differential diagnosis: Polycystic kidney disease; solitary cyst of kidney; adrenal tumor; retroperitoneal tumor; carcinoma colon.

Diseases of kidney	Features
Horseshoe kidney	
Developmental anomaly where there is failure of complete ascent of kidneys with the fusion of upper or lower poles (common); common in males; commonest in front of 4th lumbar vertebra; *isthmus*, the part that communicates the two poles lies in front of aorta, has blood supply that communicates with one kidney	Fixed, nonmobile form mass in midline at the level of 4th lumbar vertebra, resonant on percussion, more prone for infection, stone formation, hydronephrosis, tuberculosis. IVU—medialization of calyces, curving of ureter as *flower vase*
Polycystic kidney disease (PCKD)	
Adult PCKD, inherited as autosomal dominant disease. Grossly contains multiple cysts with clear or brownish fluid (due to hemorrhage) Cyst formation occurs at the junction of distal tubule and the collecting duct **Other associations:** Polycystic disease of liver (18%), pancreas, lungs, Berry's aneurysm in the circle of Willis	Presents in third decade, with loin pain hematuria (25%), infection, hypertension (75%), uremia (due to renal failure). Bilateral palpable renal mass, which is lobular, firm, mobile moves with respiration, ballotable with dull renal angle and resonant band in front. **Investigations**: IVU—*spider leg* pattern; blood urea, serum creatinine; urine specific gravity <1.010 **Differential diagnosis:** Renal cell carcinoma; hydronephrosis; solitary renal cyst
Solitary renal cyst	
Never congenital; It is due to earlier trauma/infection resulting in blockage of tubule leading to cyst formation	Usually unilateral, present as renal mass which is smooth, often tender if infected or hemorrhagic
Duplication of renal pelvis	
Most common congenital anomaly of upper urinary tract. Associated with duplication of ureter (3%). This duplication is partial where two ureters join at lower third or complete where upper ureter opens into the bladder at lower level, lower ureter opens into the bladder at upper, normal ureteric orifice—**Weigert-Meyer law**	Usually unilateral, common on left side. When associated with partial duplex ureters, there is renorenal reflux, resulting in infection, stone formation, hydronephrosis **Investigations**: IVU—diagnostic; US—for complications; cystoscopy—to look for double ureteric orifice

Diseases of kidney	Features
Retrocaval ureter	
Developmental defect of IVC; ureter passes behind IVC causing right sided HN, with upper third hydroureter	Presents as features of hydronephrosis. IVU—Reverse J sign. CT is confirmative
Ureterocele	
It is cystic enlargement of intramural portion of ureter. It is due to congenital atresia of the ureteric orifice. Its wall contains only mucous membrane **Stephen classification**: Stenotic/sphincteric/sphincterostenotic	Common in females, often bilateral; causes hydronephrosis, infection, calculi formation. IVU—*Adder head/cobra head* appearance; cystoscopy—thin walled translucent cyst surrounding the ureteric orifice
Perinephric abscess	
Causes: Infection of perinephric hematoma; perforation through renal capsule from pyonephrosis/renal carbuncle; tuberculous perinephric abscess extension from cortical abscess; hematogenous spread; extension from appendicular abscess	High fever; fullness; rigidity, tenderness in loin; scoliosis with concavity towards abscess. **Investigations:** Total count raised; plain X-ray KUB—obliteration of psoas shadow, elevation of hemidiaphragm IVU—downward displacement of kidney is not seen in erect film—*Mathe's sign; CT is ideal*
Renal tuberculosis	
Commonly secondary, primary being in the lung; common in males; common on right side. **Clinical features:** Frequency; polyuria; *sterile pyuria*—urine is pale, and opalescent with presence of pus without organism in acid urine (*abacterial aciduria*); painful micturition with often terminal hematuria, renal pain and suprapubic pain; fever; impotence; infertility Kidney is rarely palpable; prostate and seminal vesicles are thickened; vas thickened and beaded; epididymis thickened	**Investigations:** Three consecutive early morning samples of urine (EMSU); Ziehl-Neelsen staining; culture (L-J media) plain X-ray KUB—calcification; IVU—hydrocalyx, narrowing of calyx, multiple strictures of ureter with dilatations in between. RGP—very useful; cystoscopy—reveals multiple tubercles, bladder spasm, edema of ureteric orifice eventually forming "Golf-hole ureter"
Renal carbuncle	
A localized inflammatory necrotic mass of tissue involving renal parenchyma *caused by Staphylococcus aureus, coliform* organisms; source of which is cutaneous infections like boil or carbuncles	Ill-defined swelling in the loin, with pyrexia, leukocytosis Staphylococci isolated from the urine IVU—obliteration of group of calyces mimicking renal cell carcinoma

CONDITIONS OF URINARY BLADDER, PROSTATE, URETHRA

Bladder Tumors

Classification: (1) *Primary*: (a) Epithelial: *Transitional cell carcinoma* (TCC; 90%); *adenocarcinoma*, arising from urachal remnant or in exstrophy bladder or from glandular metaplasia (2%); *squamous cell carcinoma* originates from bilharzial infection (5%) or calculus. (b) Connective tissue tumor: Myoma, angioma, fibromas, sarcomas, extra-adrenal pheochromocytoma. (2) *Secondary*: From adjacent organs like sigmoid colon, rectum, uterus and ovary, prostate.

Bladder tumor can be papilloma (benign) or malignant *(TCC)*. Benign is always papilliferous villi like; presents with recurrent hematuria, clot retention. Cystoscopy and biopsy is a must to rule out malignancy.

Transitional cell arcinoma (TCC): It is the commonest type of bladder tumor. Etiology: *3C's*—Chemical carcinogens [2-Naphthylamine, aminobiphenyl, benzidine, chloro-O-toluidine, chloroaniline (occupational)]; Cigarette smoking; Cyclophosphamide.

TCC can be—nonmuscle invasive with or without involving lamina propria; muscle invasive or concomitant in situ. TCC also can be superficial bladder tumor or muscle invasive or carcinoma in situ.

Sites: Lateral wall—commonest (35%). Trigone—next common (32%).

Clinical features: (1) Painless hematuria. (2) Features of cystitis, with suprapubic pain, frequency, dysuria. (3) Hydronephrosis can occur when tumor obstructs the ureteric orifice. (4) Pain in groin, back, perineum, when tumor invades the pelvic wall.

Investigations: Urine microscopy shows RBC's and malignant cells. Blood: Hb%, blood urea, serum creatinine. IVU: shows filling defect with distortion and often hydronephrosis. Cystoscopy is diagnostic.

Bimanual examination under general anesthesia—to stage the tumor. US abdomen is done to see extension into bladder wall, pelvis, liver, lymph nodes. CT scan is done to evaluate the level of extension.

Benign Prostatic Hyperplasia (BPH)

It is benign enlargement of prostate which occurs after 50 years, usually between 60–70 years.

Theories: (1) It is involuntary hyperplasia due to a disturbance of the ratio and quantity of circulating androgens and estrogens. (2) BPH is a benign neoplasm called as *fibromyoadenoma.*

Pathology: BPH usually involves median and lateral lobes or one of them. It involves adenomatous zone of prostate, i.e. submucosal glands. Median lobe enlarges into the bladder. Lateral lobes narrow the urethra causing obstruction. Urethra above the verumontanum gets elongated and narrowed. Bladder initially takes the pressure burden causing trabeculations, sacculations and later diverticula formation. Enlarged prostate compresses the prostatic venous plexus causing congestion termed as vesical piles leading to hematuria. Incrimination of BPH as the source of hematuria before excluding other causes is termed as *Decoy prostate.* Backpressure causes hydroureter and hydronephrosis. Secondary ascending infection can cause acute or chronic pyelonephritis. Often severe obstruction can lead onto obstructive uropathy with renal failure. BPH causes impotence.

Clinical features: Frequency occurs due to introversion of sensitive urethral mucosa into the bladder or due to cystitis and urethritis. Other features are urgency; overflow and terminal dribbling; difficulty in micturition with weak stream and dribble; pain in suprapubic region and in loin due to cystitis and hydronephrosis, respectively; acute retention of urine; retention with overflow; hematuria; renal failure. Prostatism is a combination of symptoms like frequency both at day and night, poor stream, delay in starting and difficulty in micturition. Tender area in suprapubic region with palpable enlarged bladder due to chronic retention is also seen. Hydronephrotic kidney may be palpable. Per rectal examination shows enlarged prostate. It should be done when bladder is empty. Features of urinary infection like fever, chills, burning micturition, etc. are also seen.

Differential diagnosis: Stricture urethra; bladder tumor, carcinoma prostate; neurological causes of retention of urine like diabetes, tabes, disseminated sclerosis, Parkinson's disease.

Investigations: Urine for microscopy and C/S; Blood urea and serum creatinine; US abdomen; residual urine assessment; urodynamics; cystoscopy; acid phophatase; prostate specific antigen (PSA); IVU; serum electrolytes.

Carcinoma Prostate

It is the *commonest malignant tumor* in men after 65 years. Carcinoma prostate occurs in peripheral zone in prostatic gland proper, i.e. *commonly in posterior lobe.* So prostatectomy for BPH does not confer protection against development of carcinoma prostate.

Types of carcinoma prostate: (a) Microscopically latent—tumors incidentally found either by transurethral resection of the prostate (TURP) or by prostatic surface antigen (PSA) estimation. (b) Early localized carcinoma. (c) Advanced local prostatic carcinoma. (d) Metastatic carcinoma either into the bone commonly or other organs.

Histology: It is an adenocarcinoma, where there is loss of the myoepithelial cell layer which normally surrounds the prostatic glands (Gleeson). Glands here appear in confluence. Grading of carcinoma is based on dedifferentiation as proposed by Gleeson.

Local spread: Upward into seminal vesicles, bladder neck, trigone, later into both ureters causing anuria, etc. Downward extension into distal sphincter.

Blood spread: Into the bones commonly, pelvic bones, lumbar vertebrae, femoral head, ribs, skull in that order. Secondaries in bone are *osteoblastic* due to serum alkaline phosphatase. Pathological fractures can occur in long bones and vertebrae. Paraplegia may occur if spine is involved. Rarely spread to liver and lung can occur.

Lymphatic spread: Into the obturator lymph nodes, then to internal iliac lymph nodes. Through seminal vesicles, spreads into external iliac and retroperitoneal lymph nodes. Eventually mediastinal, and left supraclavicular lymph nodes get involved.

Clinical features: Commonly asymptomatic. May present with bladder outlet obstruction and so retention of urine. Other features are hematuria, frequency, pelvic pain, back pain, arthritic pain in sacroiliac joint. On per rectal examination, prostate feels hard, nodular, and irregular often with loss of median groove. It may be incidental carcinoma after TURP or after PSA analysis. It may present with features of renal failure, anemia which may be secondary to extensive bone marrow invasion or due to renal failure.

Differential diagnoses: Differential diagnoses are other causes of retention of urine and other causes of back pain.

Investigations: Hb%, Peripheral smear. Prostatic specific antigen (PSA): More than 10 nmol/mL is diagnostic. Prostatic fraction of acid phosphatase is increased. Blood urea, serum creatinine, liver function tests. Trans rectal ultra sound (TRUS) is very useful. Transrectal prostatic biopsy. Plain X-ray KUB may show *dense coarse sclerotic* secondaries. Osteolytic or combination of lytic and sclerotic lesions are also often seen. Technetium radioisotope bone scan to see secondaries. US abdomen to see the extension into the bladder and to look for hydronephrosis in kidneys.

Note: Osteoblastic secondaries are also occasionally seen in carcinoma breast.

Acid phosphatase: It is the enzyme that splits organic phosphates. It is found in many human tissues, but more concentrated in prostate. It is active at pH 5. Acid phosphatase secreted by prostate drains into the urethra through prostatic ducts and so blood levels of this enzyme remains low. Serum acid phosphatase estimation should be done *in empty stomach* because heavy meals can alter the level of the acid phosphatase. Normal value is *0–5 King Armstrong units per 100 mL of serum*. It is raised significantly in carcinoma prostate with metastases. *It does not increase in BPH*. Slight increase in acid phosphatase level occurs in acute prostatitis, Paget's disease of bone and hepatic cirrhosis. Prostatic fraction of acid phosphatase is more relevant in carcinoma prostate. Osteosclerotic osseous metastases in carcinoma of prostate are due to alkaline phosphatase.

Prostate-specific antigen (PSA): It is a protease produced from the prostatic epithelium secreted in the semen to cleave and liquefy the seminal coagulum formed after ejaculation. PSA is organ specific. *Normal value is 4 ng/mL of plasma. More than 10 ng/mL is significant.* PSA elevation occurs not only in carcinoma but also in prostatic hyperplasia and prostatitis. But level of increase is much more in carcinoma than in benign conditions.

Conditions of bladder	Features
Ectopia vesicae	
It is embryological origin where there is incomplete development of infraumbilical part of anterior abdominal wall and anterior wall of the bladder; associated with spina bifida; common in males (4:1) **Problems:** Repeated soakage; ulceration; pain; recurrent pyelonephritis; renal failure; metaplastic changes in mucosa leading to adenocarcinoma	Red mucous membrane of the posterior bladder wall protrudes out with visible urine efflux from the ureteric orifice Umbilicus is absent; separation of pubic bones In males—epispadias, rudimentary prostate, seminal vesicles; normal testis; bilateral inguinal hernia In females—defective external genitalia
Cystitis	
Inflammation of the bladder mucosa due to different causes—**acute** bacterial cystitis; **chronic** cystitis due to tuberculosis, syphilis, interstitial cystitis, radiation cystitis, cystitis due to schistosomiasis; postmenopausal atrophic cystitis **Organisms**—E. coli; Klebsiella; Pseudomonas; Staph. aureus; Staph. albus; Proteus; Candida albicans	***Predisposing factors***—congenital urinary anomalies; short urethra in females; catheters; instrumentation; bladder stone; BPH; carcinoma prostate; cystocele; bladder diverticulum; stricture urethra; bladder neck obstruction; bladder tumors; pregnancy; CNS diseases; spinal injury ***Features:*** Painful micturition; frequency; strangury; incomplete emptying; retention; occasionally hematuria; burning urine, discolored foul smelling urine, fever, chills, rigors, suprapubic pain; tenderness and often loin pain
Interstitial cystitis (Hunter's ulcer/Elusive ulcer)	
Common in Western psychic females. There is pancystitis with severe inflammation of all layers of the bladder with fibrosis and linear ulcers in the bladder mucosa	Pain, decreased bladder capacity, pain increases with bladder distension, frequency and often hematuria Bladder capacity eventually decreases (*systolic/thimble*) up to 30–60 mL
Urinary bilharziasis/endemic hematuria	
Schistosoma haematobium is the causative organism. Man gets infected through breach in skin following contact with water containing cercariae released following death of infected fresh water snail (intermediate host). These cercariae develop into male and female worms in liver which undergo fusion; reaches bladder wall and submucosa through vesical venous plexus; ova are released into urine and excreted out *Clinical features:* Initially cutaneous lesion—urticaria develops which lasts for few days. After 4–8 weeks, fever, along with features of eosinophilia, eventually, intermittent painless terminal hematuria	***Differential diagnosis***: Tuberculosis, recurrent cystitis, malignancy ***Pathological lesions***: Bilharzial pseudo-tubercles; nodules; sandy patches (calcified dead ova with overlying degenerated epithelium); granulomas, ulcerations and nodules; fibrosis and thimble bladder. *Squamous cell carcinoma* develops in due course of time; ureteral/urethral stricture, urinary fistula, bladder calculi, recurrent UTI
Thimble/systolic bladder	
Inability of the bladder to relax, distend and dilate and retain the urine as required **Causes:** Tuberculous cystitis; *Schistosoma haematobium*; interstitial cystitis; radiotherapy; malignancy; previous bladder surgery	Bladder is fibrotic and contracted; capacity is reduced <100 mL Frequency; recurrent cystitis **Investigations:** Cystoscopy; IVU, cystography, urine C/S; other specific diagnostic test

Contd...

Contd...

Conditions of bladder	Features
Residual urine	
It is the amount of urine retained in the bladder after voiding. Normal 30 mL; if more than 50 mL it is significant. **High residual urine**—BPH; obstruction to urethra; neurogenic bladder. It precipitates infection	***Assessment of residual urine***—inserting red rubber catheter after the act of voiding; USG; IVU (post-micturition film)
Malakoplakia	
Usually associated with chronic cystitis of unknown etiology causing grayish patches in bladder mucosa. *It is not premalignant condition*	***Microscopy:*** Shows submucosal infiltration with lymphocytes, plasma cell, large multinucleated malakoplakia giant cell with concretions called—*Michaelis Gutmann bodies*
Prostatitis	
Very distressing condition; often difficult to diagnose. **Types:** Acute; chronic. **Acute**— Due to instrumentation; ascending/descending infection. E. coli; streptococci/gonococci are common bacteria involved. **Clinical features:** Pain, frequency, fever, retention of urine, perineal heaviness, pain in defecation; rectal examination—firm tender prostate; initial part of urine turbid. **Complications:** Prostatic abscess; chronic prostatitis; urinary retention	**Chronic**— Associated with posterior urethritis; epididymitis. Presentations: Back pain, perineal pain, leg pain, fever, sexual dysfunction. **Prostatic massage**—extracts prostatic gleet for cytology; **three glass urine test**—first glass prostatic threads
Prostatic abscess	**Urethritis**
It is infection, suppuration and abscess formation in prostate gland. **Clinical features:** Fever, rigors, perineal pain, urinary disturbances and tender soft fluctuant swelling in the prostate. Often presents with retention of urine. **Investigations:** Total count increased. Urine C/S; US—diagnostic	**Causes:** (a) Infection—Gonococcus/non-Gonococcus; LGV; Mycoplasma; Trichomonas; (b) Trauma—catheter, cystoscope, stones; (c) Chemical urethritis; (d) Reiter's disease. **Clinical features:** Urethral discharge; dysuria; burning micturition; hematuria; increased frequency; other features—perineal pain; tenderness; suprapubic pain and tenderness
Posterior urethral valve	
They are congenital symmetrical valves in the posterior urethra just below the verumontanum. **Features:** Child finds difficult in micturition—poor urinary stream. Often associated with vesicoureteric reflux—infection; hydronephrosis. MCU is diagnostic. **Differential diagnosis:** Marion's disease; neurogenic bladder	***Pathology:*** It allows the passage of catheter but obstructs the outflow of urine. Proximal urethra—enormously dilated. Bladder shows obstructive pathology—trabeculations; sacculation; becomes thickened hypertrophied and easily palpable as a firm mass in suprapubic region—"*cricket ball bladder*"
Urethral calculi	
Stone from bladder if small commonly passes out through urethra but can impacted due to stricture or urethral diverticulum. **Sites of impaction:** Prostatic urethra; bulbous urethra; fossa navicularis; external meatus	Painful micturition; urine flow is thin and forked. Other features—urinary retention; lower UTI; hematuria; pain the penis and perineum; stone may be palpable when it is bulbar or penile urethra. **Complications:** Bleeding; stricture uretha; infection
Stricture urethra	
Etiological classification: a. Congenital b. Inflammatory—post-gonococcal (70%)—multiple, common in roof of the bulbous urethra c. Tuberculous d. Traumatic—common e. Post-instrumentation—catheter; dilator, cystoscope f. Postoperative—prostate surgery; urethrostomy **Features:** Located in proximal (bulbous urethra) or distal (congenital) urethra. Can be single or multiple (gonococcal commonest; proximal stricture narrowest). Can be in the roof/floor; catheter can/cannot be passed. Poor urinary stream; forking/spraying of urine; incomplete emptying; frequency; dysuria; retention with overflow; pain burning micturition. It can be felt as a thickening/button like crescentic feeling in bulbar urethra	***Investigations:*** USG abdomen; ascending urethrogram—to see the site, type, extent, false passages; urodynamic studies; urethroscopy. **Complications:** Retention of urine; urethral fistula; infection (urethritis, cystitis, pyelonephritis); urethral diverticula; periurethral abscess; bilateral hydronephrosis; stone formation; renal failure; due to straining (hernia, hemorrhoids, rectal prolapse)

Contd...

Contd...

Urinary fistulas	
Causes: a. Congenital—patent urachus; ectopia vesicae; in association with anorectal malformation (rectovesical fistula) b. Acquired—trauma during perineal surgery; vesicovaginal fistula due to obstructed labor; bladder injury during hysterectomy or anterior colporrhaphy; radiation induced; infiltration by carcinoma cervix c. Specific causes like tuberculosis, staghorn calculus can cause fistula after nephrostomy d. Surgery to renal pelvis, ureter, bladder in presence of distal obstruction like stricture urethra e. Crohn's disease of renal pelvis	**Features:** Passage of urine per vagina; dribbling of urine can be visualized on per speculum examination. Methylene blue test/swab test will be positive

CASE DISCUSSION

A 35-year-old male presented with dragging pain over the right loin with hematuria of 15 days duration. Hematuria is intermittent, occurred at the end of the act. There is no burning urination, frequency or fever. His blood pressure is normal; other general examination is normal. On inspection, in sitting position from behind, fullness is seen on the right loin at right renal angle compared to opposite side. On palpation in lying down, mass of 8 × 6 cm sized is palpable in right lumbar region which moves on respiration and is nodular, hard, nontender, bimanual palpable and ballotable. Liver is not palpable. Palpation in sitting position from behind showed mild tenderness in right renal angle. On percussion, there is a resonant colonic band in front in lying down position in right lumbar region; right renal angle is dull on percussion in sitting position. Opposite loin and lumbar region is normal on palpation. There is no free fluid in the peritoneal cavity. Respiratory system, skull and spine are normal.

What is your diagnosis and why?
It is probably right sided renal cell carcinoma. It is kidney because it is vertically placed in the right lumbar region, moves downwards with respiration, bimanually palpable and ballotable. It is carcinoma because of history of hematuria, dragging pain, nodular, hard kidney.

What are the differential diagnoses?
Hydronephrosis is smooth and soft. Polycystic kidney disease is nodular and firm and is usually bilateral. In adrenal tumor, loin will be normal; it does not move with respiration and does not have intrinsic mobility. Colonic mass has to be ruled out; colonic mass will have bowel symptoms and loin will be normal; mass is intra-abdominal.

What investigations are done?
USG abdomen; CT abdomen; renal function tests, hematocrit, chest X-ray or CT chest to rule out lung metastasis.

27 Approaches and Examination in Hand Diseases

Competency: SU6.1; AN12.10.

■ HISTORY

Following Points to be Noted

History of swelling, number, position, duration, onset (spontaneous or traumatic), progress (increasing or decreasing), swellings in other hand.

History of deformity and loss of function is enquired. It may be congenital or traumatic. Trauma may be fracture or dislocation where deformity appears suddenly. In conditions like Dupuytren's contracture, deformity appears gradually.

History of pain, its site—whether palm, digit, joint; nature (continuous, throbbing); whether it is more during day or night. Pain of carpal tunnel syndrome increases during midnight. Pain of vascular origin is continuous burning pain in fingers. Pain may increase with specific movements—in inflammatory condition, pain is better with elevation but worsens by making hand dependent. Pain of tenosynovitis increases during movements of the hand. Pain may radiate to arm from hand in conditions like carpal tunnel syndrome. Pregnancy worsens the pain of carpal tunnel syndrome.

History of trauma is important as often neglected trauma will lead into severe deformity later.

History of fever, its type, mode of onset, progress, presence of chills and rigors.

History of redness, irritation at some parts, discharge, discoloration, ulcer in the hand when present should be detailed properly; on which part redness is present, dorsum or ventral; fingers or only hand or entire length is involved.

History of weakness of the finger or fingers or hand partly or entirely; history of altered sensation either absent, decreased or hyperesthetic should be asked for.

History suggestive of associated diseases such as carpal tunnel syndrome, myxedema, cirrhosis, epilepsy, Dupuytren's contracture.

Family history related to the conditions like gout and rheumatoid arthritis.

Past history of similar episodes, treatment by drugs or surgery undertaken, its recovery, any long-term drug intake should be asked for.

■ EXAMINATION

Inspection

Attitude of the hand—always compare to opposite side **(Figs. 27-1 and 27-2)**.

Swelling—redness, localized or diffuse, size, shape and extent.

Deformity, its type, site and extent should be noted. It may be congenital like syndactyly, polydactyly, traumatic (mallet finger). Wrist drop is obvious on inspection in radial nerve injury **(Fig. 27-3)**.

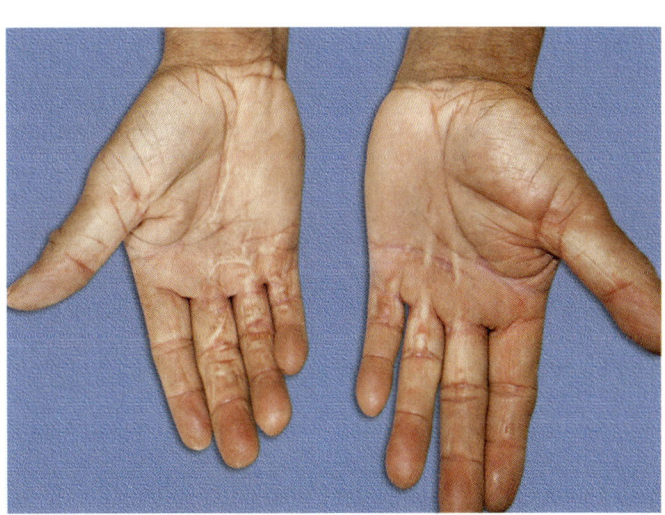

Fig. 27-1 *Dupuytren's contracture* both hands.

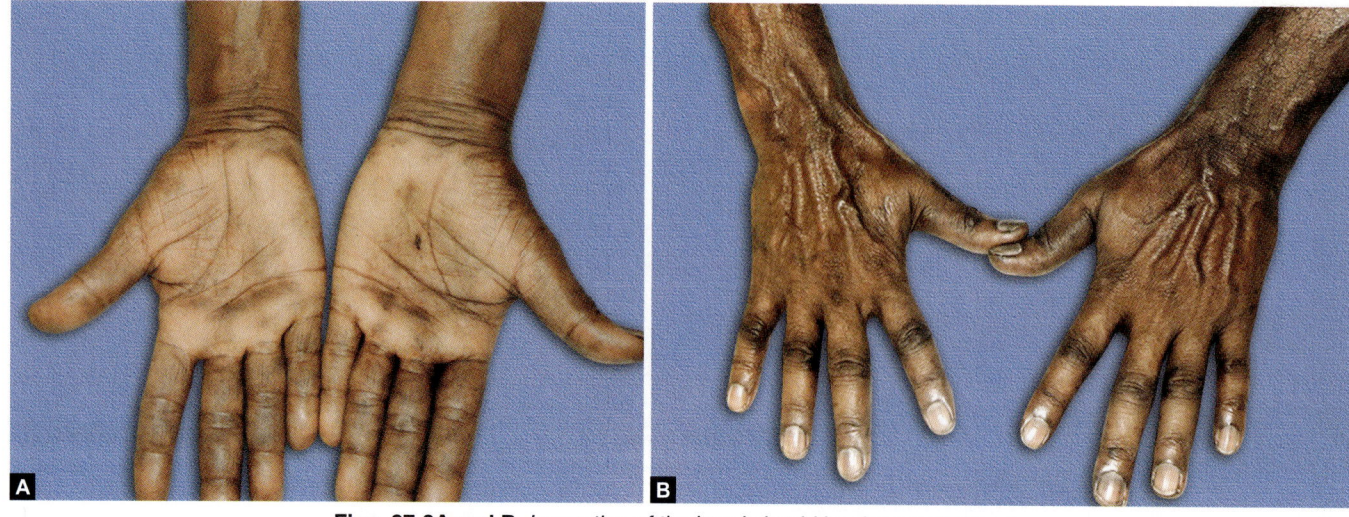

Figs. 27-2A and B *Inspection of the hand should be done* meticulously.

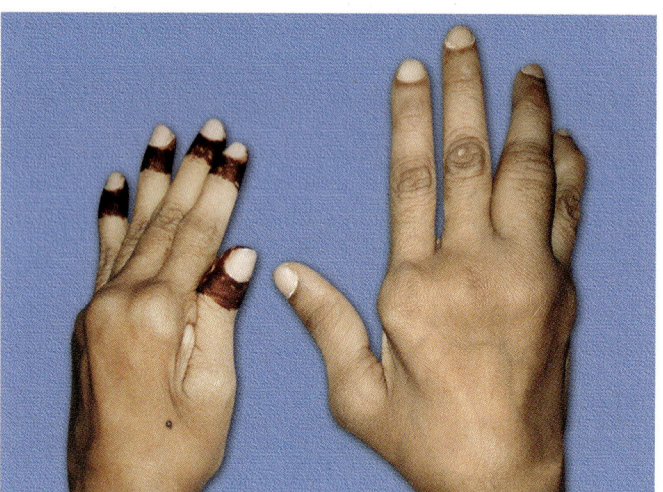

Fig. 27-3 *Deformity of the hand should be noted.*

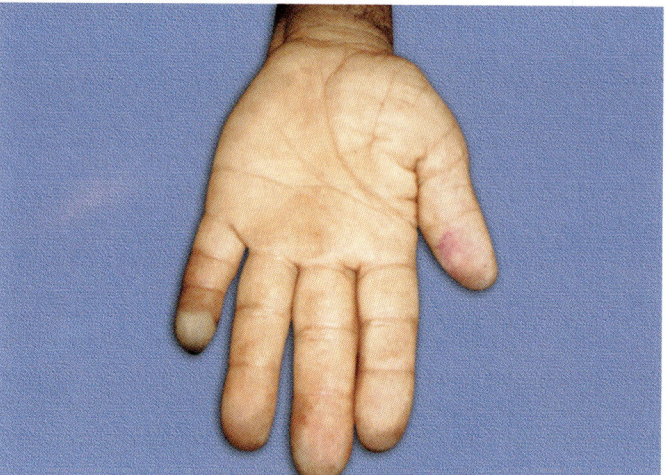

Fig. 27-5 *Blebs in finger tips.*

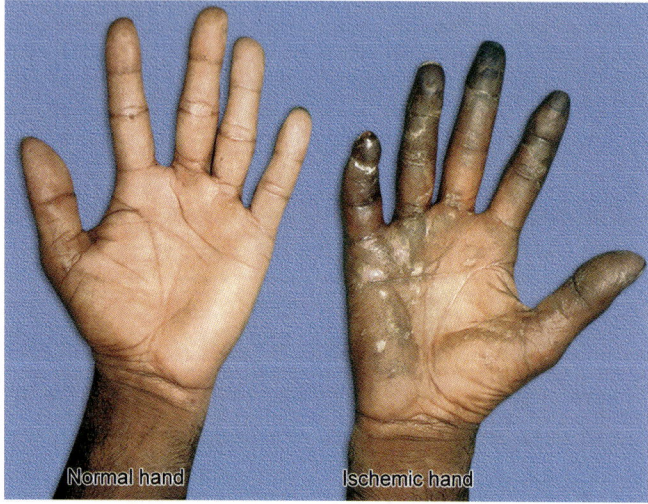

Fig. 27-4 *Ischemic hand should be compared to normal hand. Discoloration is typical.*

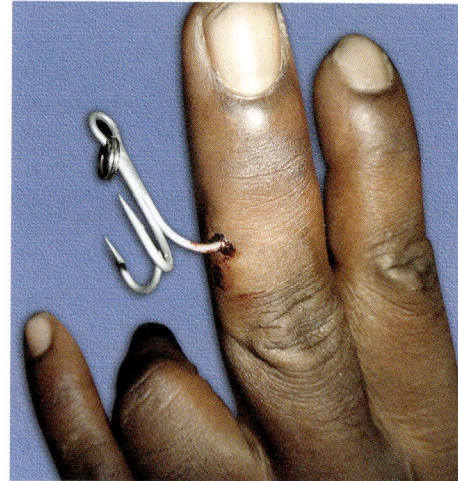

Fig. 27-6 *Fishing hook stuck in the finger.*

Wasting of thenar, hypothenar eminences and interossei between the metacarpals. Thin and pointed pulp of the finger suggests ischemic atrophy **(Fig. 27-4)**.

Presence of ulcers, blebs, gangrene over the finger tips and color changes to be noted **(Fig. 27-5)**.

Presence of foreign body should be observed carefully using proper light source; examples – thorn, pin, stone piece, sharp objects, etc. **(Fig. 27-6)**.

Changes in the forearm and arm should be noted such as swelling, wasting, redness, etc.

Axilla should be inspected for any enlarged visible nodes; in acute infection and tuberculosis, axillary nodes may be enlarged.

Palpation

Each finger, palm and dorsum of the hand should be palpated meticulously. There is local rise of *temperature* in hand infections—superficial or deep; in the joints. Fingers will be cold in ischemic conditions like cervical rib syndrome.

Tenderness may be present over the swelling and other areas. Specific point tenderness is typical in certain type of hand infections. **Kanavel sign** is typical of suppurative tenosynovitis. Cellulitis, fasciitis, abscess and arthritis can cause tenderness.

Swelling should be examined like swelling any where—size, location, shape, surface, consistency, mobility, fixity.

Pulses should be checked. Radial and ulnar pulses should be checked. Allen's test should be done **(Fig. 27-7)**.

Sensations: There may be hyperesthesia, paresthesia (tingling, numbness, pins and needles sensation), decreased sensation (blunting) or anesthesia (absence of sensation). Cotton, needle, tuning forks, and cold and warm water tubes are used to check various sensations. Sense of position of joints are also checked. Sensory distribution in hand should be checked properly. Sensations in the distribution of radial, ulnar and median nerves should be checked (Refer Chapter 9). Both superficial (light touch, pain and temperature) and deep (deep pressure) sensations should be checked in each digit, palm and dorsum of the hand and fingers.

Muscle tenderness should be checked in thenar and hypothenar eminences and in forearm muscles. Palmar aponeurosis should be palpated for thickening and nodules (*Dupuytren's contracture*).

Radial and ulnar arteries should be palpated always; it gives fair idea about the adequacy of the blood supply of the hand. Allen's test is done to check the capillary circulation. Specific clinical examination for Raynaud's phenomenon should be done.

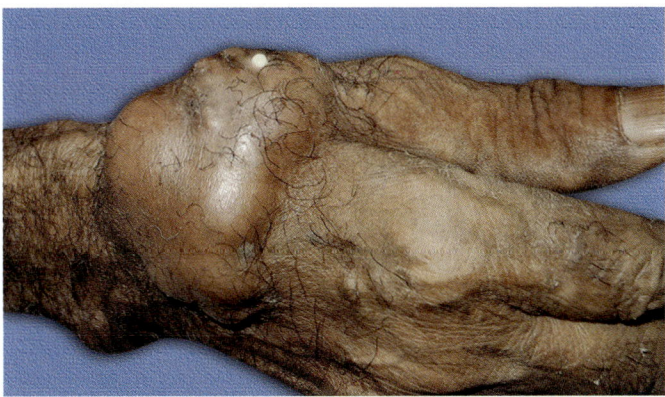

Fig. 27-7 Swelling in the hand—could be *implantation dermoid* or *cold abscess*.

Movements of the fingers and wrist joint should be checked. Flexion (midcarpal joint), extension (radiocarpal joint), abduction (midcarpal joint), adduction (radiocarpal joint) and circumduction (flexion → adduction → abduction → extension) should be checked. Thumb shows flexion, extension, abduction, adduction and opposition movements at carpometacarpal joint. Fingers at metacarpophalangeal joints show flexion, extension, abduction and adduction. Flexion and extension are the only movements in interphalangeal joints of fingers. Both **active** (by the patient) and *passive* (by the examiner) movements of the joints should be checked. Wrist joint is radiocarpal synovial joint between lower end of radius and articular surfaces of the scaphoid, lunate and triquetral bones. Other joints of the hand are intercarpal, carpometacarpal, intermetacarpal, interphalangeal joints. Movements of the wrist are—flexion is 70–80°; extension is 80–90°; adduction is 35°; abduction is 25°. Extension is checked by Indian method of salutation by keeping both the hands in contact. Flexion is checked by placing back of hands in contact. Abduction and flexion mainly occurs in midcarpal joint; extension and adduction mainly occurs in radiocarpal joint. Pronation and supination takes place at inferior radioulnar joint. In arthritis of the wrist joint, **all movements** are painful and restricted **(Figs. 27-8A and B)**.

Proximal joints (elbow and shoulder) should be examined.

Reflexes of upper limb should be checked—biceps, triceps and supinator.

Functions related to three nerves should be checked. Median nerve lesions causes—wasting of thenar eminence; absence of opposition and abduction of the thumb; absence of flexion of interphalangeal joint of index finger (pointing index); loss of sensation of lateral 3½ fingers. Ulnar nerve lesions causes—wasting of hypothenar eminence and intermetacarpal spaces; absence of abduction and adduction of fingers; absence of flexion of the little and ring fingers; ulnar claw hand; loss of sensation of medial 1½ finger. Radial nerve lesions causes—wrist drop; absence of extension of wrist, thumb and metacarpophalangeal joints of fingers; absence of extension of interphalangeal joint of the thumb.

Opposite upper limb should also be examined.

Percussion

It is only useful in carpal tunnel syndrome—percussion on flexor retinaculum may induce pain.

Auscultation

Bruit can be heard in case of arteriovenous malformations or vascular tumors.

Examination of Lymph Nodes and Other Systems

Epitrochlear and axillary lymph nodes should be examined.

Neck should be examined for thrill, bruit, swelling in detail. Cervical rib, neck mass may be found.

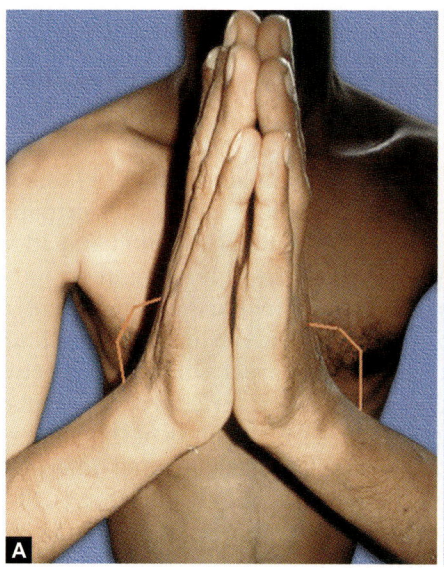 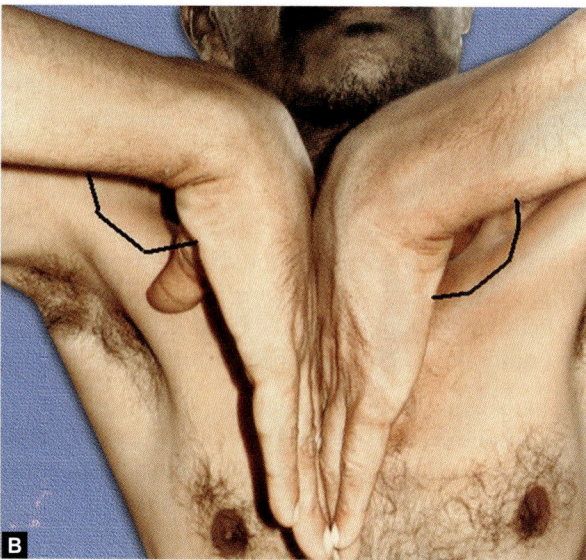

Figs. 27-8A and B *Extension* (radiocarpal) and *flexion* (midcarpal) of wrist.

Cervical spine should be looked for tenderness, spasm, restricted movements.

Respiratory system and central nervous system should be examined for relevant findings.

■ INVESTIGATIONS

<u>Blood:</u> ESR, total count, blood sugar, peripheral smear, Mantoux skin test, relevant tests for autoimmune diseases when suspected.

<u>Discharge study:</u> Microscopy, cytology, culture; FNAC of swelling and lymph node; excision biopsy of swelling are needed for tissue diagnosis.

<u>Imaging:</u> X-ray of the part, chest X-ray, X-ray of cervical spine, CT angiogram, digital subtraction angiogram (DSA) of hand, arterial Doppler study.

<u>Nerve conduction study (NCS) and electromyography (EMG)</u> is done in neuromuscular diseases and carpal tunnel syndrome.

Classification of Hand Diseases:

Deformities

Congenital: Polydactyly, syndactyly, macrodactyly, ectrodactyly.

Acquired: Post-traumatic: Skin contracture and implantation dermoid; mallet finger, boutonniere deformity, mallet thumb; *Volkmann's ischemic contracture* (of forearm), *Bunnell's ischemic contracture* (ischemic contracture of the intrinsic muscles of the hands with involvement of the deep thenar muscles and the interossei on the radial side of the hand); claw hand, wrist drop; spinal cord lesions; malunited fractures of wrist and carpus, joint diseases and stiffness. Post-inflammatory: Large ulcers with scarring; acute and chronic tenosynovitis; tuberculous dactylitis, rheumatoid arthritis, gout, Dupuytren's contracture, trigger thumb, claw hand, myopathies and neuropathies.

Traumatic

Lacerations of skin and soft tissues, subungual hematoma, avulsion of nail, injuries to muscles, nerves, vessels, tendons, fracture and dislocations.

Inflammatory

In the finger—acute-subcuticular purulent blister, subcutaneous abscess, paronychia, onychia, apical space infection, pulp space infection (felon), suppurative distal finger (whitlow), proximal pulp space or web space infection; suppurative tenosynovitis, acute osteomyelitis, acute arthritis. Chronic paronychia, ulcers, osteomyelitis, verrucal necrogenica (Butcher's wart), rheumatoid arthritis.

In the palm—subcuticular abscess, ulcers, superficial palmar space infection, collar stud abscess, deep (subaponeurotic) palmar space (midpalmar and thenar) infection; tenosynovitis of tendon sheaths (radial and ulnar bursae).

Dorsum of hand—skin boil/lymphangitis, cellulitis, abscess, carbuncle, deep abscess (subaponeurotic); osteomyelitis, arthritis, gout, leprosy, granuloma, actinomycosis.

Neoplastic

Benign—moles, fibromas, lipoma, schwannoma, glomus tumor, xanthoma of tendon sheath, enchondroma, osteoma, osteoid osteoma.

Malignant—malignant melanoma, squamous cell carcinoma, liposarcoma, fibrosarcoma, osteogenic sarcoma.

Others

Ganglion, implantation dermoid, compound palmar ganglion, carpal tunnel syndrome, arterial diseases.

Modified Verdan zone system in the hand injuries (Tendon zones)

Zone I

From the fingertip up to the attachment of flexor digitorum superficialis (Middle of middle phalnx). It contains flexor digitorum profundus.

Zone II

It begins proximal to metacarpophalangeal joint at distal palmar crease and extends distally up to the attachment of flexor digitorum superficialis at the middle of the middle phalanx. It is called as *'No-man's-land'*. Here flexors are tightly enclosed within a fibro-osseous tunnel. It is the ***most dangerous*** zone in hand injuries **(Critical zone).**

Zone III
It begins at the distal end of flexor retinaculum (base of the palm) and ends at the transverse crease of the palm. It contains lumbricals attached to flexor digitorum profundus.

Zone IV
It begins at the proximal end and ends at the distal end of flexor retinaculum.

Zone V
It extends from the proximal end of flexor retinaculum proximally up to distal third of the forearm.

HAND INFECTIONS

Hand is a compact actively functioning unit. It contains neurovascular bundles, muscles, bones and ligaments. Infection can occur due to minor injuries, or by hematogenous spread.

Precipitating causes: Diabetes; Immunosuppression; Trauma; HIV infection; Steroid therapy.

Common organisms: *Staphylococcus, Streptococcus,* Gram-negative organisms such as *E. coli, Klebsiella, Pseudomonas*. Occasionally fungal infection causes chronic paronychia, Madura hand due to Nocardia group of fungi, viral infection like *ORF (Parapox virus infection causing contagious pustular dermatitis of hand)* can occur.

General features of hand infection: Infection spreads faster in all areas. It causes edema over the dorsum of hand due to lax skin and more lymphatic network even though infection per se is more over the volar aspect. It looks like *frog hand*. There are restricted movements of fingers and hand. The hand functions such as *hook, pinch, grip and grasp* are lost. Severe pain and tenderness with fever are other features. Tender palpable axillary lymph nodes are often present.

Different types of hand infections: Acute paronychia; Chronic paronychia; Terminal pulp space infection (*Felon*); Subungual infection; Web space infection; Mid-palmar space infection.; Thenar space infection; Deep palmar abscess; Acute suppurative tenosynovitis; Chronic tenosynovitis of flexor tendon sheath of palm and forearm—Compound palmar ganglion. Lymphangitis of the hand.

Investigations: Pus for culture and sensitivity; blood sugar; urine sugar and ketone bodies; X-ray of the part.

Complications of hand infections:
- Stiffness of digits and hand (ankylosis)
- Deformity and disability
- Bacteremia and septicemia
- Osteomyelitis of bones depending on location of abscess like metacarpal bones, terminal phalanx
- Suppurative arthritis of joints
- Paralysis of median nerve

Other Infections of Hand

Infection type	Features
Acute paronychia	
Most common infection in hand, occur in subcuticular area under the eponychium **Commonest cause**—minor injury; infection tracks around the skin margin and spreads under the nail causing *hang nail/ floating nail*. Organisms—*Streptococcus; Staphylococcus aureus*	Severe throbbing pain and tenderness (*dependent throbbing*) with visible pus under the nail. Nail is very tender on touch
Chronic paronychia	
Commonly due to fungal infection	Itching in the nail bed; recurrent pain; discharge; secondary bacterial infection
Terminal pulp space infection (Felon)	
Terminal pulp space contains fat and is partitioned by septae which attaches skin to periosteum of terminal phalanx. As proximally the deep fascia is attached to the base of the terminal phalanx; it is a closed compartment It is the second most common hand infection, occurs following needle prick	Pain, tenderness, swelling in the terminal phalanx, tender axillary lymph nodes **Complications:** Any infection increases the pressure within the space causing thrombosis of the terminal artery leading to osteomyelitis of the terminal phalanx
Infection of web space	
There are three triangular web spaces between volar and dorsal skin filled with fat. Infection originates from abrasion, extension from infection of proximal spaces, callosities **Bacteria:** *Staphylococcus, Streptococcus,* Gram-negative organisms	Fever, pain, tenderness; oedema on dorsum of hand; maximum tenderness is on volar aspect; even though pus is in volar it points out dorsally, 'V' sign—separation of fingers. Untreated infection spreads to other spaces
Deep palmar space infection	
There are two deep palmar spaces— **Midpalmar space**—bound in front by palmar aponeurosis, behind by medial three metacarpals, laterally by a vertical line from lateral margin of the middle finger. Contains flexor tendons, lumbricals and neurovascular bundles. **Thenar space**—lies anterior to lateral two metacarpals **Causes:** Trauma; spread from finger and web spaces, hematogenous spread, spread from tenosynovitis	Pain, tenderness in the palm; oedema of dorsum of hand (*frog hand*); loss of concavity of palm; painful movement of metacarpophalangeal joint (IP joint movements are free and painless); fever; palpable tender axillary lymph nodes. Pus may eventually come out of palmar aponeurosis–*collar stud abscess*, sinus formation **Complications:** Osteomyelitis of metacarpals, stiffness of hand extension of infection into other spaces

Contd...

Contd...

Acute suppurative tenosynovitis	
It is the bacterial infection of flexor tendon sheath *Radial bursa*—flexor sheath of flexor tendon of thumb *Ulnar bursa*—flexor sheath of medial four flexor tendons which extends to the digit of fifth finger **Common bacteria**—*Staphylococcus, Streptococcus,* Gram-negative organisms	Symmetrical swelling of entire finger; flexion of finger—"*hook sign*"; severe pain on extension; tenderness over the sheath; oedema of whole hand *In ulnar bursa infection*, pain and tenderness extends into little finger but not much into other fingers; *in radial bursa infection*, thumb is swollen with pain and tenderness **Complications:** Spread of infection proximally into forearm; stiffness of fingers and hand; suppurative arthritis; osteomyelitis; median nerve palsy; bacteraemia and septicaemia
Apical subungual infection	
It is infection of the space between subungual epithelium and the periosteum. Occurs after minor trauma or after formation of subungual hematoma	Excruciating tenderness with small visible pus under the tip of the nail. Pus comes to the surface beneath the free edge of the nail Osteomyelitis is not common
Compound palmar ganglion	
Chronic tenosynovitis of flexor tendons due to tuberculosis or rheumatoid arthritis **Pathology**: Flexor tendon sheath on either side of flexor retinaculum is involved. Swelling contains fluid with typical melon seed bodies	Unilateral/ bilateral (rheumatoid arthritis); Swelling in the volar aspect of palm and forearm which is smooth, soft, nontender, fluctuant, cross fluctuant across flexor retinaculum; transilluminant; wasting of hand and forearm muscles matted axillary lymph nodes with primary focus in lungs
Spina ventosa	**Milker's nodules**
It is phalangeal tuberculosis; so called because of its appearance as "*air-filled balloon*"	Viral infection of hand seen in cow handlers

■ HAND INJURIES

Classification

Tidy injuries: They are clean incised wounds and are usually treated by primary suturing and also depends on the tissues involved such as nerves, tendons and muscles.

Untidy injuries: They are lacerated wounds and treated by debridement and later by delayed primary or secondary suturing.

Compartment injuries.

Degloving injuries

Indetermined injuries which could not be assessed.

Assessment of Injury: Should include—number, extent, depth, deformity—disability, neurovascular injuries, tendon injuries, muscle injuries bone and joint injuries.

■ SYNDACTYLY

It is *webbing or fusion* of fingers. *Causes:* Congenital and hereditary – Common; Traumatic like burns. *Types: Cutaneous; Fibrous; Bony*–complex. *Features:* It can be unilateral or bilateral. Often there will be webbing of toes also. If bony type is suspected, X-ray of the part should be taken.

28 Approaches and Examination in Foot Diseases

Competency: SU6.1.

■ HISTORY

History of pain is asked. Location of pain, whether over second metatarsal, bone or between third and fourth metatarsals, has to be noted. Pain in the heel may be due to plantar faciitis.

Type and severity of *deformity* should be asked. Whether it interferes with patient's walk or not is noted.

History of *swelling*, duration, mode of onset, progress should be asked.

History of *fever*, redness, and impairment of function, weakness or paralysis of parts of or entire foot, stiffness should be asked.

Past history of similar episodes, treatment taken should be asked in detail.

■ EXAMINATION

Inspection

Inspection is done in **standing position;** both feet should be inspected. Affected leg is inspected for deformity, position, wasting, ulcers, proximal parts of the limb, etc. Ulcer may be trophic.

Further inspection is done **in sitting** or **lying down** position properly for deformity, sinus, ulcer and swelling. Feet should be examined both from front and behind; standing, sitting, lying down and if possible while walking. Dorsum and plantar aspect should be examined for, corn **(Fig. 28-1)**, abscesses, ulcers, callosities, swelling, discharging sinus, and color changes.

Gait should be checked to look for shape of feet and toes, contour of the longitudinal arches, different changes like flat foot, hollow foot (pes cavus), dropped transverse arch (splay foot), clawing of toes, overriding of toes, hammer toes, hallux

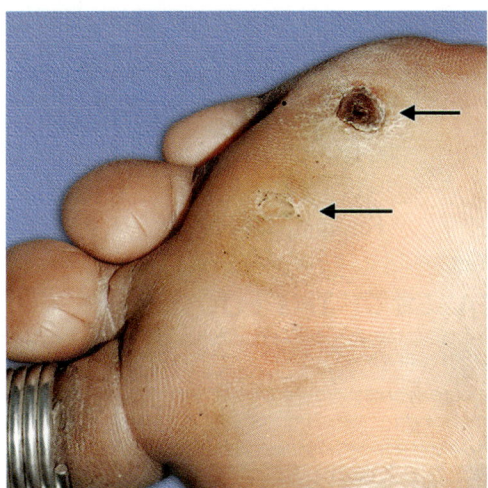

Fig. 28-1 *Corns* in the plantar aspect of foot.

valgus, hallux varus. In Achilles tendon injury, affected leg is grounded and heel is made to raise to identify the rupture of Achilles tendon.

Palpation

It is done for swelling and ulcer. In detail each of these should be examined **(Figs. 28-2 and 28-3)**.

Movements and Gait

Movements occurring at ankle joint (dorsiflexion and plantar flexion) and subtalar joint (inversion and eversion) should be checked. In *dorsiflexion*, front of leg is approximated to dorsum of foot with reduction in the angle between two. In *plantar flexion*, toes point downwards; heel is raised with increased angle between foot and leg in front. *Inversion* takes place in subtalar joint with plantar aspect of foot

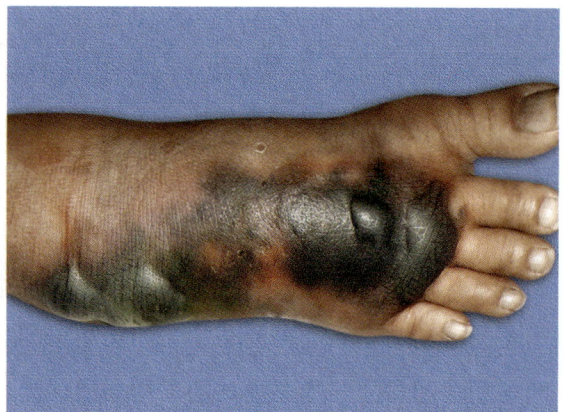

Fig. 28-2 *Necrotizing fasciitis* foot; limb is going for gangrene.

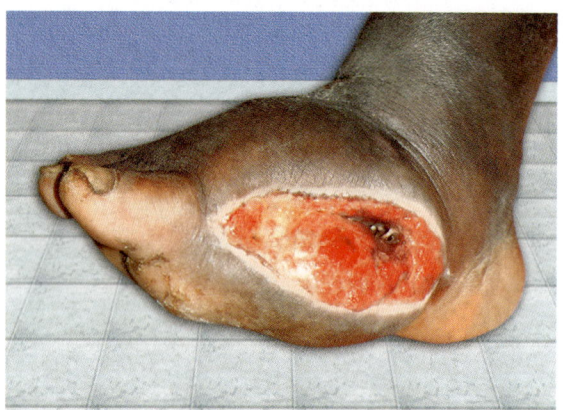

Fig. 28-3 *Osteomyelitis foot.*

facing medially; in *eversion*, plantar aspect of the foot faces laterally. Dorsiflexion is by tibialis anterior; plantar flexion is by gastrocnemius and soleus. Inversion is by tibialis anterior and tibialis posterior. Eversion is by peroneus longus and peroneus brevis.

Muscle Power, Sensations, Reflexes and Gait

Proper neurological examination should be done.

Measurements

Length of the foot is measured from tip of the medial or lateral malleolus to the head of the 1st or 5th metatarsals.

Examination of Knee, Hip and Spine

Knee, hip and spine should be examined. Often spina bifida is an association of talipes equinovarus. Genu valgum and coxa vara are often associated with deformity of foot.

Examination of Inguinal Lymph Nodes

Proper examination of inguinal lymph nodes is to be done.

Systemic Examination

Central nervous system should be examined in detail.

INVESTIGATIONS

X-ray foot; MRI foot; X-ray spine (if needed) are the needed investigations.

DISEASES OF THE FOOT

Flat foot/Pes planus	Pes cavus
It is flattening of longitudinal arches of foot **Components:** Flattening of normal concavity on the inner aspect of the foot with prominent navicular bone; limitations of movements of tarsal joints; tender spring ligament **Causes:** Genu valgum; outer rotation of tibia; forefoot varus; congenital/infantile; obesity; postural (weak intrinsic foot muscle); spasmodic (peroneal muscle); chronic illness	Also called as hollow foot **Components:** Thick splayed forefoot with claw toes and high arch; weak intrinsic muscles; prominent metatarsal heads; callosities with osteoarthritis of tarsal joints **Causes:** Can be familial; may be associated with spina bifida; May be due to poliomyelitis; or idiopathic (commonest)
Talipes equinovarus/club foot	**Ingrowing toe nail (Onychocryptosis)**
Here foot is turned inwards with sole directed medially **Components:** Inversion of foot; adduction and inward deviation of forefoot; plantar flexion/equines. There is subluxation of talonavicular joint with navicular bone lying more medially There is poor development of calf muscle **Causes:** Usually congenital; common in boys; commonly bilateral Acquired variety is seen in infantile paralysis and is unilateral	• Also called as embedded toe nail • There is inward curving of side of nail causing it to form lateral spike resulting in repeated irritation, infection and overhanging tissues in the nail fold **Causes:** Tight shoes; improper cutting of nails (very short convexly) **Clinical features:** Common in great toe, often bilateral; both medial and lateral sides of the toe can be involved. Pain; swellings of the margin of the toe; tenderness; often with foul smelling discharge
Talipes calcaneovalgus	**Hammer toe**
It is opposite of talipes equinovarus. Foot being everted and dorsiflexed. Rare congenital deformity	It is fixed flexion deformity of interphalangeal joint; usually of proximal interphalangeal joint of 2nd toe
Onychogryphosis (*Hooknail*)	**Athlete's foot**
It is curving of nail upwards (*Ram's horn nail*). Thickened, curved, over grown nail looks like an ox's horn; seen in bed ridden patients; may be due to fungal infection **Onychomycosis:** It is the fungal infection of the nail of great toe; nail becomes brittle, discolored and splits longitudinally	• It is fungal infection of skin between toes—*Tinea pedis* • Fungi enter the skin through cracks; survive due to moisture in between toes **Clinical features:** Itching; deep cracks; pain discharge are common; Skin is swollen, red, with sticky fluid, macerated with blisters

Contd...

Contd...

Hallux valgus	Hallux rigidus
Great toe is deviated laterally at metatarsophalangeal joint. It may be due to persistent lateral force or occasionally hereditary **Clinical features:** Common in females; there is outward deviation of big toe with medial deviation of the metatarsal head **Complication**: Thick-walled bursa (**bunion**) over the medial aspect of the head of the first metatarsal bone	It is osteoarthritis of metatarsophalangeal joint of great toe; with forced dorsiflexion; with bunion/ bursa over the joint. There is pain, restricted movement, narrowed joint spaces with sclerotic bones; osteophytes in the margin
Morton's metatarsalgia	**Stress/March/Fatigue metatarsal fracture**
• It is plantar digital neuritis due to fibrous thickening/neuroma of third digital nerve of foot just proximal to its division between 3rd and 4th space • Common in middle aged females; pain in 3rd interdigital space which radiates on the 3rd and 4th toes with localized tenderness and often swelling	It is hairline fracture of 2nd/3rd metatarsal bone near the neck which later during spontaneous healing forms a large callous around the fracture site mimicking tumor; Begins after unusual long walk or marching causing pain and tenderness in the forefoot
Freiberg's disease	**Kohler's disease**
It is partial necrosis and fragmentation of usually 2nd or 3rd metatarsal head which gets deformed leading to osteoarthritis of adjacent joint. It could be due to metatarsal osteochondritis dissecans; seen in adolescent girls	• It is osteochondritis of navicular bone; which becomes denser • Presents in child <5 yrs; with pain, limp, thickening of navicular bane
Sever's disease	**Other infections**
It is calcaneal apophysitis seen in children at the attachment of posterior apophysis. Earlier thought to be due to osteochondritis	Tuberculosis, syphilis, Madura foot can involve foot causing swellings and multiple discharging sinuses

Talipes:
- *Talipes equinus*—walk on toes
- *Talipes calcaneus*—walk on heel
- *Talipes varus*—walk on lateral margin with sole looking medially
- *Talipes valgus*—walk on medial margin with sole facing laterally
- *Talipes equinovarus*—inverted plantar flexed foot
- *Talipes calcaneovalgus*—everted dorsiflexed foot

Causes of painful heel:
- Calcaneal diseases
- Subtalar arthritis
- Calcaneal tendon rupture
- Calcaneal paratendinitis
- Calcaneal bursitis
- Calcaneal apophysitis
- Tender heel pad
- Calcaneal spur, plantar fasciitis
- Osteochondritis of bones
- Morton's metatarsalgia
- March fracture
- Hallux valgus/rigidus/hammer toe

29 CHAPTER

Approaches and Examination of Face and Head

Competency: SU19.1; SU19.2.

■ INTRODUCTION

Many specific and peculiar conditions pertaining to face and head occur. Because of their individuality, they are being discussed as a separate chapter. History taking, examination methods are same as in chapters—Ulcer (Chapter 3), Swelling (Chapter 4), Neck (Chapter 15) and Oral Cavity (Chapter 11). Student should refer specific chapters for method of examination (Figs. 29-1 and 29-2).

■ CLEFT DISORDERS

Face develops from different processes, defect in fusion leads into cleft disorders. Causes are – familial; vitamin deficiency; Rubella infection; radiation; chromosomal abnormalities; drug induced (during pregnancy. Often cleft disorders are associated with other anomalies also).

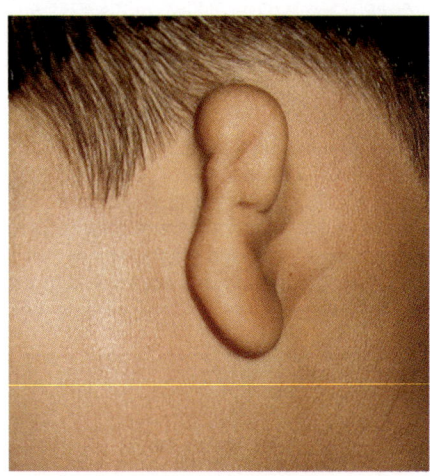

Fig. 29-1 Underdeveloped ear—*anomaly*.

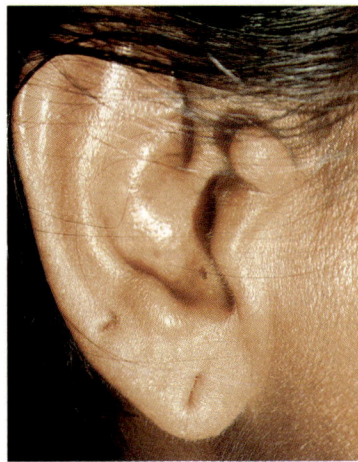

Fig. 29-2 *Accessory ear*. An accessory auricle is a protruded postero-lateral part of the face with cartilage, fibrous tissue and skin covering. It is commonly cylindrical erect in front of the tragus. It is sequestration of an island of cartilage from the mandibular arch during closure of first branchial cleft.

Cleft Palate (Fig. 29-3)

It is due to failure of fusion of the two palatine processes; defect in fusion of lines between premaxilla (developed from median nasal process) and palatine processes of maxilla one on each side

Types:
(*Type I cleft palate*)—When premaxilla and both palatine processes do not fuse, it leads into *complete cleft palate*
Incomplete fusion of these three components can cause incomplete cleft palate beginning from uvula towards posteriorly at various lengths
Type IIa— Bifid uvula
Type IIb—Bifid soft palate (entire length) or Type IIc—Bifid soft palate and posterior part of hard palate (but anterior part of hard palate is normal)

Problems: Small maxilla with crowded teeth, absent/poorly developed upper lateral incisors. Bacterial contamination of upper respiratory tract with recurrent infection is common. Chronic otitis media with deafness may occur. Swallowing difficulties to certain extent and speech problems can occur; cosmetic problems can occur.

LAHS classification of cleft disorders:
- 'L' for lip, 'A' for alveolus, 'H' for hard palate, 'S' for soft palate
- Capital 'LAHS' for 'complete' type
- Small letters 'lahs' for 'incomplete type'
- Asterisks 'lahs' for microclefts
- 'LAHSHAL' for bilateral clefts

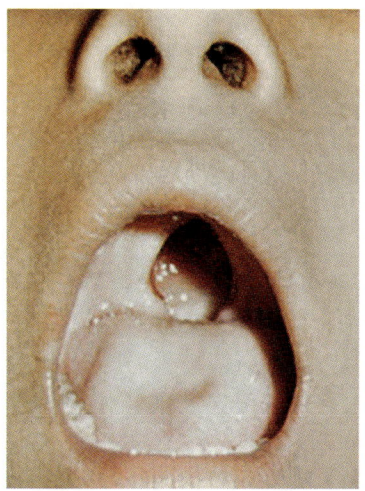

Fig. 29-3 *Cleft palate only.* Lip is normal. Premaxilla is not involved.

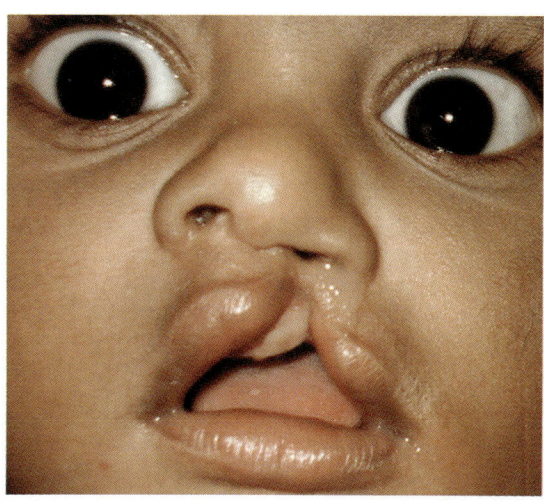

Fig. 29-4 *Unilateral cleft lip*, lateral type which is commonest.

Cleft Lip (Fig. 29-4)

Types: • *Central*: Rare. In upper lip. Between two median nasal processes (Hare lip) • *Lateral*: Maxillary and median nasal process, commonest; can be unilateral or bilateral	**Problems in cleft disorders:** Difficulty in sucking and swallowing. This is commonly observed in cleft palate than in cleft lip; speech is defective especially in cleft palate, mainly to phonate B, D, K, P, T and G
• *Incomplete* cleft lip does not extend into nose • *Complete* cleft lip extends into nasal floor • *Simple* cleft lip is only cleft in the lip • *Compound* cleft lip is cleft lip with cleft of alveolus	Altered dentition or supernumerary teeth; recurrent upper respiratory tract infection; respiratory obstruction (in Pierre–Robin syndrome); chronic otitis media, middle ear problems; cosmetic problems; hypoplasia of the maxilla; problems due to other associated disorders

Other Conditions

Bifid nose: One-half of the frontonasal process remains isolated from rest **Macrostoma**: Size of the mouth is more than the normal due to imperfect union of maxillary process with mandibular arch **Mandibular cleft**: Mandibular arch of one side fails to unite with mandibular arch of opposite side	**Congenital short frenum of upper lip**: It is seen with a wide gap between the permanent incisor teeth **Congenital fistulae of lower lip** are two rare blind pits one on either side of the midline containing wide open mucus secreting glands **Facial cleft:** Lateral nasal process fails to unite with maxillary process causing a fissure from upper lip to the inner canthus of the eye alongside of the nose

Hydrocephalous

It is dilatation of ventricles due to blockage of flow of cerebrospinal fluid (CSF).

Classification I:
1. Communicating type: Ventricles communicate freely into the subarachnoid space. Here there is defective absorption of CSF following any inflammation, subarachnoid hemorrhage or trauma
2. Noncommunicating type: Obstruction is in the ventricle or its exit due to any tumors or any inflammatory process

Classification II:

Congenital: It is associated with spina bifida/ myelomeningocele. There is failure of formation of CSF pathway. It is associated with Arnold-Chiari syndrome, congenital stenosis of aqueduct of Sylvius

Clinical features: Widening/separation of suture lines; bulged tense fontanelle; engorged scalp veins; sun setting eye; decreased cortical thickness; enlarged head

Acquired: It may be unilateral or bilateral. It is due to chronic meningitis, trauma, subarachnoid hemorrhage, brain tumors, colloid cyst of third ventricle, arachnoid cysts

Meningocele

Meningocele is protrusion of the meninges. It contains clear fluid—CSF. It is brilliantly transilluminant; shows impulse on coughing or crying. *Meningo-encephalocele* is protrusion of brain also along with meninges. It is transilluminant. *Encephalocele* is protrusion of brain. It is not transilluminant. There may be neurological deficits, incontinence of urine and feces. These conditions are seen in midline—root of the nose, occiput, anterior fontanelle region. Often it is associated with spina bifida

Preauricular Sinus

Ear develops from *six tubercles*. Failure of fusion of anterior tubercles of the auricle creates preauricular sinus. This sinus opens at the root of the helix or on tragus. Sinus track runs downwards and ends blindly. Often sinus opening gets sealed forming a preauricular cyst which gets infected forming an abscess. Sinus can get infected repeatedly discharging pus through its opening. It is often multiple. Sinusogram and study of discharge is needed. It often mimics cold abscess or sebaceous cyst

Problems of Face and Head Trauma

Head, faciomaxillary injuries are discussed in detail in *Chapter 12: Examination of Jaw* and *Chapter 30: Examination of Intracranial Diseases*.

Hematoma scalp	Subperiosteal hematoma
It is very common traumatic swelling observed; common in 2nd layer connective tissue dense or 4th layer galea aponeurotica. Hematoma in 2nd layer is localized, tender and tense swelling. Hematoma in the 4th layer is often diffuse and extensive. In front it may extend into the root of nose and eyelids as galea aponeurosis is not attached to any bone in front. Fracture of underlying skull bone should also be thought of. Neurological deficits should be assessed using Glasgow coma scale. Fracture in the line of venous sinuses can be dangerous and life-threatening.	Also called as **cephalhematoma**. It is collection of blood under the pericranium; common in newborn after forceps delivery. It is common in parietal region; localized, smooth, soft, fluctuant swelling limited to the suture lines of the particular bone; gradually disappears in few months **(Fig. 29-5)**.

Problems with Infective Lesions of Face and Head

Cavernous sinus thrombosis: Infection from face and scalp may extend through various routes to cavernous sinus causing its thrombosis. Routes are—along angular vein to ophthalmic vein; along pterygoid plexus of veins which communicate deep facial vein to cavernous sinus across foramen ovale and foramen lacerum. Patient develops toxicity, proptosis, squint, ocular muscle paralysis specifically lateral rectus which is supplied by abducent nerve which is situated within the cavernous sinus. *Dangerous zone* in the face is located in the area of nose and upper lip as infection in this area is more prone to develop cavernous sinus thrombosis. Any boil, cellulitis, erysipelas, abscess in this zone can cause this complication. It is due to *communications* between facial vein and cavernous sinus through *deep facial vein* from pterygoid plexus; and through the *communicating vein* between supraorbital and superior ophthalmic veins.

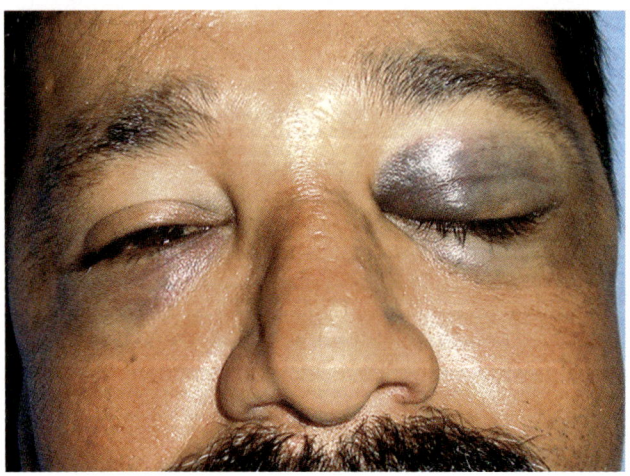

Fig. 29-5 Traumatic eyelid *hematoma*.

Note: Refer Chapters 4, 11, 12 for Pott's puffy tumor, cancrum oris, lupus vulgaris, actinomycosis of mandible.

Benign swellings of the face and head	Malignant conditions of face and head
Papilloma, lipoma, hemangioma, sebaceous cyst, Cock's peculiar tumor due to sebaceous cyst, dermoid cyst, osteoma, cirsoid aneurysm, mucus cyst of lips can occur. **Cirsoid aneurysm**: It is seen only in face in the forehead affecting the superficial temporal artery, as dilated interwoven artery and its branches. It feels like a *'bag of pulsating earthworms'* with thinned out overlying skin and loss of hair; often ulceration and severe bleeding can occur. Intracranial extension is known to occur into extradural space. X-ray skull shows bone erosion **Osteoma**: It is common in skull bone which is *compact or ivory type and is sessile type*. It affects the outer table of the skull bone—frontal, parietal or occipital bones. Painless bony hard nonmobile swelling in the skull bone is the presentation. It does not turn into malignancy **Paget's disease of bone**: Paget's disease of bone causes progressive enlargement of the skull with thickened skull bones with systolic bruit on auscultation due to vascularity	Malignant conditions like basal cell carcinoma (rodent ulcer), squamous cell carcinoma of lip or skin, malignant melanoma, secondaries in skull, osteosarcoma can occur. Secondaries in skull can occur from primaries from thyroid, kidney, lungs, adrenals, breast, etc. It is hard, tender and multiple; can be solitary also. Soft, localized warm vascular pulsatile secondaries are seen in metastasis from follicular carcinoma of thyroid **Cylindroma**: Often called as *turban tumor* occurs in the scalp involving entire scalp area as red, lobulated, slow growing, relentless, rare tumor which is locally malignant with alopecia in the affected area. It should be differentiated from plexiform neurofibromatosis and temporal arteritis

EXAMINATION OF CRANIAL NERVES

Cranial nerve palsies that commonly present in head and face are being discussed in this chapter.

Cranial nerves are olfactory; optic; oculomotor; trochlear; trigeminal; abducent; facial; auditory; glossopharyngeal; vagus; accessory; hypoglossal nerves. (Mnemonic—On Old Olympus Towering Tops A Finn And German Picked Some Hops) (Refer Chapter 30: Approaches and Examination in Intracranial Diseases).

Accessory Nerve Injury

It is 11th cranial nerve having cranial and spinal roots. Cranial part begins at nucleus ambiguous and is distributed through vagal branches to muscles of palate, pharynx and larynx. Spinal root begins from long spinal nucleus of the spinal cord between C_1 and C_5. It emerges as 5 roots from the spinal cord join to form spinal root of accessory nerve. It runs upwards to reach the foramen magnum (enters it behind the vertebral artery); joining cranial root which again gets separated. Cranial root after separation joins vagus below inferior vagal ganglion. Spinal root prior to separation from cranial root runs upwards and laterally along with 9th and 10th cranial nerves crossing jugular tubercle reaching the jugular foramen and leaving the cranium through it. Nerve descends between internal jugular vein and internal carotid artery, deep to parotid and styloid process, reaching between angle of mandible and mastoid process, reaching deep of sternomastoid muscle superficial to internal jugular vein. It is crossed by occipital artery and accompanied by sternomastoid branch of occipital artery. At the junction of upper 1/4th and lower 3/4th it pierces the anterior border of the sternomastoid muscle, emerging through the posterior border into the posterior triangle; entering the anterior margin of the trapezius 5 cm above the clavicle. It is communicated with spinal nerves on the deep surfaces of both sternomastoid and trapezius muscles through $C_{2,3}$ and $C_{3,4}$ roots. Nerve supplies sternomastoid and trapezius muscles. Nerve may be affected in advanced secondaries in neck; block dissection (radical) of the neck (Figs. 29-6A and B). Clinically, there will be wasting of trapezius muscle; drooping of the shoulder; inability to elevate the shoulder against resistance. Sternomastoid also can be checked for power by turning the patient's neck to opposite side against resistance.

Hypoglossal Nerve Injury

It is 12th cranial nerve arising from hypoglossal nucleus of medulla in the floor of the 4th ventricle as 10–15 roots which soon joins to form 2 bundles which later join to form single trunk. It comes out of the skull through hypoglossal canal/anterior condylar canal of occipital bone; it travels initially deep to internal jugular vein, later between internal jugular vein and internal carotid artery, descending in relation to front of vagus, deep to parotid, styloid process, and posterior belly of digastric, stylohyoid, posterior auricular and occipital arteries. Near lower margin of the posterior belly of digastric, it curves anteriorly hooking lower sternomastoid branch of occipital artery; crossing internal and external carotid arteries, loop of lingual artery; running deep to posterior belly of digastric reaching submandibular salivary gland. It passes on the hyoglossus and geniglossus deep to submandibular salivary gland and mylohyoid to reach the tongue. It is communicated by fibers from C_1 spinal nerve. It supplies all intrinsic and extrinsic muscles of the tongue except palatoglossus which is supplied by cranial part of accessory nerve through vagus. C_1 component gives meningeal branch supplying the meninges of anterior part of posterior cranial fossa. C_1 also supplies thyrohyoid and geniohyoid muscles; its descending hypoglossi branch forms upper root of ansa cervicalis. Nerve can be affected in advanced neck secondaries, malignant submandibular salivary gland, radical neck dissection and submandibular salivary gland excision surgery. When it is involved, there will be wasting of the tongue on that side; while protruding outwards, tongue will deviate towards *same* side (Fig. 29-7).

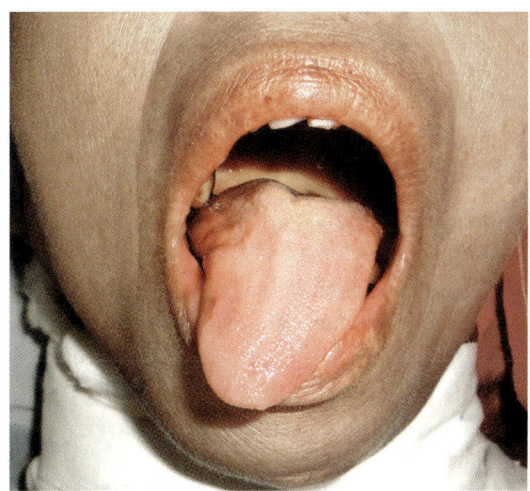

Fig. 29-7 *Hypoglossal nerve palsy*. Here tongue deviates towards same side. Wasting of tongue muscles on the same side is evident.

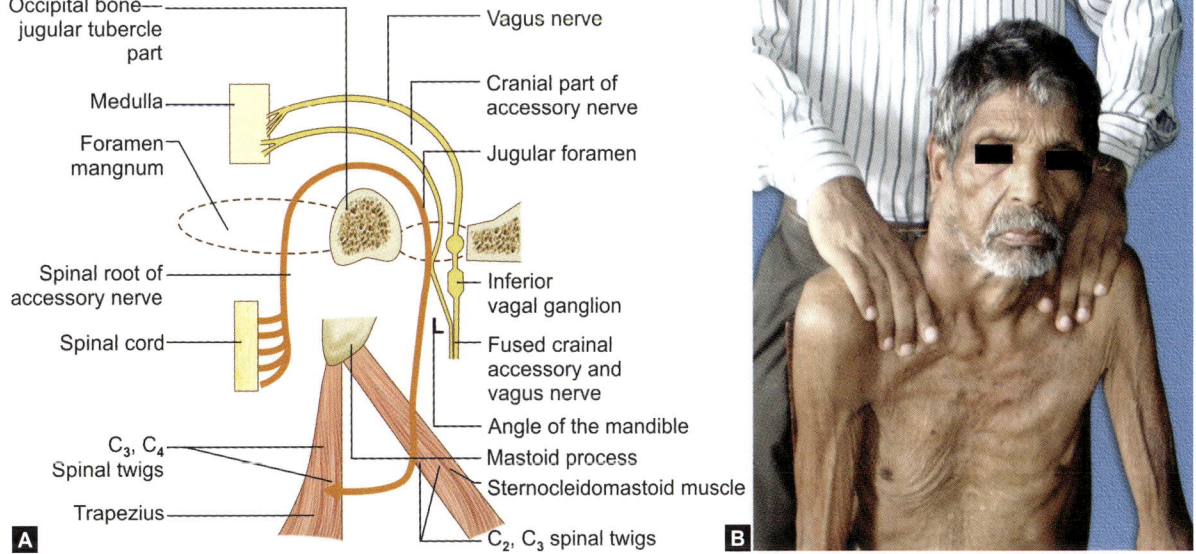

Figs. 29-6A and B *Accessory nerve anatomy* (11th cranial nerve). Wasting of trapezius and inability to shrug the shoulder are the typical features of accessory nerve injury.

30. Approaches and Examination in Intracranial Diseases

Competency: AN30.1; AN30.2

HISTORY

Medulloblastoma, glioblastoma affects younger individuals. Acoustic neuroma occurs after 30 years.

History of trauma earlier may cause late subdural hematoma or intracranial abscess causing convulsions, localizing features.

Frontal sinusitis, otitis media can cause intracranial abscess later. Such history is reliable.

History of convulsions, nature of its occurrence in detail should be asked.

History of loss of sensation, weakness in the limb suggests neurological deficit. It suggests cerebral pathology on opposite side.

In coordination on the affected side (walking) suggests cerebellar disease.

Change in the personality, retarded features, loss of memory and concentration are features of frontal lobe syndrome or tumor.

Headache (initially early morning, later generalized) is the common feature in intracranial tumors. It is unilateral on the side of the lesion. Posterior lesions show occipital headache which radiates to neck. Pituitary tumors cause bitemporal headache.

Early morning vomiting is usual without any nausea, and is aggravated by straining.

Change in the vision may occur in many tumors as part of papilledema, pituitary and, temporal tumors.

Drowsiness, neck stiffness, severe headache, vomiting, are the features of possible coning.

GENERAL EXAMINATION

Gigantism, acromegaly, Cushing's syndrome are features of pituitary tumor. Bradycardia, hypertension are features of raised intracranial pressure.

NERVOUS SYSTEM EXAMINATION

Detailed nervous system examination is needed. Mental status, speech, coordination, orientation, vision should be checked in detail. Cranial nerves should be checked properly.

EXAMINATION OF CRANIAL NERVES

Cranial nerve palsies that commonly presents in head and face is being discussed in this chapter.

Cranial nerves are: Olfactory; Optic; Oculomotor; Trochlear; Trigeminal; Abducent; Facial; Auditory; Glossopharyngeal; Vagus; Accessory; Hypoglossal nerves (Mnemonic—On Old Olympus Towering Tops A Finn And German Picked Some Hops).

Olfactory: Sense of smell is tested with cloves, peppermint, etc. Meningioma of olfactory groove or of base of frontal lobe causes *anosmia*; *parosmia* or perversion of sense of smell is due to uncinate process lesion.

Optic: *Visual acuity* (ability to read), *visual fields* (peripheral vision to be checked in one eye and compared to examiner's), *Color vision* using charts. Blindness in one half of visual field is called as *hemianopia*. If it is seen in same half of each visual field, it is called as homonymous hemianopia (optic tract lesions and radiotherapy effects). In optic chiasmal lesion bitemporal hemianopia (outer half of each field is affected) is seen. It may be due to pituitary tumor or suprasellar cyst. Pituitary tumor presses chiasma from below causing upper quadrantic hemianopia; whereas suprasellar cyst pressing from above causes lower quadrantic hemianopia.

Oculomotor: It supplies all extrinsic muscles of eyeball except superior oblique (trochlear), lateral rectus (abducent), levator palpebrae superioris and muscle of accommodation. In oculomotor nerve palsy eye looks downwards and outwards with ptosis (drooping of upper eyelid) and fixed pupil. Superior rectus—to look up; medial rectus—to converge; inferior rectus—to look down; inferior oblique—to look up and out. Complete paralysis causes—ptosis (paralysis of levator palpebrae superioris); exteroinferior squint (due to unopposed action of external rectus and inferior oblique); inability to move eyeball inwards and outwards; dilatation pupil; loss of light and accommodation reflexes; diplopia **(Fig. 30.1)**.

Trochlear: It supplies superior oblique muscle. When it gets damaged turning eye downwards and outwards is defective and patient looks inwards with diplopia below the horizontal line.

Trigeminal: Sensory supply is to entire one side of the face by three divisions—ophthalmic—upper; maxillary—middle; mandibular—lower. Ophthalmic division also supplies conjunctiva. Maxillary branch supplies mucous membrane of nose, pharynx, roof of mouth, soft palate and tonsil; mandibular division to tongue, lower teeth, mucous membrane of the mandible. Sensations should be checked in this place. Conjunctival reflex, palatal reflex will be altered. In trigeminal neuralgia there is hyperesthesia with touch becoming pain. During the period of neuralgic attack entire area is hyperesthetic. **Only certain trigger zones of Patrick** is hyperesthetic in between attacks. Motor supply to masseter, pterygoids and temporalis is from mandibular branch. Clenching the teeth will confirm the same. While opening the mouth widely jaw deviates towards the affected side due to weakness of pterygoids. Taste from anterior 2/3rd is through lingual nerve via chorda tympani from geniculate ganglion. Sweet (sugar), sour (acid), salt (salt) and bitter (quinine) tastes are checked. Salt and sweet in the tip of the tongue (through chorda tympani); sour is in lateral margin of tongue through trigeminal nerve; bitter is in posterior tongue through glossopharyngeal nerve.

Abducent nerve supplies the lateral rectus muscle of the eye. Turning of eye outwards is defective in its paralysis and attempt to look side will cause diplopia.

Facial: It supplies muscles of facial expression. It is motor nerve. Supranuclear palsy causes lower facial palsy; infranuclear palsy causes entire facial nerve palsy. Features includes—eyelids cannot be closed; whistling is defective; angle of the mouth deviates; wasting of the muscles of that side; wrinkling of eye is defective; inability to close the eyes properly **(Fig. 30-2)**.

Auditory: It supplies cochlea and semicircular canals. **Weber's tuning fork test** is used to rule out conductive deafness. After placing the tuning fork on the forehead louder sound is heard on the side of conductive deafness. Tuning fork is placed on mastoid to get louder sound in conductive deafness in **Rinne's test**. In sensory deafness there is no change in sound appreciation. Assessing the response to changes in temperature in the external meatus—**calorie test** is used to check the sensitivity of the vestibular apparatus.

Glossopharyngeal: It is sensory to posterior third of the tongue (and also carries bitter taste checked by using quinine) and to mucous membrane of pharynx. It is motor to middle constrictor. **Gag reflex** can be elicited by stroking the back of oropharynx.

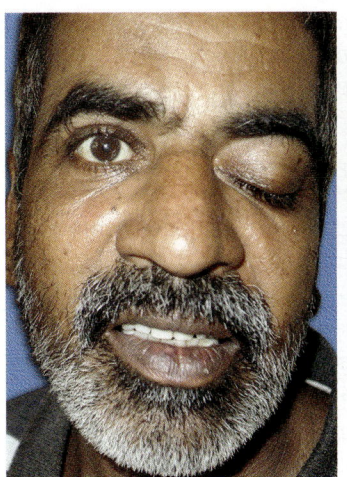 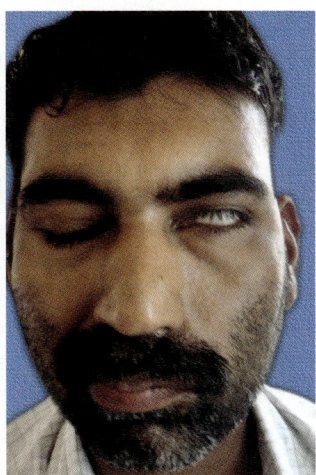

Fig. 30-1 *Oculomotor nerve (3rd cranial) palsy.* **Fig. 30-2** Features of *facial palsy.*

Vagus: It is motor to soft palate, pharynx and larynx and sensory to gut, heart and lungs. After opening the mouth patient is asked to say 'Aahh'. Soft palate arches upwards symmetrically. In paralysis of one side, it will not arch symmetrically and uvula gets pulled towards functioning *(opposite) side*. Change in voice, inability to cough and vocal cord palsy in indirect laryngoscopy are the other features.

Spinal accessory: Wasting of sternomastoid and trapezius is obvious. When chin is pushed towards opposite side against resistance weakness can be appreciated; shrugging of the shoulder against resistance is defective when checked from behind.

Hypoglossal nerve: It is motor to tongue. When it is paralyzed, wasting of tongue is seen on the same side; tongue deviates towards *same side* while protruding out.

Nystagmus

It is involuntary oscillations of eyeball. It is due to cerebellar lesions or vestibular lesions. Eyes persistently turning towards one side is called as conjugate deviation. In cerebral pathology, eyes are directed towards paralyzed side and away from the irritating side. In pontine lesions eyes are directed towards irritative side, away from paralytic side. Skew deviation of eye is one eye looking upwards and other downwards—is seen in some cerebellar pathology.

Cerebellar Lesion

It is checked by many methods—(1) Extended arm with forefinger is brought to tip of the nose with patient closing his eyes. (2) Walking in a straight line. (3) Rapid pronation and supination with forcarm at right angle is not possible—*adiadochokinesia*. (4) With eyes closed patient is asked to stand with feet very close together; patient sways towards the side of the lesion—*Romberg sign*. (5) Nystagmus. Muscle tone, rigidity, flaccidity should be checked. Power of muscle should be graded. Wasting of muscle should be observed. **Neck rigidity** is an important sign (*Kernig's sign*) to be confirmed.

Tics, athetosis, tremors of hands should be checked. **All skin sensations;** joint position sense; size, shape, form of objects given (*stereognosis*) should be checked.

Reflexes

Ankle jerk (S_1, S_2) is checked by gently stroking the Achilles tendon with foot dorsiflexed which causes sudden contraction of calf with rapid plantar flexion of the foot.

Knee jerk ($L_{2,3,4}$) is checked by a blow on patellar ligamentum of the knee which is kept over opposite knee or held by the examiner will cause brisk contraction of the quadriceps. Knee/ankle jerks are exaggerated in pyramidal tract lesion.

Triceps jerk (C_7) is checked by tapping above the olecranon with the elbow flexed causing contraction of triceps.

Biceps jerk ($C_{5,6}$) is checked by holding patients elbow with left hand and placing thumb over biceps tendon and tapping over the thumb will elicit the jerk.

Cremasteric reflex (T_{12}) is done by scratching the skin over upper inner part of thigh to draw testis upwards. It is absent in pyramidal tract lesion.

Abdominal reflexes ($T_{7,11}$) are elicited by strokes over the abdomen parallel to costal margins and iliac crests causing umbilical movements. It is absent in pyramidal tract lesion.

Ankle clonus ($S_{1,2}$) is checked by sudden dorsiflexion of foot with knee flexed slightly and heel off the ground causing oscillations of foot.

Patellar clonus ($L_{2,3,4}$) is checked with knee extended and pushing patella downwards by holding it between the thumb and fingers to develop continuous clonic movements of patella.

Relevant Other Examinations

Ear, nose and mouth should be examined. Respiratory system, abdomen should be examined.

INVESTIGATIONS

- Blood—hemoglobin, ESR, total count.
- Chest X-ray.
- CT scan to see the lesion, extent, size. Often MRI may be needed.
- Lumbar puncture: It should not be done if there is papilledema. Normal pressure is 120 mm of H_2O. If it is more than 160 mm of H_2O, cerebrospinal fluid (CSF) fluid collected should be very limited, otherwise coning due to herniation of temporal lobe through tentorium cerebelli or medulla through foramen magnum can occur. CSF is analyzed for cells (normal cells are <50; it is raised more than 100 in gliomas); proteins (normally it is 20–30 mg %), it is raised in meningiomas, cerebral abscess.
- X-ray skull: It is replaced by CT and MRI. Earlier X-ray and angiogram were essential investigations. *Features of increased intracranial pressure* are—separation of all sutures in children; silver beaten appearance of skull; thinning of posterior clinoid fossa. Erosive, hypertrophic and sclerotic features with vascular grooves and calcification are typical of meningioma. Astrocytoma, 40% oligodendrogliomas, 50% craniopharyngiomas and tuberculomas show calcification. Widening of sella tarsica with patchy calcification is seen in suprasellar cyst. Calcified pineal body shift is a feature of displacement by large tumor.
- Combined carotid and vertebral angiography is useful investigation to find out vascularity, extent, etc.
- Ventriculography, encephalographies were used earlier; now not used.
- Biopsy using Dandy's brain cannula after doing burr hole is useful to have histological confirmation.
- Radioisotope scan of brain using technetium^{99m} or I^{131} is useful to identify primary tumors, metastatic tumors, brain abscess, inflammatory pathologies, assessing the blood flow. It has got 80–90% sensitivity without any morbidity.

INTRACRANIAL DISEASES

Intracranial Abscess

Types
Extradural abscess: Caused by—osteomyelitis of skull, middle ear infection, frontal sinusitis. *Pott's puffy tumor* is infection and inflammation of the scalp. There is acute localized headache and tenderness in the skull, localized pitting edema of the scalp usually in the frontal region. ***Subdural abscess***: Is caused by septic thrombophlebitis from the frontal sinusitis or other infections. It is often very severe with extension into the venous sinuses
Intracerebral abscess: Is caused by (1) Extension from middle ear or sinuses, (2) Blood born infection, (3) After intracranial injuries. *Common sites*: Temporal lobe, cerebellum, frontal lobe. It can be: (a) **Acute**—There is acute septic encephalitis without pus formation. It may cause ventriculitis or localized abscess formation. (b) **Subacute**—Commences at 3 weeks, by the formation of a glial wall, i.e., thickness is more near the cortex and less towards ventricle. (c) **Chronic**—Occurs in 6 weeks with thick wall which may persist and may get enlarged behaving like a space occupying lesion. (d) **Metastatic**—Abscess in brain occurs either in cerebrum (parietal or temporal lobes) or in ventricles (Ventriculitis is more dangerous and often fatal)
Clinical features: Evidence of focus of infections are seen, i.e., middle ear (CSOM), sinusitis. Focal neurological features are seen, depending on the location of abscess. In temporal lobe abscess there will be dysphasia, contralateral hemiparesis; in cerebellar abscess, all cerebellar symptoms are seen; Epilepsy; *features of raised intracranial pressure*: (a) slow pulse, (b) rising BP, (c) headache, and vomiting, (d) papilledema, (e) deterioration in level of consciousness, (f) visual disturbances are other features
Differential diagnosis: (1) Intracranial tumor, (2) Tuberculoma, (3) Meningitis. *Lumbar puncture should be avoided in acute abscess as coning can occur*

Subarachnoid Hemorrhage

It is a type of intracranial hemorrhage where bleeding occurs into the subarachnoid space usually from basal cisterns; usually spontaneous
Causes: Intracranial aneurysms—commonest cause (50%). Hypertension; AV malformations; Blood dyscrasias; Anticoagulant drugs; Brain tumors (malignant)
Clinical features: Sudden onset of severe headache with vomiting. Features of raised intracranial pressure; Photophobia; Neck stiffness; Focal neurological deficits: Hemiplegia, dysphasia; eye changes: ptosis, dilated pupil, changes in the eyeball movements. Sudden loss of consciousness; Features of brain edema and cerebral ischemia. In 40% of recovered patients, rebleeding occurs in 6–8 weeks which is commonly fatal
Differential diagnosis: Meningitis; coning due to any cause

Intracranial Aneurysms

Types:
(1) **Subclinoid** type occurs in the internal carotid artery within the cavernous sinus. It causes ptosis, defective external ocular movements, and 5th nerve palsy. It can cause *caroticocavernousfistula*.
Presentations: Subarachnoid hemorrhage; pressure effects; convulsions; eye and pupillary signs.
(2) **Supraclinoid** type is common type.
(a) Berry's aneurysms: A congenital type occurs in circle of Willis in relation to internal carotid artery [40% (most commonly at the origin of posterior communicating artery)], anterior communicating artery, middle cerebral artery, vertebrobasilar artery. It occurs due to weakness in the media of major arteries.
(b) Acquired aneurysms due to atheromas, hypertension, etc.
(c) Mycotic aneurysms occur due to infection in the wall of cerebral vessels as a result of any bacteremia. *Common sites* are peripheral branches of middle cerebral artery

Intracranial Tumors

Secondaries are the commonest malignant tumor in the brain. Metastasis occurs usually from lung (commonest), nasopharynx or from any other organ in the body.

Primary Brain Tumors

Gliomas (43%): (a) *Astrocytomas* are the commonest type. They are usually malignant. They can occur anywhere in the cerebral hemispheres, medulla, and brainstem. They can be *diffuse, solid, or cystic*. They contain star-shaped cells resembling adult neuroglial cells. Astrocytic gliomas are graded as *Grade I, II, III, and IV as per the quantity of adult and primitive cells.* (b) Oligodendrogliomas. (c) *Spongioblastoma polare* arises from the primitive spongioblasts affects optic chiasma, third ventricle, hypothalamus, etc. They are irremovable but are radiosensitive. (d) *Medulloblastoma* occurs in children, affecting vermis of the cerebellum which grows rapidly with seedling elsewhere in the brain. (e) *Ependymomas*: Cells here resemble ependymal cells. It can occur throughout the cerebral hemispheres.

Meningiomas (18%): They are usually globular, arising from the arachnoids. Tumor gets attached to the dura. It gets blood supply from dural arteries and veins, from emissary veins, veins of diploe and scalp. Tumor cells invade the bone along these veins, causing bone destruction and reactive hyperostosis. Meningiomas can be *calcified, fibroblastic, endothelial and angioblastic.*
Sites: (1) Parasagittal, (2) Frontobasal, (3) Posterior fossa, (4) Choroid plexus.
Microscopic: It contains whorls of spindle cells, with central hyaline material, with Psammoma bodies.
Schwannoma (8%): Common in auditory nerve also called as *acoustic neuroma*. It occurs in the internal auditory meatus which projects into the cerebellopontine angle (C-P angle), compressing 5, 6, 7, 8th nerves. It presents with compressive features like unilateral deafness, trigeminal neuralgia, squint, cerebellar compression syndrome.
Pituitary tumors (12%), Craniopharyngiomas (5%), Blood vessel tumors (2%).

Clinical Features

Initial period of silent growth; Focal syndromes with epilepsy; Raised intracranial pressure with headache, vomiting, deterioration of level of consciousness, altered vision, slow pulse, high BP, papilledema; Brain displacement and stage of coning.

Specific Features

Frontal lobe tumors: Personality and emotional changes, epilepsy of generalized type, contralateral facial weakness.
Parietal lobe tumors: Jacksonian epilepsy, progressive hemiparesis, astereognosis, acalculia.
Occipital lobe tumors: Aura of flashing of light in contralateral field, homonymous hemianopia.
Temporal lobe tumors: Progressive aphasia, visual, auditory, smell and taste hallucinations, hemiparesis, superior quandrantic hemianopia.
Midline tumors: Produces bilateral hydrocephalus.
Tumors of the third ventricle (colloid cyst is common): Causes bilateral hydrocephalus, progressive cerebral atrophy, dementia, sexual precocity, endocrine disturbances.
Pineal tumors: Causes precocious puberty.
Cerebellar vermis tumors: Usually medulloblastomas, occur in young children, presents with progressive hydrocephalus and features of herniation of cerebellar tonsils through foramen magnum.
Cerebellar hemisphere tumors: Commonly are astrocytomas, produce cerebellar syndromes, nystagmus, etc. (Fig. 30-3).

Pituitary Tumors

Classification I

Eosinophil (Acidophil) adenomas: Tumor is usually small. Rarely it causes compressive features. It secretes excess growth hormone causing acromegaly in adults and gigantism in children.

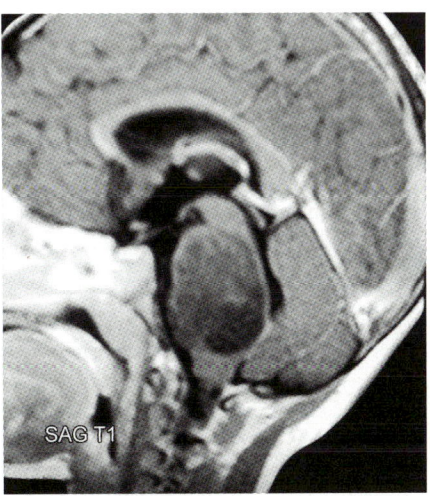

Fig. 30-3 MRI showing *pontine tumor*.

Chromophobe adenomas: Are common in females and in the age group (20–50 years). Initially it is *intrasellar* and after sometime becomes *suprasellar*. Later it extends *intracranially* often massively, causing features of intracranial space occupying lesion. It presents with myxedema, amenorrhea, infertility, headache, visual disturbances, bitemporal hemianopia, blindness, intracranial hypertension, epilepsy. *Differential diagnosis:* Meningiomas, aneurysms. CT scan, Angiogram, X-ray skull are diagnostic.

Basophil adenomas: Are usually small. They secrete ACTH and presents as Cushing's disease with all its features.

Prolactin secreting adenomas: Causes infertility, amenorrhea and galactorrhea.

Craniopharyngiomas

They are large masses with cystic cavities, lined by ciliated epithelium containing cholesterol crystals. Areas of calcifications may be present and coral-like masses may be formed. They are adherent to the basal arteries and adjacent nerves. They are *irremovable*. They are tumors of sellar region.

Clinical features: Intrasellar craniopharyngiomas inhibits sexual maturation causing obese, impotent dwarf with bitemporal hemianopia (due to compression of optic chiasma)—*Frolich's syndrome*. Suprasellar craniopharyngiomas produces Frolich's syndrome; pressure on hypothalamus which controls sleep and water metabolism (causes somnolence and diabetes insipidus). *Massive intracranial extension* causes intracranial hypertension and also hydrocephalus by obstructing CSF flow.

Approaches and Examination of Chest Diseases

CHAPTER 31

Competency: SU26.3; SU26.4.

This chapter is important for systemic management of surgical problems. Preoperative respiratory assessment and postoperative respiratory care is very important. Complications such as pneumonia, collapse of lung, empyema, aspiration, ARDS (Acute respiratory distress syndrome), pulmonary embolism, pneumothorax, hemothorax, pleural effusion, lung abscess, postoperative cardiac problems like myocardial infarction should be remembered.

Per se patient may be having bronchogenic carcinoma, mediastinal pathology, pulmonary tuberculosis, asthma, bronchitis, bronchiectasis and so detailed history taking, clinical examination, relevant investigations should be done.

■ HISTORY

Chest pain: It is the commonest symptoms in most of the lung and cardiac diseases. It may be heaviness in chest in early carcinoma lung or pain in shoulder, intercostal region (intercostal neuralgia) in advanced disease.

Fever, dyspnea, hemoptysis, cough (dry or with sputum), nature of sputum, productive or not, foul smelling or not. Tuberculosis is the commonest cause of hemoptysis in India.

Loss of weight and appetite are the features of tuberculosis and carcinoma of lung.

Swelling chest wall: It could be cold abscess, empyema necessitans, and tumor.

Discharging sinus formation could be tuberculosis or actinomycosis.

Previous history of tuberculosis, pneumonia, hospitalization, surgery are important.

Smoking history is very relevant in lung diseases.

■ GENERAL EXAMINATION

Assessment of anemia, clubbing, dyspnea, nutritional status is important.

■ LOCAL EXAMINATION

Inspection

Shape of the Chest Wall

(1) *Scoliosis*, thoracic kyphoscoliosis reduces the pulmonary ventilatory capacity. (2) *Funnel chest* also called as *pectus excavatum* is a condition wherein there is posterior concavity of sternum from above downwards, anteroposteriorly and side to side of the chest. (3) *Flat chest* where transverse diameter is more than anteroposterior diameter. (4) *Barrel chest* where anteroposterior diameter is more than transverse diameter. (5) *Ricketic chest* with bead-like prominences at costochondral junction—*Ricketic rosary*. (6) *Pigeon chest/Pectus carinatum/chicken breast* where sternum is prominently bowing forward with costal cartilages; ribs indrawn along with symmetrical Harrison's sulci/grooves. It is seen as congenital deformity or as a sequel of childhood respiratory diseases. (7) Swelling or sinus in the chest wall should be examined in detail.

Respiratory movements: Rate, equality, character, type should be observed.

Apex beat: Apex beat is lower and outermost point of cardiac impulse with a maximum perpendicular thrust. It is located 1 cm medial to midclavicular line or 10 cm lateral to midsternal line at left 5th intercostal space. It is confined to one intercostal and has an area of 2.5 cm². Apex beat of the heart is palpated. Apex beat will be reduced in obesity, acute myocardial infarction, pleural effusion, pericardial effusion, constrictive pericarditis; it may be absent in normal site in dextrocardia or if it is underneath the rib.

Neck veins: Neck veins may be engorged in congestive cardiac failure, pulmonary hypertension, pericardial effusion, mediastinal tumor.

Swelling/s: Swelling in the chest wall, if any, should be inspected like any other swelling. Swelling of the neck is important as it may be lymph node enlargement due to chest diseases such as bronchogenic carcinoma.

Palpation

Respiratory movements are checked by placing fingers of each hand on each side of the chest wall of the patient with thumbs placed at the center and tips of thumbs touching each other. Patient is asked to take deep breath. Defective movements are appreciated.

Position of the trachea whether shifted or not is noted.

Vocal fremitus is noted by placing flat of fingers over chest wall. It is reduced in effusion/pneumothorax; increased in consolidation.

Swelling over chest wall should be palpated in detail. Impulse on coughing is due to empyema necessitans. **Ribs and relation of swelling** to them should be assessed. Expansile pulsation may be due to an aneurysm. Sinus also should be examined for all features in detail.

Percussion, auscultation are very essential methods to elicit all findings in respiratory (effusion, consolidation, pneumothorax, emphysema, etc.) and cardiac systems.

Palpation of neck nodes and spine is done for any significant pathology.

INVESTIGATIONS

- **Chest X-ray, bronchography (using neohydriol contrast into the bronchial tree), barium swallow (to see compression) (Fig. 31-1).**
- ***Bronchoscopy*** **to look for tumor in the bronchus (not in the periphery of lung), to take brush biopsy/direct biopsy, to do bronchial wash, look for vocal cord palsy by tumor infiltration of nodes.**
- **Mediastinoscopy by making a small incision above the sternum.**
- **Laryngoscopy to see vocal cord palsy.**
- **CT chest is essential investigation. CT guided biopsy can be done.**
- **Pleural tap is simple easier good investigation.**
- **Scalene node biopsy.**
- **Lung function tests.**
- ***Thoracoscopy is*** **very useful method.**
- **Metastatic work up for carcinoma lung towards brain, liver, bones.**

DIFFERENT CHEST DISEASES

Empyema thoracis

It is collection of pus in thoracic cavity **Causes**: *From chest wall*—wounds, osteomyelitis of ribs *From lung*—pneumonia, abscess, bronchiectasis tuberculosis, growth *Postoperative*—after thoracotomy *From esophagus*—perforations, carcinoma *From below diaphragm*—subphrenic abscess **Pathology**: The initial serous fluid collected in the pleural space eventually becomes purulent; intrapleural clotting of pus occurs with thickening of pleura; formation of fibrinous adhesions resulting in *empyema*. The pus may perforate through the intercostal space—*empyema necessitans*	**Organisms**: Initially staphylococci, streptococci, pneumococci, later *E. coli, Pseudomonas*, drug resistant staphylococci **Clinical features:** Pain in the chest; tenderness, fever, difficulty in breathing Toxicity—in acute cases Dullness on percussion, absent breath sounds, decreased chest wall movements (due to frozen chest) ***Empyema necessitans***—bulge in intercostal space with tenderness, impulse on coughing, restricted movements and dullness without breath sounds

Lung abscess

It is localized suppuration in the lung with tissue necrosis. It is end stage of suppurative pneumonitis with thrombosis of the associated artery **Etiology:** *Infection*—pneumonia (Streptococcus, Staphylococcus, Pneumococcus, hemophilus, anaerobic bacteria). *Bronchial obstruction*—due to tumors/ foreign body *Chronic upper respiratory infection*—sinusitis/ tonsillitis *Septicemia*	**Clinical features:** Acute onset of fever, recurrent in nature; cough with expectoration; hemoptysis; foul smelling sputum; associated with chronic debilitating illness **Complications**: Spread into other areas of lung; metastatic cerebral abscess; empyema thoracis; torrential hemorrhage following necrosis of the vessel in the abscess wall

Mediastinal tumors (Figs. 31-2A and B)

Occurs at any age group; 50% are commonly asymptomatic; picked up by routine chest X-ray **Classification**: a. Superior mediastinal tumor—retrosternal goiter; b. Anterior mediastinal tumor—retrosternal goiter; thymic tumors; teratomas and dermoids; pleuro-pericardial cyst c. Midmediastinal tumors—lymphadenopathies of all causes; foregut duplication cyst; lipoma d. Posterior mediastinal tumors—neurofibromas; ganglioneuromas	**Presentations**: Chest pain, back pain; respiratory distress, venous congestion; hoarseness of voice (recurrent laryngeal nerve compression); Dysphagia (esophageal compression); Horner's syndrome (compression of sympathetic chain); Scabbard trachea; later diaphragmatic paralysis; pleural effusion; hemorrhage (due to erosion into vessels by malignant tumor); myasthenia gravis (thymoma)

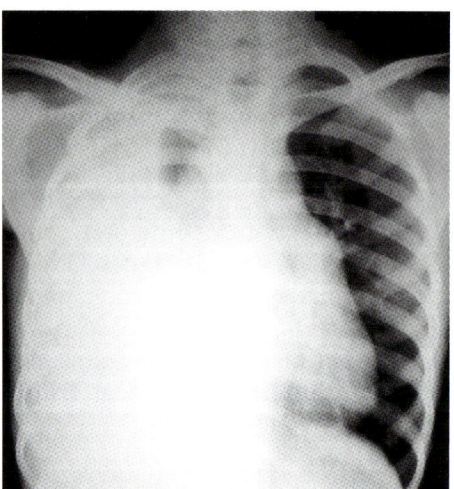

Fig. 31-1 *Massive malignant pleural effusion right sided—in a chest X-ray.*

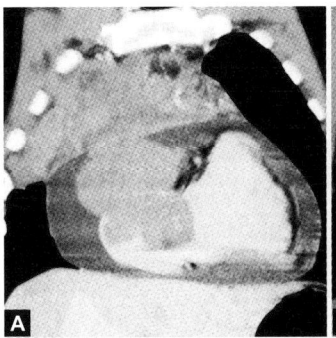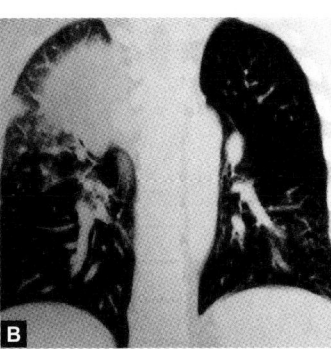

Figs. 31-2A and B CT pictures showing *mediastinal tumor*.

Pulmonary embolism

It is due to deep venous thrombosis (DVT) which gets dislodged into circulation and thereby enter into pulmonary circulation. It may be femoro-popliteal/ilio-femoral in origin

Types:
Small emboli—causes pulmonary hypertension
Medium sized emboli—sudden chest pain, severe dyspnea, shock, raised venous pressure, sudden death
Large sized emboli—chest pain, hemoptysis, dyspnea

Investigations:
Chest X-ray (hyperlucency in an area of oligemia—*Westermark sign*)
CT scan; MRI
Pulmonary angiography—diagnostic (100%)
Arterial blood gas analysis; isotope radionuclide ventilation perfusion scanning
Doppler study and venography—to rule out DVT

Shock lung (stiff lung)

Causes: Major chest trauma; septicemia; massive blood transfusions; DIC
Pathogenesis—development of microthrombo-embolism of small lung vessels following extensive intravascular coagulation leading into pulmonary consolidation which reduces the lung compliance

Features: Severe depression in gas exchange in lung; lung cannot expand at all—*stiff lung*; high mortality

Pulmonary complications in post-operative period

Precipitating factors—common in infants and elderly; common in males; common in smokers; common in patients with asthma, tuberculosis, chronic bronchitis, COPD; postoperative pain; DVT; obesity
Type of surgery—common in thoracic and upper abdomen surgeries
Septicemia; paralytic ileus; anesthetic complications, aspiration

Complications:
Bronchopneumonia, lung collapse, bronchitis, lung abscess, adult respiratory syndrome, respiratory failure, alkalosis, pleural effusion, empyema

Carcinoma lung (Figs. 31-3A and B)

Originates from primary, secondary bronchus or peripheral lung tissue. Squamous cell and small cell carcinoma are usual types
Etiology: Smoking, industrial toxins, old lung scar
Features: Chest pain, hemoptysis, hoarseness of voice (recurrent laryngeal nerve palsy), weight loss, cachexia, metastases to lymph nodes in mediastinum, axilla, neck; spread to bones, brain, liver
Investigations: Chest X-ray; CT chest, CT- guided biopsy

Pancoast tumor: It is a peripheral lung carcinoma arising from apex of lung (5%); invades brachial plexus, sympathetic chain, upper ribs, and vertebra **(Figs. 31-4A and B)**
Features: Intractable pain in upper chest and arm
Pancoast syndrome—lower brachial plexus palsy; Horner's syndrome, rib erosion, apical shadow, superior venacaval obstruction
CT guided biopsy—confirmatory

Pericarditis

Types
Acute: Usually by bacteria (*Staph. aureus, H. influenzae*, streptococci, Neisseria)
It is uncommon at present because of availability of good antibiotics. Here pus collects in pericardial space with decreased cardiac function and toxicity

Chronic constrictive pericarditis (Pick's disease): Tuberculous pericarditis is the commonest cause other—viral, after surgery, trauma. Here pericardium is thickened, fibrosed and calcified. Heart is encased in a rigid cavity which decreases cardiac function and decreases venous return
Features: Tachycardia, dyspnea, cyanosis, raised JVP, hepatomegaly, ascites and edema feet

Cardiac tamponade

It is due to accumulation of fluid or blood in the pericardial space causing increase in the intrapericardial pressure
Causes: Trauma; progressive pericardial effusion due to tuberculosis, viral, bacterial infections; uremia

Clinical features: Widened cardiac dullness; **Beck's triad** (*Hypotension; Muffled or decreased heart sounds; Raised JVP due to increased venous pressure*); pulsus paradoxus. In severe cases–as heart is unable to expand leads to shock and sudden death

Diaphragmatic hernia

It is herniation of abdominal content through diaphragm into the chest. It may be congenital or acquired (traumatic or esophageal hiatus hernia). Congenital may be associated with malrotation with *Ladd's band*

Types
1. **Eventration**: It is weakening of diaphragm due to atrophy and loss of muscle part or all of one leaf of the diaphragm, with thin fibrous tissue formation covered with pleura and peritoneum on either side. This thin diaphragm is raised and immobile. It is actually not a true herniation. But features mimic hernia. *Differential diagnosis* is diaphragmatic hernia through foramen Bochdalek. Condition causes respiratory embarrassment
2. **Hernia through the foramen of Morgagni**: The defect lies between the sternal and costal attachments of the diaphragm and is situated in front and towards right. Colon is the commonest content. Usually, it is symptom free
3. **Hernia through foramen Bochdalek** (through left sided pleuroperitoneal canal): This is a developmental defective condition where there is failure of fusion of pleuroperitoneal canal leaving a direct communication between pleura and peritoneum on left side. This allows herniation of contents of abdomen into the left side thorax. In 80% cases hernial sac is absent. Common content is colon; occasionally small bowel and stomach may be the contents
   Clinical features: Respiratory embarrassment, scaphoid abdomen, bowel sounds in left side of chest, mediastinal shift towards right side, occasionally features of intestinal obstruction. Pulmonary hypoplasia with persistent fetal circulation is the cause and is associated with respiratory acidosis
   Investigations: Chest X-ray, barium enema (common) or barium meal.
4. **Esophageal hiatus hernia**: Can be congenital or acquired (common)

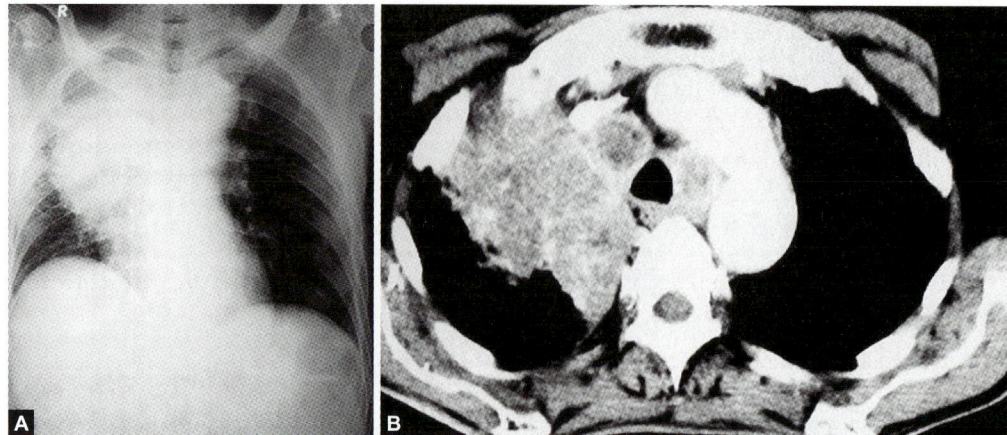

Figs. 31-3A and B Chest X-ray of *carcinoma of lung showing chest wall involvement*. CT picture showing carcinoma of lung.

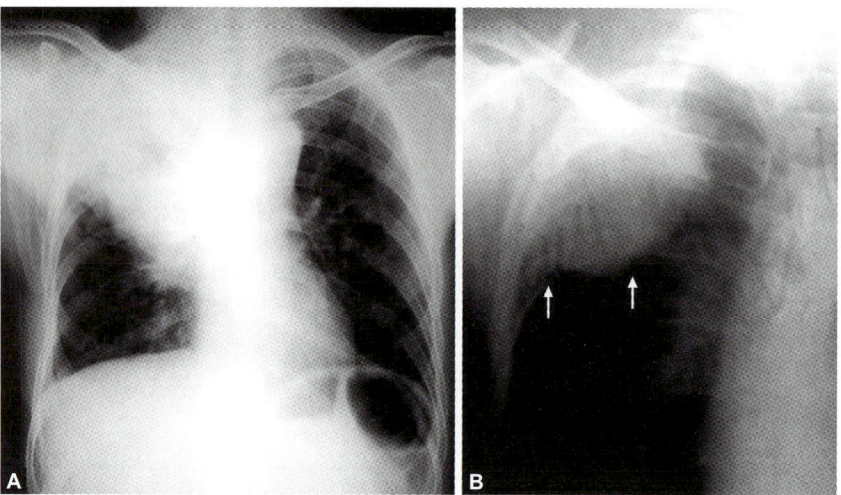

Figs. 31-4A and B X-rays showing right-sided *Pancoast* tumor in two different patients.

Chest Wall Tumors

Tumors arising from the chest wall components like muscles or ribs. They can be benign or malignant. Commonest benign tumor is chondroma arising from ribs. Malignant tumors are secondaries (commonest), chondrosarcoma arising from ribs (common among primary malignant tumors), rhabdomyosarcoma from muscles, fibrosarcoma from ribs/muscles/other soft tissues, Ewing's sarcoma and invasion from other tumors like from pleura or lungs or breast.

Benign tumors are slow growing, nonmobile, painless and usually from the rib cartilage, near costochondral junction. X-ray is diagnostic, shows rib expansion with intact cortex. One or more ribs can be involved.

Primary malignant tumor has got all features of sarcoma—progressive rapid enlargement, attaining large size, warm, vascular, nonmobile, often extends into the thoracic cavity or with skin ulceration. Secondaries in *lung/brain/liver* can occur. Chest X-ray, CT chest, US abdomen should be done to see secondaries. CT scan can also give idea about the tumor extension and operability. Open incision/trucut biopsy is essential for histological confirmation.

Solid swellings of chest wall:
- Tumors arising from ribs—chondroma, chondrosarcoma
- Tumors arising from nerve—neurofibroma
- Costochondritis at the junction of the bony part and cartilage part of the rib

Cystic swellings of the chest wall:
- Cold abscess
- Empyema necessitans—it is common in 3rd to 6th intercostal spaces; shows impulse on coughing
- Hernia of the lung—a rare entity which is seen in the root of the neck behind the clavicle; it is cystic, tympanic and reducible completely

Sinus in the chest wall:
- Tuberculous sinus
- Sinus due to chronic empyema—due to persistent underlying lung disease
- Sinus due to actinomycosis—are usually multiple, induration, puckering of skin is common; it is usually secondary with primary actinomycosis elsewhere in the body; discharge is specific—sulphur granules

Section 4: Examination in Trauma

CHAPTER 32: Approaches and Examination in Head Injuries

Competency: SU17.4; SU17.5; SU17.6.

HISTORY

Detailed history of an accident should be taken from the attender as patient may be unconscious or may be in shock and so unable to narrate the history. Type of trauma—road traffic accident, assault, fall from height is asked. Slipping and falling, etc. may also be the mode of injury.

History of vomiting is important as it may indicate that there is intracranial injury. It is usually repetitive and projective. Vomitus may contain blood in fracture of middle cranial fossa. Often it may be a sign of recovery also.

History of convulsion suggests intracranial injury. It may be due to hemorrhage or cerebral injury. Time, type, duration of convulsion should be asked. In middle meningeal hemorrhage, it is unilateral (*Jacksonian*) starting from toes going upwards towards face.

Level of consciousness: Patient may be conscious initially but later becomes unconscious. How long after the trauma, patient remained unconscious should be assessed. Duration of unconsciousness, recovery should be asked. Patient may become unconscious initially then recovers soon and after certain period of time becomes unconscious again. In the interval, patient behaves normally. This time interval of relative conscious period is called as '*lucid interval*'. It is usually seen in extradural hemorrhage.

Post-traumatic amnesia (PTA): It is to be noted that how long after trauma, patient was suffering from loss of memory. It is confirmed from patient's attender. ***Grading of PTA:*** *Grade 1* (slight)—less than 1 hour; *Grade 2* (moderate) 1-24 hours; Grade 3 (severe) is 1-7 days; *Grade* 4 (fatal) is more than 7 days. **Headache:** It is important sign in head injury. It suggests slowly progressive hematoma inside.

Swelling in the scalp may suggest scalp hematoma with a fracture underneath. It may be progressive also.

Bleeding from the nose, ear, and mouth suggests injury to the base of skull. Watery discharge from these places suggest CSF leak.

Other earlier history of blood pressure, diabetes, history of smoking and alcohol intake, intake of drugs and sedatives, history of epilepsy or receiving any other treatment are to be noted. Family history of epilepsy is also important.

EXAMINATION
General Examination

Pulse (tachycardia, *bradycardia*), respiration, presence of shock has to be noted; other systems should be examined for associated injuries which may be of priority in such occasions (abdomen bleed, hemothorax). Tachycardia is seen in cerebral concussion, slow bounding pulse with hypertension is a feature of cerebral compression to maintain cerebral circulation. Irregular pulse suggests poor prognosis.

Temperature: Hyperpyrexia is common in pontine hemorrhage, intraventricular hemorrhage and brainstem injury. Initially in cerebral concussion, temperature may be low. In brain compression, it raises. Temperature may be more by 1–2°F on the paralyzed side—***Victor Horsley's sign***. Systolic hypertension is common.

Respiration: It is slow and deep in compression; shallow in concussion. Blowing of lips and cheeks with each breathing; relaxed soft palate and tongue fall causing airway obstruction with snoring suggest compression of medulla suggesting poor prognosis. *Cheyne-Stokes respiration* suggests poor prognosis. Crepitations and altered breath sounds may suggest aspiration often with pneumonia.

LOCAL EXAMINATION

Scalp

Scalp hematoma may be subcutaneous (superficial, mobile), subaponeurotic (extends beyond skull bone suture lines), subpericranial (limited to one cranial bone by suture line).

Wound: Superficial/deep, deep with gaping if galea is injured. Its extent, number, depth, presence of deeper bone fracture—should be checked. Boggy swelling in the temporal region may suggest temporal bone fracture often with extradural hematoma. Ecchymoses appearing near the tip of the mastoid process in 3–4 days (*Battle's sign*) suggests posterior cranial fossa fracture behind the foramen magnum.

Position

Fully unconscious patient will lie flaccid and relaxed. May remain curled to one side in cerebral irritation; Restless with changing positions are also common.

Level and Depth of Consciousness

It should be checked according to coma scale. Patient's response is checked by pressing over the glabella and looking for facial expression. Absence of corneal reflex and urinary/fecal incontinence are significant. Grading of response to pain stimulus—*Grade I:* Avoid and push the stimulus with attempt; *Grade II:* Simple grunt; *Grade III:* Reflex decerebrating posture.

Bleeding from Nose, Ear and Mouth

Bleeding from nose suggests fracture of anterior cranial fossa; bleeding from mouth and ear suggests fracture in middle cranial fossa; CSF leak along with blood makes it watery. Facial palsy, deafness and meningitis can develop. Occipital bone sinuses may get torn in fracture of posterior cranial fossa causing dilated nonreactive pupil, Cheyne-Stokes breathing.

Neurological Deficits

One should check for sensation if patient is conscious; muscle power, rigid or flaccid paralysis; plantar reflex (*Babinski's sign*), abdominal reflexes. Joint jerks (Knee, ankle, biceps, and triceps) should be checked. Reflexes are useful in unconscious patient to identify paralysis. Complete neurological examination should be done.

Neck rigidity is an important sign to be looked for. It suggests subarachnoid hemorrhage, fracture dislocation of cervical spine or meningismus or meningitis. ***Ataxia and nystagmus*** are features of cerebellar injury.

Cranial Nerve Examination

All cranial nerves should be examined (**See Chapter 29**). Oculomotor nerve is most important. During initial period of cerebral compression, nerve gets irritated causing constriction of same side of pupil. Eventually nerve paralysis occurs causing pupil dilatation.

Examination of Eye

In fracture of anterior cranial fossa, extravasation of blood and ecchymoses occur after 24 hours first at lower (by gravity) than at upper eyelid—limiting to orbital margin. *Subconjunctival hemorrhage* (is deep to conjunctiva and does not move with conjunctiva) pointing towards the cornea with invisible posterior limit with conjunctival edema can occur. Eyeball may be pushed forward with limitation of movements.

'*Black eye*' is due to local injury around orbit with appearance of ecchymoses early/immediately which spreads beyond orbital margin into the cheek, nose and forehead. *Superficial conjunctival hemorrhage* is confirmed by its mobility with the conjunctiva and visibility of its posterior limit.

Pupils in cerebral concussion are equal, react to light and may be slightly dilated. *Hutchinson's pupil* is a feature of progressive cerebral compression showing three stages—
Stage I: Irritation of oculomotor nerve causing constriction of the pupil on injured side with normal sized pupil on opposite side.
Stage II: Oculomotor nerve paralysis causes dilatation of pupil on injured side with irritation of opposite oculomotor nerve causing constriction of pupil on opposite side.
Stage III: Both side pupils are dilated and fixed, not reacting to light.

Pin point pupil (fixed); pyrexia; paralysis are the (triad) features of *pontine* hemorrhage.

Examinations of Other Systems

It is mandatory to examine chest, abdomen and limbs. Often life-threatening injury and hemorrhages in the abdomen and thorax may be missed or ignored and patient may succumb to that. If there are such injuries, they take priority as otherwise hemorrhage may be life-threatening.

Reassessment of the patient by repeated examinations is needed.

INVESTIGATIONS

- **Hemoglobin, PCV, electrolytes and blood gas analysis depending on the clinical requirement.**
- **CT scan is ideal investigation to identify intracranial injuries. Usually plain CT is done in emergency situation (Fig. 32-1).**
- **Carotid angiography is done to see the site of bleeding and displacement of cranial vessels.**
- **MRI is very useful and sensitive.**

Mechanism of head injury	Effects of head injury
Distortion and mobility of brain	Brain edema
Rough surface of interior of skull	Brain ischemia and necrosis
Deceleration injury	Extradural/subdural/intracerebral/intraventricular hematoma
Acceleration injury	
Cerebral concussion	Coning and Kernohan's notch effect
Cerebral contusion	Respiratory failure
Cerebral laceration	Hyperpyrexia
Coup and contrecoup injury	CSF rhinorrhea/otorrhea
Raised intracranial pressure	Fluid and electrolyte imbalance

Chapter 32: Approaches and Examination in Head Injuries

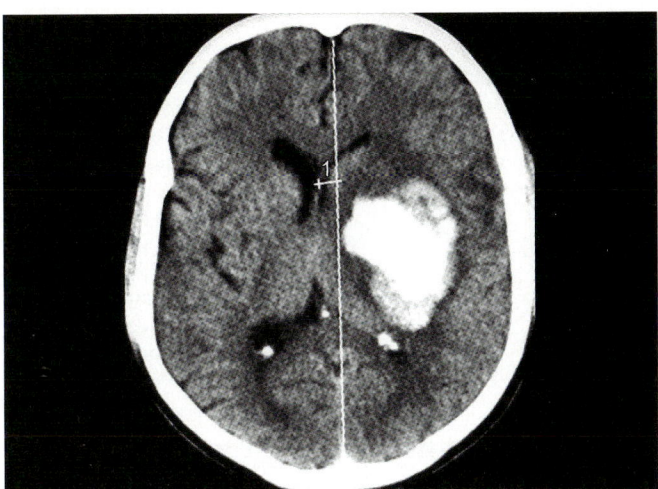

Fig. 32-1 *Intracerebral hematoma*—CT picture.

Glasgow Coma Scale

Eye opening		Verbal response		Motor response	
Spontaneous	4	Oriented	5	Obeys commands	6
To Speech	3	Confused	4	Localizes pain	5
To Pain	2	Inappropriate words	3	Flexion to pain	4
None	1	Incomprehensible words	2	Abnormal flexion	3
		None	1	Extension to pain	2
				None	1

Total score—15
Mild head injury: Score 13–15
Moderate head injury: 9–12
Severe head injury: Less than 8 (3–8)

Score 1—dead or dying. Score 2—vegetative state. Score 3—severe disability. Score 4—moderate disability. Score 5—good recovery

Adelaide Coma Scale:
It is used in children. Scores for eye opening and motor responses are same as Glasgow coma scale. But *verbal response score differs*—Oriented—5. Words—4. Vocal sounds—3. Cries—2. Nil—1. Orientation cannot be evaluated below 5 years of age. For first 6 months, the best verbal response is CRY.

Indications for admission: Any altered level of consciousness; Skull fracture; Focal neurological features; Persistent headache, vomiting, systolic hypertension, bradycardia; Alcohol intoxication; Bleeding from ear or nose; Associated injuries.

Complications of head injuries: Early: (1) Brainstem injury—due to coning. (2) Compression over cerebellum and medulla. (3) *CSF rhinorrhea*: It is due to communication between intracranial cavity and the nose. There is a tear in the dura following the fracture involving the sinuses—frontal, ethmoid, sphenoid sinuses. Meningitis is the common complication of CSF rhinorrhea. (4) Meningitis —common. (5) Pituitary damage and endocrine failure—require high-dose of hydrocortisone 200 mg 6th hourly. (6) Aerocele. (7) CSF otorrhea. (8) Depressed fractures will often cause injury to dural venous sinuses and may lead to torrential hemorrhage which may be life-threatening. So such depressed fractures should never be elevated. *Late:* Chronic subdural hematoma; post-traumatic epilepsy. Late post-traumatic epilepsy is due to scarring and gliosis of cerebrum; Post-traumatic amnesia. Post-traumatic hydrocephalous; Post-traumatic headache.

Extradural Hematoma (Fig. 32-2)

It is collection of blood in the extradural space between the dura and skull. Usually associated with fracture of temporoparietal region. Can be unilateral or bilateral

Vessels commonly involved— middle meningeal veins; anterior branch of middle meningeal artery; posterior branch of middle meningeal artery

Mechanism of injury: Direct blow like from cricket ball or road traffic accidents or fall and impact

Pathology: Fracture of thin temporal bone—bleeding following tear of vessels— hematoma under scalp and temporalis muscle on outer aspect; extra dural hematoma due to gradual stripping of dura from skull on inner aspect—in 6–12 hours intracranial tension raises leading to *coning*—herniation of supratentorial compartments through tentorial hiatus— midbrain shift towards opposite side which gets injured by sharp edge of the tentorial cerebelli → corticospinal tract before decussation on opposite side gets injured → So hemiparesis and pupillary changes occur on the same side of hematoma → this effect is called as **Kernohan's notch effect**

Clinical features: History of transient loss of consciousness following a blow or fall. Patient soon regains consciousness and again after 6–12 hours start deteriorating (**Lucid interval**— it is the golden hour/crucial time gap which is un-noticed and often missed—time taken for the intracranial pressure to raise). Later the patient presents with confusion, irritability, drowsiness, and hemiparesis on same side of the injury. Initially pupillary constriction and later pupillary dilatation occurs on the same side, finally becomes totally unconscious. Death can occur if immediate surgical intervention is not done. Features of raised intracranial pressure like high blood pressure, bradycardia, vomiting is also seen. Occasionally convulsions may be present. Wound and hematoma in the temporal region of scalp may be seen

CT scan—head is diagnostic. *Extradural hematoma shows biconvex lesion*

Subdural Hematoma (Fig. 32-3)

Types:
Acute subdural hematoma: It is a collection of blood between the brain and dura (subdural space) following injury to the cortical veins and often due to laceration of cortex of brain which bleeds forming a hematoma. Here hematoma is extensive and diffused. There is no lucid interval. There is a severe primary brain damage. Hematoma may be coup and contre coup type. Loss of consciousness occurs immediately after trauma and is progressive. Convulsion is common. Features of raised intracranial pressure are obviously seen—high BP, bradycardia, vomiting, etc. Focal neurological deficits or hemiparesis can occur. CT scan shows concavoconvex lesion

Chronic subdural hematoma: It is due to the rupture of veins between dura and brain (cerebral hemispheres), causing gradual collection of blood in subdural space. Commonly seen in elderly people following any minor trauma like fall, slipping, etc. (which might have gone un-noticed). Blood collects gradually over 2–6 weeks. Plasma and cellular components get separated and eventually cellular part gets absorbed leaving only fluid component called as *subdural hygroma*. Usual hematoma collection is 60–120 mL. It is bilateral in 50% of cases

Clinical features: Patient presents with confusion, disorientation, gradually with altered level of consciousness and drowsiness.

Contd...

Contd...

| | Later convulsions, features of intracranial hypertension, features of coning develop. Extensor plantar response and pupillary changes develop eventually
Differential diagnosis: Electrolyte imbalance, intracranial space occupying lesion
CT scan shows concavoconvex lesion | **Depressed Skull Fracture**
It is a common neurosurgical problem among the head injuries where in fracture depression is more than the depth of the inner table of skull | **Problems**: Tear in the dura beneath; hematoma in the deeper plane; injury to the cerebrum; injury to the venous sinuses—may cause life-threatening hemorrhage; fracture should not be elevated in such occasion as it itself can precipitate bleeding; convulsions; meningitis |

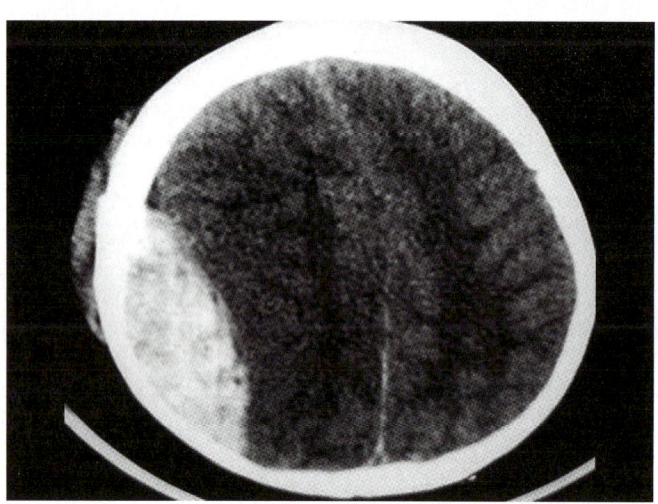

Fig. 32-2 *Extradural hematoma*. Note the biconvex configuration of the hematoma.

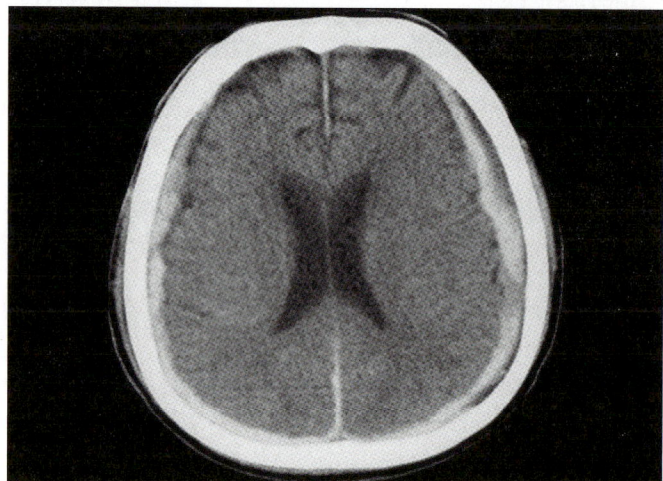

Fig. 32-3 *Subdural hematoma*. Note the concavoconvex configuration of the lesion.

33 Approaches and Examination in Chest Injuries

Competency: SU17.8; SU17.9; SU 17.10.

■ HISTORY

Detailed history of trauma should be asked. History of breathlessness, chest pain, hemoptysis/cough with blood (lung trauma), airway block should be asked. Pain in the ribs may be due to rib fracture. Excruciating pain on deep breathing suggests rib fracture.

■ EXAMINATION

General Examination

Pulse, blood pressure, cyanosis, tachypnea and features of shock should be checked. Abdomen, limbs, head and neurological systems should also be examined.

Inspection

Chest, abdomen and neck should be exposed for proper inspection. Ecchymoses, bruises in the skin over chest wall should be inspected. Wound may often look small superficially but may be deep penetrating into the thoracic cavity. Air may be bubbling through the wound with noise. Blood clot may be present in such wounds. Such patient often may need emergency resuscitation to maintain adequate ventilation.

Type of breathing—abdominal or thoracic and its character should be checked. Hyperpnea, dyspnea and altered breathing should be observed. Collapse of chest wall during inspiration and distension of part of chest wall during expiration suggest *flail chest* with paradoxical breathing, mediastinal flutter and pendular movement of the air. Tension pneumothorax causes sudden distress in breathing and sudden respiratory arrest. Emergency chest tubing or needle drainage of air from the thoracic cavity is needed.

Localized swelling due to hematoma may be evident. Diffused puffy look suggests surgical emphysema. It may be in the chest wall, abdomen, and on neck both sides.

Palpation

Rib tenderness, bone irregularity and crepitus should be checked. It suggests fracture rib. With the patient standing and keeping his hands over the head, examiner keeps his one hand over the sternum and other on the spine; applying compression over thoracic cage anteroposteriorly causes pain at the site of fracture—**Compression test.**

Sternum should be examined for fracture. When such fracture is displaced upper fragment over-rides lower. Spine should be examined for fracture as fracture sternum is commonly associated with fracture spine.

Flat of the hand is placed over the chest wall whenever there is diffuse swelling to feel for crepitus under the fingers. It suggests **surgical emphysema**. If it appears at the rib fracture site first, it is due to rib fracture. If it is rapidly spreading over neck, chest, abdomen, then it is due to injury to bronchus or esophagus—*mediastinal emphysema* (Figs. 33-1A to C).

Features of pneumothorax/hemothorax should be checked.

Percussion

Resonant on percussion in case of pneumothorax and dullness in hemothorax are observed. Liver dullness is obliterated in right-sided pneumothorax. Cardiac dullness is obliterated in left-sided pneumothorax. Cardiac dullness is widened in hemopericardium.

Auscultation

Breath sounds are reduced in pneumothorax or hemothorax. Vocal resonance is also reduced. Heart sounds are not heard in hemopericardium.

■ INVESTIGATIONS

- Chest X-ray to see fracture ribs, pneumothorax, hemothorax and hemopneumothorax.
- Pleural tap is often needed.

Section 4: Examination in Trauma

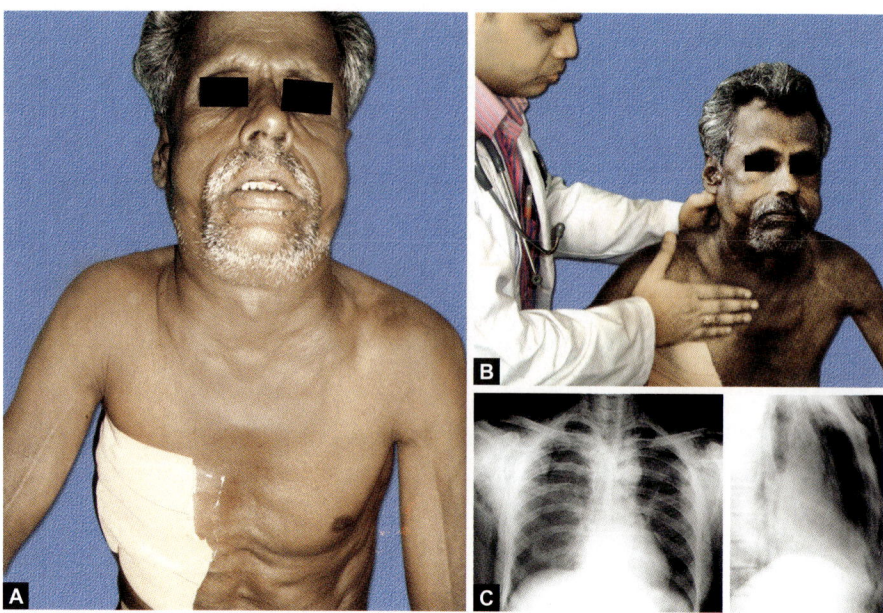

Figs. 33-1A to C Patient with puffiness of face and neck with *surgical emphysema*. X-ray showing surgical emphysema.

- US of chest wall to confirm fluid/blood/air.
- Arterial blood gas analysis (ABG) is needed to diagnose respiratory failure.
- Plain CT chest and abdomen is ideal and essential nowadays.

CHEST INJURIES

Types: (1) Crush injuries involving lung, pleura, and ribs. (2) Single rib fracture. (3) Two or more rib fractures. (4) *Steering wheel injury*—causes multiple rib fractures bilaterally often with flail chest, with fracture dislocation of upper end of sternum. (5) Stove in chest or flail chest. (6) Traumatic pneumothorax. (7) Hemothorax, hemopneumothorax, with fracture ribs. (8) Tension pneumothorax. (9) Pericardial and cardiac injuries and rupture of bronchus. (10) Associated injuries in liver, spleen, diaphragm and major vessels.

Causes: Road traffic accidents, industrial accidents, blast injuries, crush injuries and stab injuries. In children, ribs are malleable and so fracture ribs are rare. In elderly as the ribs become rigid, fracture is common. First and second ribs are protected by clavicle and so fracture is uncommon. 11th and 12th ribs are floating ribs and so fracture is rare.

Factors and pathophysiology of chest injuries: Hypoxia, hypercarbia, acidosis, hypovolemic shock, pulmonary contusion syndromes, tracheo-bronchial injuries, bilateral chest injuries, chest wall injuries, diaphragmatic injuries, cardiac injuries, hemopericardium and ARDS.

Complications: Infections—empyema, lung abscess, pneumonia, septicemia; Respiratory failure; Traumatic asphyxia; Traumatic shock lung; Disseminated intravascular coagulation (DIC). ARDS (Adult/Acute respiratory distress syndrome).

'Deadly dozen' threats to life from chest injury	
Immediately life-threatening	**Potentially life-threatening**
• Airway obstruction • Tension pneumothorax • Pericardial tamponade • Open pneumothorax • Massive hemothorax • Flail chest	• Aortic injuries • Tracheobronchial injuries • Myocardial contusion • Rupture of diaphragm • Esophageal injuries • Pulmonary contusion

Flail chest and stove in chest	
It is fracture of two or more consecutive ribs with each rib having two or more fracture sites. Such segment is called as **flail segment.** **Pathophysiology**: Flail segment moves separately, when compared with adjacent thoracic cage. During inspiration flail segment moves inwards (unlike normal thoracic cage which moves outward), and during expiration segment moves outwards (unlike normal cage which moves inward) causing pathophysiological derangements. This **paradoxical respiration** causes reduction in ventilatory lung surface and so respiratory dysfunction. **Mediastinal flutter**: Back and forth movement of tissues and organs of mediastinum during different phases of respiration, often cause kinking of great vessels and sudden cardiac arrest. **Pendular movement of air** from one lung to other occurs thus preventing atmospheric air to get into both injured and other side normal lung leading to respiratory failure.	All these derangements get aggravated by hemothorax, pneumothorax and other associated injuries **Types**: • Anterior—near costochondral junction • Lateral—in rib shafts • Posterior—safer **Problems:** Cardiac arrest; respiratory failure; hemothorax; infection; ARDS ***Note: Stove in chest** is depression of a portion of chest wall due to severe chest injury.*

Pneumothorax

It is presence of air between the layers of the pleura.

Classification: Pneumothorax, hydropneumothorax, pyopneumothorax, hemopneumothorax, artificial pneumothorax and tension pneumothorax.

Causes:
Traumatic
Spontaneous— (1) Tuberculous, (2) Non-tuberculous: (a) Emphysematous bullae; (b) Solitary lung cyst; (c) Honeycomb or cystic lung; (d) Idiopathic
Spontaneous pneumothorax can be acute, chronic or recurrent.

Clinical features: Hyperresonant, absence of breath sounds and tracheal deviation.

Chest X-ray reveals: Radiolucency on the affected side; absence of lung markings; collapsed lung margin.

Tension Pneumothorax: During inspiration, air is pumped into the pleural cavity through a valvular opening in the visceral pleura. Lung collapses first and as air continuously collects in the pleural cavity, mediastinum shifts towards opposite side, decreasing the volume of the functioning lung. Further increase in the pleural pressure, reduces the venous return, atrial filling, and ventricular filling and so cardiac output and cardiac function. It causes sudden death and hence emergency treatment is required.

Clinical features: Tachypnea, decreased breath sounds, resonant on percussion with severe mediastinal shift and cyanosis. *Once clinically diagnosed, immediately place a wide bore needle in the second intercostal space in midclavicular line*, and a sterile glove is kept on the hub (blunt) end of the needle to create a valve so as to prevent inward sucking of air from outside.

Hemothorax

It is blood collected in pleural cavity; causes pain, shock, and also very irritant to pleural cavity. It is a good culture media for bacteria and so infection is quite common.

Causes: Trauma; postoperative: pulmonary, cardiac, esophageal surgeries, cervical sympathectomy; leak from CVP monitor line; tumors of lung, mediastinum, pleura; leaking aneurysms and spontaneous. There may be rib fractures in traumatic hemothorax.

Clinical features: Pain in the chest, tenderness, difficulty in breathing, dullness, diminished breath sounds and features of shock.

Complications: Infection and empyema.

Triage: Triage means *'to sort'* in *'French'*. Triage by committee of Trauma of the American College of surgeons. ***Assessing four components:*** Physiologic response; Anatomical injury; Biomechanical injury; Comorbid factors. Triage algorithm contains steps 1, 2, 3 and 4. Primary management consists of A, B, C, D, E and F.

A—Airway:
- Chin lift
- Jaw thrust
- Nasal airway
- Oral airway
- Endotracheal intubation
- Tracheostomy (Assess airway patency)

B—Breathing:
- 100% oxygen
- Assess bilateral chest raise
- Assess breath sounds
- Use pulse oximetry
- Treat flail chest, pneumothorax
- Intercostal tube drainage

C—Circulation:
- Monitor vitals
- Heart sounds
- ECG
- IV fluids
- Blood transfusion
- Control of external bleed
- Use two IV lines—14G/16G

D—Disability evaluation:
- Neurological examination
- Glasgow coma scale
- Pupillary reaction
- Treatment of shock

E—Expose the patient fully:
- Undress the patient
- Hypothermia assessment
- Assess injuries
- Examine joints, bones, abdomen and other systems
- Look for identification marks

F—Fingers and tubes:
- Examine all orifices like P/R, P/V, etc.
- Use required tubes like catheter, Ryle's tube

34 Approaches and Examination in Abdominal Injuries

Competency: SU17.8; SU17.9; SU 17.10.

Abdominal injuries are of manifolds. It may be closed injury or open injury. It may be blunt, stab or abdominal wall injury. Open injury is obvious on examination. Closed injuries may be missed sometimes unless abdomen is carefully examined. Pelvic injuries often can cause life- threatening torrential bleed which may be difficult to manage. High velocity injury, compression injury, fracture spine, pelvis, penetrating injuries, gun- shot injuries are different types which often can cause extensive damage. **Seat belt injuries** are common in western countries. Seat belt compresses the visceral structure like bowel and mesentery causing injury. It is usually a closed/blunt injury of abdomen. History of hematuria, distension of abdomen, severe pain in abdomen, bruising over the abdomen, inability to pass urine, difficulty in breathing are all important to be considered in abdominal injuries. Often in **blunt injury**, initially patient feels comfortable as no external wound is detected but after sometime he develops distension, pain in abdomen suggesting internal organ or hollow viscus injury. Associated chest/head/limb injuries should also be assessed by history. **Referred pain** to left shoulder suggests splenic injury due to irritation of the left phrenic nerve by clot under left-sided diaphragm—**Kehr's sign**.

GENERAL EXAMINATION

Features of shock, restlessness, respiration, temperature, blood pressure should be checked. Tachycardia, tachypnea, hypotension, pallor are features of hemorrhagic shock.

Inspection of Abdomen

Patient is asked to point where exactly is the pain (*pointing sign*) and that area is inspected first. Abrasions, lacerations, bruising should be checked. Localized abdominal wall hematoma may be evident. Bruising in the abdominal wall/imprint of cloth or seat belt suggests crushing injury of bowel against vertebral column—**London's sign** (Peter S London, Birmingham). Parallel lines (two) drawn to the line of mesentery in the abdomen divides it into upper, middle and lower parts of small bowel injury—**Monks localization** method where bruising in these zones indicates respective (proximal, middle, distal) part of the small bowel injury.

Abdominal distension whether localized or generalized should be observed which indicates generalized or localized hemoperitoneum.

Movements with respiration may be reduced in hemoperitoneum or peritonitis.

Protrusion of umbilicus suggests distension of abdomen by blood, pus or fluid.

Stab injury should be inspected carefully for presence of omentum, blood, and intestine. Its location, direction, margin and edge, depth should be inspected using a proper light source **(Fig. 34-1)**.

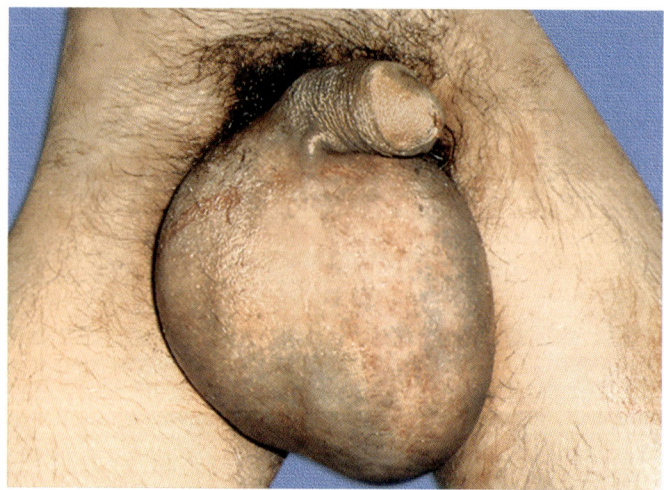

Fig. 34-1 *Urethral injury*—blood in the external meatus; extravasation of urine.

Perineum and urethra should be inspected for swelling, blood in the urethra suggesting perineal injury with extravasation.

Palpation

Abdomen should be palpated for tenderness, rebound tenderness, guarding, rigidity (sign of peritonitis/irritation). Swelling in the abdomen may be localized hematoma of abdominal wall or distended bladder, paralytic ileus, localized hemoperitoneum.
Fluid thrill suggests free fluid in the abdomen.
Repeated examination is needed.

Percussion and Auscultation

Obliteration of liver dullness (bowel injury), shifting dullness, and dullness lower abdomen for urinary bladder should be checked. Dullness in the left flank which is not shifting suggests splenic injury—**Ballance's sign.**
Auscultation showing absence of bowel sounds indicates peritonitis.
Rectal and vaginal examination should be done when needed.
Other systems should be examined for associated injury—thorax, limbs, and head.

■ INVESTIGATIONS

Blood parameters—hemoglobin, packed cell volume, serum electrolytes are essential.

Plain X-ray abdomen to look for gas under diaphragm, ground glass appearance, obliterated psoas shadow, localized mass lesion (hematoma) which are significant. Chest X-ray is also to be taken.

US abdomen is essential in all abdomen traumas. It gives rapid assessment of the abdomen for hemoperitoneum and organ injuries.

Focused assessment with sonography for trauma (FAST): It is rapid, noninvasive, portable bedside method of investigation focusing on pericardium, splenic, hepatic and pelvic areas. Blood more than 100 mL in cavities can be identified. It is not reliable for bowel or penetrating injuries. It often needs to be repeated.

CT scan abdomen and chest should be done whenever needed.

Note: eFAST is Extended FAST wherein additional ultrasound scanning of thorax is done.

Four quadrant aspirations using 19 gauge needle is done and fluid is analyzed for blood, amylase, proteins, bacteria. Negative finding is of no value to rule out intra-abdominal injury.

Diagnostic peritoneal lavage (DPL): It is done in case of blunt injury abdomen. Through a subumbilical lavage catheter one liter of saline is infused into the peritoneal cavity. Patient is changed to different positions side to side and later fluid content is aspirated for analysis. 10 mL or more blood; RBC count more than 100,000/cu mm; WBC count more than 500/cu mm; amylase level in the fluid more than 175 IU/dL; presence of bile bacteria, food—are the positive criteria. It is the procedure of choice in physiologically unstable patient. It is contraindicated in pregnancy, previous laparotomy, obesity.

Diagnostic laparoscopy is a valuable investigation.

Mesenteric angiography is needed occasionally to localize the site of bleeding.

Liver injury	
Causes: It can be due to blunt injury, stab, and gunshot injury. **Types**: It can be contusion, laceration, avulsion, extension into thorax, biliary tree; associated with other organ injuries (spleen, kidney, duodenum, bowel, IVC); associated with fracture ribs. **Clinical features**: Features of shock due to severe torrential bleeding (pallor, hypotension, tachycardia, sweating). Distension of abdomen with dull flank, guarding, tenderness and rigidity are other features seen. Oliguria; tachypnea, respiratory distress and often cyanosis is seen; rupture of right lobe is more common than left lobe leading to hemoperitoneum; occasionally can cause localized hematoma which will go for an abscess formation.	**Complications and sequelae of liver injury**: Shock and hemorrhage; liver abscess or septicemia; bile leak, biliary peritonitis, biliary fistulas; disseminated intravascular coagulation; hepatic artery aneurysm, arteriovenous and arteriobiliary fistulas; complications of massive blood transfusion; electrolyte imbalance; respiratory complications; liver failure; late sequelae of liver trauma is CBD stricture causing obstructive jaundice. **CT is diagnostic tool.** *Hematocrit; liver function tests; PT INR should be done*. Liver injury is graded depending on involvement of hepatic veins, portal system, biliary system and duodenum. Often high-grade liver injury also can be managed non-operatively.
Splenic injury (Rupture spleen)	
Splenic injury is common in case of road traffic accidents, and other blunt injury abdomen. Most often associated with fracture of left lower ribs, hemothorax, injury of liver (left lobe commonly, occasionally both lobes), bowel, tail of pancreas, left kidney. *Spontaneous rupture of spleen* can occur in malaria and infectious mononucleosis **Types of injury**: (1) Splenic subcapsular hematoma: After initial injury patient remains asymptomatic, but this hematoma later ruptures after few days causing torrential hemorrhage. (2) Clean incised wound over the surface. (3) Lacerated wound. (4) Splenic hilar injury causes torrential hemorrhage, may even cause death. (5) Splenic injury associated with other injuries.	Clot collected under the left side of the diaphragm irritates it and the phrenic nerve causing referred pain in the left shoulder (Kehr's sign); *Saegesser's tender point* is between left sternomastoid and scalenus medius. There may be left sided hemothorax with fracture of ribs *Delayed presentation* is also possible due to formation of subcapsular hematoma which later gives way. Initially gets temporarily localized by greater omentum/blood clot temporarily seals off the bleeding which later dislodged causing severe gets bleeding. This time period in between is called '*latent period of Bandet*'. Features of other abdominal organ injuries like of left lobe of liver, tail of pancreas, left kidney, left sided colon, small bowel, may be present. Diaphragm and left-sided lung injury, fracture ribs may be other associations.

Contd...

Contd...

Presentation: *Rapid development of shock* and *fast deterioration* can occur. Even death can occur sometime, which is often due to splenic hilar vessel injury, where emergency surgery and splenectomy is mandatory. In other types, *features of shock* (pallor, tachycardia, restlessness, hypotension), pain, tenderness, and abdominal rigidity in left upper quadrant is seen. Later there will be abdominal distension due to hemoperitoneum. There is dullness in the left flank which does not shift, as the collected blood gets clot—*Ballance's sign*

Plain X-ray shows—obliteration of splenic outline and left-sided psoas shadow; indentation of fundic gas shadow; fracture ribs; elevated left side diaphragm. US abdomen and CT are diagnostic
Complications of splenic injury: Hemorrhagic shock; DIC; sepsis; splenic artery pseudoaneurysm; splenic arteriovenous fistula; pancreatitis

Injuries to Kidney

Commonly due to a blunt injury. Often associated with other abdominal injuries of liver, spleen, bowel, mesentery, etc. Per se renal injury is extraperitoneal
Types: Small subcapsular; large subcapsular; cortical laceration; laceration with perinephric hematoma; medullary laceration with bleeding into the renal pelvis; corticomedullary complete rupture; hilar injury (most dangerous)
Clinical features: Features of shock; hematuria—may be mild to profuse depending on the type of injury; clot colic; bruising, swelling and tenderness in the loin; paralytic ileus with abdominal distension occurs due to retroperitoneal hematoma implicating splanchnic nerves

Investigations: *US abdomen*: Done to see the type of injury, amount of hematoma and other associated injuries in the abdomen. US should be repeated at regular intervals to see the progress (at 12–24 hourly). **CT scan is very useful and recommended always.** *IVU used to be important tool earlier to find out the functions of the both kidneys. Blood urea and serum creatinine* should be repeated again at regular intervals. Blood grouping and cross matching for blood transfusion
Complications: Clot retention in the bladder and may go for renal failure; pararenal pseudohydronephrosis; infection; perinephric abscess; aneurysm of the renal artery; renal failure

Pancreatic Trauma

It is rare because of its anatomical location— retroperitoneum. Its injury is usually associated with injuries to liver/duodenum/spleen/portal system/biliary system/kidney. Deep force in epigastrium may cause crushing of body of pancreas against vertebra—closed injury. Penetrating injury may cause direct sharp injury of pancreas
Types: Parenchymal contusion/laceration without duct disruption; parenchymal injury with duct disruption; complete transection of pancreas; massive destruction of pancreatic head

Features: Pain in epigastrium; features of associated injuries; features of shock; rise in serum amylase level is common
Investigations: CT scan is diagnostic; endoscopic retrograde cholangiopancreatography (ERCP) to confirm duct disruption; assessment of blood loss and other injuries
Complications: Hemorrhage; septicemia; pancreatitis—acute/recurrent; pseudocyst formation; pancreatic fistula; pancreatic abscess

Rupture Bladder

Causes: Blow, kick or fall; road traffic accidents; stabs, gunshot injuries; endoscopic trauma; diathermy; instrumentations
Types:
Type I: Intraperitoneal rupture—20% common. It occurs in fully distended bladder due to blow, kick, or fall
Clinical features: Sudden pain in suprapubic region. Shock and syncope; diffuse abdominal pain. Urine leaks into the abdominal cavity causing distension of abdomen; presents with features of peritonitis, with guarding, rigidity, tenderness and rebound tenderness, dull flank. Patient does not have the desire to micturate
Investigations: (1) Plain X-ray shows ground glass appearance. (2) Peritoneal tap to collect urine. (3) After passing a small catheter gently per urethra, water soluble iodine dye is passed to visualize the tear in the bladder and entry of the dye into the free peritoneal cavity. This can be done now through 'C-arm image' intensifier easily. (4) US abdomen to look for other injuries in the abdomen
Complications of rupture bladder: Cystitis and pyelonephritis; peritonitis; pelvic abscess; fistula formation (vesicovaginal or rectovesical); paralytic ileus; hemorrhage. Without surgery mortality is 100%

Type II: Extraperitoneal rupture—80% common. It is due to road traffic accidents, golf playing, fall over the manhole. Its features and management are same as rupture of posterior (membranous) urethra
Clinical features: There is collection of urine and blood in the extraperitoneal space in front, with fullness, diffuse pain and tenderness in lower abdomen. Swelling is seen in the scrotum or labia, and abdominal wall. Strangury, inability to pass urine and often blood in the external meatus; features of shock and other associated injuries
Investigations: Plain X-ray pelvis shows fracture. Cystogram shows leak from the bladder. During cystoscopy: (1) Bladder cannot be distended. (2) Endoscopy light may be shining through the abdominal wall. (3) Irrigating fluid cannot be retrieved back. Other associated urethral injury is looked for. Bladder injury can also occur during hysterectomy (both abdominal and vaginal), surgery of colon or rectum, repair of direct inguinal or femoral hernias

Urethral Injury (Fig. 34-2)

It can be *rupture of the membranous / bulbous urethra*. Depending on circumference of the urethral wall involved it can be *Complete/Incomplete rupture*. Depending on the thickness of the urethra involved it can be *Total/Partial*

Investigations: X-ray pelvis to see for fracture. US abdomen to see pelvis and other injuries. Urethrogram is done to see the site and type of tear (often reserved to do at later stage)
Complications: Urinary incontinence; impotence; stricture urethra; infection

Contd...

Contd...

Rupture of membranous urethra (Prostatic urethra/Posterior urethra)—
Causes: Usually associated with pelvic fracture, commonly due to road traffic accidents. Injury can also occur during instrumentation, calculus passage and catheterization; in prolonged labor due to long standing fetal head pressing on the urethra. Prostate is attached to pubis by puboprostatic ligament and disruption of puboprostatic ligament with complete rupture of urethra can lead to *floating prostate*. Injury can lead to incomplete rupture of urethra or may be associated with extraperitoneal rupture of bladder
Clinical features: (1) Blood in external meatus. Failure or difficulty in passing urine. (2) Extravasation of urine to scrotum, perineum and abdominal wall. (3) Shock with pallor, tachycardia and hypotension. (4) Features of associated injuries like head injury, thorax and or abdominal organs which take priority in initial phases of management. (5) On P/R examination, prostate may be felt high or may not be palpable at all. It signifies floating prostate
Investigations: X-ray pelvis to see for fracture. US abdomen to see pelvis and other injuries. Urethrogram is done to see the site and type of tear (often reserved to do at later stage) **(Fig. 34.3)**.
Complications: Urinary incontinence; impotence; stricture urethra; infection.

Rupture of bulbous urethra (anterior urethra)—
Usually due to a fall astride a projecting object, like in sailing ships, cycling, over loose manhole cover, gymnasium
Clinical features: Triad—(1) Blood in external meatus (Urethral hemorrhage). (2) Perineal hematoma. (3) Retention of urine
Investigations: X-ray pelvis, and US abdomen or CT pelvis. Condition is diagnosed clinically
Complications: Infection; extravasation of urine; stricture urethra

Abdominal Compartment Syndrome

There is sudden increase in intra-abdominal pressure which causes decreased venous return to heart (pressure more than 12 mm Hg). It leads into increased peak inspiratory pressure, hypoxia, hypercarbia, decreased urine output, hypotension due to decreased venous return to heart.

Abdominal compartment syndrome (ACS)		
Causes	**Features**	**Intra-abdominal pressure grading (Burch) in cm of water**
• Postoperative ileus • Acute abdomen • Acute gastric dilatation • Laparoscopic procedures • Intestinal obstruction	• Hypoxia, hypercarbia • Decreased urine output • Hypotension • Tense abdomen-distended • Decreased venous return • Bowel ischemia • Cardiac arrest	I—10–15 cm H_2O II—15–25 III—25–35 IV—more than 35

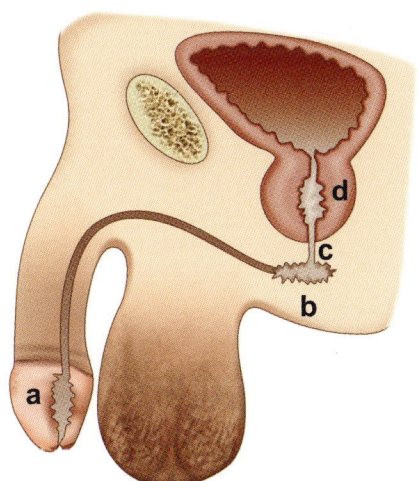

Fig. 34-2 *Common sites of urethral injuries.* Membranous and bulbar urethra are common sites.

a. Penile urethra
b. Bulbar urethra
c. Membranous urethra
d. Prostatic urethra

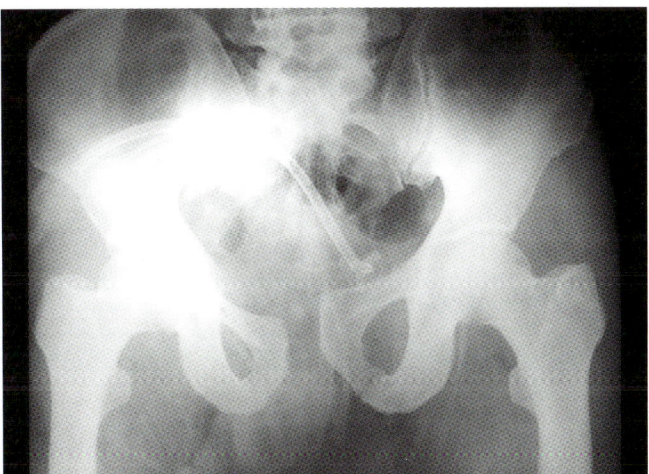

Fig. 34-3 *Pubic bone fracture* with SPC—Malecot catheter.

Section 5:
Clinical Methods in Orthopedics

CHAPTER 35

Approaches and Examination of Bone and Joint Injuries

Competency: OR2.1; OR2.15; OR2.16.

■ HISTORY

Age: Fracture bone can occur at any age group. Fracture clavicle and humerus is common in newborn due to birth injuries. Likewise pulled elbow and **Greenstick fracture** is seen in younger children, epiphyseal separation and supracondylar fracture is common in older children; dislocations in adults, **Colle's** fracture and fracture neck of femur in old age due to osteoporosis.

Sex: Colles' fracture (4:1; female to male ratio) and fracture neck of femur is more common in females.

Occupation: Avulsion fracture is more common sportsmen (athletes, footballers, skiers, ice-hockey players). March fracture is more common in soldiers, policemen, bikers.

History Pertaining to Injury

Mode of onset—it could be accidental or fall from a height or hit by a weapon or instrument. If trauma is due to a weapon, then nature of the weapon (sharp/blunt/gunshot) should be asked (**Fig. 35-1**).

History of condition of patient at the time of injury (whether walking/standing/drunk/sitting) is very essential as it gives lot of information regarding the **nature of violence** (direct/indirect/ muscular); **amount of force** that resulted in the bone injury (trivial in pathological fracture); direction of force that helps to determine the type of fracture—(a) **direct force** may be of *tapping type* causing transverse/oblique fracture or *crushing type* causing comminuted fracture (fracture with multiple fragment); (b) **indirect force**—that can result in spiral fracture due to twisting nature of the force; whereas bending type of force can lead to transverse or oblique fracture; (c) **combined**—fall from height can cause direct injury like fracture calcaneum and indirect injury like fracture of lumbar vertebra.

Fracture of patella, olecranon and lesser trochanter of femur may result due to sudden **violent muscular contraction**, as in athletes, which needs to be asked for (**Fig. 35-2**).

History of **duration of injury** is very important to be noted whether it is a recent injury/old injury as the mode of management of the injury varies.

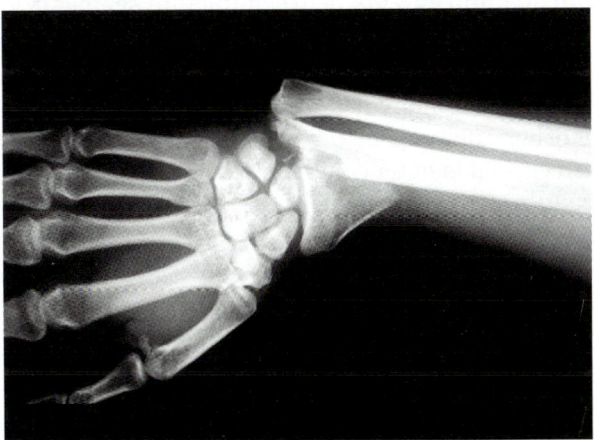

Fig. 35-1 *Fracture lower radius* after trauma.

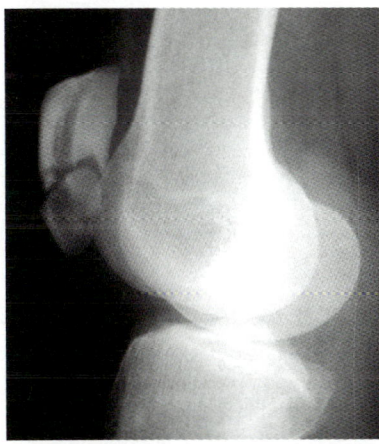

Fig. 35-2 *Fracture patella*—may be due to violent muscular contraction or direct trauma.

History of *unaccustomed repeat exercise* is seen in fractures like of neck of second metatarsals—*march fracture*.

Specific Complaints

Pain: It is present at the site of fracture, may be less severe than sprain. It is much more unbearable in dislocation of the joint. Exact site, nature (constant dull ache or severe), aggravating factors like movement can aggravate the pain in complete but to less extent in incomplete fracture.

Swelling at the site of fracture is common due to soft tissue contusion/displaced bone fragment/ hematoma. It may be small in recent injury but may be extensive involving the whole limb in those presenting late. So, exact site and nature of progress is to be asked.

Deformity is common, depends on the type of fracture. Fracture leads to deformity of that part, e.g. shoulder dislocation leads to flattening of the shoulder, *Colle's* fracture causes *'dinner fork deformity'.*

Loss of function of the part depends on the site of the fracture. Inability to move the limb, sit, walk, do joint function is seen in fracture/dislocation of the joint.

History of fever may be due to inflammation.

History of color change is due to hematoma.

■ EXAMINATION

Vital signs should be checked for any evidence of shock, especially in trauma of recent onset. Other more life-threatening injuries like of head, thorax or abdomen should not be missed.

Attitude of the patient on bed as well as *gait* of the patient on walking is noted.

Local Examination

Inspection

Swelling: Swelling is due to soft tissue injury or hematoma. Its site, size, extent should be noted. Edema at fracture site is common. Displaced fracture segment may be felt as bony swelling or projection. Size of the swelling is misleading as the swelling may be small in fracture neck of femur but can be large in muscular sprain.

Skin overlying swelling or fracture site: There may be ecchymoses, bruising, discoloration, discharge, and blood in the wound. Fracture may communicate outside with skin and soft tissue disruption—called as *compound/open fracture*. Fracture which is not communicating out to the skin surface is called as *simple closed fracture.*

Wound: Wound when present should be explored with all aseptic precautions preferably under anesthesia. The length, breadth and depth of the wound to be noted. Deeper tissues may be muscle, tendons/bones have to be noted. The color of the exposed muscle and nature of the discharge is noted. Exposed muscle may be green/black in color with foul-smelling serosanguineous discharge in suspected gas gangrene.

Deformity: Deformity is specific for specific fractures. For example, there will be flexion, internal rotation, adduction of hip in posterior dislocation of hip.

Attitude of the limb: There are specific attitudes for various fractures. Externally rotated limb is seen in fracture neck of femur.

Shortening of limb: It is due to overlapping of fracture segments.

Palpation

Local bony tenderness is elicited with utmost gentleness and initially asking the patient to locate the site of pain. The entire length of the bone is palpated by exerting gentle pressure through the uninjured soft tissue. In case of joint injuries, the maximum point of tenderness may be at the site of attachment of tendons or on joint line in meniscal injury or over the capsule of the joint in hemarthrosis. *Indirect method of eliciting bony tenderness*: (a) Gently rotating the injured arm/ forearm/thigh. (b) Gently squeezing the bone away from the site of injury (*springing the radius/fibula*) (c) applying axial pressure along the line of the bone as in fracture of metacarpals and metatarsals.

Bony irregularity is checked for elevation/gap/depression. It is a definitive sign of fracture.

Abnormal movements between fracture segments are a definitive sign but one should be gentle while eliciting it. It is useful in old fractures.

Crepitus is sensation of grating felt or heard when two cut ends of bone move against each other and is painful. Crepitus is also elicited in other conditions like surgical emphysema, osteoarthritis, tenosynovitis.

Absence of transmitted movements is typical of fracture. This helps to assess the integrity of long bones like femur, humerus, and radius. It is performed by rotating the lower part of the bone with one hand, meanwhile palpating the upper part of the bone with the other. Absence of transmitted movements suggests fracture except in impacted fracture.

Wounds when present should be palpated under aseptic precaution to see the depth, contents in the floor.

Mode of injury/mechanism of injury will give the indication of the bone involved.

Mode of injury	Injury
• Fall on a outstretched hand	Fracture clavicle/around the elbow
• Fall with spine forced in particular direction	Flexion/extension injuries of spine
• Slipping in washroom	Fracture neck of femur
• Dashboard injury	Posterior dislocation of hip.

Various conditions that can result in pathological fracture:

Infants	Osteogenesis imperfecta
Children	Solitary bone cyst, rickets, scurvy
Adolescence	Osteogenic sarcoma
Adults	Giant cell tumor, march fracture
Elderly	Osteoporosis, secondaries

Swelling when present should be described by size, site, nature (bony swelling may be due to fracture fragments or dislocated bone). Swelling in the joint may be due to hemarthrosis.

Palpation of distal vessels—pulsations may be absent due to compression or spasm.

Measurements

Both longitudinal and circumferential measurements are checked to assess the shortening/lengthening, wasting/swelling. Sound normal limb should be kept in the same position as affected limb prior to measurement. Sound limb should be measured first. *Length of the limb* is measured between two definite bony landmarks, marking with a pen and measuring with a tape. *Circumference of the limb* should be measured at the same level from a bony point and compared with the other limb.

Movements

Both active and passive should be checked, first on the healthy side, later on the diseased side. Range of movement that occur without distress/pain is noted. Good range of active and passive movement means there is no bone or joint injuries. It is lost in joint dislocation and restricted in fracture. *Abnormal movement* at the site of injury is elicited very gently which is *pathagnomonic of fracture*. It is also commonly elicited in nonunion of fracture.

Associated injuries should be looked for. Often that is more important than fracture itself, like vessel, nerve injury, and major internal organ injuries.

Features of shock due to hemorrhage, pain should be checked.

Pathological fractures needs special mention as cause for fracture is something else but may be precipitated by minor trauma. Examples are—osteogenesis imperfecta (***brittle bones***); osteopetrosis (***marble bones***) in infants; ***osteomyelitis*** and solitary bone cyst in children; osteosarcoma in young; multiple myeloma, ***hyperparathyroidism***, osteoclastoma in adults; secondaries, old age, ***Paget's disease*** in elderly. Keeping in mind the pathology here, various bone have to be examined to look for any additional fracture.

■ INVESTIGATIONS

- X-ray of Site/Part
- Both AP and lateral view should be taken. Fracture/displacement (forward or backward, upward or downward) tilt/twist should be looked for. *Oblique view* in scaphoid fracture; *stereoscopic view* for skull and pelvis; *special axial radiograph* for calcaneum are the other special views for specific sites.
- In joint injuries, X-ray of the joint along with the opposite joint in the same film has to be taken for comparison.
- In pathological fracture, X-ray of the part as well as other suspicious parts has to be taken.
- In injuries of forearm and leg, to avoid fallacy, X-ray should include joint above the fracture as well as joint below. In certain conditions like fracture scaphoid fracture line may not be visible immediately after the injury. So may have to repeat the X-ray after 10 days.

> **Reading of an X-ray should include:**
> a. Exact site of fracture, whether joint is involved or not.
> b. Type of fracture (complete/incomplete; transverse/oblique/spiral).
> c. Displacement of fracture fragment—shift/ tilt (sideward/backward/forward)/twist.
>   Look for evidence of any gas shadows indicative of gas gangrene.
>   In X-ray of old fracture, look for callus which normally appears in 2–3 weeks; signs of union; signs of non-union indicated by sclerosis at the ends of the fragments; malunion.
>   In X-ray of joint injuries, one should mention the direction of displacement, whether associated with fracture or not (**Figs. 35-3 and 35-4**).

Blood/serum for calcium, acid phosphatase, alkaline phosphatase, tumor markers for specific diseases. Immunoglobulins are analyzed in multiple myeloma.

Radioisotope bone scan using strontium (^{85}Sr) and radioactive Tc^{99m} is very useful method to detect bone secondaries, aseptic necrosis, abscesses, arthropathies.

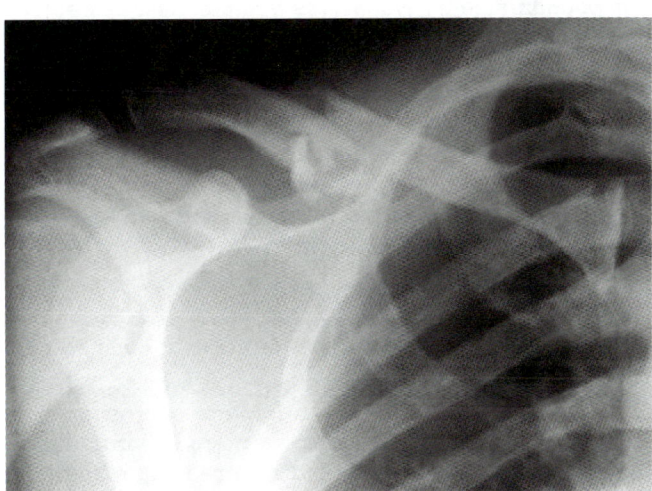

Fig. 35-3 Right-sided *clavicle fracture*.

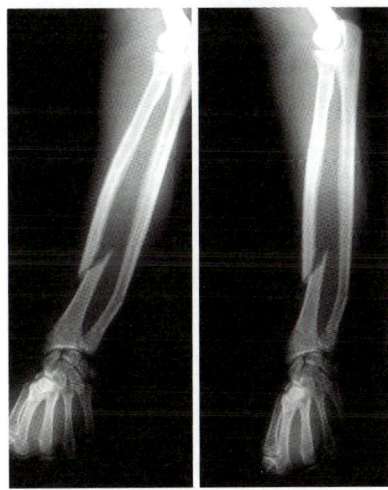

Fig. 35-4 X-ray showing *fracture lower end of radius and ulna*.

Arthroscopy is very useful to detect joint injuries by direct vision like in knee joint to detect meniscal injuries. *Arthrography* is injection of contrast into the joint and taking X-rays.

MRI is the investigation of choice for joint injuries. It clearly delineates the injuries.

■ FRACTURE

'Fracture' is defined as break in continuity of the bone.

Causes of fracture: (1) Trauma is the commonest cause. (2) Pathological: It is due to underlying pathology like malignancy, secondaries in bone, osteoporosis, osteomyelitis, multiple myeloma, hyperparathyroidism, and rickets. Stress fracture: It is due to repeated minor trauma leading to repetitive stress to the bone causing fracture. It is common in second metatarsal of foot, occurs due to repeated marching and stamping. It is also called as 'March fracture'.

Types of fracture: Greenstick fracture: It is seen in children wherein bone breaks incompletely and partially keeping cortex intact. *Closed fracture*—wherein fracture does not communicate outside. *Open fracture*—wherein fracture communicates outside to skin through soft tissues exposing the bone, and allowing infection to get in. It is also called as 'compound fracture'. *Transverse fracture, oblique fracture, spiral fracture* are other types of fractures based on fracture line; *Comminuted fracture*—here bone is broken into more than two fragments. *Stellate fracture*—begins at one point and radiates towards periphery as a star. It is common in patella and skull. *Avulsion fracture* occurs due to powerful contraction of muscle. *Depressed fracture* is common in skull. *Complicated fracture* is fracture associated with injuries to vessels, nerves, joints.

Complications of Fracture

Immediate shock; injury to other structures; compartment syndrome.

Delayed: Fat embolism: Due to fracture microscopic fat globules from the bone marrow enters the circulation and reaches the lung, brain and skin causing respiratory distress, drowsiness and petechial hemorrhage. Often it is life-threatening.

Stages of healing of fracture (Fig. 35-5)	Factors affecting fracture healing
• Stage of hematoma formation • Stage of granulation tissue formation • Stage of fibrocartilaginous callus • Stage of callus formation • Remodeling phase	• Improper immobilization • Infection • Interposition of soft tissues • Inadequate blood supply • Old age • Deficiencies of vitamin C, proteins • Anemia • Diabetes, HIV, steroid therapy

Other complications are infection, delayed nerve injury, disability, Volkmann's contracture.

Myositis ossificans is common in elbow causing stiffness due to hematoma formation under the stripped periosteum—organization—calcification in front of the elbow joint, common in children.

Late: Malunion—common in Colle's fracture; Nonunion; Osteomyelitis of the bone; stiffness and contracture; osteoarthritis of the joint, Sudeck's osteodystrophy, avascular necrosis (Bone will be denser on X-ray; occurs 3 months after fracture; common in fractures of neck of femur, scaphoid, neck of talus). Deformity of the bone and part of the limb can occur as a sequelae which may lead into shortening of the limb (Fig. 35-6).

Non-union: It is failure of bony union of the fracture segments even after consecutive three months of specified expected time of union. Causes are—infection, interposition of soft tissues, poor blood supply, wide separation of fracture segments, improper immobilization. Site forms a pseudojoint with *painless abnormal mobility*. X-ray shows sclerosis of bone ends with a gap. It is common in—fracture of waist of scaphoid, neck of femur, neck of talus, and lower third of tibia. *Non-union can be* hypovascular/avascular (true non-union) or hypervascular types.

Clinical features of fracture:
- Pain
- Deformity
- Swelling
- Local bony tenderness
- Shortening of the limb
- Abnormal mobility
- Crepitus
- Loss of function
- In fractures of femur, tibia there will be features of shock
- Features of associated injuries

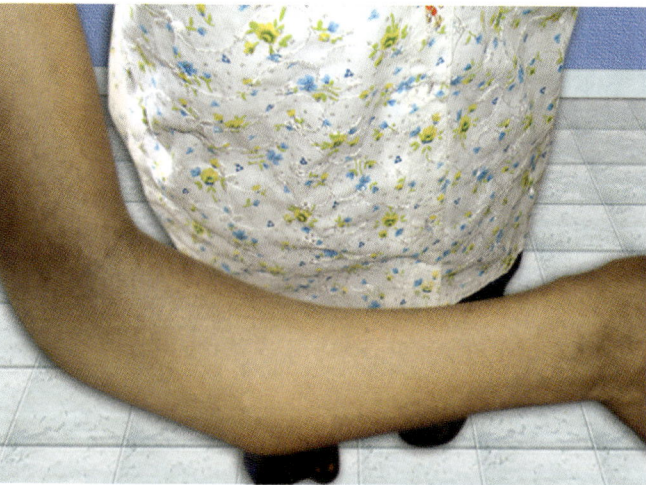

Fig. 35-6 *Deformity of the forearm* as late sequelae of the fracture radius and ulna.

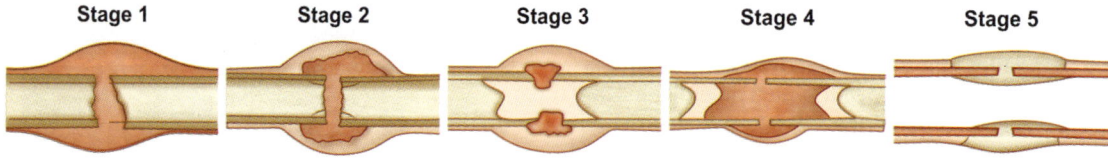

Fig. 35-5 *Stages of healing of bone* after injury.

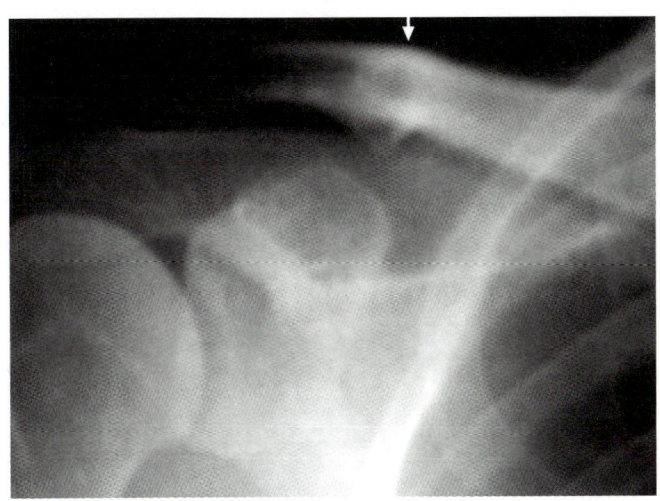

Fig. 35-7 X-ray showing *malunion in clavicle fracture*. Note the site of fracture—lateral 1/3rd.

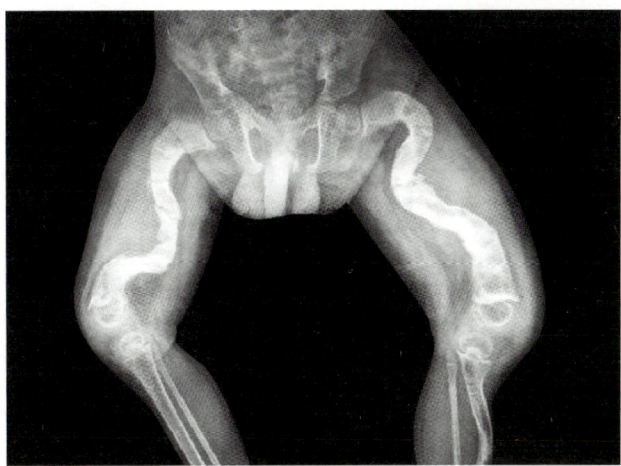

Fig. 35-8 *Shepherd Crook deformity*; it is due to recurrent fractures of long bones (femur) of baby in fibrous dysplasia. (*Courtesy*: Dr Harsharaj, Consultant orthopedician, Mangaluru, Karnataka, India).

Delayed union: It is undue delay in the process of complete union. X-ray shows callus but inadequate. There is *painful abnormal mobility*.

Malunion: It is union of fracture in defective position with anatomical malalignment—angulation, rotation, over-riding. It is due to improper reduction, redisplacement, and growth disturbance by epiphyseal injury. It is common in (cancellous bone) Colles', supracondylar (humerus), condyles of tibia fractures. *Features* are—deformity, no abnormal mobility; X-ray shows deformity with bridging callus (Figs. 35-7 and 35-8).

Sudeck's osteodystrophy (Paul Hermann Sudeck—German surgeon): It is post-traumatic painful osteoporosis with pain, swelling and marked stiffness of hand or foot of the injured limb. It may be due to abnormal activation of pain pathway with exaggerated inflammatory and immune responses. Features appear 2 months after trauma as— severe pain, swelling, hyperemia, obliterated skin crease, glossy look, atrophied nails, impaired metacarpophalangeal and interphalangeal joint movements (frozen hand) with marked stiffness. X-ray shows spotty osteoporosis with rarefaction.

DISLOCATION

Here one bony component of the joint completely looses its contact with other bony component. In subluxation, there is partial loss of contact between the joint surfaces. *Dislocation* can be traumatic, pathological, paralytic (poliomyelitis) or congenital (congenital dislocation of hip).

Approaches and Examinations in Injuries of Various Joints

CHAPTER 36

Competency: OR2.4; OR2.5; OR2.6; OR2.7; OR2.8; OR2.9; OR2.10; OR2.11; OR2.12; AN2.5; AN8.6; AN10.12; AN17.2; AN17.3; AN18.6.

EXAMINATION IN INJURIES AROUND SHOULDER JOINT AND ARM

***Shoulder girdle* consists of clavicle, scapula and shoulder joint along with sternoclavicular joint, acromioclavicular joint. *The shoulder (glenohumeral) joint* is a ball and socket type of synovial joint between glenoid cavity of scapula and head of humerus. Glenoidal labrum is fibrocartilaginous rim covering the glenoid margin to increase the depth of the cavity. Subacromial, subscapularis, infraspinatus are different important bursae around the shoulder joint.**

History

Fall on an outstretched hand is the commonest cause for the injuries around shoulder joint especially fracture of clavicle and anterior dislocation of the shoulder. However scapular fracture and fracture shaft of humerus is caused by direct blow. History of fall on point of shoulder or point of elbow is also seen in injuries around the shoulder joint.

Patient comes with the history of pain and swelling in the region of shoulder joint, limitation of movement, and inability to lift the limb.

Local Examination

Inspection

It should be done from front, behind and sideward with the patient being exposed from neck to tip of the fingers, seated on a stool. Opposite limb also should be exposed for comparison. The limb must be kept freely hanging by the side of the chest.

Attitude: The position of the neck, the shoulder joint, the position of the arm should be noted. Often the attitude itself will say the diagnosis. Patient with ***fracture clavicle*** will incline his neck to affected side, support the elbow with opposite hand, keep the arm by the side of the chest. **In *anterior shoulder dislocation*,** patient is seen supporting the flexed elbow of injured side with other hand but keeps the arm away from the chest.

The bony parts around the shoulder joint are the clavicle, acromion process of the scapula, spine of the scapula. Any irregularity or swelling, abnormal, pulsation and wasting have to be noted.

- From front, the relation of clavicles on both sides with respect to sternum, sternoclavicular and acromioclavicular joints, anterior deltoid bulge, supra and infraclavicular fossae, pectoral bulge, anterior axillary line and fold, contour of shoulder are noted.
- From behind, spines, medial border of scapula, scapular fossae, level of inferior angle of scapulae, posterior axillary fold are observed for any swelling or irregularity.
- From above acromioclavicular line, angle of acromion, bulge of the shoulder is noted.

The arm also should be inspected from front, sides and behind.

Deformity: Swelling and prominences along the length often at the junction of lateral 1/3rd and medial 2/3rd is seen in fracture clavicle. Undue swelling over the sternal/acromial end of the clavicle suggests dislocation of sternoclavicular/acromioclavicular joint respectively. Abnormal swelling in deltopectoral groove with lowered anterior axillary fold is seen in subcoracoid dislocation (commonest type) of shoulder. Drooping of shoulder occurs in fracture neck of scapula. There will be obvious angular deformity in fracture shaft of humerus.

Contour of shoulder: Loss of roundness of the shoulder is seen in subcoracoid dislocation (commonest type) of shoulder as well as in fracture neck of scapula whereas in fracture neck of humerus, there is undue fullness of shoulder **(Fig. 36-1)**.

Palpation

All bones involved in the shoulder girdle are examined carefully. Patient is made to sit on a stool and the surgeon

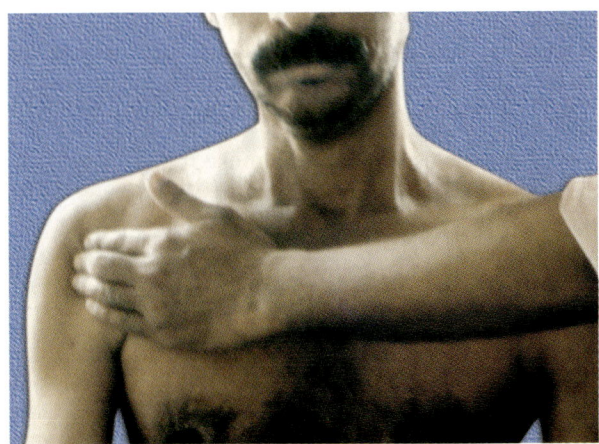

Fig. 36-1 *Loss of roundness* below the acromion is a feature of shoulder dislocation.

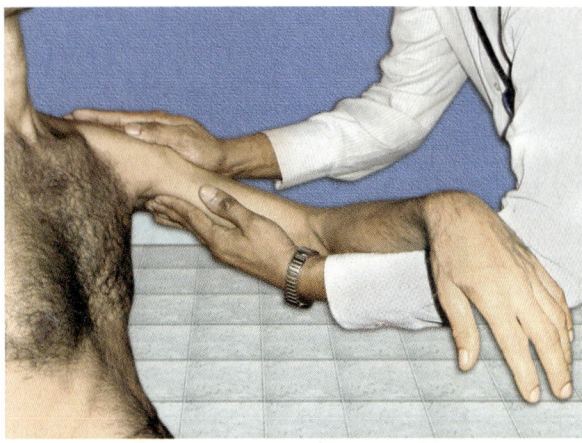

Fig. 36-2 *Bimanual palpation* of upper end of humerus across axilla and deltoid.

stands behind the patient, begins to examine from medial to lateral end systematically.

Palpation begins medially from sternoclavicular joint proceeded laterally along the length of the clavicle, to lateral end of the clavicle, acromioclavicular joint, spine of scapula, border of the scapula, upper end of the humerus.

Clavicle is palpated from behind beginning from sternal end towards acromion. Any discontinuity, abnormal projection, point of tenderness is noted. Sharp irregular edge of the fragments can be felt projecting beneath the skin. In sternoclavicular joint dislocation, clavicle is often dislocated anteriorly (backward dislocation is rare) whereas in acromioclavicular subluxation the lateral end of the clavicle is only pulled upwards.

The tip of the coracoid process, acromial end of clavicle and greater tuberosity of humerus are palpated and their relative position is compared on both sides. In acromioclavicular dislocation, the acromial end of clavicle comes close to the head of the humerus but away from the tip of coracoid process and on applying slight pressure over the prominence imparts a springboard like sensation to the examining finger. In fracture of greater tuberosity of humerus there is marked tenderness below the acromion.

Upper end of the humerus is initially felt from behind with patient in sitting position. From the acromion process of both sides, palpation is done using both hands downwards to feel greater tuberosity of humerus. It is not felt and there is no resistance in shoulder dislocation. Fingers are slowly slid downwards to feel the shaft of humerus for fracture. Tenderness and irregularity suggests fracture.

In dislocation of shoulder joint, head may be palpated in the infraclavicular fossa (anterior type), just posteroinferior to acromion or spinous process (posterior type) or in subglenoid region.

Bimanual palpation of the upper end of humerus is done from the side with one hand in the axilla and other over the shoulder. It is better felt through the axilla. Features of fracture should be looked for. In humerus the medial epicondyle points the direction of head of the humerus whereas lateral epicondyle points to the greater tuberosity of the humerus. But this relation is lost in fracture of neck/shaft of humerus (Fig. 36-2).

Palpation of scapula: Posteriorly subcutaneous portion of scapula is palpated first, followed by vertebral border and inferior angle. The spine and acromion process is better felt when arm is gently hyperabducted. Coracoid process is palpated 1.5 cm below the clavicle at the junction of medial 1/3rd and lateral 1/3rd. Glenoid cavity is palpated for tenderness. Tenderness medial to glenoid cavity will help in diagnosis of fracture neck of scapula. Coracoid process, acromial end of the clavicle and greater tuberosity are palpated for any deviation.

Movement

Both active and passive movements of the shoulder joint are checked. Serious injury to the shoulder girdle is ruled out if the patient is able to move the limb vertically up above the head and lower it down gently.

When the transmitted movement at head of humerus does not occur when the shaft is rotated by limited gentle circumgyration of the flexed forearm, then it suggests fracture neck of humerus.

Fracture of neck of scapula is suspected when patient's arm is grasped in such a manner that his forearm rests over the examiner's forearm and abnormal mobility and crepitus is seen when the whole upper extremity is raised and lowered gently provided the clavicle is intact.

Measurement

Both limbs must be kept in identical position.

Arm length is measured from angle of acromion (point where scapular spine bends forward to become acromion process) to lateral epicondyle of humerus. Length is increased in subglenoid dislocation and fracture of scapular neck; it is shortened in subcoracoid dislocation, fracture neck and shaft of humerus (Fig. 36-3).

Circumferential measurements are taken around the arm on both sides equidistant from angle of the acromion. The vertical circumference around the shoulder joint, i.e. from base of axilla to tip of the shoulder is taken and compared.

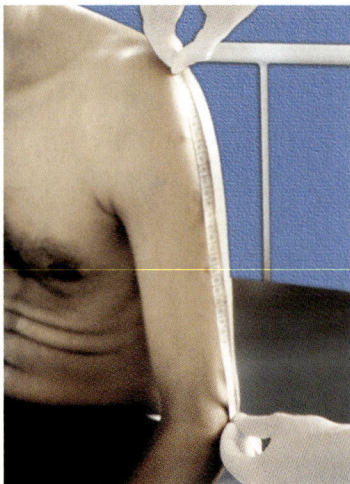

Fig. 36-3 *Length of the arm* is measured from angle of acromion to lateral epicondyle.

Vertical circumference of the axilla is increased in shoulder dislocation, fracture of upper end of humerus, fracture of neck of scapula—***Callaway's test***.

Measurements of the anterior and posterior axillary folds are done by abducting the shoulder to 90 degrees and measuring the axillary folds from their junction with the trunk to their junction with the arm. ***Bryant's sign*** is elongated and lowered anterior axillary fold seen in anterior dislocation of shoulder.

Special Tests

a. ***Hamilton ruler test:*** A straight ruler is placed along the line of acromion process and lateral epicondyle. Normally it is not possible to place the ruler due to prominent greater tuberosity. In dislocation of shoulder and fracture neck of scapula, it is possible as tuberosity is displaced medially.
b. ***Dugas' test:*** Patient is asked to touch the opposite shoulder with the hand of the affected side keeping the elbow to the side of the trunk. It is not possible if there is shoulder dislocation **(Fig. 36-4)**.

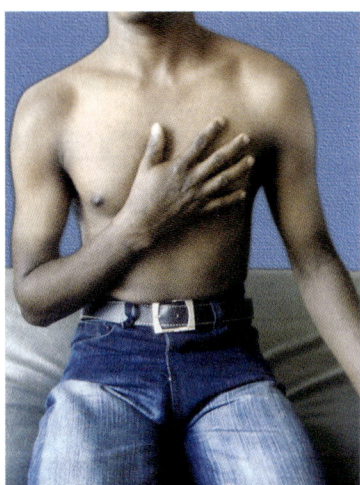

Fig. 36-4 *Dugas test*—it is inability to place hand of the injured side on the opposite shoulder.

Sensation over the skin on the lower part of deltoid should be checked to find out axillary nerve palsy. Radial nerve may get injured (neuropraxia) in the fracture of the shaft of humerus.

X-ray: AP view is essential to diagnose fracture/dislocation around the shoulder joint. In fracture of humerus, X-ray of whole arm with shoulder and elbow joint is essential.

Different Injuries of the Shoulder Joint

Fracture of clavicle	*Acromioclavicular dislocation*
Mechanism of injury—fall on outstretched hand; common in children. Fracture site is at the junction of lateral third and middle third ***Features***: Pain tenderness, swelling. It can be displaced/undisplaced. Medial fragment is displaced and tilted upwards by pull of sternocleidomastoid; lateral fragment is pulled downwards by weight of the arm	***Mechanism of injury***—results from an injury over the point of shoulder or fall on the outer aspect of shoulder ***Features:*** Acute severe pain, swelling on the outer aspect of clavicle, with restricted shoulder joint movement. It is rare, often subluxation occurs
Shoulder dislocation	***Fracture of humerus***
Mechanism of injury—fall on outstretched hand ***Types*** a. *Anterior subcoracoid*—commonest, head lies below the coracoid process. ***Features:*** Injured elbow is flexed and supported by the opposite hand, held away from the chest wall; loss of round contour of the shoulder with flattening; bulge at deltopectoral grove; patient cannot touch the opposite shoulder with diseased side hand—*Dugas test. Hamilton ruler's test shows that ruler can easily be placed;* anterior axillary fold lowered down; axillary girth increased; pseudo-lengthening of the arm seen b. *Subglenoid*—head lies below the glenoid cavity c. *Posterior dislocation*—very rare; occurs in fully abducted and forcible internal rotation ***Recurrent dislocation***—more common in anterior type; here capsule is striped off from the anterior margin of the glenoid rim. Dislocation develops when patient abducts his arm at right angle and externally rotates it **(Figs. 36-5A and B).**	***Types*** a. *Fracture of greater tuberosity*—*contusion fracture* due to direct injury or *avulsion fracture*—due to avulsion of supraspinatus tendon. It can cause *painful arc syndrome* and shoulder stiffness b. *Fracture neck of humerus*—due to fall on shoulder. It may be *impacted* (patient may able to move so often missed)/*displaced* (abnormal mobility seen) c. *Fracture of shaft of humerus*—traumatic/pathological in origin; transverse/oblique/spiral/comminuted/segmental. Lateral angulation due to abduction of the proximal fragment by deltoid muscle. Wrist drop—due to radial nerve injury ***Complications***—nonunion, delayed union.
Fracture of scapula	***Sternoclavicular dislocation***
Occurs due to direct injury over the back; difficult to diagnose; causes drooping of shoulder and undue lengthening of arm	***Mechanism of injury***—fall on shoulder point/outstretched hand. Sternal end of the clavicle dislocates forward (common) rarely backward

Chapter 36: Approaches and Examinations in Injuries of Various Joints

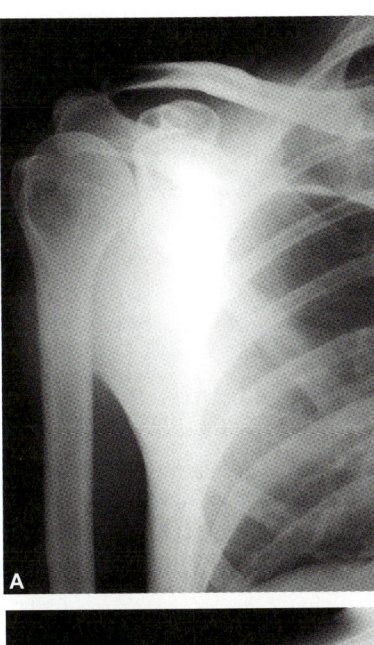
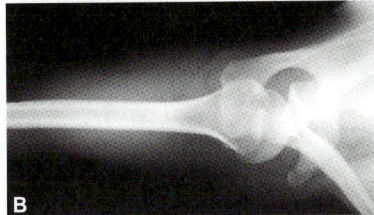

Figs. 36-5A and B *X-ray in two planes* to be taken in shoulder dislocation.

EXAMINATION IN INJURIES OF ELBOW JOINT AND FOREARM

The elbow joint is a synovial hinge joint between lower end of humerus and the upper end of radius and ulna bones. Joint line is 2 cm below the line joining the two epicondyles with medial slope having carrying angle. Upper articular surface is capitulum and trochlea; lower are upper surface of head of radius (to capitulum) and trochlear notch of ulna (to trochlea of humerus). Ligaments are capsular, anterior, posterior, ulnar collateral, radial collateral. Movements are flexion (by brachialis, biceps and brachioradialis) and extension (by triceps and anconeus). Both movements—155° range from elbow straight and vice versa. Rotation of forearm occurs in superior and inferior radioulnar joints. Both supinations (85°, palm up) and pronation (80°, palm down) are rotations. Rotation movements should be checked with elbow flexed at right angle to eliminate shoulder rotation.

History

History of fall on outstretched hand is seen in supracondylar fracture, posterior dislocation of elbow, fracture of head of radius. Whereas fracture of olecranon results due to direct violence.
History pertaining to swelling, pain, inability to move the elbow, is asked.

Local Examination

Inspection

Elbow is examined from front and back sides. Both sides are examined, compared, and looked for the change in attitude and any deformity.

Observe whether the elbow is held in extended/flexed position; supinated/pronated position. Position of the olecranon must be observed from back and sides.

Attitude: Elbow usually appears swollen and held in flexed position in injuries of the joint. In fracture of forearm bones, the patient supports the forearm and hugs it to the body.

Normal outward deviation of extended supinated forearm (from axis of arm) is called ***carrying angle*** (10°–15°; more in women). It disappears in flexed and pronated elbow. When it is exaggerated, it is ***cubitus valgus;*** when reduced is ***cubitus varus*** (Fig. 36-6).

Deformity: Olecranon becomes unduly prominent with anteroposterior broadening of the elbow in posterior dislocation of elbow (common in adults); medial or lateral displacement of olecranon along with anteroposterior broadening of the elbow is seen in supracondylar fracture (common in children). Swelling in the front of upper part of ulna is seen in ***Monteggia fracture***. In complete fracture of forearm bones, there is angular deformity at the site.

Swelling, if present, is to be examined accordingly. Localized swelling may be seen at the site of fracture, e.g, fracture of head of radius may present with a swelling on the radial aspect of elbow whereas fracture of olecranon may produce a swelling on posterior aspect of elbow.

Palpation

The bones palpated in the elbow joint are lower end of humerus, upper ends of radius and ulna. The relationship of

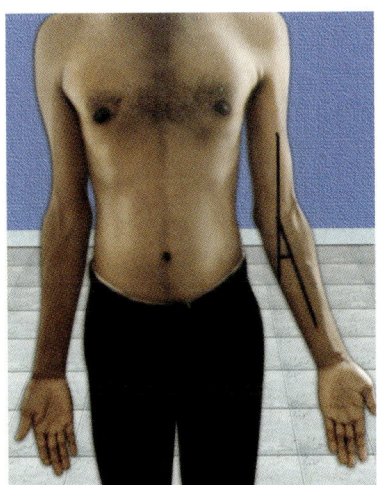

Fig. 36-6 *Normal carrying angle* is 15° outwards in an extended supinated forearm. It disappears on flexion.

three bony points—olecranon, medial and lateral epicondyle of humerus has to be noted in particular.

Bones are palpated for local tenderness, irregularity, undue mobility, and crepitus should be checked.

Tenderness is elicited either by direct palpation. Indirect method of eliciting tenderness is used in fracture head of the radius—when the radius and ulna are held together and squeezed at lower end of the forearm, pain is felt at the upper end at the fracture head of radius—***springing the radius*** (Fig. 36-7).

Palpation of lower end of humerus: It is palpated with thumb and four fingers for the two epicondyles. Any condylar fracture/separation/displacement is looked for. The epicondyles can be better palpated with elbow in semiflexed and forearm in supinated position where they stand out prominently. After palpating the epicondylar tips, proceed further along the shaft of the humerus in midplane of the arm to feel the supracondylar ridge. Any irregularity and tenderness are noted. Holding the upper part of humerus in one hand, the lower part is gently moved. Any abnormal mobility and crepitus are looked for. There will be undue broadening of the lower end of humerus with distortion of condyles in fracture (T/Y shaped) **(Fig. 36-8)**.

Palpation of head of radius: When the forearm is supinated and pronated with elbow in semiflexed position, the head of the radius is felt in the lower part of the depression below the lateral condyle of humerus. In fracture of head of radius, tenderness and irregularity are felt during rotation of radius. The head of the radius is looked for any displacement, often forward displacement, associated with **Monteggia fracture (Fig. 36-9)**.

Palpation of upper part of ulna: The subcutaneous border of ulna is easily palpable, any irregularity, swelling or any breach in continuity of the bone are looked for.

Palpation of olecranon: Olecranon is palpated on the posterior aspect of elbow joint for any irregularity, tenderness, gap in the bone, all suggestive of fracture olecranon, which occur due to direct violence. In complete fracture of olecranon, there will be wide separation of fragments due to contraction of triceps. Patient will not be able to extend the flexed forearm. Olecranon is abnormally projected posteriorly in posterior dislocation of elbow and supracondylar fracture.

Measurement

Measurement of arm and forearm is taken and compared with normal side.

Length of the arm: It is measured from angle of acromion to lateral epicondyle of the humerus.

Length of forearm: It is measured from lateral epicondyle to radial styloid process. If lateral epicondyle is not discernible as in comminuted fracture, then alternate fixed bony points like radial head, medial epicondyle, olecranon tips are considered for measurement.

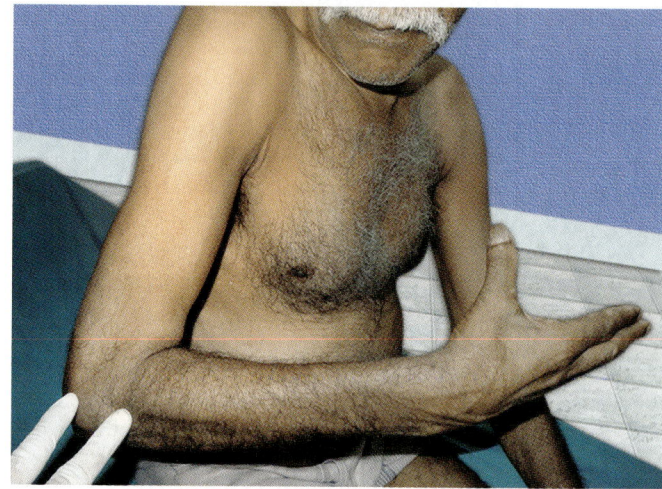

Fig. 36-8 Index is used to *feel lateral epicondyle* and middle finger is used to feel head of radius.

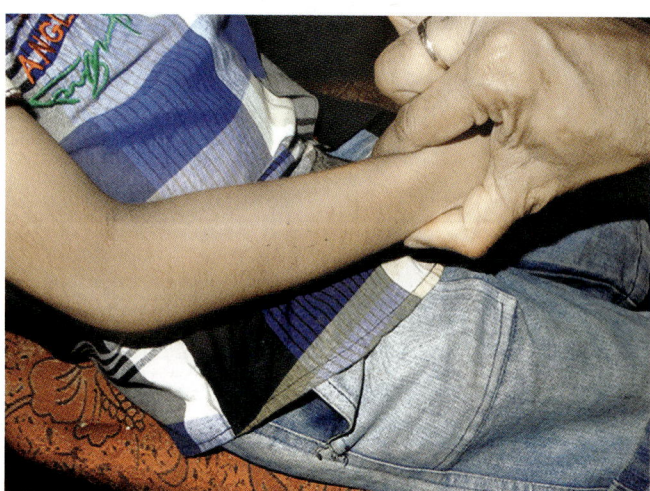

Fig. 36-7 *Springing of radius* is elicited by squeezing the radius and ulna together at the lower end of the forearm to elicit the pain at the fracture sit of upper end of radius.

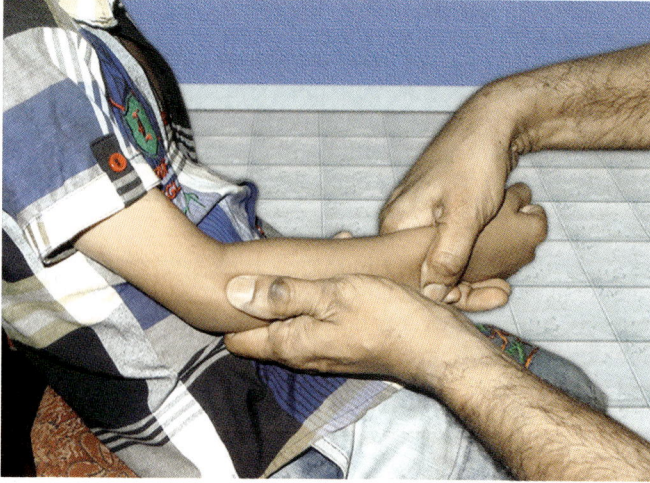

Fig. 36-9 Head of radius is felt by *pronating and supinating the forearm in flexed elbow.*

Shortening of the arm: It is seen in supracondylar fracture whereas shortening of the forearm is seen in posterior dislocation of elbow.

Three bony points relationship: The two epicondyles of humerus and tip of olecranon from the three bony points; thumb and middle fingers are placed over epicondyles while index finger is placed over tip of olecranon. In elbow flexed at 90 degrees, these three points form a near isosceles triangle whereas in fully extended elbow these three points lie in a straight line. Alternatively these points can be marked by skin pencil; sides of the triangle formed by these points are measured. These measurements are compared with that of normal side and any abnormality, if present, is noted. In posterior dislocation of elbow, the olecranon is found above the line joining the epicondyles. In supracondylar fracture the relationship between the bony points is maintained. In T/Y shaped fracture the epicondyles are widely set apart **(Figs. 36-10A to C)**.

Measurement of carrying angle: It is the angle formed between the long axis of arm and the long axis of forearm. Normal—10° in males, 20° in females. Both upper limbs are extended at elbow and supinated at forearm. The line joining the midpoint of intercondylar line at elbow and midpoint of interstyloid line at the wrist is the central axis of forearm. Central axis of the arm is obtained by joining the midpoint of intercondylar line and midpoint of transverse line drawn outwards from the point where the anterior axillary fold meets the arm to the outermost bulge of arm. This central axis of arm is prolonged downwards. And the angle formed between these two axes is ***carrying angle***. Carrying angle can be measured only when the elbow can be fully extended and forearm fully supinated **(Fig. 36-11)**.

Measurement of girth of forearm and arm: If there is any swelling, circumference of arm and forearm should be checked at a specified distance from a bony point and is compared to opposite side at the same level; it is important whenever there is a swelling of the arm or forearm.

Movement

Flexion is around 145°–160°. ***Flexion and extension*** should be checked against resistance. Flexion is by brachialis, biceps, brachioradialis; extension is by triceps, anconeus. Patent is asked to touch his shoulders with the flexed elbows to check active flexion.

Pronation and supination occur in vertical axis from head of radius to ulnar side of articular disc of radius. In pronation, hand faces downwards; in supination, hand faces upwards ***(King pronates, begger supinates)***. Supination is antigravity and is powerful. Normal pronation is 80°; supination is 85°. Both are checked in flexed position with arm beside the patient.

Both active and passive movements are checked. If the patient can flex and extend the elbow, pronate and supinate the forearm with elbow in flexed position without pain and limitation, then fracture or dislocation around elbow can be ruled out.

Also any abnormal mobility and absence of transmitted movements are checked.

Other Examinations

Examination of radial pulse is done, which may be absent due to spasm in supracondylar fracture.

Examination of three nerves—radial, ulnar, median as they may be injured in injuries around elbow. Cubitus valgus deformity may involve ulnar nerve due to undue stretching.

Investigation

X-ray of elbow region both AP/lateral view for fracture/dislocation around elbow. Similarly, X-ray AP/lateral view of forearm is taken to see the site of fracture, displacements of the fragments.

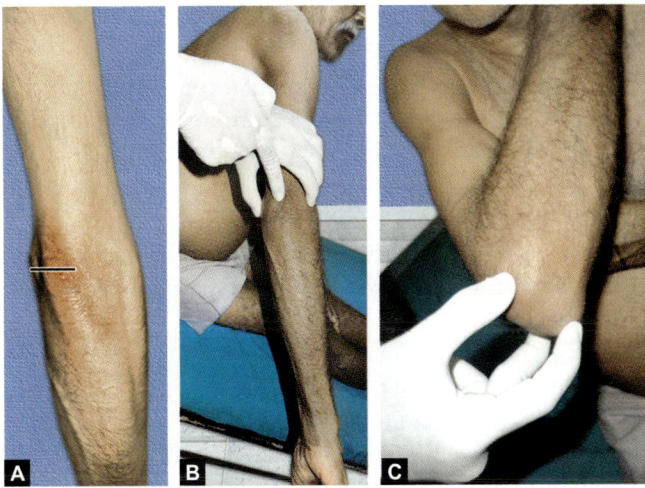

Figs. 36-10A to C *Three bony points* form a straight line while elbow in extended position; form a triangle, while elbow in flexed position.

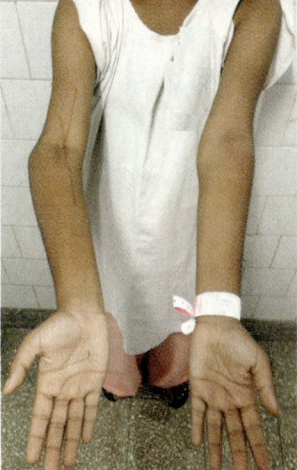

Fig. 36-11 *Cubitus varus* showing change in the carrying angle.

Different Injuries of the Elbow Joint

Supracondylar fracture	Posterior dislocation of elbow
Types: a. *Backward displacement*—fall on outstretched hand with flexed elbow. Commonest injury around elbow in children; distal fragment is displaced backwards, upwards with internal rotation b. *Forward displacement*—fall on outstretched hand with extended elbow. It is rare, arm is shortened; the relationship of three bony points on posterior aspect of elbow is not disturbed; active movements disturbed due to pain **Complications:** Malunion; cubitus valgus/varus; injury to brachial artery; nerves; myositis ossificans; Volkmann's ischemic contracture **(Fig. 36-12)**	It occurs by fall on outstretched hand with slightly flexed elbow Associated with fracture of coronoid process and lateral displacement Dislocation of elbow, fracture of coronoid process and radial head—"*Terrible triad of elbow*" **Features**: Common in adults; shortening of forearm; posterior displacement of olecranon; absence of abnormal mobility and crepitus palpable; triceps stand out prominently; movements of elbow are markedly restricted. Relationship of three bony points is disturbed **Complications**—myositis ossificans
T/Y fracture of elbow	**Subluxation of head of radius**
Fall on the point of elbow drives the olecranon upwards splitting the epicondyles. The elbow is enormously swollen and supported by the opposite hand. Movements extremely painful	Seen in children while pulling the forearm forcibly in supinated position (*pulled elbow*). Head of radius is below and lateral to normal
Fracture of head and neck of radius	**Monteggia fracture dislocation**
Fall on pronated outstretched hand. Tenderness below the lateral epicondyle with restricted rotational movement of forearm	It is fracture of upper third ulna with anterior displacement of upper fragment of ulna and anterior displacement of head of radius with angulation, tenderness, swelling in upper part of forearm **Reverse Monteggia fracture:** Here there is posterior displacement of upper fragment of ulna and posterior displacement of head of radius

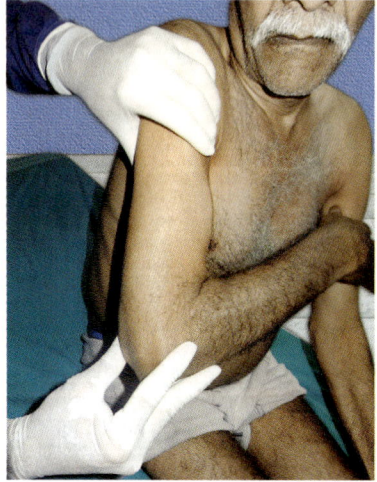

Fig. 36-12 *Abnormal mobility* is checked in supracondylar fracture.

EXAMINATION IN INJURIES OF WRIST AND HAND

Wrist joint is synovial ellipsoid radiocarpal joint between lower end of radius and three lateral bones of proximal row of carpus (scaphoid, lunate, triquetrum). Ligaments of the joint are palmar ulnocarpal, radiocarpal; dorsal radiocarpal, radial and ulnar collateral. Flexion (80 degrees), extension (90 degrees); adduction (ulnar deviation, 35 degrees); abduction (radial deviation, 25 degrees) occurs in radiocarpal joint and intercarpal joints. Intercarpal joints are integral part of the wrist joint.

History

History of fall on outstretched hand is often seen in Colle's fracture. Incidence is more in females, 4:1. The common cause for fracture of metacarpals is fall on the hand or blow upon the knuckles as in boxing.

Local Examination

Inspection

The wrist and hand is observed from dorsal and ventral aspect. Presence of swelling, bruises are looked for over the wrist and hand.

Attitude and Deformity

Dinner fork deformity, where there is dorsal prominence 2.5 cm above the wrist joint, is a feature of Colles' fracture whereas in ***garden spade deformity*** of Smith's fracture, there is ventral prominence 1" above the wrist joint. In dislocation of lunate bone, there is an abnormal slight anterior projection of the wrist.

In ***Madelung's deformity/congenital manus valgus,*** seen in adolescent girls, the hand is deviated laterally due to forward/ulnar curving of the lower end of radius resulting from growth disturbances at the ulnar aspect of distal radial physis.

Any deformity in the hand is looked for resulting from fracture/dislocation of interphalangeal/metacarpophalangeal joints. Patient is asked to make the fist and the knuckle line is observed for any obvious deviation which occurs in fracture of metacarpophalangeal joints.

'***Mallet finger***' is persistent flexion of terminal phalanx due to rupture of the extensor tendon at its insertion at the base of terminal phalanx resulting from sudden flexion violence.

Palpation

All features typical of any fracture should be looked for—***local bony tenderness, irregularity, displacement, and crepitus*** should be checked.

Lower End of the Forearm

Lower end and posterolateral surface of the radius and the lower end of ulna are palpated for bony irregularities, temperature, and tenderness. As the lower end of the radius is covered by muscles and tendon, direct palpation of the bone is not possible. However, the lower end of radius is curved smoothly concave forwards. It is palpated all along to look for any irregularity. The rounded outer aspect of radius is palpated all along to see for any fracture which causes the palpating finger to *step over* the distal fragment which is also appreciated on the dorsal aspect of the forearm. There is **posterior 'step up' in Colle's fracture** (as the distal fragment is displaced backwards), **'step down'** (as the distal fragment is displaced forwards) *in Smith's fracture*. Tenderness can be elicited either by direct palpation or by indirect method—Springing the radius' where the upper end of radius and ulna are held together and squeezed to elicit pain at the fracture site at the lower part of forearm. Lower end of ulna is relatively subcutaneous making the palpation easy for irregularity and tenderness.

Method of palpating styloid process—with the patient's forearm in pronated position, wrist in neutral position, examiner's index finger is placed over the snuff box and thumb distal to the head of ulna. By gently squeezing and slightly shifting the fingers proximally the pointed bony projections of styloid processes can be felt.

Palpation of Joint Line
The patient's wrist is supported with one hand, and with tip of index or middle finger of other hand, palpation is done in interstyloid line. The gap of the joint is felt which opens and closes during palmar/dorsiflexion of hand.

Assessment of Inferior Radioulnar Joint
Ballottement test—done to assess the stability of distal radioulnar joint. Supporting the patient's wrist in one hand, the ulnar head is pressed with the thumb anteriorly and released. The ulnar head recoils back. The anteroposterior extrusion range is compared on both the sides, found to be more and painful on the side affected with instability.

Palpation of Carpal, Metacarpal, and Phalangeal Bones
Scaphoid bone is palpated in the anatomical snuff box, whose fracture is of importance as it is often misdiagnosed for sprain, often goes for nonunion and avascular necrosis giving rise to a painful wrist. The thumb is extended and abducted as far as possible (*thumb-up position*). The wrist is supported from ulnar side. The floor formed by scaphoid bone is palpated by pressing deeply between the prominent tendons for tenderness suggestive of fracture. Percussion over the head of the 2nd metacarpal will produce pain at the anatomical snuff box indicating fracture of scaphoid bone.

Any abnormal bony protrusion in front of the wrist is palpable in fracture lunate.

The base of the metacarpals is palpated for fracture/dislocation. Also the shaft and the head are palpated for irregularity or tenderness. Here bony tenderness is elicited either by direct palpation, or indirectly by applying gentle axial pressure or applying traction along the axis of the bone.

Measurement
Measurement of forearm length (already described in previous topic)—shortening is seen in Colle's fracture/Smith's fracture. Measurement of forearm girth—taken at mid-forearm level.

Measurement of Level of Styloid Process
The forearm is kept in pronated position. The tips of styloid processes of ulna and radius are marked. A line is drawn between the points. Normally styloid process of radius is 1 to 1.25 cm below that of ulna. If the styloid process of radius is at or above the level of that of ulna, it is suggestive of Colle's fracture (**Fig. 36-13**).

Movement
Movements at the wrist joint are extension (dorsiflexion, 90°); flexion (palmar flexion, 80°); radial deviation (abduction, 25°); ulnar deviation (adduction, 35°) and circumduction. The range of movements is compared on both sides. Both active and passive movements are done and compared on both the sides. *Extension is checked*—The patient places the palms and fingers of the two hands in contact in vertical plane lifting the elbow while keeping the hands together; and angle between hand and forearm on the dorsum is measured (Indian salutation technique). *Flexion is checked*—Reverse method; the patient places the backs of the hands together with fingers directed vertically downwards and elbows are lowered properly; angle between forearm and hand on the ventral part is measured on both the sides (**Refer Chapter 27: Approaches and Examination in Hand Disease**).

Both active and passive movements of the metacarpophalangeal and interphalangeal joints are checked.

Any abnormal mobilities are checked.

Examination of Radial, Median and Ulnar Nerves and Distal Pulsation (Capillary Pulsation)
Features suggestive of distal nerve injuries should be examined; motor and sensory—both as needed (**please refer Chapter 9: Examination and Clinical Approach to Peripheral Nervous System**).

Investigation
X-ray is Diagnostic: **Both X-ray-AP/lat views are taken for diagnosis of fracture at wrist joint and hand. For scaphoid (*Skaphos—boat*) fracture, oblique view is essential. Often fracture may be identified only when X-ray is repeated after 10 days. Often MRI may be needed to identify scaphoid fracture.**

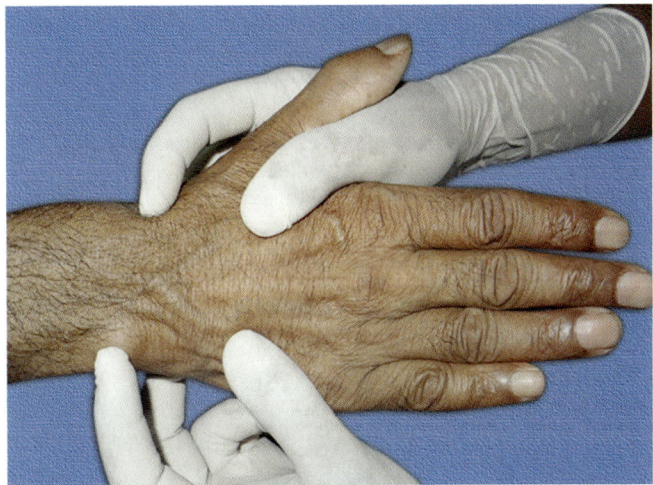

Fig. 36-13 *Tip of radial styloid process* is 1 cm lower than tip of ulnar styloid process.

Different Injuries of the Wrist Joint

Colles' fracture (Fig. 36-14)	Scaphoid fracture
It occurs following a fall on an outstretched hand. It is fracture of radius 2 cm proximal to distal articular surface of the radius with posterior, lateral and proximal displacement of distal fragment—*dinner fork deformity*	It is due to fall on outstretched, dorsiflexed radially deviated hand resulting in impact of scaphoid against radial styloid **Investigation**: Oblique scaphoid view X-ray, which needs to be repeated after 10 days; MRI **Features**: Fullness in the anatomical snuff box, tenderness especially when actively extending the thumb with medially deviated wrist **Complications**: Non-union; avascular necrosis of proximal part; osteoarthritis of wrist
Smith's fracture:	**Lunate dislocation**
It is a true reversed Colle's fracture with transverse fracture of lower end of radius 2 cm proximal articular surface with anterior, lateral, proximal displacement of the distal fragment—*garden spade deformity* **Features**: Deformity; swelling; irregularity; loss of normal concavity of radius; radial styloid process from its normal lower position becomes equal or higher than ulnar styloid process **Complications**: Stiffness; malunion; manu valgus; Sudeck's osteodystrophy; causalgia; rupture of extensor hallucis longus tendon; carpal tunnel syndrome. Neglected cases—stiffness of shoulder and hand—*"shoulder hand syndrome"*	It is due to fall on outstretched hand where entire carpus displaces backwards. Lunate bone is displaced anteriorly and rotated 90° horizontally. Lateral view X-ray—confirmatory **Complications:** Median nerve injury; avascular necrosis (*Kienbock's disease*)
Galeazzi fracture	**Madelung deformity**
It is fracture of lower end of radius (1/3 or 1/4) with dislocation or subluxation of inferior radioulnar joint. It is due to rotational force causing swelling in lower forearm; prominent head of ulna; ulnar nerve injury	It is dorsal subluxation of lower end of ulna. Probably due to delayed growth of radius as a result of repeated trauma but continuous growth of ulna forces it to subluxate dorsally. Seen in young girls with weak wrist; congenital/acquired; present with prominent dorsum of wrist
Chauffeur's fracture	**Barton's fracture**
Fracture of radius just above the styloid process. Occurs when a recoiling car handle hits directly over the radial styloid process	It is anterior marginal fracture of radius with subluxation of both wrist and inferior radio-ulnar joint, with forward displacement of carpus along with the hand. Wrist joint movements are markedly painful
Bennett's fracture dislocation	*Fractures occurring due to fall with outstretched hand*
Oblique fracture occurring at the base of 1st metacarpal bone with subluxation of the carpometacarpal joint. Triangular fragment of the bone remains in position. If fracture is T/Y—*Rolando's fracture*	• Fracture of clavicle • Fracture neck or shaft of humerus • Supracondylar fracture of humerus • Posterior dislocation of elbow • Fracture of radius and ulna • Colles' fracture; scaphoid fracture

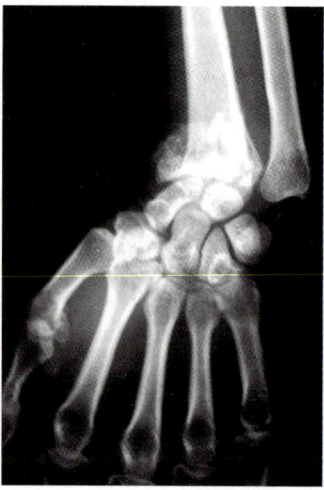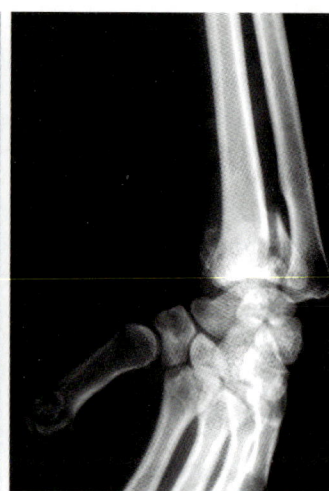

Fig. 36-14 *Colles' fracture.*

EXAMINATION IN INJURIES TO PELVIS

Pelvis is formed by two hip bones—sacrum and coccyx behind with articulations. Superior aperture is called as pelvic inlet or pelvic brim. Upper part is greater or false pelvis is formed by two iliac fossae and posterior abdominal wall. Lower part is called as lesser or true pelvis containing pelvic viscera. Pelvic inlet is bounded posteriorly by the sacral promontory, anteriorly by the superior margin of the pubic symphysis; on each side linea terminalis (ala of the sacrum, the arcuate line, lower medial border of ilium, pectinate line, pectin pubis and pubic crest. Pelvic outlet is formed posteriorly by coccyx, on each side by ischiopubic rami, ischial tuberosities and sacrotuberous ligaments; anteriorly by inferior pubic ligament. Hip bone is made up of three parts—ilium above; pubis anteroinferiorly; ischium posteroinferiorly; the three bones are joined to each other at acetabulum. Two hip bones form the *pelvic girdle*. The pubis and ischium are separated by a large opening called as obturator foramen. All three components join at acetabulum. Acetabulum is a deep cup-shaped hemispherical cavity in the lateral aspect of the hip bone. It has got horse-shaped lunate articular surface with acetabular notch inferiorly.

External rotation force, compression force, vertical shear are the types of forces which cause pelvic injury.

History

Pelvis gets injured in crush injury, direct run-over by automobile, direct or indirect violence.

Shock, severe pain, inability to sit/walk or move the pelvis is typical. Patient may have associated pelvic organ injury like that of bladder, uterus and rectum. There may be associated damage to urethra and genital tract (in females). Patient may give history of not able to pass urine or hematuria.

Local Examination

Inspection

The patient is made to lie in supine position.
The symmetry and levels of anterior superior iliac spines of both sides are noted and compared. Iliac crest, symphysis

pubis, groin folds, Scarpa's triangle are observed on both the sides. Contour of abdomen, level of umbilicus are noted. ***Ecchymoses, bruising,*** swelling in lower abdomen, perineum, scrotum and penis are common. Look for extravasation of urine in scrotum, labial region, groin and lower abdominal wall. It is difficult to turn the patient to side or to prone as it is painful. If possible, then note the symmetry, any bulge of iliac crest or in gluteal region, internatal clefts, back of thighs.

Any bleeding from urethra/rectum/vagina is observed. A large superficial hematoma in the inguinal region or scrotum or thigh is called as ***Destot's sign.***

Palpation

The symphysis pubis is palpated for symmetry, regularity of surfaces between the two halves. In disruption and fracture-dislocation of symphysis, one can insinuate one or more fingers into the gap whereas in subluxation, a step may be felt. The inlet and outlet of pelvic margins are palpated. The outer aspect and back of the pelvis, alignment and tenderness over the sacroiliac joints, ischial tuberosities, and posterior iliac spine are noted. Fracture of sacrum and coccyx can cause severe tenderness.

Palpation of urethra: Urethra is palpated backwards from penile part to membranous part.

Per-rectal and per-vaginal examination is very essential. Ischiopubic rami, coccyx, sacroiliac joint can be palpated. Condition of the prostate in males and any soft tissue swelling and tenderness is assessed.

Earle's sign: A bony prominence or large hematoma as well as tenderness on rectal examination.

Auscultation over abdomen for bowel sounds—may be absent in paralytic ileus due to peritonitis which may be associated with pelvic fracture.

Associated injuries of lower limbs, abdomen, and thorax also should be confirmed.

Measurement

Roux's sign: Decrease in the distance from the greater trochanter to the pubic spine on the affected side is seen in lateral compression fracture.

Movement

Compression test: Patient is made to lie supine, flat on bed, with legs approximated. The examiner with his both hands compresses both iliac crest towards each other. Fracture/dislocation in pelvis will elicit pain by this forceful compression **(Fig. 36-15)**.

Distraction test: Same as above but here the examiner presses the anterior superior iliac spine from inner aspect so as to push away from each other which elicits pain at the fracture site **(Fig. 36-16)**.

Pump handle test: In supine position, for right sided sacroiliac joint disease, clinician places his left hand over the left shoulder of the patient; patient keeps his right lower limb fully extended, clinician with his right hand flexes left side (*unaffected side*) knee and hip joints of the patient towards right shoulder of the patient which will cause pain in the right (diseased) sacroiliac joint **(Fig. 36-17)**.

Gaenslen's test: With patient in supine position, knee and hip joints of the *unaffected side* of the patient are fully flexed while clinician with his opposite hand hyperextends the hip to elicit pain in the affected sacroiliac joint due to pelvic rotation **(Fig. 36-18)**.

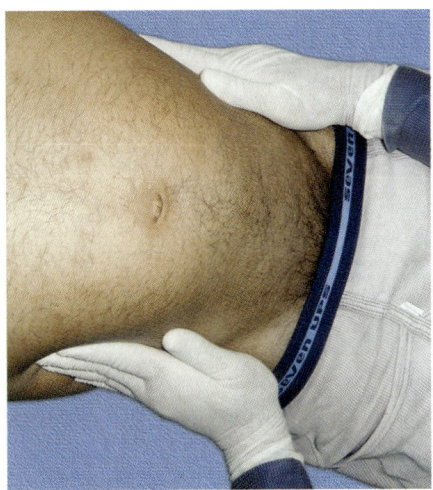

Fig. 36-15 *Compression test.*

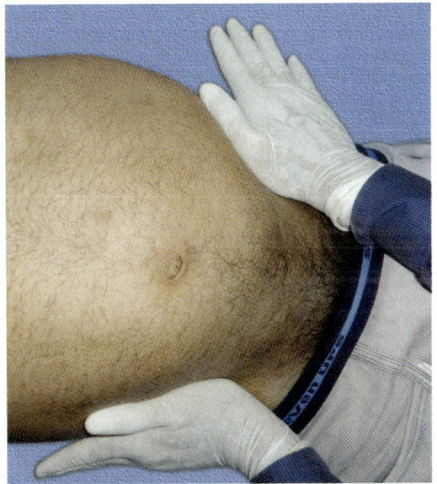

Fig. 36-16 *Distraction test.*

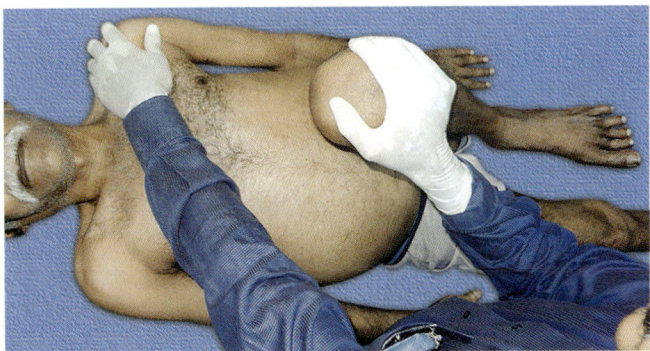

Fig. 36-17 *Pump handle test.*

Laquer's sign: When hip joint on the *affected side* is forced to flex, abduct and externally rotate, the patient feels pain in diseased sacroiliac joint **(Fig. 36-19)**.

Goldthwaite's sign: Lower limb of the *affected side* with its fully extended knee is flexed strongly at hip to tense the hamstrings and so to create rotation strain which leads into the pain at sacroiliac joint on the same side **(Fig. 36-20)**.

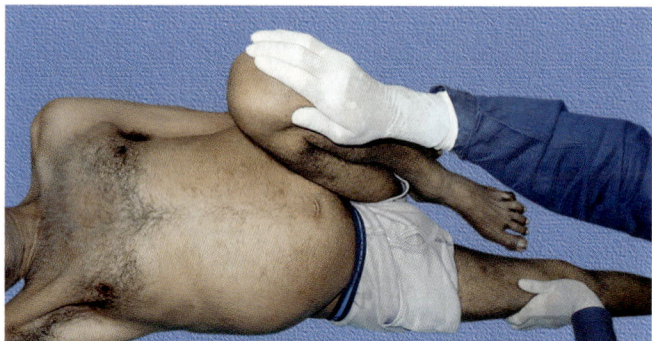

Fig. 36-18 *Gaenslen's test.*

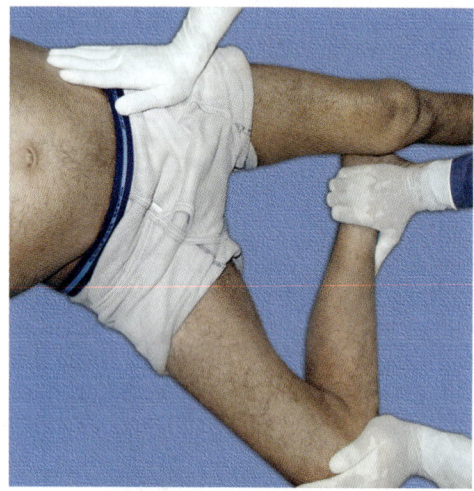

Fig. 36-19 *Laquer's sign.*

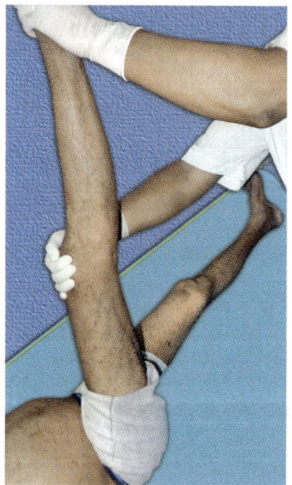

Fig. 36-20 *Goldthwaite's sign.*

Hip joint movements are not much affected except in terminal range, may produce stress pain over the fracture site.

Neurovascular Examination

Neurovascular examination of lower limb has to be done as injury to major vessels and injury to lumbosacral plexus are known to occur in pelvic fractures.

Investigation

X-ray pelvis with lumbosacral spine both anteroposterior and lateral. CT pelvis with lumbar spine is a must.

Classification of Pelvic Fractures

Stable fracture of pelvic ring: It is isolated fracture with no/minimal displacement and does not disrupt the integrity of pelvic ring, e.g. fracture of superior or inferior ischiopubic rami, fracture of ilium, or ischium due to fall, stress, avulsion fracture of ischial tuberosity. Here problems are less with minimum complications.

Unstable fracture of pelvic ring: Here fracture occurs at approximately two opposite points with separation and disruption of pelvic ring. Anterior injury with fractures through both ischiopubic rami with separation/disruption of pubic symphysis is common type. It is often associated with complications like rupture of uerthra/urinary bladder, sciatic nerve injury, hemorrhage in pelvis, shock and paralytic ileus.

Lateral wall fracture: Acetabulum fracture that is displaced/undisplaced.

Sacrococcygeal fracture: Results from blow on posterior aspect or vertical fall on the 'tail'.

Avulsion fracture: It is due to strong muscle contraction that tears away a fragment of bone, e.g. Sartorius from anterior superior iliac spine; rectus muscle from anterior inferior iliac spine, hamstring from ischial tuberosity.

Malgaigne fracture: It is a fracture through rami or symphysis pubis with disruption of posterior arch through sacrum/sacroiliac joint/ilium causing unstable anterior as well as posterior arch failure. **Complications**: Paresthesia of lower limb; severe limp; severe back/groin pain; pelvic obliquity; neurologic problems, changes in leg length.

Complications of pelvic injury: Rupture of bladder; rupture of the urethra with extravasation of urine; injury to rectum; injury to major vessels causing torrential hemorrhage; injury to lumbosacral plexus nerves; acetabular fracture with osteoarthritis.

■ EXAMINATION IN INJURIES OF HIP AND THIGH

History

Fracture of femoral neck, dislocation of head of femur is the common injuries around hip. Nature of injury should be asked as it will predict the type of fracture. Fall from height with feet first, motor car dashboard injury, falling of a heavy weight on the back of a stooping worker—all these may result in dislocation of hip. Sometimes injuries can be trivial like tripping on a step, fall in a bathroom which may cause fracture of neck of femur especially in elderly individuals with osteoporosis. Fracture/ traumatic dislocation of hip is rare below 5 years of age.

Fracture shaft of femur can occur at any age. Commonest cause is motorcycle accident.

History of pain—severe in traumatic fracture neck of femur and traumatic dislocation of hip.

History of disability to walk/stand after injury should be asked—patient with unimpacted fracture cannot walk/stand but with impacted fracture can do it with strain. Patient with dislocation of hip may not be able to walk initially but in long-standing unattended cases can do it with limp and deformity.

History of swelling in the hip region is seen in extra-capsular fracture of neck of femur.

Examination

Features of shock should be looked for especially in fracture of neck and shaft of femur as the femoral and popliteal vessels may get torn causing torrential bleeding.

Local Examination

Inspection

Attitude and Deformity

Patient (often elderly) is seen lying on the bed with externally rotated lower limb in fracture neck of femur. This range of external rotation will give an idea whether it is extracapsular (low fracture of neck)—where there is 90 degrees outward rotation (outer part of the foot is seen touching the bed) or intracapsular (high fracture neck) where the outward rotation is 45 degrees.

Limb is seen in adduction, internal rotation and slight flexion in posterior dislocation of hip (common in young). Limb is seen in external rotation, abduction, slight flexion in anterior dislocation of hip which is rare.

In impacted fracture neck of femur, patient may not present with any particular attitude or deformity.

Swelling on the lateral aspect of upper thigh is seen in fracture of extracapsular neck of femur whereas no swelling in intracapsular neck of femur. Bruising on the posterolateral aspect of thigh is seen in fracture of extracapsular neck of femur—**DA Patel sign**.

Hollowness in Scarpa's triangle is seen in posterior dislocation of hip. In fracture shaft of femur, there is abnormal swelling and angular deformity in the thigh. If it is an open fracture wound is present which needs to be examined with aseptic precaution (**Fig. 36-21**).

Palpation

The pelvic bones: Ilium, pubis and ischium; upper end of femur—head, neck and greater trochanter, full length of shaft of femur are palpated for swelling, irregularities, tenderness and crepitus.

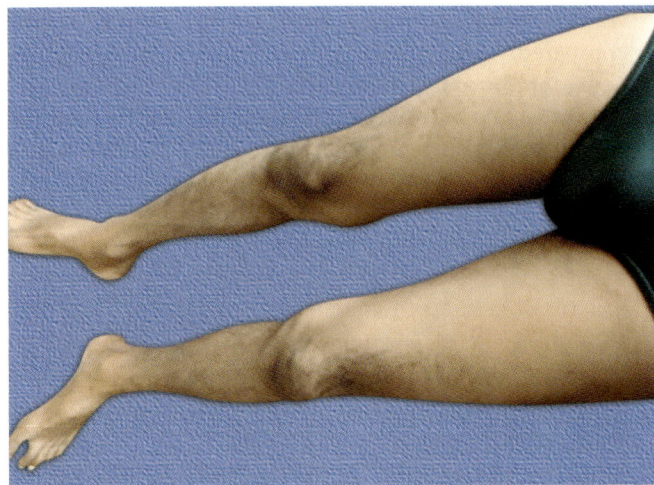

Fig. 36-21 *External rotation of hip* (left side) is a feature of fracture of neck of femur.

Tenderness can be elicited by direct palpation or indirectly by moving the lower thigh.

The head and greater trochanter of femur are assessed for their relative position with the pelvis.

Position of Greater Trochanter

Can be assessed by putting the thumb finger of one hand over the anterior superior iliac spine (ASIS), middle finger over the tip of greater trochanter and index finger over an imaginary point at the intersection of two perpendiculars—one dropped from ASIS to bed and other from the tip of greater trochanter to the above (points of **Bryant's triangle**). The three fingers of the other hand are placed similarly on the other side and compared for the position of the greater trochanter. If the position of middle finger on the affected side is displaced upwards, it indicates fracture of femoral neck or posterior dislocation of thigh. In subtrochanteric fracture, this position of middle finger is unaffected but there is external rotation of the limb.

Position of Head of the Femur

Dislocated femoral head is palpable as rounded hard mass in gluteal region in posterior dislocation, in the groin in anterior dislocation, in the perineum in obturator type. It is confirmed as head by its relation to the trochanter and its movement on moving the thigh. *In fracture of shaft of femur* the proximal fragment is flexed abducted and externally rotated by the muscles attached to it whereas the distal fragment is adducted.

Measurements

(Details of measurement are discussed in diseases of hip).

Both the limbs are placed in identical position with anterior superior iliac spine lying in a horizontal line.

a. **Linear measurement of the limb** is necessary to assess the degree of shortening in the limb. Both *apparent* (distance from central fixed point on the trunk, e.g. suprasternal notch/, umbilicus to bony point on medial malleolus) and *true measurement* (distance from anterior superior iliac spine to bony point on medial malleolus) are taken with patient lying in supine position on both sides and compared.

b. **Segmental measurement**—leg length (from medial knee joint line to medial malleolus), thigh length (from anterior superior iliac spine to medial knee joint line in flexed knee position). Measurement is taken on both sides. Helps to assess which part is shortened and how much.

In all fractures and dislocations there are shortening of the limb except in obturator type of dislocation.

Fracture of shaft of femur is also associated with limb shortening.

c. **Bryant's triangle**: Patient lies in supine position. The tips of greater trochanter and ASIS are marked on both sides. A perpendicular line is dropped from ASIS. Another line perpendicular to the above is drawn from greater trochanter (forms the base). A line is drawn to join the ASIS and tip of greater trochanter (forms the hypotenuse). This forms a right-angle triangle the components of which are compared on both the sides.

Any shortening of the base indicates riding up of trochanter that occurs in dislocation of hip, central fracture-dislocation of hip, destruction of head/acetabulum or both, fracture neck of femur, malunited intertrochanteric fracture, coxa vara deformity. Any shortening of the perpendicular line drawn from ASIS to bed indicates anterior sliding/tilting/internal rotation of greater trochanter as it occurs in posterior and central dislocation of hip. Any shortening in hypotenuse indicates approximation of trochanter towards the body that occurs in central dislocation of hip, old fracture neck of femur, absence of head due to disease or surgery **(Figs. 36-22A and B)**.

d. **Nelaton's line**: With patient lying down on his sound side with knee and hip bent at 90 degrees, a line is drawn from ischial tuberosity to tip of anterior superior iliac spine. In normal individual, this line touches the tip of greater trochanter. Any upwards displacement of greater trochanter can be easily detected **(Fig. 36-23)**.

e. **Schoemaker's line**: Patient lies in supine position. The line from the greater trochanter to anterior superior iliac spine on both sides is extended upwards which will intersect at or above the umbilicus in midline. Line shifts below the umbilical level if greater trochanter is elevated and it meets its counterpart on opposite side. In bilateral congenital dislocation of hip, they meet in the midline but below the umbilicus.

f. **Chiene's test**: A tape joining the tips of greater trochanters is parallel to another tape joining the two anterior superior iliac spines. Two will converge towards diseased side when trochanter is elevated.

g. **Morris bitrochanteric test**: Using pair of graduated calipers, distance between outer margin of greater trochanter and pubic symphysis is measured and compared on both the sides. If the trochanter is externally rotated, this distance is increased on that side and vice-versa.

h. **Circumferential measurement**: It is taken at mid-thigh level on both the sides to identify any swelling or wasting

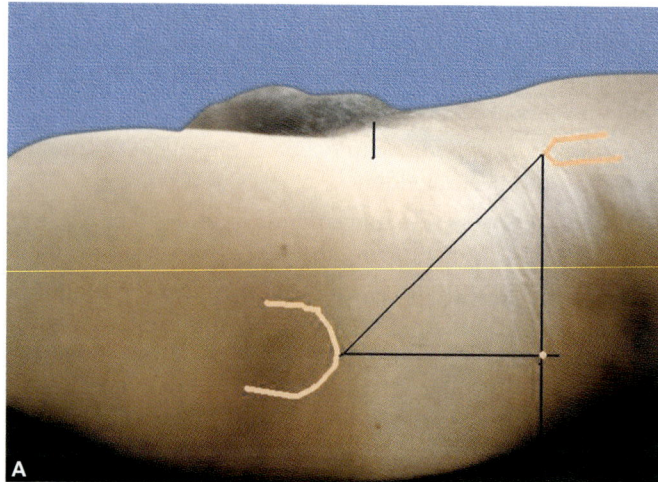
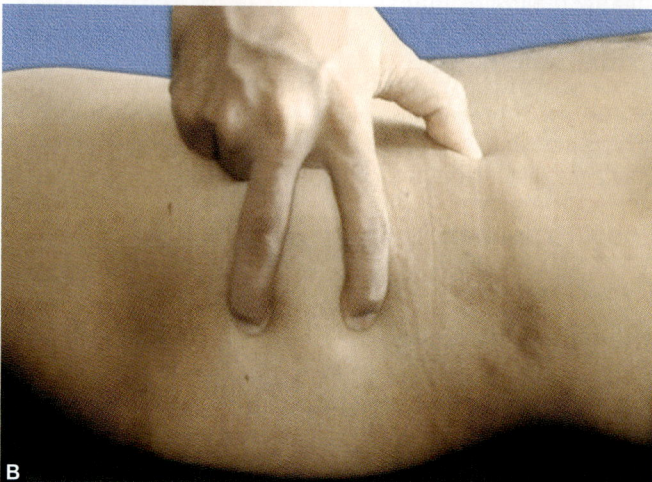

Figs. 36-22A and B Method of drawing *Bryant's triangle* and feeling its points.

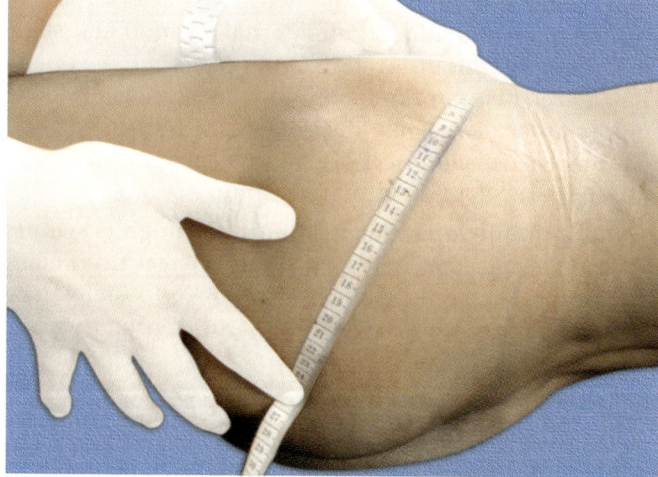

Fig. 36-23 *Nelaton's line.*

in the thigh. It is taken from equidistant from a fixed point like 10–15 cm above the apex of patella.

Movement

Movements at the hip joint should be checked. Normal flexion is 110°; extension is 30° from neutral; abduction is 50°;

adduction is 30°; internal rotation in flexion is 45°; external rotation in flexion is 45°; external rotation in extension 45°; internal rotation in extension is 35°.

Both active and passive movements are checked on both the sides:

a. ***Straight leg raising test:*** Lying in supine position, the patient is asked to raise the leg off the bed actively with knee extended which normally can be done up to 90 degrees. If the patient is able to do this movement, then serious injury at the hip except impacted fracture of the neck of femur is ruled out.

b. ***Test for any abnormal mobility (telescopic test):*** Patient lying down in supine position with knee and hip flexed at 90 degrees, the examiner holds the patient's hip with open hand over the greater trochanter and buttock. With the other hand, examiner grasps the lower end of femur, pushes down and pulls up the thigh. Meanwhile amount of mobility at the greater trochanter is felt by the other hand which is marked in old untreated dislocation of hip.

Abnormal mobility is also seen in fracture of shaft of femur. There is absence of transmitted movement—when shaft is moved, its movement is not felt at greater trochanter.

Other Examinations

Rectal examination reveals palpable head of femur within the pelvis in central dislocation. By rotating the limb, the rotation of the head can be appreciated by the finger in the rectum.

Palpation of vessels: Femoral artery pulsation may not be felt in posterior dislocation of hip as it has lost the support posteriorly (***Narath's sign***). In fracture of shaft of femur pulsation of dorsalis pedis and posterior tibial should be checked.

Examination of nerves: Sciatic, femoral, and obturator nerves are involved in posterior, anterior, or central dislocation respectively.

Investigation

X-ray of hip AP/lateral view are *very* useful. Lines of fracture, type of displacement are to be looked for.

Pauwel's angle (i.e. the angle formed by fracture line in neck of femur to horizontal plane, more the angle less is the prognosis); position of lesser trochanter (often partly visible in normal X-ray; if clearly visible then femur is externally rotated, not visibly in internally rotated femur), **Shenton's line** (the lower margin of the neck of femur and superior ramus of the pubis form the part of same arc which is disrupted in dislocation of hip and fracture of neck of femur); acetabulum, are the points to be assessed.

X-ray of femur in fracture of shaft—fracture line may be in upper third, mid-third, or in lower third. It can be transverse or spiral or oblique or green stick in children.

Different Injuries of the Hip Joint

Dislocation of hip (Fig. 36-24)	*Fracture of shaft of femur*
Types: **a. Posterior dislocation:** Commonest type; causes flexion, adduction, internal rotation of hip with shortening, impalpable femoral artery pulse (*Narath's sign*) **b. Anterior dislocation**: Occurs while stepping into a boat with abducted limb; limb takes the attitude of flexion, external rotation and abduction of hip. Head is adjacent to pubis symphysis (*pubic type*) or under adductor muscle (*obturator type*); obturator type causes lengthening of limb **c. Central dislocation:** Head of femur is forced through fractured acetabulum into the pelvis making it to be palpated per rectally	• Includes subtrochanteric fracture, fracture midshaft, distal femur including supracondylar fracture. As femur is surrounded by powerful muscles, there will be displacement of fractured segments. In upper third fracture—proximal fragment is drawn upwards (iliopsoas) into abducted position (gluteus maximus and minimus). • In mid third—the distal fragment is displaced medially and upward (adductors). • In distal third—the distal fragment is pulled upwards (gastrocnemius)
Fracture neck of femur	*Avulsion fracture of lesser trochanter*
Common in elderly and in females. **Types**: Subcapital (70%); basal (10%); transcervical (10%). It can be incomplete; complete with or without displacement **Features**: Patient not able to move the limb or get up; flexion, abduction, and external rotation are the attitudes with tender mid-inguinal point; shortening of limb	It is due to violent contraction of the iliopsoas muscle **Ludloff's sign:** Inability to flex the stretched leg once the patient is seated
Intertrochanteric fracture	*Subtrochanteric fracture (Fig. 36-25)*
It is extracapsular fracture between greater and lesser trochanter of femur. It can be undisplaced/displaced, two fragments, or three fragments or four fragments or reverse oblique. It unites readily with fewer complications **Features:** Marked pain, tenderness, and ecchymoses and hematoma over the trochanteric region with abduction, external rotation, and shortening	• It is fracture femur occurring up to 5-7.5 cm below the lesser trochanter. It is difficult fracture as it is a cortical bone as it an area of greater stress and force • Proximal segment is flexed (iliopsoas), abducted (gluteus medius); distal segment is adducted (adductors). Bleeding and hematoma are common

■ EXAMINATION IN INJURIES OF KNEE JOINT AND LEG BONES

The knee joint is the complex and largest joint in the body. It is formed by fusion of lateral femorotibial, medial femorotibial and femoropatellar joints. It is a compound joint with two joints between condyles of the femur and tibia and one saddle joint between femur and patella. Ligaments of knee joint are—ligamentum patellae, medial collateral,

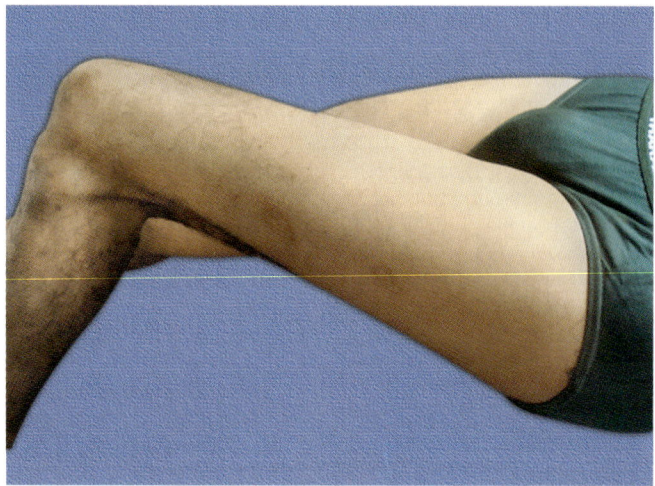

Fig. 36-24 *Posterior dislocation* of left hip.

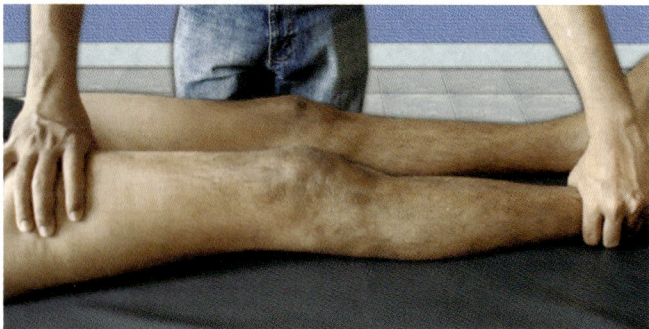

Fig. 36-25 Shaft of the femur when moved greater trochanter will be immobile in *subtrochanteric fracture*.

lateral collateral, oblique popliteal, arcuate popliteal, anterior cruciate, posterior cruciate and transverse ligaments; medial and lateral menisci. Bursae around knee joint are—in front—subcutaneous prepatellar, subcutaneous infrapatellar, deep infrapatellar, suprapatellar; laterally—deep to lateral head of gastrocnemius, between lateral collateral ligament and biceps femoris, between lateral collateral ligament and popliteus tendon, between popliteus tendon and lateral condyle of the tibia; medially—deep to medial head of gastrocnemius, bursa anserina between sartorius, gracilis, semitendinosus and tibia and medial collateral ligament, bursa deep to medial collateral ligament, bursa deep to semimembranosus. Movements are—flexion, extension, rotator movements, slight abduction and adduction, locking and unlocking movements. Flexion and extension movements are associated with rotations of the knee joint. Medial rotation of the femur occurs in last 30 degrees of extension and lateral rotation of femur occurs during initial stages of flexion. When foot is off the ground, tibia rotates in opposite direction. Locking is a mechanism which keeps the knee in a position of full extension as in standing; locking is due to medial rotation of femur. Unlocking of the locked knee occurs only by lateral rotation of the femur which is brought by the action of the popliteus muscle. Injuries around the knee joint may involve ligaments in and around the knee joint or the articular bones of the knee joint.

History

Nature of Violence

Injuries to medial collateral ligaments are common in sportsman (ball games and skiing) where a forceful valgus bending of the knee results in its tear.

In dashboard injury where the front passenger is thrown forward hitting the tibia results in tear of the posterior cruciate ligament.

When a twist in the knee joint occurs with flexed knee and weight bearing, as seen in football players and coal miners, it results in tears of meniscus (medial is more common than lateral).

Violent contraction of quadriceps that occurs while stumbling on a stair or catching the foot while walking or running results in traction injuries of the tibial tuberosities in adolescents, rupture of ligamentum patellae in young adults, transverse fracture of patella in middle age, rupture of quadriceps in elderly people.

Bony injuries result from direct violence, by fall on knee joint.

Pain: Duration, site (on the lateral aspect in tears of collateral ligament and meniscus; front—bursitis, tendon irritability of quadriceps and ligamentum patellae; posterior aspect in Baker's cyst, meniscal tear), nature of pain (continuous/intermittent acute onset); association with activities are asked.

Swelling: Swelling in and around the knee joint may be due to effusion, hemarthrosis, dislocation of patellae (here swelling is on lateral aspect of femoral condyle). Duration of swelling should be asked—immediate onset of swelling is seen in cruciate ligament tear or fracture of patella; delayed in meniscal tear, ligament sprain.

Locking of knee: It is inability to bend or straighten the leg. It could be due to meniscal tear or loose bodies in the joint cavity. ***Pseudolocking*** is due to pain where normal activity is limited.

Instability/giving way: Especially while climbing—common in cruciate ligament injury; Intermittent instability of knee joint with sudden severe pain is seen in meniscal tears.

Disability: Inability to walk/stand—partial in ligament sprain/tear, complete in supracondylar fracture.

Local Examination

Inspection

Examination is done with patient in lying down position, exposing from pelvis to toes. Both limbs are kept together in identical position for comparison.

Attitude: Knee commonly assumes an attitude of 30 degrees flexion in all traumatic conditions as it is the position of ease and rest.

Deformity: The joint should be examined carefully whether it is abnormally abducted (genu valgum), adducted (genu varum), hyperextended or displaced backwards. Normally the midinguinal point, midpoint of patella and midpoint of ankle all fall in a straight line (axis of leg) which when prolonged, pass through the 2nd web space. Outward deviation of this axis from midpoint of patella—*genu valgum*; inward deviation is *genu varum*.

Knee is examined from front, back and from sides.

From front, knee is examined for normal contour; position, size and shape of patella; patellar ligament, supra and infrapatellar fossae; anterolateral and anteromedial tibial flares; tibial tubercle; shin of tibia. Any swelling, sinuses, if present, are noted.

Swelling: It could be due to effusion, hemarthrosis causing typical *horse-shoe* look—around superior and lateral aspect of the patella, obliterating the normal parapatellar depression. Patellar dislocation causes swelling on lateral aspect over femoral condyles.

Wasting of quadriceps, sometimes, is common after knee injury. Normal contour is looked for from the lateral aspect of the knee. Any abnormal shift or prominence of fibular head is noted. The contour of the knee must be examined from popliteal aspect. Any collection in knee joint or pathology in posterior aspect of knee manifests as obliteration of popliteal fossa. Any swelling, pulsations have to be looked for.

Palpation

Temperature over the knee joint is noted.

Muscles and tendons are palpated for tenderness. Quadriceps muscle and tendon, ligamentum patellae, vastus medialis and lateralis are palpated for tenderness and wasting.

Tenderness anterior to the medial collateral ligament (it is elicited on flexed knee using thumb pressing at this point and knee is gradually extended) suggests a bucket-handle tear. Tenderness over the medial collateral ligament at the level of joint line indicates injury to medial meniscus. Tenderness posterior to medial collateral ligament indicates tear of the posterior horn of medial meniscus.

Medial collateral ligament injury causes tenderness at its femoral attachment.

Bones are palpated for irregularities and tenderness—patella, medial femoral and tibial condyle, lateral femoral and tibial condyle, fibular head and neck, tibial tuberosity.

The supported knee is extended and the quadriceps is relaxed, the patella is pushed to the other side and with the other hand the articular surfaces are palpated, which is repeated in the other direction. *Patella is palpated* for tenderness, gap, irregularity (bruising over the surface is common in patellar fracture). Injury to extensor mechanism of knee (quadriceps, patella, ligamentum patellae) makes patient unable to lift the extended leg. ***Patellar tap*** should be done to check for any fluid. Minimal and massive effusion will give negative result for patellar tap **(Discussed in detail in Chapter 39: Approaches and Examinations in Pathologies of Individual Joints)**.

The femoral condyles are palpated by gradually flexing the knee to the fullest extent. The articular surfaces of the tibial condyles are palpated in 90 degrees flexed position of the knee.

In supracondylar fracture, lower end of femur will be directed backward and upper end will be directed forward. Lateral tibial condyle is commonly fractured than medial. Squeezing the lower part of tibia and fibula will cause tenderness in fibular fracture site (upper end of fibula—*springing of fibula*—indirect method of eliciting tenderness) **(Fig. 36-26)**.

In suspected fracture, shaft of fibula is better elicited as follows—the patient is made to lie on the couch. Examiner stands on the medial aspect of the affected limb. The knee is grasped in one hand and the heel in another. Using the examiner is knee against the medial aspect of mid leg, limb is pressed which will open up the crack in fibula with tenderness—***springing of fibula.***

Similarly in suspected stress fracture of tibia where only the cortex is involved, clinician stands on the lateral aspect and does the above test. On pressing the lateral aspect of mid-leg against the examiner's knee causes opening up of the fracture site on medial aspect of tibia—***springing of tibia.***

Measurement

Both thigh and leg length are taken and compared with normal side to assess the shortening. Circumference of thigh and leg are taken from fixed bony points and compared for any muscle wasting. Breadth of lower end of femur and upper end of tibia is measured with calipers.

Movement

Active and passive movements at the knee joint are checked. In fracture of tibial spine, there is limitation of last few degrees of extension. There is 0–135 degrees of flexion, extension from 135 degrees to 0 degree; at 90 degrees flexion there is some amount of abduction, adduction, medial rotation and lateral rotation. Any abnormal mobility at the injured site is checked.

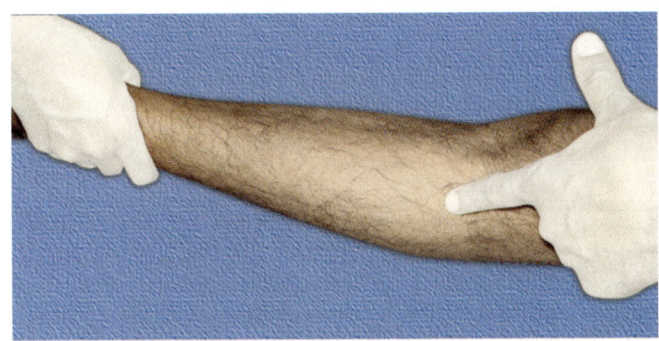

Fig. 36-26 *Springing of fibula.*

Specific Tests

McMurray's test: It is used to detect the integrity of posterior half of medial and lateral meniscus. With the patient lying in supine position, the examiner stands by the side of injured limb. Knee joint is flexed till the foot touches the buttocks. With one hand, knee is steadied and with other hand, foot is grasped. *While the foot is laterally rotated, leg is slowly extended and abducted.* Patient develops *pain and click* due to injury to *medial meniscus*. Pain and click, if develops in the beginning, means injury to posterior part of medial meniscus, in the middle of extension means injury to middle of meniscus; at the end of extension means injury to anterior end of meniscus. *Lateral meniscus* is checked similarly by *medial rotation* of foot and *adduction of leg* **(Fig. 36-27)**.

Apley's grinding test: This test helps to differentiate collateral ligament injury from meniscal injury. Patient lies on a couch on his face with affected knee towards the side of the couch. The examiner stands with his flexed knee leaning over the patient's ham in order to fix the femur. The foot is held and knee is flexed to 90 degrees. Compression is applied over the femoral condyles by pressing with the body weight over the tibial plateau. With *compression,* the leg is *laterally rotated*. If patient complains of pain, it indicates tear of *medial meniscus*. Similarly, if pain appears on *compression* and *medial rotation* of leg, it indicates tear of *lateral meniscus* **(Figs. 36-28A and B)**.

Apley's distraction test: Similar to the above, with the patient lying on his face on a couch with knee flexed to 90 degrees patient's ham steadied by examiner's knee, if patient develops pain on pulling the leg *upwards* and *rotated laterally* indicates injury to *medial collateral ligament*. Likewise if pain develops on *upwards* pull and *medial rotation* of leg indicates injury to *lateral collateral ligament*.

Tests for Abnormal Mobility (Stability)

a. **Abduction and adduction tests for lateral mobility:** With patient seated and knee fully extended, foot is held up with one hand, other hand is kept behind the knee in the upper part of popliteal space. Leg is abducted to feel any abnormal opening of the joint on the medial side in case of medial collateral ligament injury. When adducted, joint opens laterally in lateral collateral ligament injury. This movement is compared with the other joint **(Fig. 36-29)**.

b. **Drawer sign:** Patient sleeps on his couch with knee flexed (right angle) and foot resting on the bed. Foot is fixed by the examiner with one hand f or by sitting on foot. Upper end of tibia is moved with the other hand anteroposteriorly to check increased mobility. Increased anterior mobility of tibial condyles over the femur means it is anterior cruciate ligament injury; increased posterior movement of tibial condyles over femur means it is injury of posterior cruciate ligament **(Figs. 36-30 and 36-31)**.

Other Examinations

Palpate the dorsalis pedis and posterior tibial artery pulsation as the popliteal artery is often involved with supracondylar fracture.

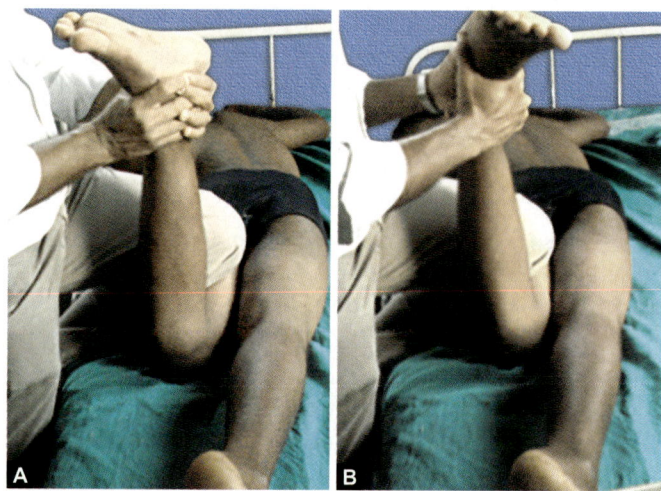

Figs. 36-28A and B *Apley's* grinding test.

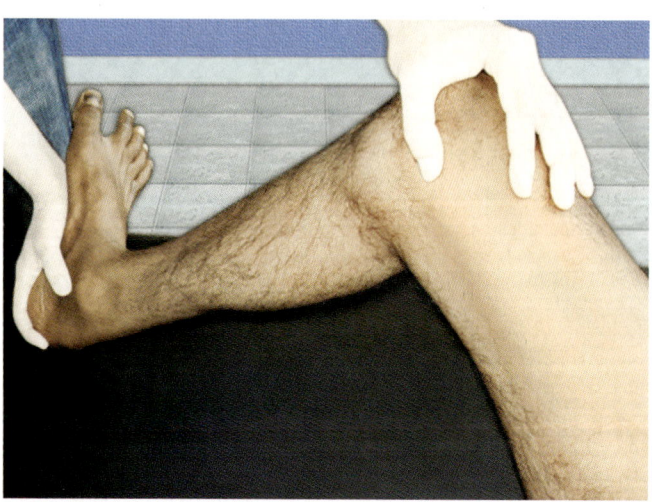

Fig. 36-27 *McMurray's* test.

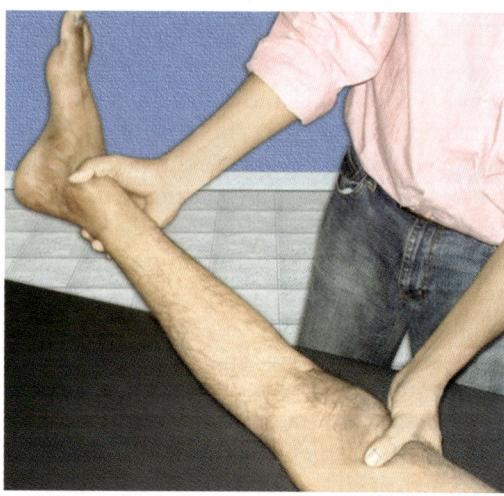

Fig. 36-29 *Abduction of knee* to confirm medial collateral ligament injury.

Chapter 36: Approaches and Examinations in Injuries of Various Joints

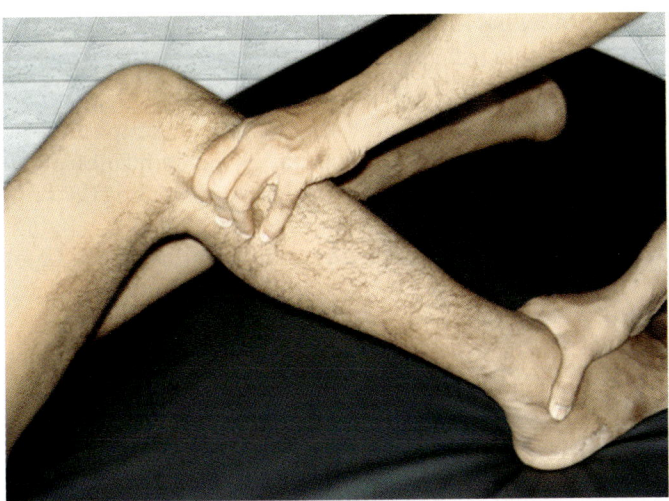

Fig. 36-30 *Drawer sign.* Forward push is done to check anterior cruciate ligament; backward push for posterior cruciate ligament.

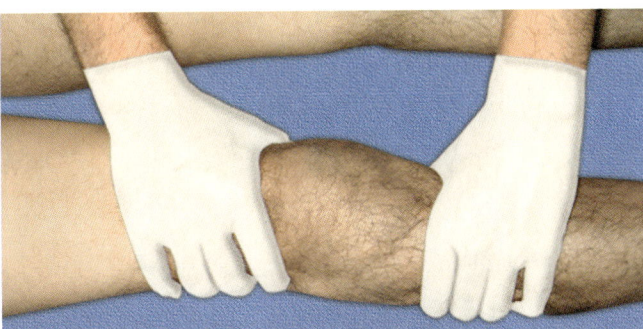

Fig. 36-31 *Checking the stability of cruciate ligaments* by moving upper end of tibia on femur.

Checking for complications: Popliteal artery injury, venous edema, hematoma of calf, compartment syndrome, nerve injuries (lateral peroneal nerve in fibular injury) can occur. Lateral popliteal nerve may get involved in the fracture of neck of fibula.

Different Injuries of the Knee Joint

Patellar fracture (Fig. 36-32)	**Medial semilunar (Meniscus) ligament**
It occurs by direct/indirect trauma (by violent muscular contraction); direct trauma results in comminuted fracture/indirect results in transverse fracture **Feature**: Swelling of the knee, effusion or blood are the features. With separation of fragments in transverse fracture of patella, the knee is in semiflexed position and the patient is unable to extend the leg actively **Recurrent dislocation of patella:** Common in females with tendency for genu valgum and small sized patella. Knee suddenly gives way with patient falling on the ground. Each attack painful. Wasting of vastus medialis and excessive lateral mobility of patella seen	Injury to meniscus occurs in flexed position of the joint; rotational force with forcible abduction is required. Medial meniscus is more commonly injured than lateral as it is fixed to medial collateral ligament. Lateral meniscus injury is rare as popliteus protects from being crushed between the articular surfaces **Features**: Common in football players and mine workers. It can be anterior horn/ posterior horn or bucket handle tear. Joint gets locked and suddenly gets unlocked and gives way. Joint line tenderness, effusion, positive McMurray's test, Apley's grinding test
Cruciate ligament injuries	**Pellegrini- Stieda's disease**
It is due to severe trauma. Causes joint's instability confirmed by *Drawer's sign*. Hyperextension of knee is common in anterior cruciate ligament injury	It is calcification of medial collateral ligament after partial avulsion from medial femoral condyle
Supra-condylar fracture	**Femoral condylar fracture**
Seen in adults; swelling above the patella, extreme tenderness, not able to move the limb. Lower fragments displaced backwards. **Complications**: Popliteal vessel injury	One condyle may be drawn up. Both condyles may be wedged apart by T-shaped fracture
Fracture of lateral tibial condyle—"Bumper fracture"	**Loose bodies in knee joint**
It may be caused due to hit by car bumper on lateral aspect of leg. Fall with knee extended and bent medially is the commonest mode of injury. Often seen in individuals of >50 years. Lateral condyle is depressed associated with valgus deformity. Hemarthrosis is present. Often associated with tear of medial collateral ligament with or without tear of anterior cruciate ligament	**Types** • Fibrous: Traumatic, tuberculosis, syphilis, osteoarthritis • Fibrinous: Traumatic, tuberculosis, chronic synovitis • Cartilaginous: Meniscal injury • Osteocartilaginous: Osteochondritis dissecans, osteophytes detached, sequestrum, synovial chondroma, fracture of tibial spine • Others: Foreign body, lipoma, carcinoma **Diagnosis:** Locking; X-ray, arthroscopy, MRI
Stress fracture of tibia	**Fracture of shaft of tibia**
Common in athletes, ballet dancer compelled to give up intensive training due to repetitive gnawing type of pain. Incomplete fracture involving only the cortex often on medial aspect	Direct blow/ kick—mode of injury. Transverse/ oblique fracture, often with a open wound **Features**: Young patient not able to stand and take weight one side after a fall **Fracture of distal third**: More prone for non-union/ malunion due to poor blood supply because of few muscular attachments

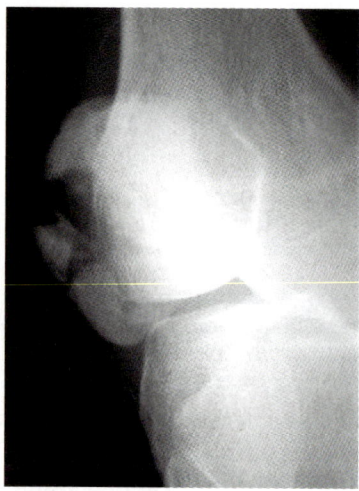

Fig. 36-32 *Patellar fracture.*

EXAMINATION IN INJURIES OF ANKLE JOINT AND FOOT

Ankle joint is a synovial hinge type with upper articular surface formed by lower end of the tibia including medial malleolus, lateral malleolus and inferior transverse tibiofibular ligament; inferior articular surface is formed by articular areas on the upper, medial and lateral aspects of the talus. Fibrous capsule, deltoid ligament and lateral ligaments are the ligaments of the ankle joint. Medial deltoid ligament is a very strong triangular ligament which has got superficial and deep parts; above it is attached to medial malleolus as common apex; lower attachments of superficial part are—tibionavicular, tibiocalcaneal and posterior tibiotalar and deep part are attached below to the anterior part of the medial surface of the talus as anterior tibiotalar ligament. Lateral ligament has got three parts—the anterior talofibular ligament; the posterior talofibular ligament; the calcaneofibular ligament.

Subtalar joint is talocalcanean joint between talus and calcaneum. Posterior part is the actual talocalcanean subtalar joint; anterior part is talocalcaneonavicular joint; two components are separated by sinus tarsi; but for all practical purposes, both components together termed as subtalar joint. Subtalar joint is a synovial joint causing *inversion and eversion* (each 20 degrees) of the foot. During inversion, medial border of the foot is elevated with sole facing medially. In eversion, lateral border of the foot is elevated with sole facing laterally. Inversion is accompanied by plantar flexion of the foot and adduction of the forefoot. Eversion is accompanied by dorsiflexion of the foot and abduction of the forefoot. Inversion is freer than eversion. Inversion is produced by tibialis anterior and tibialis posterior. Eversion is produced by peroneus longus, brevis and tertius.

History

History of tripping; falling or landing awkwardly after a jump; walking or running on uneven surfaces as the basket ball, volleyball players; a sudden impact such as a car crash; twisting or rotating or rolling the ankle are seen in ankle joint injuries.

Pain: It may be very severe and immediate in onset. The location of pain will give an indication as to which ligaments are injured.

Swelling: Most ankle joint injuries are accompanied by swelling. The site of the swelling may give an indication of the location of the pathology, but the degree of swelling does not always give a reliable indication of severity.

History of not able to put any weight on the injured foot should be asked.

Local Examination

Inspection

Observe the attitude or deformity, i.e. relation of the foot to the ankle—could be normal/equines/calcaneus/valgus/varus.

Swelling, bruising, open wound exposing the bones, shape, posture should be observed.

The relation between the two malleoli to be noted—usually the lateral malleolus lies 1 cm below and behind the medial malleolus. Medial or lateral malleolus becomes prominent if the foot is displaced laterally or medially.

The fossae in front of malleoli are observed—may become full in swelling of the ankle.

Ankle appears to be excessively broadened in *Dupuytren's fracture*—dislocation where the inferior tibiofibular joint is avulsed by the wedging of talus.

Posteriorly tendo-Achilles, any irregularity, swelling in its relation is noted.

Foot is observed for any swelling over the dorsum, any bruising, wound over the sole.

Palpation

The lower part of tibia, fibula and the two malleoli, head of talus and calcaneum is palpated for irregularity, swelling, tenderness and crepitus. Bony tenderness is elicited either by direct palpation or indirectly by rotating the foot. Squeezing of upper part of fibula and tibia together may elicit tenderness at the fracture site at lower end of fibula or lateral malleolus—*springing of fibula.*

The calcaneum is palpated with thumb and finger and is compared with the opposite limb for and discrepancy in thickness which is indicative of fracture; also, looked for tenderness.

The talus bone is difficult to be palpated unless when it gets dislocated in front of ankle.

Collateral ligaments are palpated on anterolateral aspect of ankle joint for any tenderness in ankle sprain.

Posteriorly tendo-Achilles is palpated for any rupture which is revealed by a gap in the tendon approximately 5 m above its insertion.

Test for rupture of tendo-Achilles: Patient is asked to stand on tip of toes. When there is rupture of tendo-Achilles, there will be a lag on lifting the heel.

Thompson's test: Patient is asked lie prone with the foot beyond the table. On squeezing the calf muscle, plantar flexion of foot is observed in normal individuals and also with those with partial rupture whereas with complete rupture there is no plantar flexion of the foot.

The tarsal and metatarsals are palpated for bony irregularities, tenderness, swelling and crepitus. Tenderness in metatarsals can be elicited by exerting pressure along the axis of the bones.

Measurement

Distance between medial malleolus to the head of first metatarsal bone and distance between lateral malleolus to the head of the 5th metatarsal bone and distance between malleoli and point of heel are taken on both sides and compared. These measurements give the idea about the displacements.
Length of leg is measured from medial knee joint line to medial malleolus. From the sole aspect, distance between the prominent point on heel to tip of greater toe and from prominent point on heel to tip of 5h toe is taken.

Movements at Ankle and Foot

Dorsiflexion (extension) at ankle* is 25°; *plantar flexion at ankle is 35°. Left hand is placed behind the lower leg; right hand is placed over hindfoot (not over forefoot as movements of midtarsal and subtalar joints are to be eliminated). Dorsiflexion and plantar flexion is checked with knee slightly flexed and heel off the ground.

> **Note:**
> **Forefoot** is metatarsal and phalanges;
> **Midfoot** is navicular, cuboid, 3 cuneiforms;
> **Hindfoot** is calcaneum and talus.
> **Subtalar joint** is between talus and calcaneum.
> **Midtarsal joint** (Chopart's) is between hindfoot and midfoot.
> **Lisfranc's joint** is between midfoot and forefoot.

Inversion and eversion is checked at ***subtalar*** joint (between talus and calcaneus). Patient lies supine and lower leg is supported by holding the ankle firmly with one hand to fix the talus; with other hand calcaneum is grasped to move over the fixed talus—turning in of the heel is inversion and turning out is eversion. Normal range is of 20°.

Abduction and adduction occurs in midtarsal joint (between hindfoot and midfoot—Chopart's). Calcaneum is held firmly with one hand; midfoot is grasped near bases of metatarsals and forefoot is deviated inwards to demonstrate adduction and outwards to demonstrate adduction. Normal range of each is 20°.

All active and passive movements are checked. Any abnormal, lateral or medial mobility is checked which indicates fracture of lateral/medial malleolus or lateral/medial collateral ligament.

Stress Test to Check the Abnormal Mobility: The ankle is placed in neutral position. With one hand the lower leg is held firmly from the front. With the other, the foot is held at the talus. By forceful inversion of foot, the integrity of lateral collateral ligament and by forceful eversion, the integrity of medial collateral ligament are checked. The yielding of foot, gap in front/behind/beneath the malleoli and point of maximum tenderness are noted.

Movements at the Foot

All active and passive movements of subtalar joint, metatarsophalangeal, interphalangeal joints are checked **(Figs. 36-33 to 36-37).**

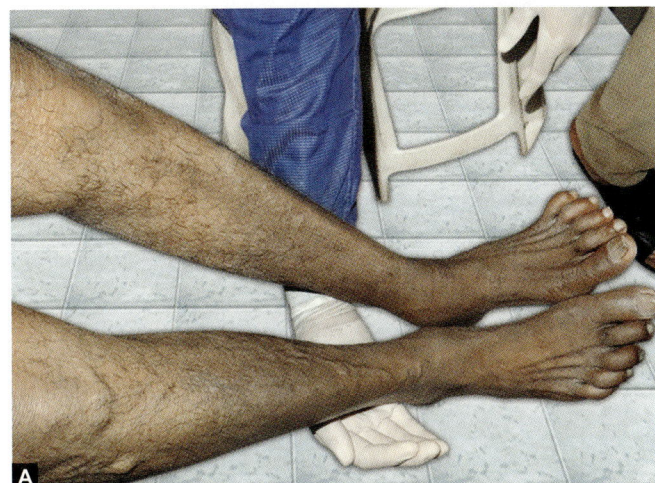
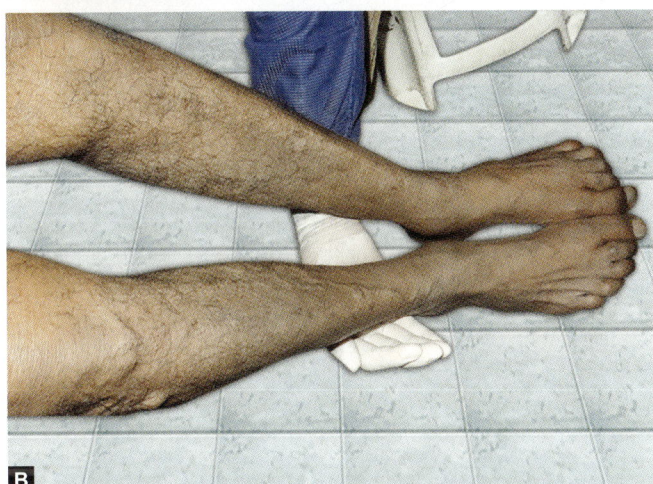

Figs. 36-33A and B (A) *Active dorsiflexion* ankle joint; (B) *Active plantar* flexion of the ankle joint.

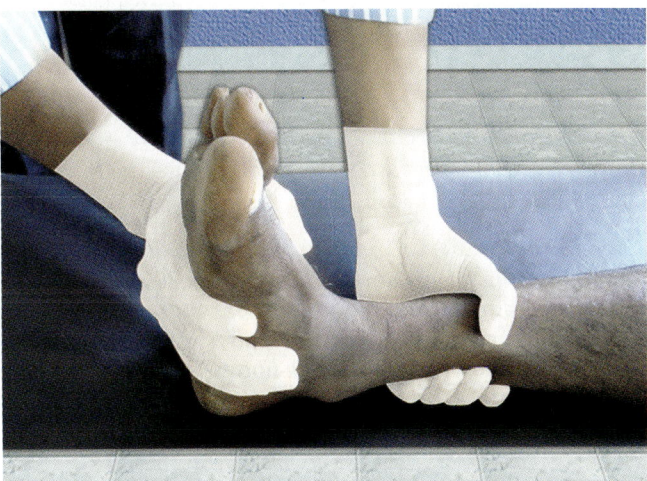

Fig. 36-34 Eliciting ankle joint movements—*dorsiflexion and plantar flexion.*

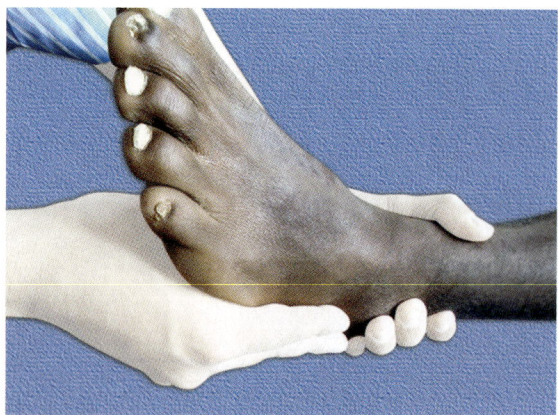

Fig. 36-35 Eliciting subtalar joint movements—*inversion and eversion.*

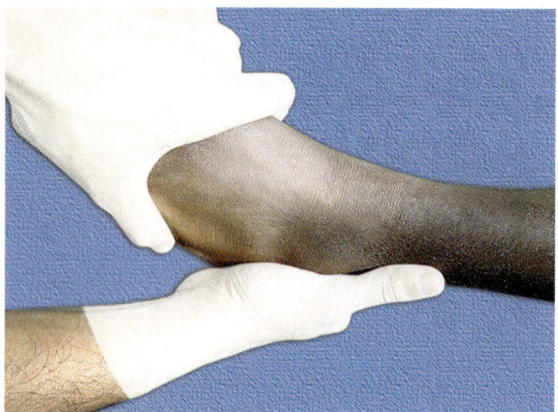

Fig. 36-36 Eliciting midtarsal joint movements—*abduction and adduction.*

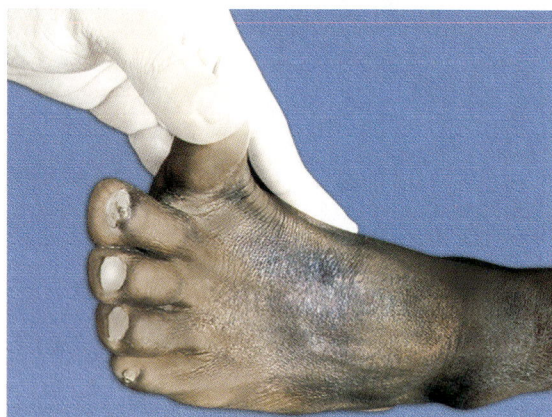

Fig. 36-37 *Normal dorsiflexion* of great toe is 90°.

Abduction injury: Transverse fracture of fibula 5 cm above ankle, avulsion of medial malleolus, avulsion of inferior tibiofibular joint with upwards displacement of talus.

Adduction injury: Vertical fracture of the medial malleolus, avulsion of tip of fibula.

Vertical compression injury: Fracture of anterior margin of lower end of tibia, displacement of foot upwards and forwards.

Different Types of Fractures of the Ankle

Chopart's injury	Fracture dislocation of midfoot involving calcaneum, talus and navicular bones
Lisfranc's injury	It is fracture dislocation between midfoot and fore foot involving metatarsals, often cuneiform and cuboid
Jone's fracture	Transverse fracture of base of 5th metatarsal bone by indirect violence
March fracture	Stress fracture that occurs at the neck of second metatarsal bone. History of unaccustomed walking/marching; pain and swelling on dorsum of foot
Tillaux fracture	Fracture of lateral malleolus with lateral displacement of talus
Pott's fracture	Fracture of both malleoli with displacement of talus
Dupuytren's fracture	Diastasis of inferior radioulnar joint
Trilamellar fracture/Cotton fracture	Posterior marginal fracture of tibia
Calcaneal fracture (Lover's fracture/Don Juan fracture) (Fig. 36-38)	It is usually due to fall from height. It can be split/crush fracture; can be displaced/undisplaced. Often associated with compression fracture of spine. Fracture often extends into subtalar joint. In compression fracture, upper surface of calcaneum is flattened. The angle between the subtalar joint with upper surface of the calcaneal tuberosity (normal is 35–40 degrees) is flattened to form a straight line

Investigation

Anteroposterior/lateral view X-ray foot and ankle is necessary. *Tuber joint angle* formed by a line passing over the nonarticular surface of the calcaneum and another line over the articular surface of talus which is normally 25–40°. MRI foot is often needed.

Injuries Around Ankle

External rotation injury causing spiral fracture of fibula, avulsion of medial malleolus, avulsion of posterior fragment of tibia with tibiofibular diastasis.

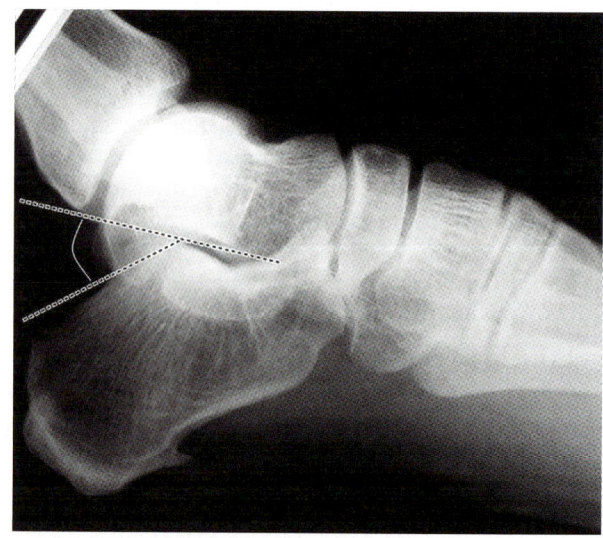

Fig. 36-38 *Tuberosity joint angle*—normal here. It gets reduced in compression fracture of the calcaneum.

37 CHAPTER

Approaches and Examination in Bone Diseases

Competency: PA33.1; PA33.2; PA33.4; OR10.1; OR7.1.

■ HISTORY

Age of onset of disease: Secondaries in bone and Paget's disease of bone occur in old age; multiple myeloma between 40 and 50 years of age; osteoclastoma 30-40 years; osteosarcoma 15-30 years; benign tumors of bone, fibrous dysplasia occur in adolescents; solitary bone cyst, acute osteomyelitis and osteogenesis imperfecta tarda occur in children; osteogenesis imperfecta congenita (brittle bone) occurs at birth.

Sex: Ewing's sarcoma and osteogenic sarcoma is more common in males.

Complaints and History

Swelling

Mode of onset: Spontaneous in benign bone tumor and chronic inflammatory condition (**Brodie's abscess**) whereas it is sudden in acute osteomyelitis.

History of trauma may be seen in osteomyelitis (acute/chronic) whereas in osteosarcoma any trauma may draw attention to the swelling.

Duration and progress: Swelling is of short duration and progresses rapidly in acute osteomyelitis; where it takes months in chronic osteomyelitis but years in benign bone tumors. Malignant bone tumors progresses rapidly with short duration of onset.

Pain

It is typical in acute osteomyelitis and malignant tumors. The *site and nature of pain* is asked—throbbing type in acute osteomyelitis but dull ache in malignant tumors. Benign tumors are painless, become painful on turning to malignant. Pain precedes the swelling by weeks to months in osteosarcoma but occurs simultaneously with the swelling in acute osteomyelitis. ***Often pain may be a first symptom in osteosarcoma before swelling appears***.

Fever

Fever is typical of acute osteomyelitis, where it is high grade with features of toxemia. Patient here is really sick. Low grade fever is seen in malignant tumor and chronic osteomyelitis.

Ulcer/Sinuses

Onset, duration and nature of discharge is asked.

History of similar swelling in other areas is asked—often multiple swellings are seen in diaphyseal aclasis.

History of disability: Inability to walk/stand/sit.

History of deformity: Shortening of limb, pigeon chest, manus valgus/varus, genu valgum/varum, enlargement of skull in Paget's disease.

History of loss of appetite, loss of weight: In secondaries in bone, tuberculosis.

Past History

Ear/skin/respiratory infections or typhoid, measles or tuberculosis or pneumonia should be asked.

Family History

Bone diseases like achondroplasia, diaphyseal aclasis, Marfan's syndrome run in families.

■ EXAMINATION

General Examination

Features of anemia/malnutrition/cachexia are looked for especially in secondaries and tuberculosis of bone. Features of syphilitic stigma is looked for. Features of toxemia: Fever, tachycardia, hypotension, rapid respiration are looked for in acute osteomyelitis.

Local Examination

Affected limb is adequately exposed under good light.

Epiphysis	Metaphysis	Diaphysis
• Epiphysitis • Osteoclastoma	• Acute osteomyelitis • Brodie's abscess • Tuberculosis • Osteoma • Chondroma, osteosarcoma • Bone cyst	• Syphilis • Ewing's tumor • Multiple myeloma

Inspection

Swelling: The number/site/(epiphysis/metaphysis/diaphysis) should be noted; which bone is involved; shape—pedunculated in exostosis/diffuse in infection/globular in malignant growth; surface appears regular in benign but irregular in chronic inflammatory condition and malignancy; any visible pulsations are looked for. Ewing's sarcoma, multiple myeloma and syphilis occur in diaphysis; acute osteomyelitis, tuberculous osteomyelitis, bone cyst and osteosarcoma occur in metaphysis; osteoclastoma occurs in epiphysis. Exostoses are pedunculated with a stalk towards the bone.

Ulcer/sinus: Note the site/number/edge/margin/discharge—bony chips from sinuses in chronic osteomyelitis with **sprouting granulation tissues**; blackish granules in actinomycosis. Discharge may be foul smelling. **Undermined edge with bluish edge** of neoepithelialization is seen in tuberculosis.

Overlying skin: *Red congested* edematous skin is seen in acute osteomyelitis; *tense, shiny, with dilated veins* in osteosarcoma; *multiple sinuses* with sprouting granulation in the skin are due to chronic osteomyelitis or with **undermined edge** in tuberculosis; *multiple healed scars* suggest previous osteomyelitis. **Deep and puckered scar** suggests earlier disease which has healed with time. Wasting of the muscle in relation to the bone or that particular limb.

Parts distal to swelling: Limb edema, *wasting of muscles*, joint above and below should be examined. Effusion is common in adjoining joints. Valgus, varus deformity can develop due to destruction of epiphyseal cartilage (knee or elbow). **Limb shortening or lengthening** can occur.

Examination of adjacent (neighboring) joints: Diaphyseal aclasis can cause deformed joints. Acute osteomyelitis can cause sympathetic effusion; or by direct spread across joint capsule can cause pyogenic arthritis. Epiphyseal destruction in children may cause shortening of the limb or deformity at joint. Valgus or varus deformities of the elbow or knee can occur.

Palpation

Local rise of temperature is seen in osteomyelitis and osteosarcoma (due to increased vascularity).

Tenderness is a feature of inflammation. Tenderness over metaphysis is seen in osteomyelitis; whereas in septic arthritis, tenderness is seen over the joint line. Tumors are nontender to begin with but later once it starts, infiltrating deeper structures become tender.

Swelling is **always fixed** to bone, **cannot be moved** apart from the bone. Its **location, size, shape** (diffused is inflammatory, pedunculated is exostosis, localized spherical may be bony tumor), **surface** (smooth in benign tumor, irregular in malignancy and chronic inflammation), **edge** (ill-defined in inflammation, well-defined in tumors) and **consistency** (is bony hard in osteoma, egg shell crackling in osteoclastoma, variable in osteosarcoma) are noted. Surrounding muscles and nerves are palpated to see for any infiltration that is seen in malignancy and sometimes in chronic inflammation. Highly vascular osteosarcoma, aneurysmal bone cyst, bone hemangioma, vascular secondaries (from follicular carcinoma of thyroid and renal cell carcinoma) are often **pulsatile. Thrill** may be felt through palpating fingers (it should be auscultated for bruit also). In acute inflammatory conditions of the bone, there will be surrounding soft tissue edema which pits on pressure; often due to severe pain and tenderness, it is difficult to feel the bone proper in such situation.

Detailed palpation of **ulcers or sinuses** should be done. Ulcer base should be palpated for induration, fixity/mobility.

The bony surface is palpated using thumb (gently run the thumb on the surface) to see for any gap due to **pathological fracture. Bony irregularity** should be checked which is common in osteomyelitis (pyogenic/syphilitic/tuberculous/Brodie's abscess).

Distal pulses, neurological examination (sensory, motor), *muscle power* both distally and proximally should be checked. Tumor neck of fibula can cause pressure over lateral popliteal nerve resulting in foot drop.

Percussion and Auscultation

Bony tenderness can be elicited by **gentle percussion** with finger or fist in long bones, skull, sternum and spine. Auscultation for *bruit* should be done in pulsatile or vascular tumors.

Measurements

Limb length and circumference are measured on both sides. Shortening occurs in epiphyseal destruction. Hyperemia in metaphysis causes lengthening. Muscle wasting is confirmed by measuring circumference and comparing to opposite side. Wasting is common in tuberculosis.

Movements

Both active and passive movements of joints, above and below should be checked. Joints are examined for sympathetic effusion, stiffness, any type of restricted movements. **Gait** should be checked.

Other Bones

Other bones in the body should be examined for generalized skeletal lesions (multiple exostoses, diaphyseal aclasis, osteitis fibrosa cystica of hyperparathyroidism, multiple myeloma, secondaries and rickets).

Lymph Node Examination

Drainage lymph nodes should be palpated. Its number, size, surface, consistency, fixity should be checked. It is significant in osteomyelitis and certain tumors which may spread to regional lymph nodes like Ewing's sarcoma; even though usual spread of malignant tumors is through blood (*commonest site is lungs*).

Other Relevant Examinations

Skin, mouth (teeth/tonsils), ear, sinuses are examined for infective foci.

Systemic Examination

Lungs should be examined for pulmonary tuberculosis or secondaries (malignant bone tumors commonly spread through blood to lungs); abdomen should be examined for similar reasons. Site for primary (***thyroid, kidney, breast, lungs, prostate, testis, GIT***) if bony lesion is to be suspected due to secondaries should be looked for. Spine should be examined.

■ INVESTIGATIONS

Blood and Urine

Total count (increased in osteomyelitis), ESR, serum calcium (raised in hyperparathyroidism, secondaries, sarcoidosis, myeloma), alkaline phosphatase (raised in osteosarcoma and Paget's disease), acid phosphatase (increased in secondaries due to carcinoma prostate), serum phosphorus, total serum proteins including serum globulins (multiple myeloma) are done in different situations.
VDRL, Kahn test for syphilis, blood culture in acute osteomyelitis, serum calcium, calcitonin, parathormone estimation in primary hyperparathyroidism.

Urine for albumin, Bence Jones proteins (urine of myeloma patient is heated and when temperature reaches 55°C it shows coagulation and on further heating beyond 80°C, coagulum disappears; events reappear while cooling also). But only 50% of myeloma patients show Bence-Jones proteins; false positive can occur in secondaries, leukemia and nephritis.

X-ray

Plain X-ray of the affected part both AP/lateral, sometimes oblique views are taken. It is not useful in acute osteomyelitis up to 10 days of onset of disease. It is useful in chronic osteomyelitis and all bone tumors, Paget's disease, Rickets, myeloma, hyperparathyroidism. In generalized disease, X-rays of multiple bones (rickets, generalized osteitis fibrosa, multiple myeloma) are taken.

> **X-ray bone should be commented on following aspects:**
> *General appearance:* (a) Shape (bent in malunited fracture, rickets, sabre tibia where there is faulty growth due to epiphyseal damage). (b) Density (increased in fluorosis, marble bones; decreased in osteomalacia, osteoporosis). (c) Architecture (soap bubble appearance in giant cell tumor, alternating areas of increased density with rarified area in chronic osteomyelitis)
> *Periosteum:* Usually not seen except in premature infants, periosteal hematoma without fracture, acute/chronic osteomyelitis, osteosarcoma where a typical Codman's triangle is formed, onion peel appearance of Ewing's sarcoma
> *Cortex:* Thickened in chronic osteomyelitis, Paget's disease; thinned out in benign tumor, aneurysm, cyst
> In Brodie's abscess, there is localized area of thickening around an area of translucency
> *Medulla:* Look for areas of rarefaction (single—in Brodie's abscess, solitary cyst, chondroma, osteoclastoma; multiple in multiple myeloma, carcinomatosis, fibrous dysplasia, tuberculosis); areas of increased density (single area—chondroblastoma, osteosarcoma, aseptic necrosis; multiple areas—secondaries from prostate carcinoma, hypoparathyroidism)
> *Calcified areas outside the bone:* Myositis ossificans, calcification in lipoma, fibroma

Chest X-ray is needed to see lung secondaries. But chest X-ray may miss 30% of secondaries where X-ray looks normal; if chest X-ray shows cannon ball secondaries often with effusion then it is confirmation of secondaries. If chest X-ray is normal still there could be metastatic disease in lungs and in such situation, CT chest is a must.

Other Relevant Investigations

1. Open biopsy is *ideal for bone tumors*. FNAC is done only in spine tumors. Even in spine tumors, especially secondaries and localized myeloma diseases, open biopsy is better.
2. Bone marrow study (*aspiration/biopsy* from iliac crest) is needed in multiple myeloma for plasma cells.
3. Discharge for culture, AFB, cytology is necessary.
4. CT scan or MRI: CT or MRI scan of the *local part* is very useful in identifying the extent of the disease in osteomyelitis or mainly in bone tumors. In malignant bone tumors, *CT chest and often CT abdomen* to identify metastases in lungs liver (systemic spread).
5. Angiography is needed in malignancy to identify the vascular invasion/encasement and in Paget's disease of bone. CT angiogram is ideal.
6. Radioactive bone scan: It is used in infective as well as neoplastic conditions. 10 µci ^{99m}Tc phosphate is injected intravenously. Scan is done in 4 hours (using gamma camera) to get the picture. Bladder should be empty while scanning pelvis. It is commonly used in assessing bone secondaries.

DIFFERENT CONDITIONS OF THE BONE

Conditions of the bone	Features
Acute osteomyelitis It is acute bacterial infection of bone caused by Gram-positive staphylococci, streptococci, Gram-negative bacteria like *Klebsiella, Pseudomonas*. Infection may occur through traumatic wound or hematogenous spread from a distant septic focus **Pathology**: Bacteria spreads to metaphysis of bone through metaphyseal vessels, releasing toxins, evoking inflammation — increases pressure in the metaphysis, compressing vessels which are end arteries resulting in suppuration and pus formation The pus spreads longitudinally into diaphysis; across the joint capsule causing septic arthritis; spread outward to reach subcutaneous plane – forms a swelling, which bursts resulting in discharging sinuses	Common in young boys, high grade fever, toxicity, pain in the metaphysic of bone, tender swelling, effusion in the adjacent joint, inability to move the limb **Investigations: X-ray**—no changes in initial two weeks; later widening of cortical margin with new bone formation; joint effusion seen; TC, ESR—raised; blood culture; MRI **Sequelae**: Septicemia, pyogenic arthritis, chronic osteomyelitis, limb shortening, disability, recurrent infection, chronic discharging sinuses. *Garre's nonsuppurative sclerosing osteomyelitis—rare with sclerosis* (Fig. 37-1) *Note:* Bone gets infected by Gram-positive and Gram-negative bacteria, *Mycobacterium tuberculosis*, brucellosis, typhoid and syphilis. Infection of the bone along with bone marrow is called as *osteomyelitis*. It can be acute or chronic
Chronic osteomyelitis (Fig. 37-2) It is chronic, recurrent bacterial infection and inflammation of bone and bone marrow usually of long bones; occurs due to trauma or sequelae to acute osteomyelitis **Pathology**: There is new bone formation (*involucrum*) with discharging sinuses with bone spicules in sinuses. Dead part of the bone within the infected bone is separated by granulation tissue (*sequestrum*)	Swelling with discharging sinus; bone pain and tenderness; thickening of bone; limb shortening; restricted mobility; and deformity **Problems**: Deformity; malignant change—*squamous cell carcinoma*; amyloid deposition; recurrence ***Brodie's abscess***—localization of pus in metaphysis; common in upper end of tibia and humerus; causes localized tenderness; swelling in the bone; can lead to pathological fracture; requires open drainage and curettage
Paget's disease of bone (Fig. 37.3) Also called as *"Osteitis deformans"* **Pathology**: Here there is increased blood supply to bones (vascular phase) due to which bone enlarges more than normal with laying of coarse layered abnormal bone (sclerotic phase). Though the bone is thick it is not strong, vulnerable for fracture. Common in femur, tibia, spine and skull. These bones are more prone for osteogenic sarcoma	Common in elderly male; thickening and increase in size of the bone; dull continuous pain; often pathological fracture; CCF due to hyperdynamic circulation resulting from increased vascularity in bone; paraplegia if vertebra involved; deafness due to middle ear sclerosis **Investigations:** Raised serum alkaline phosphatase; elevated urinary hydroxyproline; X-ray—dense sclerotic bone; bone scan-confirmatory
Rickets Here bone contains uncalcified bone matrix called *"osteoid"* **Causes**: *Vitamin D deficiency* prevents calcium absorption from gut. *Renal rickets*—excessive excretion of calcium in the kidney leads to less available calcium for bone calcification	Seen in infants; *ricketic rossary* in costochondral junction; bosselated frontal bone; triradiate pelvis; bowing of long bones; stunted growth. X-ray—confirmatory; serum calcium; serum phosphatase estimation. *Osteomalacia*—vitamin D deficiency seen in adults
Bone disease of hyperparathyroidism (von Recklinghausen's disease) Increased parathormone secretion by hyperfunctioning parathyroid glands or parathyroid adenoma causes calcium resorption from the bone replacing bone with fibrous tissue often with cystic spaces—also called as *osteitis fibrosa cystica*	Common in phalanges, jaw bones, skull bones; pathological fracture common; serum calcium raised; serum phosphorus lowered; serum alkaline phosphatase increased; serum PTH raised. Thallium scan shows hyperfunctioning parathyroids. CT neck/MRI –nodule in parathyroid. X-ray skull, hand and jaw—*salt and pepper* lesion
Osteoporosis It is reduction in skeleton bone mass leading to thinning of cortical margins, less dense cancellous bone. **Cause**: After menopause in women; old age; disuse due to lesser activity	**Problems:** They are more prone for fractures by minor trauma which is often unnoticed. *Common fractures*—Colle's fracture, fracture neck of femur, compression fracture of vertebra, intertrochanteric fracture
Scurvy Deficiency of vitamin C causes defective endochondral ossification with more unossified cartilages leading to hemorrhages and swelling in the epiphyseal region	Present with hemorrhages, swelling, pathological fractures
Osteogenesis imperfecta (Brittle bones) It is congenital inherited (recessive) disease with defective collagen synthesis leading to brittle bones which are more prone for multiple fractures in multiple bones	Multiple fractures, sclerosed ears (otosclerosis); blue eyes (blue sclerosis); ligament laxity; blood chemistry normal; bone histology normal *Osteogenesis imperfecta tarda*—occurs in puberty–autosomal dominant

Contd...

Contd...

Diaphyseal aclasia (Multiple exostosis)	
It is a growth disorder due to defective endochondral ossification with failure of remodelling of bone ends; commonly familial; Dwarfism is common	Exostosis is peduncle with cartilage as cap with bursa in between; grows away from the joint surface; common in lower end of femur and upper end of tibia, humerus
	Complications: Bursitis; compression of neurovascular bundle, restriction of joint movement; turns into *chondrosarcoma* (5%)
Achondroplasia (Fig. 37.4)	
It is familial congenital disease (autosomal dominant) where there is failure of normal ossification of long bones and skull bones	Long large head; normal trunk; short proximal part of the limb; lumbar lordosis; *trident hand and wide pelvis* side-by side. Mental impairment not present
Enchondromatosis (Oilier's disease)	
There is abnormal proliferation of cartilage cells of the growth plate into the metaphysis of long bones	It is often seen in bones of fingers, toes and other long bones. It also can turn into chondrosarcoma (5%)
Inborn defects of mucopolysaccharide metabolism	
Morquio-Brailsford disease: Flat vertebra, distorted hip, undue lax ligaments, keratin sulfate in urine	*Hurler's disease:* Mental retardation; cardiac and respiratory complications; derman and heparin sulfate in urine
Marfan's syndrome	
Defect in elastin/collagen formation; autosomal dominant trait; when associated with homocystinuria it is autosomal recessive	Tall undue lengthening of distal body segment, scoliosis arachnodactyly, high arched palate, dislocation of ocular lens, aortic aneurysm
Cysts of the bone	
Unicameral bone cyst (solitary bone cyst): Seen in children/adolescents; in long bones (proximal humerus) occasionally scaphoid/lunate. Cyst in the center of the metaphysis, vertically oval contains clear fluid	**Aneurysmal bone cyst:** Occurs in adolescents as a blown-out disease of bone of unknown etiology. It is a misnomer as it is not related to artery. Cyst is eccentric, expands under periosteum often under soft tissues containing connective tissues, vascular spaces and blood in fluid status
Features: Pain, discomfort, pathological fractures	**X-ray**—eccentric blown out look is typical and pathological fracture
Differential diagnosis: Brodie's abscess, aneurysmal bone cyst, hyperparathyroidism, secondaries	

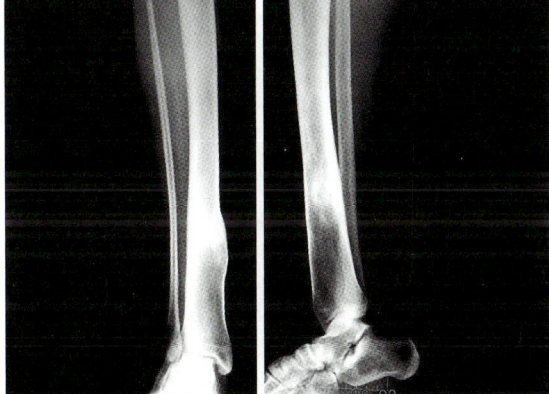

Fig. 37-1 *Garre's nonsuppurative* sclerosing osteomyelitis.

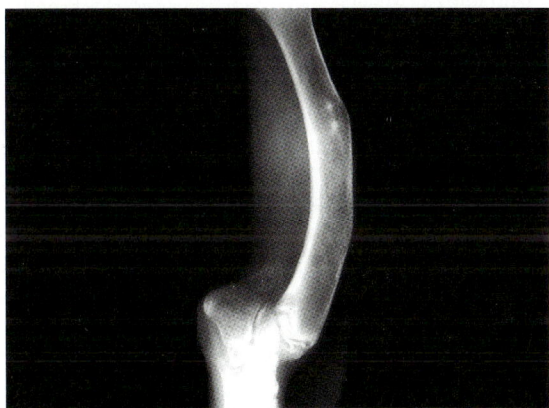

Fig. 37-3 *Paget's disease of bone*—tibia.

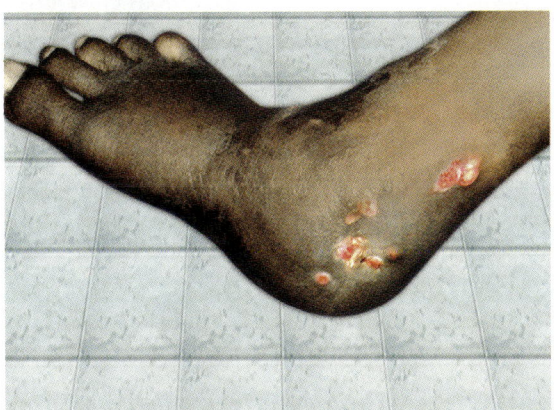

Fig. 37-2 Osteomyelitis leg and foot with *multiple discharging sinuses*.

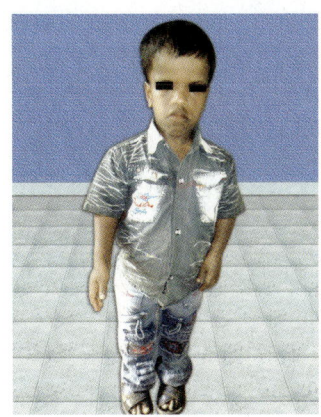

Fig. 37-4 *Achondroplasia*.

BONE TUMORS

It is either benign or malignant. Malignant can be either secondaries or primary. **Secondaries are the commonest malignant bone tumor.** Osteochondroma is the commonest benign bone tumor

Benign bone tumors

Osteoma
It is a benign tumor arising from the surface of a long/flat/skull bone.
Types:
1. *Ivory osteoma* is hard compact; usually occurs in skull bone like frontal bone/parietal bone; present like localized bony hard swelling which is nontender, nonmobile, with free skin over the surface; does not turn into malignancy; can be left alone

Indication for surgery: If cosmetically troublesome, frontal bone osteoma if extends into frontal sinus or orbital cavity

Differential diagnosis: Dermoid cysts or secondaries. (2) *Cancellous osteoma* is usually arising from spongy bone with a localized swelling. Features are similar to ivory osteoma

Chondroma
It is a tumor arising from cartilage.
Types:
1. *Ecchondroma* grows outwards from the bone; common in flat bones like scapula/ ilium or bones of hands and feet. In flat bones, they often reach large size. Occasionally may turn into malignancy as chondrosarcoma
2. *Enchondroma* is more common in bones of hands and feet. The affected bone expands from within with thinning of the bone cortex. Pathological fracture can occur. If this type is not troublesome, it can be left alone
3. *Multiple chondromas* in major long bones are called as *dyschondroplasia/multiple chondromatosis or Ollier's* disease. Begins in childhood as enchondromatosis in the region of the growing epiphyseal cartilages of many bones. There will be interference of the growth of the epiphyseal plates which causes shortening and deformity

Osteochondroma
It is the **commonest benign tumor** of the bone; begins in childhood from the growing epiphyseal cartilage plate. It grows outwards like a mushroom with stalk and the proximal part being bony but distal part cartilaginous like a cap often with a bursa in between. As the bone grows, tumor is left behind and therefore appears like migrating towards the shaft of the bone. Usually single but it can be multiple. Multiple osteochondromas involving several long bones is called as *diaphyseal aclasis/multiple exostoses*. Osteochondroma should be excised only after completion of the development of the bone.
Complications: It often can compress neurovascular bundle. Only cartilaginous component turns into malignancy —chondrosarcoma; Osseous part will not turn into malignancy

Osteoclastoma (Figs. 37-5 and 37-6)
It is often termed as *giant cell tumor*, occurs in ends of long bones from epiphyses often extends into the joint cavity; also, can occur in jaw either mandible or maxilla. It can be benign/intermediate or malignant (10%). *Malignant osteoclastoma* spreads into lungs through blood; forms an expanding tumor with localized swelling which is bony hard. It has got typical loculated appearance. Histologically, contains typical spindle cells with osteoclastoma giant cells. It can cause pathological fracture

Investigations: X-ray/incision biopsy and CT/MRI

Malignant bone tumors:

Primary malignant bone tumors:
Osteosarcoma (Figs. 37.7 and 37.8): It is the commonest primary malignant tumour of the bone; common in children/adolescents. Common sites—lower end of femur/upper end of tibia/upper end of humerus; arises from metaphysis expands outwards extending into adjacent soft tissues; spreads into lungs commonly through blood. Very aggressive tumor causing extensive destruction of bone with rising of periosteum with new bone formation
Features: Pathological fracture is common. Localized pain, swelling which is warm, hard, and vascular are the features.
Investigations: X-ray shows tumor in the end of the long bone with cortical destruction, *Codman's triangle, 'sun-ray'* appearance, pathological fracture; open incision biopsy; MRI of the lesion and CT chest to see secondaries

Ewing's sarcoma: It is highly malignant endothelial sarcoma of bone arising from bone marrow. It is soft, vascular tumor arising commonly from shafts of femur/ tibia/humerus; expands outwards with successive layer by layer of new bone formation; commonly spreads through blood into lungs
Features: Commonly occurs in children; presents as soft, vascular, firm, fusiform swelling in the shaft of long bones with warm skin over the tumor
Investigations: X-ray is typical *'onion-peel'* appearance

Contd...

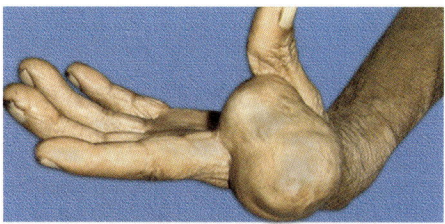
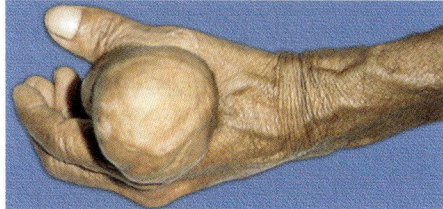

Fig. 37-5 *Osteoclastoma* of base of 1st metacarpal bone.

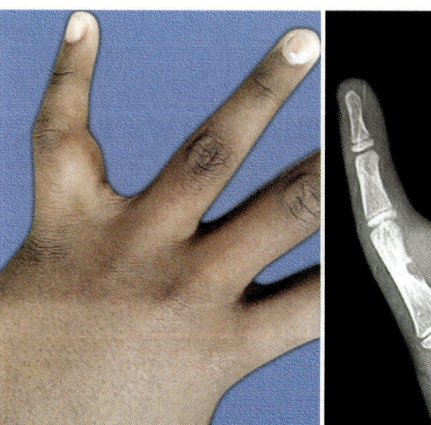
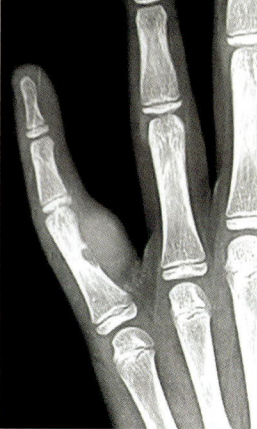

Fig. 37-6 *Giant cell tumor* of the flexor tendon.

Contd...

Multiple myeloma: It is an aggressive malignant tumor arising from plasma cells of the bone marrow. It mainly involves spine, skull, flat bones and ends of long bones

Features: Generalized pain and illness, anemia, bone pain, pathological fracture, neurological deficits often with paraplegia are the features

Investigations: X-ray shows multiple radiolucent areas in spine, pelvic bones, and skull bones; blood smear shows cart-wheel shaped plasma cells; *Bence-Jones proteins* are positive in urine of the patient; specific immunoglobulin will be elevated and is diagnostic; bone marrow biopsy is essential; radioisotope study of bone is useful

Chondrosarcoma: It is common in flat bones like ilium and ribs.

Features: Swelling which is slowly progressive attaining enormous size with dull aching pain is the usual presentation.

Investigations: X-ray shows lytic lesion or often with calcifications. It spreads to lungs through blood

Common primaries causing secondaries in bone are	Common bones involved:-	Types
• All sarcomas • Carcinoma kidney (RCC) • Carcinoma breast—70% cases in females • Follicular carcinoma thyroid • Carcinoma prostate • Carcinoma lung	• Vertebral bodies • Ribs and sternum • Pelvis • Upper end of femur and humerus	Osteolytic—common Osteosclerotic—carcinoma prostate Combined osteosclerotic and osteolytic **NOTE:** *In the bone; in the liver; in the brain – secondaries are the commonest malignant tumor*

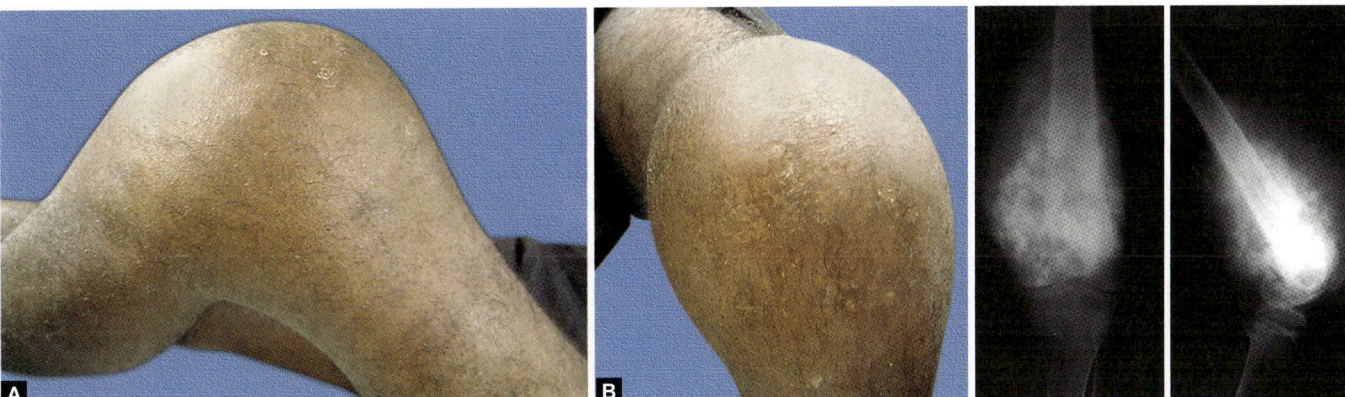

Figs. 37-7A and B *Osteosarcoma* of femur.

Fig. 37-8 X-ray femur showing features of osteosarcoma.

38

Approaches and Examination of Pathological Joint

Competency: OR5.1; AN18.7; MI4.2; IM7.10.

■ HISTORY

Age: Tuberculous arthritis is common in children and adolescents. Rheumatoid arthritis is seen in adults (30–40 years); gonococcal arthritis is seen in children, whereas osteoarthritis is seen in old age.

Sex: Rheumatoid arthritis, is common in females gout and gonococcal arthritis in males.

Occupation: Osteoarthritis is common among manual laborers.

History of Present Illness

Swelling

Exact site—when it was first observed;

Mode of onset—traumatic origin/spontaneous; it can be acute in onset with severe constitutional symptoms/gradual in onset with mild constitutional symptoms.

Duration of swelling is asked, it may be days in acute arthritis/weeks in tuberculous/months to year in osteoarthritis.

Progress of swelling has to be asked, it may be progressive in osteoarthritis/regressive in tuberculous arthritis or stationary.

Whether there are swellings in other joints.

Pain

Most pathological joints are painful, except Charcot's joints.

Site—exact site of pain, whether it is localized to one joint (acute arthritis), fleeting from one joint to another (rheumatoid arthritis).

Nature of pain—throbbing in nature in acute suppurative arthritis, dull in nature in chronic osteoarthritis, shooting in nature when it is neurogenic cause. In tuberculous arthritis the pain may be dull to begin, but in later disease with typical history of **'night cry'** in child which is sudden severe cramp like pain due to friction between the eroded articular cartilages in relaxed state of sleep. During day time, the movements are restricted due to muscle spasm, so not much of pain. Tightening type of pain in leg/**'girdle' pain** in trunk is seen in **Charcot's joint** (tabes dorsalis, syringomyelia, cauda equina syndrome, leprosy). Whether the pain is persistent type (neoplastic origin)/subsides after sometime (traumatic origin)/with remissions and exacerbation (as in rheumatoid arthritis). Whether the pain from a joint ***radiates*** to other part, e.g. from shoulder to arm, hip to front of thigh and knee. ***Relation to movement*** to be asked. Generally the pain increases with movement but pain in osteoarthritis decreases with movement. Here the patient complains of 'early morning pain and stiffness' which reduces with activities as the joint gets lubricated by the synovial fluid. Pain may be ***referred*** from one joint to another as the pain in hip joint is referred to knee joint.

Fever

High grade in acute suppurative arthritis; low grade in tuberculous arthritis/rheumatoid arthritis.

Skin Changes

Redness of skin is seen in acute inflammatory arthritis/acute suppurative arthritis.

Disability/Impairment of Function

Inability to walk/sit/stand is asked. Locking of joints is asked. Patient may also complain of limp which may be painless [poliomyelitis, coxa vara, congenital diaphragmatic hernia (CDH)] or painful (all traumatic, inflammatory condition of the limb).

Deformity

Flexion contracture/valgus/varus deformity in limbs.

Stiffness

Limitation of movements is seen in osteoarthritis/tuberculosis/rheumatoid arthritis.

In early stage of the disease it is due to protective muscle spasm but later it is due to intra and extra articular adhesion.

Past History

Past history of tuberculosis, syphilis, trauma, gonorrhea, diabetes should be asked.

Family History

Family history of hemophilia, gout, tuberculosis should be asked.

■ EXAMINATION

General Examination

Features of anemia, malnutrition, cachexia are looked for especially in tuberculosis of joints. Features of syphilitic stigmata are looked for.

Features of toxemia—fever, tachycardia, hypotension, rapid respiration are looked for in acute suppurative arthritis.

Gait is observed for any abnormalities. Gait may be '***antalgic***' type in arthritis where the limp is towards normal side, '***Trendelenburg***' type in unilateral congenital dislocation of hip and *coxa vara* where limp is towards affected side, 'waddling' type in bilateral congenital dislocation of hip and bilateral *coxa vara*.

Local Examination

Inspection

Affected joint should be inspected carefully and compared with that of normal side. Joints proximal and distal to the affected joint should be inspected. Inspection should be done from all sides.

Swelling of the joint: when present is inspected from all sides. It can be generalized (as in effusion) or localized (bursa or ganglion) swelling of the joint. The number, site, shape, size, surface, margin and extent are noted. Obliteration of fossae around knee, elbow and ankle indicates joint swelling whereas if the swelling extends beyond the joint, it suggests juxta-articular disease like cellulites. Fullness may be due to synovial thickening of the joint also.

Position of the joint/attitude: The joint may attain a position (normal/abnormal) in relation to the body due to pathological process. Joint when filled with fluid, takes the *position of ease/rest* so as to accommodate maximum fluid without tension/pain. It is plantar flexion and inversion for ankle joint; slight flexion for knee; slight flexion, external rotation and abduction for hip; slight flexion for wrist; flexion and slight pronation for elbow; slight flexion, adduction and internal rotation for shoulder.

Deformity (Fig. 38-1): The joints may acquire varus (adduction)/valgus (abduction) deformity (elbow—cubitus, hand—manus, hip—coxa, knee—genu, ankle—talipes) which is observed early in rheumatoid arthritis and tuberculous arthritis but late in osteoarthritis/neuropathic arthritis.

Note: Valgus—outward angulation from the midline of the body; *Varus*—inward angulation from the midline of the body.

Overlying skin: The skin overlying the joint is red, tense and glossy in pyogenic arthritis. Any scar/ ulcer/ sinus are observed especially in tuberculous arthritis.

Structure above/below the joint: Muscular wasting is marked in rheumatoid arthritis, tuberculous arthritis. In knee joint lesion wasting of quadriceps muscle, in hip joint lesion wasting of gluteal muscle is seen. Any swelling edema, deformities are observed.

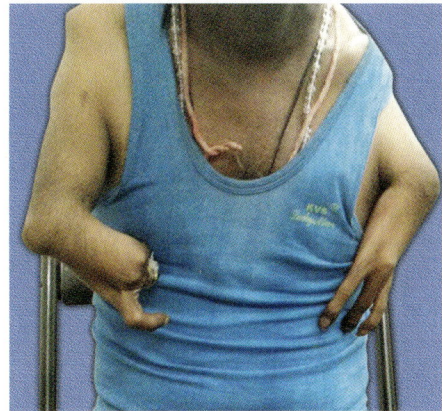

Fig. 38-1 Deformity of upper limbs in *bilateral radial club foot* with absence of thumb and radius. *Courtesy:* Dr Harsharaj, Consultant Orthopedician, Mangaluru, Karnataka.

Palpation

Temperature: It is checked over the joint using back of the hand, first on sound joint then on diseased joint. It is warm in acute suppurative arthritis and hemophilic arthrosis.

Tenderness: Whether it is uniformly tender all along the joint line (in acute pyogenic arthritis), over tendon sheath (in tendinitis), over bony attachments of ligaments (in sprain), articular end of bone (in fracture), should be checked.

Swelling: Palpate for the surface (smooth/irregular); edge (well defined/ill defined); consistency (soft in effusion, synovial thickening is confirmed by elastic/boggy/spongy nature); shape (joint effusion takes the form of the joint); fluctuation (can be elicited in the joint effusion). A cyst communicating with the joint is reducible (Baker's cyst). The synovial membrane which is often not palpable gets markedly thickened in rheumatoid arthritis/tuberculous arthritis, the edge of which can be rolled under palpating finger. The articular ends of the bone are palpated for tenderness, irregularity, crepitus, thickness. Loose bodies may be palpable in osteoarthritis.

Movements

Normal side should be examined first. Both active (by the patient) and passive (by the examiner) movements should be checked. When movements are checked, confirm whether it is painful or not; if so which movement is painful, angle in which pain appears and at which angle it disappears (if at all); presence of any protective muscle spasm (suggests active disease); presence or absence of restriction of movements, if present whether all movements or only certain movements are restricted; presence of any crepitus during joint movements (osteoarthritis) should be seen. Full range of all possible movements and if any abnormality in that is noted. Limitation of all movements is a feature of acute arthritis, whereas in Charcot's joint there is excess movement in all direction. Selective limitation in one direction suggests mechanical derangement, excess mobility in one direction suggest—rupture tendon/ligament.

Measurements

Length of each segment of the limb and circumference of the limb should be checked. It should be compared to opposite side. This helps in assessing the lengthening/shortening; wasting/ swelling of the limb.

> **Tests for stability of joint:**
> - For hip: Trendelenburg test; telescopic test.
> - For knee: Drawer test; abduction and adduction test.

Other Examinations

Auscultation: Crepitus of joint can be auscultated also.

Lymph node examination: Regional lymph nodes should be examined. In upper limb joints axillary and neck nodes; in knee and ankle inguinal nodes; in hip joint external iliac nodes are affected.

Other joints in the limb, and on opposite side and other parts of the body also should be examined to rule out polyarticular disease.

Systemic examinations like of respiratory system (tuberculosis), cardiac system (rheumatic fever), neurological (CNS) system (in Charcot's joint with tabes dorsalis or syringomyelia) should be done, urogenital examination to rule out gonococcal urethritis.

■ INVESTIGATION

Blood: Total count is increased in acute infection. ESR is raised in tuberculosis. Bleeding time, clotting time is altered in hemophilia.

X-ray of joint: To see articular surfaces, widening of space, loose bodies.

Joint fluid aspiration: For culture, cytology, AFB.

Synovial biopsy is very useful.

Arthroscopy is very useful and is diagnostic. It is not done in acute suppurative arthritis.

Gallium or technetium isotope scan is used in inflammation.

MRI of joint is very useful investigation.

Other tests: Blood uric acid, VDRL/Kahn test for syphilis; Rose Waaler test for Rheumatoid arthritis; Mantoux test for tuberculosis; FNAC of lymph node.

Diseases of the Joint

Diseases	Features
Acute pyogenic arthritis	
• It is acute infection of a joint caused by *Staphylococcus, Streptococcus, Pneumococcus* organisms either through hematogenous spread from distant focus or trauma. • Exudates may be serous, serofibrinous or purulent depending on the severity of infection. • Pus formation in the joint leads to destruction of articular cartilage which may track through the soft tissues and skin causing abscess and sinus. Often severe virulent infection causes septicemia and if not treated properly death may ensue. • Pneumococcal arthritis occurs in children due to spread from ear, throat, lungs, common in knee joint, often painless purulent joint is the presentation, aspirated pus is creamy green. **Chronic pyogenic arthritis:** It is due to chronic recurrent infection of the joint by gram positive or other bacteria Causes deformity, disability and eventually bony ankylosis of the joint.	Pain and swelling in the joint; restricted joint movement, diffuse tenderness, warmness, redness, and fullness over the joint; joint is in maximum ease position; spasm of the muscles adjacent to the joint. Active movement are absent and passive movement are painful. **Complications**: Destruction of joint surfaces leading to *bony ankylosis* (fusion of joint). *Arthritis* can occur in infants, in patients with gonococcal infection and also syphilis. *Gonococcal arthritis* is acute, polyarticular, occurs as blood borne infection after 3 weeks after primary infection (or once urethral discharge has stopped). **Reiter's disease:** Acute polyarthritis (with sacroiliac joint), nonspecific urethritis, conjunctivitis.
Rheumatoid arthritis	
Pathology: It is an autoimmune connective tissue disorder involving many systems including skeletal system. In joints, it causes inflammation of the synovial membrane which gets thickened, edematous, and vascular. Eventually, articular cartilage also gets involved in inflammatory process leading to formation of granulation tissue called as **pannus**. Pannus eventually extends to capsule, periarticular tissue and deeper bone surfaces. Finally joint ankylosis, muscle atrophy occurs. Common in women; It has many phases with remissions and exacerbations. Small joints of hand and feet are first involved followed by proximal joints.	Typical morning stiffness and pain; symmetrical joint involvement; restricted painful movements of the joints with effusion and swelling occur; flexion deformity of fingers and toes occurs often with "*buttonhole*" or "*swan neck*" deformity. In severe cases patient may be permanently crippled. Patient may present with carpal tunnel syndrome, tennis elbow, plantar fasciitis, rheumatoid subcutaneous nodules, vasculitis with ischemia or gangrene of fingers or toes, pleural effusion, pericardial effusion, muscle wasting. **Investigations**: X-ray shows narrowed joint space with subchondral cystic areas; high ESR; *IGM rheumatoid factor* is positive; synovial fluid shows high cell count (>10,000) and high protein (>5 g%); synovial biopsy is diagnostic; arthroscopy is very useful.

Contd...

Contd...

Osteoarthrosis	
It is a degenerative disease of the joint wherein there is degeneration of articular cartilage due to wear and tear. As there is not much of inflammatory reaction it is better called as *osteoarthrosis* not as osteoarthritis. There is fragmentation and fibrillation. Cartilage gets thinned out exposing the bone surface. Reactive hypertrophy is observed in peripheral margins of the bone surfaces which forms *osteophytes*. Ankylosis of joint is not common. **Types**: (a) *Primary osteoarthrosis* occurs in weight-bearing joints like knee, hip and spinal joints; common in old age, women, and obese individuals. (b) *Secondary osteoarthrosis* is due to other diseases in the joint like avascular necrosis, trauma and so on. It is due to mechanical incongruity of the articular surfaces; common joints involved are knee and then hip.	Osteoarthritis is a morbid condition; pain, stiffness, difficulty in squatting; muscle wasting, position of ease; restricted movements, disability; joint effusion and swelling; crepitations over the joint. **Investigations**: X-ray reveals narrowed joint space with subchondral sclerosis and osteophytes over the margins of the articular surfaces.
Tuberculous arthritis	
It is usually secondary to primary pulmonary or urogenital tuberculosis. Lower limb joints are commonly involved (hip/ knee). Disease can be osseous (hip) or synovial (knee) or combined (spine).	Common in children; night cry due to absence of protective muscular spasm during night sleep; all movements restricted due to protective muscle spasm; muscle wasting; cold abscess/sinus formation. Synovial thickening is common. **Investigations**: X-ray, fluid aspiration, ESR, Mantoux test, synovial biopsy. **Complications**: Fibrous (common)/bony ankylosis (if joint has secondary infection); disability, shortening of limb, cold abscess/sinus formation occurs later.
Ankylosis	
It is stiffness of joints. It can be intra-articular, true ankylosis or extra-articular, false ankylosis. It can be painless/painful ankylosis. **True ankylosis**: (1) *Fibrous*: It is due to fibrosis of two articular surfaces; seen in —acute or tuberculous or gonococcal arthritis, intra-articular hemorrhage. (2) *Bony*: Severe destruction of articular cartilages causes formation of bony trabeculae between the articular ends; seen in rheumatoid arthritis, suppurative arthritis, tubercular arthritis.	**False ankylosis**: It is due to fibrosis of extra-articular tissues near the joint causing limitation of joint movement. It can be due to—skin involvement (burns contracture); muscle contracture (Quadriceps/Volkmann's/myositis ossificans traumatic); fascial contracture (Dupuytren's); contracture of capsule and ligaments (fibrosis following prolonged immobilization); bony (excessive callous deposits causing bony block).
Gouty arthritis	
There is high serum uric acid due to more production or poor excretion. Urate crystals deposited causes acute painful arthritis. Later osteoarthritis of joint sets in.	First metatarsophalangeal joint (**great toe**) is commonly involved, later other toes, fingers, wrist and ankle. X-ray shows tophi in the joints and different parts of the body.
Clutton's joint	
It is seen in congenital syphilis with interstitial keratitis.	It is painless symmetrical synovitis commonly of both knee joints with wasting of thigh muscles.

Osteochondritis
Crushing osteochondritis:
Avascular necrosis of epiphysis of unknown cause.
Pain, spasm, irritability, deformity are the features.
1. Hip (humeral head)—Perthes' disease
2. Thoracic spine—Scheuermann's disease
3. Lunate bone—Kienbock's disease
4. Navicular bone—Kohler's disease
5. 2nd metatarsal—Freiberg's disease

Splitting osteochondritis dissecans:
Trauma causing avascular segment—splitting— loose bodies.
Common in adolescents.
1. Knee joint is commonest site. Medial femoral condyle is the site. Pain, tenderness, locking due to loose bodies is the features
2. Elbow is second common site. Capitulum of radial head is affected
3. Ankle is rare site. Upper surface of talus is affected

Traction osteochondritis:
Occurs at site where tendon is attached to epiphysis/apophysis.
1. At the attachment of ligamentum patella to tibial tubercle—Osgood Schlatter's disease
2. At the attachment of tendo-Achilles to calcaneum—Sever's disease
3. At the lower part of patella attaching to ligamentum patella—Johansson-Larsen disease

39 Approaches and Examinations in Pathologies of Individual Joints

Competency: IM7.13; IM24.12; IM7.5.

EXAMINATION OF PATHOLOGICAL SHOULDER JOINT

History

Pain: The nature, site, relation with activities, diurnal variation of pain and radiation of pain should be asked. The pain from the shoulder may radiate to neck, arm, forearm, and hand. Care should be taken to elicit any cardiogenic origin of pain which typically radiates through the shoulder along the inner aspect of the upper limb. Pain in the shoulder can also be supradiaphragmatic, subdiaphragmatic, and diaphragmatic in origin.

Stiffness of movements: Diurnal variations, seasonal variation and amount of restriction are all asked.

Swelling: History of joint swelling, its duration, progress should be asked.

Inspection

The patient should be stripped till waist exposing both the joints.

Attitude/Position

In effusion, the affected joint may be held by the side of the chest in the position of rest, i.e. slight flexion, adduction and internal rotation. In periarthritis, shoulder is held in adducted position whereas in deltoid fibrosis in abducted position. In Sprengel's shoulder, the shoulder girdle appears elevated due to high scapula.

Contour of the Shoulder

The roundness or contour of the shoulder is due to head of humerus and bulk of deltoid muscle. The deltoid bulge is examined from front side and behind. **Loss of contour** or **flattening** of **shoulder** is due to dislocation of head or deltoid muscle wasting as it occurs in rheumatoid arthritis, tuberculous arthritis, and rotator cuff lesions. Joint becomes more prominent and **rounded** in joint **effusion** (swelling extends beyond the anterior and posterior margins of deltoid and along long tendon of biceps, also fullness is seen in axilla) or **subdeltoid/subacromial bursitis** (a cystic swelling that lies only beneath the deltoid with normally palpable humeral head). It may also be due to old injury or tumor in the region of the shoulder where the swelling is localized to one side **(Fig. 39-1)**.

Skin Over the Swelling

Skin stretching, engorged veins, abnormal pulsation and healed or active sinuses especially over the axilla have to be looked for.

Any wasting of pectoral bulge is looked for.

Anterior/posterior axillary line and fold are observed for any deviation as they occur in dislocation of shoulder.

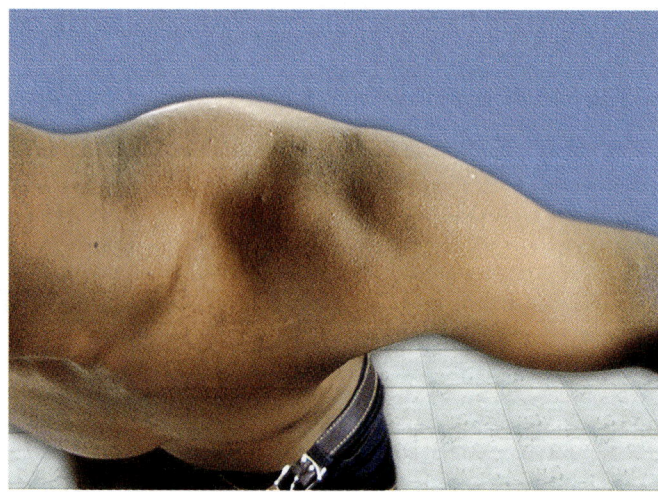

Fig. 39-1 Shoulder should be *inspected from all around*.

Opposite Side

Opposite shoulder, arms, elbows, axilla and neck should be inspected.

Palpation

It is done with patient *sitting* on a stool, keeping his arm beside the chest wall **(Fig. 39-2)**. It is best done by *Codman's method*—Left hand of the examiner rests on the right shoulder of the patient (and vice versa) and examiner stands behind the patient. Posterior part of the shoulder is palpated using the thumb placed along the depression below the spine of scapula. Index finger is placed just anterior to acromion (near insertion of supraspinatus tendon) to palpate the superior and part of anterior part of the joint. Other three fingers are used to hold the clavicle. Patient's flexed elbow is held with right hand and flexion and extension movements are done while palpating the shoulder. Tenderness in the joint and crepitus can be best elicited with this method **(Figs. 39-3A and B)**.

Examination of axilla: Examination of shoulder joint is complete only after palpation of axilla with fingers directed laterally, and going as high as possible in the axilla where the subglenoid synovial pouch of shoulder joint is reached. In joint effusion, fullness can be felt here.

Temperature: Local rise of temperature is observed in acute arthritis.

Tenderness: It is felt below the acromion process in supraspinatus tendinitis; in painful arc syndrome below the acromion process only during adduction; tenderness over coracoid process may be felt in certain other joint pathologies.

Crepitus over joint suggests osteoarthritis.

Palpation of subcutaneous tissue for any swelling is important. A cystic swelling beneath the acromion with normal axilla is suggestive of subdeltoid bursitis.

Swelling should be palpated and confirmed by palpating across axilla.

Effusion of the joint is fluctuant, bursa communicating with the joint is reducible.

Bony points: Tip of coracoid process (in front), tip of acromion (above and behind) and greater tuberosity clavicle should be felt.

Surrounding muscles are palpated for wasting and spasm.

In paralytic shoulder, as the deltoid mass is thinned out, the head of the humerus stands out prominent below the acromion, thereby a *'step'* is felt by the palpating fingers between the acromion and head of humerus.

Movement

Movements should be examined both from front and behind and compared to opposite side. Both active and passive movements are checked on both sides and compared. The shoulder joint movements are abduction (normal range 180°), adduction (neutral position as the movement is restricted by the chest wall), flexion (normal range is 90°), extension (is 45°), medial rotation (up to 90°), lateral rotation (up to 70°) and all movements together form circumduction. In flexion arm is carried forward and medially; in extension it is backward and laterally, in abduction laterally and slightly forwards. These movements occur at glenohumeral scapulothoracic joints, controlled by deltoid and musculotendinous cuff. Plane of body of scapula is not in the coronal plane of the body but 30° to this plane. Abduction and adduction occur in the plane of the body of the scapula whereas extension and flexion occur at right angles to this plane **(Fig. 39-4)**.

Active Movement

Abduction: Patient is asked to raise the hand sideways until it points the ceiling **(Fig. 39-5)**. Whether the patient shrugs the shoulder at the beginning of the act is noted which usually occurs in rupture of supraspinatus tendon. Beginning 30° of abduction is by the action of supraspinatus and it is difficult if this *tendon is ruptured completely*. If the arm is assisted

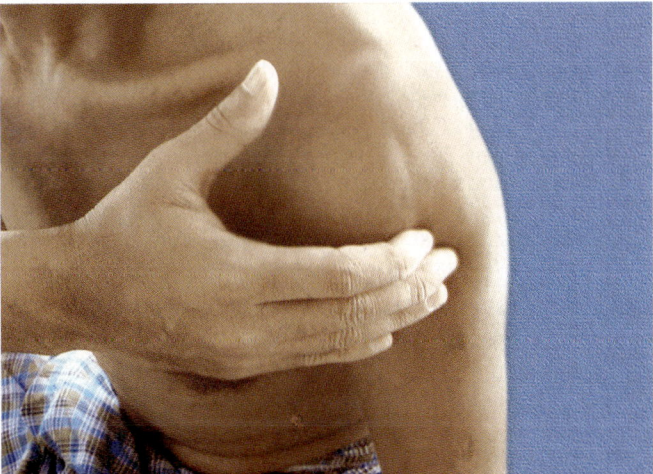

Fig. 39-2 Shoulder is palpated in *sitting position with arm on the side of the chest wall.*

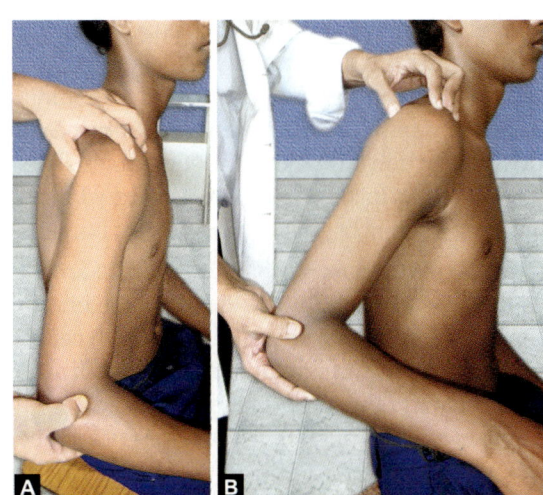

Figs. 39-3A and B *Codman's method* of shoulder joint palpation.

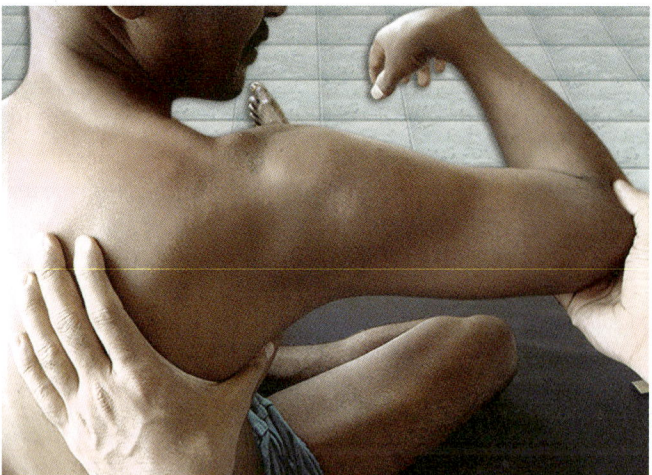

Fig. 39-4 *Passive movement* of the shoulder joint is done by fixing the scapula with one hand.

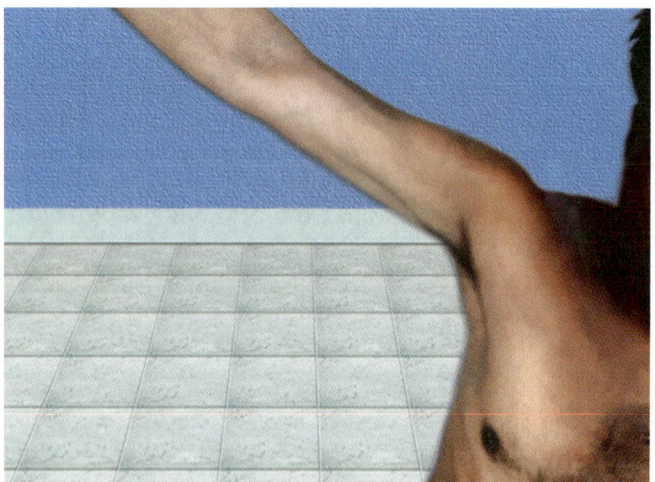

Fig. 39-5 *Abduction* of shoulder joint.

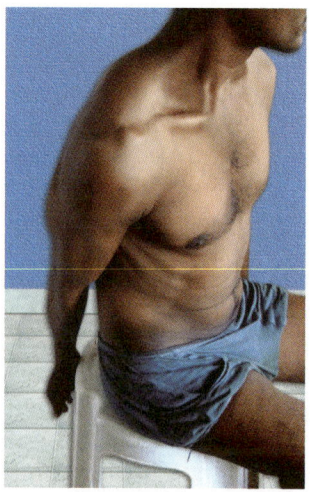

Fig. 39-6 *Adduction* of shoulder joint.

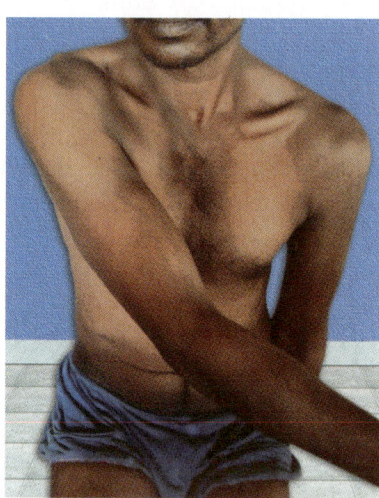

Fig. 39-7 *Flexion* of shoulder joint.

passively for this part's movement patient can then continue the remaining abduction actively beyond 30°, which is done by deltoid.

Mid-range abduction (60°–120°) is affected and painful in *chronic supraspinatus tendinitis* as degenerated tendon impinges between under surface of acromion and greater tuberosity of humerus—***painful arc syndrome***. Beginning and end of abduction is painless. It is sometimes also seen in subdeltoid bursitis, incomplete rupture of the supraspinatus tendon, crack fracture of greater tuberosity of humerus.

Entire range of abduction is painful in acute arthritis and acute supraspinatus tendinitis (localized degeneration of supraspinatus tendon in young adult often with calcification and acute edema causing painful abduction which disappears once calcified part bursts into subdeltoid bursa).

Sharp pain appears only when the arm is raised above the shoulder level (90°) in case of arthritis of acromioclavicular joint.

Note:
- In abduction, initial 30° movement is by shoulder joint alone; further up to 120°, for every 15° movement, 10° is from genohumeral and 5° from scapular movement. A good range of movement in the shoulder is still possible in presence of stiffness by the rotation of the scapula and clavicle. During abduction, scapula should be held firmly to find out the range of movement at the glenohumeral joint. Abduction and external rotations are most *commonly* affected in shoulder joint pathologies.
- *Arm-drop sign:* The examiner abducts the patient's arm to 90°, with other hand stabilizing the scapula. Now the examiner leaves the hold from the patient's hand, asking him to hold it in that position in air. In case of complete rotator cuff tear, the patient is unable to balance the arm and immediately drops it down.

Adduction: Patient is asked to move his arm across the front of the body **(Fig. 39-6)**.

Flexion: Patient is asked to bring the arm backwards **(Fig. 39-7)**.

Extension Patient is asked to move the arm backwards as far as possible **(Fig. 39-8)**.

External rotation: Patient is asked to flex his elbow to 90° and tuck it to the side of the body and then asked to separate the forearm **(Fig. 39-9)**.

Internal rotation: It is checked by asking the patient to scratch opposite scapula from behind **(Fig. 39-10)**.

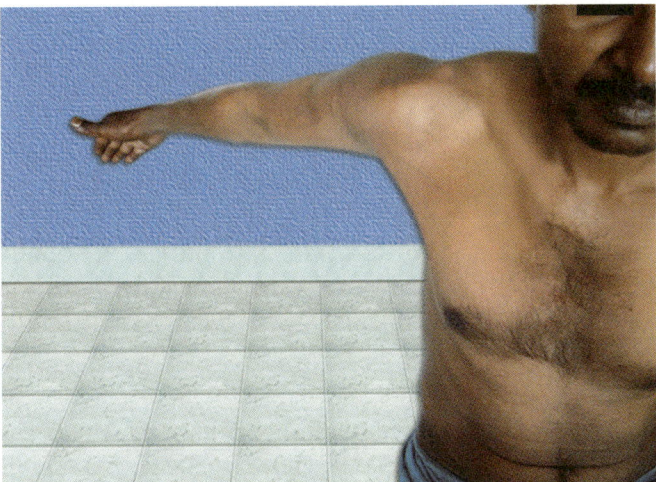

Fig. 39-8 *Extension* of shoulder joint.

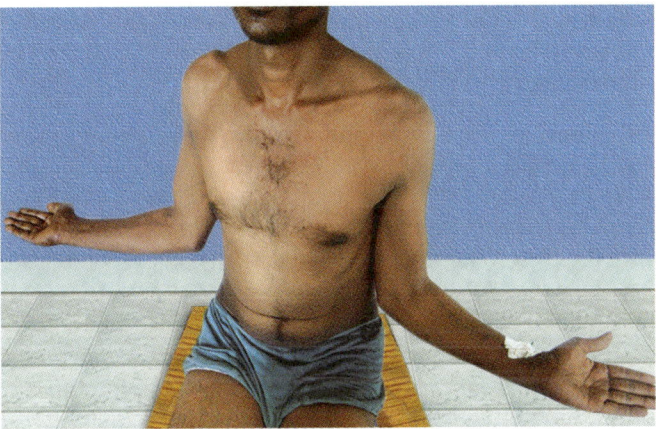

Fig. 39-9 *External rotation* of shoulder joint.

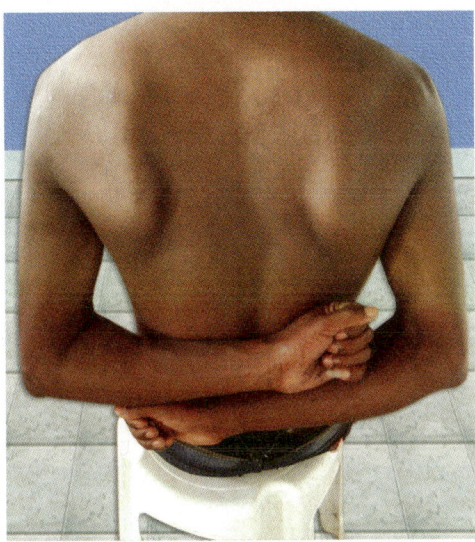

Fig. 39-10 *Internal rotation* of shoulder joint.

Passive Movements

This is especially done in patient who is not able to do the active movements specifically abduction. The initial active abduction is grossly limited in partial/complete tear of supraspinatus tendon and fracture of greater tuberosity where the passive movement is free and painless. The shoulder is anchored with other hand to check the movement occurring at glenohumeral joint. Passive abduction to nearly 90° is still possible even in completely arthrodesed joint.

Measurement

The linear and circumferential measurement of arm are done.

Examination of Acromioclavicular and Sternoclavicular Joints

The patient is asked to elevate the arm or asked to brace the shoulder backwards and forwards.

Investigation

X-ray of shoulder girdle along with upper third of arm—both AP/lateral view.
Aspiration of joint in effusion and the fluid are sent for cytological, biochemical and cultural analysis. Arthroscopy—to study the condition of synovium and articular surface.

Diseases of the Shoulder

Tuberculosis of shoulder joint	Rotator cuff
Causes restriction of shoulder joint movement is called as *'caries sicca'*. Often there will be cold abscess or sinuses called florid type	It is a tendinous cuff formed by subscapularis in front, supraspinatus above, infraspinatus and teres minor behind which fuse with shoulder joint capsule. Its injury restricts the abduction
Frozen shoulder	**Painful arc syndrome**
It is common in elderly women. There is adhesion between synovial membrane and joint capsule. • *Stage I*: There is pain more at night and with gradual progressive stiffness with restriction • *Stage II*: Pain gradually subsides but stiffness persists • *Stage III*: Disappearance of stiffness and regaining normal shoulder movements. Each phase lasts 6–8 months with total duration of 2 years	*Commonest causes* are—chronic suppurative tendinitis, incomplete rupture of supraspinatus tendon, subacromial bursitis and crack fracture of greater tuberosity. It is commonly seen in aged individuals, where there is *pain in mid-range of abduction (60°–120°)*. Pain is aggravated by movements; tenderness just below the acromion process is elicited. During mid-abduction a characteristic jerk is elicited. X-ray may show calcification just above the greater tuberosity

■ EXAMINATION OF PATHOLOGICAL ELBOW JOINT

Pain, stiffness and deformity are the main problems.

Inspection

Patient is asked to keep the arm by the side of the body with elbow extended and forearm supinated.

Attitude and deformity: The *carrying angle*, i.e. angle between the long axis of forearm and long axis of arm at the central point of extended elbow is noted. Exaggeration in carrying angle (*cubitus valgus*) or reversal of carrying angle (*cubitus varus, gunstock deformity*) are noted. The elbow attains the position of ease (slight flexion) in effusion. The joint may show varying degrees of flexion in different pathologies **(Figs. 39-11A to C)**.

The joint is inspected from front, back and sides. Biceps and forearm muscle bulge, cubital fossa are inspected from front. Any fixed flexion deformity and muscle wasting are noted. From back, triceps bulge, olecranon process, antecubital fossa, paraolecranon depressions are noted. Paraolecranon depressions are obliterated by joint effusion whereas fullness may be seen in the antecubital fossa in large effusion. Localized swelling over the olecranon is noted in olecranon bursitis **(miner's bursa/student's elbow)**. Any sinuses and scars are noted.

Palpation

Temperature: around the joint is raised in inflammatory condition—acute arthritis, olecranon bursitis.

Tenderness: Bony tenderness over the lateral and medial epicondyle is elicited by holding the patient's elbow at 35° and with thumb and middle fingers the two epicondylar areas are pressed. In lateral epicondylitis **(tennis's elbow)** and medial epicondylitis **(golfer's elbow, pitcher's elbow, baseballer's elbow)**, maximum tenderness is elicited at anteroinferior portion of epicondyles.

Palpation of the bone: The lower end of humerus, upper end of radius and ulna, olecranon are all palpated for any thickness, irregularity. On the posterior aspect, the relationship between the three bony points, i.e. medial and lateral epicondyle and olecranon are observed (they form a triangle in flexed elbow but fall in a straight line when elbow is extended).

Joint effusion first obliterates the concavity on each side of olecranon (as synovial cavity is nearest at this region and posterior ligament is thin and lax), eventually swelling is noticed over posterolateral part of elbow over radiohumeral joint eliciting *cross-fluctuation* when elbow is held in semiflexed position. In *triceps bursitis* two identical sacculation on either side of triceps is identified when elbow is held in 45° flexion.

Supratrochlear lymph node should be examined for enlargement—is checked in front of medial intermuscular septum 1–1.5 cm above the medial epicondyle with elbow in flexed position (90°). Unilateral enlargement may be due to infection but bilateral enlargement is seen in syphilis. Biopsy of the node is useful for diagnosis.

Ulnar nerve is palpated above the medial epicondyle, its thickening, beading and tenderness are to be noted. The elbow is held in semiflexed position and the pulp of middle finger is gently rolled above the medial epicondyle. The ulnar nerve is palpable as a slippery cord.

Surrounding muscles are palpated for wasting and spasm.

Movement

Movement at the elbow joint occurs at: (a) **Humeroulnar joint**—flexion (normal range 140°, where the soft tissues of forearm and arm touch each other), extension (where the arm and forearm almost lie in a straight line; in individual with lax elbow, there may be hyperextension of 15°–20°); (b) **Superior radioulnar joint**—supination (90°), pronation (90°). Flexion and extension are compared with that of sound side. Degree of limitation of movements, pain during movement any abnormal movements and are noted. Supination and pronation are checked by keeping the elbow at 90° by the side of the chest, wrist extended and fingers opened. Ask the patient to turn the palm towards sky (supination) and towards ground (pronation).

Snapping elbow: It is snap that is audible or palpable while flexing the extended elbow and vice versa, due to recurrent dislocation of ulnar nerve or medial head of triceps over medial epicondyle. This is due to hypermobile ulnar nerve or shallow groove over medial epicondyle.

Measurement

Linear and circumferential measurements of forearm and arm are taken from a fixed bony point on both sides and compared. Assessment of carrying angle—**already discussed in Chapter 36** (normal—10° in males, 20° in females).

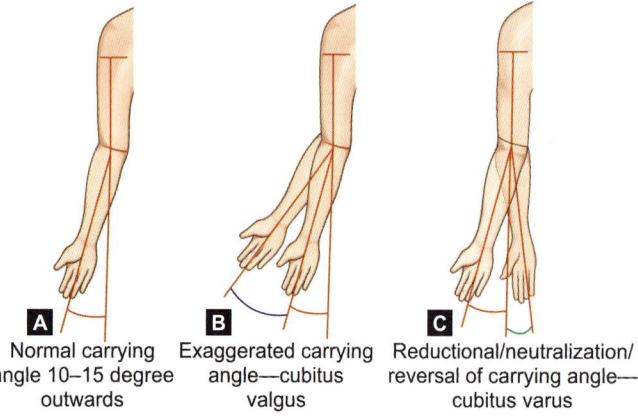

Figs. 39-11A to C *Carrying angle.* (A) Normal; (B) Cubitus vulgus; (C) Cubitus varus.

Diseases of the Elbow

Tennis elbow (Figs. 39-12 and 39-13)

It is **lateral epicondylitis** involving common extensor origin. It is due to repetitive stress, caused by overloading of *origin of the wrist extensor against resistance at the lateral epicondyle region*. Presents with pain, and tenderness that aggravates on dorsiflexion of wrist
Wringing test—the patient is asked to wring a towel which results in pain at the lateral epicondyle
Chair test—pain is felt at the lateral epicondylar region when the patient is asked to get up from the chair with both hands firmly gripping and pressing the arms of the chair.

Cozen's test—the examiner stabilizes the patient's elbow with his/her thumb while palpating the lateral epicondyle. The patient is then asked to actively make a fist, pronate the forearm as well as radially deviate and extend the wrist against resistance. Severe pain is felt near the lateral epicondyle
Mill's maneuver—while the elbow kept firmly straight and wrist flexed, patient complains of severe pain at common extensor origin when his forearm is pronated

Golfer's elbow (Baseballer's elbow)

It is rare, but similar to tennis elbow due to repetitive stress disorder **on medial epicondyle** at common flexor origin.

The test is similar to Cozen's test, but here the patient is asked to extend the elbow and supinate the forearm and later flex the clenched wrist against resistance leading to severe pain at medial epicondyle

Cubitus valgus

It is *increase in carrying angle* more than normal (male–10°; female–15°) with extended forearm showing excessive abduction in relation to arm.

Causes—previous fracture of lower end of humerus or capitulum with malunion, injury or infection of lateral aspect interfering with lateral epiphyseal growth. It causes angulation of the ulnar nerve medially with repeated friction of nerve leading into ulnar nerve palsy

Cubitus varus (Fig. 39-14)

It is opposite of valgus showing decreased or *reversed carrying angle* in extended elbow.
Causes—supracondylar fracture of humerus with malunion; epiphyseal growth interference on medial side.

It is less troublesome than valgus. It causes **gunstock deformity** in extended elbow with abducted shoulder. Internal rotation of radius over ulna may be limited

Elbow tunnel syndrome

It is a rare condition where the ulnar nerve is trapped as it passes between the two heads of triceps in or just below the ulnar groove especially in osteoarthritis of the elbow joint

Patient complains of tingling and numbness over the ulnar distribution area and considerable wasting of hypothenar muscles. Keeping the elbow tightly flexed for few minutes will precipitate the symptoms if the tunnel is tight—**elbow flexion test**

Students/Miner's elbow: It is effusion of the bursa over the olecranon process, whose pyogenic inflammation results in olecranon bursitis

Refer chapter 4—swelling

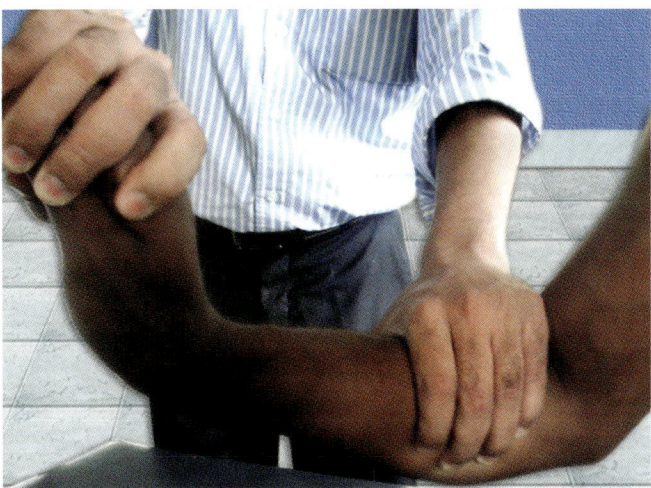

Fig. 39-12 *Cozen's test* in tennis elbow.

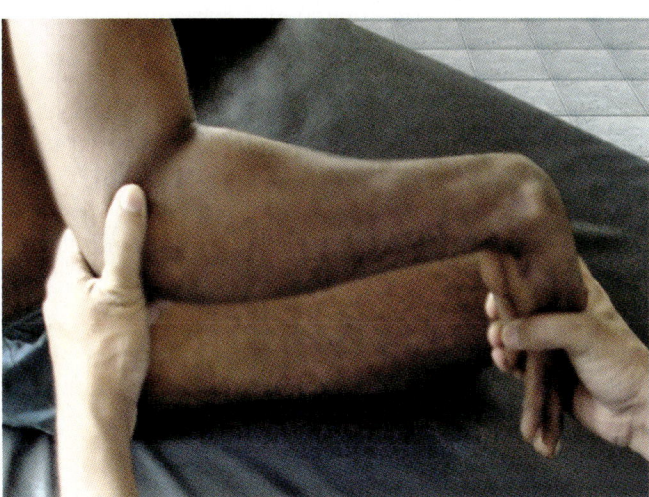

Fig. 39-13 *Mill's maneuver* used in tennis elbow.

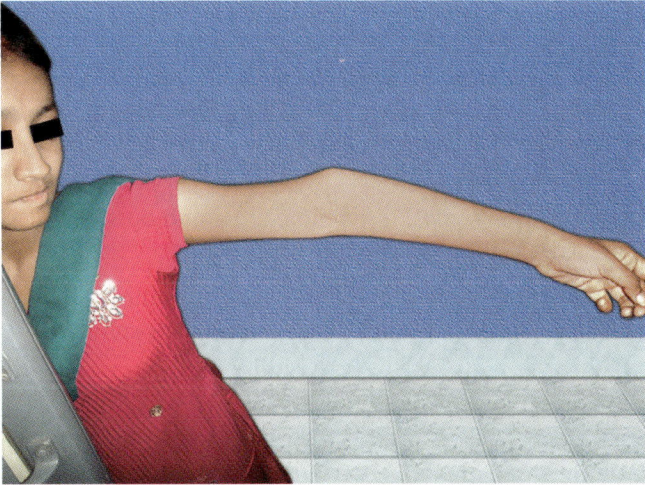

Fig. 39-14 *Gunstock deformity* in cubitus varus.

EXAMINATION OF PATHOLOGICAL WRIST AND JOINTS OF HAND

Patient may come with complaints of pain and swelling in wrist and fingers.

Inspection

Attitude and Deformity

In effusion, wrist attains a *position of ease*, i.e. flexion. In rheumatoid arthritis, there is flexion with mild ulnar deviation of wrist and fingers. In Volkmann's ischemic contracture, there is flexion contracture of wrist and fingers. In tendon sheath infection, fingers assume semiflexed position.

In congenital conditions of fingers, certain deformities are obvious—*polydactyly* (reduplication of finger, radial side is common), *syndactyly* (jointed finger), *arachnodactyly* (in the form of spider), *megalodactyly* (congenital hypertrophy), *macrodactyly* (enlarged digits) and *microdactyly* (small digits).

In rheumatoid arthritis, there may be radial/ulnar deviation of wrist with fingers, *swan neck* deformity (flexion at distal IP joint and hyperextension of proximal IP joint), *Boutonnierre* deformity, finger drop and hooding deformity in fingers.

Claw hand—due to ulnar—median nerve paralysis; hyperextension of metacarpophalangeal joints and flexion of interphalangeal joints.

Wrist drop—due to radial nerve paralysis.

Benediction attitude—due to median nerve paralysis; when patient is asked to make a fist the index finger remains prominently extended.

Swelling

It may be due to *effusion* in the wrist joint or in the tendon sheath. In the former, the swelling is present both in front and back of wrist and does not extend beyond the joint line whereas in latter the swelling is present on one side and extends beyond the joint line along the tendon. A compound palmer ganglion is a swelling on palmer aspect (sometimes on dorsum) extending beyond the retinaculum presenting as an hourglass swelling. A ganglion is a small round swelling on the dorsum sometimes on the ventral aspect of the wrist joint.

Any ulcer, sinus, scars visible in palmer and dorsal aspects of the wrist joint are noted.

Any bony prominence in the lower end of radius which is a typical site of deQuervain's disease and giant cell tumor is noted.

Spindle shaped swelling seen in proximal inter-phalangeal joint due to rheumatoid arthritis, gout; spindle shaped swelling along phalanx—*dactylitis* is seen in tuberculosis, pyogenic infection, enchondroma, syphilis and Madura hand.

Bulbous appearance of tips of fingers is seen in osteomyelitis, whitlow and hyperparathyroidism; nodular swellings on the dorsum of interphalangeal joints (*Heberden's node*) are seen in osteoarthrosis and Ollier's disease.

Palpation

Any elevation of **temperature** is noted suggestive of inflammation.

Tenderness along the joint line indicates arthritis.

Bony landmarks—styloid processes of radius and ulna are palpated for any swelling and bony projections.

Tenderness along the tendon sheath is seen in tenosynovitis.

Effusion in the wrist and compound palmer ganglion is cross-fluctuant. Ganglion when tensely cystic is not fluctuant and feels firm to hard in consistency.

The palmar and dorsal surface of the hand and fingers and webs are palpated for skin texture, tenderness and stretchability. Any nodules along the tendons are palpated.

Phalen's test (wrist flexion test): It is done for carpal tunnel syndrome. Flexing the wrist for 1–2 minutes causes the exacerbation of symptoms with paresthesia; but symptoms disappear once wrist is straightened. *Reverse Phalen's test* is similar but wrist is placed in extension position. **(For details about carpal tunnel syndrome, refer Chapters 9 and 10).**

Movement

The movement at wrist joint occurs at (a) *Radiocarpal joint*—flexion (70-80°), extension (80-90°), ulnar deviation (35°), radial deviation (25°); (b) *Inferior radioulnar joint*—supination (85°) and pronation (80°) *(Refer Chapter 27).*

Testing the dorsiflexion: Patient is asked to appose the palms and fingers of both hands as in Indian method of salutation *'namasthe'* and lift the elbow as high as possible keeping the hands apposed to each other. Angle on both sides are noted.

Testing palmar flexion: Patient is asked to appose back side of the hand and lower the elbow as far as possible. The angles on both sides are compared.

All movements are painful and limited in arthritis.

Diseases of the Wrist and Hand

de Quervain's stenosing tenosynovitis: It is degenerative thickening, inflammation and later stenosis of abductor pollicis longus and extensor pollicis brevis in middle aged women near radial styloid process in anatomical snuff box under common synovial sheath. Localized tender swelling may be present with painful thumb extension against resistance. Passively adducted wrist or ulnar deviated thumb causes pain. With the flexed thumb in the palm covered by fingers firmly, hand is passively deviated medially to cause pain at radial styloid process which shoots below to thumb and above to elbow—*Finkelstein's test*.

EXAMINATION OF PATHOLOGICAL HIP JOINT

History

Age: Congenital dislocation of hip occurs at birth; Perthes' disease from 5–10 years of age; slipped femoral epiphysis from

10-15 years of age; tuberculosis of hip at any age group can occur; rheumatoid arthritis—15-35 years of age. Degenerative osteoarthrosis and secondaries— in elderly.

Complaints

Pain: In front of the thigh, or groin, often radiating to knee, thus, misleading. Pain may be constant dull aching or night *cry* where the pain is severe at night due to absence of protective muscle spasm in relaxed state of night, as it occurs in tuberculous arthritis. Pain of short duration may be due to acute infection, arthritis or trauma whereas pain in chronic condition may be of longer duration with history of remission and exacerbation. Onset and progress of pain along with history of trauma, physical stress, infection preceding the pain should be asked which is often seen in rheumatoid arthritis. Exaggerating and relieving factors in particular to physical activity should be asked as they give an idea of nature of disease. Prolonged period of standing or walking may bring the pain.

Limp: A very important early symptom, can be associated with pain (tuberculosis hip, osteoarthritis)/painless (coxa vara).

Inability to squat: Due to painful spasm of the muscle around the joint or adhesions within the joint.

Inability to walk: Due to pain or structural failure (fracture neck of femur, polio).

Examination

Patient is exposed from mid thorax so that entire hip, pelvis and spine and visualized and examined under good light.

Inspection

Gait

If the patient is able to walk then the walking pattern should be observed which helps in diagnosis of the condition as the gait of the patient is altered in certain diseases of the hip.

Antalgic gait—seen in painful hip condition where the patient not able to bear the weight on affected side quickly takes the weight off the affected limb, and so he keeps the affected limb for a short time on the ground.

Trendelenburg gait—seen in hip with ineffective abductors, where the patient in order to avoid falling tilts the torso to the affected side. If the case is bilateral the gait becomes *waddling* type.

Short–limb gait—if the limb shortening due to some pathology is less than 1.5 cm, it will be compensated by pelvic tilt; shortening up to 5 cm is made up by equinus (walking on the forefoot and toes); if the shortening is more than 5 cm then the patient dips his body onto the affected side resulting in 'up and down' movement of that half of the body.

Stiff hip gait—patient walks without the normal 20° flexion at the hip, raising the pelvis and semicircumducting the limb.

Circumduction gait—in apparent lengthening of the limb as seen in hip in fixed abduction, the limb is taken in 'round about' fashion.

a. Patient should be observed initially in standing position from front, side and back

Attitude and deformity: Any flexion, adduction, abduction, lateral/medial rotation deformity of the hip is observed. Any compensatory mechanism of lumbar spine like increased lumbar lordosis to compensate fixed flexion deformity, pelvic tilt to compensate abduction and adduction deformity (as noted by the position of anterior superior iliac spine) is noted. In bilateral congenital dislocation of hip, there is undue protuberance of abdomen due to lumbar lordosis. Slight flexion of diseased hip is common. Patient bears his weight on sound side in arthritis. Any shortening of the limb is observed where there is flexion of the knee on the sound side or plantar flexion of ankle on affected side.

Swelling: Any visible **swelling on gluteal region**, groin and in the region of greater trochanter is observed. Its size, surface and edge number are noted. In hip joint effusion, there is fullness in the upper part of the femoral triangle. Cold abscess, sinuses and scar of tuberculous origin may be seen in groin, buttocks, and back of the thigh. Their exact location and number are noted.

Skin over the joint: Any asymmetrical skin grooves with additional grooves between the labia and thigh/duplication of gluteal fold is observed which is often seen in congenital dislocation of hip.

Wasting of the muscle (gluteal, thigh and leg) and muscular spasm are noted along with obvious lengthening and shortening of the limb.

Trendelenburg test: This test is done to demonstrate instability in the hip joint due to inefficiency of the abductor mechanism of the hip joint. Abductor mechanism comprises head of the femur with its socket which acts as a fulcrum, the length of the head and neck of femur that acts as a lever and the gluteus medius muscle that acts as a power. Inefficiency in any of these components leads to instability in the joint. Normally while standing both the legs bear equal weight of the body. While walking when one leg is lifted off the ground, the other leg bears the weight and there is inclination of the trunk towards weight-bearing side which is brought about by the abductors which thereby prevent dropping of the pelvis to the other side by gravity. Patient is first asked to stand on normal leg and lift the affected leg off the ground. There will be normal tilting up of the pelvis on the unsupported side. Now patient is asked to stand on the affected side and lift the normal leg off the ground. **The Trendelenburg test is said to be positive when there is sagging/dropping of the pelvis on unsupported side.** This test becomes positive in congenital/pathological dislocation of hip; destruction of head as in Perthes' disease, tuberculous arthritis, septic arthritis; fracture neck of femur; coxa vara; anterior poliomyelitis and muscle dystrophies where the abductors are weak.

b. **Patient is made to lie down on a couch as straight as much as possible and observed for:**

Fixed flexion deformity (*Hugh Owen Thomas* test): When limb is fixed in flexion, there will be lumbar spine lordosis and patient extends the limb by bending lumbar spine forward. The aim of this test is to remove this lumbar lordosis so that the flexion deformity becomes obvious and measurable. The patient is asked to lie supine on a hard surface with legs straight. This becomes possible in spite of flexion deformity by producing excessive lumbar lordosis which is confirmed by easily passing the hand behind the patient's lumbar spine. Now the sound hip with flexed knee of the patient is flexed towards abdomen until lumbar lordosis disappears which is confirmed by inability to pass hand behind the lumbar spine. As this is done diseased hip will automatically flex and form which angle between the flexed limb with the bed, is considered as *angle of fixed flexion deformity*. Forcible maneuver has to be avoided as it may lead to exaggeration of deformity. The test has to be repeated on opposite side **(Figs. 39-15A and B)**.

Fixed abduction or adduction deformity: Limb when fixed in abduction there will be scoliosis of lumbar spine with convexity towards affected side with downward tilt of pelvis and apparent lengthening of the limb. Limb when fixed in adduction, there is scoliosis of lumbar spine with convexity towards normal side with upward tilt of pelvis and apparent shortening of the limb. Line joining two anterior superior iliac spines (ASIS) is normally horizontal and right angle to midline. This line will be at lower level in affected side in abduction, deformity; higher in affected side in adduction deformity. **In abduction deformity**—the affected leg is held just above the foot, and is abducted till interspinous line becomes horizontal and angle at which line becomes horizontal is ***actual angle of fixed abduction deformity***. Similarly angle of fixed adduction deformity is checked by adducting the limb until line becomes horizontal **(Fig. 39-16)**.

Fixed medial or lateral rotation deformity: Normally lower limb is in slight lateral rotation with patella facing 5–10°

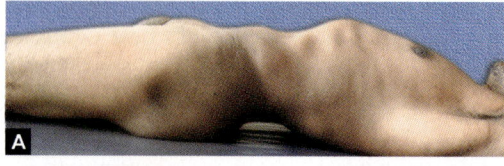

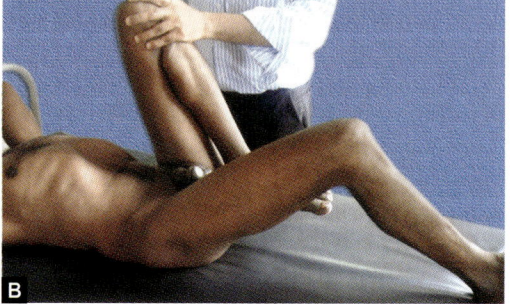

Figs. 39-15A and B *Fixed flexion deformity* of hip is compensated by lumbar lordosis. Angle of fixed flexion deformity is checked by flexing the normal knee and hip over the abdomen.

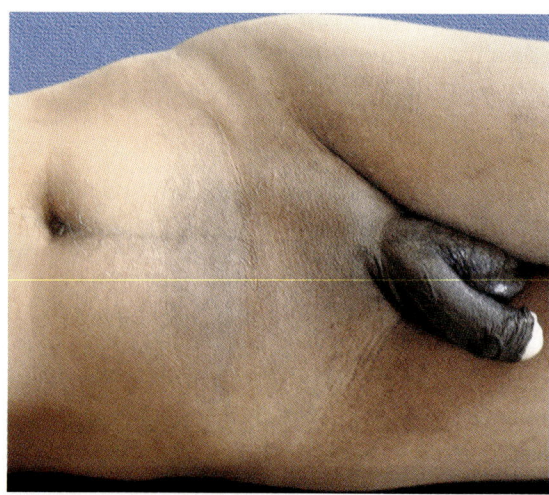

Fig. 39-16 *Interspinous line* should be made horizontal by adducting or abducting the limb depending on the adduction/abduction deformity to make the interspinous line horizontal.

outwards. It is clinically assessed by looking at the anterior surface of the patella or toes with foot at right angle to leg. If it is pointing towards the ceiling (i.e. facing inwards) it means there is medial rotation.

Palpation

Temperature: Rise of temperature over the groin or any swelling suggestive of active inflammation.

Tenderness: It may be elicited in and around the joint in inflammatory conditions. As the joint is thoroughly covered by muscles, direct access to the joint is not possible. By applying gradual pressure over the greater trochanter, tenderness can be elicited in the joint. In acute arthritis, tenderness can be elicited at a point lateral to femoral artery below the inguinal ligament that corresponds to neck of femur.

Swelling: when present has to be examined in similar way as any swelling—size, shape, margin, consistency, fixity to bone, tenderness, etc.

Fluctuation can be elicited in huge synovial effusion as in septic arthritis and cold abscess of tuberculous arthritis. Effusion presents as fluctuant swelling below the mid-inguinal point. ***Sites of cold abscess around hip joint***—medial to greater trochanter, medial to femoral vessels, in ischeorectal fossa that has come from central perforation of acetabulum towards pelvis later gravitated downwards to form sinus or fistula; gluteal region.

Palpation of femoral head: Normally located head is difficult to be palpated; however, it can be palpable below the inguinal ligament lateral to femoral vessels in anterior dislocation of hip; in the gluteal region in posterior dislocation of hip.

Palpation of greater trochanter: The shaft of the femur is palpated and the hands are moved up to feel the most prominent bony structure at the proximal end of the thigh which can be confirmed by moving the thigh. Often it is difficult to palpate in obese individuals. Dislocated head, myositis mass around the hip is often confused for greater trochanter. In malunited intertrochanteric fracture, trochanteric bursitis greater trochanter is thickened. Both sides are compared for the level by placing thumb over ASIS and index finger over greater trochanter and noting any difference between the two points. Bryant's triangle and Nelaton's line test also help in identifying any displacement of greater trochanter.

Palpation of muscle: Muscles of thigh and hip are palpated for any spasm and tenderness.

Palpation of femoral pulse: Femoral artery pulsation is felt against the neck of femur, which is absent in posterior dislocation of hip (*'vascular sign of Narath*).

Movement

Pelvis has to be steadied before checking the movement. Both active and passive movements are checked. Movements are checked first on healthy side then on the affected side.

Flexion: With the knee extended (tensed hamstrings), flexion of hip is up to 90°. With the knee flexed, flexion of hip is possible up to apposition of thigh to abdomen—140°. Flexed knee is held with the one hand and with other hand pelvis is grasped firmly over ASIS to prevent pelvic tilt and hip is flexed to assess the range without any movement at the pelvis. In fixed flexion deformity, Thomas test is done initially to find out the angle of fixed flexion. The patient is asked to hold the normal knee flexed and examiner keeps his hand below the lumbar spine. The affected hip is further flexed gently beyond the angle of deformity. This arc of motion from deformed position to the position of possible flexion is the range of free flexion of the diseased side. When hip flexion becomes limited, the pelvis starts tilting as the hip is forced beyond the limit of flexion which can be made out by the hand under the lumbar spine that feels the movement of spine. Completely fused hip can still show 30–40° of flexion which actually takes place at spine.

Extension: Normal range of extension at hip is 15°. When fixed flexion deformity is absent, extension can be tested by asking the patient to lie in prone position. The pelvis is steadied first and the hip is extended by lifting the limb. In the presence of fixed flexion, extension of hip is totally absent **(Fig. 39-17)**.

Abduction: The range of abduction is more in children—about 80°; it diminishes with age. It is about 45°.

Abduction in extension—in adults it is checked by holding patient's iliac crest with one hand, and with other hand, the leg is gently abducted; the range of abduction is noted without the movement of pelvis.

In children, the pelvis is first fixed by placing the fingers over anterior superior iliac spine (ASIS). Both the ASIS are brought to same level. The sound hip is abducted until the pelvis starts moving. It is placed at that position and the diseased hip is abducted until the pelvis starts moving. The difference in range of abduction in the hips can easily be assessed.

Abduction in flexion—the patient lies straight supine, with the lower limb placed together. Both the hips and knee are flexed simultaneously and the heels are brought towards the buttocks such that the soles rest comfortably on the couch. Now the patient is instructed to let his knees fall apart on both sides. The range of abduction is noted on both sides **(Fig. 39-18)**.

Adduction: normal range is about 30°. Patient is asked to lie on a hard couch. After steadying the pelvis, the patient is instructed to carry his affected limb over the other, first at lower third, next mid third later at upper third of the opposite leg. Normally it should cross the mid third of opposite leg **(Fig. 39-19)**.

Rotation: Normally there is internal rotation of 45° and external rotation of 40°. It can be checked as follows: When the hip can be extended—the limb is rolled laterally and medially by placing the hand over lower thigh. Or the extended limb is held at the ankle and rotated internally and next externally. By observing the patella the extent of rotation can be assessed. When the limb cannot be extended then the hip and knee are flexed at 90° and rotated internally and externally by rotating the foot **(Figs. 39-20 to 39-22)**.

All the movements are noted in detail along with which movements are restricted or exaggerated has to be observed. In coxa vara there is exaggeration of adduction and external rotation but restriction of abduction and internal rotation. In

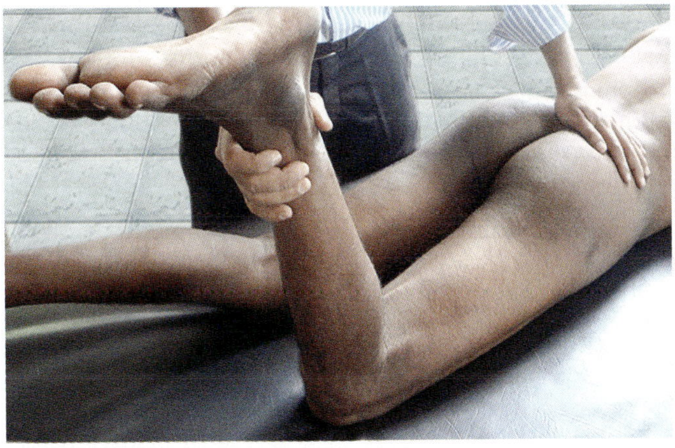

Fig. 39-17 *Hip extension* is checked in prone position with knee flexed (done when there is no fixed flexion deformity).

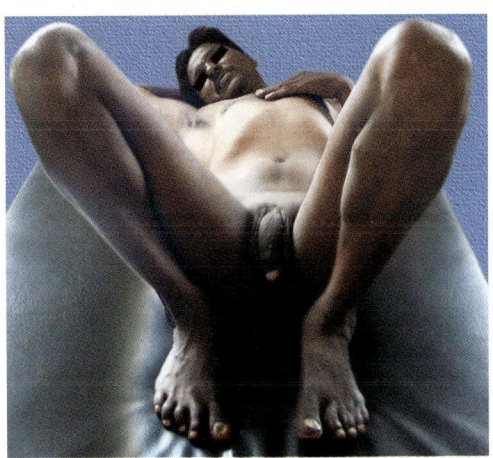

Fig. 39-18 *Abduction* of hip with flexed knees.

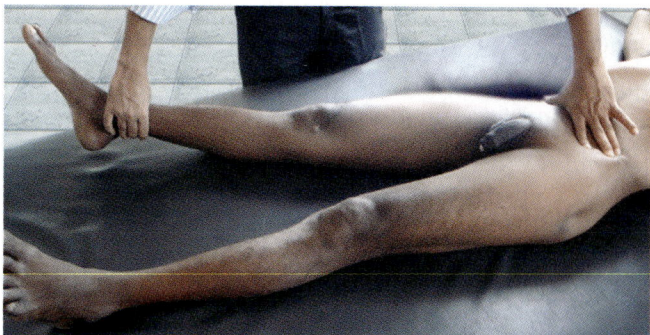

Fig. 39-19 *Checking abduction* and adduction of hip with extended knee.

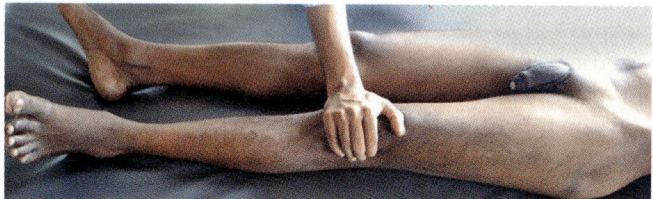

Fig. 39-20 *Checking the rotation* of hip with hip and knee in extended position.

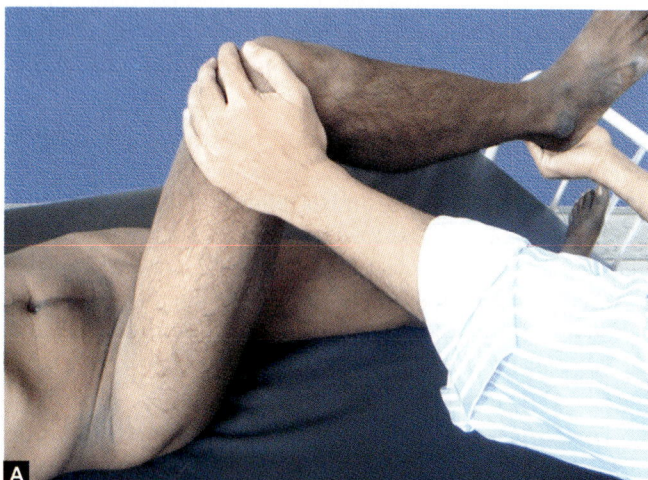

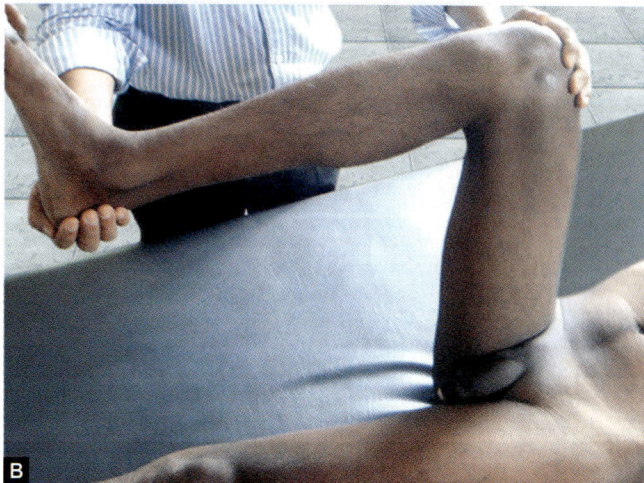

Figs. 39-21A and B *Checking the rotation of hip* in supine position with hip and knee flexed at right angle. This method is used in fixed flexion deformity.

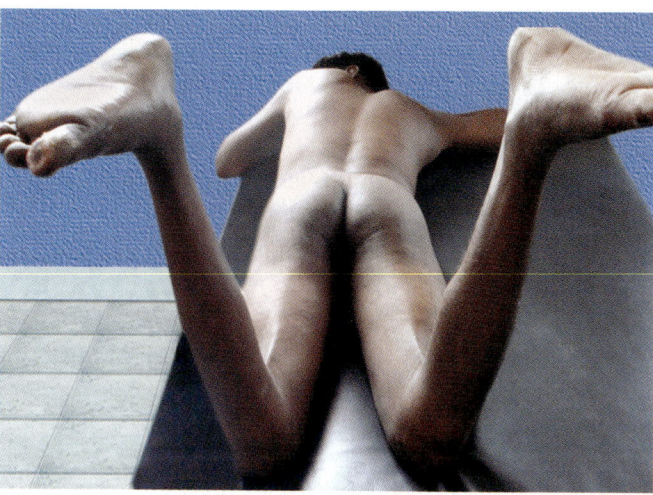

Fig. 39-22 *Checking the rotation of hip in prone position* with knee flexed at right angle, this method cannot be used when there is fixed flexion deformity.

Perthes' disease, there is limitation in abduction and internal rotation but other movements not affected. In CDH, there is excessive adduction, free flexion/extension but painless limitation of abduction. In arthritis, there is painful limitation of all the movements in hip.

Measurements

Length and girth of both limbs are measured.

Length: Both apparent and real lengths are measured. **Apparent shortening** means that the limb *looks* short due to fixed flexion deformity but is not really short. **Real shortening** means there is true shortening of the limb due to bone/joint/both components.

Measuring apparent length of limb: Both limbs are kept straight in bed and apparent length is measured as the distance between fixed point in the midline (umbilicus/xiphisternum) and tips of both medial malleoli irrespective of position of spine, pelvis or joints or the limb.

Measurement of real length of limb: Before measuring the real length of limb, both the limbs should be kept in identical position so that position of pelvis, spine or joints of limb should not affect the limb length. It is measured as the distance between two bony points—anterior superior iliac spine and medial malleolus. Whatever degree of flexion deformity and abduction deformity is present in diseased limb, the other limb also should be placed in that identical position before measuring the real length.

Segmental measurements of thigh and leg are to be taken. Length of thigh alone is measured from ASIS to medial joint line or adductor tubercle or upper border of patella **(Fig. 39-23)**.

Note:

- By flexing both the hips and knees to 90° limb shortening can be assessed by observing the level of knees.
- Shortening above the greater trochanter may be measured by drawing Byrant's triangle, Nelaton' line, Shoemaker's line's (**already discussed in Chapter 36 under injuries of hip joint**).

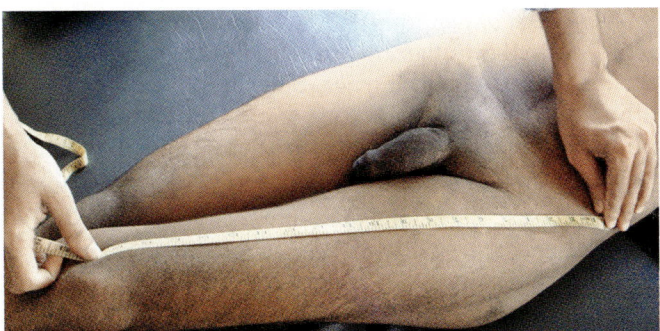

Fig. 39-23 Thigh is measured from *anterior superior iliac spine to the inner aspect of the joint line of knee.*

> **Shortening above the greater trochanter occurs in:**
> - Dislocation of hip (CDH/traumatic)
> - Coxa vara, (slipped femoral epiphysis)
> - Erosion of head of femur as in suppurative arthritis, osteoarthritis, Perthe's disease, tuberculous arthritis-3rd stage.

Circumference of the thigh is measured at a specific distant from anterior superior iliac spine and opposite side is also measured at the same level. It is done to assess muscular wasting.

Tests for Stability of Hip Joint

Telescopic test: Patient lies supine. Hip and knee are flexed to 90°. Pelvis is fixed with one hand closely adapting the greater trochanter with fingers over the buttock. With the other hand knee is grasped to push the thigh posteriorly along the axis of femur. The exaggerated posterior movement of greater trochanter is felt in unstable hip. This positivity is felt in dislocations of hip—Charcot's hip, old unreduced posterior dislocation, and loss of neck/head of femur **(Fig. 39-24)**.

Ortolani's test: It is done in neonates to diagnose congenital dislocation of hip. The child lies supine and both the hips are flexed to 90° and knees are kept in flexed position. Both thighs are gradually abducted and externally rotated and the spread up fingers press inwards and medially over the greater trochanter. A 'click of entrance' as the femoral head slips into the acetabulum and 'click of exit' while releasing the compression as it comes out is felt.

Barlow's test: It is done in infants to diagnose early cases of CDH and acetabular dysplasia. Both hips are flexed at 90° and knees completely flexed. Both lower limbs that are folded are held with both hands, placing fingers over the greater trochanters. Limbs are adducted completely with pressure exerted downwards along the axis of the bone to feel a clear click of dislocation of femoral head from the posterior margin of the acetabulum. Limbs are now gradually abducted with fingers applying inward pressure over the trochanter to feel a click again due to reduction of femoral head into the acetabulum.

Other Examinations

External iliac lymph nodes are palpated in hip joint pathology.

Rectal examination should be done to look for pelvic abscess in tuberculosis of hip.

Systemic examinations like that of respiratory system and abdomen should be done.

Investigation

X-ray: Both AP/lateral views are essential—helps to assess the condition of head, neck, acetabulum, neck-shaft angle, axial rotation of the head, and length of the neck.

Shenton's line—upper curved part of obturator foramen and the lower border of neck of femur form a continuous arched line. It is altered in pathological dislocation of hip, disruption of neck of femur, Perthes' disease and tuberculosis of hip.

Perkin's line, acetabular angle, Von Rosen femoral lines (See Congenital Dislocation of Hip) are useful in congenital dislocation of hip.

Diseases of the Hip

Congenital dislocation of hip

Disease is common in girls; common in Europe and Japan; rare in Negroes. Bilateral disease more common than unilateral (7 times).
Features: There is marked lordosis, anterior protrusion of abdomen, buttock protruding behind, and broadened space below the perineum in bilateral disease. *Waddling gait* is observed in bilateral case; *Trendelenburg gait* with pelvis lurching towards disease side is seen in unilateral case. If it is unilateral, grooves between thigh and labia are asymmetrical with additional skin crease which will be present on the medial side of the thigh. Abduction and rotations are limited; flexion and extension are normal; adduction is in excess

Stability of hip joint is lost here (*telescopic test, Ortolani's test and Barlow's test* are positive). Movements are painless. *Vascular sign of Narath* is present. In **X-ray**, *Perkin's line* helps in assessing the displacement (upper femoral epiphysis is above the horizontal line of triradiate cartilage and outer to vertical line along the outer margin of acetabulum), *acetabular angle* (widened from normal 22° to 45°), *Von Rosen femoral lines* (line of femoral shaft extending upward which normally touches acetabular roof will be displaced above into the pelvis) are useful.

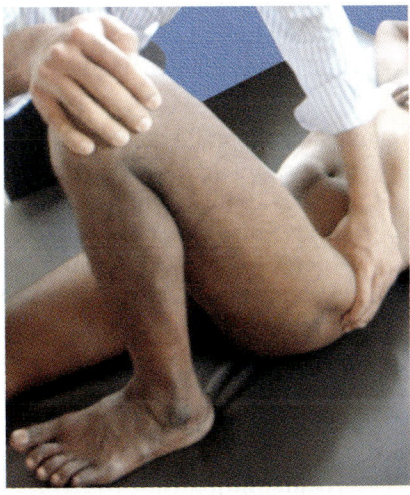

Fig. 39-24 *Telescopic test* for stability of hip.

Contd...

Contd...	
Slipped femoral epiphysis (adolescent coxa vara)	
It is common in boys between 10–15 years of age. Trendelenburg sign is positive. There is increased external rotation with adduction; but limitation of internal rotation and abduction. In **X-ray**, line from upper part of neck passes above the head instead of passing on superior margin of head as in normal (*Trethowan's sign*)	Metaphysis lies lateral to posterior acetabular margin instead of normal medial location (*Capener's sign*). Epiphysis is displaced backwards and downwards; *neck shaft angle is reduced* (normal in child 150°, in adult 127°). Lesser trochanter is prominent
Tuberculosis of hip	
It is 2nd common site of joint tuberculosis after spine. Pain radiating to knee, night cry, and limp are typical **Note:** Abduction is the first movement to be restricted in tuberculosis of hip. *Babcock's triangle* on the lower margin of neck close to head is affected first	**Stage I**: There is joint effusion with position of ease being flexion, abduction, external rotation with downward tilt of pelvis and apparent lengthening of the limb **Stage II**: Involvement of articular cartilage is seen with spasm of adductors and flexors causing flexion, adduction, and internal rotation and upward tilting of pelvis along with apparent shortening of the limb **Stage III**: There is erosion of upper part of acetabulum with dislocation of femoral head with spasm of adductors causing wandering acetabulum with true/real shortening of the limb with similar attitude like stage II
Perthes' disease	
Exact etiology not known. There is avascular necrosis of femoral head; common in boys of 5–10 years of age. Painless limp present, muscular wasting slight, shortening is trivial	Here abduction and internal rotation are restricted. Other movements are normal. Positive Trendelenburg sign; deformity, 10% are bilateral
Avascular necrosis of femoral head (AVN)	
When intraosseous microcirculation of femoral head is disturbed due to prolonged ischemia, it leads to osteonecrosis of femoral head	**Etiology**—after trauma, high doses of steroid therapy, renal transplant, cirrhosis, lipid lowering drugs, sickle cell disease, collagen vascular disorder, SLE, radiation therapy and cancer chemotherapy
Osteoarthritis of hip	
Here pain, stiffness, limp, wasting of glutei, limitations of all movements with *X-ray showing osteophytes* is the presentation	Causes are—trauma, Perthes' disease, tuberculosis, slipped epiphysis, etc.

■ EXAMINATION IN PATHOLOGICAL KNEE JOINT

History

Pain, stiffness, swelling, deformity, limp, locking, feeling of give away and click are the commonest complaints in knee joint pathologies.

Mode of onset of symptoms: Traumatic (fracture or ligament injury)/infective/inflammatory/spontaneous. In recurrent swelling of knee in young age, one should ask the history of bleeding disorders. History of pain simultaneously in other joints has to be asked (gout/rheumatoid arthritis). In traumatic cause, the nature of violence should be asked.

Duration—usually of long duration.

Progress of symptoms—intermittent, gradually progressive, gradually regressive.

Deformity—most deformities associated with arthritis are painful, painless deformity occurs in polio and cerebral palsy. Deformity in arthritis is flexion, however, varus/valgus deformity can do occur. Recurvatum deformity occurs in polio and fracture in the knee region.

Examination

Inspection

Whole limb is exposed from pelvis to toes. Patient is examined in standing and lying down position.

Gait: Recurvatum deformity is best appreciated when patient walks.

Hand-knee gait—patient with weakness in quadriceps supports his knee on the front with his hand when he takes weight on the body.

Both knee joints are inspected from all sides, first in supine then in prone position.

Deformity and attitude: Knee joint assumes the position of ease in painful conditions—moderate flexion, which is due to spasm of hamstring muscle but later due to contracture of the capsule and other structure around the joint.

Typical deformities of genu varum (abnormal adduction) or valgum (abnormal abduction) or recurvatum (hyperextension) are observed. **The typical triple displacement**—flexion, posterior subluxation and lateral rotation of tibia occur in neglected case of tuberculous arthritis or septic arthritis. Position of patella is a good indicator of the deformity.

Locking: It is flexion deformity in the knee joint; true locking—terminal 15–20° of extension is not possible (due to miniscal tear), pseudo-locking—locking due to hamstring muscle spasm, osteoarthritis, loose bodies. Locking due to loose body occurs at different position of the knee.

Swelling: Joint effusion obliterates all hollowness around the patella causing horseshoe-shaped swelling. Bilateral knee joint effusion is seen in Clutton's syphilitic joint, hemophilia and bilateral trauma. Localized painless swelling in the popliteal fossa which becomes prominent and tense on extension—*semimembranous bursa*. Other extra-articular swellings like prepatellar bursa (*housemaid's knee*—between skin and patella), infrapatellar bursa (*Clergyman's knee*—between skin and lower part of patellar ligament), **Morrant Baker's cyst** (posterior herniation of synovial membrane through oblique popliteal ligament in midline at lower part of the popliteal fossa, below the joint line which is more obvious on extension and disappears on flexion, is due to underlying osteoarthritis with effusion). ***Cyst of the lateral semilunar cartilage*** is on only one side (lateral) of ligamentum patellae. ***Suprapatellar bursa,*** as it communicates with the joint, becomes prominent during joint effusion.

Muscle wasting above (quadriceps) and below (calf muscles) the knee joint has to be observed.

Any obvious shortening of the leg is noted.

The skin around the knee joint is observed for sinuses, ulcers, scars of sinuses and wound. The skin is stretched and shiny in effusion and inflammation.

Palpation

Temperature: The skin over the joint is felt for raise of temperature often seen in inflammatory condition.

Tenderness: The joint is also palpated for *tenderness*. Diffused tenderness is present in infective arthritis. In meniscus tears and osteoarthritis, tenderness is elicited on medial/lateral aspect of the joint line. Tenderness is elicited systematically by palpating the patellar tendon, medial and lateral collateral ligament and different parts of the bone.

Swelling: It may be due to fluid accumulation or synovial thickening, or bony thickening. It is examined as any other swelling for surface, edge and consistency.

Consistency: Inflammatory swelling pits on pressure. Cystic swelling and effusion are soft in consistency.

Cross-fluctuation: This helps to detect effusion in the joint. When there is adequate fluid in the joint, it fills up the suprapatellar pouch. By applying constant downward and backward pressure over the suprapatellar region with one hand, impulse will be felt by the fingers and thumb kept on either side of patella or ligamentum patellae **(Fig. 39-25)**.

Patellar tap: The knee is fully extended and suprapatellar pouch is emptied by pressing it with one hand. The fluid now comes to lie between the patella and femoral condyles and, thus, lifts the patella .When patella is sharply pressed or tapped downwards, one can feel it hitting the femoral condyles and spring back. However, this becomes negative in massive effusion where the patella fails to hit the condyles or when effusion is too minimal to lift the patella.

In case of small effusion, pressure is applied over the obliterated hollow on the one side of the patella and the filling on the other side is watched. On release of the pressure, the refilling of the hollow by the fluid occurs **(Figs. 39-26A and B)**.

Note:
Fluid in the joint may be due to effusion, blood or pus. Hemarthrosis builds up quickly, whereas effusion slowly. Pus in the joint cavity shows signs of inflammation.

Transillumination test is useful in case of clear fluid as in bursa, Morrant Baker's cyst. It is negative in the presence of blood and pus.

Compressibility/reducibility: Cysts that communicate with the joint cavity like Morrant-Baker's cyst and those that communicate with the vessel like popliteal aneurysm are compressible and reducible.

Palpation of Other Components

Synovial thickening is a boggy swelling on either side of patella which can be fluctuant but without patellar tap. It is commonly seen in tuberculosis. Hypertrophied synovium feels like a rubbery/ boggy swelling, the edge of the thickened synovium can be rolled under the palpating fingers **(Fig. 39-27)**.

Bony swelling may be all around due to osteophytes or may be localized to one condyle, due to bony tumor. By careful palpation the difference in thickness and smoothness can be appreciated. The lower end of femur and upper and of tibia-fibula is palpated for any irregularities and tenderness.

Position of the patella is checked. Displacement often takes place upwards or laterally. Mobility is tested in extended knee by moving it sideways.

Joint line is palpated for irregularity, tenderness. Any loose bodies, palpable are noted.

Popliteal artery is palpated in the popliteal fossa in the position of flexion **(Fig. 39-28)**.

Muscles of the thigh and calf muscles are palpated for any spasm and wasting.

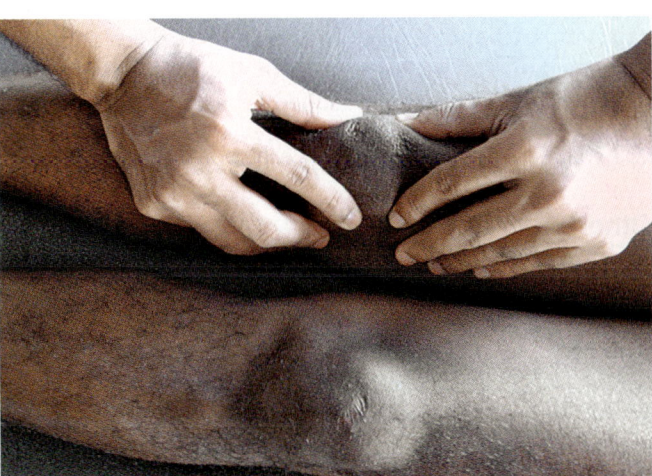

Fig. 39-25 *Fluctuation in knee joint effusion* is checked using fingers of both hands in an extended knee.

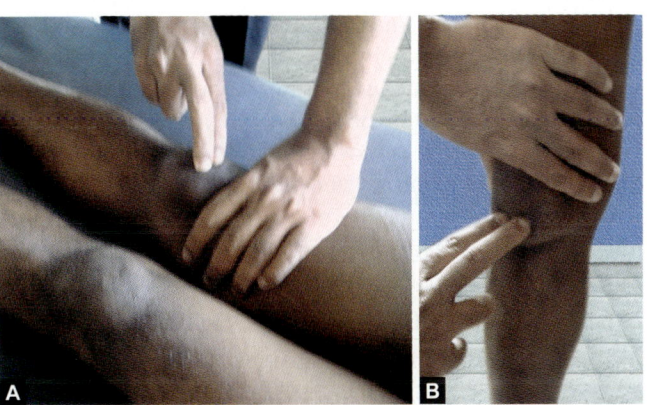

Figs. 39-26A and B *Classical method of eliciting the patellar tap* in lying down position in extended knee. Small effusion can be checked as 'patellar tap in standing'.

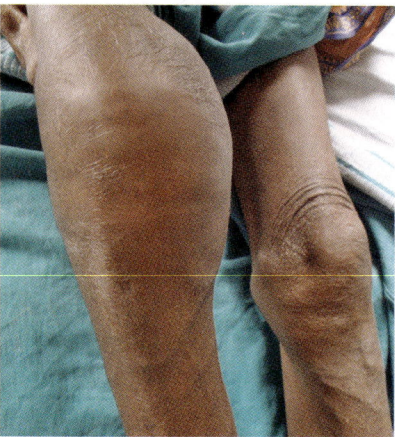

Fig. 39-27 *Tuberculosis of the knee joint.*

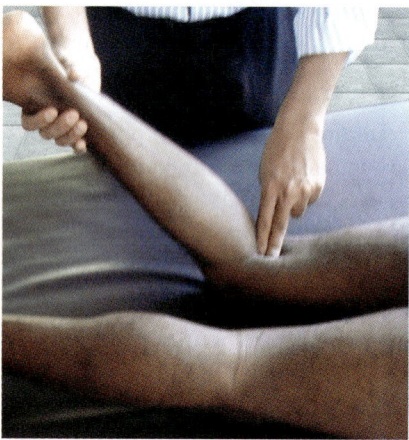

Fig. 39-28 *Popliteal fossa should be examined* in knee joint pathology.

Examination in Prone Position: In prone position the joint is palpated for tenderness along the attachments of ligaments, swellings—(Morrant-Baker's cyst, lymph nodes, and popliteal artery).

Movement

Flexion: At full flexion, when calf touches the posterior aspect of the thigh—150°. Limitation of flexion at knee occurs due to quadriceps tightness; quadriceps contracture; or quadriceps adhesion. Quadriceps tightness can be assessed by making the patient to lie prone on the table and passively flex the knee to bring the heels towards the buttocks. Normally there should be no resistance in this movement. If there is any resistance then the distance of the resisted heel from the buttock is noted which gives the proportion of contracture. 0°–90° range of movement at the knee is the most useful range of which 0°–30° motion at the knee is critical arc required for walking.

Extension: It is about 180–190° at knee joint.

Abduction/adduction: Negligible.

Rotation: Few degrees of rotation is seen in flexed knee.

All active and passive movements are checked on both sides and compared.

Any type of abnormal mobility is noted. In Charcot's joint, joint can be moved in any abnormal direction. ***Tests for abnormal mobility***—(already discussed in **Chapter 36 under knee joint injuries**). It helps to assess the integrity of medial and lateral collateral ligaments and cruciate ligaments. **(a)** *Abduction and adduction tests for lateral mobility*. **(b)** *Drawer sign.*

Abnormal Sounds during Movement: By repeated passive flexion and extension, click can be heard in meniscal tear and crepitus may be felt in degenerative arthrosis and neuropathic joints by placing hand over the knee. Intra-articular painful click is significant and is commonly seen in osteoarthritis. A 'thud' especially on anterolateral aspect indicates discoid lateral meniscus. In habitual dislocation of patella, with flexion and extension of knee, a 'snap' is felt while the patella slips out laterally and relocates back.

Measurements

Measurement of entire limb and measurement of each segment is taken and compared with that of opposite side. Any shortening of the length is noted.

Normally, a line passing from the midinguinal point, center of the patella, when extended passes through the mid-ankle joint. This line when prolonged passes through the second web space. Deviation of this axis outwards is called valgus and inwards is varus. Alternatively, the line joining ASIS (anterior superior iliac spine) to the center of patella when extended passes through the medial malleolus. But in genu valgum, it passes medial to the medial malleolus, and in genu varum, it passes lateral to medial malleolus.

Girth of the thigh and calf muscles are taken to look for muscle wasting or any swelling.

Assessment of Varum/Valgum

Patient is asked to sit at the edge of the couch with legs extended, and asked to approximate both malleoli to touch each other. Normally, the malleoli must touch before the medial surface of the knee come to touch each other. Normally, there will be a gap of 0.5 cm between the medial surface of the knee when the malleoli touch each other. If this gap is more, then it is **genu varum (bow leg)** and the gap is expressed roughly as finger breadth. If the medial surface of the knee touch before the malleoli then it is **genu valgum (knock knee)** and the distance between the two malleoli is measured in centimeters or finger breadths.

Other Examination

Popliteal and inguinal lymph nodes are to be examined. Abdomen and respiratory systems are examined.

Investigation

Plain X-ray—AP view/lateral view/oblique/tangential view.

CT scan and MRI are useful.

Aspiration and synovial biopsy: This is useful in suspected tuberculosis, arthritis, etc.

Arthroscopy: It is used for direct visualization of articular surfaces of patella, femur, joint capsule, cruciate ligament, loose bodies and synovium. The findings are to be photographed or video-recorded.

Arthrography: By injecting radiopaque dye into the cavity meniscal tear, cruciate ligament tear, and space occupying lesions are identified.

Diseases of the Knee Joint

Tuberculosis of knee joint (tumor alba/white knee)	Knock knee (Genu valgum) (Fig. 39-29)	Bow leg (Genu varum)
It is secondary synovial type causing synovial thickening, pannus formation, and later only becomes osteoarticular. **Features**: Pain, night cry, fever, gait changes, loss of weight, joint effusion, thickening of synovium, thigh muscle wasting, triple deformity—posterior subluxation and lateral rotation of tibia. Arthroscopy and synovial biopsy are diagnostic	It is abnormal abduction of the knee. **Causes**: Rickets, metabolic causes and epiphyseal diseases. It is assessed in standing position by measuring distance between medial malleoli. Pathology on the lateral aspect of tibial or femoral condyles causes abnormal increase in abduction and genu valgum. If it is femoral component, deformity disappears on flexion but not if it is due to tibial component **Complication**—Later osteoarthritis	It is abnormal adduction due to all causes mentioned for knock-knee wherein there is pathology on the medial aspect of the articular surfaces of tibial or femoral condyles. **Blount's disease** is an epiphyseal dysplasia seen in West Indies involving posteromedial aspect of proximal tibial epiphysis resulting in bow leg. *Physiological bow leg* is common in newborn which disappears spontaneously in 3 years

■ EXAMINATION OF PATHOLOGICAL ANKLE JOINT AND FOOT

History

Pain, swelling, limp, deformity and instability are the common complaints of the pathology around the ankle joint.

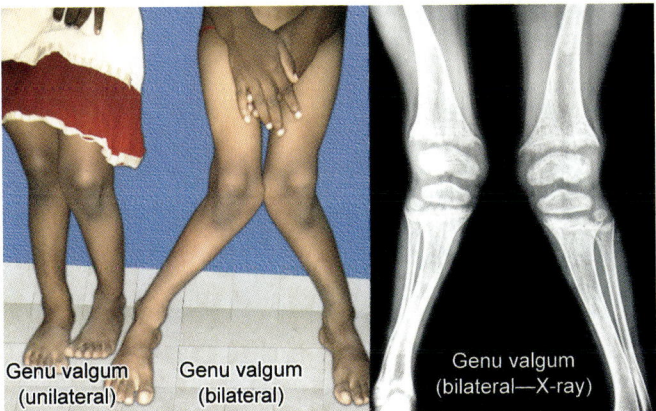

Fig. 39-29 *Genu valgum (Knock knee)*; here it is due to rickets; typical X-ray features— widening of epiphysis; splaying of metaphysis.

Local Examination

Inspection

Swelling—may be due to effusion in the ankle joint which may be seen as fullness across the front of the joint and on either side of the tendo-Achillis. Swelling due to effusion in the tendon sheath extends beyond the joint into the leg along the long axis of the tendons. The size, shape, surface and consistency are noted.

Ulcer, sinuses, if present, are noted, with respect to its site, size, surface and margin. They are due to tuberculosis, Madhura foot, Kaposi's sarcoma, tropical ulcer.

Attitude and deformity: Plantar flexion is the position of ease that joint attains at the time of effusion.

Note:

- *Equinus foot:* Entire weight is borne by the forefoot and the hind foot remains off the ground. It is due to contracture of gastrocnemius and or soleus. If the deformity disappears after flexing the knee by 90° then it is due to gastrocnemius contracture; if it persists even after flexing then it is due to soleus.
- *Calcaneus foot:* Here the weight is borne by the hind foot, with forefoot having below normal capacity of bearing the weight.
- *Varus foot:* The weight is borne by the outer side of the foot.
- *Valgus foot:* Weight is borne on inner side of the foot.
- *Inverted foot/everted foot.*
- *Pes cavus:* The normal proportion of medial longitudinal arch is accentuated so that medial side of the foot tends to assume a shape of high arch.
- *Pes planus:* It is due to collapse of the medial longitudinal arch leading to medial convexity on weight-bearing and flat foot.
- *Clawing of toes:* Hyperextension of metatarsophalangeal joint and plantar flexion of interphalangeal joints.
- *Hammer toe deformity:* Acute plantar flexion contracture at the proximal interphalangeal joint, flexion/extension of distal interphalangeal joint.
- *Hallux valgus:* The long axis of the great toe deviates outwards at the metatarsophalangeal joint.
- *Hallux varus:* Adduction of the hallux with medial subluxation of first metacarpophalangeal joint.
- *Digitus quintus varus:* Deviation of long axis of the little toe medially.
- *Wind sweep deformities of toes:* Valgus deformity of big toe, varus deformity in other toes seen in rheumatoid arthritis.
- *Bunionette:* Lateral prominence of fifth metatarsal accompanied by moderate quintus varus.

Muscle wasting, edema and *venous engorgement* are noted.

Inter-relation of the malleoli is noted where the lateral malleolus is 1 cm below and behind the medial malleolus.

Palpation

Temperature around the ankle and foot are found to be elevated in inflammatory condition.

Any *tenderness* around the ankle and foot is noted.

Fluid in the ankle joint presents as swelling on posterolateral, posteromedial; anterolateral, anteromedial aspects.

Cross-fluctuation test: Ankle joint is plantar flexed as far as possible so that dorsal tendon forms tight longitudinal strap-like across the joint. Index fingers of both hands are placed in front of both malleoli. When pressure is applied by one finger the contralateral finger will feel the impulse when there is effusion in the joint. Minimal effusion will not elicit cross-fluctuation. Similarly cross-fluctuation can be elicited in posterolateral/posteromedial swellings by dorsiflexing the ankle and pressing on either side of tendo-Achilles.

Malleoli are palpated for thickening, tenderness and irregularity. Individual tendons around the ankle joint are palpated and assessed for their position, thickening, and irregularity. Any tenderness, synovial thickening and ganglion along their course are noted. Posteriorly soft to firm swelling in relation to tendo-Achilles—anterior (*pre-Achilles bursitis*, which lies in relation to Achilles tendon and calcaneum), posterior to the tendo-Achilles (post-*Achilles bursitis; also* termed as **pump bump**) may be seen.

Palpation of calf muscles for spasm/wasting.

Palpation of arteries: **Anterior tibial artery** pulsation is palpated midway between the malleoli; *posterior tibial artery* pulsation is felt 1 fingerbreadth behind the medial malleolus.

Movement and Measurement

Already discussed in 'Chapter 37 under injuries of ankle joint and foot'. Dorsiflexion, plantar flexion at ankle joint; inversion and eversion at subtalar joint (**Figs. 39-30A and B**).

Diseases of the Ankle Joint

Calcaneal spur	Tuberculosis of the ankle
It is prominent projection of calcaneal bone on its inferior aspect causing friction and pain in heel. Pain and tenderness is typical. Often fasciitis can occur underneath	Swelling around the ankle with doughy feel due to synovial thickening, painful limp with tenderness in the joint line; sinuses in posteromedial/posterolateral aspect; all movements restricted, equinus/equinovarus deformity; fibrous ankylosis in late cases
Tailor's ankle	Villonodular synovitis
Persons regularly sitting in crossed leg position develop adventitious bursae over lateral malleolus	Chronic synovitis in young adults (males), soft nodular swelling with effusion. Aspirated fluid is thick orange brown colored containing large amount of cholesterol which is pathognomonic
Congenital talipes equinovarus (CTEV/club foot)	
It is common in boys. It is subluxation of talonavicular joint causing navicular bone to lie on the medial aspect of the head of the talus; soft tissues on the medial side of	the foot are under developed; foot is adducted, inverted at subtalar/midtarsal and anterior tarsal joints; plantar flexion of foot (equinus) at ankle; underdevelopment of calf and ankle muscles

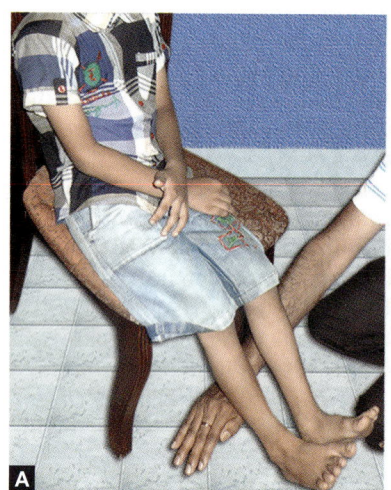 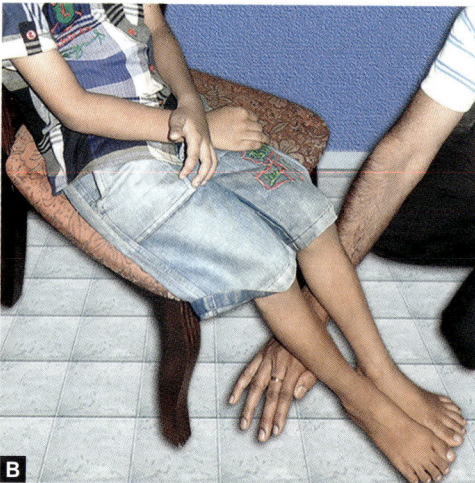

Figs. 39-30A and B *Active movements of the* joint (ankle) are done by the patient in sitting in a chair/stool with surgeon supporting loosely from behind at lower leg; Active dorsiflexion of the ankle joint; Active plantar flexion of the joint.

Approaches and Examinations in Spine Injuries and Diseases

CHAPTER 40

Competency: OR4.1; OR6.1; OR12.1; AN50.4; PM7.1; PM7.3.

SPINAL INJURIES

History

Nature of injury: Road traffic accident/fall/hit by a weapon. Severity can be assessed from the history. Fall from height, severe violence can cause fracture dislocation of cervical spine. Seat belt injury can injure lumbar vertebra **(Fig. 40-1)**.

Pain: Back pain more in dorsolumbar region, neck, legs should be asked. History of girdle pain (sense of constriction around the trunk) should be asked.

Swelling/deformity may be seen due to fracture. Dislocation is not common in thoracic/lumbar vertebra. Indirect violence causes injury commonly at C_6 and L_1 vertebrae.

History of numbness, paresthesia in limbs after injury is important and its onset whether immediate or late is asked.

History of paralysis: Inability to walk/sit and move the limbs may be seen in spinal injuries. Paraplegia/quadriplegia may occur from spine injury. Exact time and mode of onset should be noted because compression of spinal cord or crushing injury of spinal cord due to fracture or hemorrhage in the cord can cause sudden paralysis. Rapidly progressing paralysis in upwards direction occur in extramedullary hemorrhage.

Disturbance of bowel and bladder is very important history, especially in lower spinal injuries. History of incontinence of urine and feces/retention of urine should be asked.

Examination

Vital examination: It includes pulse, temperature, blood pressure, respiration (thoracoabdominal/abdominal to be noted).

LOCAL EXAMINATION

Inspection

Whole of the neck, back, chest, and abdomen must be exposed. Examination of spine includes from atlanto-occipital region to coccyx including the sacroiliac joints. Patient is examined in standing, sitting on a stool, or lying down, especially in paralytic patient.

Attitude

Observe the attitude of entire body, upper and lower limbs.

In case of suspected spinal cord injury, utmost care has to be taken while shifting the patient to the hospital. Unnecessary movements should be strictly avoided as it may worsen the injury or precipitate the paralysis. If paralysis is already present, then it is not advisable to unnecessary turn the patient to side **(Figs. 40-2A to C)**.

- **When there is no evidence of neurological deficit,** the patient can be examined in sitting/standing/lying down position; but with very cautious way and gently.
- ***Any swelling/ulcer/bruise in*** spinal and paraspinal region are observed.

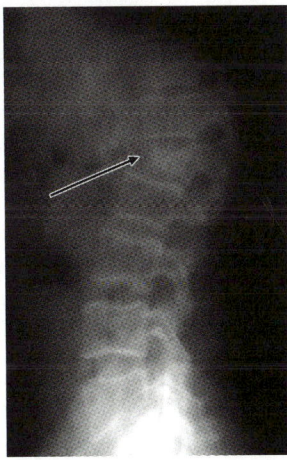

Fig. 40-1 *Burst fracture spine*; it is usually caused by fall from height.

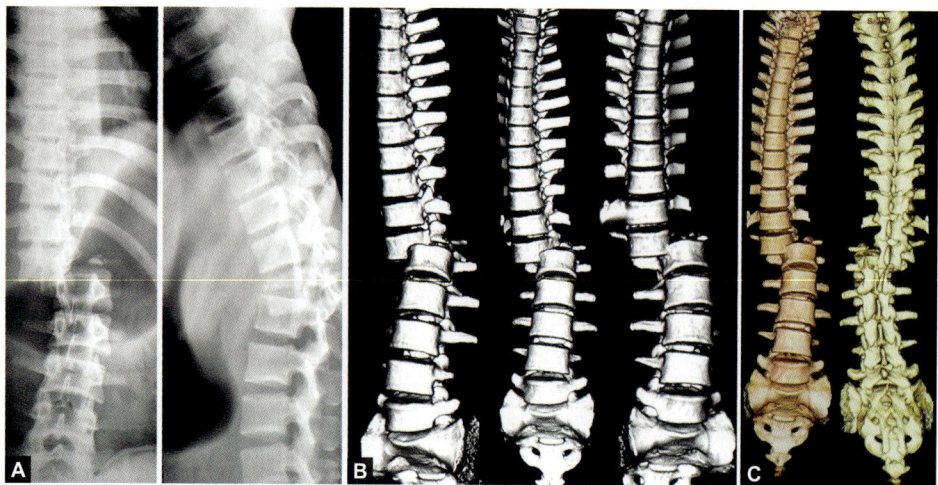

Figs. 40-2A to C X-ray and CT images of *transection of the spine* causing complete paralysis.

- ***Injury above C_5 causes immediate death*** due to paralysis of phrenic nerve.
- ***Injury at C_5*** causes completely immobile paralyzed body.
- ***Injury at C_6*** causes paralyzed body with partially closed hands held above the head with elbow flexed, arm abducted (spasticity of deltoid and supraspinatus) and externally rotated (infraspinatus and teres minor); forearm flexed and supinated (spasticity of biceps) **(Fig. 40-3)**.
- ***C_7 lesion*** causes upper extremity immobile with slightly abducted internally rotated arm and with forearm flexed and pronated (spasticity of serratus anterior, part of pectoralis major and pronators) **(Fig. 40-4)**.
- ***C_8, T_1 lesion*** causes paralysis with ***claw hand***-like deformity.
- Below T_1 up to T_{10} level, chest, lower limbs are flaccidly paralyzed corresponding to the level of injury.
- Below L_1 level, ***cauda equina*** is injured causing flaccid paralysis below knee level with loss of sensation around perineum, back of legs with retention of urine.
- In injury above T_2, breathing is ***abdominal*** as all intercostal muscles are paralyzed.

Palpation

By running the thumb over spinous and transverse processes and exerting mild pressure, the exact area of ***tenderness*** can be made out.

Holdsworth test: Fingers are run over the spinous processes, any gap in the interspinous space is indicative of unstable fracture due to tear of interspinous ligament.

Any abnormal prominence in the line of spinous process has to be noted which may be due to fracture.

In fracture dislocation spinous process will be prominent *below* the displaced vertebra. Vertebra *above* the injured one will be having prominent spine in compression fracture. *Fluctuation* can be elicited in the presence of hematoma.

Note: Abnormal mobility and movements of the spine *should not be checked* in spinal injuries unless one is sure that there is no fracture.

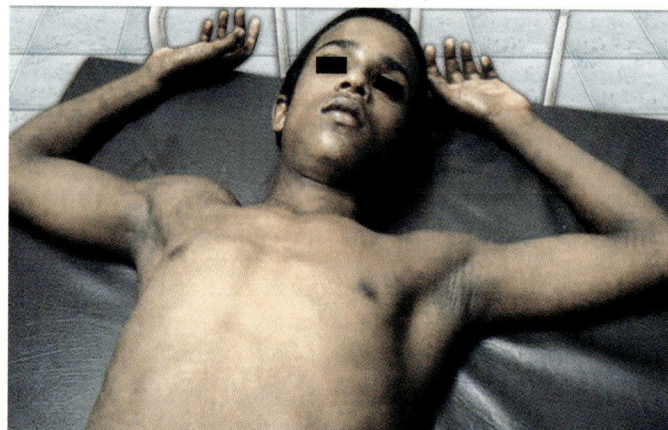

Fig. 40-3 Attitude in C_6 spine injury.

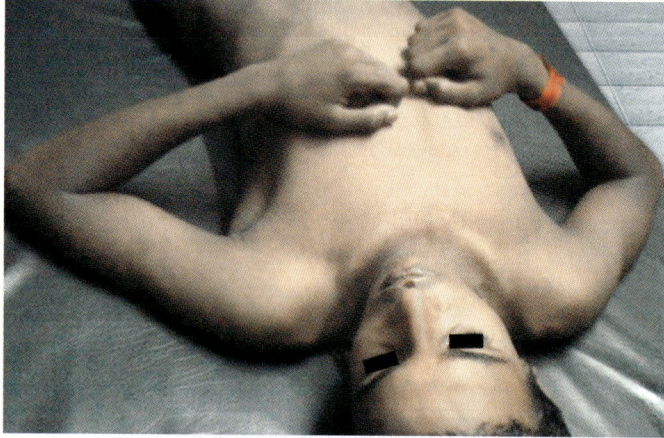

Fig. 40-4 Attitude in C_7 spine injury.

Percussion

It is done gently with tip of fingers over the spinous processes which will elicit tenderness in site of fracture.

Systemic Examination

Respiratory system: Fracture ribs and sternum should be looked for. Lungs and heart are to be examined for any trauma.

Abdomen: Distension may be present due to paralytic ileus, retention of urine. Any intra-abdominal organ injury has to be ruled out.

Rectal examination is done to detect fracture coccyx. Other skeletal injuries of limbs have to be ruled out.

Sensation are checked with help of a pin (pain), wisp of a cotton (light touch), test tubes containing hot water (temperature). The level of hypoesthesia, hyperesthesia (intervening zone) and normal sensation are noted which depends on the level of lesion. In complete injury of spinal cord, there will be total loss of sensation below the level.

Muscle power—of both upper and lower limb muscles are checked. **A person who can walk has no spinal injury.** If a person is not able to move all the four limbs—*quadriplegia*—lesion is at cervical level. If he cannot move the lower limbs—*paraplegia*—lesion is at thoracolumbar level. In supine position, patient is asked to move his toes and ankle against resistance; lift the legs one after another. If the patient is able to do it satisfactorily then there is sufficient muscle power. Upper limb muscles are also checked in similar way against resistance.

Reflexes: Initially all reflexes will be lost due to spinal shock but gradually many of them reappear in 3 weeks depending on level of injury. If it fails to occur in 3 weeks it indicates complete transection of the cord.

■ FRACTURE SPINE

Stability of spine is maintained by *anterior component* (anterior half of body of vertebra, anterior part of annulus fibrosus, anterior longitudinal ligament), *middle component* (posterior part of annulus fibrosus, posterior longitudinal ligament, posterior half of the vertebral body), and *posterior component* (posterior bony arches and posterior ligament complex). Posterior ligament complex maintains the stability of the spine (supra, interspinous ligaments).

Fracture spine can be *stable* without spinal cord injury where further displacement between the vertebral bodies does not occur because of the intact mechanical linkages, or *unstable* where further displacement can occur due to serious disruption of the structure responsible for stability, with or susceptible cord injury. When one component is disrupted (wedge compression fracture) the stability is not at threat, still it is stable. When two or more components are disrupted (burst fracture, dislocation of one vertebra over the other), the spine is unstable (Figs. 40-5A to C).

Types of Fracture Spine

Burst fracture	Extension injury
It is unstable vertical compression fracture that may result from a blow on the top of the head by some object or fall from a height vertically downwards in head-down position. Vertebral body is crushed and a piece may get displaced to cause compression to the cord.	It is stable fracture in atlas/axis (anterior ligament is torn)/lumbar region (fracture lamina). For example, forehead striking against the windscreen forcing neck into hyperextension resulting in chip fracture of anterior rim of vertebra.
Flexion injury	**Shearing force injury**
Commonest spinal injury. Here body of vertebra fractures with intact posterior ligaments causing stable fracture. It is common in lumbar vertebra but rare in neck.	Here there is flexion with rotation during the injury; unstable injury causing fracture of vertebra and posterior facet. *Worst type of spinal injury*; where one vertebra is twisted off in front of the one below it so that the upper vertebra takes a slice of the body of the lower vertebra with it.
Incomplete fractures	**Jefferson fracture**
These are fractures of spinous processes, transverse processes and laminae due to direct injury. Spinous process fractures are common in thoracic spine; transverse process fractures are common in lumbar region.	It is *burst fracture of C_1* (atlas) without neurological deficit but vertebral artery may get involved causing Wallenberg syndrome (involvement of same side cranial nerves, Horner's syndrome, ataxia, loss of pain and temperature sensation on opposite side).
Hangman fracture (Wood–Jones)	**Clay Shoveler's fracture (Australia)**
It occurs in judicial hanging with distraction fracture of C_2 (axis).	It is avulsion injury of spine of C_7 vertebra.
Chance/jack-knife seat belt injury	**Whiplash injury**
It is due to forced forward flexion causing transverse fracture of posterior element with compression fracture of vertebral body. If posterior injury causes failure of ligament complex it becomes unstable.	Neck is forcibly hyperextended and flexed due to rear end collision. It causes injury of soft tissues, ligaments and nerve roots. **Features**: Pain and stiffness in neck; limitation of neck movements; headache; hoarseness of voice due to recurrent laryngeal nerve injury; dysphagia; radiating pain in back and shoulder, paresthesia.

■ SPINAL CORD INJURIES

Spinal shock due to concussion: It causes initial complete paralysis but later complete recovery.

Contusion of cord: It causes partial damage of the cord and features of same.

Root transaction: It is due to nerve root or cauda equine injury. Flaccid paralysis may recover.

Complete transaction of the spinal cord: It causes total loss of spinal cord function below the level.

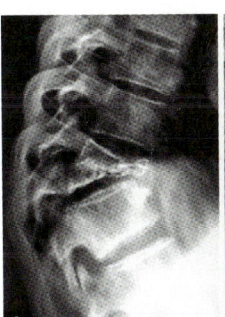 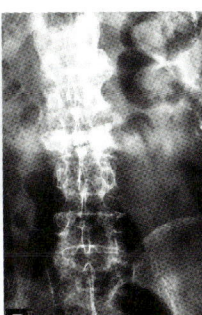 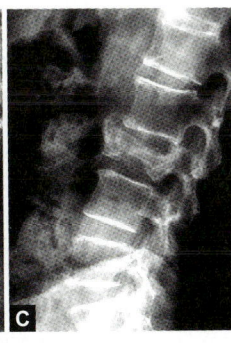

Figs. 40-5A to C X-rays showing *spine fracture*.

Intraspinal hemorrhage: **Hematomyelia** is bleeding into the cord can cause paralysis. **Hematorrachis** is bleeding in extramedullary region which causes initial spinal irritation, later progressive spinal cord damage from below upwards.

Incomplete injury to spinal cord (partial trisection) causes various syndromes: (1) *Anterior cord syndrome:* There is complete motor loss, loss of pain, temperature below the level of injury; but intact deep touch, position and vibration sense. (2) *Central cord syndrome:* It is due to hyperextension injury in cervical spine involving central part of the spinal cord. It shows 50% gradual recovery. (3) *Brown-Sequard syndrome:* Here transaction one half of the cord causes ipsilateral complete paralysis; hypoesthesia of opposite side.

SPINAL DISEASES

History

Age: *Spina bifida* occurs in newborn. *Tuberculosis spine* is common in children. *Ankylosing spondylitis* seen in adults; *disc prolapse* occurs in middle-aged. *Secondaries* in spine and *osteoarthritis* occur in aged.

Sex: Disc prolapse, ankylosing spondylitis are common in males; osteomalacia, osteoporosis are common in females.

Complaints

Pain

Site of pain: Cervical, thoracic, lumbar or lumbosacral is asked.

Mode of onset: Traumatic/inflammatory/following unaccustomed strain or exercise such as lifting heavy weight in stooping position as in intervertebral disc prolapse/spontaneous.

Nature: May be dull aching (inflammatory condition)/sudden, sharp intermittent (disc prolapsed)/continuous throbbing as in case of an abscess or osteomyelitis; intermittent and dull in case of spondylolisthesis. In secondaries of spine, pain is mild in nature but gets aggravated with movements of spine.

Night pain is common in tuberculosis. Pain of ankylosing spondylitis is more in the morning with stiffness of spine.

Progression of pain: Whether progressive/regressive/constant.

Radiation of pain: Pain may get radiated along the nerve to the limbs due to compression of their roots (prolapsed disc, extramedullary spinal tumors, osteophytes). In tuberculosis of cervical spine, pain is referred to occiput and arm; thoracic spine referred along the intercostal nerves; 'girdle pain' is seen in thoracolumbar tuberculosis; from lumbar spine, it is referred to hip and leg. Pain in ankylosing spondylitis occurs along the course of sciatic nerve alternating one side and other.

Aggravating and relieving factors: Pain due to intervertebral disc prolapse as well as secondaries in spine can get aggravated by coughing, sneezing, defecation. Movements of spine can increase the pain in caries, fracture spine. Most pain lessens with complete rest.

Fever: Seen inflammatory conditions, osteomyelitis spine.

Other Complaints

Swelling in meningocele, fibrolipoma, nevolipoma; *dimple/tuft of hair* in lumbosacral region in spina bifida occulta; deformities like scoliosis/kyphosis/lordosis; *ulcer or sinuses* in tuberculosis. The duration, mode of onset of each complaints should be asked.

Impairment of function: Inability to stand, sit, walk due to weakness of back muscles; weakness or paralysis of one or both limb; painful standing and walking in anterior spinal stenosis; paresthesia/ loss of sensation due to compression over nerve roots; impairment of bowel and bladder function in cauda equina lesions, Pott's paraplegia; stiffness of back in ankylosing spondylitis, tuberculosis, disc prolapsed; loss of weight—tuberculosis, secondaries spine.

Past History

History of tuberculosis, intervertebral disc prolapse, primary malignancies of breast, thyroid; pelvic inflammatory disease are to be asked which are the causative factors in backache. History of trauma/fall on spine in the past; history of drugs like corticosteroids, hormones are important in osteoporosis.

Personal History

Dietary history including vitamin D and calcium intake is important in osteomalacia. Menstrual history is taken that tries to rule out any gynecological cause for back pain.

General Examination

To look for anemia, cachexia, malnutrition as seen in secondaries spine, tuberculosis spine.

Gait—high stepping gait in foot drop; ataxic gait in tabes dorsalis; spastic gait in spinal tumors or cerebral palsy.

Local Examination

Inspection

Entire back should be examined from behind and from sides. Patient is examined in sitting, standing, lying down positions. Examination includes from atlanto-occipital region to coccyx along with sacroiliac joints.

Attitude: Posture of the patient while standing/walking has to be noted. In tuberculosis of cervical spine, child supports the head with both hands under the chin and when asked to look sideways he turns his entire body to that side and when asked to stand he leans forwards with stiff back supporting the body weight on something with the help of hands. *A fixed statue-like* with stooping posture is characteristic of ankylosing spondylitis; standing with legs crossed and with tendency for equinus position is seen in cerebral diplegia; swaying of the body while standing with feet close together is seen in cerebellar lesions.

Patient is asked *to stand as erect as much* as possible. Positions of head, levels of shoulders, margins of body from axilla to iliac crest, iliac crests, scapulae, curvatures of spine should be noted from side and behind. The midline furrow—is the normal longitudinal depression which contains the knob-like projections of the spinous processes. The paraspinal muscles produce bulge on either side of this furrow which stands out prominently in case of muscle spasms. They look increasingly prominent in early caries spine. The seventh spinous process of the cervical spine stands out prominently as vertebral prominence.

Any deviation in the normal spinal curvature, central furrow, any change in scapular position (elevated/depressed), fullness below and above the iliac crest, any change in levels of anterior superior iliac spine. Whether the head is deviated to one side (torticollis), any change in curvature of the back from axilla to iliac crest (scoliosis), any bulge in loin region should be noted.

Deformity: Patient is examined in standing, sitting, bending and supine position. Structural deformity of spine persists in all positions whereas the deformity due to postural defect disappears on lying down; deformity due to defect in the lower limb disappears on sitting.

1. **Kyphosis (gibbus/hump):** There is abnormality in the anteroposterior curvature of spine as the result of which there is forward bending or increased backward convexity of spine. In advanced kyphosis, there will be forward bending of sternum and crowding of ribs.
   Types:
   a. Knuckle—due to collapse of one vertebra (tuberculosis, fracture, secondaries, Kummel's disease).
   b. Angular/hunch back—collapse of two or more vertebra (late stage of tuberculosis spine, multiple secondaries in spine).
   c. Round type—due to involvement of several vertebras (senility, osteomalcia, ankylosing spondylitis, Scheuermann's disease in adolescents).
2. **Lordosis:** It is abnormal anterior convexity of spine usually at lumbar region. Here the abdomen looks protuberant, with central furrow deeper than normal. Often it is due to flexion deformity of one or both hips. Other causes are pregnancy, rickets, obesity, cretinism, spondylolisthesis (here the central furrow shows a sudden depression to give an impression of a 'step' due to slipping of one vertebra over the vertebra below and there may be a prominent sacrum with depression above it). Loss of lordosis can happen in Koch's spine, ankylosing spondylitis, acute disc prolapse.
3. **Scoliosis:** Here the spine bends sideways producing lateral curvature along with rotation of spine.
   The site, number of curvatures and persistence or absence of curvature on forward bending (functional scoliosis due to leg length discrepancy, sciatica disappears on forward bending), upper and lower limit of curvature and side of convexity are to be noted. Curves are primary (major) or secondary (compensatory). Any associated other deformity like kyphosis, and chest wall abnormality are to be noted.
4. **Combined:** It occurs in two planes with both forward and lateral tilt of spine (Fig. 40-6).

Swelling: It should be assessed for all features like size, shape, and impulse on coughing. It may be cold abscess, lipoma, neurofibroma, spina bifida, meningocele/menigomyelocele in lumbosacral region, sacrococcygeal teratoma, etc.

Dimpling/sinus: May be present at the lumbosacral region, due to spina bifida occulta. It may present with tuft of hair, dilated vessels along with fibrofatty tissue.

Ulcers, if present, have to be described in similar way.

Neurological deficit: Paraplegia is evident on inspection that can occur in tuberculous thoracic spine.

Palpation

It should be done in *standing/sitting as well as in prone position.* Patient should keep his hand across the chest with back as straight as possible.

Whole of the back from occipital protuberance to tip of coccyx should be palpated. Central furrow, paraspinal bulges, sides of chest, loin, iliac crest, sacroiliac joints, buttocks must be palpated in order. The spinous processes are palpated in the central furrow. Any prominent process is noted along with its site, shape, size and tenderness.

Tenderness: It is elicited by applying direct pressure with the thumb in midline over spinous processes from cervical region to sacral region from above downwards. Alternatively, it can be also elicited by pressing the side of the spinous process so as to rotate the vertebra **(Fig. 40-7)**. If both these methods fail to elicit tenderness as it occurs in chronic disease, gentle blows with ulnar side of the fist on the side of the spine may elicit tenderness **(Fig. 40-8)**. *Anvil test:* Sudden jerk applied over the head of the patient causes pain/tenderness in the spinous process (this should be done cautiously). Tenderness can be also elicited by percussion over spine **(Fig. 40-9)**.

Paraspinal muscles are palpated for spasm/tightness; wasting, where it is thinned out so that the posterior portion of ribs may become palpable.

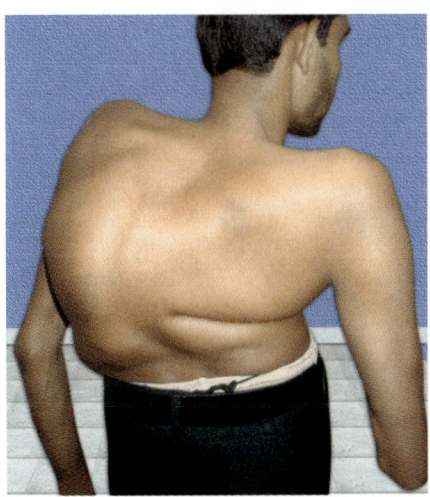

Fig. 40-6 *Kyphoscoliosis.*

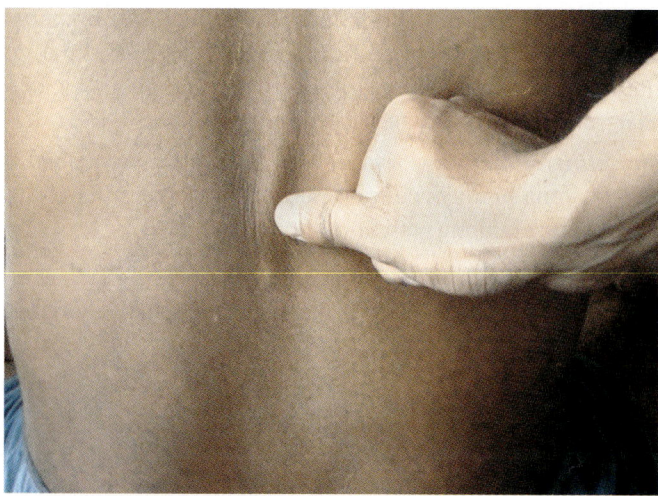

Fig. 40-7 Gentle blows can be used to *elicit tenderness.*

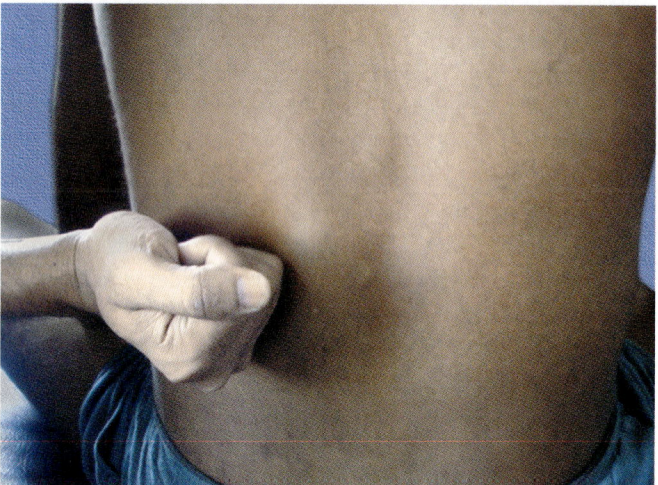

Fig. 40-8 Pressing the lateral margin of the spine causes *rotation and tenderness.*

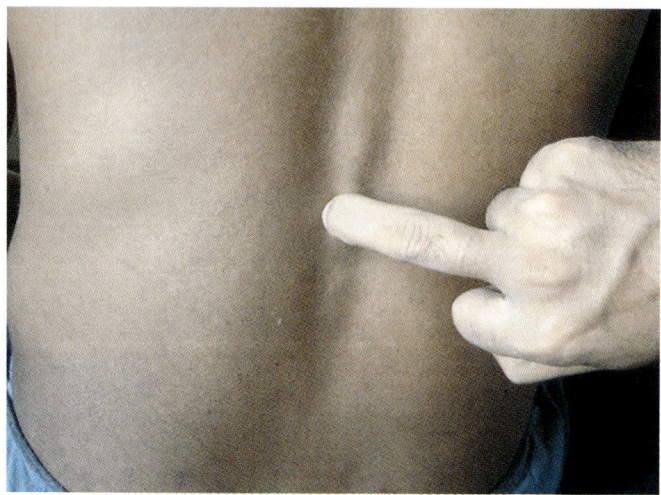

Fig. 40-9 *Percussion* also is used to elicit tenderness.

Anterior convexity *(lordosis),* lateral convexity *(scoliosis),* posterior convexity *(kyphosis)* are palpated by sliding the fingers over the spinous process. *The 'step'* at lumbosacral region in spondylolisthesis can be felt by sliding fingers over the spinous processes.

Swelling: As in any swelling, temperature, tenderness are checked. Paraspinal abscesses are warm and tender. Cold abscess may occur in neck, mediastinum, thoracic wall, psoas region, pelvis, etc. Cold abscess of chest and loin may show impulse on coughing. Meningocele in spina bifida may be present in occipital and lumbosacral region. It also shows *impulse on coughing*. In children, when the meningocele is pressed the impulse may be felt by the fingers placed over the anterior fontanelle.

Movements

Cervical Spine

Patient is asked to sit erect on stool and the shoulders are fixed from behind in a horizontal plane. The patient is asked to touch the front of the chest with the chin keeping the mouth closed (for flexion) and then take back the head as far as possible (for extension); to touch the ear to the top of the shoulder (lateral rotation); to look towards right and left shoulder (for rotation). Movements are restricted when atlantoaxial joint (rotation of the head) and atlanto-occipital joints (nodding) are affected. Movements are to be cautiously performed when the lesions are suspected at atlas and axis so as to avoid sudden dislocation of the atlantoaxial joint that will result in sudden death as it compresses the vital center. Movements are not restricted when lower cervical vertebrae are affected.

Thoracolumbar Spine

Flexion: It is maximum in lumbar region (90°) up to the extent of obliteration of lumbar convexity but least in thoracic region. It is checked by asking the patient to lean forward and touch the toes with knees kept straight while the examiner keeps his hands over the spine to note the spine movements. In children, it is tested by asking the child to pick up a coin from the ground without bending the knees *(Coin test)*. In tuberculosis spine, the child is not able to stoop without flexing his knees and hip and while rising he will successively put his hands for support on legs, knees and thigh.

Extension: It is less in thoracic region but occurs in lumbar region (25–30°). Patient standing erect is asked to lean backwards as far as possible as if to look at the ceiling. In children, lumbar spine has got more mobility, especially extension. Child is asked to lie down on the bed in prone position. Examiner places one hand over the dorsal spine to fix it and with other hand lifts the legs together to elicit the range of extension in lumbar spine. When patient complains of pain and not able to bend while lifting the vertebral column, it indicates that lesion is in the lumbar vertebra.

Lateral flexion: It occurs with rotation of the vertebra in thoracic part. It is checked in standing position. Examiner stabilizes the pelvis of the patient by holding it firmly then patient is asked to bend sideward so as to slide his hand with extended elbow along the thigh. In children it is tested as follows—the child is asked to lie down on the bed in prone position. Examiner places one hand over the dorsal spine to fix it and with other hand lifts the legs together and turns one side and next to other side to elicit lateral flexion.

In ankylosing spondylitis, there is marked restriction of all movements with rigidity of spine.

Rotation: It occurs in thoracic spines. Patient is asked to sit on a chair so that his pelvis is fixed and is asked to rotate his trunk right and left to demonstrate rotation. This can be done passively by moving the shoulders **(Fig. 40-10)**.

Measurement

Length of lower limbs are measured to see any shortening as the cause for scoliosis.

Chest expansion is measured by measuring girth of chest in full inspiration and expiration. Normal expansion is approximately 8 cm. It is markedly restricted in ankylosing spondylitis.

Special Tests

Straight leg raising test (SLR): It is performed on normal side first and later on the affected side. Both by active (by the patient) and passive (by the examiner) methods, it should be checked. Patient is asked to lie supine on the bed. He is asked to lift his leg with knee straight until he develops pain. In passive SLR, the patient is made to lie supine completely relaxed without any compensatory lordosis. The ankle is grasped with one hand and other hand is placed in front of the thigh so as to keep the knee straight. The leg is now raised until the patient experiences pain. Normally it can be raised up to 90° without experiencing pain. If angle at which he develops pain is 40°, it is due to impingement of protruded intervertebral disc over nerve roots. If pain develops beyond 40°, it is due to tension on the nerve root which may or may not be due to disc prolapse. ***Lasègue's sign:*** The angle at which patient develops pain, ankle is now passively dorsiflexed by the examiner which will aggravate the pain in case of disc prolapse or spine lesions but not in case of sacroiliac joint disease or sciatica (where SLR may be positive but not Lasègue's sign) **(Figs. 40-11A and B)**.

Femoral nerve stretch test: Patient is made to lie in prone position, the other leg is kept extended and on the affected side knee is flexed to 90°. Patient will complain of pain in front of the thigh along the distribution of femoral nerve if L_2, L_3 disc is protruded causing stretching of femoral nerve root.

Naffziger's test: Pressure on the jugular vein increases the pain of disc prolapse.

Lhermitte's sign: Neck and hips are simultaneously flexed with the knees in extended position. Patient will experience sharp pain down the spine into extremities due to irritation of spinal duramater by intervertebral disc prolapse or extradural spinal tumor **(Fig. 40-12)**.

Aired test for malingering: Patient is asked to touch the toes in standing and if he is unable to do, so he is asked to touch toes in sitting position, which if he can means he is malingering.

Magnuson's test for malingering: Patient is asked to pinpoint the site of pain which is marked. Patient's attention is diverted by throat, neck, and other examinations and once again is asked to show the site of pain. If he shows different site then he is malingering.

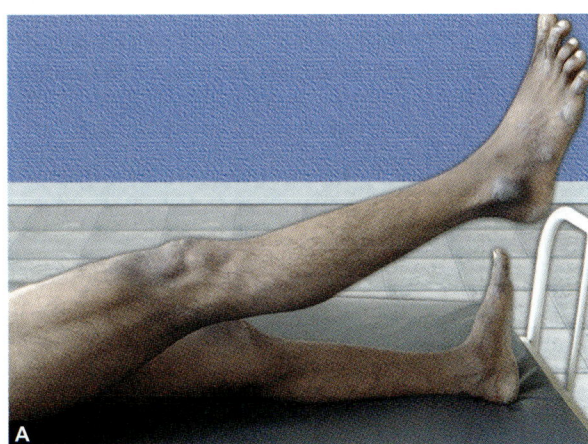

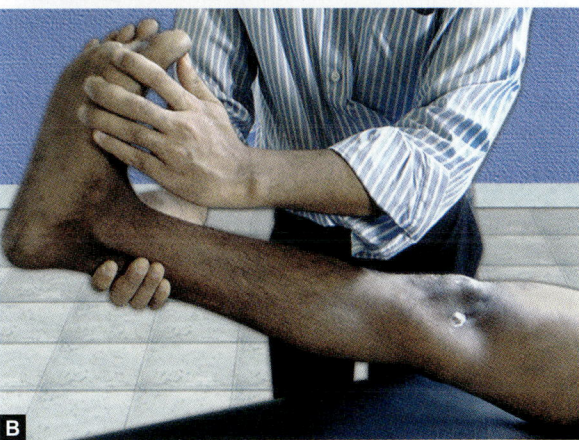

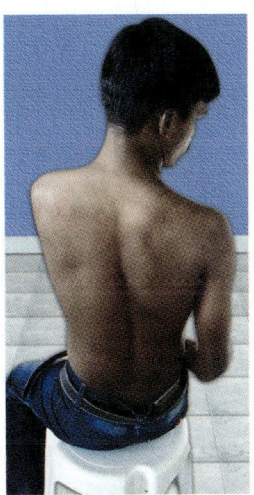

Fig. 40-10 *Rotation movement of spine* checked in sitting position so that to fix the pelvis.

Figs. 40-11A and B (A) *Straight leg raising* (SLR): Active; (B) SLR *Lasègue's sign* eliciting: Passive.

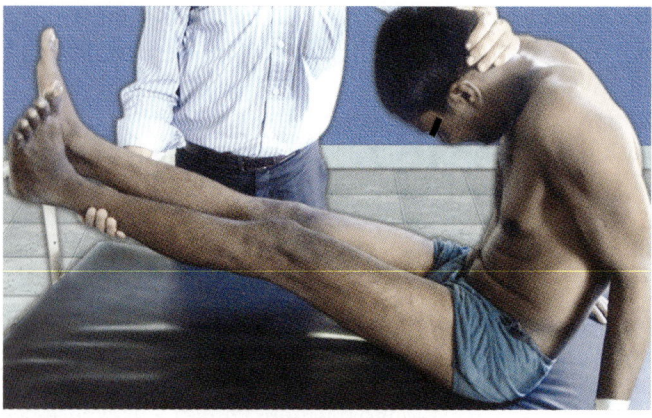

Fig. 40-12 *Lhermitte's sign.*

Reflexes

Biceps and supinator ($C_{5,6}$); triceps jerk ($C_{7,8}$); knee jerk ($L_{3,4}$); ankle jerk and clonus (S_1); abdominal reflexes; cremasteric reflexes (L_2); plantar reflexes (S_2) are checked on both sides.

Sensations

Sensations are checked for temperature, touch, pain and vibration sense.

Tests for Sacroiliac Joint

Tenderness in this joint is elicited by pressing with the thumb over the dimple situated just medial to the posterior superior iliac spine while the patient is bending forwards. It can also be elicited by compressing the iliac crest with the patient lying in supine position.

Movements: Forward bending and rotatory movements are painful in standing but not in sitting position.

Gillie's test: Patient is asked to lie prone on a bed. Pelvis is fixed by keeping hand over the unaffected sacroiliac joint when affected leg is hyperextended the patient may complain of pain if the sacroiliac joint is affected **(Fig. 40-13)**.

Gaenslen's test: The patient is asked to lie on the affected side and pelvis is fixed by flexing the hip and knee of the affected side. The unaffected leg is held and hip is hyperextended to give rotational strain over the sacroiliac joint meanwhile other hand is placed over the lumbar spine to steady it. If patient complains of pain, it indicates that sacroiliac joint is affected **(Fig. 40-14)**.

Pump handle test: Patient is asked to lie supine. Sound side is examined first, later the diseased side. The limb is grasped below the knee and the hip and knee joint are flexed fully. The flexed knee is directed towards the opposite shoulder, meanwhile pressure is applied downwards on the same side of shoulder. The test is positive if patient complains pain near sacroiliac joint **(Figs. 40-15A and B)**.

Both active and passive SLR is done. *Lasègue's sign of SLR* will be negative in sacroiliac joint disease.

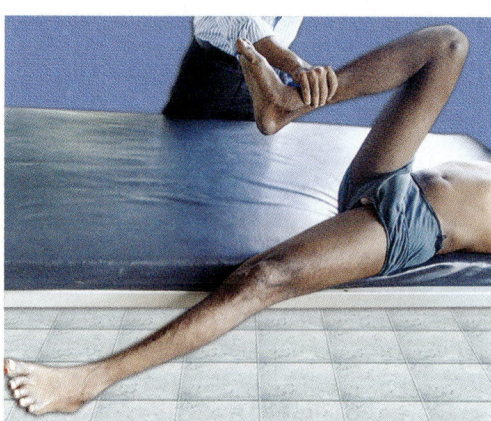

Fig. 40-14 *Gaenslen's test.*

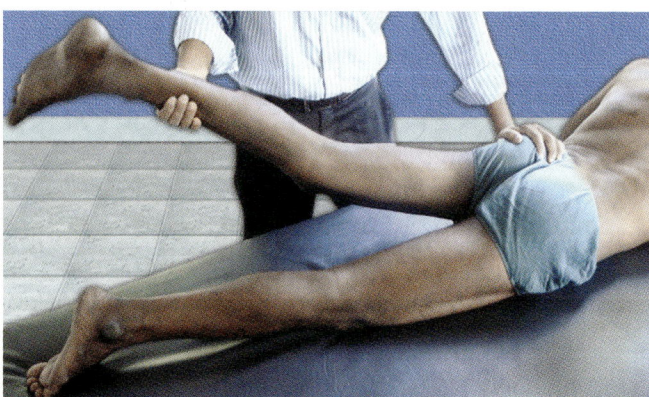

Fig. 40-13 *Gillie's test.*

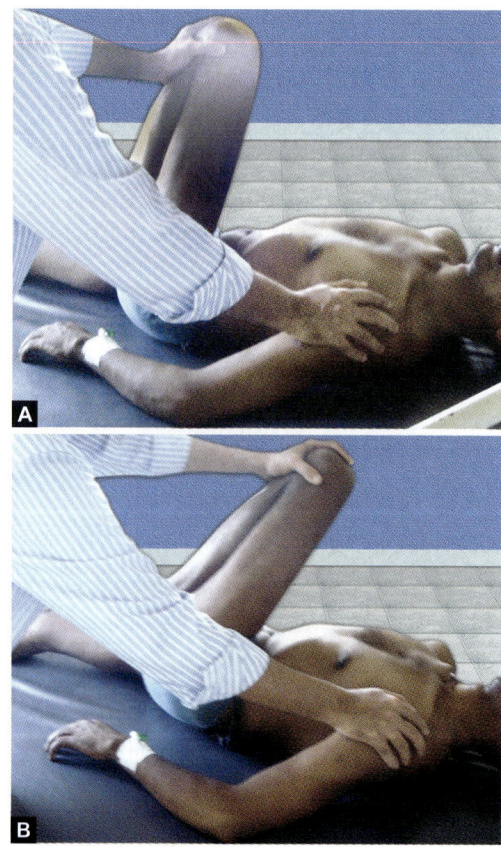

Figs. 40-15A and B *Pump handle test.*

Chapter 40: Approaches and Examinations in Spine Injuries and Diseases   607

Lymph nodes—axillary lymph nodes, inguinal nodes are checked for enlargement.

Neurological examination including motor, sensory system and reflexes are checked.

Systemic examination—breast, thyroid, lungs, kidney, prostate are examined for primary. Chest should be examined to rule out tuberculosis, carcinoma lungs.

Other joints should be examined for arthritis.

INVESTIGATIONS

X-ray spine and X-ray chest.

Blood tests: ESR, tumor markers. Relevant investigations are done depending on the condition suspected—peripheral smear, spine biopsy.

MRI is very useful. Myelography to see the disc prolapse or spinal diseases. Discography, epidurography are other investigations.

CT chest, CT abdomen if secondaries or tuberculosis is suspected.

Diseases of the Spine

Ankylosing spondylitis (Poker's back or Marie-Strumpell arthritis)	
It is a chronic, progressive disease of spine and sacroiliac joints, which is genetically predisposed as HLA-B27. There is progressive restriction of movements of all joints in the spine. Patient cannot bend with total stiffness and calcification of ligaments of the spine (*Bamboo spine*).	Aortic valve disease, urethritis are other associations. Pain radiating to right and left lower limbs alternatively is typical. Patient stands with kyphosis with knees bent. Costovertebral ankylosis causes poor chest expansion (< 5 cm) leading into pulmonary complications.
Spondylolisthesis	
It is defined *as slipping forward of one vertebra over the next lower vertebra*, usually seen in L_4–L_5 or L_5–S_1 junction. It can be congenital (75%); degenerative (20%); traumatic (5%). Pars interarticularis of L_5 is defective with fibrous tissue component.	**Features**: It causes sudden severe pain with lumbar lordosis and step-like depression over the sacrum. Short trunk, flat buttock, prominent sacrum with a depression above, transverse furrow encircling body between ribs and iliac crest are the features. X-ray oblique of spine shows *decapitated Scottish terrier sign*.
Kyphosis	
It means there is an exaggerated curvature of thoracic spine with obliteration of lumbar lordosis. There is excessive posterior convexity of thoracic spine. **Causes**: Tuberculosis of spine— angular—Gibbus type; adolescent kyphosis; post-traumatic (Kummell's), ankylosing spondylitis, osteoporosis, secondaries, Paget's disease, eosinophilic granuloma of vertebra (Calve's disease).	**Types**: 1. *Angular—knuckle*—where one spine is prominent due to collapse of one vertebra. 2. *Angular— gibbus*—one or two vertebrae are involved. 3. *Rounded*—many vertebrae are involved. *Postural kyphosis* is seen in girls with flat foot, obesity. *Compensatory kyphosis* is seen in lumbar lordosis, fixed flexion deformity of hip, CDH. **Scheuermann's disease** is osteochondritis of vertebral epiphysis in adolescents involving T6 to T10. Epiphyses contain small, translucent Schmorl's nodes. *Senile kyphosis* is due to old age degeneration of the disc.
Scoliosis (Figs. 40-16A and B)	
It is *lateral curvature of the spine* usually associated with rotational deformity; common in thoracic spine. It can be thoracolumbar or lumbar; can be transient, mobile, non-structural or can be structural. Condition may be associated with cardiac anomalies.	On X-ray, *Cobb's angle* between margins of vertebrae is assessed for severity. Completion index is assessed by fusion of apophysis with iliac bones (*Reisser's sign*).
Types: **Structural scoliosis**: Here body rotates towards convexity of the curve; spine towards concavity. It progresses till the cessation of growth. Main curvature is called as *primary curve* with compensatory *secondary curvatures* above and below. Rib hump appears on flexion of spine. Chest opposite to posterior convexity is more prominent. It can be: (1) Idiopathic: It begins in infancy, childhood, adolescents. It may resolve or progress. Progressive type leads into ugly type deformity with rib hump in thoracic spine. (2) Congenital—hemivertebrae, fused vertebrae, absence ribs, fused ribs. (3) Paralytic—poliomyelitis, cerebral palsy, muscle dystrophy. (4) von Recklinghausen disease of neurofibromatosis is associated with scoliosis (33%).	*Transient scoliosis*: (1) Postural: It is commonest non-structural type seen in girls with mild convex curve towards left. It disappears while bending forward. (2) Compensatory: It is to compensate pelvic tilt in short leg or hip disease which disappears on sitting. (3) Sciatic: It is due to pain of intervertebral disc prolapse.
Intervertebral disc prolapse (IVDP) (Fig. 40-17)	
It is *herniation of the nucleus pulposus of the disc through the nucleus fibrosus of the disc*, commonly at posterolateral direction in one or both sides. It is common in L_4–L_5 or L_5–S_1 region. Prolapse of L_4–L_5 disc compresses the lower nerve root—L_5. Prolapse of L_5–S_1 compresses the S_1 nerve root.	X-ray shows findings only at late stage. Myelograms, MRI are diagnostic. It is the commonest cause of back pain. Always possible neurological deficits should be looked for. SLR test will be positive.

Contd...

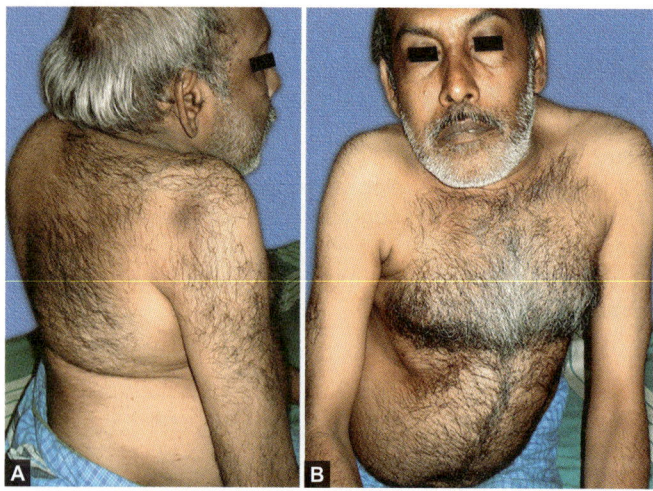

Figs. 40-16A and B *Structural* kyphoscoliosis.

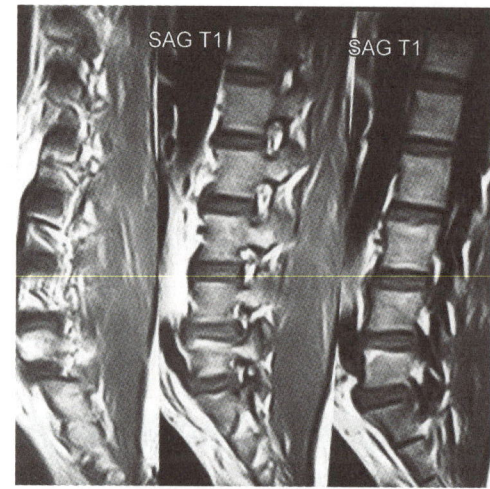

Fig. 40-17 MRI is the *ideal investigation* for IVDP.

Contd...

Spina bifida (Fig. 40-18)	
It is failure of enfolding of nerve elements within the spinal canal during developmental period. It is usually seen in lumbosacral region. There is failure of fusion of the one or more posterior vertebral arches. It is often associated with other anomalies. **Sites**: (1) Lumbosacral; (2) Thoracolumbar. **Types**: **Spina bifida occulta**: There is dimpling of skin with dermoids, lipomas in the site. Impulse on coughing can be seen. Initially there is no neurological deficit but later tethering, traction on dura, infection can lead onto neurological deficits, a fibrous band between skin and spinal theca will be present.	**Spina bifida aperta**: Here neurological deficit is present. It may be *myelomeningocele* wherein spinal cord and nerve roots are in the sac or *meningocele* wherein sac consists of meninges and fluid only. Meningocele is brilliantly transilluminant. Myelomeningocele is not transilluminant. *Syringomyelocele* shows dilated central canal of spinal cord which lies within and is adherent to the sac. *Myelocele* has central canal of spinal cord opened into the skin discharging CSF. It is commonest and is not compatible with life. Paralysis, incontinence, sepsis sets in soon. **Clinical features**: Motor paralysis; sensory paralysis; visceral paralysis with incontinence of urine and feces; swelling at the site of the lesion may be lipoma or dermoid with impulse on coughing; bony defect at the site; later hydrocephalous.
Tuberculosis of spine (Pott disease of spine)	
It is the commonest type of joint tuberculosis (40%). It is common in children and adolescents; usually secondary type. *Commonest area is thoracolumbar region (T_{10})*. Common site is paradiscal part of the vertebra. Occasionally central body, anterior surface, pedicle, lamina, spinous process may be involved. It is commonly hematogenous in origin. There is destruction of bone, *caseation, and cold abscess formation*. Caseating fluid may trickle along the neurovascular bundle or along fascial planes leading to formation of cold abscess at different sites like psoas area (psoas abscess), paraspinal area. Destructed bone, granulation tissue, cold abscess may compress the spinal cord leading to early onset paraplegia (*paraplegia in flexion*). It can be reversed by treatment. Longitudinal gliosis, destruction of spinal cord will lead onto late onset paraplegia—*paraplegia in extension*. It is irreversible type.	**In cervical vertebra**: C_6, C_7 is commonly involved. Neck pain, rigidity, brachial neuralgia, rust sign, tenderness and paraspinal spasm, restricted neck movements, retropharyngeal or posterior triangle cold abscess are the features. **In thoracic vertebra:** Tuberculous metaphysitis is the commonest type. **Pathology:** Once intervertebral disc gets destructed, vertebral bodies collapse, causing **kyphosis** (forward bending of the spine). It is commonly angular type called as **gibbus**. If many vertebrae are involved then it is called as **rounded kyphosis**. **Clinical features:** *Typical military attitude* with raised shoulder; pain and tenderness in the spine; paraspinal spasm confirmed by positive coin test; restricted spine movements; deformity like gibbus; cold abscess in different locations; neurological deficits and paraplegia **(Figs. 40-19 to 40-21)**.
Spinal cord tumors	
Extradural: Here commonest is *secondaries*. Primary may be bronchus, breast, prostate or kidney. **Intradural**: (1) *Extramedullay (75%)*: Neurofibroma is the commonest type (males) from posterior nerve roots. Spinal meningiomas are seen in females. (2) *Intramedullary*: Diffuse gliomas are commonest type. Ependymoma and vascular lesions are others. Common site is cervical region.	**Clinical features:** Paraplegia, neurological deficits, pain and urinary disturbances. Compression of spinal cord can occur. X-ray, myelography, MRI are investigations. CSF below the block may be yellow and proteinaceous—*Froin's syndrome*. **Secondaries in spine (metastases)**: Secondaries in spine is one of the common malignancies in spine. Primary may be from carcinoma of breast, GIT, prostate, lungs, kidney, etc. It causes back pain, restricted mobility and later neurological deficits. CT scan/ MRI/bone biopsy and evaluation for primary should be done.

Chapter 40: Approaches and Examinations in Spine Injuries and Diseases 609

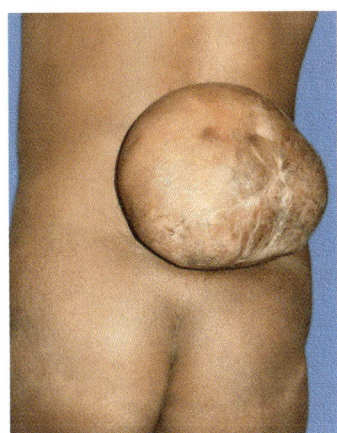

Fig. 40-18 *Spina bifida.*

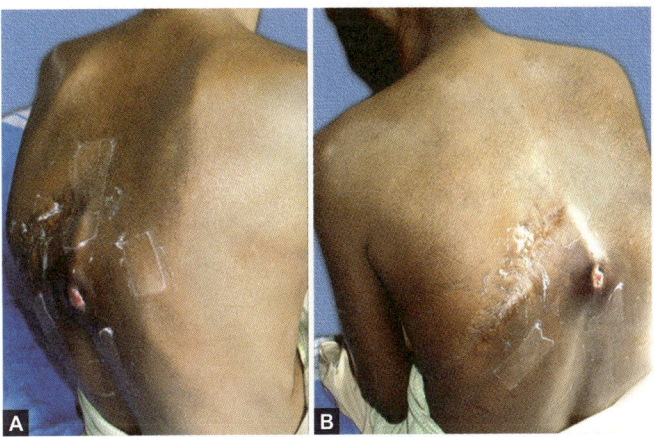

Figs. 40-20A and B *Gibbus type of ankylosis* in tuberculosis of thoracic spine.

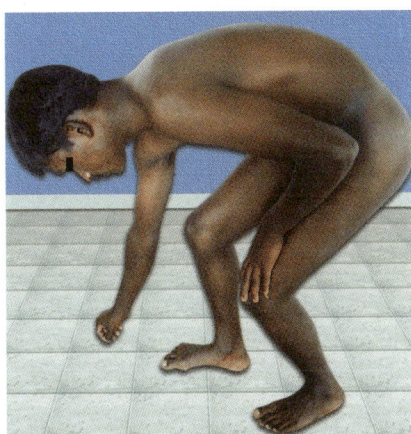

Fig. 40-19 *Coin test* in tuberculosis. Paraspinal spasm prevents proper spine functioning.

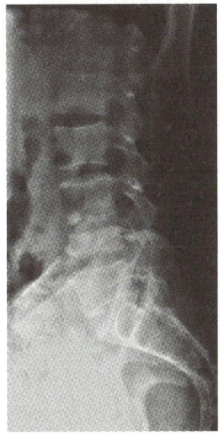

Fig. 40-21 *Tuberculosis of spine* L_4, L_5 lateral view X-ray.

Section 6: Miscellaneous

CHAPTER 41

Instruments

Competency: SU14.2; SU14.3.

Surgical instruments are essential for any surgery, whether minor or major. All instruments should be sterilized prior to use to prevent infection.

Parts of an instrument:
- Two finger bows for holding
- A ratchet or lock
- A pair of shaft or body
- Joint either box type (with a slot) or pivot (attached by a screw)
- Pair of blades at terminal part

FORCEPS

Cheatle's Forceps

It is used to pick sterilized articles like instruments and drapes so to avoid touching of the instruments while transferring them from one tray/table to other. It is kept dipped in antiseptic solutions like Savlon/Cidex. It does not have lock. It is heavy metallic forceps with curved blades with serrations. One blade of proximal handle has got rounded ring for finger and other blade has got free hook to have proper grip (Fig. 41-1).

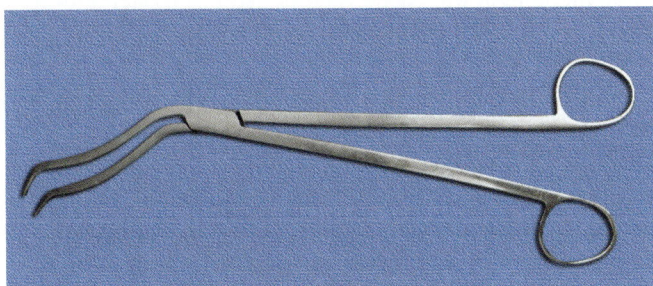

Fig. 41-1 Cheatle's forceps.

Sponge Holding Forceps (Rampley's)

It has got fenestrated, serrated flat distal end. It is used to clean the operative field. Because of the length, the surgeon's hand will not get contaminated while cleaning the patient, it is also used to swab the cavities, to mop the oozing area, to hold gallbladder or cervix or tongue or bowel or stomach during surgeries, for blunt dissections or as ovum forceps. It can also be used to dry the operative field using gauze (Fig. 41-2).

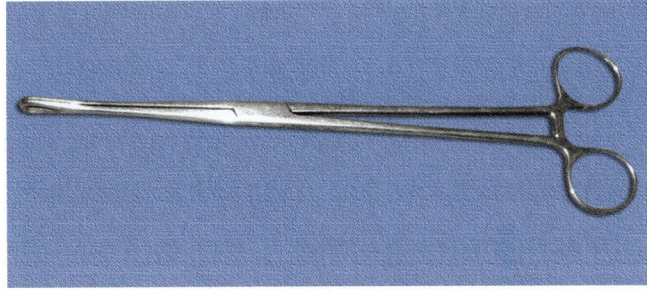

Fig. 41-2 Sponge holding forceps- (Rampley's) both curved and straight.

Artery Forceps–(Hemostat)

Types

- <u>Based on size</u>—large, medium or small sized/mosquito artery forceps (*Mosquito forceps* is so called because of its fine tip which even can catch the proboscis of a mosquito).
- <u>Based on shape</u>—straight artery forceps; curved artery forceps.
- <u>Features of artery forceps</u>—distal blades are having transverse serrations which are well apposed; lock in the proximal part.

Uses: To catch bleeding points; to open the facial planes in different surgeries; to pass a ligature and to hold it; to hold fascia, peritoneum, aponeurosis; to hold sutures; to drain an abscess like a sinus forceps; to hold gauze as pea-nut; to crush the base of the appendix; to clamp a catheter in between the hinge and ratchet of the hemostat; to catch prepuceal skin in circumcision; mosquito forceps is used in pediatric surgery/microsurgery/cleft surgery/plastic surgery. Instrument can also be used to catch arteries/veins/capillaries

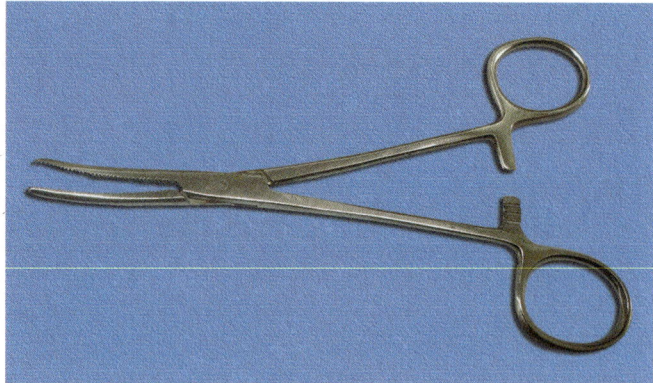

Fig. 41-3 Curved medium sized artery forceps (hemostat).

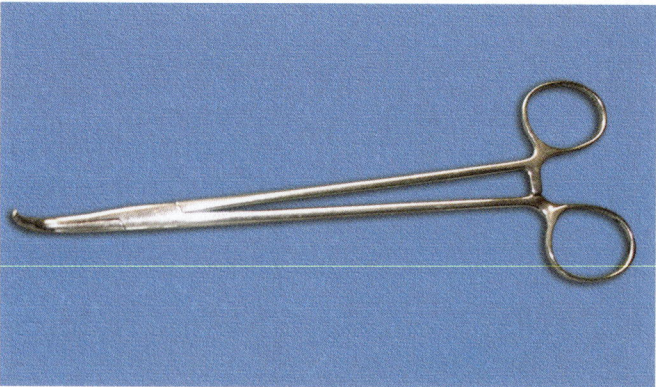

Fig. 41-5 Meigster right angled forceps.

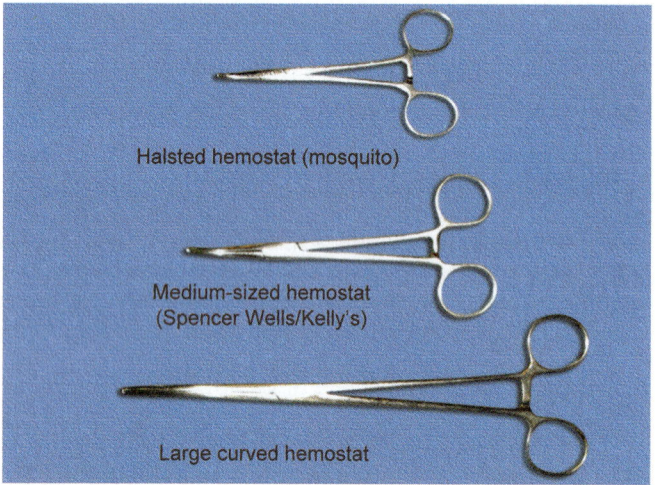

Fig. 41-4 Different types of hemostats. It can be small, medium or large sized; it can be curved or straight.

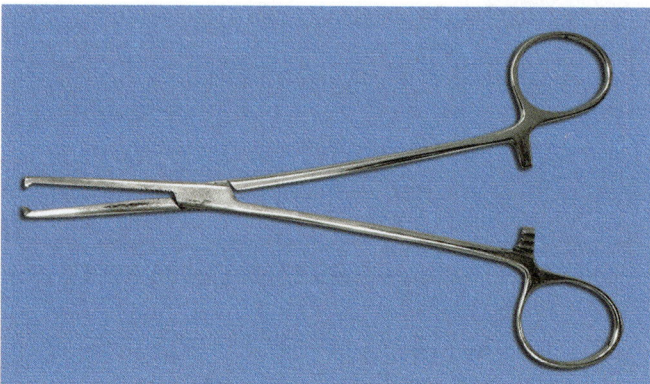

Fig. 41-6 Kocher's forceps.

and so ideally should be called as *hemostat*. But common word used is artery forceps. Hemostat has got serrations on the distal half of the each blade. (In pedicle clamp entire blade has got serrations). Medium sized, curved half serrated hemostat is called as Kelly's artery forceps (Fig. 41-4).

Right Angle Forceps – Meigster's/Lahey's/Mixter's

It has got 90° curves in terminal 1 cm part of the blades. Blades are *longitudinally* serrated. It has got a ratchet. Tip is blunt. It is used to dissect pedicles and to pass ligatures, to dissect the vagus and ligate in vagotomy, to hold bleeding vessels in depth, to dissect major vessels, to dissect and pass ligatures to cystic duct and cystic artery in cholecystectomy and in thyroid, biliary, splenic, gastric, renal and pelvic surgeries (Fig. 41-5).

Kocher's Forceps

It has got serrations in the distal blades and apposing tooth in the tip. It holds the tissues/pedicle well and prevents slippage of the tissues and retraction of the vessels/bleeders. It can be straight or curved; small or medium sized. It is used to hold pedicles, tough structures, cut ends of the muscles like - in thyroidectomy/hemorrhoidectomy/mastectomy/polypectomy/hysterectomy. It is used to hold tough/fibrous structures like in palms/soles/scalp to prevent retraction of vessels during surgery. It is used to hold peanuts (gauze pellets of 3-4 mm sized used in blunt dissection). It is used to hold gauze for blunt dissection, to hold resected bowel, to hold ribs during rib resection. *Emil Theodor Kocher* (1912)–from Switzerland is the first surgeon to get Nobel Prize (Fig. 41-6).

Allis' Tissue Holding Forceps

Here distal blades are not apposing each other. Tip has got teeth in each blade which are apposing. It has got lock. It is used to hold skin flaps, fascias, fibrous tissue, aponeurosis, galea (in craniotomy) and bladder wall. It is essential instrument in any surgery whether major or minor. It can be small/medium/large. Large Allis is used in hysterectomy to hold vaginal wall and tough structures (Fig. 41-7).

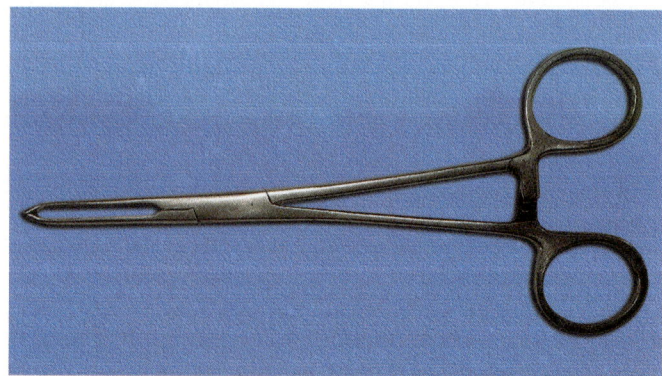

Fig. 41-7 Allis' tissue holding forceps.

Babcock's Forceps

Their distal parts of distal blades are curved with triangular fenestra in it which allows soft tissues to bulge out. Tip is non-traumatic with transverse serrations/ridges on it. It has got a lock. It is used to hold any part of the bowel, fallopian tubes, appendix, urinary bladder, ureter, cord, lymph node (Fig. 41-8).

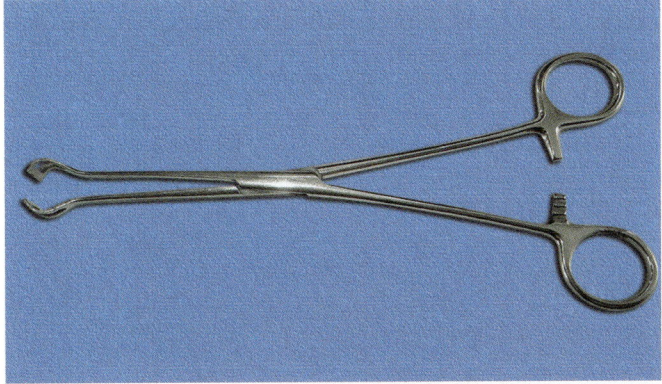

Fig. 41-8 Babcock's forceps.

Lane's Tissue Holding Forceps

It has got thick, stout distal blades with oval fenestra in each blade with a curvature at the end. It has got apposing tooth in the tip. It has got lock. It is used to hold bulky and tough structures (like to hold breast during mastectomy; to hold salivary glands while excising), to hold lymph nodes, to hold tumor tissue. It is also used as towel clip or as sponge holding forceps (Fig. 41-9).

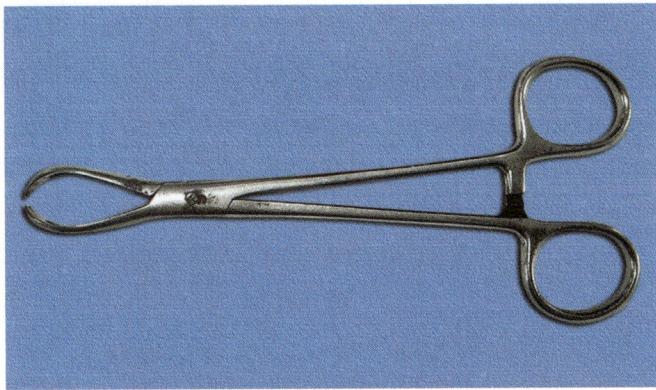

Fig. 41-9 Lane's tissue holding forceps.

Moran-Baker's Appendix Holding Forceps

It is like Lane's forceps but with apposing serrations proximal to the tooth. These serrations give a good grip on mesoappendix while holding appendix in appendicectomy. Its use is replaced by Babcock's forceps (Fig. 41-10).

Dissecting Forceps

Plain non-toothed dissecting forceps: It is used to hold delicate soft, friable structures like peritoneum, vessels, bowel, nerves, and tendons. It cannot be used to hold skin or tough structures. During surgical dissection it is used to hold/fix/steady/stretch the structures as needed. It is also used to hold bleeding points, to cauterize small vessels.

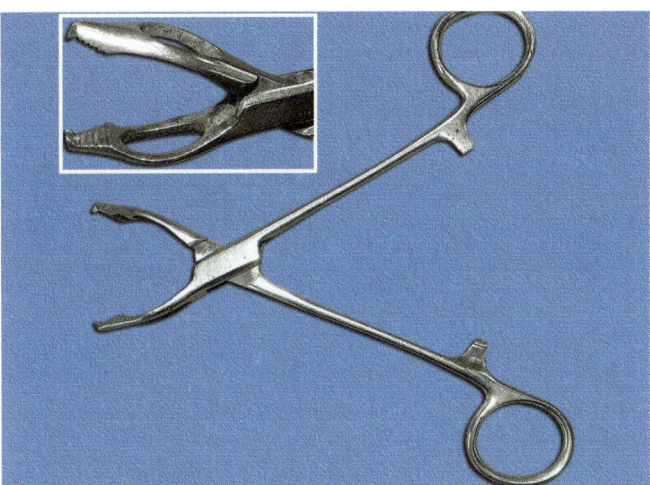

Fig. 41-10 Moran-Baker's tissue holding forceps.

Toothed-dissecting forceps: It is used to hold skin and tough structures like fascia, aponeurosis. It is not used to hold delicate structures like bowel/vessel/nerve. It can have one in two teeth or two in three teeth. Small, fine forceps used for fine works is called as Adson's forceps. *Adson's forceps can be toothed or non-toothed* (Fig. 41-11).

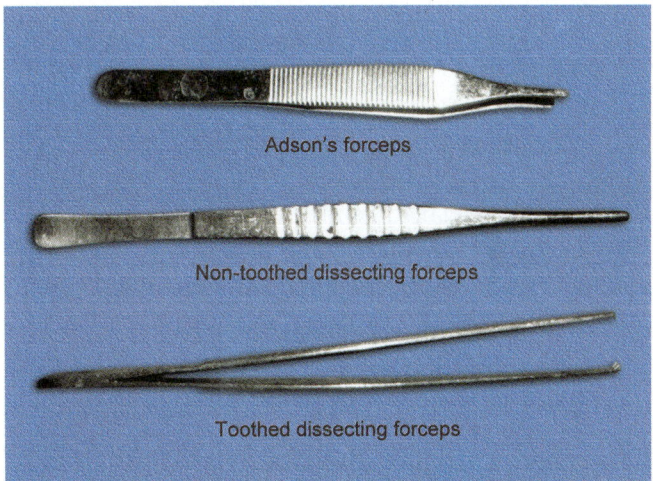

Fig. 41-11 Different types of dissecting forceps.

Sinus Forceps (Lister's)

It has got straight, long blades with serrations in the tip; does not have lock. It is atraumatic. It is used to drain pus from abscess cavity (Hilton's method); it is initially originated to pack the sinus cavities hence the name; also used to pack nasal cavity and ear. It is less traumatic (Fig. 41-12).

■ CLAMPS

Bowel Occlusion Clamps

It is used in gastrointestinal surgeries. *Moynihan's occlusion clamp (gastric):* It has got long distal blades with transverse serrations with a longitudinal fenestration one on each blade. It may be straight or curved. It is non-traumatic, non-crushing

Section 6: Miscellaneous

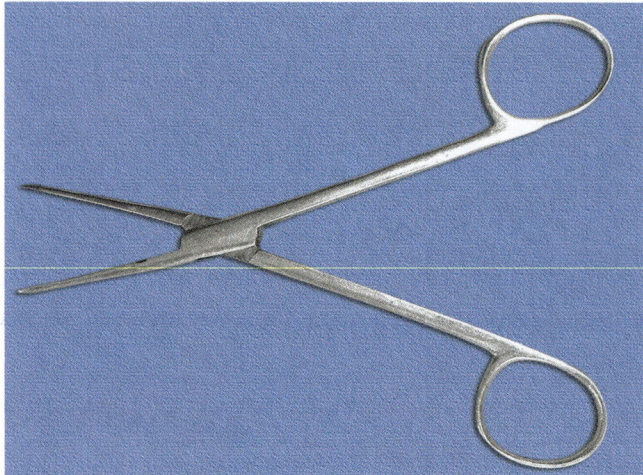

Fig. 41-12 Lister's sinus forceps

type. It occludes lumen of the bowel/stomach and so prevents spillage of the content of the bowel. It also occludes the vessels in the wall of the bowel and so prevents bleeding during surgery. It is used during anastomosis of the stomach and other parts of the bowel. *Doyen's intestinal occlusion clamps (straight or curved)*—it has got longitudinal serrations with apposing blades (Figs. 41-13 and 41-14).

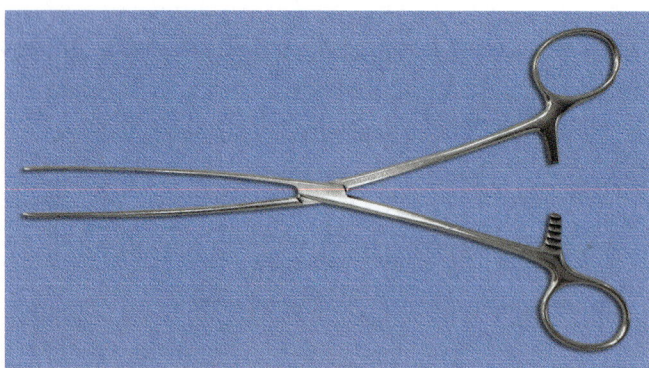

Fig. 41-13 Moynihan's occlusion clamp. It has got transverse serrations.

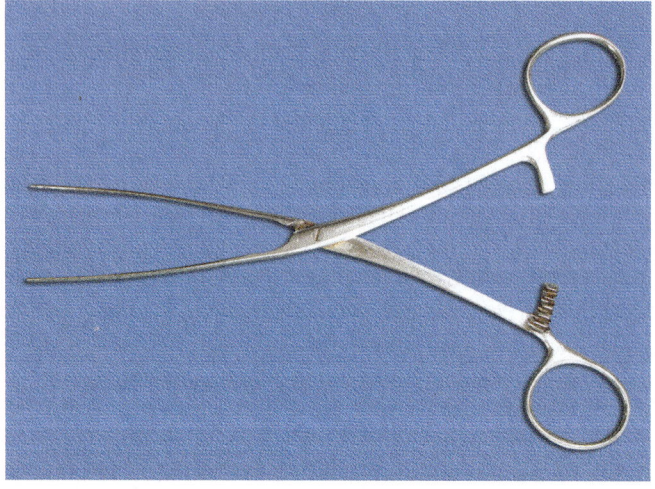

Fig. 41-14 Doyen's occlusion clamp. It has got longitudinal serrations.

Bowel Crushing Clamps (Fig. 41-15)

Crushing clamps are usually strong, stout which holds tissues firmly. *Payr's crushing clamp (Fig. 41-18) – gastric/intestinal/appendix crushing clamp*—it is stout and heavy instrument with double lever in the handle with longitudinal serrations. Once applied it crushes the bowel. So before applying it, line of resection of stomach/bowel should be assessed properly. It is applied to the part which has to be removed. Viability of the bowel is lost once it is applied. It is used in gastrectomy, resection and anastomosis of the bowel.

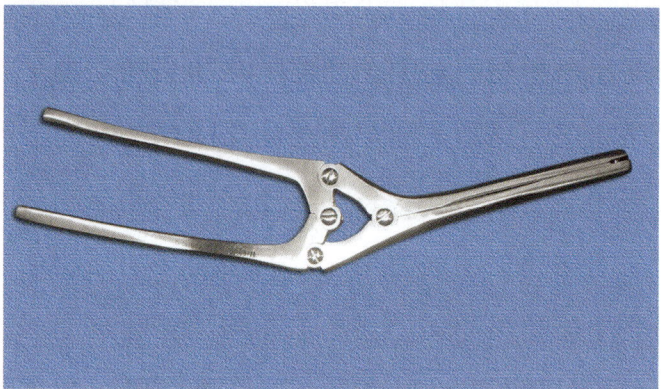

Fig. 41-15 Payr's gastric crushing clamp.

RETRACTORS

A retractor is an instrument used to retract tissues away from the operating field, to expose surgical field properly, to carry out surgery precisely and also to prevent damage to adjacent structures while conducting operation. It also prevents the unnecessary handling of the adjacent tissues.

> **Uses of retractors**
> - Retraction of cut edges of the incision
> - To hold important structures like liver/spleen, etc. away from surgical field
> - To steady the tissues
> - To control bleeding
> - To avoid inadvertent trauma to adjacent structures

Langenbeck's Retractor

It has got a long handle and a small solid blade. It is used in hernia surgery or any superficial surgeries to retract skin, fascia and aponeurosis, etc. It can be single bladed or double bladed (Fig. 41-16).

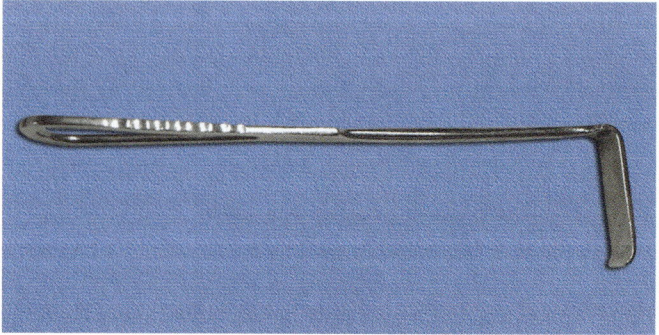

Fig. 41-16 Langenbeck's retractor.

Czerney's Retractor (Hernia Retractor)

This retractor has got thick, small blade on one side and biflanged hook on the other side in opposite directions. It is used in surgeries like hernia, laparotomy especially during closure. Bleeders in the edge can be identified and cauterized easily (Fig. 41-17).

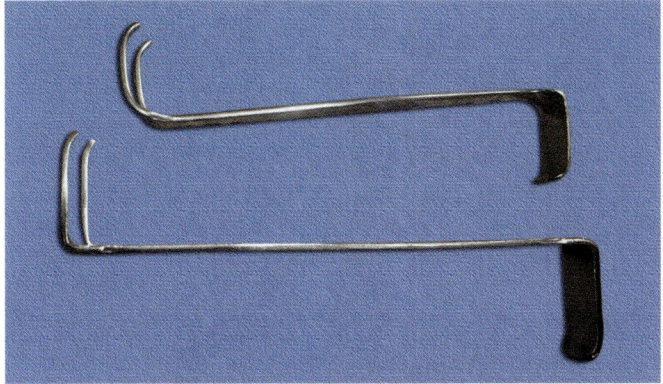

Fig. 41-17 Czerney's hernia retractor.

Morris' (Abdominal Wall) Retractor

It may be single blade type or double blade type. It has flat transversely curved blade. There is a blunt projecting ridge with backward projection to have a better hold. It is used to retract abdominal wall incisions/loin incisions/subcostal wounds/any wider wounds in depth (Fig. 41-18).

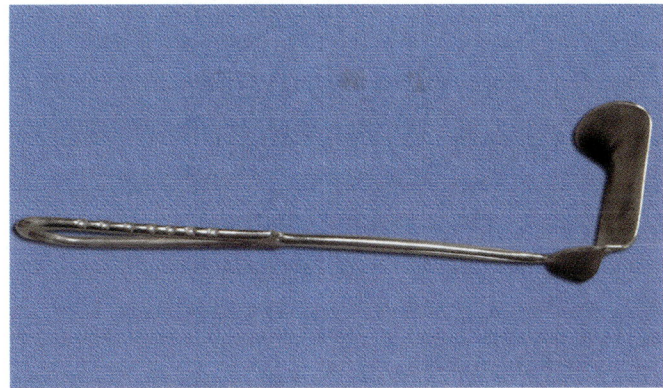

Fig. 41-18 Morris retractors-single blade (one sided).

Deaver's Retractor

It is an instrument like a question mark (?). It is stout but atraumatic and gives adequate exposure of the surgical field. Its action is *levering* of the tissues not by push or pull or traction. Moist mops should be kept underneath prior to placing this retractor. It is a retractor with a broad, gently curved blade. It is used to retract the abdominal wall, liver, spleen and other abdominal viscera. All major abdominal surgeries like vagotomy, cholecystectomy, gastrectomy, pancreatic surgeries, colonic surgeries, kidney surgeries, anterior resection/abdomino-perineal resection, bladder surgeries need this instrument (Fig. 41-19).

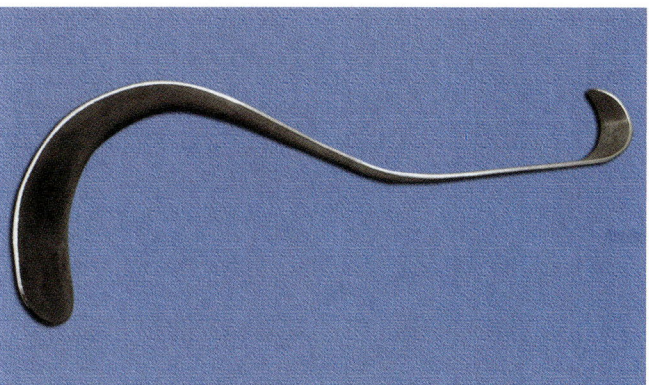

Fig. 41-19 Deaver's retractor (manual).

Doyen's Retractor

It is used in pelvic surgeries and in laparotomies. It has a curved blade with convex edge with a long handle. It is used to retract urinary bladder during hysterectomy, during cesarean section (Fig. 41-20).

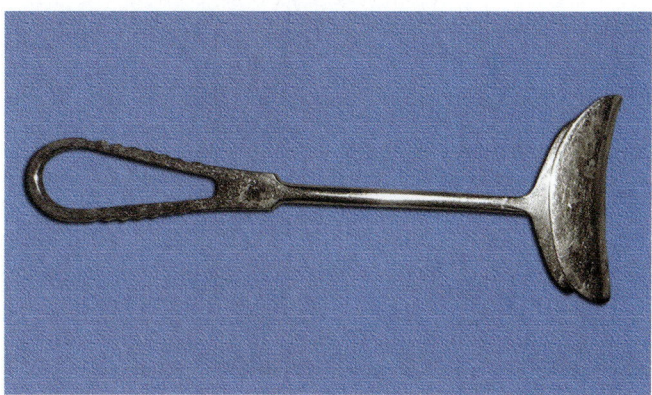

Fig. 41-20 Doyen's Retractor.

Balfour's Self-retaining Retractor

It has got different adjustable blades so as to retract abdominal wall and tissues during surgery. It has got quadrangular metal frame. Two side heavy blades are hook shaped to fit into the wound sides. There is a detachable third blade to retract the viscera. One of the side blades has got screw to adjust the width of the retraction by side blades. Detachable blade is also fixed through an adjustable screw with a slot. Closed instrument is inserted into the wound and adequately widened as required to have its use. Tissues/bowel/organs should not be trapped while widening and adjusting (Fig. 41-21).

Joll's Thyroid Retractor

It is a self-retaining retractor specifically used for thyroid/parathyroid surgeries. It is a semi-circular retractor with two blades attached with a handle. End of the blades are sharp like a towel clip with a catch/ratchet on it. Handle has got a screw by which instrument can be opened or closed. Upper

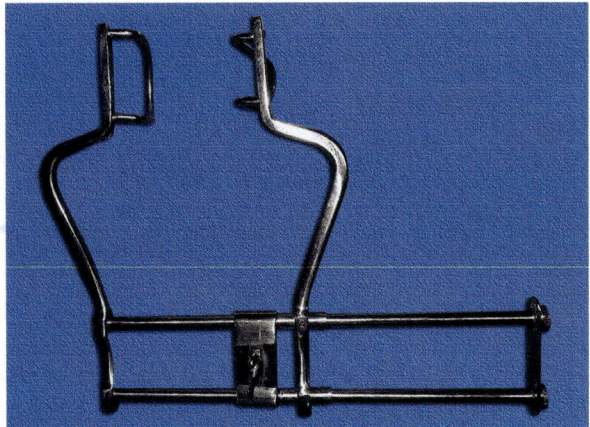

Fig. 41-21 Balfour's self-retaining retractor.

and lower skin flaps in thyroid surgery is retracted well using this instrument (Fig. 41-22).

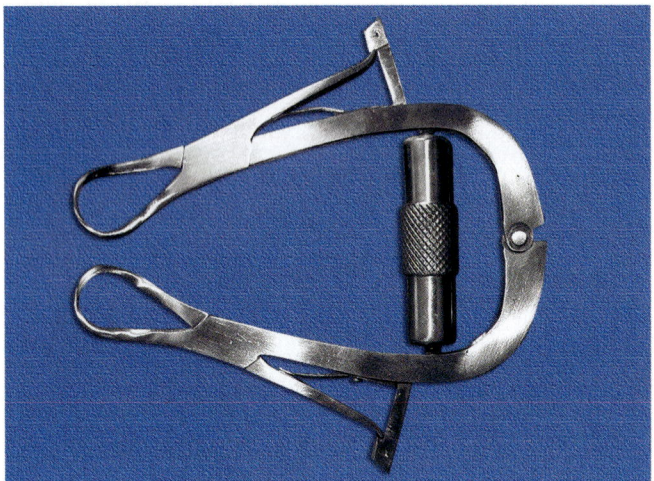

Fig. 41-22 Joll's thyroid retractor.

SCISSORS

Scissors has got various purposes in surgical field like dissection, cutting tissues, cutting suture materials, opening tissue planes, venesection, cutting bandages, corrugated/tube drains and dressing, ophthalmic or microsurgeries, etc. It can be straight, curved, small, medium or long scissors (Fig. 41-23 to 41-26).

Different scissors are:
Mayo's scissors – are long and stout scissors. It can be blunt tipped/pointed tip/straight or curved.
McIndoe scissor – is having fine small blade. It is used mainly for dissection and in cutting delicate structures.
Metzenbaum scissor – has got long blades in comparison to shaft. It is used in depth dissection like vagotomy, cholecystectomy, pelvic surgeries, etc.
Heath suture cutting scissor – has got long shaft, small curves angled blades with tip is having fine serrations which ensures the proper grip of the suture material to be cut. Suture is held with dissecting forceps and is cut using heath's scissor between knot and skin where suture enters **(Fig. 41-24)**.

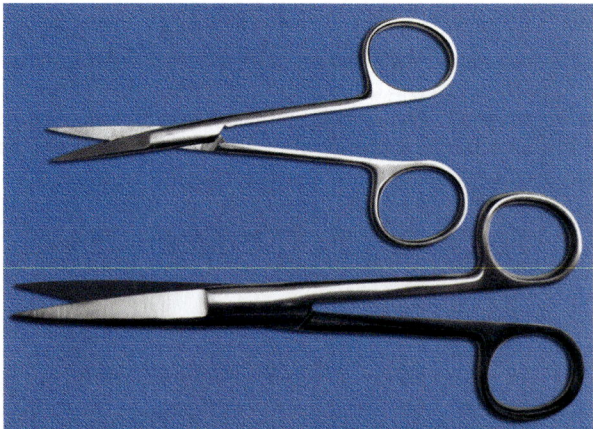

Fig. 41-23 Different scissors used in surgical practice.

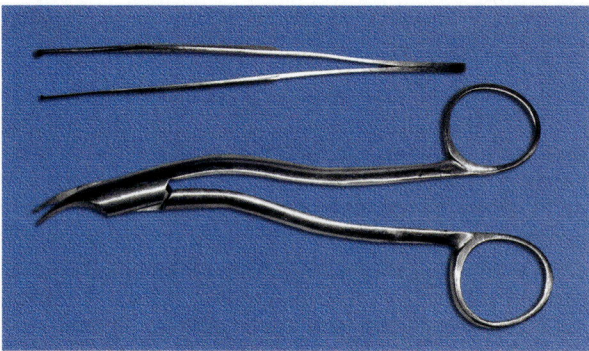

Fig. 41-24 Heath's scissor with toothed forceps.

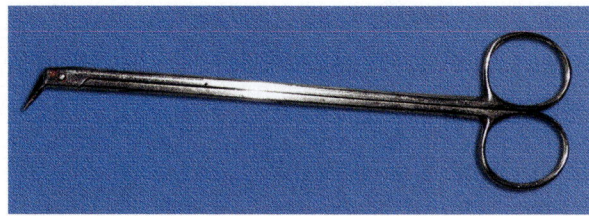

Fig. 41-25 Pott's Smith scissor. It is useful in cutting tubular structures like ureter, bile duct, vessels in various surgeries. Its anglulation makes it easier to cut as per need.

Steele's scissor is like Metzenbaum scissor with similar use.
Lister's bandage/dressing cutting scissor has got flat lower blade to avoid damage to skin. Lower blade has got a knob at the terminal **(Fig. 41-26)**.

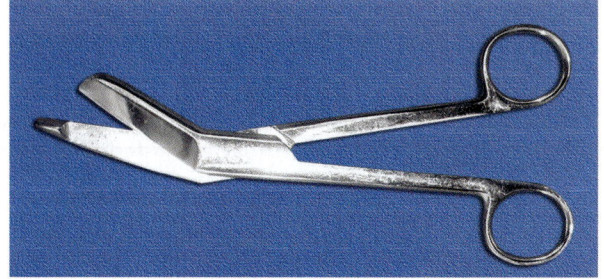

Fig. 41-26 Lister's bandage cutting scissor.

SUCTION INSTRUMENTS

These are essential instruments needed in all surgical practice to suck out blood from the surgical field, pus, infected fluid, fluid in peritoneal/thoracic/cranial cavities. It has got a *suction tip* of varying type, *suction tube* which connects tip to the *suction apparatus* and suction creating system, either central suction system *or* power suction system with two suction glass bottles connected to each other *or* manual suction apparatus (now not used). Suction tip has got a long bent tube with openings at one end to suck the fluid, with a stout handle which has got a proximal ridged part at the other end to which suction tube (rubber or plastic) is attached, which is in turn is connected to suction apparatus. Suction tip and suction tubes should be sterile. They are sterilized by autoclave.

Types of suction tips – Adson's fine suction tip – it is angled with a vent/thumb rest to control the suction as needed (Fig. 41-27). It is a fine suction tip which is used in meticulous surgeries like plastic, vascular and reconstructive surgeries. It cannot be used when large quantity of blood/pus/fluid/clot needs to be sucked out. Yankauer suction tip – it is large suction tip used mainly in peritoneal cavity after lavage, in haemoperitoneum, in peritonitis, in pelvis, in thoracotomy, etc. It has got central hole with outer small multiple holes. It creates strong suction and so may suck omentum; bowel wall, etc. (Fig. 41-28) and so with one hand bowel and omentum should be pushed aside while sucking the fluid. Often its tip is supported by a rubber tube. When it is present, care is taken to see that it is not left inside the peritoneal cavity by inadvertent slippage. Poole's multi-perforated suction tip – it has got outer and inner tubes – one inside the other (Fig. 41-29). Outer tube has got multiple holes with blunt closed tip so that bowel/tissues will not be sucked inside. Inner tube has got one terminal and another proximal side holes. Inner tube will be inside the outer tube attached with a screw on proximal aspect. It acts by sump action principle.

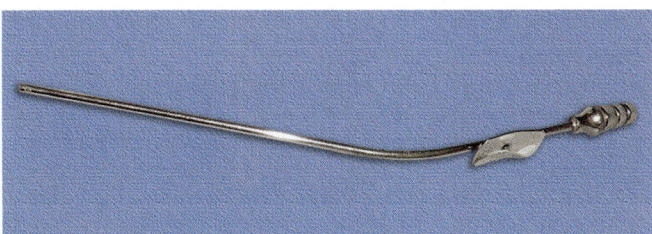

Fig. 41-27 Adson's suction tip.

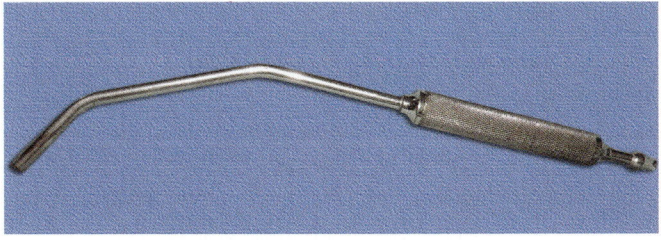

Fig. 41-28 Yankauer suction tip.

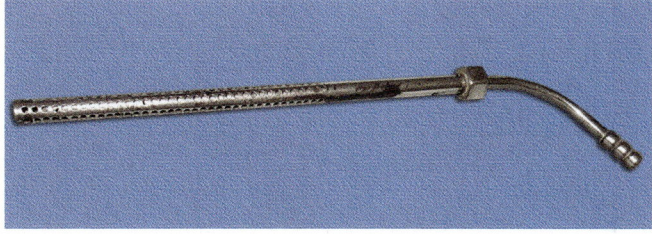

Fig. 41-29 Poole's suction tip.

DRAINS

A drain is a created channel which allows any collected fluid to come out after closure of the main wound (Figs. 41-30 to 41.32).

Types: (1) *Corrugated rubber drain:* It drains by capillary action and gravity. It is cheaper and technically easier. But it allows soakage of dressings and causes discomfort to the patient (Fig. 41-30). (2) *Tube drains:* Malecot catheter can be used as tube drain; Penrose soft latex rubber tube; multiple perforated tubes; (3) *Closed suction tube drain system.* (4) *Glove drain.* (5) *Wick drain* is a gauze drain to drain pus, discharge, etc.

Indications for drains: In drainage of an abscess; in bleeding surgical conditions like trauma, per-operative bleed; in hemo, pyo or pneumothorax; in acute abdominal conditions like peritonitis, hemoperitoneum; in major abdominal surgeries like of pancreas, biliary tree, stomach, etc.; in thyroid surgery; in hydrocele surgery.

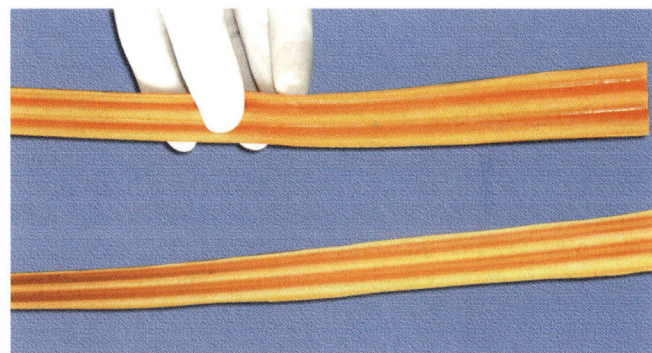

Fig. 41-30 Corrugated rubber drain.

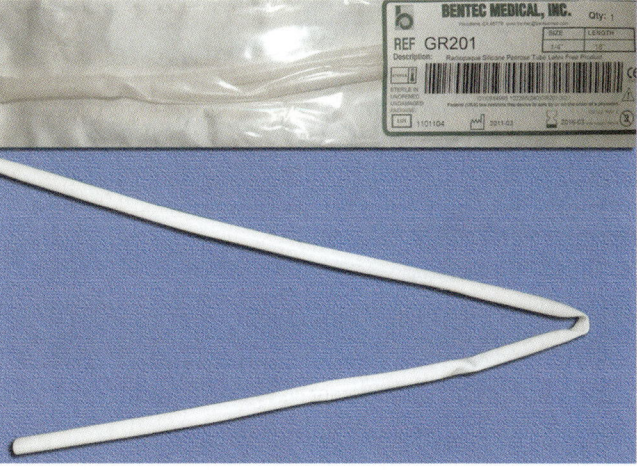

Fig. 41-31 Pen rose drain.

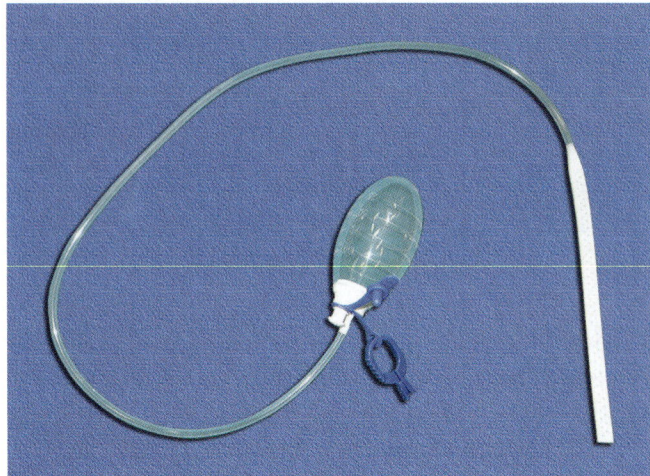

Fig. 41-32 Jackson Pratt suction drain.

Problems in drains: Infection through the drain; displacement.; it may not drain adequately and can give a false information; it may interfere with healing process inside. A drain should be placed always in most dependent position and should be brought out through shortest straight route with a separate stab incision. It should be anchored to skin securely. Corrugated drain should be kept with adequate length otherwise it may get into the abdominal cavity during phases of respiration. In tube drain – quantity of drain can be measured; can be kept longer; patient will be comfortable without excoriation; removal easier and less infection. Problem is tube get clogged giving false impression of less drain quantity.

■ CATHETERS

They are hollow tubes used to relieve urinary retention, obtain urine for analysis, irrigate bladder and to instill drugs into bladder. They are made up of India rubber, latex rubber, metal, polyethylene, gum elastic materials.

Types (Fig. 41-33)– (1) *Non-self-retaining catheter:* Simple red rubber catheter. (2) *Self-retaining catheter:* Foley's catheter, Malecot's catheter, Gibbon's catheter, De-pezzer catheter.

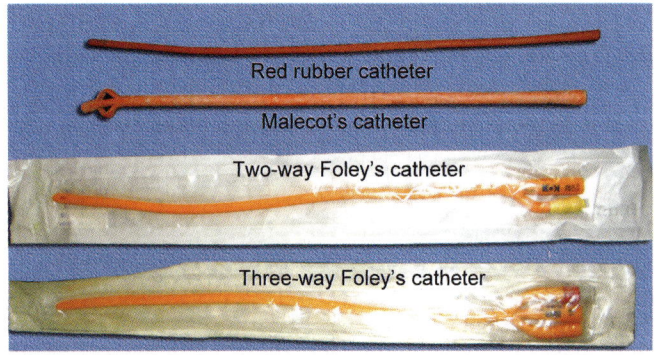

Fig. 41-33 Different types of catheters.

Foley's Catheter (Fredrick Eugene Basil Foley–American Urologist)

It is a *self-retaining* urinary catheter made up of *latex*. It has got a balloon near the tip into which distilled water is infused to make *itself retainable*. Usually Foley's catheter is kept for 7 days. It is *sterilized* by γ radiation. Size: Adults–16 F; Children–8 F or 10 F. (F-*French unit, Charriere unit, where each unit equals 0.33 mm*). 16 F means circumference of the catheter is 16 mm. (Diameter is one third of circumference). Different sized Foley's catheter is identified number labeled and color strap near two or three way end. *Types:* (1) Two-way Foley's; (2) Three way Foley's—To give bladder irrigation, e.g. following TURP; (3) Silicon coated Foley's—To reduce reaction and so as to keep for longer period (3 months).

Procedure: After cleaning under strict asepsis, lignocaine gel is lubricated into the urethral meatus. Catheter is passed into the urethra. Sometimes *Maryfield introducer* is used to pass Foley's catheter. Once catheter is in the bladder, urine will flow out. It is now connected to an *urosac bag*. Balloon is inflated with 20-30 mL (amount is written on the catheter) of distilled water to make itself retainable. During removal of the catheter same amount of water should be removed from the balloon before pulling out the catheter.

Uses:
- To pass per urethrally in retention of urine of any cause [BPH, stricture, trauma)
- To measure the urine output in renal failure, postoperative patients, and terminally ill patients, and patients under critical care
- After prostatectomy or TURP – three way catheter is used for irrigation also. Here it is also used as hemostatic by inflating more distilled water into the balloon and giving traction causing tamponade effect
- Paraplegia/neurogenic bladder – initially Foley's catheter is used later condom drainage is better
- To give bladder wash in hematuria, infection, etc.
- Percutaneous suprapubic cystostomy
- Cholecystostomy
- To drain fistulas
- To control bleeding from nostrils/post hemorrhoidectomy secondary hemorrhage
- In children to give enema or to do barium/contrast enema X-rays

Complications
- Infection; encrustation; bleeding; stone formation; blockage, false passage; stricture
- Difficulty in removal of the catheter due to blockage of the balloon channel. Here bulb of Foley's can be punctured from above under ultrasound guidance or injection of ether into the balloon so as to burst it but it may cause chemical cystitis or passing a stilette into the channel.

Malecot's Catheter

It is self-retaining urinary catheter with an umbrella or flower at the tip. It is made of red rubber, contains sulphur and so it is radiopaque. *It is never introduced per urethral*. It is sterilized by boiling.

Uses: (1) Suprapubic cystostomy (SPC). In case of urinary retention when Foley's catheterization fails (after two trials); For diversion of urine following bladder, prostate or urethral surgeries. (2) To continuous drainage of abscess cavities – perinephric abscess, pyonephrosis, subphrenic abscess, amebic liver abscess. (3) Cabot's nephrostomy. (4) Cholecystostomy. (5) Infected pseudocyst of the pancreas. (6) Gastrostomy, cecostomy (tube type).

Advantages: Malecot's catheter can be kept for a long period of time (3 months); it drains fluid adequately; less infection rate; removal is easier (gentle pull with pressure).

Disadvantage: Surgery (open method) is required to insert the catheter. Now percutaneous tubes are available.

Simple Red Rubber Catheter

It is a non-self retaining urinary catheter. It is stiffer than Foley's catheter. Its tip is rounded and blunt. Opening is only on the side wall (In flatus tube opening is present on both sides and also at the tip). Here English unit is used to number – diameter is 1 + catheter number/2.

Uses: (1) Used to drain urine from the bladder temporarily in retention of urine. (2) To find out residual urine. After passing urine, catheter is introduced into the bladder. The amount of retained urine is measured. If it is more than 30-50 mL it signifies obstruction. It often increases more than 200 mL in conditions like BPH and indicates significant obstruction that needs surgical intervention like TURP. (3) While doing cystography to infuse dilute iodine dye into the bladder. (4) Single gentle passage of the red rubber catheter is tried as a diagnostic method to identify the urethral/bladder/renal injuries. Hematuria signifies urinary tract injury. Measured normal saline is infused into the bladder and return volume is collected; if it is less, then it indicates injury to bladder. (5) For administration of intravesical chemotherapy or therapeutic BCG infusion in to the bladder per urethral in bladder carcinoma. (6) To collect urine from the bladder for culture and sensitivity. (7) To identify the urethra in perineal surgery/urethral surgery/penectomy. (8) To dislodge and push back the calculus impacted in the urinary meatus or in the urethra. (9) Other uses like—to administer nasal oxygen; for suction of throat/endotracheal tube/tracheostomy tube; as a tourniquet for venesection and surgeries of fingers and toes; used as a sling in many places like to hold cord, to hold vagus, to hold pedicles, to hold esophagus/bowel/ureter; to irrigate and clear the pus after opening the abscess cavity/or any other cavities in depth; to irrigate common bile duct after choledochotomy; to irrigate ureter/renal pelvis after stone removal.

■ URETHRAL DILATORS

Lister's Urethral Dilator

It has got olive tip with a rounded handle. Handle is rounded with numbers marked. Denominator is circumference in mm at the base of the Lister's dilator. Numerator signifies circumference just proximal to the olive tip (narrowest point). Difference between denominator and numerator is 3 mm. So each dilator is narrowed for 3 mm from base to proximal end of olive tip. Circumference of olive tip is equal to circumference in the base. Numbering is based on English scale (diameter in mm = Number/2 + 1 (Fig. 41-34).

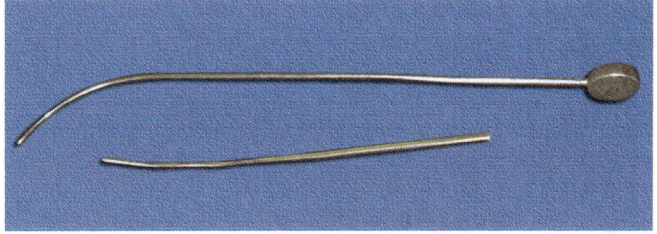

Fig. 41-34 Lister's urethral dilator.

It is used dilate stricture urethra; to pass catheter by open rail road technique in rupture urethra. With all aseptic precautions urethral dilatation is done (proper cleaning and draping).

Clutton's Dilator

It is a long metallic instrument with a curve and blunt tip at the end. Handle is violin shaped. It is numbered in English units. Denominator of the part signifies the circumference in the base and numerator suggests the circumference in the tip. Difference between denominator and numerator is 4. Numbers are like 6/10; 8/12; 10/14—so on (Fig. 41-35).

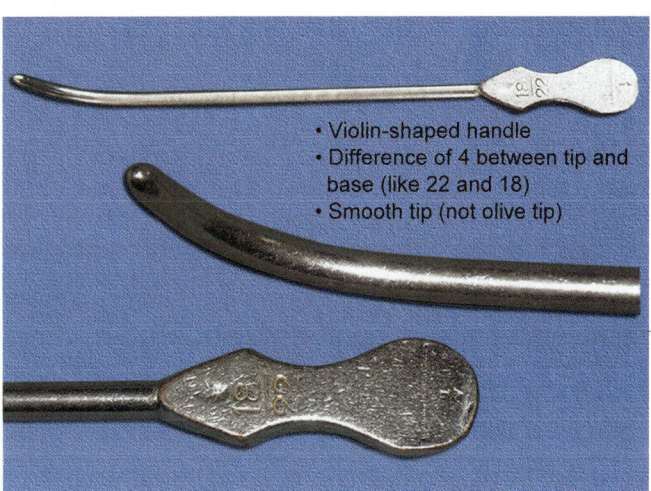

- Violin-shaped handle
- Difference of 4 between tip and base (like 22 and 18)
- Smooth tip (not olive tip)

Fig. 41-35 Clutton's urethral dilator.

■ NASOGASTRIC TUBE/RYLE'S TUBE

It is one meter long which is made up of red rubber or plastic. Original Ryle's tube was made up of moulded red rubber (Fig. 41-36). Presently used nasogastric tubes are made up of polyethylene or portex. Tip is blunt without opening.

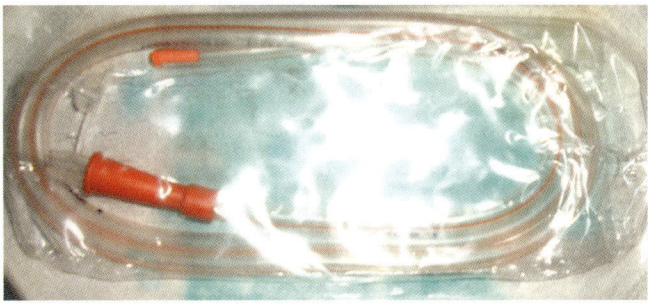

Fig. 41-36 Ryle's tube.

Subterminal multiple openings are present on all the sides. It is sterilized by gamma rays. It has got three lead shots in the tip which makes it radiopaque. It also facilitates easy passage of the tube through the esophagus. Once tube is inside the stomach, bile/gastric juice will come out of the proximal end, often confirmed by aspiration. Stethoscope is placed over the stomach; syringe with air is pushed into the tube; if tip of the tube is in the stomach air entering into the stomach can be heard through the stethoscope. It is passed through one of the nostrils using xylocaine 2% jelly. Under anesthesia it is passed using Magill's forceps. It should be fixed securely to the nostrils otherwise it may get displaced or come out. It should be replaced with new tube in 2 weeks. Intermittent suction or continuous open drainage can be done depending on requirement. In postoperative period it is removed once patient passes flatus; adequate bowel sounds are heard; content in the tube is reduced to less than 50 mL.

It has got markings at different levels: At 40 cm distance indicates the level of gastroesophageal junction. At 50 cm distance, indicates the level of body of the stomach. At 60 cm distance, indicates the level of the pylorus. At 65 cm distance, indicates the level of the duodenum.

Indications

(1) *Diagnostic:* For gastric function tests. To assess free acid and total acid – in gastric/duodenal ulcers; pyloric obstruction/carcinoma stomach (exfoliative cytology); achylia; Zollinger – Ellison syndrome; pernicious anemia; saline load test to confirm gastric motility and outlet obstruction; small bowel enema; Hollander's test for completion of vagotomy; to diagnose tracheoesophageal fistula; Baid test for pseudocyst of the pancreas. (2) *Therapeutic:* In acute abdominal conditions like peritonitis/obstruction, etc. In abdominal trauma; after abdominal surgeries; in pyloric stenosis; in upper GIT bleeding; in paralytic ileus, gastric dilatation to decompress the bowel; for feeding purpose in comatose patients, faciomaxillary injuries, major head and neck surgeries, head injuries, pharyngolaryngeal surgeries.

Complications

Injury to nostrils and bleeding; pharyngitis/rhinitis; discomfort/unacceptancy; ulceration in the pharynx/esophagus; aspiration pneumonia as lower sphincter is kept open – dangerous complication – may cause death also; perforation of esophagus. *Nasogastric tube is contraindicated in corrosive esophageal burns in initial phases for 2 weeks.*

SURGICAL NEEDLES

It is classified as –

Based on curvature: Straight needle. Curved needle. Half circle; 5/8 circle etc.

Based on existence of the eye: *Atraumatic needle* is eyeless. Here suture material is attached to the needle by *swaging* (Mr Merson of England). Size of the suture material and that of needle is same and so tissue trauma is less. Needle once used is disposed (not reusable). It is available as sterilized pack. These needles can be round body or cutting. *Traumatic needle:* It is eyed needle. Needle in the eye area is wider than the body of the needle and so tissue trauma is more. These needles are re-usable.

Types (Fig. 41-37)

Based on the Edge

- *Round body needle:* It is round and smooth on cross section. It is used to suture muscles/intestines/soft tissues/vessels/nerves/tendons/peritoneum.
- *Conventional cutting needle:* Here needle is triangular on cross section with apex facing inward. It is used to suture skin/aponeurosis/tough structures.
- *Reverse cutting needle:* Here needle is triangular (reverse) on cross section with apex facing outward. It increases the strength and is less likely to bend while suturing.
- *Taper cut needle:* Here tip of the needle is reverse cut in section but eventually tapers into the body as round in section. It improves the penetration of needle but minimizes the trauma.

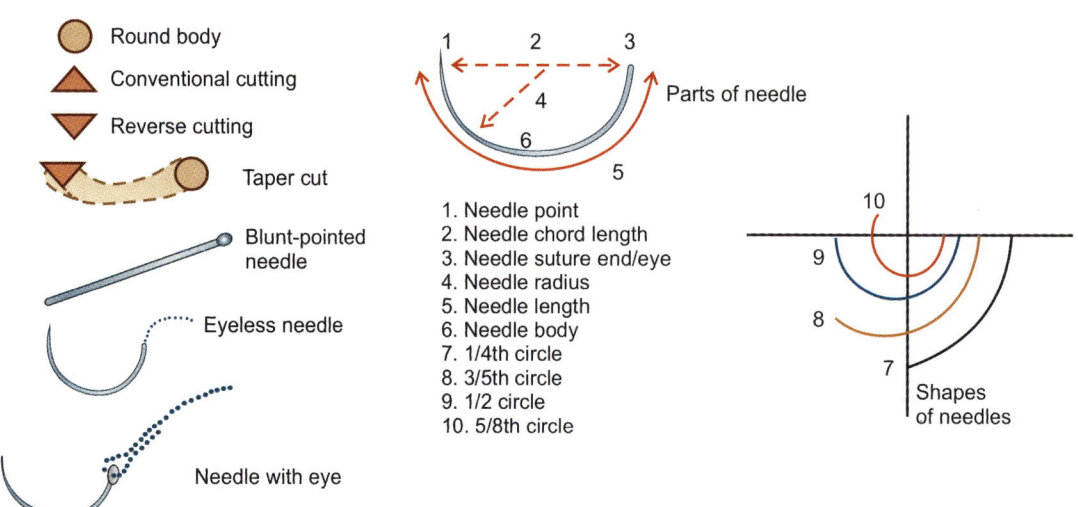

Fig. 41-37 Different types of needles. Diagram also shows the eyeless/eyed needles and gives the meanings of 1/4th, 1/2, 3/8th and 5/8th circle needles.

Needle Holder

Smaller distal blades with criss-cross serrations often with a groove in the middle are the features of a needle holder. Often there is a longitudinal groove in the middle of the distal blade between serrations. Ratio of length of handle to blades is 4:1. It may be straight or curved. It may be available in different sizes. While holding a needle in a needle holder one should get a good control and good grip. This is achieved by placing the needle at junction of proximal 2/3 and distal 1/3 of the blade. Needle holder should be held between thumb and ring finger. Curved needle holders are available to hold the needles and work at the depth like in pelvis/thoracic cavity for better maneuverability and visualization. Needle holder is sterilized by autoclave. Tungsten – carbide inner surface coated needle holder is available which has got longer duration of life due to reduced wear and tear of the instrument because of tungsten coating (Fig. 41-38).

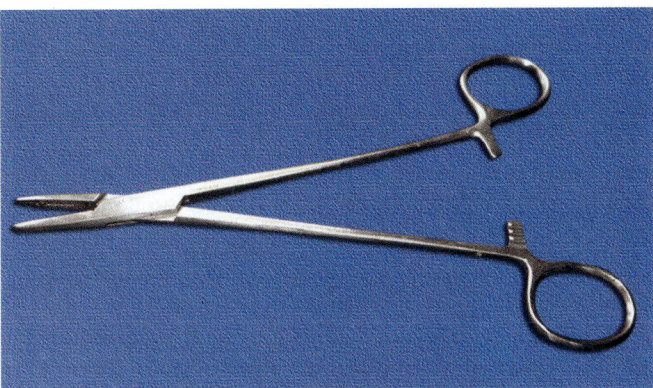

Fig. 41-38 Needle holder (driver).

Bard Parker's Handle (BP Handle)

Bard Parker's handle is a flat stainless steel instrument with a slot on narrower side on both surfaces to attach scalpel blade. 3, 4, 5 and 7 numbered blades are available. Number 4 handle is wider. Scalpel blades 10, 11, 12, and 15 fit into Bard Parker handle numbers 3, 5 and 7. Scalpel blades 18, 19, 20, 21, 22, 23 and 24 fit into slot of Bard Parker's blade number 4. New blade is used into the slot of the handle for each patient and so sharpness of the blade is maintained. BP handle is sterilized by autoclave (Fig. 41-39).

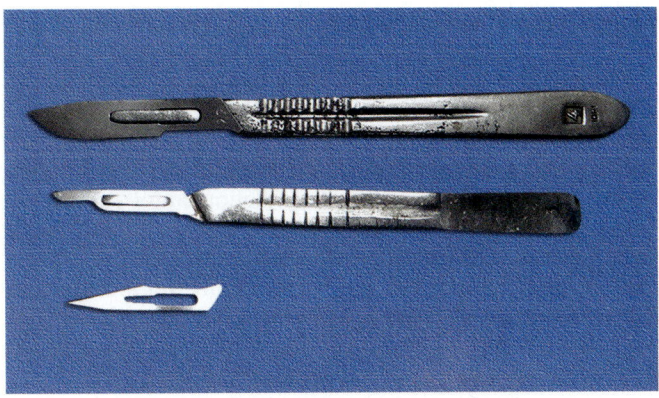

Fig. 41-39 Bard Parker's handles and blades.

Surgical Blades

They are detachable blades. Number 11 blade is stab knife blade which is used in incision and drainage of an abscess and in making small incision like for drains. Number 12 blade is curved one, used for tonsillectomy. Here cutting edge faces surgeon. Number 15 is used in plastic surgery, head and neck surgery, face surgeries. Numbers 20, 22 and 24 used in skin incisions of major surgeries like laparotomy, thoracotomy, craniotomy, incisions in limb. Blades are sterilized by gamma radiation with aluminum foil packing. Commonly blades are used only once and then disposed. If sterilization is needed it is done using Cetrimide/Lysol immersion (not autoclave or boiling).

Suture Materials (Fig. 41-40)

Features of ideal suture material
- Adequate tensile strength
- Good knot holding property
- Should be least reactive
- Easy handling property
- Should have *less memory*. Recoiling tendency of the suture material after removal from the packet is called as memory of suture material. Suture material should have poor memory. More memory causes recoiling, difficulty in handling and knotting.
- Should be easily available and cost effective

Absorbable Suture Materials

(1) <u>Catgut:</u> *It is natural absorbable monofilament suture material.* It is 99% collagen derived from the submucosa of jejunum of the sheep or serosa of beef (Kit means cattle/sheep). After washing, intestine is slit longitudinally into four strands; muscle and fat are removed using water spray–slimming. Chemical bath saponification is also used to remove fat. Strands are spun together, dried with tension and electronically polished. It is absorbed by inflammatory reaction and phagocytosis. *Plain catgut* is yellowish white in

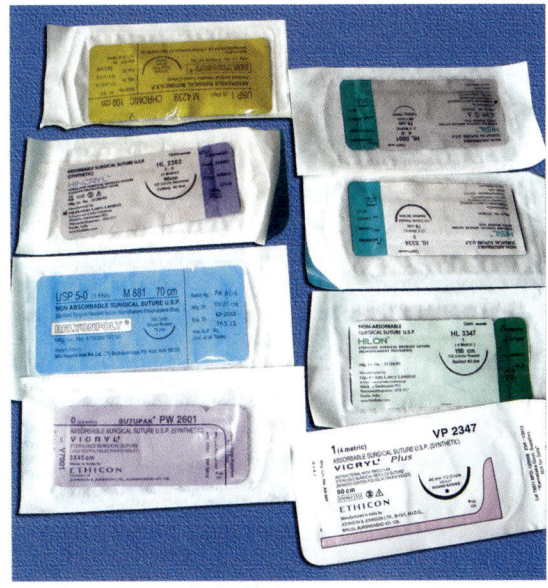

Fig. 41-40 Photograph showing different types of suture materials (with pack).

color. Absorption time is 7 days. It is used for subcutaneous tissue, muscle, circumcision in children. *Chromic catgut* is catgut with chromic acid salt. 20% chromium salt in water with 5 parts of glycerine is used to treat the catgut. It is brown in color. Its absorption time is 21 days. It is used in suturing muscle, fascia, external oblique aponeurosis, ligating pedicles, etc. Atraumatic sutures are manufactured either by swaging or by entangling the suture material into the grooved proximal part of the needle by mechanical pressure. Wound suture material in a support card is packed in a foil envelope with isopropyl alcohol. It is sterilized by gamma radiation. (2) Polylactic acid/polyglactin 910/vicryl: It is *synthetic braided multifilament absorbable*. It is synthetic absorbable suture material – copolymer of glycolide and lactide. It has got excellent tensile strength, long tensile half life, low reactivity, less memory, easy handling and knotting. It gets absorbed in 90 days. Absorption is by hydrolysis. It is violet in color. Coating consists of 50% calcium stearate which acts as a lubricant. It is multifilament and braided. It is very good suture material for bowel anastomosis, suturing muscles, closure of peritoneum. It is sterilized by ethylene oxide. Vicryl plus is vicryl coated with antibacterial material (triclosan). Vicryl rapide is low molecular weight vicryl with rapid absorption of suture material. It is used in circumcision and in subcuticular suturing. (3) Polyglycolic acid/Dexon/Synthetic polymer of glycolic acid is multifilament absorbable suture material (braided) like vicryl. Usually it is colored green/natural beige. It is sterilized by two stage ethylene oxide process. It is not affected by infection. Its knot security is poor and so at least 5 knots should be placed for security. (4) Polyglyconate/Maxon is a monofilament absorbable copolymer of glycolic acid and trimethylene carbonate. It has got good knot holding/security; suppleness and flexibility. It is used in soft tissues and skin. It cannot be used in cardiac/vascular/neural/opthalmic surgeries. It can be colorless or green colored. (5) Polydioxanone suture material/PDS is synthetic monofilament absorbable suture material. It is cream/blue/violet/in color or colorless with properties like vicryl. It is costly but better suture material than vicryl. It is relatively inert. (6) Polyglecaprone 25/Monocryl is monofilament containing 75% glycolide and 25% caprolactone. It has got smooth surface, excellent handling property, good knot security and adequate tissue compatibility. *Uses of absorbable suture materials*—In bowel anastomosis like gastrojejunostomy, resection and anastomosis vicryl (2 or 3 zero); in cholecysto-jejunostomy (CCJ), choledocho-jejunostomy (CDJ), pancreatico-jejunostomy – (3 zero vicryl); in suturing muscle, fascia, peritoneum, subcutaneous tissue, mucosa; in ligating pedicles, e.g. ligation of pedicles during hysterectomy-1 – zero chromic catgut or vicryl are used; in circumcision usually 3-zero plain or chromic catgut or vicryl rapid are used. Absorbable suture materials should not be used in suturing tendon, nerves, vessels (vascular anastomosis) or in hernia surgery where tissue approximation under stress is needed.

Nonabsorbable Suture Materials

(1) Silk is natural multifilament braided nonabsorbable suture material derived from cocoon of silkworm larva. It is black in color, a coating got from a vegetable dye. It is coated suture material to reduce capillary action. Serum proofing of the suture material is also done to reduce the capillary attraction. It has got less memory; good knot holding property; easy handling ability. (2) Cotton is twisted multifilament natural non-absorbable suture material. It is white in color. (3) Linen is derived from bark of cotton tree (natural non-absorbable twisted multifilament suture material). It is made from flax and cellulose in nature. It has got excellent knotting property and is commonly used as ligatures. (4) Polyamide is monofilament synthetic non-absorbable polymer. Nylon (New York and LONdon) is a polyamide. Multiple pre-cut nylons are available for skin suturing/ligatures. It has got less tissue reaction, easy handling ability, inertness, adequate elasticity and can be used in presence of infection. Ethilon/surgidek/dermalon/sutupak pre-cut sutures are different polyamides. Memory is high like that of polypropylene and so causes problem. (5) Polypropylene (Prolene) is synthetic monofilament suture material. It is blue in color. It has got high memory. (Prolene mesh used for hernioplasty is white in color). It is inert, flexible, strong and least reactive. It can be re-sterilized by autoclave once or twice. (6) Polybutester–Novafil is monofilament, blue colored, synthetic suture material which has got adequate flexibility, suppleness and strength.

Uses of non-absorbable suture materials; In herniorrhaphy for repair; for closure of abdomen after laparotomy; for vascular anastomosis (6—zero), nerve suturing, tendon suturing; for tension suturing in the abdomen; for suturing the skin.

> Suture materials can be—(1) *Natural:* Catgut, silk, cotton, linen; (2) *Synthetic:* Vicryl, Dexon, PDS, Maxon, Polypropylene, polyethylene, polyester, polyamide.
>
> Suture materials can be—(1) *Braided:* Polyester, polyamide, Vicryl, Dexon, and Silk; (2) *Twisted:* Cotton, Linen.
>
> Suture materials can be – (1) *Monofilament:* Polypropylene, Polyethylene, PDS, Catgut, Steel; (2) *Multifilament:* Polyester, Polyamide, Vicryl, Dexon, Silk, Cotton.
>
> Suture materials can be— (1) Coated; (2) Uncoated.

TRACHEOSTOMY AND ENDOTRACHEAL TUBES AND RELATED INSTRUMENTS

Tracheostomy Tubes

(1) *Fuller's bivalved tracheostomy tube:* It has got outer tube and inner tube. Outer tube is biflanged and so insertion is easier. Inner tube is longer with an opening on its posterior aspect. Inner tube can be removed and re-inserted easily whenever required (Fig. 41-41). (2) *Jackson's tracheostomy tube:* It has got outer tube and an obturator (Fig. 41-42). (3) *Red-rubber tracheostomy tube.* (4) *PVC tracheostomy tube.*

Modern tracheostomy tubes are made of plastic. They are soft, least irritant and disposable. They have inflatable cuff which makes it easier to give assisted ventilation. Cuff should be deflated at regular intervals to prevent tracheal pressure necrosis (for assisted ventilation endotracheal tube can be kept for 7 days. Beyond that period patient needs tracheostomy for further ventilation).

Indications for tracheostomy: In head, neck and facial injuries; tetanus; tracheomalacia after thyroidectomy; laryngeal edema/spasm; major head and neck surgeries like commando's operation, block dissection, etc.

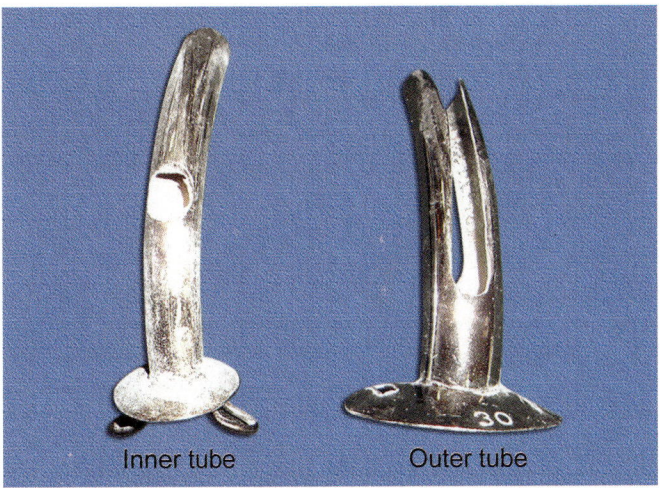

Fig. 41-41 Fullers biflanged tracheostomy tube.

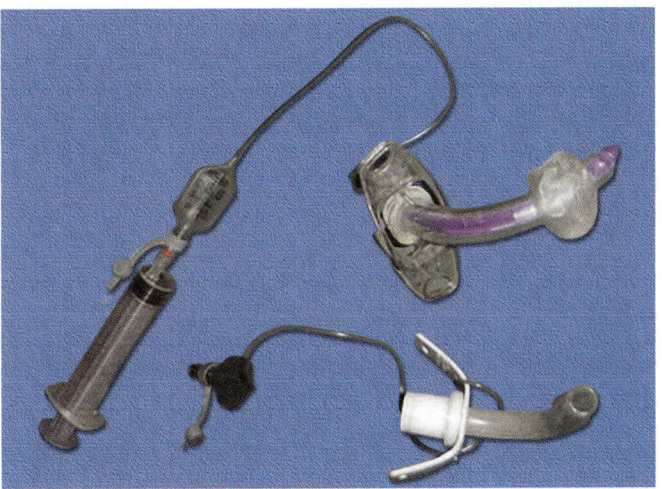

Fig. 41-42 Jackson's tracheostomy tube.

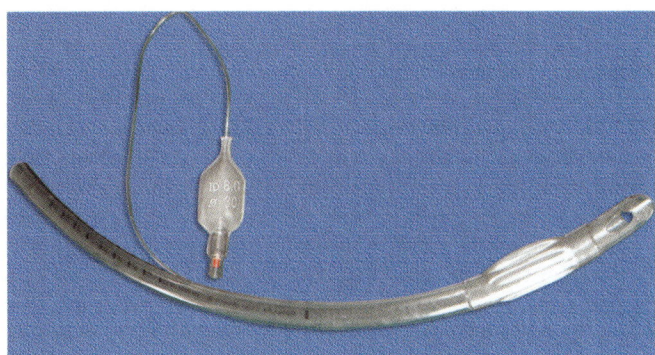

Fig. 41-43 Endotracheal tube.

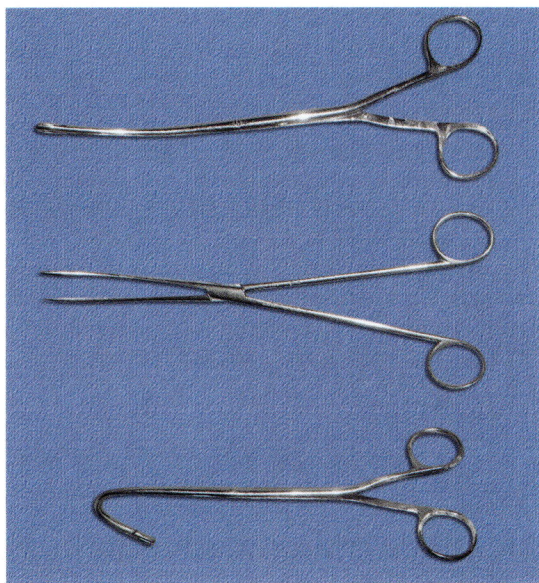

Fig. 41-44 Desjardin's choledocholithotomy forceps.

Endotracheal Tube

It is a gently curved tube used to pass into the trachea via the nasal/oral route. It is made up of India rubber or portex. It may be cuffed or non-cuffed (plain). Cuff is present on the distal part of the tube which is inflated using air through a fine tube present on the body of the endotracheal tube. Small pilot balloon on the proximal part is present to check the tension of the cuff. Cuff prevents aspiration and air leak. Capacity of the cuff is 4 mL. and often tip is radiopaque. When non-cuffed tube is used, ribbon gauze should be packed around it to protect air way from aspiration. Its distal end is beveled – 38 degrees towards left as tube is passed from the right angle of the mouth of the patient. It has got a thick black mark which should pass just beyond the vocal cords. Cuff should be 3 cm beyond vocal cords in adult and 1 cm beyond vocal cords in infants.

Different sized tubes are available depending on age of the patient. Number 6.5 to 8.0 in females and 8.0 to 9.5 in males are used. Styllet is often used while passing the endotracheal tube for easy intubation (Fig. 41-43).

It is used in general anesthesia, to maintain airway in emergency in patients with trauma, in patients with respiratory distress, in cardia arrest. It is a life saving tube used during resuscitation. It is usually kept for 7 days. If patient needs further continuation of artificial ventilation then tracheostomy is done.

Complications are—esophageal intubation; trauma to airway; one lung ventilation; displacement; laryngeal edema; vocal cord dysfunction; infection.

OTHER INSTRUMENTS

Desjardin's Choledocholithotomy Forceps

It has got long distal blades with smooth serrations and fenestra in the tip. It does not have lock and so accidental damage to CBD mucosa or crushing of the CBD stone are avoided. It is used for choledocholithotomy (removal of CBD stones). Length and curve facilitate the stone extraction better. In laparoscopic cholecystectomy, to make easier delivering of the gallbladder it can be used to remove stones from gallbladder by passing through the 10 mm port. Disadvantage is the instrument may dilate the CBD significantly while manipulating (Fig. 41-44).

Kehr's 'T' Tube

It is used after opening of CBD (choledochotomy). CBD is closed with 'T' tube in situ. It is made up of latex or red rubber. 'T' tube has got horizontal part which is kept in the CBD and vertical part which is allowed to come out to drain bile. Amount of bile draining is measured daily. Before removal of 'T' tube, patency of CBD should be confirmed. *It is done by following methods:* The vertical limb (done in 10–14 days) is clamped and observed for development of pain, fever and jaundice in 24 hours. If normal then one can presume that there is no obstruction in the CBD. Water soluble iodine dye is injected through the tube to visualize biliary tree and free flow of dye into the duodenum (Post-operative 'T' tube cholangiogram). It is done in 10-14 days which is the time required to develop fibrous track. Once there is free flow tube is removed and track gets closed on its own (Fig. 41-45).

Flatus Tube

It is made up of India rubber, 45 cm in length. There is *one opening in the tip* and another on the side proximal to the tip. (Urinary catheter like red rubber catheter has no opening on the tip, only side opening is present). It is used in sigmoid volvulus to decompress and derotate; in paralytic ileus; in subacute intestinal obstruction. It is passed per anal into the recto-sigmoid area. Proximal end is connected to water container to observe the quantity of air bubble which signifies the amount of gas getting deflated (Fig. 41-46).

Trocar and Cannula

Trocar has got stout handle with a sharp pointed distal end. Trocar passes through the cannula of different sizes and snugly fits in to proximal end of cannula. Trocar with sheath is punctured into the needed place and trocar is removed. Through sheath fluid is evacuated. Through the sheath Foley's catheter can also be passed to keep in place. It is used in per cutaneous cystostomy, draining hydrocele fluid, draining pus from gallbladder, pleural cavity, maxillary antrum, etc. (Fig. 41-47).

Humby's Knife

It is used to take split skin graft from donor site. Usually, it is taken from thigh. Often it can also be taken from arm, leg, and forearm. Humby's knife has got stout handle, two flat leaves in blade, one of which is fixed and other can be rotated. Disposable skin grafting blade is passed between the rods into the flat leave which has got three knobs which fits exactly into the openings of the blade. Front leaf has got slots which when pushed gets fixed over the blade. Using firm constant pressure with sawing action split skin is harvested from the thigh. Punctuate bleeding over the donor area confirms the proper skin harvesting. Donor graft is placed over the sterile wooden board. Multiple small window cuts are made to prevent formation of seroma. Skin is placed over the recipient bed and fixed using polypropylene sutures or skin staples. Dressing is placed and part is immobilized (Fig. 41-48).

Volkmann's Scoop

It is spoon shaped strong stout instrument with serrations in the middle; ends are spoon shaped with cups. Spoons on the ends are of different sizes. It is used to scoop granulation tissue, slough, ulcer bed, to scoop cavities, curette sinus tracts (Fig. 41-49).

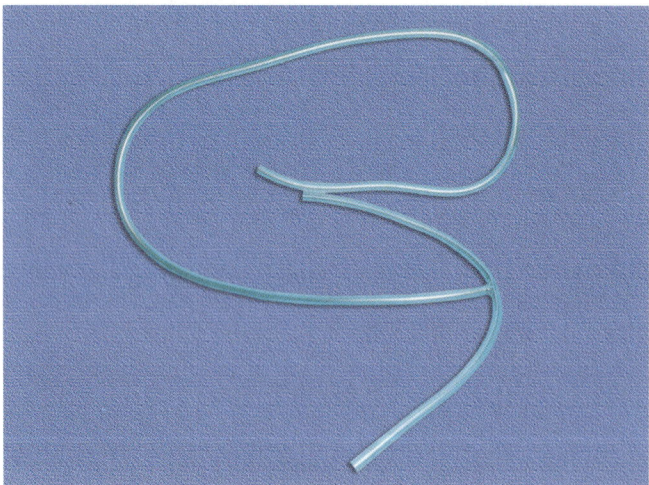

Fig. 41-45 Kehr's 'T' Tube.

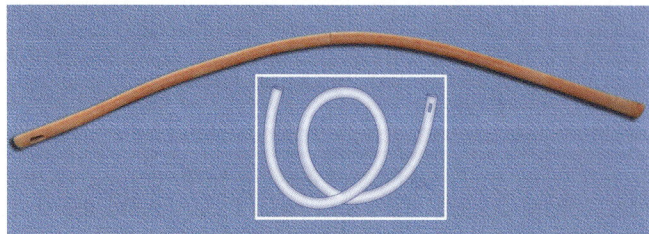

Fig. 41-46 Flatus tube.

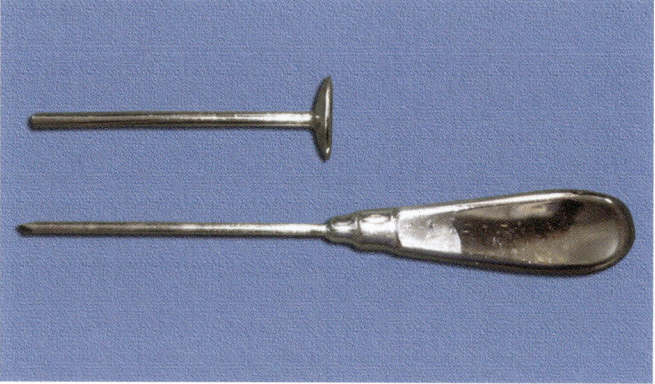

Fig. 41-47 Trocar and cannula.

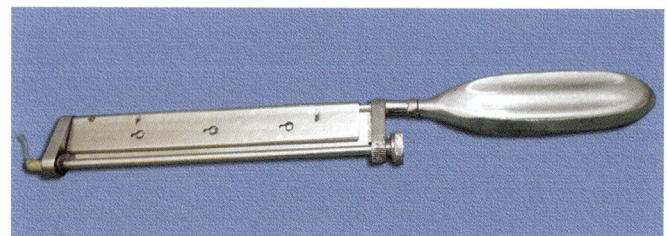

Fig. 41-48 Humby's knife to harvest skin graft.

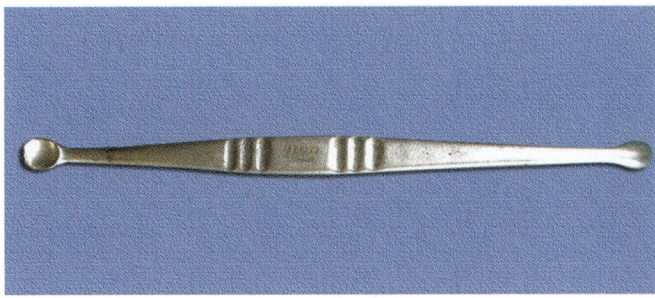

Fig. 41-49 Volkmann's scoop.

Towel Clips

Towel clip is used mainly to keep the draped towels in place in surgical field; it is also used to fix suction tubes, diathermy wires, and laparoscopic cables in operative table. It is used to fix ribs in flail chest. It can be used to hold cord in hernia or to hold tongue if specific instruments are not available. It can be used to hold dental wiring; patella during patellectomy; in faciomaxillary fractures. *Different towel clips are—Mayo's towel clip; Backhaus' towel clip; Moynihan's tetra towel clip; Doyen's towel clip.* It is a short instrument with curved ends with sharp points. Handles join at proximal ends. When handles are pressed tips open and when handles are released tips close and firmly grip the towels (Figs. 41-50 and 41.51).

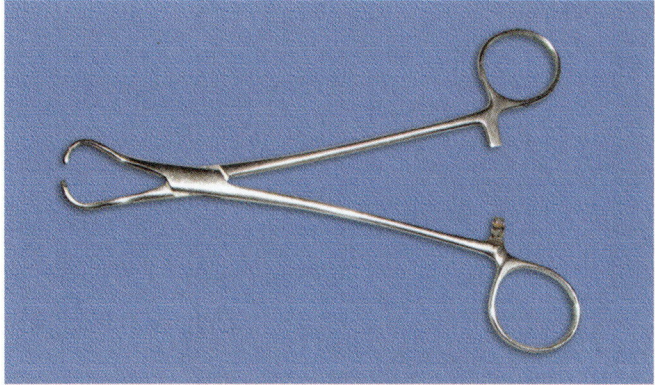

Fig. 41-50 Mayo's towel clip.

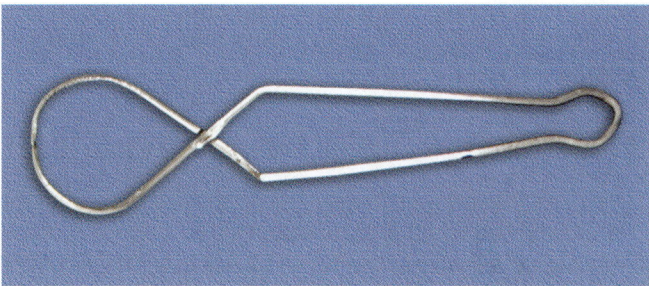

Fig. 41-51 Doyens towel clip.

42 X-rays

Competency: SU9.1; SU9.2.

X-rays are usually a part of the examination for undergraduates as well as postgraduates in surgery. Students should have fair idea about common X-rays, their findings and significances. However computed tomography (CT) and magnetic resonance imaging (MRI) have taken over X-rays in places of diagnosis, X-rays are still commonly used and in certain occasions it is the compulsory method of investigation.

X-rays may be plain or contrast. Plain X-rays of abdomen/chest/bone or skull are being used for diagnosis. Contrast X-rays are barium studies/angiograms/urograms/cholangiograms, etc.

PLAIN X-RAY ABDOMEN

Plain X-ray abdomen is often taken in acute abdomen/to see stones in pancreas/gallstones or any calcifications. It is also used to see viscus perforation/multiple air-fluid levels/ground-glass appearance and so on.

Plain X-ray abdomen is usually taken in standing position (erect X-ray). Often X-ray side to side is taken in left lateral decubitus (right side up) position.

Proper plain X-ray abdomen is taken with low penetration X-ray exposing diaphragm, upper part of the pelvis, bowel shadows, liver shadow and peritoneal outline. Calcifications due to pancreatitis (parenchymal/ductal stone), radiopaque gallstones (10%), calcifications in liver/spleen/kidney/meconium ileus/ovarian teratodermoids/gallstone ileus/phleboliths/vascular calcifications of aorta, renal or splenic arteries/calcified fibroid/calcified amebic liver abscess/calcified hydatid cyst/calcified lymph node may be seen. Gas under diaphragm is diagnostic of bowel perforation; here chest X-ray with upper abdomen in erect posture is ideal. Multiple air-fluid levels are features of intestinal obstruction.

Gas Under Diaphragm (Fig. 42-1)

It is due to:
- Perforated anterior duodenal ulcer (anterior DU perforates; posterior DU bleeds). It is the commonest cause of perforation. Acute ulcer or chronic ulcer with acute exacerbation perforates commonly. Perforation may be precipitated by nonsteroidal anti-inflammatory durgs (NSAIDs), alcohol.
- Gastric ulcer perforation- both benign and malignant ulcer can perforate. But large gas leak is more likely to be due to malignant ulcer perforation. Gas leak can occur posteriorly into lesser sac causing abscess in lesser sac.
- Jejunal perforation—rare.
- Ileum is another common site of perforation. It causes fecal peritonitis and is more dangerous. It could be typhoid ulcer perforation/Crohn's disease perforation/roundworm perforation/amebic ulcer perforation (in terminal ileum)/tuberculous ulcer perforation (commonly it causes stricture–intestinal obstruction–necrosis–perforation)/small bowel malignancy like lymphoma or adenocarcinoma or carcinoid perforation.
- Colonic perforation is due to amebic ulcer/toxic megacolon/carcinoma/ischemic colitis.

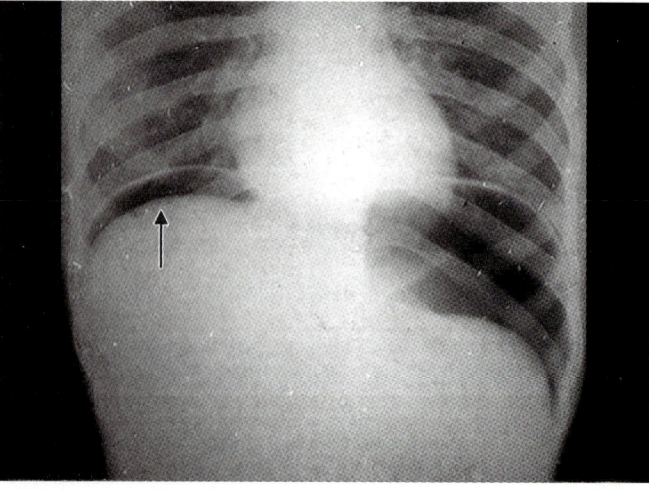

Fig. 42-1 Chest X-ray with plain X-ray abdomen *in erect posture* showing gas under the diaphragm.

- Traumatic perforation may be due to either stab injury causing direct penetrating injury of bowel or due to blunt injury abdomen. In blunt injury abdomen sudden shearing force causes traction of either duodenojejunal junction or ileocecal region causing perforation or transection of the bowel.
- Perforation can occur following surgical/diagnostic procedures like laparoscopic/open laparotomy/tubal insufflation.

Multiple air-fluid levels: It is due to intestinal obstruction; it is checked in plain X-ray abdomen in erect posture (Fig. 42-3).

Causes of Intestinal Obstruction (Figs. 42-4 and 42-5)
- Hernia (commonly inguinal hernias but can be any hernias) and adhesions are the commonest causes. In Western countries adhesions and bands, either congenital or postoperative are the common causes. In Asian countries hernia is the common cause of intestinal obstruction.
- Intussusception.
- Roundworm bolus obstruction.
- Stricture ileum—either tuberculosis or Crohn's disease.
- Carcinoma small bowel/carcinoma colon when it is stricture type (left sided colonic growth).
- Volvulus of colon/small bowel.

Normally, three fluid levels can be seen in plain X-ray film—at fundus of stomach, at duodenum and often at cecum. Maximum caliber of jejunum is 3.5 cm; of ileum is 2.5 cm; of cecum is 9 cm and of transverse colon is 5.5 cm. Dilatation of transverse colon more than 6 cm is

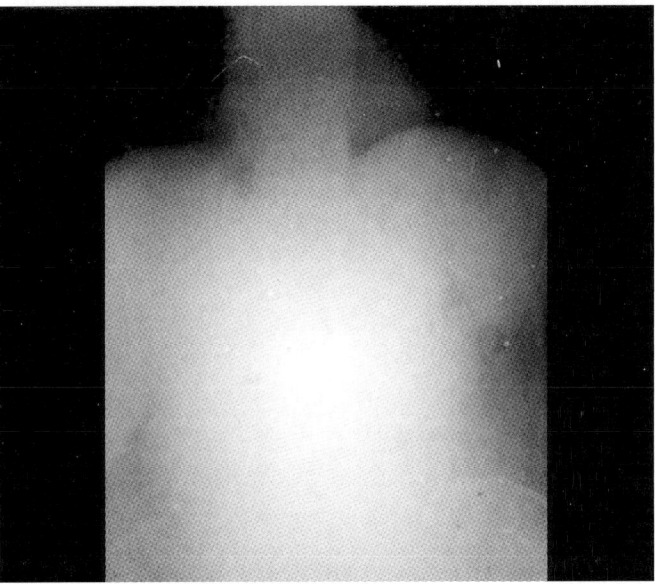

Fig. 42-2 Plain X-ray abdomen showing *ground-glass appearance*—feature of peritonitis.

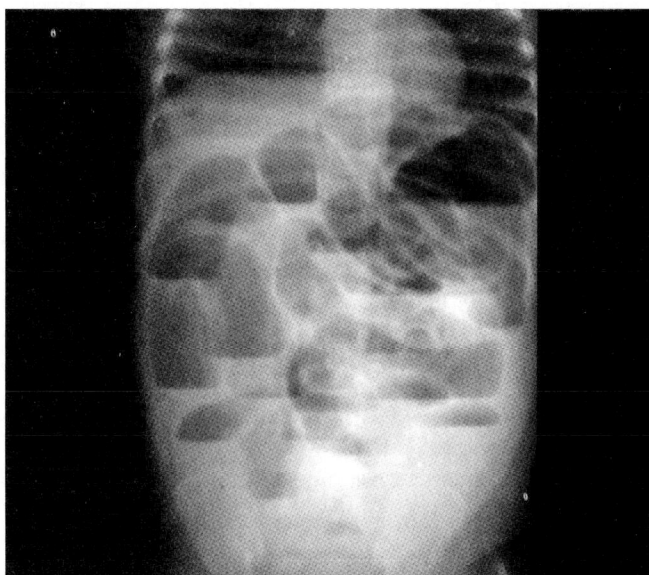

Fig. 42-4 Plain X-ray abdomen showing *air-fluid levels* with dilated colon. Probable site of obstruction is distal colon. It could be due to growth in the colon.

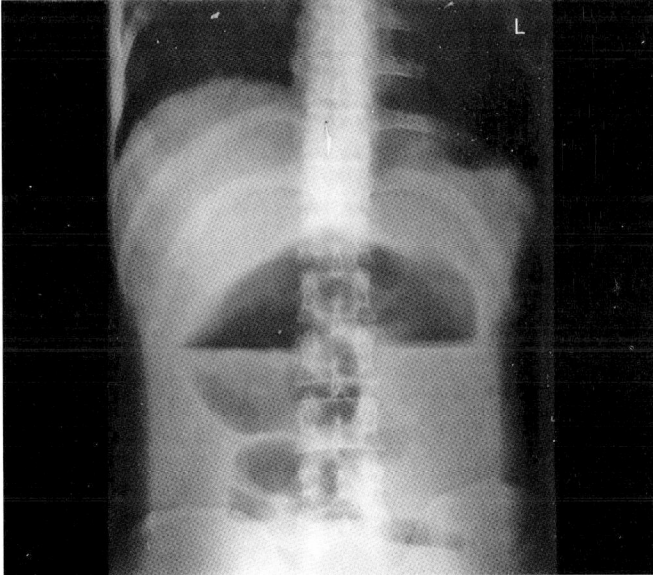

Fig. 42-3 Plain X-ray abdomen showing *multiple air-fluid levels* due to intestinal obstruction.

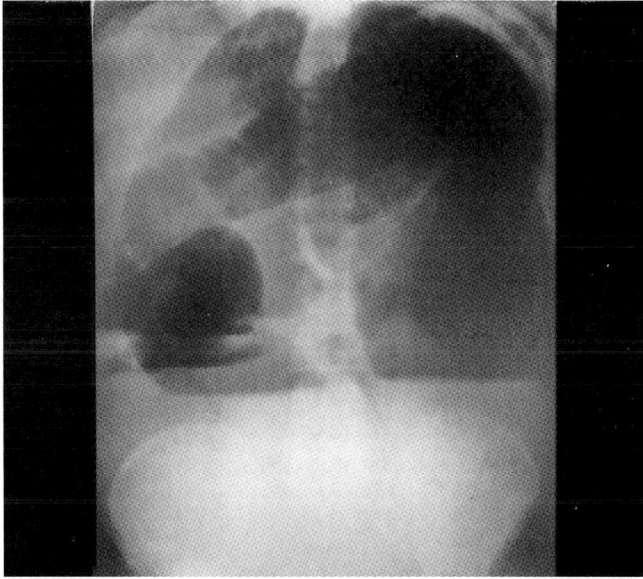

Fig. 42-5 Intestinal obstruction with *colonic dilatation*. It is due to distal colonic obstruction may be due to growth (carcinoma).

called as *megacolon*. Cecum can dilate up to the diameter of 15 cm. Cecal dilatation more than 15 cm diameter is a sign of impending perforation. Competent ileocecal valve aggravates the chances of colonic dilatation and perforation because of the closed loop obstruction which increases the intra-colonic pressure significantly.

- *Jejunum shows concertina effect due to valvulae conniventes.*
- *Ileum is smooth and characterless (Wangensteen).*
- *Large bowel shows haustration.*
- Note: Barium enema and meal is contraindicated in acute intestinal obstruction. CT scan abdomen is very reliable type of investigation.

Sigmoid volvulus: In plain X-ray abdomen it shows—Omega sign/coffee-bean sign/bent inner tube sign is also observed. Dilute barium or water-soluble contrast study shows tapering of the upper end into a spirally twisted sigmoid colon—*bird-beak sign/ace of spades* appearance. CT scan shows typical whirl pattern. Volvulus is twist/abnormal rotation of the loop of the bowel on its own mesenteric axis. It occurs in sigmoid colon commonly (65%). Sigmoid volvulus is anticlockwise—65% common in males; cecal volvulus is clockwise ('C' for cecum—clockwise)—30%—common in females (Fig. 42-6).

Plain X-ray abdomen showing pancreatic stones: Pancreatic stones are commonly radiopaque and multiple. It can be pancreatic parenchymal calcification or ductal stones. In ductal stones ductal dilatation is common (more than 3 mm). Often it will be 10–20 mm diameter. Ductal stones are reasonably better than parenchymal calcification. Essential investigations are MDCT scan, ERCP (*chain of lake appearance*) and often MRCP (Fig. 42-7).

Plain X-ray abdomen showing gallstones (Fig. 42-8):

Remember
- Presently ultrasound is ideal investigation for gallstones.
- Mixed stones are commonest—90%.
- '*Gallstone is a tomb stone erected to the memory of the organism within it*'—Moynihan's aphorism.
- **Saint's triad**: Gallstones—colonic diverticulosis—hiatus hernia.
- **Complications of gallstones**: Acute cholecystitis, chronic cholecystitis, empyema gallbladder, mucocele of gallbladder, perforation and peritonitis, secondary CBD stones, cholangitis, pancreatitis, Mirizzi syndrome, gallstone ileus, pericholecystitic abscess and carcinoma of gallbladder.

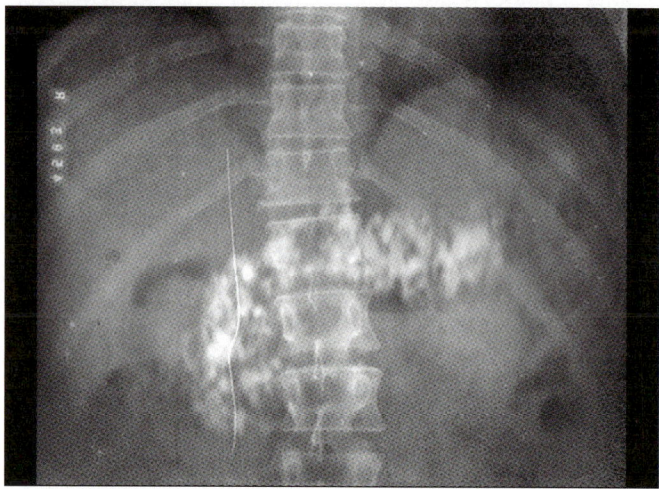

Fig. 42-7 Pancreatic parenchymal calcification in *chronic pancreatitis*.

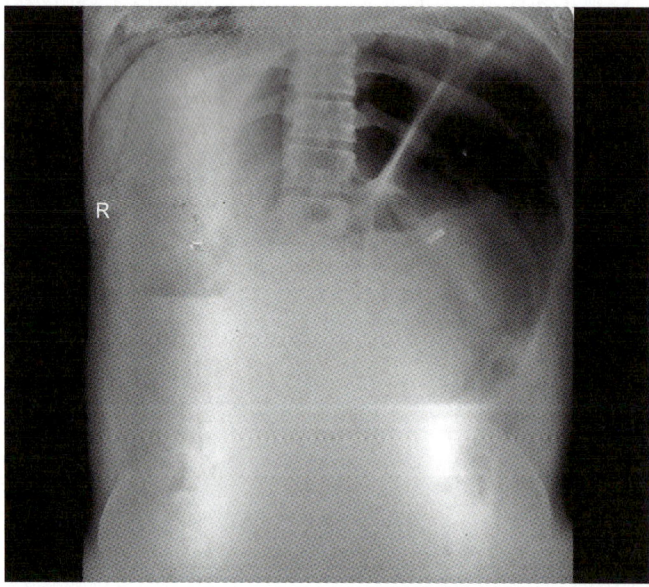

Fig. 42-6 Plain X-ray abdomen showing sigmoid volvulus—*dilated sigmoid colon*.

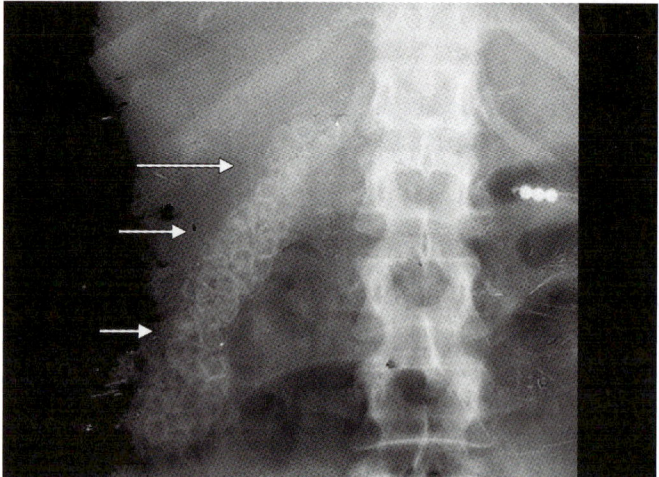

Fig. 42-8 Multiple gallstones in a plain X-ray. *Only 10% gallstones are radiopaque*. Often they are faceted each other because of compact and equal pressure. Center of the gallstone is often found radiolucent and is called as Mercedes Benz sign/Seagull sign.

CHEST X-RAYS (FIGS. 42-9 TO 42-13)

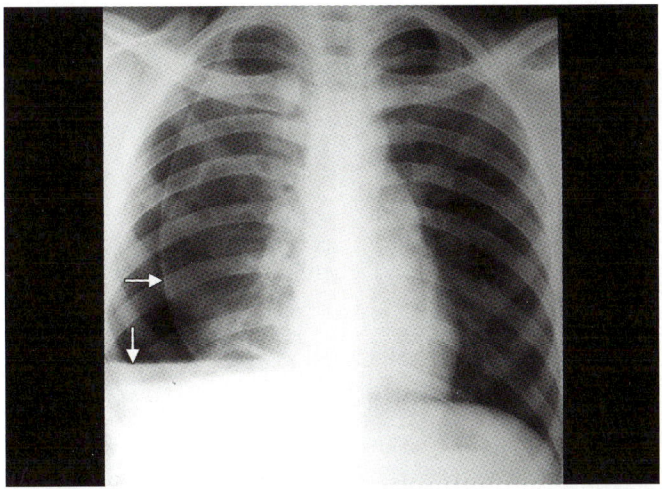

Fig. 42-9 Chest X-ray showing *hydropneumothorax* with collapsed lung margin and fluid level. It could be due to trauma, ruptured bullae or tuberculosis.

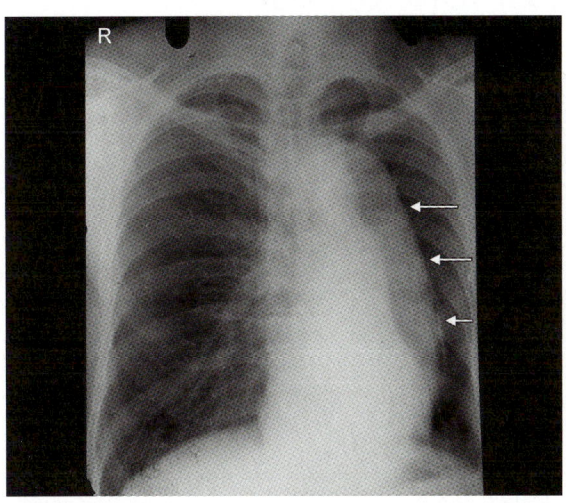

Fig. 42-12 *Thoracic aortic aneurysm* (descending thoracic aorta).

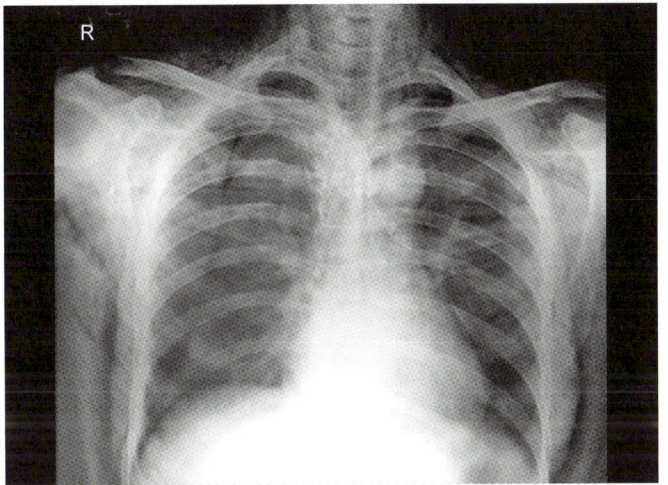

Fig. 42-10 Chest X-ray posteroanterior view showing *subcutaneous emphysema* as dark multiple streaks/lines.

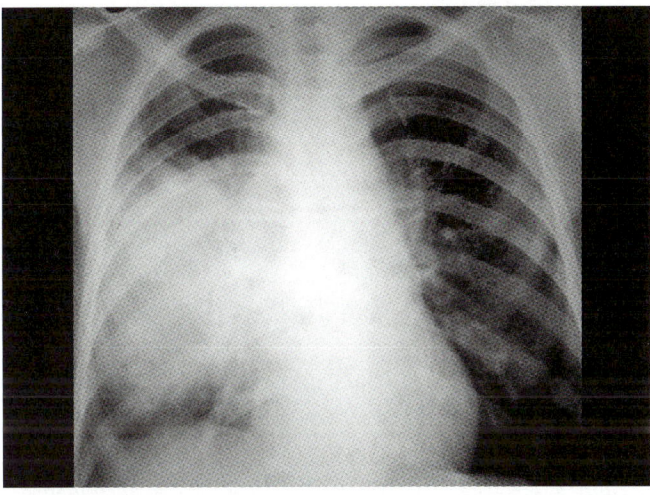

Fig. 42-13 Chest X-ray PA [6 feet (180 cm) from patient] and lateral view showing *mediastinal tumor*—probably lymph nodal mass. It may be lymphoma/secondaries.

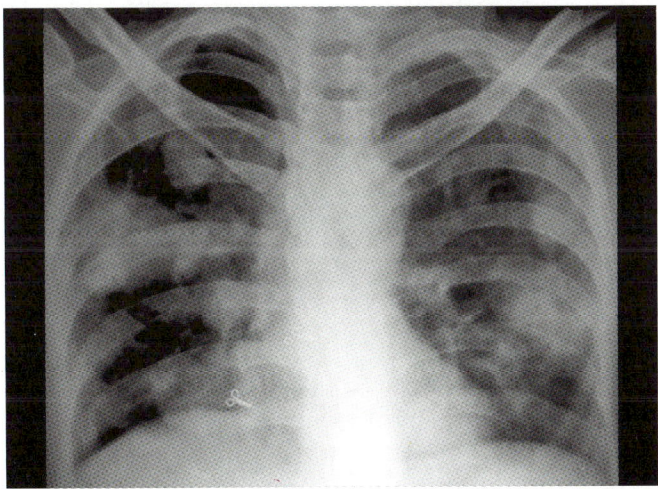

Fig. 42-11 Chest X-ray showing *cannon ball secondaries*. Often there may be pleural effusion/consolidation also. Early secondaries may be missed by chest X-ray as only 60–70% of the lung can be seen in chest X-ray. So contrast (HRCT) is ideal to pick up lung secondaries. Secondaries in the lung are usually multiple, smooth and rounded. It is because secondaries arise from the single primary spread into different places of the lung that occurs at same time with similar cellular mitotic activity. It is smooth because of the lung resistance. Common primaries causing secondaries in lungs are—all sarcomas, carcinomas from breast, thyroid, kidney, testis and prostate.

X-RAY BONES (FIGS. 42-14 TO 42-16)

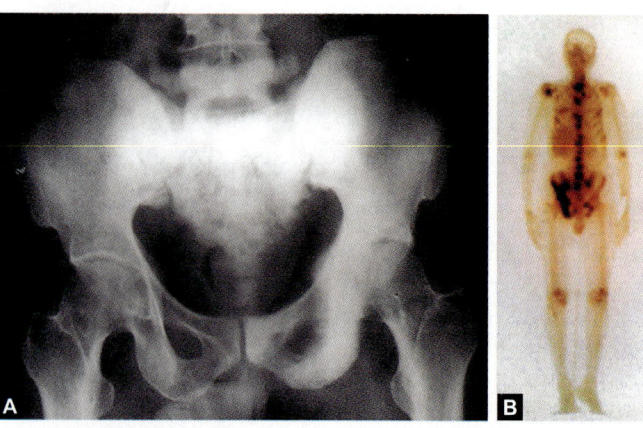

Figs. 42-14A and B X-ray pelvis showing *osteoblastic secondaries in ilium, ischium and sacrum* (pelvic bones)—primary is from prostate. Radioisotope bone scan is ideal to identify bone secondaries.

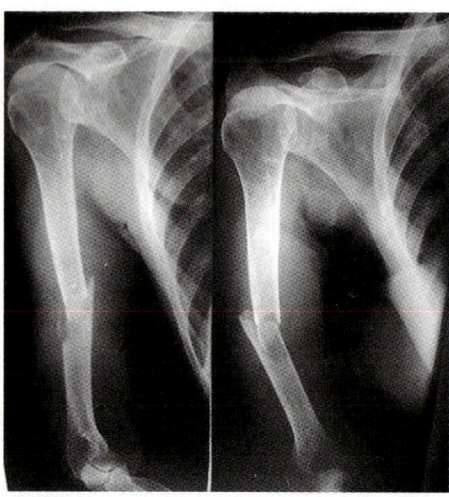

Fig. 42-15 X-ray humerus showing *pathological fracture in humerus* due to secondaries from carcinoma breast.

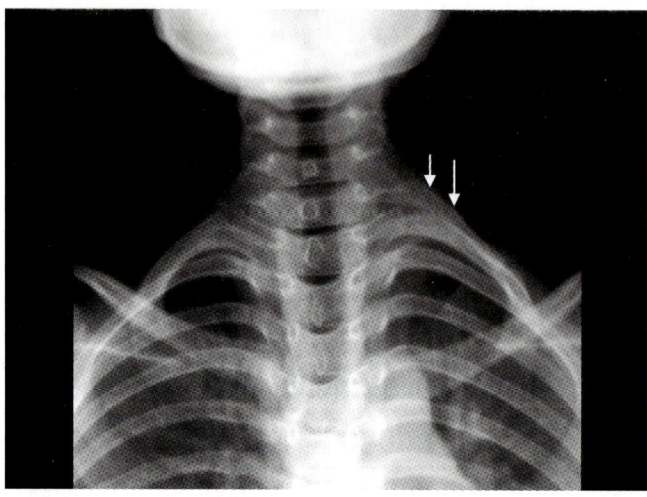

Fig. 42-16 X-ray neck with upper chest showing *cervical rib on left side*. It is of complete type.

OTHER PLAIN X-RAYS (FIGS. 42-17 TO 42-19)

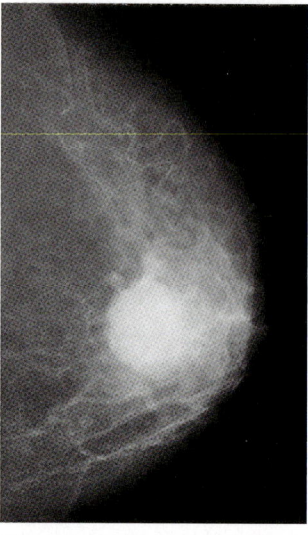
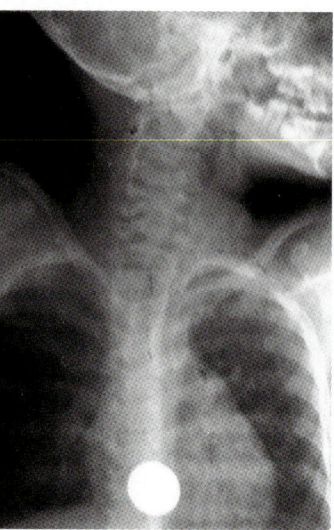

Fig. 42-17 *Mammography*. It is plain X-ray of breast. Craniocaudal and medio-lateral films are taken. Microcalcification; smooth/irregular soft tissue shadow; speculations are the findings to be looked for.

Fig. 42-18 *Foreign body (coin) in the lower esophagus*. Usually it can be removed by an endoscope. Common foreign bodies are—Coins, dentures, pins, fish or meat bones. Fish or meat bones are more dangerous because of their ragged sharp edges which often perforate the esophagus causing mediastinitis, empyema and septicemia.

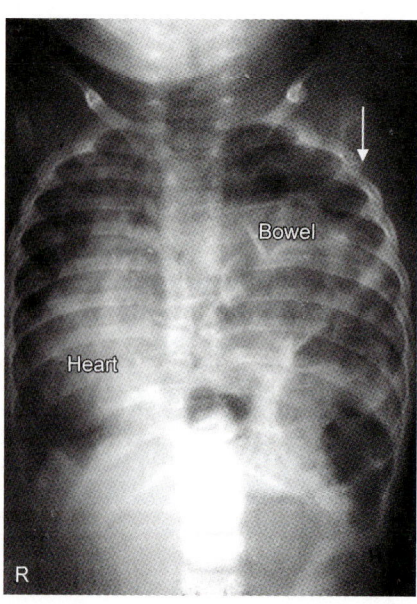

Fig. 42-19 X-ray showing *diaphragmatic hernia* with bowel shadow on the left side of the chest and heart shadow on right side.

Plain X-ray KUB/KUBU (Kidney, Ureter, Bladder, Urethra)

For detail Refer Chapter 26 (Fig. 42-20 to 42-22).

Barium Swallow X-ray

Thick solution/paste of barium sulphate is given to the patient to swallow. Under fluoroscopy (dynamic study) while barium is descending along the esophagus slowly, esophagus is observed for any mucosal changes, alteration in motility and block/narrowing. Once suspected area is identified required films are taken as needed. Usually oblique films are taken. Indications are—any patient with dysphagia/odynophagia (painful swallowing) for more than 3 weeks is an indication for barium swallow/esophagoscopy like—achalasia cardia, carcinoma esophagus, esophageal strictures—corrosive, extrinsic compression—mediastinal mass, tracheoesophageal fistula, pharyngeal pouch and esophageal diverticula, esophageal varices, hiatus hernia, esophageal webs, leaking esophageal anastomosis. Barium is radiopaque and so it is used. Barium sulphate is inert and in sulphate media, it will not get absorbed into circulation. Barium phosphate (barium in phosphate media) gets absorbed and barium is neurotoxic. Barium phosphate is commercially used rat poison. Water soluble contrast like gastrograffin is used for identifying leak, perforation or fistula.

Barium swallow X-ray achalasia cardia: Pencil shaped narrowing of the esophagus at its lower end—*bird beak appearance;* proximal dilatation of the esophagus—*mega/sigmoid esophagus; a*bsence of fundic gas shadow; no mucosal irregularity (Fig. 42-23).

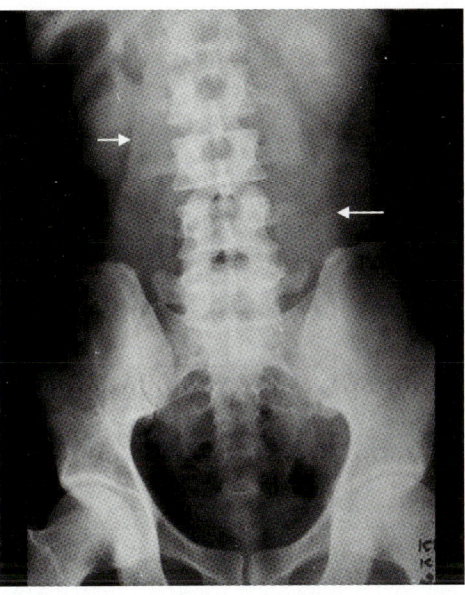

Fig. 42-20 Plain X-ray KUB/KUBU *(Kidney; Ureter: Bladder: Urethra). Note the psoas shadow.*

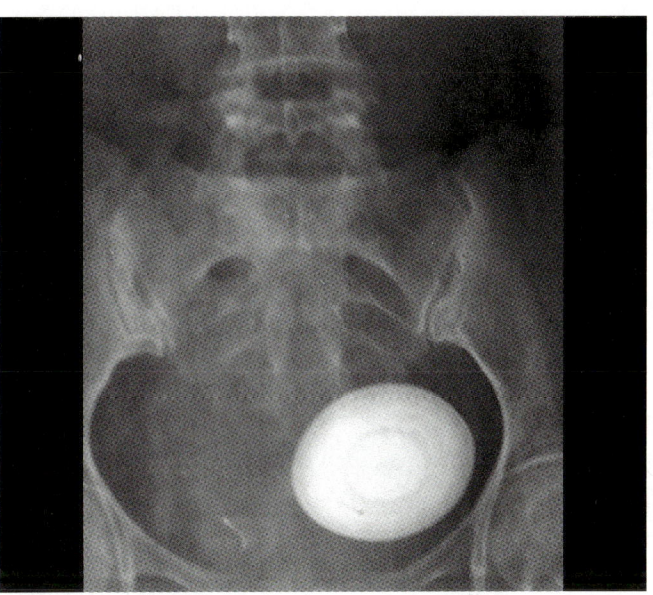

Fig. 42-22 *Large vesical calculus.* It is radiopaque; phosphate/triple phosphate stone with laminations. It is secondary bladder stone (which is secondary to infection).

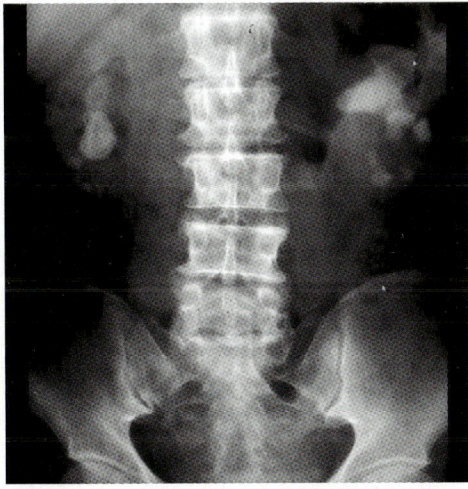

Fig. 42-21 Plain X-ray KUB showing *bilateral staghorn calculi.* Patient may be presenting with renal failure.

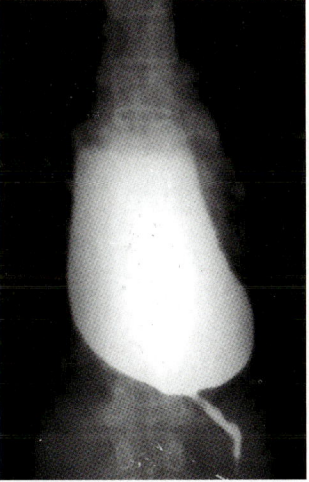

Fig. 42-23 Barium swallow X-ray in *Achalasia cardia* showing pencil narrowing of distal esophagus near O–G junction with proximal dilatation.

Barium swallow X-ray in carcinoma esophagus: Irregular filling defect; *shouldering sign* at the beginning of the tumor; narrowing; *rat tail lesion* in fluoroscopy—normal esophagus shows horizontal movements/oscillations in fluoroscopy. This is absent in carcinoma and so it looks as stiff area like rat tail (Fig. 42-24).

Barium Meal X-ray

Refer Chapter 21

Barium meal X-ray features of benign gastric ulcer: *Niche* on the lesser curve with *notch* on the greater curvature (Fig. 42-25).

Barium meal X-ray in duodenal ulcer: *Absence of duodenal cap or deformed first part of the duodenum* is the classical feature of chronic duodenal ulcer.

Barium meal X-ray of gastric outlet obstruction: Absent duodenal cap, if it is due to cicatrized chronic duodenal ulcer; greater curvature is below the level of iliac crest; mottled stomach due to retained food particles which gives coated/mosaic appearance; barium will not pass into the duodenum; dilated stomach (Fig. 42-26).

Barium meal X-ray of carcinoma stomach: Irregular filling defect; margin of the lesion projects outward from the ulcer/lesion into the gastric lumen—*Carmanns meniscus sign*; distorted and altered gastric folds with asymmetry; Kirklin complex; if growth is in the stomach, features of gastric outlet obstruction due to narrowing may be observed; in linitis plastica, there is small shrunken stomach with diffuse mucosal changes—*leather bottle stomach*; carcinoma stomach is common in greater curvature.

Small Bowel Enema—Enteroclysis

Refer Chapter 21 (Fig. 42-27).

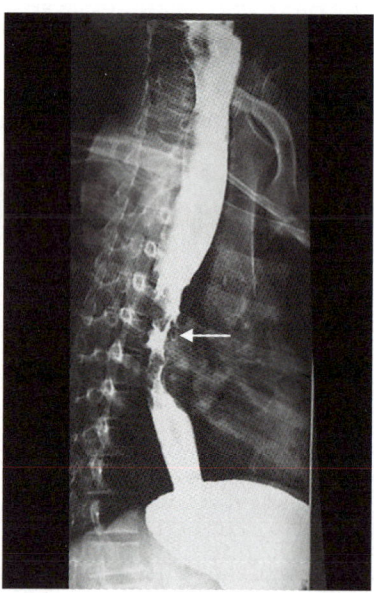

Fig. 42-24 Barium swallow X-ray showing *irregular filling defect and shouldering sign* of carcinoma esophagus.

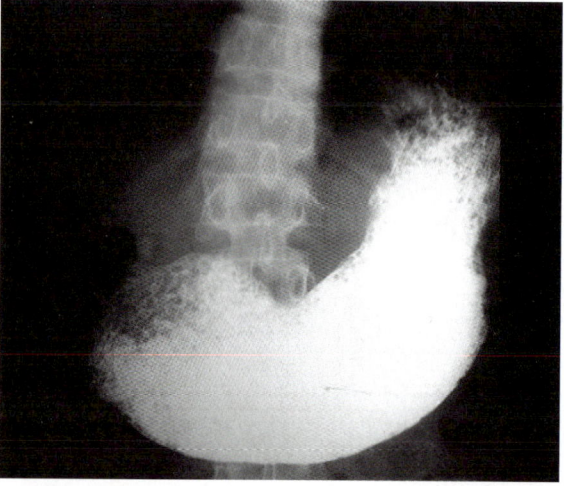

Fig. 42.26 Barium meal X-ray showing *gastric outlet obstruction*. It is due to scarred chronic duodenal ulcer (commonly)/or due to growth in the pylorus.

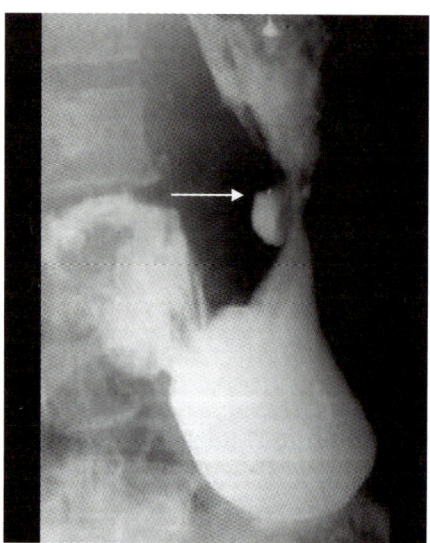

Fig. 42-25 Barium meal X-ray showing *niche and notch in gastric ulcer*.

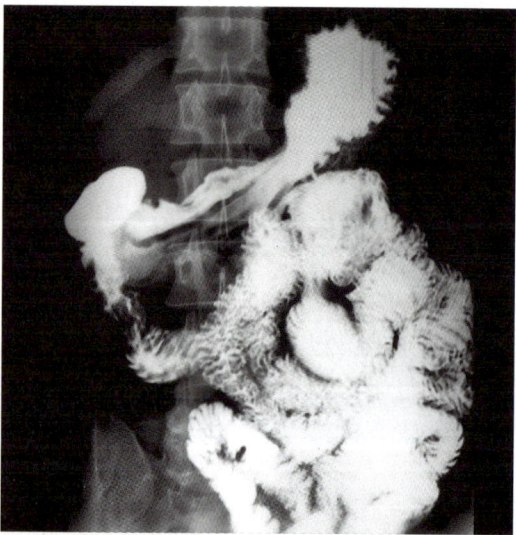

Fig. 42-27 *Enteroclysis/small bowel enema X-ray*. Nasojejunal tube should be seen in proper enteroclysis.

Barium Enema X-ray

Refer Chapter 21.
Refer Chapter 21 (Figs. 42-28 to 42-30).

Intravenous Urogram (IVU) (Intravenous Pyelogram–IVP—Older Terminology) (Figs. 42.31 and 42.32)

Refer Chapter 26

Retrograde Pyelography (RGP) and Renal Angiogram (Refer Chapter 26)

Micturating cystourethrography (MCU).
Ascending urethrogram (Fig. 42-33) Refer Chapter 26.
Endoscopic retrograde cholangiopancreatography (ERCP) (Fig. 42-34) Refer Chapter 21.

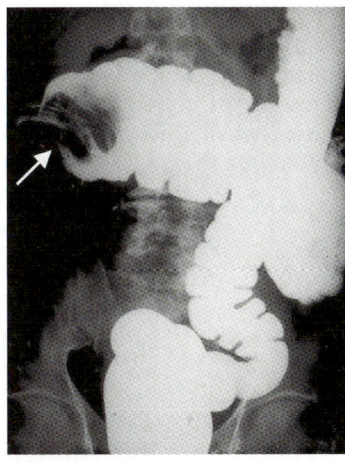

Fig. 42-30 Barium enema X-ray showing *typical claw sign/coiled spring sign*—in transverse colon—ileocolic type—commonest type.

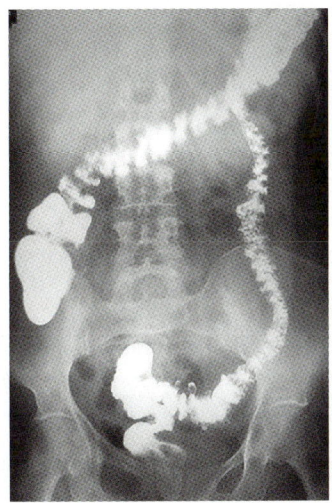

Fig. 42-28 Barium enema X-rays taken *after complete filling and evacuation of barium sulphate enema solution*. Air is insufflated per anum into the colorectum which delineates the mucosa better to visualize small ulcers/small polyps.

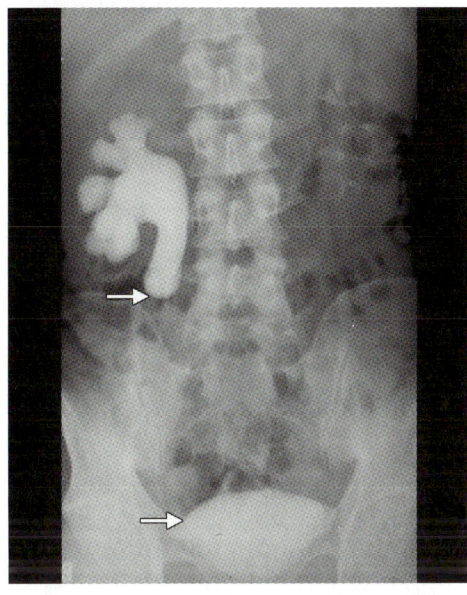

Fig. 42-31 IVU showing right-sided hydronephrosis and proximal hydroureter. *Note the clubbing of calyces.*

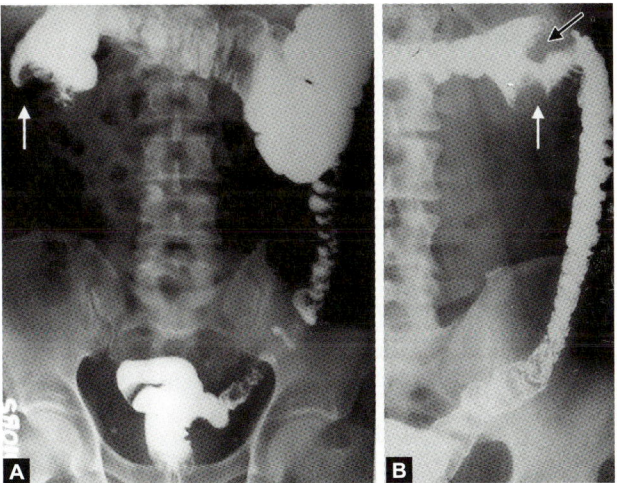

Figs. 42-29A and B Barium enema X-ray showing *irregular filling defect in hepatic flexure* with intussusception in one X-ray and *in splenic flexure in other X-ray* (carcinoma colon). Note growth in splenic flexure is narrow—stricture/ obstructive type (*apple—core lesion*). X-ray of hepatic flexure growth presented as intussusception.

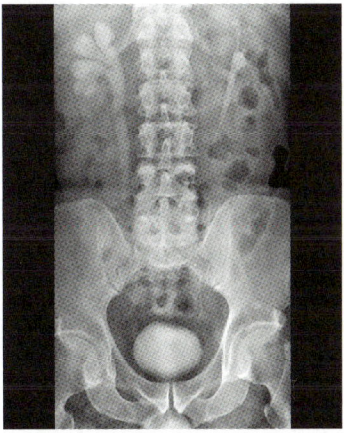

Fig. 42-32 IVU showing right sided hydronephrosis. Note the clubbing of the calyces with hydroureter also. *Secretion is normal on left side (cup-shaped calyces are normal).*

Postoperative T-tube cholangiogram: After choledochotomy, Kehr's T-tube is placed in CBD. After 10–14 days water soluble dye is injected into the tube and X-ray is taken. Initially T tube is flushed with 20 mL of normal saline to flush out any air bubble. Air bubble, when present will be dense black area which shifts with change in position. 3 mL of urograffin is injected into the T-tube. Under guidance, X-ray film is taken. Complete free flow of dye into the duodenum indicates that there is no blockage. T-tube can then be removed safely. Usually T-tube is removed by gentle traction without any anesthesia. Block indicates presence of residual CBD stones (Fig. 42-35).

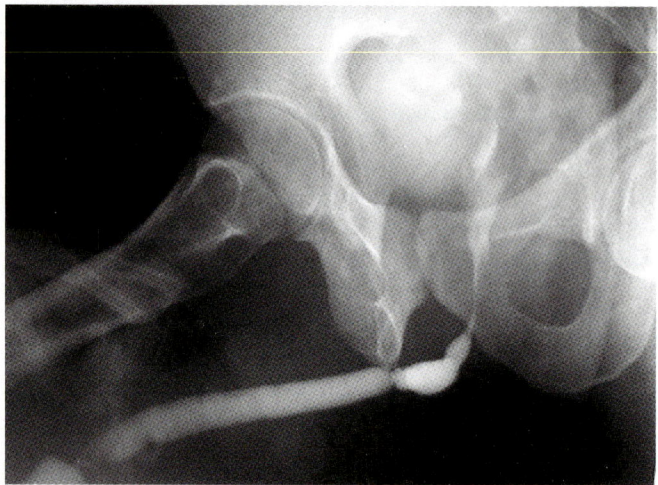

Fig. 42-33 Ascending urethrogram showing *multiple stricture urethra*.

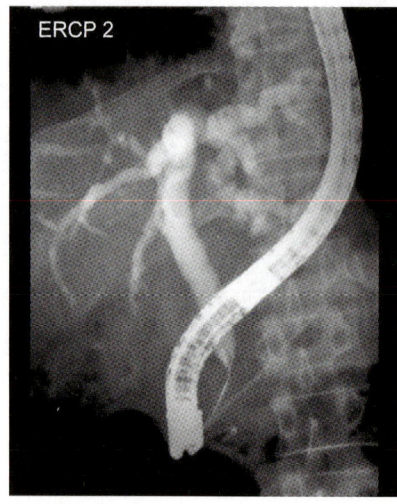

Fig. 42-34 *ERCP being done*. Note the gastroduodenoscope with injection of dye. There is dilatation of biliary radicles with CBD and hepatic ducts.

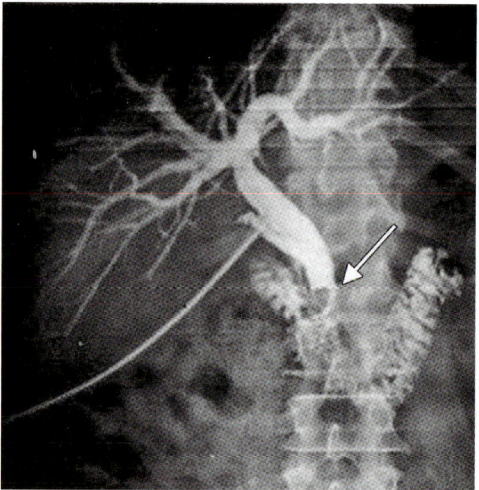

Fig. 42-35 Plain X-ray showing *T-tube in place in postoperative period*. Once dye is injected.

43

Surgical Pathology

Competency: SU9.1.

Surgical pathology is indeed important and interesting aspect, to know how exactly a diseased area looks like and also to think its possible causes and prognosis. Specimen should be sent properly, labeled with markers. Suspected area should be marked. Whenever nodes are removed it should be sent by mentioning in detail of its location and nature. In many centers specimen moulds/keeping trays are used for particular organs. Detailed history and clinical findings should be sent to the pathologists.

Specimen of stomach—Benign gastric ulcer and "Hour glass contracture"

Specimen of stomach (identified by the mucosal pattern and rugae) showing deep ulcer near lesser curvature. Margin of the ulcer is clear, not everted with gastric mucosal folds converging towards the base of the ulcer. 95% of benign gastric ulcer occurs towards lesser curve. Benign gastric ulcer is more common in lesser curvature, as it takes more burden of passage of food and so more of wear and tear. Benign gastric ulcer is rare in greater curvature, fundus and cardia. Gastric ulcer >3 cm is giant gastric ulcer. It has got 6–23% chances of turning into carcinoma.
Histologically, it shows destruction of epithelial lining; proliferation of margin; destruction of the part of the muscle layer; granulation tissue in the floor; infiltration with chronic inflammatory cells; endarteritis and fibrosis in the base.

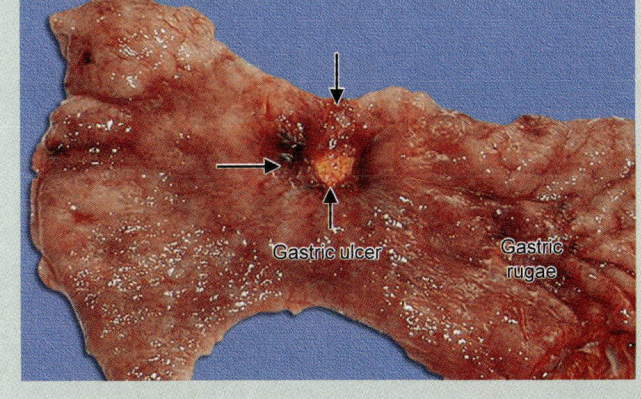

"Hour glass contracture" of stomach– complication of benign gastric ulcer.

Specimen of stomach—carcinoma stomach

Specimen of stomach showing *thickening of the wall of stomach at pylorus*—might be causing obstruction. It could be *localized linitis plastica*. In Asian countries pylorus is the commonest site. In Western countries proximal stomach is the commonest site.
Histological types: Adenocarcinoma—commonest. It could be *intestinal* (well differentiated), papillary, tubular/glandular. It can be *diffuse*—poorly differentiated. *Mucinous* or *signet ring* type can occur.

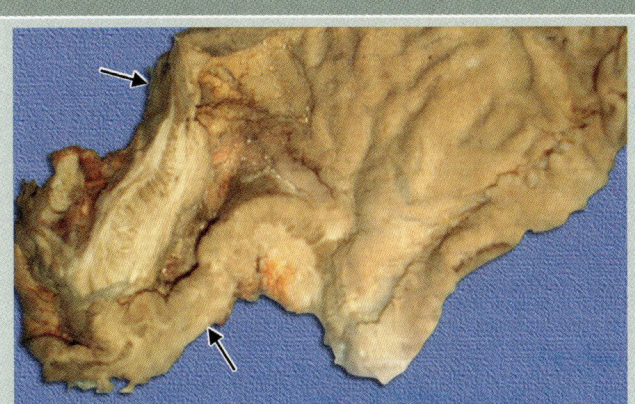

Gross types: Cauliflower type; ulcerative type; leather bottle (linitis plastica) which is more aggressive.

Carcinoma colon

Specimen of cecum, ascending colon, ileum showing large proliferative lesion with narrowing—feature of carcinoma colon. *Adenocarcinoma—commonest type.*
Gross types: Annular → Tubular → Ulcerative → Cauliflower like.
Annular (stenosing) type: It is more common on left side. Here the growth spreads round the internal wall and so it often presents with intestinal obstruction.
Ulcerative type: It is common on right side; *can present with primary* carcinomas in different parts of the colon at same time, i.e. *synchronous* (5%). Patient can present with growth in different parts of the colon in different periods, i.e. *metachronous* (2–5%).

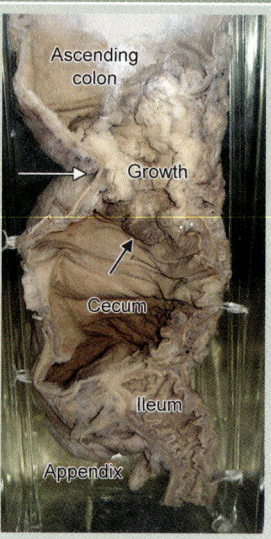

Carcinoma rectum

Specimen showing rectum, anal canal and sigmoid after abdominoperineal resection (APR) with ulceroproliferative / proliferative growth in the rectum. Note the lower part of anal skin. Patient needs permanent end colostomy in left iliac fossa. Digital examination of the rectum (P/R) is the important method of diagnosis (90%).
Presentation of carcinoma rectum are usually as bleeding per rectum; tenesmus; altered bowel habits; pain; backache (sacrum / sacral nerves are involved); urinary symptoms; features of bowel obstruction; features of secondaries. MRI of pelvis is useful to see rectal wall, pararectal tissues and pelvis. Nodal status is better assessed by contrast CT scan. Transrectal ultrasound is very useful to find out local spread. APR; sphincter saving operations (anterior resection); total mesorectal excision (TME) are various treatment strategies. Adjuvant radiotherapy and chemotherapy are beneficial. Laparoscopic mobilization of rectum is very useful.

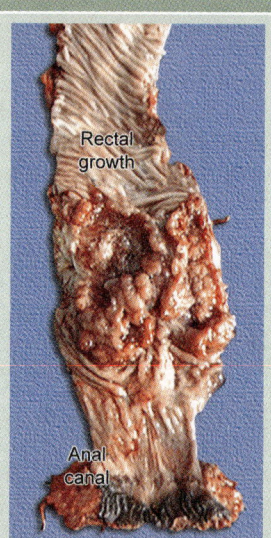

Specimen of intestine with intussusception

It is the telescoping of one segment of bowel into the adjacent segment. Ileo-colic is the most common type. It occurs in children commonly during weaning period. *Red currant jelly stool, sausage-shaped resonant mass, appearing and disappearing of mass, empty right iliac fossa are the features.* Barium enema shows **claw sign**; ultrasound shows **target sign / pseudokidney sign**. Therapeutic enema using barium or air is tried. If it fails, laparotomy, resection and anastomosis is done. **Parts are** – apex; intussuscepiens; intussusceptum.

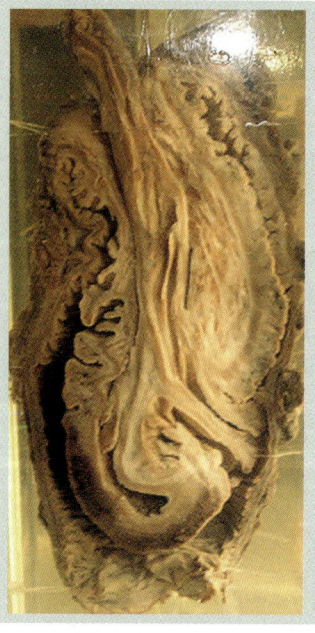

Chapter 43: Surgical Pathology   637

Specimen of colon—Multiple polyposis of colon

Colectomy specimen showing multiple colonic polyps.
Classification of intestinal (colonic) polyps:
a. *Inflammatory*
b. *Hyperplastic*: Metaplastic
c. *Hamartomatous*: Peutz-Jeghers' polyp, juvenile polyp, Cronkhite Canada syndrome
d. *Adenomatous*: (Neoplastic). Tubular (pedunculated), tubulovillous, villous (sessile), FAP
e. *Others*: Hemangioma, lipomas

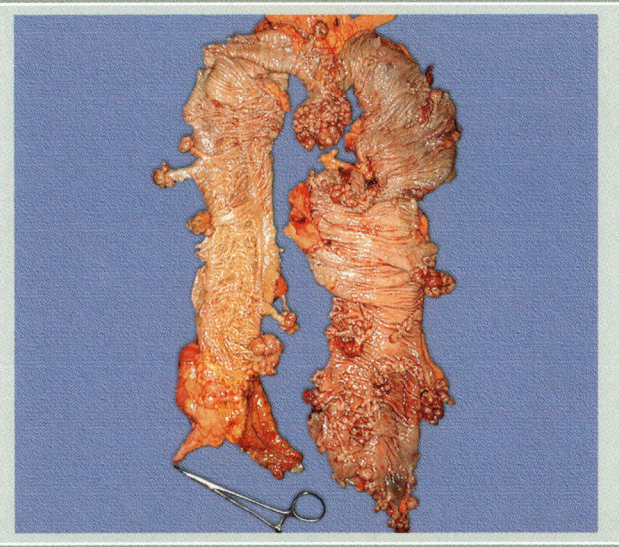

Gallbladder specimen with stones

Note the faceting nature of the multiple stones. Faceting is due to equal pressure of the stones. Mixed stones are the commonest type—90%. They contain cholesterol; calcium bilirubinate; calcium palmitate; calcium phosphate and calcium carbonate. Pigment stones can be black or brown. Black stones are usually calcium bilirubinate stones—
they are commonly seen in gallbladder in association with hemolytic diseases; can also occur independently. Brown pigment stones are commonly observed in biliary tree—CBD, hepatic ducts and ductules. These stones are commonly associated with bacterial infection like *E.coli* as the nidus. Other components may be calcium palmitate and cholesterol.

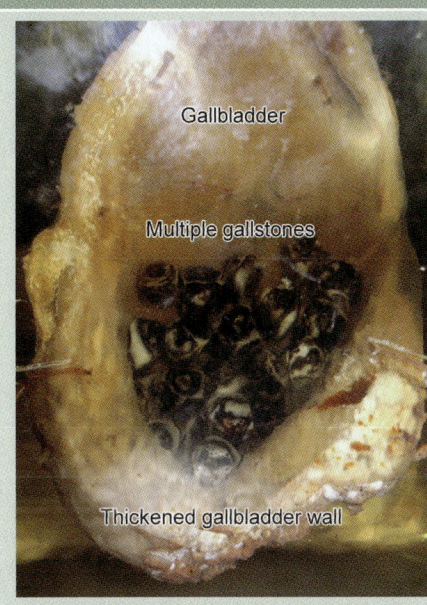

Specimen of staghorn calculus of kidney

Staghorn calculus occupies the major and minor calyces. It presents as recurrent pyelonephritis, pyonephrosis and if bilateral renal failure. If kidney function is adequate which is confirmed by DTPA radioisotope scan then nephropyelolithotomy is done. Often initial nephrostomy is needed.

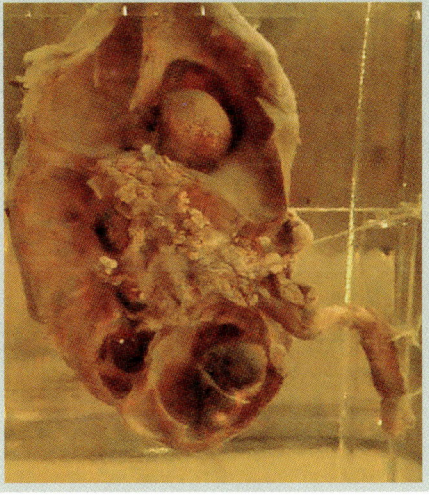

Specimen of kidney showing hydronephrosis

Specimen of *kidney showing dilated thin renal pelvis which is extrarenal*; dilated calyces; and thin renal parenchyma. Here hydronephrosis is due to congenital PUJ obstruction. Nephrectomy is done if the thickness of renal parenchyma is less than 2 cm, if DTPA scan shows less than 15% function, or hydronephrosis is infected. Nephrectomy is also done if kidney function does not improve after pyeloplasty or surgical correction.

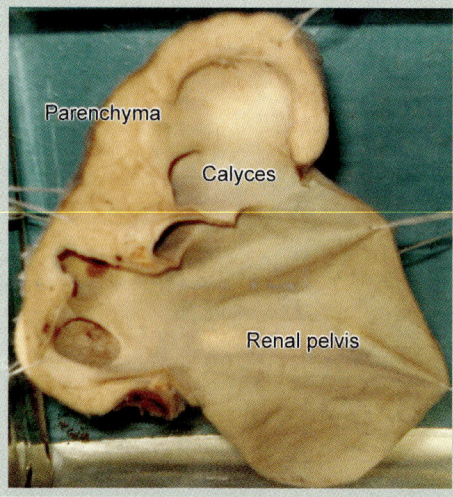

Specimen of testicular tumor

Gross and cut section of testicular tumor. Note the cystic spaces with solid tissues and cartilages which signify the feature of teratoma of testis. Teratoma arises from totipotent cells in rete testis. 99% of testicular tumors are malignant. 10% of testicular tumors are associated with undescended testis. Measurement of tumor markers (b-hCG, AFP, LDH) are important. AFP and hCG are elevated in nonseminomatous germ cell tumors (teratomas). Raised AFP always indicate teratomatous feature of the tumor.

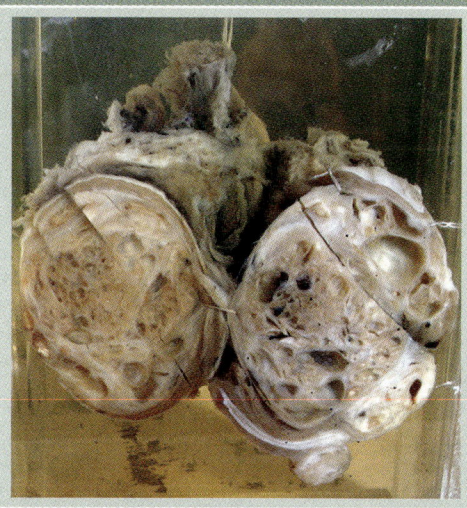

Specimen of transitional cell carcinoma (TCC) of urinary bladder

Specimen of urinary bladder showing multiple *papillary / polypoid transitional cell carcinoma*. It is the commonest type of bladder tumor.
Etiology: 3C's— chemical carcinogens; cigarette smoking; cyclophosphamide.
Types of bladder tumors: (a) *Superficial bladder tumor*; (b) *Muscle invasive TCC*; (c) *Carcinoma in situ*.
Sites: Lateral wall—*commonest*; (35%); trigone—next common (32%).

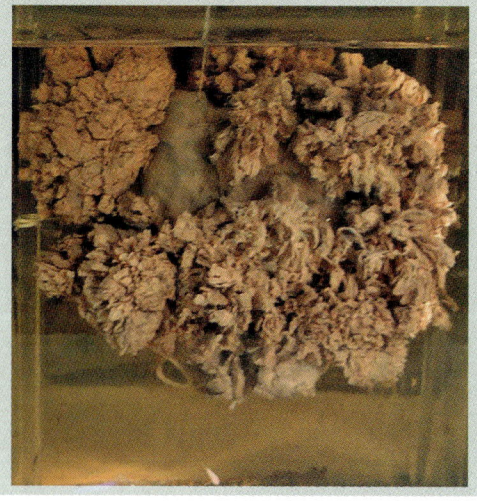

Specimen of hydatid cyst of liver

Specimen of hydatid cysts of liver during extraction from the liver.
Pathology: It has got 3 layers—*Adventitia (pseudocyst, pericyst)*: Is an inseparable fibrous tissue due to reaction of the liver to the parasite. *Laminated membrane (ectocyst)*: Formed of the parasite itself, is whitish, elastic, contains hydatid fluid, which can be peeled of readily from the adventitia. *Germinal epithelium* is the only living part, lining the cyst *(endocyst)*. This layer secretes *hydatid fluid, brood capsules with scolices (*heads of future worms).

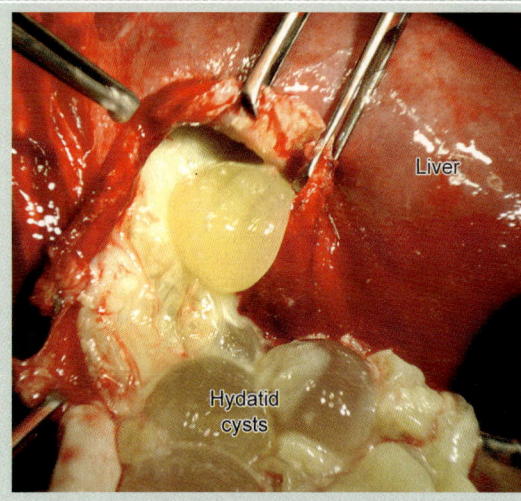

Specimen of carcinoma of breast

Cut section of breast showing gritty whitish tumor area without any capsule surrounded by normal breast tissue. It is scirrhous carcinoma of breast. Histologically, it shows spheroidal ductal malignant epithelial cells with abundant fibrous stroma. Medullary carcinoma is soft, encephaloid, bulky showing malignant columnar cells, with intense lymphocytic infiltration.

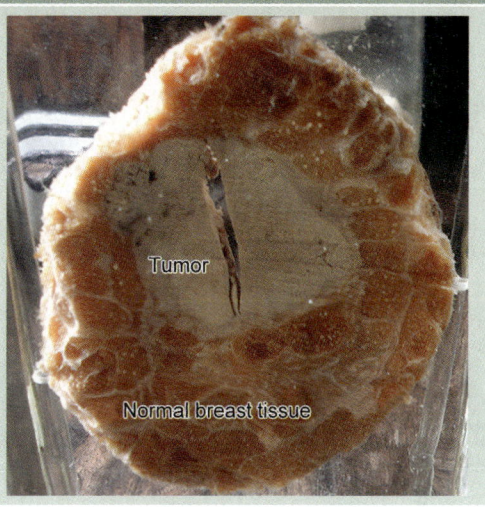

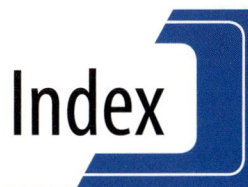

Index

A

AAGSV 198
Abacterial aciduria 506
Abdomen, auscultation 423
Abdomen, contour 435
Abdomen, deep palpation 417
Abdomen, deep palpation, two hand method 417
Abdomen, dilated veins 449
Abdomen, inspection 415
Abdomen, local examination 435, 448
Abdomen, palpation 416
Abdomen, palpation, dipping method 418
Abdomen, palpation, Grainger's method 417, 418
Abdomen, percussion 422, 458
Abdomen, shape/contour 415
Abdomen, skin over 415
Abdomen, standard method of palpation 417
Abdomen, tender spot 418
Abdomen, tenderness 418
Abdomen, visible peristalsis 416
Abdomen, visible pulsation 416
Abdomens, quadrants in 446, 447
Abdomens, regions in 446
Abdominal aneurysms 178
Abdominal compartment syndrome 543
Abdominal crisis 445
Abdominal reflexes 526
Abdominal wall abscess 470
Abdominal wall tumors 469
Abdominal wall, Meleney's progressive gangrene 470
Abducent nerve 525
Abduction and adduction test 566
Abduction in shoulder joint 583
Abductor pollicis brevis 225
ABPI 35
Abscess drainage, Hilton method 613
Abscess, alveolar 274
Abscess, amebic liver 442
Abscess, anorectum 486
Abscess, appendicular 466
Abscess, Brodie's 571-574
Abscess, cold 140, 300, 301, 304, 313, 316
Abscess, complications 140
Abscess, dental 274
Abscess, external 139
Abscess, extradural 526
Abscess, injection 90, 91
Abscess, internal 140
Abscess, intracerebral 526
Abscess, intracranial 526
Abscess, ischiorectal 486
Abscess, lung 530

Abscess, parapharyngeal 316
Abscess, pelvirectal 486
Abscess, perianal 486
Abscess, perinephric 465
Abscess, peritonsillar 276
Abscess, pyemic 140
Abscess, pyogenic 139, 140
Abscess, retropharyngeal 310, 316
Abscess, subdural 526
Abscess, submucous 486
Abscess, subphrenic 460
Accessory auricle 38
Accessory ear 520
Accessory nerve injury 522
Accessory nerve, function 289
Accessory parotid 296
Acetabular angle 593
Achalasia cardia 491
Achilles tendon reflex 332
Achondroplasia 575
Acid phosphatase 508
Acinic cell tumor 295
Acoustic neuroma 527
Acquired cyst 118
Acrocyanosis 178
Acromegaly 16
Acromioclavicular dislocation 552
Actinic cheilitis 242
Actinomyces israelii 150
Actinomycosis 150
Actinomycosis jaw 274
Actinomycosis of the mandible 302
Actinomycosis, right iliac fossa 467
Acute abdomen, causes 432
Acute abdomen, causes, both sexes 432
Acute abdomen, causes, children 432
Acute abdomen, children 432
Acute abdomen, extra-abdominal causes 432
Acute abdomen, intra-abdominal causes 432
Acute abdomen, investigation 439
Acute abdomen, pain 433
Acute appendicitis 440
Acute cholecystitis 441
Acute cholecystitis, acalculous 441
Acute cholecystitis, calculous 441
Acute compartment syndrome 176, 177
Acute lymphadenitis 216, 218
Acute lymphangitis 218
Acute pancreatitis 441
Acute pancreatitis, Trapnell's classification 441
Acute parotitis 280, 284, 295
Acute peritonitis 441
Acute retropharyngeal abscess 316
Acute submandibular sialadenitis 290

Acute suppurative tenosynovitis 516
Adamantinoma 273
Addictions 6
Adductor pollicis 227
Adelaide coma scale 535
Adenoid cystic carcinoma 295
Adenoid facies 16
Adenolymphoma 280, 294, 295
Adenoma, basophil 528
Adenoma, chromophobe 528
Adenoma, eosinophil 527
Adhesions and bands 444
Adiadochokinesia 525
Adiposis dolorosa 124
Adolescent coxa vara 594
Adrenal mass 465
Adrenal tumor 462
Adson's forceps 613
Adson's test 167, 168
Adventitious bursae 4, 124
Aggravating and relieving factors 433
Aggressive fibromatosis 126, 470
Ainhum 179
Air embolism 177
Air plethysmography 196
Aird test 605
Alcohol abuse 6
Alcohol intake 5
Alcohol intake classification 5
Allen's test 168, 169
Allis' tissue holding forceps 612
Alopecia 28
Alopecia androgenic 28
Alopecia areata 28
Alopecia totalis 28
Alopecia universalis 28
Alpha maneuver 484
Alvarado scoring 441
Alveolar abscess 274
Alveolar mucosa 245
Amastia 365
Amazia 365
Ambiguous tumor 124
Ambosexual hair 27
Ambulatory venous pressure (AVP) 196
Amebic liver abscess 443, 461
Amebic liver abscess, complication 442
Amebic point 418
Ameloblastoma 273
American Society of Anesthesiologist (ASA) physical status classification 55
Amoebiasis cutis 442
Amoeboma 467
Anagen 27
Anal canal and perianal area 476
Anal canal carcinoma 477-479
Anal canal palpation 479

Anal canal, malignant tumors 486
Anal fissure 485
Anal fissure, acute 485
Anal fissure, chronic 486
Anal fissure, types 485
Anal groove 479
Anal incontinence 487
Anatomical bursa 123
Anchovy sauce 147
Anemia, causes 17
Aneurysm mycotic 178
Aneurysm, Berry 527
Aneurysm, cirsoid 137
Aneurysm, dissecting 178
Aneurysm, intracranial 527
Aneurysm, intracranial, subclenoid 527
Aneurysm, intracranial, supraclenoid 527
Aneurysmal bone cyst 575
Aneurysms 177
Aneurysms, abdominal 178
Aneurysms, peripheral 178
Angel's sign 400
Angiogram, aortic 174
Angiogram, renal 501
Angiogram, retrograde transfemoral 174
Angiogram, retrograde transfemoral, complications 174
Angiography 174
Angioma, cherry 137
Angle, lovibond 22, 23
Angle, Pauwel's 563
Angular stomatitis 264
Ankle brachial pressure index 35, 173
Ankle clonus 526
Ankle flare 185
Ankle jerk 526
Ankle joint 568
Ankle joint, cross-fluctuation 597
Ankle perforators 198
Ankle pressure 35
Ankle reflex 332
Ankyloglossia 39, 248, 249, 261
Ankylosing spondylitis 607
Ankylosis 581
Ankylosis, bony 581
Ankylosis, false 581
Ankylosis, fibrous 581
Ankylosis, true 581
Anomalies of vitellointestinal duct 469
Anorchism 399
Anorectal abscess 486
Anorectal malformations (ARM) 487
Anorectal ring 480
Anorexia 11, 414
Anosmia 524
Anovaginal bidigital examination 482
Antalgic gait 579, 589
Antegrade pyelogram 501
Anterior accessory great saphenous vein (AAGSV) 198
Anterior rhinoscopy 278
Anterior tibial artery 163, 164
Anteverted testis 396
Antibioma of breast 364
Anti-thyroglobulin antibodies 336

Anti-thyroid peroxidase antibody 336
Anti-TSH receptor antibody 336
Anuria 493
Anvil test 603
Aortic aneurysm 457, 463
Aortic aneurysm ruptured 445
Aortic angiogram 174
Aorto-iliac block 154, 156
Ape thumb deformity 222, 230
Apex beat 529
Aphagia 488
Aphthous stomatitis 264
Aphthous ulcer 241
Apical subungual infection 516
Apley's distraction test 566
Apley's grinding test 566
Apoplectic cyst 118
Apparent shortening of limb 592
Appendicitis, acute 440
Appendicitis, acute non-obstructive 440
Appendicitis, acute obstructive 440
Appendicitis, recurrent 440
Appendicitis, subacute 440
Appendicular abscess 440, 441, 466
Appendicular mass 466
Appetite 414
Appetite and weight 6
Apple jelly nodule 82
Apple-core lesion 633
APUD cell 337
Arachnodactyly 588
Arcus cornealis 36
Arcus senilis 36
Areola, palpation 354
Argyll Robertson pupil 36
Arm-foot venous pressure 196
Arterial diseases, classification of 175
Arterial diseases, examination 153
Arterial diseases, investigations 173
Arterial occlusion, acute 176
Arterial pile 485
Arteries, diseases of 175
Arteriosclerosis 175
Arteriovenous fistula 179
Arteriovenous fistula, acquired 179
Artery, anterior tibial 163, 164
Artery, axillary 166
Artery, brachial 166
Artery, common carotid 166
Artery, dorsalis pedis 163, 164
Artery, facial 166
Artery, femoral 165, 174
Artery, peroneal 163
Artery, popliteal 163
Artery, posterior tibial 163, 164
Artery, radial 165
Artery, subclavian 166
Artery, superficial temporal 166
Artery, ulnar 165
Arthritis, gouty 581
Arthritis, rheumatoid 580
Arthritis, tuberculous 581
Arthroscopy 548, 597
Ascending urethrogram 502, 633, 634
Ascites, grading 422

Askanazy cells 338
Assessment of specific symptoms 7
Associated symptoms 5
Astereognosis 222
Astrocytoma 527
Atheroma 175
Atherosclerosis 175
Athlete's foot 518
Atrophic scirrhous carcinoma breast 362
Attitude of the patient 14
Auditory nerve 527
Auscultation 40
Auscultopercussion test 423, 454
Avascular necrosis of femoral head 594
Avulsion fracture lesser trochanter 563
Axillary artery 166
Axillary lymph nodes 209
Axillary lymph nodes, Berg's levels 209
Axillary nerve injury 231
Axillary nodes examination 209
Axillary tail of Spence 350, 358
Axillary vein thrombosis 199
Axonotmesis 229
Azotemia 493

B

Babcock's forceps 613
Babcock's triangle 594
Backwash ileitis 430
Bacteremia 142
Bag of worms 393, 397, 401
Baghdad sore 86
Baid test 463
Bairnsdale ulcer 85
Balanoposthitis 403, 405, 408
Baldwin's method of renal percussion 498
Baldwing's test 438
Balfour's retractor 615
Ballance's sign 541
Ballooning of prepuce 405, 406, 408
Ballooning of rectum 438
Ballottement test 557
Ballottment, kidney 497
Bamboo spine 607
Barium enema X-ray 426, 633
Barium enema X-ray, Crohn's disease 426
Barium enema X-ray, Hirschsprung's disease 426
Barium enema X-ray, ileocecal tuberculosis 426
Barium enema X-ray, indications 426
Barium enema X-ray, intussusception 426
Barium enema X-ray, required preparation 426
Barium enema X-ray, sigmoid diverticula 426
Barium enema X-ray, ulcerative colitis 426
Barium enema X-ray, carcinoma colon 426
Barium follow through X-ray 426
Barium meal X-ray 426, 632
Barium meal X-ray, benign gastric ulcer 426
Barium meal X-ray, carcinoma head of pancreas 426

Barium meal X-ray, carcinoma stomach 426
Barium meal X-ray, duodenal diverticula 426
Barium meal X-ray, gastric outlet obstruction 426
Barium meal X-ray, pseudocyst of pancreas 426
Barium meal X-ray, stomal ulcer 426
Barium swallow 490-492
Barium swallow X-ray 231
Barley water fluid 390, 401
Barlow's test 593
Barrel chest 529
Barrett's esophagus 491
Barrett's ulcer 491
Bartholin cyst 377
Bartholin duct 297
Bartholin glands 482
Basal cell carcinoma 132
Basal cell papilloma 129
Base ball finger 236
Baseballer's elbow 586, 587
Basedow's disease 336
Bassi peroforator 198
Bat ear 38
Bazin's disease 86
Bazin's ulcer 61
BCC 132
Beau's lines 20
Beck's triad 531
Bed sore 80
Bednar's tumor 132
Beefy red tongue 247
Beeturia 56
Belching 413, 488
Bells at evening pealing 423
Belly cleft 470
Bence Jones protein 577
Benedict's quantitative test 56
Benediction attitude 488
Benign gastric ulcer 635
Benign prostatic hyperplasia (BPH) 507
Benign prostatic hyperplasia (BPH), clinical features 507
Benign prostatic hyperplasia (BPH), pathology 507
Benign subepithelial nodular fibrosis 130
Bennett's fracture dislocation 558
Benzidine test 494
Berg's level of axillary nodes 357
Bernard's aphorism 443
Berry's ligament 325
Berry's sign 331, 337, 338
BI RADS 360
Biceps jerk 526
Bidigital palpation of anal canal 479
Bidigital palpation of mandible 269
Bidigital palpation of salivary gland 291, 292
Bidigital palpation of submandibular salivary gland 291
Bidigital palpation of the mandible 251
Bidigital palpation of the parotid duct 285
Bifid nose 521

Biligram 427
Billiard testis 400
Billing's gate hump 124
Bimanual examination of anorectum 481
Bimanual examination of vagina 482
Bimanual palpation, upper end of humerus 551
Biopsy 44
Biopsy oral cavity 258
Biopsy types 45
Biopsy, drill 45
Biopsy, excision 46
Biopsy, incision 46
Biopsy, lymph node 214
Biopsy, needle 46
Biopsy, open 46
Biopsy, punch 46
Biopsy, trucut 46
Biopsy, wedge 46
Bird beak appearance 631
Bird beak esophagus 490
Black eye 534
Black hairy tongue 246
Bladder mass 468
Bladder rupture 542
Bladder tumors 506
Bladder tumors, classification 506
Bladder, palpation 499
Blandin and Nuhn glands 262
Blaxland ruler test 421, 422
Bleeding per rectum 472
Bleeding per rectum, causes 472
Blind boil 140
Blood pressure 34
Blood pressure apparatus 35
Blood pressure cuff 35
Blood pressure phases 35
Bloodgood cyst 351
Blount's disease 597
Blow outs 182, 186, 188
Blue line in gums 245
Blue nail 22
Blue nevus 131
Blue toe syndrome 174
Blumberg's sign 437, 440
Blumer's shelf 424, 429, 460, 480, 481
BMI 13
Boas's sign 436
Bocca's sign 306
Body mass index (BMI) 13
Body weight 13
Boerhaave's syndrome 40
Boil 140
Boil, blind 140
Bolus obstruction 444
Bone cyst, aneurysmal 575
Bone cyst, unicameral 575
Bone disease of hyperparathyroidism 574
Bone tumors 576
Bone tumors, benign 576
Bone tumors, malignant 576
Borborygmi 423, 438, 444
Borrelia vincentii 80
Borrmann's classification 429
Bottle nose 129

Boutonniere deformity 237, 588
Bow leg 597
Bow sign 401
Bowel habit 413, 434
Bowel sounds 423
Boyd's perforator 198
Boyd's grading 154
Boyd's grading of claudication 154
Brachial artery 166
Brachial plexus injury 229
Brachioradialis 223
Bradycardia 33
Bradycardia, relative 33
Branchial cyst 298, 300, 303-305 312, 313, 315
Branchial fistula 298, 302, 315
Branding 27
Branham's sign 179
BRCA1 362
Breast examination positions 359
Breast mouse 351
Breast self-examination 359
Breast, chest wall fixity 353
Breast, colloid carcinoma 362
Breast, fixity of lump to breast tissue 351
Breast, fixity to latissimus dorsi muscle 352
Breast, fixity to pectoralis major muscle 351
Breast, fixity to serratus anterior muscle 353
Breast, fixity to skin 351
Breast, gliding test 351
Breast, lactational abscess 364
Breast, local examination 343
Breast, lump 349
Breast, medullary carcinoma 362
Breast, MRI 361
Breast, non-lactational abscess 364
Breast, palpation 349
Breast, pinching test 351
Breast, quadrants 350
Breast, Scirrhous carcinoma 362
Breast, Sentinel lymph node biopsy (SLNB) 361
Breast, skin tethering 351
Breast, swelling 349
Breast, trucut biopsy 360, 361
Brittle bones 547, 574
Broder's grading 258, 259
Brodie's abscess 571-574
Brodie-Trendelenburg test 187
Bronchoscopy 530
Brown's law 396
Brown's vasomotor index 174
Browse's classification of lymphedema 215
Bruit 113, 170
Bryant's triangle 561, 562
Bubo 86
Bubo, climatic 86
Bubo, tropical 86
Budd-Chiari syndrome 416
Buerger's angle of vascular insufficiency 161, 169
Buerger's disease 176
Buerger's postural test 161, 169
Built 13
Built and nutritional status 13

Bulla 26
Bunion 124, 519
Bunionette 597
Bunnell's ischemic contracture 514
Burkitt's lymphoma 217, 272, 273
Burns contracture of finger 236
Bursa anserina 123
Bursa olecranon 123
Bursa, adventitious 124
Bursa, anatomical 123
Bursa, porter's 124
Bursa, psoas 123
Bursa, semimembranosus 114, 123
Bursa, subacromial 123
Bursa, subhyoid 123
Bursa, tailor's 124
Bursa, weaver's 124
Bursae 122
Bursae, adventitious 124
Bursitis 123
Bursitis, infrapatellar 123
Bursitis, prepatellar 123
Bursitis, retrocalcaneal 123
Burst fracture 601
Buruli ulcer 85
Buschke-Lowenstein tumor 409
Butcher's wart 129, 514
Buttonhole deformity 580

C

C_7 lesion 600
$C_8 T_1$ lesion 600
Cabana sentinel node 408
Cabanas node 209
Cachexia 14, 94, 239
Cachexia, malignant 14
Cadaveric pallor 161
Café au lait spots 26, 125
Calcaneal spur 598
Calcaneus foot 695
Calcinosis cutis 126
Calcitonin 337
Calculus, staghorn 637
Calculus, urinary 504
Callaway's test 552
Callosity 127
Callous ulcer 60
Calorie test 525
Calve's disease 607
Campbell de Morgan spot 27, 137
Cancer en cuirasse 347-349, 355
Cancer, chimney sweep's 387
Cancer, Kangri 4
Cancer, tear 132
Cancrum oris 179, 245, 264, 265
Canker sore 241
Cannon ball secondaries 629
Capillary filling time 161
Capillary refilling 162
Capillary refilling time 162
Capillary vascular malformation 137
Caput medusa 449
Caput medusae 31, 416
Carbuncle 140, 141

Carbuncle, renal 141
Carbuncle, upper lip 242
Carcinoid facies 16
Carcinoma alveolus 262
Carcinoma breast 639
Carcinoma breast, etiology 362
Carcinoma breast, investigations 360
Carcinoma breast, pathological types 362
Carcinoma breast, spread 362
Carcinoma breast, TNM staging 363
Carcinoma cecum 466
Carcinoma cheek 243, 260
Carcinoma cheek, advanced, features 261
Carcinoma cheek, biological behavior 261
Carcinoma cheek, clinical features 261
Carcinoma cheek, precipitating factors 261
Carcinoma cheek, premalignant
  conditions 261
Carcinoma colon 431, 636
Carcinoma colon, features 431
Carcinoma colon, spread 431
Carcinoma cuniculatum 133
Carcinoma esophagus 492
Carcinoma lip 241, 261
Carcinoma lung 531
Carcinoma of breast 361, 362
Carcinoma of breast, classification 362
Carcinoma of floor of the mouth 262
Carcinoma of stomach 429
Carcinoma penis 403, 405-408
Carcinoma penis, clinical features 408
Carcinoma penis, pathology 408
Carcinoma penis, spread 408
Carcinoma penis, verrucous 409
Carcinoma prostate 507
Carcinoma prostate, blood spread 507
Carcinoma prostate, clinical features 507
Carcinoma prostate, histology 507
Carcinoma prostate, investigations 508
Carcinoma prostate, lymphatic spread 507
Carcinoma prostate, types 507
Carcinoma pyriform fossa 275, 278
Carcinoma rectum 484
Carcinoma rectum, clinical features 484
Carcinoma rectum, spread 484
Carcinoma scrotum 388
Carcinoma sigmoid colon 468
Carcinoma stomach 635
Carcinoma stomach mass 454
Carcinoma stomach, barium meal
  X-ray 632
Carcinoma tongue 261
Carcinoma tongue, features 261
Carcinoma tongue, terminal events in
  advanced 261
Carcinoma tongue, types 261
Carcinoma transverse colon 464
Carcinoma, adenoid cystic 295
Carcinoma, hard palate 262
Carcinoma, Hurthle cell 337
Carcinoma, larynx 299, 309
Carcinoma, lip 241
Carcinoma, medullary, thyroid 337
Carcinoma, nasopharyngeal 276
Carcinoma, primary branchiogenic 315

Carcinoma, verrucous 239, 261
Card test 227, 228, 230
Cardiac tamponade 531
Caries sicca 585
Carman's meniscus sign 632
Carnett's test 420, 421, 452, 453
Caroticocavernous fistula 527
Carotid artery aneurysm 300
Carotid blow out 261
Carotid body 315
Carotid body syncope 315
Carotid body tumor 298, 300, 304, 315
Carotid body tumor, Shamblin
  classification 315
Carpal tunnel syndrome 230, 235
Carpal, metacarpal, phalangeal bones 557
Carr's postulates 504
Carrying angle 553, 555, 586
Carrying angle, measurement 555
Case taking 1
Cat scratch fever 219
Catagen 27
Catgut 621
Catgut, chromic 622
Catgut, plain 621
Catheter introducer 618
Catheter, Foley's 618
Catheter, Malecot's 618
Catheter, nonself-retaining 618
Catheter, red rubber 618
Catheter, self-retaining 618
Catheters 618
Cauda equina injury 600
Cauliflower ear 38, 92
Causalgia 7, 220, 221
Causes of intestinal obstruction 627
Causes of nonhealing ulcer 79
Cavernous sinus thrombosis 138, 522
CEAP classification of varicose veins 195
Cellular study 44
Cellulitis 138
Cellulitis face 138
Cellulitis, clinical features 138
Cellulitis, orbital 138
Cellulitis, sequelae 138
Cerebellar hemisphere tumors 527
Cerebellar lesion 525
Cerebellar vermis tumors 527
Cervical lymph node 210
Cervical lymph node examination 258
Cervical rib 314, 630
Cervical rib syndrome 314
Cervical rib, types 314
Chain of lake appearance 427, 628
Chair test 587
Champagne bottle sign 186, 193
Chance injury 601
Chancre, hard 85
Chancre, Hunterian 85
Chancre, soft 86
Chancroid 403
Chancroid ulcer 65
Charcot's joint 578
Chassaignac anterior tubercle 166
Chassaigne tubercle 166

Index

Cheatle's forceps 611
Cheek, inspection 243
Cheek, mucus cyst 243
Cheek, palpation 251
Cheilosis 242, 264
Chemodectoma 315
Chemosis 322, 323
Cherry angioma 137
Cherubism 274
Chest injuries 538
Chest wall tumors 532
Chest wall, cystic swellings 532
Chest wall, shape 529
Chest wall, sinus 532
Chest wall, solid swellings 532
Chest X-ray 47, 629
Chevrier Percussion/Tap Sign 191
Chew and spit test 426
Cheyne-Stokes respiration 533
Chiba needle 427
Chief complaints 4
Chiene's test 562
Chilaiditi's syndrome 442
Chilblains 85, 179
Child's grading 462
Child's grading, Pugh's modification 462
Chimney sweep's cancer 387
Chin test 303
Cholecystitis, acute 441
Cholecystitis, emphysematous 441
Cholescintigraphy 440
Cholesterol crystals 398
Chondroma 576
Chondroma, types 576
Chondrosarcoma 577
Chordee 405, 408, 409
Chordee, dorsal 408
Chordee, ventral 408
Chordoma 127
Chromocystoscopy 502
Chromophobe adenomas 528
Chronic cholecystitis 429
Chronic constrictive pericarditis 531
Chronic lymphadenitis 216, 218
Chronic lymphatic leukemia 219
Chronic osteomyelitis 151
Chronic pancreatitis 429
Chronic pancreatitis, complications 429
Chronic retropharyngeal abscess 316
Chronic subdural hematoma 535
Chronic superficial glossitis 263
Chutta carcinoma 261
Chvostek-Weiss sign 338
Chylocele 398
Chylolymphatic cyst 465
Chyluria 56
Cimino fistula 179
Circumduction gait 589
Circumferential measurement of limb 562
Circumvallate papillae 246
Cirsoid aneurysm 137, 522
Clamps 613
Clamps, bowel occlusion 613
Clamps, Doyen's intestinal occlusion 614
Clamps, Moynihan's bowel occlusion 613

Clamps, Payr's crushing 614
Clapper in bell 400
Classification of diseases 41
Classification, Browse's, lymphoedema 215
Classification, DeBakey's 178
Classifications of neck swellings 312
Claudication distance 154
Claudication grading 154
Claudication pain 63
Claudication, intermittent 154
Claudication, neurogenic 155
Claudication, neurological 155
Claudication, venous 155
Claudio 154
Claw hand 221, 588
Claw hand deformity 230
Claw hand, median 230
Claw hand, ulnar 230
Claw sign 426, 636
Clawing of toes 597
Cleft disorders 521
Cleft disorders, problems in 521
Cleft lip 240, 521
Cleft lip, types 521
Cleft palate 240, 251, 520
Cleft palate, types 520
Clergyman's knee 4, 123, 594
Clicking of jaw 270
Climatic bubo 86
Clinical examination 1
Clinical methods 1
Clinician 1
Clinistix 56
Cloquet lymph node 208
Cloquet's, deep lymph node 407
Closed loop obstruction 444
Club foot 518, 598
Clubbing 22
Clubbing causes 22
Clubbing grading 22
Clutton's joint 85, 400, 581
Cobb's angle 607
Coccydynia 482
Cock's peculiar tumor 120
Cockett perforator 198
Codman's method of shoulder palpation 583
Codman's triangle 576
Coin test 604, 609
Cold abscess 140, 202, 207, 216, 300, 301, 304, 313, 316
Cold abscess, hip joint 590
Cold and warm water test 168
Colic, appendicular 432, 433
Colic, biliary 432, 433, 435
Colic, intestinal 432, 433
Colic, salivary 281
Colic, ureteric 432, 433, 435
Colicky pain 433
Collapsing pulse 34
Collar button ulcer 426
Colloid cyst 527
Colonic mass 463
Colonic polyps 637
Colonic tuberculosis 464

Colonoscopy 484
Common carotid artery 166
Common peroneal nerve lesion 231
Compensatory peripheral vascular disease 176
Complications of neurofibroma 125
Compound nevus 132
Compound palmar ganglion 516
Compressibility 107
Compression test 537, 559
Condyloid process 266
Condyloma 130
Condyloma acuminata 406, 477
Condyloma lata 477
Congenital anomalies of breast 365
Congenital contracture of little finger 236
Congenital cyst 118
Congenital dislocation of hip 593
Congenital fistulae of lower lip 521
Congenital manus valgus 556
Congenital short frenuium of upper lip 521
Congenital talipes equinovarus 598
Coning 535
Consistency, paradox 102
Constipation 11, 414
Constipation, grading 11
Contour of shoulder 550, 582
Contrast X-ray 47
Cope's obturator test 437
Cope's psoas test 437, 441
Cork screw esophagus 490
Corn 127
Corona phlebectatica 182
Coronoid process 266
Corrigan's pulse 34
Corrosive stricture of esophagus 492
Corrosive strictures 489
Cortisol ulcer 61
Costoclavicular compression maneuver 167
Costoclavicular space 314
Cough impulse, Morrissey's 185
Countryman's lip 238, 261
Courvoisier's law 419, 430, 462
Coxa vara 579
Cozen's test 587
Cracked lip 241
Cranial nerve, examination 522
Craniopharyngiomas 528
Creatinine clearance 500
Cremaesteric reflex 526
Crepitus 40, 103
Crepitus of bone 40
Crepitus of bursitis 40
Crepitus tenosynovitis 40
Crepitus, joint 40
Crepitus, laryngeal 306
Crepitus, subcutaneous emphysema 40
Cretinism, facies 16
Cricket ball bladder 494, 509
Cricketing approach to the abdomen 425
Crile's grading 321
Crile's method of palpation of thyroid 327
Crisis porphyria 445
Crisis, diabetic 445
Critical limb ischemia 175, 176

Crohn's disease 467
Crohn's disease, acute 467
Crohn's disease, chronic 467
Crosby Kugler capsule 45
Cross fluctuation 105, 393
Cross fluctuation, elbow joint 586
Crossed leg test 169
Crurum puellarum frigidum 178
Crust 26, 57, 69
Cruveilhier's sign of Saphena Varix 190
Cry of dying nerves 155
Cryptorchidism 390, 391, 399
CSF rhinorrhea 535
CT scan high resolution 51
CT scan imaging 50
CT scan, advantages 51
CT scan, spiral, advantages 51
Cubitus valgus 553, 555, 586, 587
Cubitus varus 553, 555, 586, 587
Curdy white tongue 247
Curtain sign 284, 285, 294
Cutaneous T cell lymphoma 217
Cyanosis 18
Cyanosis, central 18
Cyanosis, differential 18
Cyanosis, peripheral 18
Cyclical mastalgia 8
Cylindroma 522
Cylindroma, multiple 130
Cyst dermoid, ear 38
Cyst distention 118
Cyst exudation 118
Cyst of the epididymis 401
Cyst retention 118, 119
Cyst, apoplectic 118
Cyst, bloodgood 351
Cyst, branchial 298, 300, 303-305, 312, 313, 315
Cyst, clinical features 118
Cyst, congenital 118
Cyst, degenerative 118
Cyst, dental 269, 273
Cyst, dentigerous 269, 273
Cyst, dermoid 300, 303, 304
Cyst, effects 118
Cyst, epidermal 121
Cyst, false 1118
Cyst, lymph 121, 122
Cyst, Morrant Baker's 123
Cyst, mucus retention 262
Cyst, mucus, cheek 243
Cyst, parasitic 118
Cyst, periapical 273
Cyst, pilar 121
Cyst, radicular 273
Cyst, sequestration dermoid 118
Cyst, thyroid 336
Cyst, traumatic 118
Cyst, trichilemmal 121
Cyst, true 118
Cyst, unicameral bone 575
Cystadenocarcinoma of pancreas 430, 463
Cystic hygroma 137, 298, 300, 303, 304, 315
Cystic swellings of breast 359
Cystic tumors 118

Cystine calculus 504
Cystine stone 504
Cystitis 508
Cystocele 379
Cystosarcoma phyllodes 363
Cystoscopy 502
Cystoscopy, types 502
Cysts 118
Cysts of bone 575
Cysts of embryonic remnants 118
Cysts, acquired 118
Cysts, classification 118
Cytology 44
Cytology, brush 44
Cytology, exfoliative 44
Cytology, imprint 44
Cytology, sponge 44
Czerney's retractor 615

D

Dactylitis 588
Daintree Johnson classification 428
Dangerous zone of face 522
D-dimer test 196
de Quervain's stenosing tenosynovitis 588
de Quervain's tenosynovitis 234
de' Quervain's thyroiditis 336
Deaver's retractor 615
DeBakey's classification 178
Decompensatory peripheral vascular disease 176
Decoy prostate 507
Decubitus of the patient 15
Decubitus ulcer 80
Decubitus, coiled up 15
Decubitus, kneeling prayer 15
Decubitus, left lateral 15
Decubitus, right lateral 15
Decubitus, rigid dorsal 15
Decubitus, squatting 15
Deep cervical lymph nodes 306
Deep inguinal ring 378
Deep lobe of parotid 283
Deep palmar space infection 515
Deep ring occlusion test 373, 374
Deep vein thrombosis (DVT) 199
Deep venous thrombosis (DVT) 181, 199
Defecation 11
Delayed union 549
Delhi boil 86
Delphian node 332
Deltoid muscle 223
Deming's sign 400
Demodex folliculorum 119
Dental abscess 274
Dental cyst 269, 273
Dentigerous cyst 269, 273
Depressed skull fracture 536
Derbyshire neck 318
Dercum's disease 93, 124
Dermal flare 182, 184, 193
Dermal histiocytoma 130
Dermatofibroma 130
Dermatofibrosarcoma protuberans 132

Dermoid cyst 300, 303, 304
Dermoid cyst, ear 38
Dermoid sequestration 119, 122
Dermoid, external angular 119
Dermoid, implantation 90, 119
Dermoid, internal angular 119
Dermoid, submental 119
Dermoid, teratomatous 119
Dermoids 118
Dermoids, sequestration 118
Desjardin's choledocholithotomy forceps 623
Desmoid tumor 126, 470
Diabetic crisis 445
Diabetic foot 179
Diagnosis, anatomical 117
Diagnosis, pathological 117
Diagnostic peritoneal lavage 541
Diaphragmatic eventration 531
Diaphragmatic hernia 531, 630
Diaphyseal aclasia 575, 576
Diarrhea 11
Diarrhea grading 11
Diarrhea 414
Diarrhea, acute 414
Diarrhea, chronic 414
Diet 5
Dietl's crisis 496, 503
Dieulafoy's disease 412
Difference between direct and indirect inguinal hernia 381
Differential diagnosis for neck lymph node enlargement 313
Diffuse esophageal spasm 490
di-George's syndrome 338
Digital examination of anorectum 479
Digital examination of rectum 424, 438, 499
Digital examination of rectum, positions 475
Digital subtraction angiogram (DSA) 174
Digitus quintus varus 597
Dilator, Clutton's 619
Dilator, Lister's urethral 619
Dinner fork deformity 556, 558
Dip method for ascites 453
Diphtheritic desert sore 86
Diphtheritic ulcer 62
Direct hernia 379
Direct laryngoscopy 277
Disappearing pulse syndrome 169
Disappearing pulse, sign 163
Discharge, sinus 144
Disease, Buerger's 176
Disease, Dercum's 124
Disease, Eve's 273
Disease, Marvan's 195
Disease, Mondor's 200, 347, 364
Disease, Mule spinner's 387
Disease, Nonne-Milroy's 218
Disease, Peyronie's 235
Disease, von Recklinghausen of neurofibroma 125
Diseases of arteries 175
Diseases of larynx 277
Diseases of pharynx 276
Diseases of umbilicus 469

Index

Dislocation 549
Dislocation lunate 558
Dislocation of elbow, posterior 556
Dislocation of hip 563
Dislocation of patella, recurrent 656
Dislocation of shoulder 552
Dislocation of shoulder, anterior 552
Dislocation of shoulder, posterior 552
Dislocation of shoulder, recurrent 552
Dislocation of shoulder, types 552
Dissecting forceps 613
Distal run off 174
Distraction test 559
Diverticular disease colon 467
Diverticulitis 464, 468
Diverticulosis 468
Dodd perforator 198
Donovan ulcer 403
Doppler 173
Doppler effect 49
Doppler study 49
Doppler types 49
Doppler, venous 196
Dorsal interossei 227
Dorsal position 475
Dorsalis pedis artery 163, 164
Dorsiflexion 517
Double barreled aorta 178
Double hernia 385
Doyen's retractor 615
DPL 541
Dragstedt test 425
Drain, closed suction tube 617
Drain, corrugated rubber 617
Drain, glove 617
Drain, Jackson Pratt 618
Drain, tube 617
Drain, wick 617
Drains 617
Drill biopsy 45
Drinker, heavy 6
Drinker, light 5
Drinker, moderate 6
Drinker, occasional 5
Drinker, problem 5
Drinker, very heavy 6
Driver's bottom 485
Drop foot 228
Dryness of mouth 39
Ducrey's ulcer 60
Duct ectasia 364
Duct papilloma 364
Duct, Stenson's 281, 283
Duct, Wharton's 281, 290
Dugas' test 552
Dumb bell tumor 294, 315
Duodenal point 411
Duodenal ulcer 428
Duodenal ulcer, features of 428
Duplex scan 173
Duplication of renal pelvis 506
Dupuytren's contracture 235, 513
Dupuytren's fracture 568, 570
Dwarfism 13
Dyshormonogenesis 317, 320, 338
Dyspepsia, flatulent 413
Dyspepsia, non-ulcer 413
Dysphagia 488-492
Dysphagia lusoria 490
Dysphagia, causes 489
Dysphagia, evaluation of 490
Dysphagia, history taking 488
Dysphagia, sideropenic 275, 488
Dysuria 493

E

e-thrombosis 182, 199
Ear, bat 38
Ear, cauliflower 38
Ear, keloid 38
Early satiety 6
Ears 38
EAST 314
Ecchondroma 576
Ecchymosis 26
ECOG performance status 42
Ectopia vesicae 508
Ectopic gestation, ruptured 445
Ectopic kidney 467
Ectopic salivary gland 293, 297
Ectopic testis 381, 401
Ectopic thyroid 339
Edema 28
Edema eyelid 37
Edema generalized 29
Edema glottis 277
Edema localized 29
Edema, grading 31
Edge, everted 59
Edge, everted/rolled out 67
Edge, punched out 58, 67
Edge, raised and beaded 67
Edge, sloping 57, 66
Edge, undermined 67
Elbow flexion test 587
Elbow joint 553
Elbow joint movement 555, 586
Elbow joint, three bony point relationship 555
Elbow tunnel syndrome 587
Elephantiatic neurofibromatosis 125
Elevated arm stress test (EAST) 167
Elusive ulcer 508
Emboli, arterial 177
Embolism 155, 177
Embolism, air 177
Embolism, fat 177
Embolism, features 177
Embolus 175
Embolus, saddle 177
Emphysema, mediastinal 537
Emphysema, subcutaneous 629
Emphysema, surgical 537, 538
Empyema necessitans 530
Empyema thoracis 530
Encephalocele 521
Enchondroma 576
Enchondromatosis 575
Encysted hydrocele 393

Encysted hydrocele of the cord 387, 390, 392, 396, 398
Endemic goiter 318, 320
Endemic hematuria 508
Endoscopic esophageal staining 490
Endoscopic retrograde cholangiopancreatography (ERCP) 427
Endoscopy examination 47
Endosonography 490
Endotracheal tube 622, 623
Enlarged spleen 464
Entamoeba histolytica 442
Enterocele 379, 381
Enteroclysis 426, 632
Enterogenous cyst 465
Enterohepatic circulation 20
Entrapment neuropathy 220
Enuresis 493
Eosinophil (Acidophil) adenomas 527
Ependymoma 527
Epicondylitis, lateral 237
Epicondylitis, medial 237
Epidermal cyst 121
Epidermoid cyst 121
Epididymal cyst, 'Chinese lantern' pattern 395
Epididymis, cyst of 401
Epididymis, palpation of 396
Epididymitis, tuberculous 396, 400
Epididymo-orchitis, acute 396, 400
Epididymo-orchitis, filarial 396
Epigastric hernia 384
Epiphora 272
Epispadias 405, 409
Epithelioid cells 214, 219
Epithelioma 83, 133
Epitheliomatous ulcer 67
Eponychium 20
Epstein-Barr virus 217, 219
Epulis 271, 272
Epulis carcinomatous 273
Epulis, congenital 271, 272
Epulis, fibrosarcomatous 273
Epulis, fibrous 271, 272
Epulis, giant cell 271, 273
Epulis, granulomatous 272
Epulis, myelomatous 271, 272
Epulis, pregnancy 271, 272
Equinus foot 597
Erb's palsy 221
Erb's point 221
Erb-Duchenne palsy 220
ERCP 634
Eruptions nonpalpable 23
Erysipelas 139
Erysipeloid disease 139
Erythema ab agne 17
Erythema induratum 86
Erythema nodosum 18
Erythralgia 178
Erythrocyanosis frigida 61, 86
Erythromelalgia 178
Erythroplakia 243, 261, 263
Erythroplasia of Queyrat 407

Index

Esbach's albuminometer 56
Esbach's reagent 56
Eschar 175
Eskimoma 294
Esophageal candidial infection 489
Esophageal manometry 490
Esophageal motility disorder 490
Esophagoscopy 490
Esophagoscopy, fiberoptic/video flexible 490
Esophagus, 'bird beak' 490
Esophagus, 'cork screw' 490
Esophagus, carcinoma 492
Esophagus, corrosive stricture 492
Esophagus, foreign body 491, 630
Esophagus, sigmoid 631
Esthiomene 86
Estrogen receptors 361
Ethmoidal sinusitis 279
Etiology of oral cancers 239
European Hernia Society classification 379
Eve's disease 273
Eventration of diaphragm 531
Eversion 517, 568-570
Ewing's sarcoma 576
Examination by exploration 53
Examination in abdominal injuries 540
Examination in arterial diseases 153
Examination in bone diseases 571
Examination in dysphagia 488
Examination in head injuries 533
Examination in injuries around shoulder joint and arm 550
Examination in injuries of ankle joint and foot 568
Examination in injuries of elbow joint and forearm 553
Examination in injuries of knee joint and leg bones 563
Examination in injuries of various joints 550
Examination in injuries of wrist joint and hand 556
Examination in intracranial diseases 524
Examination in pathological knee joint 594
Examination in pathologies of individual joint 582
Examination in rectal and vaginal problems 472
Examination in spine injuries and diseases 599
Examination in urinary diseases 493
Examination of acute abdomen 432
Examination of anorectum 475
Examination of axillary nodes 209
Examination of bone and joint injuries 545
Examination of breast 340
Examination of cervical lymph nodes 258
Examination of chest diseases 529
Examination of chest injuries 537
Examination of cranial nerves 524
Examination of face and head 520
Examination of feces 55
Examination of foot disease 517
Examination of hand disease 511
Examination of hernia 366
Examination of inguinoscrotal and scrotal swellings 387
Examination of injuries to pelvis 558
Examination of jaw 266
Examination of larynx 276
Examination of male external genitalia 403
Examination of muscles, tendons and fasciae 234
Examination of nails 20
Examination of nasal cavities and paranasal air sinuses 278
Examination of nasopharynx 276
Examination of neck 298
Examination of oral cavity 238
Examination of pathological ankle joint and foot 597
Examination of pathological elbow joint 585
Examination of pathological hip joint 588
Examination of pathological joint 578
Examination of pathological shoulder joint 582
Examination of pathological wrist and joints of hand 588
Examination of peripheral nervous system 220
Examination of pharynx 275
Examination of pulse 33
Examination of salivary gland 280
Examination of skin and mucous membrane 17
Examination of tongue 255
Examination of thyroid 317
Examination of urine 55, 500
Examination of varicose veins 184
Examination on injuries of hip and thigh 560
Examinations in chronic abdominal conditions 411
Excessive hair growth 28
Exomphalos 470
Exomphalos major 470
Exomphalos minor 470
Exophthalmometry 336
Exophthalmos 36, 319, 321-324, 327, 336
Exophthalmos, malignant 323
Expansile impulse 100
Expansile impulse on coughing 107, 301, 302, 305, 371, 373
Expansile pulsation 107, 457, 463
Expansile pulsation, abdomen 171
Extensor muscles of the wrist 223
External angular dermoid 119
External genitalia, examination 457
Extradural hematoma 535
Extravasation of urine 401
Exuberant granulation tissue 78
Eyelid edema 37
Eyes 36

F

Face and head, benign swellings 522
Face and head, infective lesions 522
Face and head, malignant conditions of 522
Face and head, traumatic problems 522
Face lemon yellow 16
Face look 16
Face of myasthenia gravis 16
Face, in Addison's disease 16
Face, in myxedema 16
Face, in primary polycythemia 16
Face, in Wilson's disease 16
Face, mask 16
Face, moon red 16
Facial artery 166
Facial cleft 521
Facial nerve 285, 295, 525
Facial nerve palsy, clinical signs 287
Facial nerve, anatomy 296
Facial nerve, examination 286
Facies 16
Facies of congenital syphilis 16
Facies of cretinism 16
Facies of hepatic cirrhosis 16
Facies of Punch and Judy 16
Facies, adenoid 16
Facies, Ape man 16
Facies, carcinoid 16
Facies, cirrhosis 16
Facies, congenital syphilis 16
Facies, Down's syndrome 16
Facies, Hippocratica 434
Facies, Parkinsonism 16
Facies, Punch and Judy 16
Facies, tabetic 16
Faciovenous plane of Patey 286, 296
Faciovenous plane of Patey of retromandibular vein 296, 297
Factitia, thyrotoxicosis 336
Factitious ulcer 61
Falconer test 168
Falling of hair 27
Familial adenomatous polyp (FAP) 431
Family history and genetic history 6
FAP 431
FAST 541
Fat embolism 177, 548
Fatigue 11
Fatigue metatarsal fracture 519
Febrile convulsions 39
Feces examination 55
Fegan's test 190, 193, 196
Felon 515
Felty's syndrome 465
Femoral artery 165, 174
Femoral canal, surgical anatomy 383
Femoral head, palpation 590
Femoral hernia 381, 384
Femoral nerve stretch test 605
Femoral swellings 387
Ferguson Smith syndrome 133
Fetor oris 261
Fever 38
Fever causes 39
Fever grading 39
Fever, continuous 38
Fever, drug 39
Fever, glandular 219

Fever, intermittent 38
Fever, Pel-Ebstein 39, 204
Fever, relapsing 39
Fever, remittent 38
Fever, types 38
Fibroadenoma breast 363
Fibroadenoma, giant 351
Fibrocystadenosis of breast 363
Fibrocystic disease of breast 363
Fibroepithelial polyp 262
Fibroepithelioma of Pinkus 132
Fibrolipoma 124
Fibroma 126
Fibroma hard 126
Fibroma soft 126
Fibroma true 126
Fibroma, osteofying 273
Fibrosarcoma 136
Fibrous dysplasia 273
Filarial lymphadenitis 202, 203, 218
Filiform papillae 245
Final diagnosis 41
Fine needle aspiration cytology (FNAC) 46
Finger invagination test 374, 380
Finkelstein's test 588
Fish handler's disease 139
Fissure in ano 472, 473, 476, 485, 486
Fistula 143
Fistula in ano 472, 473, 476, 477, 486
Fistula, branchial 146
Fistula, causes 143
Fistula, cimino 179
Fistula, classification 144
Fistula, different discharges 147
Fistula, high level 486
Fistula, low level 486
Fistula, Park's classification 486
Fistula, salivary 282, 294
Fistula, standard classification 486
Fistulogram 148
Fixed abduction and adduction deformity of hip 590
Fixed flexion deformity of hip 590
Fixed medial or lateral rotation deformity of hip 590
Flail chest 537, 538
Flail segment 538
Flat chest 529
Flat foot 518
Flatulence 11
Flatulent dyspepsia 413
Flexor carpi ulnaris 225
Flexor digitorum profundus 224
Flexor digitorum superficialis 224
Flexor pollicis longus 224
Floating nail 515
Floating prostate 543
Floor of the mouth, inspection 249
Floor of the mouth, palpation 256
Fluctuation 103
Fluctuation, by three finger test 105
Fluctuation, cross 105, 393
Fluctuation, standard 103
Fluid collections in the skin 26
Fluid thrill 421, 458, 459

Flush venogram 502
FNAC 44, 46
FNAC breast 360
FNNAC breast 360
Focused assessment with sonography for trauma 541
Foliate papillae 246
Follicular odontome 273
Folliculitis 140
Food bolus 444
Foot drop 222, 228, 231
Foot ulcers 86
Foot, calcaneus 597
Foot, equinus 597
Foot, everted 597
Foot, flat 518
Foot, hollow 518
Foot, inverted 597
Foot, valgus 597
Foot, varus 597
Footballer's ulcer 61, 86
Foramen cecum 246
Foramen Langer 358
Forcep's, Kocher's 612
Forceps, (Lister's) sinus 613
Forceps, Adson's 613
Forceps, Allis' tissue holding 612
Forceps, artery 611
Forceps, Babcock's 613
Forceps, Cheatle's 611
Forceps, Desjardin's choledocholithotomy 623
Forceps, dissecting 613
Forceps, dissecting, non-toothed 613
Forceps, dissecting, toothed 613
Forceps, Lane's tissue holding 613
Forceps, Moran-Baker's appendix holding 613
Forceps, mosquito 611
Forceps, right angle, Meigster's/ Laney's 612
Forceps, sponge-holding (Rampley's) 611
Fordyce's disease 121
Foreign body esophagus 630
Foreign body in esophagus 491
Foreign body nose 279
Fossa of Rosenmuller 275, 276
Fournier's gangrene 391, 392, 400, 402, 405
Fovea palatini 250
Fracture 548
Fracture clavicle 550, 552
Fracture dislocation, Monteggia 553, 556
Fracture hangman 601
Fracture humerus 552
Fracture humerus, greater tuberosity 552
Fracture humerus, neck of humerus 552
Fracture humerus, shaft of humerus 552
Fracture neck of femur 563
Fracture of lateral tibial condyle 567
Fracture of nasal bone 279
Fracture of pelvic ring, stable 560
Fracture of pelvic ring, unstable 560
Fracture pelvis 482
Fracture reverse Monteggia 556
Fracture scapula 552
Fracture shaft of tibia 567

Fracture spine 601
Fracture, 'Bumper' 567
Fracture, avulsion 548
Fracture, Barton's 558
Fracture, burst 601
Fracture, calcaneal 570
Fracture, causes 548
Fracture, Chauffeur's 558
Fracture, Clay Shoveler's 601
Fracture, clinical features 548
Fracture, closed 546, 548
Fracture, Colle's 545, 546, 548
Fracture, comminuted 548
Fracture, complicated 548
Fracture, complications 548
Fracture, compound 546, 548
Fracture, Cotton's 570
Fracture, depressed 548
Fracture, Don Juan's 570
Fracture, Dupuytren's 570
Fracture, factors affecting healing 548
Fracture, femoral condyles 565
Fracture, Galeazzi 558
Fracture, Green stick 545, 548
Fracture, intertrochanteric 563
Fracture, Jefferson 601
Fracture, Jone's 570
Fracture, Lover's 570
Fracture, Malgaigne 560
Fracture, march 545, 546, 548
Fracture, oblique 548
Fracture, open 546, 548
Fracture, patella 567
Fracture, pathological 545-548
Fracture, pathological, X-ray 630
Fracture, Pott's 570
Fracture, Reading of an X-ray 547
Fracture, Rolando's 558
Fracture, scaphoid 558
Fracture, simple 546
Fracture, Smith's 557, 558
Fracture, spiral 548
Fracture, stages of healing 548
Fracture, stellate 548
Fracture, subtrochanteric 563
Fracture, supracondylar 556, 565
Fracture, T/Y 556
Fracture, tillaux 570
Fracture, transverse 548
Fracture, trilamellar 570
Fracture, types 548
Fracture, Wood Jones 601
Fracture/injury Chopart's 570
Fracture/injury Lisfranc's 570
Fractures around ankle joint 570
Fragility test 464
Free flush arteriography 174
Freiberg's disease 519, 581
Frenulum linguae 246
Frequency of urine 493
Frey's syndrome 296
Frie's test 215
Frog hand 515
Froment's sign 228, 230
Froment's test 228, 230

Frontal lobe tumors 527
Frontal sinusitis 279
Frostbite 61, 85, 179
Frozen chest 530
Frozen hand 549
Frozen shoulder 237, 585
Fruchaud's myopectineal orifice 379
Fuchsig's test 169
Functional limb ischemia 175
Fungiform papillae 245
Funicular hernia 385
Funiculitis 400
Funiculitis, filarial 400
Funiculitis, tuberculous 400
Funnel chest 529
Furuncle 140
Furunculosis 140
Fusobacterium fusiformis
    (Vincent's organisms) 80

G

Gaenslen's test 606
Gag reflex 525
Gait 517, 589
Gait of the patient 15
Gait, antalgic 589
Gait, circumduction 16, 589
Gait, festinating 16
Gait, hand-knee 594
Gait, high stepping 16
Gait, short-limb 589
Gait, stiff hip 589
Gait, trendelenburg 16, 589
Gait, waddling 16, 589, 593
Gaiter's area 183, 185
Gaiter's zone 82, 199
Galactocele 364
Galactorrhea 364
Galactorrhea, primary 364
Galactorrhea, secondary 364
Galeazzi fracture 558
Galezia triad 235
Gallbladder, surface marking 419
Gallstones 637
Gallstones, complications of 628
Gallbladder specimen 637
Gallbladder, palpable mass 461
Gallbladder, palpation 419, 453
Gallstone ileus 444
Gallstones 429
Gallstones, effects 429
Ganglion 121
Ganglion wrist 92
Ganglioneuroma 126
Gangrene 154, 156, 175
Gangrene, classification 175
Gangrene, dry 175
Gangrene, Fournier's 391, 392, 400, 402
Gangrene, gas 179
Gangrene, infective 179
Gangrene, wet 175
Gangrenous area 162
Garden spade deformity 556, 558
Gardner's syndrome 126, 431

Garre's nonsuppurative sclerosing
    osteomyelitis 574, 575
Garrod's pads 235
Gas gangrene 179
Gas under diaphragm 626
Gastric antral vascular ectasia 412
Gastric function tests 425
Gastric outlet obstruction 429, 632
Gastric outlet obstruction, features of 429
Gastric ulcer classification 429
Gastric ulcer, benign 635
Gastric ulcer, chronic 428
Gastrinoma 430
Gastroesophageal reflux disease 489, 491
Gastroschisis 470
Gastroscopy 427
General examination 11
General history 3
Generalized hyperplastic progressive
    gingivitis 245
Generalized lymphadenopathy 211, 216
Genu valgum 564, 565, 596, 597
Genu varum 565, 594, 596, 597
Geographic tongue 262
Geographical tongue 247
GERD 491
Gerhardt's test 56
Get above the swelling 392
Giacomini Cruveilhier vein 197
Giant cell reparative granuloma 273
Giant cell tumor 576
Giant fibroadenoma 351
Giant hernia 371
Gibbus 603, 607-609
Gigantism 13
Gillie's test 606
Gilmore's hernia 385
Gimbernat's ligament 384
Gingivae 244
Girdle pain 578
Glands of Blandin and Nuhn 262
Glandular fever 219
Glans 405
Glasgow coma scale 535
Gliomas 527
Globus pharyngeus 488
Glomangioma 126
Glomus tumor 126
Glossitis migrans 247
Glossitis, chronic superficial 246, 263
Glossitis, median rhomboid 247, 262
Glossopharyngeal nerve 289, 525
Glottis, edema 277
Glucagonoma 430
Godwin's tumor 294
Goiter in infancy 339
Goldstein saline load test 429
Golfer's elbow 234, 237, 586, 587
Golf-hole ureter 506
Goodsall's rule 477, 486
Goose foot 123, 286, 296
GORD 491
Gordon's biological test 215
Gornall's test 377
Gouty arthritis 581

Grading of ascites 422
Grading of trismus 244
Grading, Boyd's 154
Granulation tissue 78
Granulation tissue, exuberant 78
Granulation tissue, healthy 78
Granulation tissue, unhealthy 78
Granule 24
Granuloma pyogenicum 141
Granuloma, giant cell reparative 273
Grave's disease 320, 336
Grawitz tumor 505
Great saphenous vein 184, 185
Greater trochanter, palpation 590
Greater trochanter, position 561
Grey Turner's method 420
Grey Turner's sign 416
Groin 366
Groin abscess 377, 381
Groin hernia 378
Groin hernia, Bendavid classification 379
Groin hernia, classification 379
Groin hernia, Gilbert's classification 379
Groin hernia, Nyhus classification 379
Groin pain 368
Groin swellings, differential diagnosis 381
Groin swellings, reduce on lying down 389
Groin, lymph nodes 208
Grynfeltt-Lesshaft triangle 385
Gumma of testis 400
Gumma, syphilitc 250, 257
Gums and teeth, palpation 253
Gums, hyperplastic 245
Gums, scurvy 245
Gunstock deformity 586, 587
Gustatory sweating 296
Guttered veins 161
Guttering of vein 161
Gynecomastia 341, 364

H

Hair 27
Hairs, Lanugo 27
Hairy mole 131
Halitosis 239, 261
Hallux rigidus 519
Hallux valgus 519, 597
Hallux varus 597
Halo nevus 132
Halstead maneuver 167
Halsted nodes 356
Hamartoma 136
Hamilton ruler test 552
Hammer toe 518
Hammer toe deformity 597
Hand diseases, classification 514
Hand infections 515
Hand infections, complications 515
Hand infections, different types 515
Hand injuries 516
Hand, attitude 511
Hand-knee gait 594
Handle, Bard Parker's 621
Hang nail 515

Hard chancre 85, 403
Hard liver with multiple nodules 461
Hard palate 249
Hard swellings in the breast 359
Harvey's venous refilling test 162
Hashimoto's thyroiditis 337, 338
Hatch perforator 198
Hay's test 56
Head injury, complications 535
Head of radius, palpation 554
Head of the femur, position 561
Healy's classification of lymph nodes 306
Heartburn 11, 413 488
Heberden's nodes 236, 588
Helicobacter pylori 428
Heller's test 56
Hemangioma 136
Hemangioma, capillary 136
Hemangioma, cavernous 136
Hemangioma, oral cavity 262
Hemangioma, strawberry 136
Hematemesis 10, 412, 434
Hematemesis, causes 412
Hematocele 398
Hematocele, chronic 399
Hematocele, recent 399
Hematoma 26
Hematoma ear 92
Hematoma scalp 522
Hematoma, extradural 535
Hematoma, nasal septum 279
Hematoma, subdural 535
Hematomyelia 602
Hematorrachis 602
Hematuria 493
Hematuria, causes 494
Hematuria, diffuse 493
Hematuria, early 493, 496
Hematuria, gross 494
Hematuria, isolated 494
Hematuria, microscopic 494
Hematuria, nephronal 494
Hematuria, silent 494
Hematuria, terminal 493, 496
Hematuria, total 493, 496
Hemianopia 524
Hemoglobinuria 494
Hemorrhage, pontine triad 534
Hemorrhage, subconjunctival 534
Hemorrhage, superficial conjunctival 534
Hemorrhages, splinter 21
Hemorrhoids 485
Hemorrhoids, primary 485
Hemorrhoids, secondary 485
Hemostat 611
Hemothorax 539
Hemothorax, clinical features 539
Henoch-Schonlein purpura 26
Hepar lobatum 461
Hepatojugular reflux 32
Hepatoma 461
Her2 neu Receptor 361
Herald Style's technique 356
Hereditary spherocytosis 464
Hernia 378

Hernia examination, rules 378
Hernia orifices 436
Hernia testis 391
Hernia through foramen, Bochdalek 531
Hernia through foramen, Morgagni 531
Hernia, clinical classification 379
Hernia, deep ring occlusion test 373, 374
Hernia, diaphragmatic 531, 630
Hernia, direct 379
Hernia, double 385
Hernia, epigastric 384
Hernia, femoral 384
Hernia, finger invagination test 374
Hernia, funicular 385
Hernia, get above the swelling 372, 377
Hernia, giant 371
Hernia, Gilbert's classification 379
Hernia, history taking 368
Hernia, incarcerated 379
Hernia, incisional 382
Hernia, infantile 385
Hernia, inflamed 379
Hernia, inspection 370
Hernia, irreducibility 369
Hernia, irreducible 379
Hernia, local examination 370
Hernia, lumbar 385
Hernia, Maydl's 385
Hernia, obstructed 379
Hernia, obstruction 369
Hernia, obturator 372, 385
Hernia, occult 379
Hernia, pain 369
Hernia, palpation 371
Hernia, pantaloon 382, 385
Hernia, paraumbilical 384
Hernia, phantom 385
Hernia, precipitating factors 369
Hernia, recurrent 382
Hernia, reducibility 369, 373
Hernia, reducible 379
Hernia, Richter's 385
Hernia, rolling 491
Hernia, Romberg 385
Hernia, saddle 385
Hernia, sliding 373, 379, 385
Hernia, Spigelian 385
Hernia, strangulated 379, 385
Hernia, strangulation 369
Hernia, umbilical 384
Hernia, ventral 367, 384
Hernia, Zieman's test 373, 374
Hess, tourniquet test 464
Hesselbach's triangle 379, 380
Hiatus hernia 491
Hiatus hernia, classification 491
Hibernoma 124
Hiccough 488
Hiccup 10
Hidradenitis suppurativa 141, 147
Hidradenoma 130
High stepping gait 231
Hilton's method 613
Hip dislocation 563
Hip joint movements 560, 562

Hip, abduction in extension 591
Hip, abduction in flexion 591
Hip, adduction 591
Hip, extension 591
Hip, flexion 591
Hip, rotation 591
Hip, tuberculosis 594
Hippocrates facies 16, 442
Hirschsprung's disease 430
Hirschsprung's disease, types 430
Hirsutism 28
History of present illness 5
History taking 1, 3
HO's triangle 276
Hodgkin's lymphoma, Ann Arbor clinical staging 217
Hodgkin's lymphoma, Rye's classification 217
Holdsworth test 600
Hollander's insulin test 426
Hollow foot 518
Homan's test 191, 192
Hood sign 338
Hook nail 518
Hook sign 419, 456, 464
Hormone assay 53
Horner's syndrome 37, 206, 221, 261, 306, 313, 319, 331
Horseshoe kidney 506
Hounsfield number 50
Hour glass contracture 635
Housemaid's knee 4, 123, 594
Howship-Romberg sign 372
Human papilloma virus 239
Humby's knife 624
Hunger pain 8, 412
Huntarian chancre 403
Hunter's perforator 198
Hunter's ulcer 508
Hunterian chancre 85, 263
Hurler's disease 575
Hutchinson's condyloma 263
Hutchinson's freckle 132
Hutchinson's pupil 534
Hutchinson's sign 134
Hutchinson's teeth 244
Hydatid cyst of liver 639
Hydatid of Morgagni 401
Hydatid thrill 105, 458
Hydrocele 381, 387-394, 396-400
Hydrocele fluid 398
Hydrocele of canal of Nuck 377, 381
Hydrocele of the canal of Nuck 398
Hydrocele of the cord, encysted 387, 390, 392, 396, 398
Hydrocele of the hernia sac 398
Hydrocele, bilocular 398
Hydrocele, complications of 398
Hydrocele, congenital 398
Hydrocele, En bisac 398
Hydrocele, filarial 398
Hydrocele, infantile 381, 398
Hydrocele, post herniorrhaphy 398
Hydrocele, primary vaginal 398
Hydrocele, secondary 398

Hydrocephalous 521
Hydrocephalous, classification 521
Hydrohepatosis 419, 430, 461
Hydronephrosis 500, 501, 503
Hydronephrosis, classification 503
Hydronephrosis, clinical features 503
Hydronephrosis, specimen of kidney 638
Hydropneumothorax 629
Hydrops gallbladder 467
Hyperabduction maneuver 167
Hypercarotenemia 20
Hypernephroma 505
Hyperpyrexia 38
Hypertension 35
Hyperthyroidism 320, 336
Hypertrophic pulmonary osteoarthropathy 23
Hypertrophic scar 90, 128
Hypoglossal nerve 306, 525
Hypoglossal nerve compression 206
Hypoglossal nerve injury 523
Hypoglossal nerve palsy 223, 248, 523
Hypoglossal nerve, function 289
Hyponychium 20
Hypopharynx 275
Hypospadias 403, 405, 409
Hypospadias, classification 409
Hypotension 35
Hypothyroidism, features 320
Hypotonic duodenography 426

I

I^{131} Rose Bengal radioisotope scan 440
Ian-Arid test 196
Icterus 19, 413
Idiopathic thrombocytopenic purpura (ITP) 464
Ileocecal tuberculosis 466
Iliac lymph node mass 467
Iliopsoas abscess 467
ILS 277
Impetigo 142
Implantation dermoid 90, 119
Impulse on coughing 392
In transit nodule 134
Incarcerated hernia 369
Incisional hernia 382
Incisional hernia, local examination 382
Incontinence of urine 497
Incontinence, false 496
Incontinence, stress 496
Incontinence, true 496
Incontinence, urge 496
Indentation 103
India rubber consistency 207
Indigo stone 504
Indirect inguinal hernia 379
Indirect laryngoscopy 277
Induratio penis plastica 409
Infantile body frame 13
Infantile hernia 385
Infectious mononucleosis 216, 219
Inferior radioulnar joint, assessment 557
Inferior venacaval obstruction 449

Inflammatory carcinoma of breast 341, 344, 362
Infrapatellar bursitis 123
Infusion IVU 501
Ingrowing toe nail 21, 518
Inguinal canal, anatomy 378
Inguinal canal, boundaries and anatomy 378
Inguinal hernia 368
Inguinal hernia in females 377
Inguinal hernia, bubonocele 379
Inguinal hernia, complete 379
Inguinal hernia, direct 379
Inguinal hernia, funicular 379
Inguinal hernia, indirect 379
Inguinal hernia, indirect, types 379
Inguinal hernia, parts 368
Inguinal hernia, precipitating causes 381
Inguinal hernia, testing, in children 377
Inguinal lymphadenopathy 382
Inguinal region, land marks 371
Inguinoscrotal and scrotal swellings 387
Injection abscess 90, 91
Injuries around ankle 570
Injuries to cruciate ligaments of knee 567
Injuries to kidney 542
Injuries to medial collateral ligaments of knee 564
Injury above C_5 600
Injury above T_2 600
Injury at C_5 600
Injury at C_6 600
Inner Waldeyer's ring 306
Innervation of various joints with muscle actions 233
Inspection 40
Instruments 611
Insulinoma 430
Intercostal tenderness 418, 442
Intermittent claudication 154
Intermittent hydronephrosis 496
Internal angular dermoid 119
Internist tumor 505
Interossei, dorsal 227
Interossei, palmar 226
Interspinous line 590
Interstitial cystitis 508
Intervertebral disc prolapse (IVDP) 607
Intestinal obstruction 443, 444
Intestinal obstruction, classification 443
Intestinal obstruction, pathology 444
Intra-abdominal mass 462
Intra-abdominal pressure, Burch grading 543
Intracranial abscess 526
Intracranial tumors 527
Intradermal nevus 131
Intramuscular hematoma 236
In-transit lesion 85
Intravenous cholangiogram 427
Intravenous urogram 501
Intravenous urogram 633
Intravenous urogram, contraindications 501
Intravenous urogram, indications 501

Intussusception 464, 466, 636
Intussusception, acute 444
Inversion 517, 568-570
Inverted beer bottle sign 186
Inverted foot 597
Inverted testis 396
Invertogram 487
Investigation types 43
Investigations 43
Involucrum 151, 574
Iopanoic acid 427
Ischemia, critical limb 175, 176
Ischemia, features 175
Ischemia, features of severe 172
Ischemia, functional limb 175
Ischemia, limb 175
Ischemia, upper limb 179
Ischemic ulceration 172
Ischiorectal abscess 486
Isotope 51
Isotope lymphoscintigraphy 215
Isotope renography 502
Itching 11
IVC obstruction 31, 416, 449
Ivory osteoma 576
IVU 633
IVU finding, Adder-head appearance 506
IVU finding, Cobra head appearance 506
IVU finding, flower vase 506
IVU finding, spider leg pattern 506

J

Jack knife injury 601
Jaffe tumor 273
Jaundice 19, 413
Jaundice, obstructive 462
Jaundice, surgical 462
Jaw diseases, investigations 270
Jaw tumors 270
Jaw tumors, lower 271
Jaw tumors, upper 271
Jaw tumors, classification 271
Jaw, clicking 270
Jeep bottom 485
Jod-Basedow thyrotoxicosis 336
Johansson-Larsen disease 581
Jugular venous pressure 31
Jugulodigastric nodes 306
Jugulo-omohyoid nodes 306
Junctional nevus 131
Juvenile melanoma 132
JVP 31

K

Kangri cancer 4
Kaposi's sarcoma 136
Kaposi's sarcoma, types 136
Karnofsky performance status (KPS) 42
Kay's augmented histamine test 425
Kehr's sign 540, 541
Kehr's T tube 624
Kelly's point 487
Keloid 90, 96, 127

Keloid, ear 38
Kenawy's sign 423
Keratin pearls 258
Keratoacanthoma 129, 130, 133, 242
Keratoconjunctivitis sicca 296
Kernohan's notch effect 535
Ketone bodies 56
Kidney, ballotability 456, 457
Kidney, bimanual palpation 456, 457
Kidney, palpable mass 465
Kidney, palpation 456
Kienbock's disease 558, 581
Killian's dehiscence 315
Kingsbury test 56
Kirklin complex 632
Kissing tonsils 275
Klap sign 145
Klat skin tumor 462
Klinefelter's syndrome 13, 15
Klumpke's paralysis 221
Knee elbow position 457, 458
Knee jerk 526
Knee joint, cross-fluctuation 595
Knee joint, cruciate ligament injuries 567
Knee joint, injuries to medial semilunar lgament 567
Knee joint, locking 594
Knee joint, meniscus injury 567
Knee joint, movement 595, 596
Knee joint, synovial thickening 595
Knee joint, transillumination test 595
Knee joint, triple displacement 594
Knee-elbow position 475
Knie's sign 324
Knock knee 597
Knows in clinical practice 42
Knuckle 603, 607
Kocher's forceps 612
Kocher's test 330
Kohler's disease 519, 581
Kolionychia 21
Korotkoff's sound 34
Krukenberg tumor 424
KUB, plain X-rays 631
Kussmaul's sign 32
Kveim-Siltzbach test 219
Kyphosis 603, 607
Kyphosis, angular 603, 607
Kyphosis, compensatory 607
Kyphosis, knuckle 603, 607
Kyphosis, postural 607
Kyphosis, round 603, 607, 608
Kyphosis, senile 607
Kyphosis, types 603, 604, 607

L

Laboratory investigations 53
Lactating carcinoma of breast 341
Lactational abscess of breast 364
Ladd's band 531
Lahey's forceps 612
Lahey's method 329, 334
LAHS classification of cleft disorders 520
Lane's tissue holding forceps 613

Langhans giant cells 214, 215
Lanugo hairs 27
Laryngeal carcinoma 278
Laryngeal crepitus 306
Laryngocele 112, 298, 301-303, 305, 310, 315
Laryngopharynx 275
Laryngoscopy, direct 277
Laryngoscopy, indirect 277
Larynx, diseases of 277
Larynx, examination of 276
Larynx, external examination 276
Larynx, internal examination 277
Latent period of Bandet 541
Lateral aberrant thyroid 332
Lauren's classification 429
Law, Courvoisier's 419
Leather bottle stomach 429, 632
Ledderhose disease 235
Left hypochondrium, mass 464
Left iliac fossa, mass 467
Leg ulcers 86
Leiomyosarcoma 135
Lemierre's syndrome 316
Leriche's syndrome 154-157
Letssier-Meige's syndrome 218
Leukemia, chronic lymphatic 219
Leukonychia punctate 22
Leukonychia striata 22
Leukoplakia 243, 247, 251, 254, 261, 263
Levels of evidences 42
Lewis test 170
LGV 86
Lichen planus 247
Lid lag 323
Lid retraction 322, 323
Liebermeister rule 33
Ligament, Berry's 325
Ligneous thyroiditis 338
Limb deformity 161
Limb ischemia 175
Lime juice test 290
Limp 16
Lindsay line 21
Line of demarcation 159, 160
Line, Nelaton's 562
Line, Perkin's 593
Line, schoemaker's 562
Line, Shenton's 563
Linear measurement of limb 561
Lingual thyroid 39, 248, 322, 339
Linitis plastic 635
Linitis plastica 429
Linton's test 192, 196, 200
Lip, carcinoma 241, 261
Lip, cleft 240
Lip, countryman's 238, 261
Lip, cracked 241
Lip, inspection 240
Lip, palpation 251
Lip, upper, carbuncle 242
Lipodermatosclerosis 186, 198, 199
Lipoma 124
Lipoma arborigens 124
Lipoma clinical features 124

Lipoma of the cord 381, 382
Lipoma, complications 124
Lipoma, diffuse 124
Lipoma, localized 124
Lipoma, telangiectasis 124
Liposarcoma 135
Lisch nodules 125
Lister's sinus forceps 613
Lithotomy position 475
Litter's hernia 379
Liver dullness 422, 458
Liver dullness obliteration 438
Liver injury 541
Liver injury, complications and sequelae 541
Liver injury, CT 541
Liver, hydatid cyst 461
Liver, palpable left lobe 462
Liver, palpation 419, 453
Liver, span 453
Liver, surface marking 419
Local examination 40
Locally advanced carcinoma of breast (LACB) 362
Locking of knee 564
Long thoracic nerve injury 231
Loose bodies in knee joint 567
Lordosis 603-605, 607
Loss of weight 414
Lovibond angle 22, 23
Lower end of forearm, palpation 556
Lower end of humerus, palpation 554
Lucid interval 533, 535
Ludwig's angina 139, 298, 316
Lumbar hernia 385
Lumbar puncture 526
Lumbrical muscles 226
Lump 88
Lunate dislocation 558
Lung abscess 530
Lung abscess, complication 530
Lupus vulgaris 82
Lymph cyst 121, 122
Lymph node, biopsy 214
Lymph node, Cloquet 208
Lymph node, epitrochlear 21, 212
Lymph node, microanatomy 201
Lymph node, sigmund 211
Lymph nodes of groin 208
Lymph nodes of the neck, examination of 306
Lymph nodes, axilla 209
Lymph nodes, cervical 210
Lymph nodes, Cloquet's, deep 407
Lymph nodes, popliteal 211, 212
Lymph scrotum 401
Lymph varix 387, 389, 392, 393, 396, 397, 401
Lymphadenitis, acute 216, 218
Lymphadenitis, chronic 216, 218
Lymphadenitis, filarial 218
Lymphadenitis, reactive 218
Lymphadenitis, tuberculous 214, 216
Lymphadenopathy, generalized 211, 216
Lymphangiography 215

Lymphangioma 137
Lymphangioma ab agne 137
Lymphangioma circumscriptum 137
Lymphangioma diffusum 137
Lymphangioma, capillary 137
Lymphangioma, cavernous 137
Lymphangitis, acute 218
Lymphatic, watershed area 201
Lymphatics of head and neck, anatomy 3063
Lymphedema, Browse's classification 215
Lymphoedema 218
Lymphoedema congenita 218
Lymphoedema praecox 218
Lymphoedema tarda 218
Lymphoedema, Kinmonth classification 218
Lymphoedema, primary 218
Lymphoedema, secondary 218
Lymphogranuloma inguinale 86
Lymphoma 216
Lymphoma, Hodgkin's 217
Lymphoma, non-Hodgkin's 217
Lymphoma, WHO modified REAL (Revised European American Lymphoma) classification 217
Lymphomas, types 217
Lymphorrhagia 401
Lyre sign 315

M

Machinery murmur 113, 170
Macrocheilia 240
Macrodactyly 588
Macroglossia 39, 246
Macrostoma 521
Macule 23
Madelung deformity 556, 558
Madura foot 150
Madura hand 150
Magnetic resonance cholangio pancreatography (MRCP) 427
Magnetic resonance imaging (MRI) 51
Magnuson's test 605
Malakoplakia 509
Malgaigne bulging 376, 378
Malgaigne fracture 560
Malignant bone tumors 576
Malignant cachexia 14, 414
Malignant fibrous histiocytoma (MFH) 135
Malignant hypertension 35
Malignant hyperthermia 39
Mallet finger 236, 556
Mallet-Guy sign 420
Mallory-Weiss syndrome 412
Malunion 548, 549
Mammary dysplasia 363
Mammary fistula of Atkins 365
Mammography 360, 630
Mandible anatomy 267
Mandible, bidigital palpation of 251
Mandibular cleft 521
Mantoux test 44, 215
Marble bones 547
Marble white pallor 161

March fracture 519, 570
Marfan's syndrome 575
Marie Strumpell arthritis 607
Marion's disease 495, 509
Marjolin's ulcer 62, 133, 199
Martorell's hypertensive ulcer 61
Martorelle's ulcer 85, 86
Maryfield introducer 618
Mask face 16
Mass 88
Mass abdomen 446
Mass abdomen, intrinsic mobility 452, 453
Mass abdomen, investigations 468
Mass abdomen, mobility 452
Mass in ascending colon 465
Mass in lumbar region 465
Mass in the epigastrium 462
Mass in the hypogastrium 468
Mastalgia 341
Mastalgia chart 342
Mastalgia, cyclical 363
Mastitis 364
Mastitis carcinomatosis 341, 362
Mastitis, intramammary 364
Mastitis, retromammary 364
Mastitis, subareolar 364
Matchstick test 104
Maxillary sinusitis 279
Maxillary tumors 272
May or Kuster perforator 198
Maydl's hernia 385
McBurney's point 418
McBurney's tenderness 437
McMurray's test 566
Measurement of level of styloid process 557
Measurement, apparent length of limb 592
Measurement, arm length 551
Measurement, hip joint 592
Measurement, real length of limb 592
Meatal ulcer 410
Meckel's diverticulum 443, 469
Meckel's diverticulum, presentation 443
Meckler's triad 491
Meconium 55
Medial popliteal nerve 231
Median mental sinus 143, 150
Median nerve injury 230
Median nerve palsy, high 230
Median nerve palsy, low 230
Median nerve, compression neuropathy 230
Median rhomboid glossitis 247, 262
Mediastinal emphysema 537
Mediastinal flutter 538
Mediastinal tumors 530
Mediastinal tumors, classification 530
Medullary carcinoma of breast 362
Medulloblastoma 527
Megacolon 628
Megalodactyly 588
Megaloglossia 246
Meglumine ioglycamate 427
Meglumine iothalamate 501
Meigster's forceps 612
Melaena 55, 413
Melanoglossia 39

Melanoma 133
Melanoma, ABCDE 134
Melanoma, acral lentiginous 134
Melanoma, amelanotic 134
Melanoma, choroid 134
Melanoma, desmoplastic 134
Melanoma, juvenile 132
Melanoma, lentigo maligna 134
Melanoma, nodular 134
Melanoma, spread 134
Melanoma, subungual 134
Melanoma, superficial spreading 134
Melemesis 10
Melena 55
Meleney's ulcer 61
Melon seed bodies 516
MEN syndrome 320
Meningiomas 527
Meningocele 521, 608
Meningo-encephalocele 521
Mental status 12
Mental status, grading 12
Mesenteric cyst 465
Mesenteric lymph node mass 467
Mesenteric lymphadenitis, acute nonspecific 445
Metachronous growth 636
Metastatic carcinoma of breast 363
Methods of contractions of different muscles 110
Michaelis Gutmann bodies 509
Microalbuminuria 493
Microdactyly 588
Micrognathism 274
Micturating cystourethrography 502
Mid stream urine 500
Middleton's maneuver 419
Midline tumors 527
Midpalmar space 515
Migraine 8
Mikulicz disease 296
Mikulicz syndrome 280, 281
Mikulicz triad 296
Milian's ear sign 139
Milker's nodules 516
Mill's manoeuvre 587
Miner's bursa 586
Miner's elbow 123
Minor salivary gland 297
Minor salivary gland swellings, examination 292
Minor salivary gland tumor 293, 295
Minute IVU 501
Mirizzi syndrome 429
Mittelschmerz 8
Mixed salivary tumor 294
Mobile kidney 467
Mode of onset of symptom 5
Modified Adson's test 168
Modified Perthes test 192
Modified Roos test 314
Modified Verdan zone in hand 514
MODS 142
Mole 131
Mole, hairy 131

Mole, non-hairy 131
Molluscum sebaceum 129, 242
Mondor's disease 200, 347, 364
Mongolism 16
Monilial stomatitis 264
Monks localization 540
Monteggia fracture dislocation 556
Montgomery's gland 346
Moodley's sign 31
Moon face of Cushing's syndrome 594
Moon red face 16
Moon's molar 244
Moran-Baker's appendix holding forceps 613
Morgagni follicles infection 409
Morquio-Brailsford's disease 575
Morrant Baker's cyst 123, 594
Morris bitrochanteric test 562
Morris retractor 615
Morrisey's cough impulse 185
Morrison's kidney pouch 443
Morton's metatarsalgia 519
Morvan's disease 179
Mose's sign 191, 192, 196, 200
Moulding 103
Mouth dryness, grading 39
Movement hip joint 560
Movement with deglutition 300
Movements of ankle joint 569
Movements of cervical spine 604
Movements of elbow joint 555
Movements of knee joint 565
Movements of shoulder joint 583
Movements of thoracolumbar spine 604
Movements of vocal cord 277
Moynihan's aphorism 628
Moynihan's method 418
Moynihan's sign 418
MRI uses 51
MRI, advantages 51
MRI, disadvantages 51
Mucoepidermoid tumor 295
Mucus cyst, cheek 243
Mucus retention cyst 262
Mulberry stone 504
Mule spinner's disease 387
Multilocular cystic disease of jaw 273
Multiple air fluid levels 444, 627
Multiple chondromatosis 576
Multiple cylindroma 130
Multiple exostoses 575, 576
Multiple fissures in ano 477
Multiple fistula in ano 477
Multiple myeloma 577
Multiple neurofibromatosis 92, 93
Multiple neurolipomatosis 124
Multiple polyposis colon 637
Multiple tourniquet test 187, 189
Murphy's kidney punch 456, 497, 498
Murphy's point 437
Murphy's sign 418, 429
Murugassu's technique 487
Muscle guarding 417, 436
Muscle guarding and rigidity 436
Muscle hernia 236
Muscle power 170

Muscle power, checking 224
Muscle power, grading 170, 223
Muscle wasting 159
Myasthenia gravis, face 16
Myasthenia smile 16
Mycetoma pedis 150
Mycosis fungoides 217
Mycotic aneurysm 527
Myelocele 608
Myelomeningocele 608
Myopectineal orifice 379
Myositis ossificans 235, 236, 548
Myotic aneurysm 178
Myxedema 320
Myxedema coma 320
Myxedema crisis 320
Myxedema, features 320

N

Naevus of Ota 132
Nail 20
Nail bed infarcts 21
Nail matrix 20
Nail plate 20
Nail, anatomy of 20
Nail, blue 22
Nail, deformities 20
Nail, dry, brittle 21
Nail, in growing toe 21
Nail, red 22
Nail, white 22
Nails, examination of 20
Narath's sign 165
Nasal bone, fracture 279
Nasal cavities, paranasal sinuses, larynx, pharynx examination 310
Nasal cavity and paranasal sinuses, diseases 279
Nasal cavity, examination 310
Nasopalatine papilla 250
Nasopharyngeal carcinoma 276
Nasopharynx 275
Nasopharynx palpation 310
Nasopharynx, examination of 276
Naunyn's sign 418
Nausea 11, 412, 488
Neck lymph node enlargement, differential diagnosis 313
Neck nodes at different levels 307
Neck rigidity 525
Neck shaft angle 594
Neck swelling, brilliantly transilluminant 304
Neck swelling, causes 313
Neck swelling, classification 312
Neck swelling, transilluminant 305
Neck, dilated visible veins 301
Necrosis 175
Needle holder 621
Needle, Chiba 427
Needle, Menghini 45
Needle, Okuda 427
Needle, Travenol 45
Needle, Vim Silverman 45, 46

Needles, atraumatic 620
Needles, cutting 620
Needles, reverse cutting 620
Needles, round body 620
Needles, surgical 620
Needles, surgical, parts 620
Needles, taper cut 620
Needles, traumatic 620
Negative confirmative evidence 44
Negus esophagoscope 490
Nelaton's line 562
Neonatal thyrotoxicosis 336
Nerve of Bell 223, 233
Nerve, facial 285, 295
Nerve, hypoglossal, compression 206
Neuhof's sign 196
Neurilemmoma 126
Neurilemmoma, Anthoni type A 126
Neurilemmoma, Anthoni type B 126
Neuroblastoma 462, 505
Neurofiborma, nodular 125
Neurofibroma 125
Neurofibroma, complications of 125
Neurofibroma, disease, von Recklinghausen's of 125
Neurofibroma, generalized 125
Neurofibroma, plexiform 125
Neurofibroma, types 125
Neurolipoma 124
Neuroma 126
Neuroma, end 126
Neuroma, false 126
Neuroma, lateral 126
Neuroma, myelinic 126
Neuroma, side 126
Neuroma, true 126
Neuropraxia 229
Neurotmesis 229
Neville J Nicholson maneuver 417
Nevolipoma 124
Nevus 131
Nevus flammeus 137
Nevus of Ito 132
Nevus spilus 132
Nevus, blue 131
Nevus, compound 132
Nevus, halo 132
Nevus, intradermal 131
Nevus, junctional 131
Nevus, spider 137
Nevus, spindle cell 132
Nevus, Spitz 132
Niche and notch 632
Nicoladoni's sign 170, 173, 179
Night cramps 183
Night cry 578
Nipple destruction 345, 362
Nipple deviation 354
Nipple elevation 345
Nipple retraction 345, 362
Nipple, changes 354
Nipple, discharge 342, 363
Nipple, inspection 345
Nipple, palpation 353
No man's land in hand 514

Nocturia 493
Node, Delphian 332
Nodular goiter 336
Nodule 24
Nodule, in transit 134
Nodule, Lisch 125
Nodule, satellite 134, 135
Noma 179, 245, 264
Non-hairy mole 131
Non-Hodgkin's lymphoma, Rappaport and working classification 217
Non-chromaffin paraganglioma 315
Non-Hodgkin's lymphoma 217
Non-lactational abscess of breast 364
Nonne-Milroy's disease 218
Non-palpable eruptions 23
Non-pulsatile elevation of JVP 32
Non-specific mesenteric lymphadenitis, acute 445
Non-ulcer dyspepsia 413
Non-union 548
Nose 38
Nose, bottle 129
Nose, foreign body 279
Nose, potato 129
Nose, saddle 38
Novafil 622
Nutrition 13
Nutrition assessment 13
Nutritional assay 53
Nutritional status 13
Nylon 622
Nystagmus 525

O

Obstetrician paralysis 221
Obturator hernia 372, 385
Occipital lobe tumors 527
Ochsner Sherren regime 466
Ochsner's clasping test 225, 230
Oculomotor nerve 525
Odontomes 271
Odynophagia 488, 489
Okuda needle 427
Olecranon, palpation 554
Olfactory nerve 524
Oligodendroglioma 527
Oliguria 493
Oliver's sign 306
Ollier's disease 576
Omental cyst 466
Omental mass 463
Omentocele 379, 381
Omphalocele 470
Onion peel appearance 576
Onychauxis 22
Onychia 22
Onychocryptosis 518
Onychodermal band 20
Onychogryphosis 21, 518
Onycholysis 22
Onychomycosis 518
Onychorrhexis 22

OPG 293
Ophthalmoplegia 324
Opponens pollicis 225
Optic nerve 524
Oral cancer 238
Oral cancer, tobacco chewing 239
Oral cancers, six 'S' 239
Oral carcinoma, general features 260
Oral carcinoma, problems 260
Oral cholecystography 427
Oral submucus fibrosis 263
Oral thrush 264, 489
Orbital cellulitis 138
Orchitis 400
Orchitis, syphilis 396
Orchitis, syphilitic 400
ORF 515
Organ of Geraides 401
Oriental sore 86
Oropharynx 275
Oropharynx, examination 275
Orphan Annie eye nuclei 337
Orr Chair test 396, 401
Orthopantomogram (OPG) 259, 270, 271, 293
Ortolani's test 593
Ochsner-Mahoner test 187
Oscillometry 174
Osgood-Schlatter disease 581
Osteitis deformans 574
Osteitis fibrosa cystica 574
Osteoarthritis of hip 594
Osteoarthrosis 581
Osteoarthrosis, primary 581
Osteoarthrosis, secondary 581
Osteoblastic secondaries bone 630
Osteochondritis 581
Osteochondritis, crushing 581
Osteochondritis, splitting 581
Osteochondritis, traction 581
Osteochondroma 576
Osteoclastoma 576
Osteoclastoma, mandible 273
Osteofying fibroma 273
Osteogenesis imperfecta 574
Osteogenesis imperfecta tarda 574
Osteoid 574
Osteoma 522, 576
Osteoma, types 576
Osteomalacia 574
Osteomyelitis jaw 274
Osteomyelitis, acute 571, 574
Osteomyelitis, acute, pathology 574
Osteomyelitis, acute, sequelae 574
Osteomyelitis, chronic 145, 574
Osteomyelitis, chronic, pathology 574
Osteoporosis 574
Osteosarcoma 576
Ostial reflux 197
Other drinking habits 6
Other habits 6
Other relevant history 7
Outer Waldeyer's ring 306
Ovarian mass 468

Overwhelming postsplenectomy infection (OPSI) 142
Oxalate stone 504

P

Pachydermatocele 125
Pachyglossia 246
Pack year index 158
Paget's disease of bone 522, 574, 575
Paget's disease of breast 346
Paget's disease of nipple 362
Paget's disease of penis 407
Paget's positive 119
Paget's test 104
Pain 7
Pain hunger 8
Pain in the anus 473
Pain, acute onset 8
Pain, aggravating factor 9, 412
Pain, central 7
Pain, chronic onset 8
Pain, colicky 8, 433
Pain, constricting 8
Pain, deep 7
Pain, distension 8
Pain, duration 9
Pain, features of 7
Pain, grading 10
Pain, migration 9, 433
Pain, Mittelschmerz 8
Pain, mode of onset 8
Pain, mode of onset and progression 412
Pain, nature 8, 411
Pain, original site 8
Pain, periodicity 9, 411
Pain, progression 9
Pain, prostatic 496
Pain, psychogenic 7
Pain, radiation 9, 412, 433
Pain, referred 9, 412, 433
Pain, relation with food intake 412
Pain, relieving factors 9
Pain, renal 495
Pain, segmental 7
Pain, severity 8
Pain, shifting 9
Pain, superficial 7
Pain, ureteric 495
Pain, urethral 496
Pain, vesical 496
Painful arc syndrome 237, 552, 583-585
Painful heel, causes 519
Palate, cleft 240, 251
Palate, hard 249
Palate, inspection 249
Palate, palpation 256
Palate, soft 249, 250
Palatine raphe 250
Palatine rugae 250
Palatine tonsil 275
Pallor 17
Pallor, cadaveric 161
Pallor, marble white 161

Index

Palmar erythema 18
Palmar interossei 226
Palpable liver mass 460
Palpation 40
Palpation of axillary lymph nodes 355
Palpation of blood vessels 163
Palpation of cheek 251
Palpation of colon 420
Palpation of kidney 420, 497, 498
Palpation of palate 256
Palpation of posterior third of tongue 255
Palpation of prostate 499
Palpation of the floor of the mouth 256
Palpation of tonsils and fauces 257
Palpation tongue 253
Palpation, clavicle 551
Palpation, scapula 551
Palpation, upper end of humerus 551
Palsy, saturday night 231
Palsy, tourniquet 231
Pancoast syndrome 531
Pancoast tumor 531
Pancreas, cystadenocarcinoma 463
Pancreas, palpation 420
Pancreas, pseudocyst 463
Pancreatic mass 455
Pancreatic stones, plain X-ray 628
Pancreatic trauma 542
Pancreatic tumors 430
Pancreatic tumors, classification 430
Pancreatic tumors, endocrine 430
Pancreatic tumors, exocrine 430
Pancreatitis, acute 441
Panendoscopy 260
Pannus 580, 597
Pantaloon hernia 385
Papillae, circumvallate 246
Papillae, filiform 245
Papillae, foliate 246
Papillae, fungiform 245
Papillary cystadenolymphomatosum 295
Papilloma 129
Papilloma infective 129
Papilloma pedunculated 129
Papilloma true 129
Papilloma, anal canal 130
Papilloma, basal cell 129
Papilloma, infective 129
Papilloma, larynx 278
Papilloma, oral cavity 262
Papilloma, pedunculated 129
Papilloma, true 129
Papule 23
Para Achilian Achillean 198
Paraaortic lymph node mass 463
Paradidymis 401
Paradoxin consistency 102
Paradoxical aciduria 429
Paradoxical respiration 538
Parafollicular C cells 337
Paranasal sinuses, examination 279
Parapharyngeal abscess 316
Paraphimosis 403-405, 408, 409
Paraphimosis, complication 408
Paraplegia 601

Paraplegia in extension 608
Paraplegia in flexion 608
Paraumbilical hernia 384
Parietal lobe tumors 527
Paronychia, acute 515
Paronychia, chronic 515
Paronychium 20
Parosmia 524
Parotid abscess 296
Parotid duct 283
Parotid enlargement, differential diagnosis 289
Parotid fistula 296
Parotid gland, anatomy 296
Parotid lymphoma 295
Parotid swelling, features of 284
Parotid, palpation 289
Parotitis 295
Parotitis, acute 295
Parotitis, chronic 295
Pascal's law 103
Passavant's ridge 275
Past history 5
Patch, skin 23
Patella, recurrent dislocation 567
Patellar clonus 526
Patellar fracture 567
Patellar tap 565, 595
Patent urachus 469
Pathological fracture 630
Pathologist's wart 129
Patient 1
Paul Bunnel test 219
Pauwel's angle 563
Payr's crushing clamp 614
PDS suture 622
Peaud' orange 94, 347, 348, 351
Pectoralis minor syndrome 167
Pectus carinatum 529
Pectus excavatum 529
Pel-Ebstein fever 204
Pellegrini-Stieda disease 235, 567
Pelvic fracture, avulsion 560
Pelvic fracture, classification 560
Pelvic injuries, complications 560
Pelvic masses 467
Pelvic ring fracture, stable 560
Pelvic ring fracture, unstable 560
Pelvirectal abscess 486
Pemberton's sign 330
Pen test 225, 230
Penis, examination 391
Penis, Paget's disease of 407
Penis, prepuce 405
Penis, Ram's horn 391, 405
Pentagastrin test 425
Per vaginal examination 460
Percussion 40
Percussion, Castell's method of splenic dullness 422
Percussion, free fluid 458
Percussion, Nixon's method of splenic dullness 422
Percussion, renal angle 458

Percutaneous transhepatic cholangiography (PTC) 427
Perforated duodenal ulcer 442
Perforated typhoid ulcer 443
Perforation, stages 442
Perforator, Bassi 198
Perforator, Boyd 198
Perforator, Cockett 198
Perforator, Dodd 198
Perforator, Hatch 198
Perforator, Hunter's 198
Perforator, May or Kuster 198
Perforator, Sherman 198
Perforators, ankle 198
Periampullary carcinoma 430
Perianal abscess 486
Periapical cyst 273
Pericarditis 531
Pericarditis, constrictive 531
Perineal urethrostomy 404
Perinephric abscess 465, 506
Peripheral nerve injuries 229
Peripheral nerve injuries, causes 229
Peristalsis, step ladder pattern 416
Peristalsis, visible gastric 419
Peritonitis, acute 441
Peritonitis, primary 441
Peritonitis, secondary 441
Peritonitis, tertiary 441
Peritonsillar abscess 276
Periurethral abscess 476
Perkin's line 593
Perleche 242, 264
Perniosis 85, 179
Peroneal artery 163
Per-rectal examination 460
Persistence of sinus/fistula 145
Personal history 5
Perthes test 191
Perthes' disease 594
Pes anserinus 286, 296
Pes cavus 517, 597
Pes planus 518, 597
PET scan, uses 53
Petechiae 26
Petit's triangle 385
Peyronie's disease 235, 409
Phagedena 66, 80, 245, 264
Phagophobia 488
Phalen's test 588
Phalen's test, reverse 588
Phantom hernia 385
Pharyngeal pouch 315
Pharyngitis 276
Pharynx, diseases of 276
Phenomenon, Raynaud's 155
Philtrum 240
Phimosis 403-409
Phimosis, problems 408
Phlebography 196
Phlegmasia alba dolens 185, 200
Phlegmasia cerulea dolens 185, 200
Phosphate stone 504
Photoplethysmography 196
Physical examination 11

Physiological bow leg 597
Pick's disease 531
Picker position 397, 476, 499
Pigeon chest 529
Pigmentation of skin 17
Pigmented lesions in skin 27
Pilar cyst 121
Pile, arterial 485
Pile, sentinel 477, 486
Piles 485
Piles, classification 485
Piles, clinical features 485
Piles, complications 485
Pilonidal sinus 474, 477, 478, 485
Pilonidal sinus, pathology 485
Pin point pupil 534
Pinched skin 26
Pineal tumors 527
Pinhole meatus 403, 405, 406, 408, 410
Pinhole meatus, acquired 410
Pipe stem stool 55, 474
PIPIDA 52
Pitcher's elbow 586
Pitted nails 21
Pituitary tumors 527
Pituitary tumors, classification 527
Plain X-ray abdomen 626
Plain X-ray KUB 500, 631
Plain X-ray KUB, psoas shadow 500
Plain X-ray KUB, radiopaque shadow, differential diagnosis 500
Plain X-ray KUB, ureteric line 500
Plane of swelling 108
Plantar fasciitis 237
Plantar flexion 517
Plantar wart 129
Plaque 24
Plasma cell mastitis 364
Platynychia 21
Pleomorphic adenoma 294
Plethysmography 173, 196
Plethysmography air 196
Plethysmography, photo 196
Plica polonica 27
Plummer disease 336
Plummer's sign 321
Plummer-Vinson syndrome 488, 490
Plunging ranula 249, 256, 262
Pneumaturia 493
Pneumopyelography 501
Pneumothorax 539
Pneumothorax, tension 539
Point tenderness 437
Pointing index 222
Pointing sign 540
Pointing test 433
Poker's back 607
Policeman receiving tip 221
Polycystic kidney 465
Polycystic kidney disease 506
Polycythemia 19
Polydactyly 588
Polyglactin acid 622
Polymazia 365
Polymide 622

Polyp, vocal 278
Polypropylene 622
Polyps colon 637
Polythelia 365
Polyuria 493
Pons asinorum 481
Pontine hemorrhage 534
Popliteal artery 163
Popliteal lymph nodes 211, 212
Porphyria 56
Porphyria crisis 445
Port wine stain 137
Portal hypertension 462
Porter's bursa 124
Porter's tip hand 221
Position of ease, wrist joint 588
Position of ease/rest 579
Position, Picker 397
Positive confirmative evidence 44
Positron emission tomography scan (PET scan) 52
Positrons 53
Post phlebitic ulcer 83
Post traumatic amnesia 533
Post traumatic amnesia, grading 533
Post-Achilles bursitis 598
Posterior arch vein 184, 197
Posterior rhinoscopy 278
Posterior tibial artery 163, 164
Posterior urethral valve 509
Postoperative synergistic gangrene 81
Postoperative thrombosis 199
Post-phlebitic limb 82
Post-thrombotic ulcer 83
Postural test 279
Posture of the patient 15
Potato nose 129
Potato tumor 315
Pott's puffy tumor 141
Pott's spine 439
Pratt's test 188
Pre-Achilles bursitis 598
Preanesthetic assessment 53
Preanesthetic investigations, recommended 55
Preauricular sinus 521
Pregangrene 160, 175
Pregangrene, features 160
Prehn's sign 400
Premalignant conditions of oral cavity 263
Prepatellar bursitis 123
Pressure sore 80
Pretibial myxedema 319, 321
Prevaginal examination 438
Priapism 409
Primary brain tumor 527
Primary branchiogenic carcinoma 315
Primary syphilitic chancre 242
Probe test 148
Probing 477
Procidentia 474
Proctalgia fugax 486
Proctitis 487
Proctoscopy (Kelly's) 483
Proctoscopy, positions 483, 484

Proctoscopy, technique 483
Progesterone receptor 361
Prognathism 274
Prognathous deformity 270
Progress of the disease 5
Prolapse rectum 478
Prolapsed piles 473, 478
Prolene 622
Prostate 499
Prostate, palpation 481
Prostatic abscess 509
Prostatic massage 509
Prostatic pain 496
Prostatic specific antigen (PSA) 508
Prostatism 507
Prostatitis 509
Protein bound iodide (PBI) 334
Proteinuria 493
Proteinuria tests 56
Proteinuria, orthostatic 493
Proud flesh 78, 79
Pruritus 11, 447
Pruritus ani, causes 474
Psammoma bodies 337
Pseudoclubbing 23
Pseudocyst of the pancreas 463
Pseudodiarrhea 414
Pseudofluctuation 103
Pseudohematemesis 413
Pseudolipoma 124
Pseudolocking of knee 564
Pseudomalignancy 129
Pseudopneumoperitoneum 440
Pseudopolyposis 430, 431
Psittacosis 219
Psoriasis 24
PSP test 500
Pterygium, nail 22
Ptosis 37
Ptyalism 281
Pubo coccygeal line 487
Puddle sign 422
Pugh's modification 462
Pulled elbow 556
Pulmonary complications, post-operative period 531
Pulmonary embolism 531
Pulsatile elevation of JVP 32
Pulsatile mass 452
Pulsatility 107
Pulsation, expansile 107
Pulsation, expansile 99
Pulsation, transmitted 99, 108
Pulse 33
Pulse anacrotic wave 33
Pulse assessment 33
Pulse pressure, wide 35
Pulse volume 33
Pulse, bisferiens 33
Pulse, collapsing 34
Pulse, Corrigan's 34
Pulse, dicrotic 33
Pulse, normal 33
Pulse, unmasking 163
Pulse, waterhammer 34

Pulseless arteritis 178
Pulsus alterans 33
Pulsus bigeminus 34
Pulsus magnus 33
Pulsus paradoxus 34
Pulsus parvus 33
Pump bump 598
Pump handle test 559, 606
Punch biopsy 46
Punctum 119
PUO 39
Purplish striae 18
Purpura 18, 26
Pustules 26
Putrefaction 156, 159
Pyemia 142
Pyemic abscess 140
Pyocele 399
Pyoderma gangrenosum 81
Pyogenic abscess 139, 140
Pyogenic arthritis, acute 580
Pyogenic arthritis, acute, complications 580
Pyogenic arthritis, chronic 580
Pyogenic granuloma 79, 141
Pyonephrosis 465, 503
Pyonephrosis, triad 503
Pyrexia of unknown origin 39
Pyriform fossa 275
Pyriform fossa, carcinoma 275, 278
Pyrosis 413, 488, 491
Pyuria 493

Q

Quadrants in abdomen 446
Quadriplegia 601
Qualities of a good surgeon 1

R

Radial artery 165
Radial bursa 516
Radial nerve lesions 230
Radicular cyst 273
Radioactive bone scan, bone diseases 573
Radioactive fibrinogen test 196
Radioisotope bone scan 547
Radioisotope scanning 428
Radionuclide imaging 51
Raju test 191
Ram's horn nail 518
Ram's horn penis 391, 405, 409
Rampley's forceps 611
Ranula 249, 256, 262, 292
Rapunzel syndrome 429
Raspberry tongue 247
Raspberry tumor 469
Ray fungus 150
Raynaud's disease 176
Raynaud's phenomenon 155, 176
Raynaud's phenomenon, causes 176
Raynaud's syndrome 176
Reactive hyperemia time test 170
Reactive lymphadenitis 218
Reagent, Esbach's 56
Real shortening of limb 592
Rebound tenderness 7, 437
Rectal carcinoma 481
Rectal prolapse 485
Rectal prolapse, complete 479, 485
Rectal prolapse, partial 485
Rectum, polyp 481
Rectus sheath hematoma 470
Recurrent dislocation of patella 567
Red currant jelly 444
Red nail 22
Reducibility 106, 393
Reed Sternberg cells 217
Reflexes 526
Reflexes, tendons 228
Reflux esophagitis 491
Regaud tumor 276
Regional ileitis 467
Regions in the abdomen 446
Regurgitation 11, 412, 488
Reiter's disease 580
Related symptoms suggestive of complications 5
Renal angle 497
Renal angle tenderness 456
Renal angle, percussion 422
Renal calculus 504
Renal calculus, clinical features 504
Renal calculus, types 504
Renal carbuncle 141, 506
Renal cell carcinoma 465, 505
Renal cell carcinoma, clinical features 505
Renal cell carcinoma, investigation 506
Renal cell carcinoma, pathology 505
Renal cell carcinoma, triad 505
Renal cyst 506
Renal function tests 500
Renal mass, differential diagnosis 498
Renal mass, features 498
Renal pain 495
Renal rickets 574
Renal tuberculosis 506
Residual urine 509
Respiration 36
Respiration, Cheyne-Stokes 36
Rest pain 154, 155
Retching 488
Retention mucus cyst 243
Retention of urine 494
Retention of urine, acute 494
Retention of urine, acute on chronic 494
Retention of urine, causes 494
Retention of urine, chronic 494
Reticular varices 182
Reticular veins 182, 185, 193
Retractile testis, test for 396
Retraction of nipple 345, 362
Retractor, Balfour's self-retaining 615
Retractor, Czerney's 614
Retractor, Deaver's 615
Retractor, Doyen's 615
Retractor, hernia 615
Retractor, Joll's thyroid 615
Retractor, Langenbeck's 614
Retractor, Morris 615
Retractors 614
Retractors, self-retaining 615
Retrocalcaneal bursitis 123
Retrocaval ureter 506
Retrograde pyelography 501, 633
Retrograde Seldinger technique 502
Retromolar trigone 251
Retroperitoneal cysts 465
Retroperitoneal mass 457
Retroperitoneal tumors 465
Retropharyngeal abscess 310, 316
Retropharyngeal abscess acute, chronic 316
Retrosternal goiter 319, 339
Reverse smoking 239
RGP 633
Rhabdomyosarcoma 135
Rhagades 242
Rheumatoid arthritis 578-580
Rheumatoid arthritis of the hand 237
Rhinophyma 38, 129
Rhinoscopy, anterior 278
Rhinoscopy, posterior 278
Rhinosporidiosis 279
Rhinosporidium seeberi 279
Richter's hernia 379, 385
Ricketic chest 529
Ricketic rosary 529, 574
Rickets 574
Riedel's lobe of liver 460, 461
Riedel's thyroiditis 338
Right hypochondrium, mass 462
Right iliac fossa, mass 466
Rinne's test 525
Rippled artery 174
Risus sardonicus 16
Robertson's giant limb 179
Rodent ulcer 84, 132
Rolando's fracture 558
Rolling hernia 491
Roos test 167
Roseolar 23
Rotator cuff 585
Rothera's test 56
Rotter's nodes 356
Roundworm bolus mass 467
Rouviere zones 208
Rovsing's sign 437, 440
Rule, Goodsall's 477, 486
Rule, Liebermeister 33
Rupture bladder 542
Rupture bladder, extraperitoneal 542
Rupture bladder, intraperitoneal 542
Rupture bladder, intraperitoneal, complications 542
Rupture bladder, types 542
Rupture of tendo Achilles 568
Rupture spleen 541
Rupture urethra, anterior 543
Rupture urethra, prostatic 543
Ruptured extensor pollicis longus 236
Ruptured muscle fibers 236
Rutherford Morrison's kidney pouch 442

S

Sacrococcygeal teratoma 90
Saddle embolus 177
Saddle hernia 385
Saddle nose 38
Saegesser's tender point 541
Saint's triad 467, 628
Salivary calculus 295
Salivary colic 281
Salivary diseases, investigations 293
Salivary fistula 282, 294
Salivary gland tumor, minor 241
Salivary neoplasms 294
Salmon patch 137
Salpingitis, acute 445
Saphena 197
Saphena varix 186, 191, 193, 368
Sarcoidosis 219
Sarcoma 135
Sarcoma, Kaposi's 136
Sarcoma, synovial 136
Satellite nodule 134, 135
Satiety 11, 414, 446, 447
Satiety, early 6, 414
Saturday night palsy 231
Scab 68, 69
Scabbard trachea 330
Scalene syndrome 314
Scalene triangle 314
Scales 26
Scaphoid bone palpation 557
Scarpa's triangle 559, 561
SCC 133
Schatzki rings 492
Scheuermann's disease 581, 607
Schistosoma hematobium 508
Schmincke tumor 276
Schmorl's nodes 607
Schoemaker's line 562
Schwannoma 126, 527
Schwartz test 188
Sciatic nerve injury 228
Scintiscan 51
Scirrhous carcinoma breast 362
Scissor, Lister's bandage cutting 616
Scissor, McIndoe 616
Scissor, Metzenbaum 616
Scissor, Pott's Smith 616
Scissors 616
Scissors, Heath's suture cutting 616
Scissors, Mayo's 616
Scissors, Steele's 616
Scleroderma 16
Sclerosing angioma 130
Scoliosis 529, 603, 607
Scoliosis, structural 607
Scoliosis, transient 607
Scoliosis, types 607
Screwdriver tooth 244
Scrotal carcinoma 391
Scrotal edema 391
Scrotum syphilitic gummatous ulcer 391
Scrotum, lymph 401
Scrumpox 142
Scurvy 574
Scurvy gums 245
Seat belt injury 540, 601
Sebaceous cyst 119, 121, 122
Sebaceous horn 121
Seborrheic keratosis 27
Seborrheic wart 129
Seborrhoeic keratosis 98, 129, 133
Secondaries bone, osteoblastic 630
Secondaries in bone 577
Secondaries in lymph nodes 217
Secondaries in neck lymph nodes 313
Secondaries in neck lymph nodes, known primary 313
Secondaries in neck lymph nodes, nodal staging 314
Secondaries in neck lymph nodes, occult primary 314
Secondaries in neck lymph nodes, unidentified primary 313
Secondaries in spine 608
Secondaries lung 629
Secretomotor fibers of submandibular salivary gland 297
Secretomotor fibers parotid gland 297
Seddon's classification 229
Segmental measurement of limb 562
Segmental measurement of thigh and leg 592
Segmental pressure measurement 173
Seldinger angiography 174
Selective urine sample 500
Semimembranosus bursa 114, 123
Semimembranous bursa 594
Seminal vesicles 499
Senile keratosis 129
Sentinel pile 477, 486
Septal deviation 279
Septicemia 142
Sequestration dermoid 118
Sequestrum 147, 151, 574
Serocystic disease of Brodie 363
Serpiginous ulcer 65
Serratus anterior muscle 223
Serum calcitonin estimation 336
Serum thyroglobulin 335
Sestamibi TC ^{99m} scan 337
Sever's disease 519, 581
Severe ischemia, features 172
Severe malnutrition 13
Sezzary syndrome 217
Shambling classification 315
Shenton's line 563, 593
Shepherd crook deformity 549
Sherman perforator 198
Sherren's triangle 436
Shifting dullness 421, 422, 458
Shock lung 531
Short saphenous vein varicosity 189
Shortening above the greater trochanter 593
Short-limb gait 589
Shoulder girdle 550
Shoulder hand syndrome 558
Shoulder joint movement 552
Sialadenitis 295
Sialectasis 294, 296
Sialography 294
Sialorrhea 239
Sialosis 296
Sideropenic dysphagia 275, 488
Sigmoid esophagus 490, 491, 631
Sigmoid volvulus 432, 444, 445, 628
Sigmoidoscope, types 483
Sigmoidoscopy 483
Sigmund lymph node 211
Sign 3
Sign de Dance 444
Sign of disappearing pulse 163
Sign of indentation 103
Sign slip 124
Sign Tanyol's 415, 422
Sign, 'V' 515
Sign, 'V' of Naclerio 491
Sign, accessory 3
Sign, Angel's 400
Sign, antecedent 3
Sign, Arm-drop 584
Sign, assident 3
Sign, Babinski's 534
Sign, Balance's 541
Sign, Baldwing's 438
Sign, Ballance's 541
Sign, Ballet's 324
Sign, Battle's 534
Sign, Becker's 324
Sign, Berry's 331, 337, 338
Sign, Blumberg's 3, 437, 440
Sign, Boas's 436, 441
Sign, Bocca's 306
Sign, Boston's 324
Sign, Bow 401
Sign, Branham's 179
Sign, Bryant's 552
Sign, bull's-eye 426
Sign, Capener's 594
Sign, Carmanns meniscus 632
Sign, champagne bottle 186, 193
Sign, champagne glass of sigmoid diverticula 426
Sign, Chevrier Percussion/Tap 191
Sign, Chvostek-Weiss's 338
Sign, claw 426, 444
Sign, coffee bean 444
Sign, Cowen's 324
Sign, Cruveilhier's of saphena varix 190
Sign, Cullen's 435, 441, 449
Sign, Cupola 440
Sign, curtain 284, 285, 294
Sign, DA Patel's 561
Sign, Dalrymple's 323
Sign, Deming's 400
Sign, Destot's 559
Sign, diagnostic 3
Sign, Donder's 324
Sign, Drawer 566, 567
Sign, Earle 559
Sign, Enroth 324
Sign, Faget's 33
Sign, Fleischner's 426

Sign, Football 440
Sign, Fox 441
Sign, Froment's 228, 230
Sign, Frostberg's reverse 3, periampullary carcinoma 426
Sign, Gaur 384
Sign, Gifford's 324
Sign, Goldthwaite's 560
Sign, Goldzieher's 324
Sign, Grey Turner's 416, 436, 441
Sign, Griffith's 324
Sign, Grove's 324
Sign, Hamman's 491
Sign, hood 338
Sign, hook 419, 456, 464, 516
Sign, Howship-Romberg 372
Sign, Hutchinson's 134
Sign, inverted 'V' 440
Sign, inverted beer bottle 186
Sign, inverted umbrella 426
Sign, Jellinek's 324
Sign, Joffroy's 323
Sign, Johnston 449
Sign, Kamenchik's 441
Sign, Kanavel 513
Sign, Kehr's 540
Sign, Kenawy's 423
Sign, Kernig's 525
Sign, klap 145
Sign, Knie's 324
Sign, Kocher's 324
Sign, Korte's 441
Sign, Kussmaul's 32
Sign, Laquer's 560
Sign, Lasegue's 605
Sign, Lhermitte's 605
Sign, Loewi's 324
Sign, London's 540
Sign, Ludloff's 563
Sign, Lyre 315
Sign, Mallet Guy's 420
Sign, Mathe's 506
Sign, Mayo Robson's 441
Sign, Mean's 324
Sign, Milian's ear 139
Sign, Moebius 323
Sign, Moodley's 31
Sign, Mose's 191, 192, 196, 200
Sign, Moynihan's 418, 454
Sign, Murphy's 418, 429, 454
Sign, Naffziger's 323
Sign, Narath's 165, 563
Sign, Naunyn's 418
Sign, Neuhof's 196
Sign, Nicolodani's 170, 173, 179
Sign, of (string) Kanter 426
Sign, Oliver's 306
Sign, omega 444
Sign, Pandiaraja'a 441
Sign, pathognomonic 3
Sign, Payne's 324
Sign, Pemberton's 330, 331
Sign, Plummer's 321
Sign, pointing 540
Sign, Prehn's 400

Sign, pseudokidney 426
Sign, puddle 422, 458, 459
Sign, Reisser's 607
Sign, release 437
Sign, reverse 'J' 501
Sign, Riglers 440
Sign, Rochin's 324
Sign, Romberg's 525
Sign, Rosenbach's 324
Sign, Roux 559
Sign, Rovsing's 437, 440
Sign, Sainton's 324
Sign, Schamroth's 23
Sign, Scottish terrier 607
Sign, shouldering 492
Sign, slik glove 375
Sign, slip 102, 124
Sign, Snellen 324
Sign, Srinivasan costal 415
Sign, Stellwag's 323
Sign, Stethoscope 441
Sign, Stierlin 426
Sign, Suker's 324
Sign, Tanyol 449
Sign, target 426
Sign, Terry's 21
Sign, thumb print 426
Sign, Tinel's 228, 229
Sign, trail 330, 334, 336
Sign, Trethowan's 594
Sign, Triangle 440
Sign, Troisier's 423, 459
Sign, Trousseau's 200, 324, 338, 430
Sign, vas deferens 397
Sign, Victor Horsley's 533
Sign, Vigouroux's 324
Sign, Volkmann's 234, 235
Sign, Wilder 324
Silent abdomen 438
Silk 622
Silk glove sign 375
Sim's position 475
Simian thumb deformity 230
Singultus 10, 488
Sinus 143
Sinus clinical features 144
Sinus, causes 143
Sinus, causes of persistence 145
Sinus, clinical features 144
Sinus, different discharges 147
Sinus, median mental 143, 150
Sinus, pilonidal 143, 146
Sinus, preauricular 146, 150
Sinus/fistula, sites 146
Sinusitis 279
Sinusitis, ethmoidal 279
Sinusitis, frontal 279
Sinusitis, maxillary 279
Sinusogram CT 148
SIRS 142
Sister Joseph Mary tumor 469
Sister Joseph's nodule 416, 429, 449, 469
Sitophobia 414, 488
Sjögren's syndrome 36, 281, 284, 294, 296
Sjögren's syndrome, primary 296

Sjögren's syndrome, secondary 296
Skin adnexal tumors 129, 130
Skin changes and eruptions 23
Skin markers 18
Skin, malignant lesions 132
Skin, pigmentatrion 17
Skin, pigmented lesions 27, 134
Skin, pinched 26
Skin, texture of 26
Skip lesions 160
Sleep habits 6
Sleeping pulse rate 321
Sliding hernia 373, 379, 385
Slip sign 102
Slipped femoral epiphysis 593, 594
Sloan Kettering Memorial Hospital 306
Sloping edge 66
Slough 59, 68, 69, 175
Small bowel enema 620, 632
Small bowel mass 456
Small saphenous vein 185, 198
Smiling umbilicus 30
Smoke screen translucency 273
Smoker classification 6
Smoker, heavy 6
Smoker, light 6
Smoker, moderate 6
Smoking 6
Smoking index 158
Smoking, reverse 239
Snail track ulcers 263
Snapping elbow 586
Snapping thumb 236
Social status 4
Sodium diatrizoate 174
Soft chancre 86
Soft palate 249, 250
Soft palate, paralysis 251
Soft sore 403
Solar keratosis 129
Solitary bone cyst 273
Solitary renal cyst 506
Solitary secondary in liver 461
Solitary thyroid nodule 336
Solitary ulcer syndrome 486
Somatostatinoma 430
Sound waves 48
Space of Burns 300
Specimen of carcinoma breast 639
Specimen of hydatid cyst of liver 639
Specimen of kidney, hydronephrosis 638
Specimen of staghorn calculus 637
Specimen of stomach 635
Specimen of testicular tumor 638
Specimen of transitional cell carcinoma 638
Speculum, Thudichum's 278
Spermatic cord, contents 379
Spermatic cord, palpation 397
Spermatocele 387, 390, 393, 398, 401
Sphincter tone 480
Sphygmomanometer 34
Sphygmomanometer, aneroid 34
Sphygmomanometer, mercury 34
Spider naevi 18
Spider nevus 137

Spigelian hernia 385
Spina bifida 90, 608
Spina bifida, aperta 608
Spina bifida, occulta 608
Spina bifida, types 608
Spina ventosa 516
Spinal accessory nerve 306, 313, 525
Spinal cord injuries 601
Spinal cord tumors 608
Spinal diseases 602
Spindle cell nevus 132
Spine, extension injury 601
Spine, flexion injury 601
Spine, Naffziger's test 605
Spine, palpation 600
Spine, Pott's disease 608
Spine, shearing force injury 601
Spitz nevus 132
Spleen, palpation 419, 455
Spleen, surface marking 419
Splenic dullness, percussion for 422
Splenic injury 541
Splenic injury, types 541
Splenic rub 423
Splenomegaly, causes 420
Splinter hemorrhages 21
Spondylolisthesis 607
Spongioblastoma polare 527
Spontaneous thrombosis 199
Sportsman's hernia 385
Springing of fibula 565
Springing of radius 554
Springing of radius/fibula 546
Springing of tibia 565
Springing the radius 554, 557
Sprouting granulation tissue 144
Spurious diarrhea 474
Squamous cell carcinoma 133
Squamous cell carcinoma, Broder's grading 83
Srinivasan costal sign 415
Stability of spine 601
Stafne bone cyst 297
Staghorn calculus 504, 637
Starch iodine test 296
Stationary ulcer 60
Stature of the patient 15
Stauffer's syndrome 505
Steatorrhea 11, 55
Steering wheel injury 538
Stenosing tenosynovitis 236
Stenosing tenovaginitis 236
Stenson's duct 281, 283, 295
Stephen's line 487
Stereognosis 526
Sterile pyuria 493, 506
Sternoclavicular dislocation 552
Sternomastoid tumor 315
Stewart-Treves syndrome 363
Stiff hip gait 589
Stiff lung 531
Stomach mass 454
Stomach mass, features 462
Stomach, carcinoma of 429
Stomach, leather bottle 429

Stomach, palpation 418
Stomach, specimen 635
Stomach, tiger stripe 412
Stomach, watermelon/tiger stripe 412
Stomatitis 264
Stomatitis, angular 264
Stomatitis, aphthous 264
Stomatitis, catarrhal 264
Stomatitis, causes 264
Stomatitis, infective 264
Stomatitis, monilial 264
Stomatitis, ulcerative 264
Stork bite 137
Stove in chest 538
Straight leg raising (SLR) 605
Straight leg raising test 563
Strangury 493
Strawberry hemangioma 136
Strawberry tongue 247
Stream of urine 496
Stress fracture 519
Stress fracture tibia 567
Stress test to check abnormal mobility 569
Stricture rectum 480
Stricture urethra 509
Stricture urethra, complications 509
Stricture urethra, etiological classification 509
Stricture urethra, features 509
Stridor 330
Stridor at rest 319
String sign of Kantor 426, 467
Struma lymphomatosa 338
Struvite stone 504
Student's elbow 4, 123, 586
Styloid process, method of palpation 557
Subacromial bursitis 582
Subarachnoid hemorrhage 526
Subclavian artery 166
Subclavian steal syndrome 178
Subconjunctival hemorrhage 534
Subcutaneous emphysema 40, 629
Subdeltoid bursitis 582
Subdural hematoma 535
Subdural hematoma, acute 535
Subdural hematoma, chronic 535
Subdural hygroma 535
Subfascial pyemic abscesses 140
Subhyoid bursitis 316
Sublingual dermoid 249, 250, 256, 262
Sublingual dermoid, lateral 262
Sublingual dermoid, median 262
Subluxation of head of radius 556
Submandibular lymph nodes 306, 307
Submandibular salivary gland 294, 297
Submandibular salivary gland enlargement, differential diagnosis 291
Submandibular salivary gland tumors 295
Submandibular salivary gland tumors, benign 295
Submandibular salivary gland tumors, malignant 295
Submandibular salivary gland, examination 290

Submandibular sialadenitis, acute 290
Submental dermoid 119
Submental lymph nodes 306
Submucosal fibrosis, oral 263
Submucous abscess 486
Subperiosteal hematoma 522
Subphrenic abscess 460
Subphrenic spaces and abscesses 442
Subtalar joint 568
Succussion splash 423, 454
Suction instruments 617
Suction tip, Adson's fine 617
Suction tip, Poole's multiperforated 617
Suction tip, Yankauer 617
Suction tips 617
Sudeck's osteodystrophy 549
Sulphur granules 150
Sunderland's classification 229
Superficial cervical nodes 306
Superficial conjunctival hemorrhage 534
Superficial inguinal ring 378
Superficial temporal artery 166
Superficial thrombophlebitis 200
Superior venacaval obstruction 449
Supraclavicular fossa, examination 168
Suprapatellar bursa 595
Suprapubic cystostomy 618
Supraspinatus tendinitis 237, 584
Supratrochlear lymph node 586
Surgical blades 621
Surgical emphysema 537
Surgical pathology 635
Suture materials 621
Suture materials, absorbable 622
Suture materials, braided 622
Suture materials, monofilament 622
Suture materials, multifilament 622
Suture materials, natural 622
Suture materials, non-absorbable 622
Suture materials, synthetic 622
Suture materials, twisted 622
SVC obstruction 32, 416
Swaging 620
Swan neck deformity 237, 580, 588
Swelling 88
Swelling adherent to muscle underneath 109
Swelling adherent to tendon underneath 109
Swelling arising from muscle 109
Swelling arising from vessels or nerves 109
Swelling inspection 94
Swelling palpation 100
Swelling recurrence 93
Swelling, congenital 88
Swelling, consistency 102
Swelling, cystic 118
Swelling, edge 98
Swelling, extrinsic mobility 110
Swelling, fixity to deeper structures 109
Swelling, fixity to skin 116
Swelling, gliding test 108
Swelling, history 88
Swelling, in subcutaneous plane 109
Swelling, inflammatory 88

Swelling, intrinsic mobility 110
Swelling, location 94
Swelling, mobility 110
Swelling, movement 98
Swelling, pinching test 108
Swelling, plane of 108
Swelling, pressure effects 100
Swelling, pulsatility 107
Swelling, reducibility 106
Swelling, skin over the 94
Swellings, brilliantly transilluminant 105, 106, 393
Swellings, classification of 117
Symbiotic effect 81
Sympathetic chain 306
Symptoms 3
Symptoms and signs 3
Symptoms, associated 5
Symptoms, related, suggestive of complications 5
Synchronous growth 636
Syndactyly 516, 588
Syndrome, Crigler-Najjar 19
Syndrome, Dubin-Johnson's 19
Syndrome, Gilbert's 19
Syndrome, Horner's 261
Syndrome, Pendred's 338
Syndrome, Pierre Robin 521
Syndrome, Rotor's 19
Syndrome, abdominal compartment 543
Syndrome, acute compartment 176, 177
Syndrome, Albright's 273
Syndrome, anterior cord 602
Syndrome, auriculotemporal 296
Syndrome, Beckwith-Weidemann 246
Syndrome, blue toe 174
Syndrome, Boerhaave's 490, 491
Syndrome, Brown-Sequerd 602
Syndrome, carpal tunnel 230, 235
Syndrome, central cord 602
Syndrome, cervical rib 314
Syndrome, Chilaiditi's 442
Syndrome, CREST 176
Syndrome, Cruveilhier Baumgarten 423
Syndrome, Cushing's 16
Syndrome, di-George's 338
Syndrome, disappearing pulse 169
Syndrome, Felty's 465
Syndrome, Ferguson Smith 133
Syndrome, Frey's 296
Syndrome, Froin's 608
Syndrome, Frolich's 528
Syndrome, Gardner's 126, 431
Syndrome, Horner's 37, 206, 221, 306, 313, 319, 331
Syndrome, Klinefelter's 13, 15
Syndrome, Klippel Trenauny Weber 137
Syndrome, Lemierre's 316
Syndrome, Leriche 154, 156, 157
Syndrome, Letssier-Meige's 218
Syndrome, Mallory-Weiss 412, 491
Syndrome, MEN 124, 320
Syndrome, MEN II 337
Syndrome, Mikulicz 280, 281
Syndrome, Mirizzi 429

Syndrome, Munchausen's 445
Syndrome, painful arc 237
Syndrome, pancoast 531
Syndrome, Paterson Kelly 247, 492
Syndrome, Pierre-Robin 521
Syndrome, Plummer Vinson 247, 488, 490, 492
Syndrome, Poland's 365
Syndrome, Rapunzel 429
Syndrome, Raynaud's 176
Syndrome, Sezzary 217
Syndrome, Sjogren's 281, 284, 294
Syndrome, solitary ulcer 486
Syndrome, Stauffer's 505
Syndrome, Stewart-Treves 363
Syndrome, subclavian steal 178
Syndrome, thoracic outlet 301, 314
Syndrome, Tietze's 365
Syndrome, Treacher Collins 274
Syndrome, Turcot's 431
Syndrome, Turner's 13, 15
Syndrome, Verner Morrison 430
Syndrome, Wallenberg 601
Syndrome, yellow nail 22
Synovial sarcoma 136
Syphilis, primary 85
Syphilis, secondary 85
Syphilis, tertiary 85
Syphilitic gumma 250, 257
Syphilitic stigmata 85
Syphilitic ulcer 85
Syphilitic, chancre, primary 242
Syringomyelia 179
Syringomyelocele 608
Systemic examination 41
Systolic bladder 508

T

T tube cholangiogram, postoperative 634
T3 resin uptake study 334
Tabes dorsalis 85
Tabes mesenterica 466
Tabetic facies 16
Tachycardia 33
Tailor's ankle 598
Tailor's bursa 124
Takayasu's arteritis 179
Takayasu's pulseless arteritis 178
Talipes calcaneovalgus 518, 519
Talipes calcaneus 519
Talipes equino varus 199, 228
Talipes equinovarus 518, 519
Talipes equinus 519
Talipes valgus 519
Talipes varus 519
Tanyol's sign 415, 422
TAO 176
Tape-like stool 474
Tardy ulnar palsy 220
Tartar 244
Taste sensation 287
Taxis 373
TBPI 36
Tc ^{99m} labeled DMSA 52

Tc ^{99m} labeled DTPA 52
Tc ^{99m} labeled sulfur 52
Tc ^{99m} labeled HMPAQ 52
Tc ^{99m} labeled HIDA 52
Tear cancer 84, 132
Technetium 99m 52
Teeth and gums, inspection of 244
Teeth, Hutchinson's 244
Teetotaler 5
Telepaque 427
Telescopic test 563
Telogen 27
Temporal lobe tumors 527
Temporomandibular joint 267
Temporomandibular joint, ankylosis 270
Temporomandibular joint, dislocation 270
Temporomandibular joint, movements 270
Tenderness 7
Tenderness, rebound 7
Tenesmus 434, 474
Tennis elbow 234, 237, 586, 587
Tension pneumothorax 539
Tension pneumothorax, clinical features 539
Terminal hair 27
Terminal hematuria 508
Terminal pulp space infection 515
Terrible triad of elbow 556
Terry's sign 21
Test Rothera's 56
Test, Adson's 167, 168
Test, Adson's, modified 168
Test, Allen's 168, 169
Test, anvil 603
Test, arid 605
Test, Baid 463
Test, Baldwing's 438
Test, Barlow's 593
Test, Benedict's 56
Test, Blaxland ruler 468
Test, Brodie-Trendelenburg 187
Test, Buerger's postural 169
Test, Callaway's 552
Test, calorie 525
Test, card 227, 228, 230
Test, Carnett's 420, 421
Test, Chair 587
Test, chew and split 426
Test, Chiene's 562
Test, chin 303
Test, coin 604, 609
Test, compression 559
Test, Cope's obturator 437
Test, Cope's psoas 437, 441
Test, Cozen's 587
Test, crossed leg 169
Test, D-dimer 196
Test, distraction 559
Test, Dragstedt 425
Test, Dugas' 552
Test, elevated arm stress test 167
Test, Falconer 168
Test, Fegan's 190, 193, 196
Test, femoral nerve stretch 605
Test, fragility 465

Test, Froment's 228, 230
Test, Fuchsig's 169
Test, Gaenslen's 606
Test, Gerhardt's 56
Test, Gillie's 606
Test, gliding 108
Test, gliding, breast 351
Test, Goldstein saline load 429
Test, Gordon's biological 215
Test, Hamilton ruler 552
Test, Harvey's 162
Test, Hay's 56
Test, head rising 420, 421
Test, Heller's 56
Test, Hess tourniquet 464
Test, Holdsworth 600
Test, Hollander's insulin 426
Test, Homan's 191, 192
Test, Ian-Arid 196
Test, Kay's segmented histamine 425
Test, Kingsbury 56
Test, Kocher's 330
Test, Kveim Siltzbach 219
Test, leg rising 420, 421
Test, Lewis 170
Test, lime juice 290
Test, Linton's 192, 196, 200
Test, Magnuson's 605
Test, matchstick 104
Test, modified Adson's 168
Test, modified Perthe's 188, 191
Test, Morris bitrochanteric 562
Test, multiple tourniquet 187, 189
Test, Naffziger's for spine 605
Test, obturator 441
Test, Ochsner's clasping 225, 230
Test, Orr Chair 396, 401
Test, Ortolani's 593
Test, Oschner's Mahoner 187
Test, Paget's 104
Test, Paul Bunnel 219
Test, pen 225
Test, pentagastrin 425
Test, Perthe's 191
Test, Phalen's 588
Test, Phalen's, reverse 588
Test, pinching, breast 351
Test, Pratt's 188
Test, probe 148
Test, pump handle 559, 606
Test, Raju 191
Test, reactive hyperemia time 170
Test, Rinne's 525
Test, Roos 167
Test, Schwartz 188
Test, straight leg raising 563
Test, telescopic 563, 593
Test, three swab 149
Test, traction 396
Test, transillumination 105
Test, Weber's tuning fork 525
Test, Wright 167
Test, wringing 587
Test, Zieman's 373, 374
Testes, Pigeon-egg 400

Testicular sensation 396
Testicular sensation, loss of 399, 400
Testicular tumor 399
Testicular tumor, Hurricane type 400
Testicular tumor, specimen of 638
Testis, anteverted 396
Testis, billiard 400
Testis, different location 399
Testis, ectopic 401
Testis, gumma of 400
Testis, inverted 396
Testis, palpation 396
Testis, position 396
Testis, seminoma 399
Testis, size 396
Testis, teratoma 399
Testis, third 390, 401
Testis, torsion 387-390, 396, 399, 400
Testis, undescended 390-392, 396, 399, 401
Tetany 337
Texture of skin 26
Thenar space 515
Thimble bladder 508
Third testis 390, 401
Thomas test 590
Thomas Wharton 317
Thompson's test 569
Thoracic aortic aneurysm 629
Thoracic inlet syndrome 314
Thoracic outlet syndrome 301, 314
Thread veins 182, 185
Thready pulse 34
Three finger test 105
Three glass urine test 500, 509
Three swab test 149
Thrill 108
Thrill, hydatid 105
Thromboangiitis obliterans (TAO) 176
Thrombophlebitis, migratory superficial 430
Thrombophlebitis, superficial 200
Thrombosed piles 480, 481
Thudicum's speculum 278
Thyroglossal cyst 338
Thyroglossal fistula 302, 320, 326, 338
Thyroid acropachy 322
Thyroid cyst 336
Thyroid diseases, biopsy 335
Thyroid diseases, imaging 335
Thyroid function test 334
Thyroid malignancy, Dunhill classification 337
Thyroid malignancy, etiology 337
Thyroid neoplasms 337
Thyroid neoplasms, classifications 337
Thyroid palpation, Crile's method 324
Thyroid palpation, Lahey's method 324
Thyroid palpation, Pizillo's method 324
Thyroid paradox 328
Thyroid scan 335
Thyroid steal 333
Thyroid storm 336, 367
Thyroid, anaplastic carcinoma 337
Thyroid, ectopic 339
Thyroid, facies 321

Thyroid, follicular carcinoma 337
Thyroid, Hurthle cell carcinoma 337
Thyroid, lingual 248, 322, 339
Thyroid, malignant lymphoma 337
Thyroid, medullary carcinoma 337
Thyroid, medullary carcinoma, familial 337
Thyroid, papillary carcinoma 337
Thyroid, radioisotope uptake study 334
Thyroid, Technetium-99m scan 336
Thyroiditis 319
Thyrotoxic crisis 336
Thyrotoxicosis 336
Thyrotoxicosis factitia 336
Thyrotoxicosis, Jod-Basedow 336
Thyrotoxicosis, neonatal 336
Thyrotoxicosis, primary 319, 336
Thyrotoxicosis, secondary 319, 336
Tietze's syndrome 365
Tiger stripe stomach 412
Tillaux's triad 466
Tinea pedis 518
Tinel's sign 228, 229
Toe brachial pressure index 36, 173
Tongue 39
Tongue anatomy 246
Tongue tie 246, 255
Tongue tremor 248
Tongue ulcers 40
Tongue, abnormal pigmentations 40
Tongue, aphthous ulcer 263
Tongue, bald 39, 247
Tongue, beefy red 247
Tongue, black hairy 39
Tongue, carcinoma 261
Tongue, chronic nonspecific ulcer 264
Tongue, congenital fissure 247
Tongue, curdy white 247
Tongue, dental ulcer 263
Tongue, dry brown 39
Tongue, fissuring 39
Tongue, furring 39
Tongue, geographic 262
Tongue, geographical 247
Tongue, inspection 245
Tongue, leukoplakia 39
Tongue, malignant ulcer 264
Tongue, palpation 253
Tongue, papilloma 248
Tongue, posterior third palpation 255
Tongue, post-pertussis ulcer 264
Tongue, raspberry 247
Tongue, strawberry 247
Tongue, syphilitic fissure 247
Tongue, syphilitic ulcer 263
Tongue, tuberculous ulcer 264
Tonsil, carcinoma 276
Tonsil, palatine 275
Tonsil, tubal 275
Tonsillar carcinoma 276
Tonsillitis 276
Tonsils and fauces, inspection 251
Tonsils and fauces, palpation 257
Tonsils, kissing 275
Tooth, dead 244
Tooth, impacted 244

Tooth, screwdriver 244
Toothpaste stool 55
Tophi 61, 581
Torsion testis 387-390, 396, 399, 400
Torticollis 301, 305, 315, 603
Tourniquet palsy 231
Tourniquet test for short saphenous vein 187
Towel clip 625
Towel clip, Backhaus' 625
Towel clip, Doyen's 625
Towel clip, Moynihan's tetra 625
Toxic dilatation of colon 430
Toxic multinodular goiter 336
Toxic nodule 336
Toxic thyroid, cardinal signs 319
Trachea, examination 306
Trachea, position 330
Tracheal tug 489
Tracheo-esophageal fistula 491
Tracheomalacia 330
Tracheostomy tube 622
Tracheostomy tube, Fuller's bivalved 622
Tracheostomy tube, Jackson's 622
Tracheostomy tube, PVC 622
Tracheostomy tube, red-rubber 622
Tracheostomy, indication 622
Traction test 396
Trail sign 330
Transcutaneous oximetry 174
Transillumination 105, 106
Transillumination test, maxillary sinus 279
Transilluminoscope 105, 393, 394
Transitional cell carcinoma (TCC) 507
Transitional cell carcinoma, clinical features 507
Transitional cell carcinomas of urinary bladder 638
Translucency 393
Transmitted pulsation 108, 457
Transpyloric plane 446
Transtubercular line 446
Trapezius 223
Traube's area 422
Traumatic fat necrosis of breast 363
Treadmill test 175
Tremor 318, 321
Tremor tongue 39
Tremors of hands and tongue 319, 339
Trench mouth 245
Trendelenburg gait 579, 589, 593
Trendelenburg test 589
Treponema pallidum 85
Treponema pertenue 86
TRH stimulation test 334
Triad, Murphy's 434
Triad, Saint's 467, 628
Triad, Tillaux's 466
Triad, Trotter's 276
Triage 539
Triangle HO's 276
Triceps bursitis 586
Triceps jerk 526
Trichilemmal cyst 121
Trichobezoar 429

Trident hand 575
Trigeminal nerve 525
Trigger finger 236
Trigger thumb 236
Trigger zones of Patrick 525
Triple ABC technique 359
Triple deformity 597
Triple endoscopy 260
Triple phosphate stone 504
Trismus 243, 270, 281
Trismus, grading 244
Trocar and cannula 624
Trochlear nerve 524
Troisier's sign 423
Trophic ulcer 61, 80
Tropical bubo 86
Tropical ulcer 61
Trotter's triad 276
Trousseau's sign 200, 338, 430
Trousseau's sign of pancreas 430
Trucut biopsy 46
Tubal tonsil 275
Tube, endotracheal 622, 623
Tube, flatus 624
Tube, Kehr's T 624
Tube, nasogastric 619
Tube, nasogastric, complications 620
Tube, Ryle's 619
Tube, tracheostomy 622
Tuber joint angle 570
Tubercle, carotid 166
Tubercle, chassaignac anterior 166
Tuberculosis of breast 365
Tuberculosis of hip 594
Tuberculosis of knee 597
Tuberculosis of shoulder joint 585
Tuberculosis of spine 608
Tuberculosis, ankle 598
Tuberculosis, colonic 464
Tuberculous arthritis 578, 579, 581
Tuberculous arthritis, complications 581
Tuberculous dactylitis 514
Tuberculous epididymitis 389, 391, 400
Tuberculous lymphadenitis 214, 216, 298, 301
Tuberculous lymphadenitis, caseating 216
Tuberculous lymphadenitis, hyperplastic 216
Tuberculous lymphadenitis, stages 216
Tuberculous sinus 145-147,150
Tubulodermoids 119
Tumor alba 597
Tumor of the third ventricle 527
Tumor, acinic cell 295
Tumor, ambiguous 124
Tumor, Bedner's 132
Tumor, carotid body 298, 300, 304, 315
Tumor, Cock's peculiar 120
Tumor, desmoid 126
Tumor, dumb bell 294
Tumor, glomus 126
Tumor, Godwin's 294
Tumor, Klat skin 462
Tumor, Krukenberg 424
Tumor, minor salivary gland 295
Tumor, mucoepidermoid 295

Tumor, pancoast 531
Tumor, potato 315
Tumor, Pott's puffy 141
Tumor, Regaud 276
Tumor, Schmincke 276
Tumor, skin adnexal 129, 130
Tumor, spinal cord 608
Tumor, sternomastoid 315
Tumor, testicular 399
Tumor, turban 130
Tumor, ubiquitous 124
Tumor, universal 124
Tumor, Warthin's 294, 295, 280
Turban tumor 93, 130
Turcot's syndrome 431
Turner's syndrome 13, 15
Tylosis 492
Tyson's gland infection 409

U

Ubiquitous tumor 124
Ulce, Marjolin's 133
Ulcer base 72
Ulcer Buruli 85
Ulcer definition 57
Ulcer discharges 63
Ulcer due to chilblains 61, 85
Ulcer grading, Wagner's 62
Ulcer non specific 61
Ulcer parts 57
Ulcer penetrating 80
Ulcer perforating 80
Ulcer syphilitic 60
Ulcer, acute 60, 62
Ulcer, aphthous 241
Ulcer, arterial 61, 82
Ulcer, assessment 78
Ulcer, Bairnsdale 85
Ulcer, Barrett's 491
Ulcer, basal cell carcinoma 65
Ulcer, base 59
Ulcer, Bazin's 61
Ulcer, biopsy, oral cavity 258
Ulcer, bone thickening 72
Ulcer, callous 60
Ulcer, carcinomatous 83
Ulcer, causes of nonhealing 79
Ulcer, chilblains 85
Ulcer, chronic 60, 62
Ulcer, classifications 59
Ulcer, common sites 64
Ulcer, cortisol 61
Ulcer, cryopathic 61
Ulcer, decubitus 80
Ulcer, depth 72
Ulcer, diabetic 61, 80
Ulcer, diphtheritic 62
Ulcer, discharge from bed 69
Ulcer, discharge study 76
Ulcer, Donovan 403
Ulcer, Ducrey's 60
Ulcer, edge 66
Ulcer, edge, punched out 58
Ulcer, edge, raised and beaded 59

Ulcer, edge, undermined 58
Ulcer, epitheliomatous 67
Ulcer, examination of adjacent joint 74
Ulcer, factitious 61
Ulcer, floor 59, 68
Ulcer, footballer's 61, 86
Ulcer, frostbite 85
Ulcer, general examination 64
Ulcer, granulation tissue 68, 78
Ulcer, gravitational 82
Ulcer, healing 59
Ulcer, history 62
Ulcer, imaging 76
Ulcer, induration 70, 71
Ulcer, ischemic 82
Ulcer, local examination 64
Ulcer, malignant 61, 65
Ulcer, margin 66
Ulcer, Marjolin's 62, 83, 84
Ulcer, Martorell's 85, 86
Ulcer, Martorell's hypertensive 61
Ulcer, meatus 410
Ulcer, melanotic 85
Ulcer, Meleney's 61, 65, 81, 86
Ulcer, neurogenic 80
Ulcer, neuropathic 61, 80
Ulcer, nonhealing 59
Ulcer, palpation 70
Ulcer, post-phlebitic 83
Ulcer, post-thrombotic 83
Ulcer, relation to deeper structures 72
Ulcer, rodent 61, 65, 84
Ulcer, serpiginous 65
Ulcer, size 72
Ulcer, spreading 59, 67
Ulcer, stationary 60
Ulcer, surrounding area 72
Ulcer, surrounding skin and area 70
Ulcer, syphilitic 85
Ulcer, syphilitic granulomatous 65
Ulcer, traumatic 61, 82
Ulcer, trophic 61, 65, 80
Ulcer, tropical 61, 80
Ulcer, tuberculous 65, 81
Ulcer, vela 62
Ulcer, venous 65, 82, 199
Ulcer, wedge biopsy 76
Ulcerative colitis 430
Ulcerative colitis, types 430
Ulcers, foot 86
Ulcers, leg 86
Ulcers, snail track 263
Ulcers, specific 60
Ulcers, tongue 40
Ulnar artery 165
Ulnar bursa 516
Ulnar drift 237
Ulnar nerve injury 230
Ulnar nerve, palpation 586
Ulnar paradox 230
Ultrasonography real time 49
Ultrasound examination 48

Ultrasound gray scale 48
Ultrasound guided core needle biopsy (USCNB) 294
Ultrasound of breast 360
Ultrasound uses 49
Ultrasound, advantages 49
Ultrasound, disadvantages 49
Umbilical adenoma 469
Umbilical fistula 469
Umbilical granuloma 469
Umbilical hernia 384
Umbilical region, mass 465
Umbilical sinus 469
Umbilicus 435
Umbilicus examination 415
Umbilicus, smiling 30
Umbolith 469
Undescended testis 381, 387, 390-392, 396, 399, 467
Undescended testis, complication 399
Unicameral bone cyst 575
Universal tumor 124
Unmasking the pulse 163
Upper end of ulna, palpation 554
Upper limb ischemia 179
Urachal cyst 469
Urachal diverticulum 469
Urachal fistula 469
Urachal sinus 469
Urate stone 504
Ureteric calculi 504
Ureteric calculi, clinical features 504
Ureteric pain 495
Ureterocele, Stephen classification 506
Urethra 499
Urethral calculi 509
Urethral discharge 496
Urethral injury 542
Urethral injury, bulbous 543
Urethral injury, membranous 543
Urethral meatus 405
Urethral pain 496
Urethral stricture 509
Urethritis 509
Urethrogram, ascending 502, 633, 634
Urethroscopy 502
Urethrostomy, perineal 404
Urgency 493
Uric acid stone 504
Urinary bilharziasis 508
Urinary bladder diverticulum 467
Urinary fistulas 510
Urinary fistulas, causes 510
Urinary frequency, increased 495
Urinary frequency, increased, causes 495
Urinary stream 496
Urine examination 55, 500
Urine microscopic examination 56
Urine pH 56
Urine protein 24 hours 56
Urine specific gravity 56
Urine, extravasation of 401

Urograffin 501
Uterine mass 468

V

V sign of Naclerio 491
VACTER anomalies 492
Vaginal examination 482
Vagus nerve 525
Valgum / varum assessment 596
Valgus deformity 579
Valgus foot 597
Valsalva maneuver 453
Valvulae conniventes 444
Varices, reticular 182
Varicocele 381, 387-390, 392-394, 396, 397, 401
Varicocele, grading 401
Varicocele, primary idiopathic 401
Varicocele, secondary 401
Varicocele, types 401
Varicography 196
Varicose vein 181, 198
Varicose veins, CEAP classification 195
Varicose veins, complications 194
Varicose veins, examination 184
Varicose veins, familial 198
Varicose veins, investigations 196
Varicose veins, signs 193
Varicose veins, symptoms 193
Varicose veins, types 182
Various positions in body 40
Varus deformity 579
Varus foot 597
Vas aberrans of Haller 401
Vas deferens sign 397
Vascular malformation 136
Vascular malformation, capillary 137
Vascular sign of Narath 591, 593
Vein, Anterior accessory great saphenous 198
Vein, Giacomini Cruveilhier 197
Vein, posterior arch 184, 197
Veins, Gaertner's 32
Veins, guttered 161
Veins, May's 32
Veins, reticular 182, 185, 193
Vela sore 62
Vela ulcer 62
Vellus 27
Venereal warts 409
Venography 196
Venous Doppler 196
Venous refilling time 161
Venous ulcer 82, 199
Venous ulcer, complications 195
Ventral hernia 367, 384
Verdan modified zone in hand 514
Vermilion border 240
Verrucous carcinoma 83, 133, 239, 261
Vesical calculus 504
Vesical calculus, types 504

Vesical pain 496
Vesicles 26
Vesicoureteric reflux 502
Vicryl 622
Victor Riddell method 351
Villonodular synovitis 598
Vin Rose Patch 27, 137
Vincent's angina 264
Vincent's gingivitis 245
Vincent's stomatitis 245
Vipoma 430
Virchow's node 423, 424
Virchow's triad 199
Virile facies 16
Virus, human papilloma 239
Visible gastric peristalsis 419
Visible gastric peristalsis (VGP) 450
Visible intestinal peristalsis (VIP) 449
Visible peristalsis 435
Visible veins 31
Visual acuity 524
Visual fields 524
Vitellointestinal duct 469
Vocal cords, movements of 277
Vocal fremitus 530
Vocal nodules 277
Vocal polyp 278
Volkmann's ischemic contracture 234, 235, 514
Volkmann's scoop 624
Volkmann's sign 234, 235
Volvulus 444
Volvulus, cecal 444
Volvulus, sigmoid 444, 628
Vomiting 10, 412, 434
Vomiting causes 10, 412
Vomiting, frequency 412
Vomiting, grading 10
Vomiting, relation to food and pain 412
Vomitus 10
Vomitus, Coffee-ground 412
Vomitus, nature and quantity 412
von Recklinghausen's disease 92, 125, 574
Von Recklinghausen's disease of neurofibroma 125
von Rosen femoral lines 593
von-Hippel-Lindae disease 505

W

Waddling gait 579, 589, 593
Waldeyer's ring 211, 306
Waldeyer-Pirogov ring 211
Wandering acetabulum 594
Wart 129
Wart, Butcher's 129
Wart, pathologist's 129
Wart, plantar 129
Warthin's tumor 294, 295, 280
Wash leather slough 68
Wasting 14
Wasting of limb muscle, assessment 173
Water brash 488
Water melon stomach 412
Water shed area 450
Waterhammer pulse 34
Watering can perineum 146, 389
Weaver's bursa 124
Web space infection 515
Weber's tuning fork test 525
Wedge biopsy, ulcer 76
Weigert Meyer law 506
Weight gain 13
Weight loss 14
Weight loss, significant 414
Weight loss, significant definition 14
Wen 119
Werner's T3 suppression test 335
Westermark sign 531
Wet chamois leather slough 68
Wharton's duct 281, 290, 291
Wheal 26
Whiplash injury 601
Whipple's triad 430
Whitaker test 503
White knee 597
White nail 22
Wilm's tumor 495-496
Wind sweep deformities of toes 597
Winging of scapula 221, 223, 231
Wingspread classification of ARM 487
Witch milk 364
Woody thyroiditis 338
Wound 57
Wound imaging 78
Wound perimeter 78
Wright test 167
Wringing test 587
Wrist drop 221, 223, 230, 588
Wrist joint line, palpation 557
Wrist joint movement 557, 558, 588
Wrist, palpation of joint line 557
Wrist, testing dorsiflexion 588
Wrist, testing palmar flexion 588
Wry neck 315

X

X-ray and imaging 47
X-ray, chest 47
X-ray, double contrast 48
X-ray bone, bone diseases 573
X-ray, barium enema 633
X-ray, plain 47
X-rays 626
X-rays bones 630
X-rays, barium meal 632
Xanthelasma 37
Xanthine stone 504
Xanthomas 18
Xerostomia 296

Y

Yaws 86
Yellow nail syndrome 22

Z

Zieman's test 373, 374
Zones of Rouviere 208